Tumors of
The Head and Neck

2nd Edition

Tumors of
The Head and Neck

CLINICAL AND
PATHOLOGICAL CONSIDERATIONS
2nd Edition

John G. Batsakis, M.D.

Professor of Pathology
The University of Michigan Medical School
Ann Arbor, Michigan

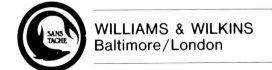

WILLIAMS & WILKINS
Baltimore/London

Made in the United States of America

Reprinted 1979
Reprinted 1980
Reprinted 1981
Reprinted 1982

Library of Congress Cataloging in Publication Data

Batsakis, John G
  Tumors of the head and neck.

  Includes bibliographical references and index.
  1. Head—Tumors. 2. Neck—Tumors. I. Title.
RC280.H4B38 1979   616.9′92′91   78-12703
ISBN 0-683-00476-X

Composed and printed at the
Waverly Press, Inc.
Mt. Royal and Guilford Aves.
Baltimore, Md. 21202, U.S.A.

DEDICATION

To my wife, Mary, and the children

Preface to the Second Edition

"A large part of abdominal work is recreation as compared with the work of what might be called the heavy surgery of the neck."

From the perspective of a surgical pathologist, this statement by C. H. Mayo in 1905 is even more applicable today. Interpreting "heavy" in modern parlance, surgery of the head and neck is indeed one of the most intellectually and technically demanding of the surgical specialties. Nearly every disease process, neoplastic or otherwise, may have a primary or secondary manifestation in the head and neck. To prepare for this challenge, the head and neck scientist-therapist must know well not only surgical judgment and skills, but also nearly the full gamut of available diagnostic (radiological, laboratory and physical) measures and therapeutic modalities. Pathology and more important, clinicopathological correlations are encountered daily by the head and neck clinician. The first and this edition of this book have been addressed to these last two aspects of knowledge.

I have completely revised or updated every chapter found in the first edition and four new chapters have been added. The book, however, remains true to its original purpose: a cento tied together by the surgical pathology of the diseases presented. Once again, I have departed from the conventional way of chapter presentations, taking, for the most part, tissue types and diseases rather than anatomical sites for many of the chapter headings.

In a field where there is constant research to achieve better therapeutic end-results, there is little reason for me to consider I have been "up-to-the-minute." I am acutely aware of this and have tried to be as contemporary as possible.

I am especially grateful for the chapters contributed by several of my colleagues: Dr. John T. Headington, Professor of Pathology and Dermatology, Dr. Kenneth D. McClatchey, Assistant Professor of Pathology, and Dr. Bertram Schnitzer, Professor of Pathology, all of the University of Michigan Medical School; Dr. Michael E. Johns, Assistant Professor of Otolaryngology, University of Virginia Medical School; and Dr. Don K. Weaver, Associate Pathologist, Williamsport Hospital, Williamsport, Pennsylvania.

I am also indebted to the many pathologists who have sent me interesting material for examination and use in the illustrations for the book. Further appreciation is extended to Craig Biddle, Medical Photographer, the Department of Pathology, University of Michigan, William Graham, Medical Illustration, University of Michigan Medical School and to MaryAnn Dutzer who typed the manuscript.

Finally, to Walter P. Work, M.D., must go my heartfelt thanks and appreciation for his spoken and unspoken encouragement and acceptance into the fraternity of head and neck physicians.

Contents:

CHAPTER 1

Tumors of the Major Salivary Glands

At the turn of the present century, despite their characteristically rather pronounced variation in histological appearance, *all* salivary gland tumors were simplistically separated only into "infiltrating" and "encapsulated" types. Serious attempts at a clinicopathological correlation were not made until the late 1940s and the early 1950s. This delay was occasioned by a combination of the relative rarity of these tumors and by a policy of expectant treatment for the tumors. McFarland,[1] for example, considered in 1933 that surgical treatment of parotid gland tumors was unnecessary. In 1942, this same pathologist concluded that postoperative prognostication for mixed tumors could not be determined with any greater accuracy than by tossing a coin.[2]

The situation remained essentially static until the fifth decade of the century, when improvement of surgical techniques, better anesthesia, transfusion services and the advent of antibiotics revived the role of surgery for both benign and malignant tumors of the salivary glands. The more aggressive surgical approach can be attributed to a more precise surgery (especially in regard to facial nerve exposure) and to a centralization of tumor treatment in medical centers.

Despite these noteworthy advances, many aspects of salivary gland tumors are either in a state of flux or continue to elude us. A major problem relates to their relative infrequency with respect to the over-all tumor load of a surgical pathology section. Another difficulty, arising from the marked variation in the histological features of the tumors, is the lack of a universally accepted classification.[3] Their rather diverse sites of origin (major and minor salivary glands) and incomplete knowledge of their histogenesis further compound the difficulties in clinical correlation.

There are considerable functional, embryogenic and morphological similarities between the exocrine pancreas and the major salivary glands. In terms of neoplastic growths, however, there is hardly a comparison. Perhaps no tissue in the body is capable of producing such a diverse histopathological expression than salivary tissue. This uniqueness may, in part, be due to the presence of the myoepithelial cell in the salivary glands; it is absent in the pancreas (Fig. 1.1). The presence of the facial nerve in the operative field further establishes the singularity of salivary gland tumors.

The biological behavior or malignancy of salivary gland tumors as a group is also peculiar. In the conservation of space, this aspect is best summarized by Ackerman and del Regato[4]: "The usual tumor of salivary gland is a tumor in which the benign variant is less benign than the usual benign tumor and the malignant variant is less malignant than the usual malignant tumor." Because of this biological behavior, expressions of local control, success of treatment and ultimate prognosis cannot be expressed in 5 or 10 year terms, but rather in 20 years.

EMBRYOGENESIS OF THE MAJOR SALIVARY GLANDS

Based on studies of lower mammalian forms, the major salivary glands have their beginnings at the end of the second week of intrauterine life. The morphosis of the parotid gland lags behind the sublingual and submandibular glands throughout the prenatal period and at birth is the least advanced.

The parotid gland of the rat and mouse is initiated approximately 24 hours later than the submandibular gland and sublingual glands with the latter lagging slightly behind the submandibular gland anlage.[5]

Embryologists remain far more indecisive about the entodermal or ectodermal origin of the salivary gland anlagen than standard textbooks appear to relate. From its location near the corner of the mouth, it is evident that the parotid gland anlage

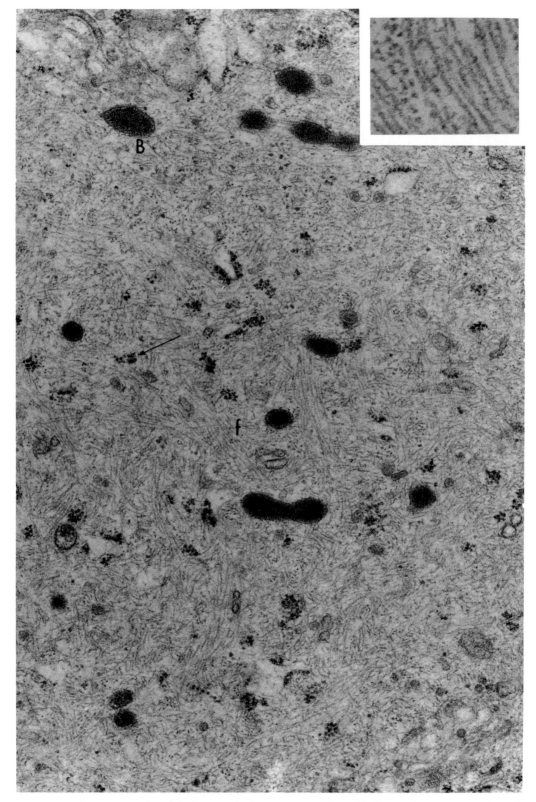

Figure 1.1. The myoepithelial cell; ultrastructural appearance. The cell is from a tumor composed nearly exclusively of myoepithelial cells. The cell cytoplasm demonstrates a haphazard arrangement of delicate fibrils (*f*). The dense bodies (*B*) likely represent a secretory material. The *arrow* points to free ribosomes (×11,000). *Inset,* a higher magnification of the cytoplasmic fibrils (×200,000). (Courtesy of J. J. Sciubba, D.M.D.)

of the rat arises from the epithelium which originates from the stomodeal ectoderm. The anlagen of the other major glands arise near the zone where the buccopharyngeal membrane once marked the junction of ectoderm and entoderm.

The parotid anlage is first seen as a club-shaped projection of epithelial cells in the buccal wall. These proliferate to form a narrow cord or stem (rudiment of Stensen's duct) and terminate in a knob or cluster of cells. The terminal clusters of the parotid "migrate" to near the angle and ramus of the developing mandible (16th to 17th day in utero). Initial signs of budding and branching of the terminal clusters appear only after this time. A system of ducts and terminal clusters resembling a tubuloacinar complex is evident by the 18th or 20th intrauterine day. At birth, the terminal clusters still consist of solid knobs of cells with centrally placed nuclei, indicating that the acinar component of the tubuloacinar complex has not definitely emerged at the end of the prenatal period of life. In contrast, the sublingual acini appear differentiated at this time and the terminal clusters of the submandibular gland are definitely at a more advanced stage of development. The branching of the primordia of all three glands is accompanied by a condensation of mesenchyme around their respective terminal clusters.

An examination of the embryogenesis and development of the acini of the submandibular gland is instructive toward an understanding of neoplastic changes occurring at the terminal end of the tubuloacinar complex.

The submandibular gland of the rat is a somewhat unique exocrine gland in that secretory differentiation occurs in both the pre- and postnatal periods. The pancreas and parotid gland, on the other hand, manifest their differentiation predominantly in the postnatal period.

In the submandibular gland, the development of acini begins at the 15th or 16th day of gestation and full differentiation is not complete until about the 6th *postnatal* week.[6-8]

In the fetal rat, the anlage of the submandibular gland is first observed as a spherical or elongated downgrowth of the oral epithelium. This epithelium is clearly separated from the surrounding mesenchyme by a thin basement membrane. As the anlage elongates, an excretory duct is formed at its distal end with the intralobular parenchyma represented by a "solid terminal bulb." Small cleavages in the terminal bulb appear on the 15th fetal day and represent the initial branching of the rudiment. By the 16th intrauterine day, 4 to 12 well-formed branches extend from the main stalk. Each branch terminates in one or two cellular

"end buds." The end buds elongate by differential growth and there is, by the 18th day, beginning lumen formation. This change gives rise to the earliest form of "terminal tubules." On the 19th day, secretory cells of the terminal tubules show an increase of rough endoplasmic reticulum and in the number of secretory granules per cell. From this time to birth, the structures remain essentially unchanged except for granule development.

By the third day after birth, the amount of rough endoplasmic reticulum in the secretory cells is greatly increased, Golgi apparatus is present, and the cells begin to assume the morphological appearance of mature acinar cells.

The submandibular gland of the rat then begins an orderly sequence of development of events in utero, culminating in mature acinar cells in the first month to 6 weeks after birth. There is a coincident appearance of a lumen and the onset of secretory granule differentiation at about the 18th or 19th day of gestation.

From a composite of morphological, histochemical and ultrastructural studies, the cells making up the proximal end of the developing submandibular gland may be identified as follows: (1) the intercalated duct cell; (2) terminal tubule cell; (3) the proacinar cell; and (4) the acinar cell.

The relevance of each type of cell to regeneration and neoplasia remains controversial. In the human, for example, the regenerative and proliferative capacity is said to reside in the intercalated duct. Some corollary for this may be found in the rat where, as the animal ages, the number of dividing secretory cells decreases and is substantially less than during the embryonic process.

Studies using partial extirpation and chemical degeneration substantiate that regeneration following injury appears analogous to embryological development.

Ethionine possesses a near selective toxicity for acinar cells, wherein the process of the passage of RNA precursors from the nucleolus appears to be inhibited. If there is *partial* destruction of acini, the recovery phase manifests *both* acinar cell proliferation and the appearance of acinar cells as the result of differentiation of the most terminal portion of the salivary duct system. In contrast, *complete* acinar destruction following ionizing radiation is followed by no evidence of regeneration as long as 75 weeks later.[9]

Hanks and Chaudhry,[10] in their study of regeneration following partial extirpation, describe the appearance of a pluripotential epithelial cell. This cell forms at least two different epithelial cell lines; one transforms into terminal tubules, the other becomes striated ducts. As in postnatal development, acini and intercalated ducts evolve from the terminal tubules. The fate of the terminal tubule cell and the proacinar cell remain elusive. Bressler,[11] capitalizing on precocious differentiation of acinar cells with the use of isoproterenal, and Yamashina and Barka,[12] using peroxidase as a marker, have come to similar conclusions. The former concludes that the terminal tubular cell and the proacinar cell of the young rat are independent cell lines. Terminal tubular cells may be a source of acinar cells after depletion of the proacinar cell population. Yamashina and Barka[12] have considered that the terminal tubule cells and proacinar cells are committed cells, the former evolving into second order intercalated duct cells and the latter into mature acinar cells.

For an understanding of our theory of the histogenesis of neoplasms of the major salivary glands, the key cells are the terminal tubule cell (intercalated duct reserve cell) and the excretory duct reserve cell (vide infra).

The submandibular gland not only serves as an experimental model to support our theory of histogenesis of salivary gland tumors, it also is ideal for the further exploration of epithelial-mesenchymal interactions. Many organs and tissues of the body, including the skin, pancreas and salivary glands seem to develop their phenotypic and morphogenetic characterization as a consequence of heterotypic interactions between epithelial and mesenchymal cells.[13, 14] The nature of the inductive influence that apparently elicits differentiation in nascent embryonic cells and determines specific cellular function is not known. What is known is that the expected epithelial configuration depends on a homologous local mesenchyme for appropriate expression and collagenous matrices mediate an organizing influence during the interaction of the two cell types. Collagen is a stabilizing influence during morphogenesis. When collagenase is added to organ cultures of salivary gland, the characteristic branching of the epithelium does not occur. Growth and random spreading of epithelium does continue. When the action of collagenase is stopped, a recovery of the normal histogenetic process begins and an epithelial organ typical of salivary gland is restored.

Salivary gland structure is then the result of an invasion intrinsic to the salivary epithelial primordia and a modulating or modeling effect of the surrounding mesodermal tissues. In addition, the acellular interface, the basement membrane between the mesodermal and epithelial masses, mediates and stabilizes the balance of histogenetic influences.

Since few, if any biological processes are iso-lated, these tissue interactions are neither more nor less important in the study of histogenesis than cell division, cell enlargement, cell synthetic processes, cell structure, membrane dynamics, DNA transcription and numerous other facets of growth and development. If neoplasia is an epigenetic process, the stroma very likely is concerned in the changes that result in its related epithelium acquiring neoplastic properties. Using culture systems, it is clear that specific salivary mesenchyme is the only obtainable inducer of salivary epithelium (neoplastic or normal).

Much more work needs to be done on both the tissue interactions mentioned above as well as on the epithelial cell derivation of salivary gland tumors. The latter is closer to definition.[15, 16]

The mature salivary gland unit is made up of serous or mucous acini that lead to an intercalated duct, which in turn is connected to a striated duct that finally empties into an extralobular excretory duct. Myoepithelial cells are located around the periphery of the acini and intercalated duct (Fig. 1.2).

Separation of the salivary gland unit into these component parts is necessary because of the specialized function and morphological characteristics of each segment. The acinar cells are highly differentiated cells, and are responsible for the production of mucinous or serous secretions. This is most readily appreciated from their ultrastructural features. Acinar cells contain well-developed rough endoplasmic reticulum and Golgi bodies and abundant secretory granules, features common to cells that are active in the production of protein (Fig. 1.3).

In the parotid gland, the acinar cells are predominantly or exclusively serous in type, resembling in some respects the zymogenic cells of the pancreas.[17] They are pyramidal in shape, enclosing with their narrow apical surfaces a small lumen

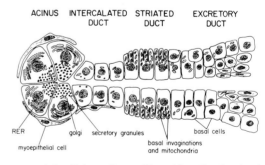

Figure 1.2. Schematic rendition of the ultrastructural components of the salivary gland unit. (RER, rough endoplasmic reticulum).

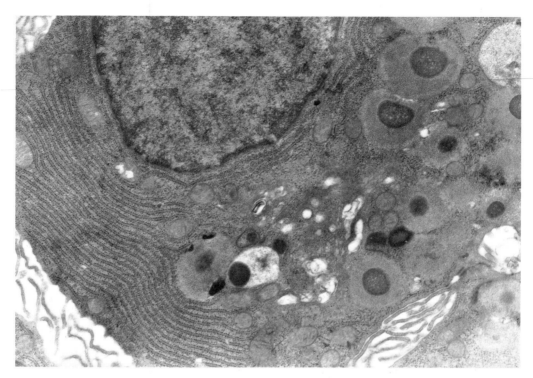

Figure 1.3. A serous secreting acinous cell of the submandibular gland. Nucleus (*top*), rough endoplasmic reticulum (*left*), Golgi vesicles (*center*), and maturing secretory granules (*right*).

lined by microvilli of variable orientation. Scattered lateral desmosomes and an apical junctional complex form the cell adhesion specializations. The cells rest on a flat and uninterrupted basal lamina. Secretion granules vary in appearance. They may be homogenous of variable density, or they may be layered with a dense outer and a pale inner zone, or with an eccentric dense core within a paler mass. The limiting membranes of the granules are tight fitting. The membrane system of the cytoplasm is highly organized and well suited for the principal function of secretion of the enzymic component of saliva. Unmyelinated nerves are commonly seen in the connective tissue surrounding the acini. Nerve terminals containing numerous synoptic vesicles are found between acinar cells indicating an autonomic innervation of the gland cells.

The acinar cells of the submandibular gland are mainly of a single type, often classified as seromucous. The granules are often poorly defined, often lack clear limiting membranes, and appear foamy or vacuolated. Secretion granules lie not only in the cell apex but also around and below the nucleus.

The mucous cells of the sublingual gland resemble those of the submandibular gland.

The salivary duct system is complex. The cu-

boidal cells of the intercalated ducts are relatively unspecialized. Cells near acini appear in some instances to have a a secretory function since they contain a number of dense apical membrane-limited granules and have a relatively prominent Golgi apparatus and a granular endoplasmic reticulum.[17] A few small microvilli may be seen at the cell apex while the cell base is flat and unspecialized. The more distal intercalated ducts have no granules and lack the cytoplasmic findings of the more proximal portions. Their lack of specialization suggests they play little part in the elaboration of saliva.[17] The cells of the striated ducts are well differentiated and show deep basal membrane invaginations and abundant mitochondria, features shared also by the proximal tubule cells of the kidney. Striated duct cells, like the renal cells, play a role in electrolyte and water transport. The pronounced specialization of the fine structure is in marked contrast to the featureless cells of the intercalated ducts. The epithelial cells of the excretory duct vary histologically from columnar cells with mucous goblet cells proximally to stratified squamous cells distally, and form collecting tubes for salivary secretions. The myoepithelial cell, first described in the parotid gland in 1898 remains a controversial cell. Its functions appear to be 3-fold: ability to contract like muscle fibers;

a transport function; and formation of basement membranes. As the name implies these cells lie at the base of the epithelial layer of the acini or at the base of the intercalated and perhaps striated duct. They exhibit a stellate cell body and, therefore, have been called "basket-cells." These cells make up some 12% of the acinar volume in the submandibular gland of the rat.

The myoepithelial cell is a two-sided cell.[18] This is expressed by their position: on the one hand it is connected with secreting epithelium and on the other it is interacting with the stroma and the secreting epithelium in the same way as a smooth muscle fiber. The cell's two-sidedness is also evident by its ectodermal origin modified by a mesenchymal potential. In spite of this intraepithelial position these cells act as smooth muscle cells and facilitate the movement of secretion down the duct system. Electron microscopy and immunofluorescence have shown that the cells are quite similar to smooth muscle cells and contain many fine fibers which are similar to myofilaments.[19-21] They further manifest the same distribution of cell organelles and the same differentiations on the cell membrane as smooth muscle cell. The myoepithelial cell is separated by a basement membrane only on the side adjacent to the connective tissue. Desmosomes connect the epithelial cells with the myoepithelial cells.

Light microscopic and histochemical reaction findings are by no means conclusive for the identification of the myoepithelial cells. Electron microscopy is required and even here is not infallible, primarily due to sampling error. In the salivary unit, the "epithelial" part of the myoepithelial cell is remarkably poor in cell organelles. The cells are linked to the secreting epithelial cells by desmosomes and to the basement membrane by hemidesmosomes (much like smooth muscle fibers). Glycogen granules and pinocytotic vesicles are present. Myoepithelia of the ducts differ in that they do not stain with any of the techniques that are characteristic of the fibrils of smooth muscle, owing to the scarcity or absence of fibrils.[18] On this part of the salivary unit, the mesenchymal components of the myoepithelia are replaced by epithelial ones. Hamperl[18] describes transition forms between the basal epithelial cells and the myoepithelial cells. When the myoepithelial cells contain few or no fibrils, they are not only difficult to distinguish from the so-called basal cells of the epithelium, but they may actually function as basal cells, in that, through division, they provide a substitute for the secretory cells.

Thus it may be seen that the myoepithelial cell exhibits a wide range of form and possible histo-chemical reactions.[22] Its identification is best done by the detection of fibrils (myo) and by positive results by methods and tests which depend on their presence.[18, 19] The reader is cautioned, however, that (1) some forms may be completely devoid of fibrils, (2) it is not clear whether the filaments should be classified as myofilaments or tonofilaments, (3) neither alkaline phosphatase nor adenosine triphosphatase reactions are specific for the cell. In the cells where no fibrils are found, their epithelial aspect is so prominent that they may appear to be basal cells or transition forms. These cells are suspect for myoepithelia because of their shape, position between basement membranes and secretory epithelium and by their ability to form basement-membrane-like substances.

The myoepithelial cell very likely plays an important role in the composition and growth of many salivary gland tumors.[18, 23, 24] Because of their intimate relationship to the epithelium, epithelial tumors of myoepithelium containing organs (breast, salivary and sweat glands) may consist wholly of epithelial cells, rarely, wholly of myoepithelial cells (see myoepithelioma) or of a mixture of both types of cells. Except for the rare myoepitheliomas, it is doubtful that the myoepithelial cell is the sole cell of *origin* for *any* salivary gland tumor. Its *participation* in the mixed tumor, adenoid cystic carcinoma and salivary duct carcinomas, among others, cannot be denied.

Three explanations have been proposed for the cellular derivation of the mixed tumor.[27] These are: (1) origin from neoplastic elements of both epithelium and mesenchymal tissues; (2) origin solely from neoplastic epithelial cells that, in turn, produce the other tissue components, either directly or by transformation into mesenchymal cells; and (3) the tumors are derived from cells that stimulate a non-neoplastic mesenchyme to undergo a metasplasia to cartilage, etc. If the mesenchymal components represent an end result of a chemical transition of epithelial secretions, no further explanation is necessary, but we do not consider this likely.

In the major salivary glands, the myoepithelium is involved in several tumors, especially in the mixed tumor and less so in adenoid cystic carcinomas. In my opinion and in Hamperl's,[18] myoepithelial cells play a determining role in mixed tumors. Mixed tumors of minor salivary glands have been shown to have duct cells as their major component.[85]

Mixed tumors manifest two types of mucin, an epithelial and a mesenchymal mucin. These may be differentiated by their different staining properties with toluidine blue and methylene blue and by their different behavior toward hyaluronidase, testicular extract and the extract of leeches. Epithelial mucus contains neutral glycoproteins with a small amount of sialuronic acid; mesenchymal mucus contains glycosamine-glycane, composed of hyaluronic acid, chondroitin-4 and/or chondroitin-sulphate.

Azzopardi and Smith[25] contend that mesenchymal mucin is a product of the myoepithelium. Hamperl[18] goes further and also includes the production of the chondroid matrix and cartilage and bone among the hidden potential of the myoepithelium. I accept this thesis and by doing so contend that the term "mixed tumor" can and should be used to designate these peculiar tumors. The tumors consist of a mixture of epithelium (glandular or squamous) and mesenchymal components and in essence represent a mixture of epithelium and pleuripotential myoepithelium.

The studies of Welsh and Meyer[27] and Quintarelli and Robinson[87] are important to this mode of histogenesis. According to these workers, who used histochemical reactions and electron microscopic observations, the mixed tumor is exactly that—not purely epithelial, but rather a *combination* of mesenchymal and epithelial elements. Similarly, the differences between an adenoid cystic carcinoma and a mixed tumor lie less in the quality than in the *quantity* and *distribution* of these structures in both cell types.[18] In the mixed tumor, the diversity of the mesenchymal differentiation prevails, proceeding to the production of even cartilage and bone; in the adenoid cystic carcinoma, mesenchymal differentiation is more regular and restricted to hyaline and mucoid material in rather specifically arranged masses. The duplex nature of the myoepithelium and the fact that the tissue of origin contains two cell types become evident in both types of tumor. With this in mind, it should not be surprising that mixed tumor-like areas may occur occasionally in adenoid cystic carcinomas and areas of adenoid cystic differentiation may appear in mixed tumors.

The foregoing represents a dualistic theory of origin for the mixed tumor. Willis,[88] the champion of the unitarians, maintains that the term "mixed tumor" is a misnomer, preferring "pleomorphic adenoma" because he believes the tumor is of epithelial origin alone. "Mixed tumor" as a diagnostic term has a considerable following and conveys to the listener or reader a clinicopathological impression that is probably lacking in "pleomorphic adenoma." The final judgment rests with the definition of the myoepithelial cells and their role in the histogenesis of these tumors. Dualists prefer "mixed tumor" and we agree; the unitarian

theorists favor "pleomorphic adenoma" or alternatively, "complex adenoma."

HISTOGENESIS OF SALIVARY GLAND NEOPLASMS

It is generally accepted that the basal cells of the excretory duct and intercalated duct cells act as reserve cells for the more differentiated cells of the salivary gland unit, both during the later stages of development and in the mature gland. The basal cells of the excretory duct give rise to the columnar and squamous cells of the excretory duct, and the intercalated duct cells give rise to the acinar cells, other intercalated duct cells, striated duct cells, and probably the myoepithelial cells. The importance of these two cells as reserve or progenitor cells in salivary gland development as well as tumor formation has been previously emphasized.[16] In the remainder of this discussion they will be referred to as excretory duct reserve cells and intercalated duct reserve cells.

Current classifications of neoplasms are based upon the ability of the neoplastic cell to mimic morphologically and functionally its cell of origin. For example, the neoplastic cells of squamous cell carcinomas resemble normal stratified squamous cells, by both light and electron microscopic examinations. They retain the ability to make basement membrane, desmosomes and tonofilaments (keratin). Similarly, the cells of osteosarcoma look like osteoblasts and make bone, and the cells in multiple myeloma resemble plasma cells and also produce globulins.

When this principle is applied to salivary gland neoplasms, two hypothetical possibilities are suggested. The first would be the genesis of neoplasms from their adult differentiated counterparts of the salivary gland unit. Under this scheme, the acinous cell carcinomas would originate from acinar cells, oncocytic tumors from striated duct cells, squamous cell carcinomas and mucoepidermoid carcinomas from excretory duct cells, and all other adenomas and adenocarcinomas from intercalated duct cells.

A second hypothetical possibility, which I favor, is more plausible since it would not require dedifferentiation of already highly specialized cells such as acinar and striated duct cells. Neoplasms under this scheme would generate from the two undifferentiated reserve cells discussed previously, the excretory duct reserve cell and the intercalated duct reserve cell. This "bicellular theory of origin" is similar to one previously proposed, which was based on light microscopic findings only.[16] Electron microscopic studies can now be added to light microscopic findings in support of this bicellular theory of salivary gland tumor histogenesis.[15]

Mixed Tumor

Ultrastructurally, two main types of cells, epithelial cells and myoepithelial cells, have been described in mixed tumors.[23, 26] Other cells such as mesenchymal cells and indeterminate cells have also been reported.[27] The epithelial cells, which vary from intercalated duct-like cells to epidermoid cells, comprise the histological majority of most tumors. Myoepithelial and myoepithelial-like cells have been described in varying numbers, depending upon the tumor studied. These cells are most commonly found in the myxoid areas of mixed tumors.

It can be further appreciated that mixed tumors represent a spectrum of lesions dependent upon the relative number of epithelial and myoepithelial cells present. At one end of the spectrum would be monomorphic adenomas that would be composed primarily of epithelial cells, and at the other end of the spectrum would be myoepitheliomas composed primarily of myoepithelial cells. In the range between these two extremes would be the mixed tumors, composed of different ratios of epithelial to myoepithelial cells.

Adenoid Cystic Carcinoma

The morphological resemblance of adenoid cystic carcinoma cells to intercalated duct cells in both light and electron microscopic examinations has been generally accepted by most investigators. The tumor cells are generally unremarkable and contain relatively few organelles. An inconsistently reported finding has been the presence of myoepithelial and myoepithelial-like cells, suggesting to some that this is the cell of origin for the adenoid cystic carcinoma.[28, 29] This apparent mixture of cells would seem analogous to the mixture seen in the mixed tumor, even though it is quantitatively different. The bicellular theory of origin would account for the appearance of both ductal and myoepithelial cells through neoplastic transformation of the intercalated duct reserve cell.

It should be noted that on occasion the adenoid cystic carcinoma (microscopically) resembles the mixed tumor. This simulation very likely results from the influence of myoepithelial cells in these tumors.

Squamous Cell Carcinoma and Mucoepidermoid Carcinoma

Theoretically all cells of the salivary gland unit carry the potential to keratinize or become squamous in type under appropriate circumstances because of their origin from surface epithelium. The cells of the excretory duct would be expected to have the greatest potential for this phenomenon because of their lack of specialization and their proximity to the gland orifice. Reactive glandular changes, associated with such stimuli as smoking or infection, result in squamous metaplasia and occasionally mucous metaplasia of the excretory ducts. (It should be remembered that mucous cells can normally be seen in the excretory duct.)

Neoplastic transformation of such metaplastic excretory ducts may result in squamous cell carcinomas or mucoepidermoid carcinomas. An analogy is the bronchogenic carcinoma induced by smoking.

Alternatively, either neoplasm can arise from direct neoplastic transformation of the excretory duct reserve cell, since this cell normally differentiates into squamous, columnar and mucous cells of the excretory duct (Fig. 1.6). A squamous cell carcinoma would result if only squamous cells were produced. A low-grade mucoepidermoid carcinoma would result if differentiation were directed more toward the production of mucous cells than squamous, and a high-grade mucoepidermoid carcinoma would result if squamous cells were favored over mucous cells. Additional support for the excretory duct reserve cell as the cell of origin comes from the observation by Eversole[16] that mucoepidermoid carcinomas do not occur as intralobular lesions.

Oncocytic Tumors

Oncocytes are cells that contain hyperplastic and pleomorphic mitochondria. These cells are generally not present in the salivary glands of younger individuals, but are commonly seen with increasing age. They may be found anywhere along the salivary gland unit, but are most frequently encountered among the intercalated duct cells and acinar cells. Oncocytes are believed to represent a form of cellular degeneration since they lack the differentiation of adjacent cells. It has also been suggested that these cells are biochemically deficient since they have reduced levels of oxidative enzymes. This deficiency is thought to trigger a compensatory mechanism at the organelle level in the form of mitochondrial hyperplasia.

Theoretically oncocytomas could originate from oncocytes anywhere along the salivary unit or from the mature ductal cell that they most closely mimic, the striated duct cell. Against the latter is the fact that oncocytoma cells do not exhibit any other feature of the striated duct cell such as extensive basal infoldings. On the other hand, cells from oncocytomas are nearly identical morphologically to oncocytes in normal glands. Also oncocytomas, like oncocytes, occur in older patients. The ultimate cell of origin for this tumor could be either the excretory duct reserve cell or the intercalated duct reserve cell. The latter cell is more likely since it gives rise to the salivary gland tissue where most oncocytes have been described.

Acinous Cell Carcinoma

Ultrastructurally, these cells contain secretory granules similar to those seen in serous acinar cells and intercalated duct cells. Since secretory granules are found nowhere else in the salivary glands, this implicates the acinar cell or intercalated duct cell as the cell of origin. Since the intercalated duct reserve cell gives rise to both these cells, it is this cell that is the hypothetical source of these neoplasms.

Adenocarcinoma

Adenocarcinomas, which cannot be further subclassified, would be expected to arise from the intercalated duct reserve cell. These tumors seen under the microscope most closely resemble the undifferentiated intercalated duct cells, and do not show the distinctive features associated with the neoplasms already described.

Given the prominent role of the duct stem cells in replenishing the epithelium of the salivary gland unit, my theory of the origin of salivary gland tumors is in concert with Pierce's[30] concept of the development of general neoplasia, i.e., a pathology of the cells involved in tissue renewal. The genome of the normal cell contains all the information necessary for the expression of the malignant as well as the normal phenotype. Malignancy is superimposed upon the process of cell renewal by stem or reserve cells. Malignant stem cells are derived from normal stem cells by a process equivalent to postembryonic differentiation. If the stem cells, capable of synthesizing DNA, are the oncogenic target, malignancy results; if well-differentiated cells, still capable of one more division, are the targets, a benign lesion results. Whether or not a benign or malignant tumor develops is dependent upon the state of differentiation of the target cell. Malignant stem cells have a capacity for proliferation and differentiation that operate on a different level of control than the normal phenotypic expression.

CLASSIFICATION OF SALIVARY GLAND TUMORS

Table 1.1 presents my concept of a working classification of the epithelial neoplasms of the

Table 1.1
Classification of Epithelial Salivary Gland Tumors

Type of Lesion	Variations
Benign	Mixed tumor (pleomorphic adenoma)
	Papillary cystadenoma lymphomatosum (Warthin's tumor)
	Oncocytoma (oncocytosis)
	Monomorphic tumors
	Basal cell adenoma
	Glycogen rich adenoma (?)
	Clear cell adenoma
	Membranous adenoma
	Myoepithelioma
	Sebaceous tumors
	Adenoma
	Lymphadenoma
	Papillary ductal adenoma (papilloma)
	Benign lymphoepithelial lesion
	Unclassified
Malignant	Carcinoma ex pleomorphic adenoma (carcinoma arising in a mixed tumor)
	Malignant mixed tumor (biphasic malignancy)
	Mucoepidermoid carcinoma
	Low-grade
	Intermediate-grade
	High-grade
	Adenoid cystic carcinoma
	Acinous cell (acinic) carcinoma
	Adenocarcinoma
	Mucus-producing adenopapillary and nonpapillary carcinoma
	Salivary duct carcinoma (ductal carcinoma)
	Other adenocarcinomas
	Oncocytic carcinoma (malignant oncocytoma)
	Clear cell carcinoma (nonmucinous and glycogen-containing or non-glycogen-containing)
	Primary squamous cell carcinoma
	Hybrid basal cell adenoma/adenoid cystic carcinoma
	Undifferentiated carcinoma
	Epithelial-myoepithelial carcinoma of intercalated ducts
	Miscellaneous (includes sebaceous, Stensen's duct, melanoma and carcinoma ex lymphoepithelial lesion)
	Metastatic
	Unclassified

major salivary glands. It is to be compared with Tables 1.2 and 1.3, which present classifications proposed by others.[31, 32] Some classifications present a listing of supporting tumors of the salivary glands in addition to the epithelial tumors. In my opinion, there is only one supporting tissue neoplasm that is unique to salivary tissues, the hemangioma of the parotid gland. All others are exceedingly rare as primary neoplasms. Most often supporting tissue neoplasms involve salivary tissue secondarily, usually by contiguity and occasionally be metastasis. Table 1.4 presents a listing of soft tissue tumors that may be found in and about the parotid area. Although the table considers all the

Table 1.2
Classification of Minor Salivary Gland Tumors*

> Benign
> > Mixed tumor
> > Oncocytoma
> Malignant
> > Adenoid cystic carcinoma
> > Tumors of duct origin
> > Mucoepidermoid carcinoma
> > Solid duct carcinoma
> > Variants of duct carcinoma
> > > Mucus adenocarcinoma
> > > Papillary-cystic carcinoma
> > > Clear cell adenocarcinoma
> > > Papillary adenocarcinoma
> > > Spindle cell carcinoma
> > > Unclassified
> Other malignant tumors
> > Malignant mixed tumor
> > Oat cell carcinoma
> > Colonic type carcinoma

* Spiro et al.[31]

Table 1.3
W. H. O. Classification of Salivary Gland Tumors*

> Epithelial tumors
> > Adenomas
> > > Pleomorphic adenoma (mixed tumor)
> > Monomorphic adenomas
> > > Adenolymphoma
> > > Oxyphilic adenoma
> > > Other types
> > Mucoepidermoid tumor
> > Acinic cell tumor
> > Carcinomas
> > > Adenoid cystic
> > > Adenocarcinoma
> > > Epidermoid carcinoma
> > > Undifferentiated
> > > Carcinoma in pleomorphic adenoma (malignant mixed tumor)
> Nonepithelial tumors
> Unclassified tumors
> Allied conditions
> > Benign lymphoepithelial lesion
> > Sialosis
> > Oncocytosis

* Thackray and Sobin.[32]

Table 1.4
Soft Tissue Tumors of the Major Salivary Glands and Paraglandular Tissues

Vascular
> Primary hemangioma of the parotid gland
> Lymphangioma
> Arteriovenous fistula (aneurysms)
> Angiosarcoma

Lymphoreticular
> Lymphoma (primary and secondary)
> Atypical lymphoreticular hyperplasia (pseudolymphoma)
> Histiocytosis
> Lymphoepithelial lesion (with or without Sjögren's syndrome)
> Benign, reactive hyperplasia

Neurogenous
> Neurofibroma
> Neurofibrosarcoma
> Neurilemmoma
> Traumatic neuroma
> Neuroepithelial tumor (sarcoma)
> Granular cell tumor
> Meningioma

Skeletal muscle
> Rhabdomyosarcoma
> Rhabdomyoma
> Infantile rhabdomyoma
> Masseteric hypertrophy

Smooth muscle
> Leiomyoma
> Leiomyosarcoma

Fibroblastic and histiocytic
> Fibrous scar or keloid
> Fibrosarcoma
> Fibromatosis
> Histiocytoma and variants

major glands, it relates almost exclusively to the parotid gland.

Most of the soft tissue lesions may simulate a parotid mass, but they usually involve the gland in an extrinsic fashion. The vascular lesions are cases in point. Lymphangiomas as localized lesions, restricted to the salivary parenchyma, have been reported but are numerically overwhelmed by those lymphangiomas that incorporate the gland as they involve neck and facial tissues.

Under the lymphoreticular category, I refer to lesions of both the intraparotid lymph nodes and the salivary parenchyma. The lymphoepithelial lesions may involve both, but the remainder are primarily disorders of the intrasalivary gland lymphoid structures.

Clearly the neurogenous lesions are of structures not of salivary origin. The granular cell tumor appears to have two histogenetic sources: the perineural supporting cells and the histiocyte. A rare meningioma may make an extracranial presentation as a parotid mass.

An extraparotid gland origin also applies for the majority of skeletal muscle, smooth muscle and fibrous tumors that may affect the salivary glands.

In a time when considerable effort is being directed to simplifying classifications, the reader may be discouraged by the subdivisions of the epithelial tumors of the salivary glands, and in that sense a declaration of a "working" classification may seem incongruous. I am fully cognizant of the possible criticisms but justify the classification for the following reasons.

Prior to 1953 and the work of Foote and Frazell,[33] many kinds of salivary gland tumors were often grouped together under vague designations such as "semimalignant." As a result, many parotid tumors were radically operated upon unnecessarily. On the other hand, many patients died of their tumors because of a false benign identification. A large portion of the fault lies in the relative infrequency of primary salivary gland tumors. This required the earlier authors to make their judgments on single cases or small series. Foote and Frazell[33] had the first opportunity to consider a large series of tumors with a correlation to their biological behavior. Since that time, the work of others has carried our knowledge further. In that respect, the monographs by Glaser,[34] Seifert,[35] Evans and Cruickshank[36] and Eneroth[37] are particularly noteworthy.

Other major handicaps in the biological appraisal of salivary gland tumors have been largely overcome. This has to do with the fortunate discreditation of enucleation and likewise limited surgical removal of these tumors, and a growing realization that 3- and 5-year survival data are inadequate to express prognosis in this group of tumors.

Criteria Employed in the New Classification. With the foregoing advances, I feel that it is now appropriate to subdivide the epithelial neoplasms into defined clinicopathological entities. Histogenesis aside, each of the entities in my classification has specific histopathological criteria that, for the most part, clearly delineate it from the other lesions in the classification. Some of these criteria are reiterated in subsequent sections of this chapter.

Although this classification may not reveal any significant difference in biological behavior, until this can be scientifically defined, there is a danger of "lumping" these entities together under vague labels that may be disadvantageous to the patient. For that reason alone, I subscribe to the subdivision of tumors into the histopathological types given in the classification.

I have studiously avoided, wherever possible, the use of the term *tumor* in the classification. In the histopathological sense this is not appropriate because it is a gross pathological designation conveying only the sense of a mass. In that respect there are mucoepidermoid carcinomas of varying grade and acinous cell (acinic) carcinomas. One cannot predict on light microscopic evidence alone the degree of malignancy of the low or intermediate grade mucoepidermoid carcinomas or of the acinous cell carcinomas, but this should not lead one to beg the issue of carcinoma. I cannot subscribe to the notion that there are only facultative malignant variants of the acinous cell carcinoma, for repeated clinical experiences belie that statement.

Specific Entities. Warthin's tumor and the oncocytic lesions are characterized by numerous, often distorted, mitochondria in their epithelial cells. The two lesions differ in that Warthin's tumor is bicellular and requires for diagnosis a lymphoreticular component as well as the oncocytes. Failure on the part of diagnosticians to require both components has led to the erroneous diagnosis of Warthin's tumor in peculiar sites such as the larynx, nasal cavity, and oral mucosa.

The monomorphic adenomas have only recently emerged from their inclusion under the heading of mixed tumors. Basal cell adenoma, glycogen rich adenoma, and other clear cell lesions are now recognized. Too short a follow-up period, however, has been recorded in these lesions to fully assess their biological potential.

I am particularly concerned with the as yet undefined biological potential of the entire group of nonmucinous clear cell tumors and, although I have separated these into two types (benign and malignant), my subjective impression is that they are probably all of low-grade malignancy. Donath et al.[38] have expressed this best and have given these lesions the designation epithelial-myoepithelial carcinomas of intercalated ducts.

Primary squamous cell carcinomas of the salivary glands are of very low frequency, yet in many clinical series they have accounted for 4 to 8% of the total number of malignant lesions of the parotid gland. Before a diagnosis of primary squamous cell carcinoma can be made, it is mandatory to exclude variants of mucoepidermoid carcinoma, necrotizing sialometaplasia and metastases to the parotid gland.[39]

Also unusual in occurrence are the benign papillomas of major salivary gland ducts. A distinction must be made between these lesions and hyperplastic infoldings and the adenopapillary carcinomas.

Adenocarcinomas not otherwise specified as adenoid cystic carcinomas deserve segregation, not only because of their distinctive histopathology, but also because this permits a separate appraisal of their behavior that is not possible when all glandular or gland-like neoplasms are grouped under the generic term "adenocarcinoma." Statistical degradation clearly follows if this term is not strictly applied.

Malignant variants of the mixed tumor (pleomorphic adenoma) are of two types: carcinoma ex pleomorphic adenoma and a biphasic malignant or so-called true malignant mixed tumor. The latter is exceedingly rare, whereas the former is being recognized with greater frequency. In carcinoma ex pleomorphic adenoma, an epithelial malignant tumor arises from the epithelial elements of the mixed tumor and metastasizes only as a carcinoma. Although any type of epithelial malignant entity may be derived from the mixed tumor, our experience indicates that it is usually a poorly differentiated ductal carcinoma.

The undifferentiated salivary carcinomas are those neoplasms whose differentiation is so low or so poor that they cannot be classified into other categories. These have been subdivided on histological grounds into spindle cell, spheroidal cell and trabecular carcinoma. I see no clinical advantage to this subclassification.

Under miscellaneous epithelial neoplasms I have placed those carcinomas that are very rare. Primary melanomas of the parotid gland do exist, but the majority are metastatic to the parotid gland and more often to the parotid nodes with secondary involvement of the salivary parenchyma. The carcinoma ex lymphoepithelial lesion is a nonkeratinizing carcinoma that takes its origin from the "epimyoepithelial" islands of the benign lymphoepithelial lesion.

Renal cell carcinomas must be singled out in the category of metastatic lesions to salivary tissue. Their clear or eosinophilic and sometimes papillary configuration may be confused with oncocytomas, acinous cell carcinomas and clear cell neoplasms. In addition, a metastasis to the head and neck from a renal cell carcinoma may be the first indication of its presence or, at the other extreme, may be a late manifestation after an apparent "curative" removal of the primary renal cell carcinoma.

A histological subclassification into high, low, and varying intermediate grades of malignancy has been attempted by several workers, including the author. While it is no difficult task to assign salivary malignancies to high and low categories, the translation of the subtyping into an indication of biological activity is usually not successful. The mucoepidermoid carcinomas are exceptions to this statement. For the remainder, there is too much inconsistency. Clinical stage and the effectiveness of *primary* therapy are far more important.

SURGICAL ANATOMY AND THE FACIAL NERVE

To perform parotid gland surgery without knowledge of the anatomy of the facial nerve and its relationship to other structures invites production of facial palsy, and in some quarters, is tantamount to malpractice. Because of this, a brief introduction to the surgical anatomy of the region is necessary before consideration of the types of neoplasms.

The major salivary glands are the parotid, the submandibular (submaxillary) and the sublingual glands.

Parotid Gland

The parotid gland is encased in a firm fascial covering derived from the anterior layer of the deep cervical fascia. It lies in a compartment whose medial wall consists of the styloid process and the transverse process of the atlas. The anterior wall is the ascending ramus of the mandible. The anterior surface of the mastoid process forms the posterior wall. The external auditory meatus and the head of the mandible, in its fossa, limit the parotid compartment in its superior aspect.

The muscular components of the compartment are as follows: medial wall; posterior belly of the digastric; and the styloglossus, stylohyoid, and stylopharyngeus muscles, which take their origin from the styloid process. Anteriorly, three muscles cover the posterior surface of the ascending ramus of the mandible. Inferiorly is the masseter muscle (normally overlapped by the superficial portion of the parotid gland). The remaining ones are the internal and external pterygoid muscles; they are somewhat overlapped by the deep portion of the gland.

Because of the bony and muscular boundries of the parotid compartment, the parotid gland assumes an irregular shape. The superficial surface is triangular, with its apex pointing downward. The base of this irregular triangle is parallel to the zygoma. The anterior border overlaps the masseter muscle and the ramus of the mandible, and the posterior border overlaps the sternocleidomastoid muscle. The deep surface lies on the styloid process and its muscles, and more posteriorly, on the digastric muscle and the internal jugular vein.

In the region of the temporomandibular joint, a portion of the normal gland may extend deep to the mandible and then be in close relation to the lateral pharyngeal wall. Involvement of this portion by tumor accounts for a pharyngeal presentation. Anteriorly, the gland is grooved by the ascending ramus of the mandible, while posteriorly it lies in contact with the external auditory meatus, the mastoid process and the sternocleidomastoid muscle.

Anterior and attached projections of the parotid salivary glands may be found along the parotid duct, as it courses toward the oral cavity.

The chief surgical consideration of the parotid gland is the presence of the facial nerve. The gland may be, *surgically speaking*, divided into superficial (80%) and deep portions (20%), as defined in terms of their relationship to the facial nerve. The lateral superficial lobe and the medial retromandibular deep lobe are connected by an isthmus. This oversimplification is of considerable surgical merit for the creation of a neurovenous plane of cleavage between the deep and superficial lobes in order to identify and isolate the facial nerve where it passes superficial to the retromandibular (posterofacial) vein. Along this neurovenous plane, the main trunk of the facial nerve divides into the temporofacial and cervicofacial divisions, which again divide into temporal, zygomatic, buccal, mandibular and cervical branches.

The anatomical concept of the facial nerve sandwiched between two lobes forms the basis for the operative procedures, subtotal superficial lobectomy and total parotidectomy.

The parotid duct (Stensen's duct) is formed by the confluens of several branches near the anterior border of the gland. It crosses the masseter muscle and pierces the buccinator muscle at the anterior border of the masseter.

Accessory glandular tissue (distinct and separate from the gland) may be found along the course of Stensen's duct. These tissues are usually on or above the duct and bound to the masseter muscle by extensions of the masseteric fascia. They appear as flattened pea- to lima-bean-sized collections. In Frommer's[40] study, 21% of parotid glands manifested these accessory tissues. The average distance of distinctly separated accessory glands from the anterior edge of the main gland was 6.0 mm. The farthest removed accessory gland rested on the buccal fat pad at the anterior border of the masseter muscle. Usually the accessory glands have one major drainage conduit into Stensen's duct. Accessory parotid tissues do not differ from the main gland in histological appearance, function and aging changes.

The fascial encasement of the gland, as indicated above, is not unique to the gland. The outer layer is that fascia which, in the cervical region and the lower face, contains the platysma muscle. The investing fascia of the masseter muscle forms the inner layer. The fused fascial layers send numerous septa into the lobules of the gland as well as accompanying the intraglandular portion of the facial nerve.

Beahrs[41] considers all surgical procedures in the parotid region as facilitated by the existence of the fascial elements.

Facial Nerve

Two quotations from Conley[42] set the stage for any surgeon wishing to perform parotid gland surgery: "A fundamental knowledge of the surgical anatomy of the parotid gland and facial nerve is the sine qua non for adequate management," and "The experience with the nerve itself is always unique and demanding."

Developmentally, the relation of the parotid gland to the facial nerve is a secondary one since the anlage of the gland migrates posteriorly from its origin in the fetal pharynx and enfolds the nerve.

The surgical approach to the facial nerve is selected by the surgeon and dependent on the point of the lesion in the parotid gland.[41, 42] However, the distribution of the peripheral branches of the nerve is variable, whereas the exit of the trunk from the stylomastoid foramen is constant. The tip of the mastoid process, the transverse process of the second cervical vertebra, the tympanomastoid fissure and styloid process are encircling bony landmarks which help in locating the trunk of the nerve. If these bony landmarks are obliterated, the neurovenous plane (where the facial nerve divides superficial to the posterior facial vein) can serve as a provisional landmark.

The facial nerve is slightly more superficial than the stylomastoid foramen, appears as a whitish cord 2 to 3 mm in diameter and runs in a posteroanterior direction into the gland.

Immediately after it emerges from the stylomastoid foramen at the base of the skull, the nerve gives off three small branches: posterior auricular, posterior digastric and stylohyoid nerves. The nerve then enters the parotid gland superficial to the external carotid artery and the posterior facial vein. At this point, the nerve usually branches into two major divisions: the temporofacial and cervicofacial portions. The bifurcation occurs 5 to 7 mm dorsal to the ramus of the mandible and 4.1 to 4.7 cm above the external angle of the mandible. The temporofacial branch is the larger of the two by far. The pattern of sub-branching from the two main trunks has no end to variation, but eight main types of configuration may be distinguished (Fig. 1.4).[43] The variations and anastomoses of the sub-branches appear to be governed, at least in part, by the shape and position of the deep lobe of the gland and the presence of the isthmus. At least five main sub-branches are present: temporal, zygomatic, buccal, mandibular and cervical. The buccal branch may take origin from the main trunk. According to Conley,[42] it is always single and always connects with temporal or cervical branches. Almost all of the branching and connections of the facial nerve occur *within* the parotid gland.

The surgeon may elect to locate a facial nerve branch by blunt dissection as it courses anterior to the gland or along Stensen's duct. Retrograde dissection of a branch will be a safe surgical procedure in order to locate the pes anserivus and the main trunk. Other surgical methods for nerve exposure are: branch identification at the site of the posterior common facial vein; incision of the superficial layer of the deep cervical fascia and then the use of blunt dissection for locating a nerve branch as it courses through the gland; identification of the main trunk at the stylomastoid foramen; and lastly, locating the main trunk in its descending bony fallopian canal. As a general rule, dissection of the nerve or nerve branch in an antegrade manner is easier and carries less hazard for injury to the nerve than a retrograde dissection. If inadvertent facial nerve injury occurs, it is repaired by neurolysis, nerve suture or nerve grafting. Nerve sacrifice is a *planned* surgical procedure. Here too, repair is by suture, graft or nerve substitution. Nerve repair must be carried out at initial surgery, or after short delay after primary surgery.

As indicated earlier, parotidectomy should be considered as dissection of the gland away from the facial nerve. Conley,[42] Beahrs,[41] Beahrs and Adson[44] and Cocke and Finley[45] have detailed this operation. Conley [42] further has presented indications for preservation and resection of the facial nerve in the treatment of tumors of the parotid gland. The relative indications for VIIth nerve resections are: (1) high grade malignant neoplasms; (2) large malignant tumors having an in-

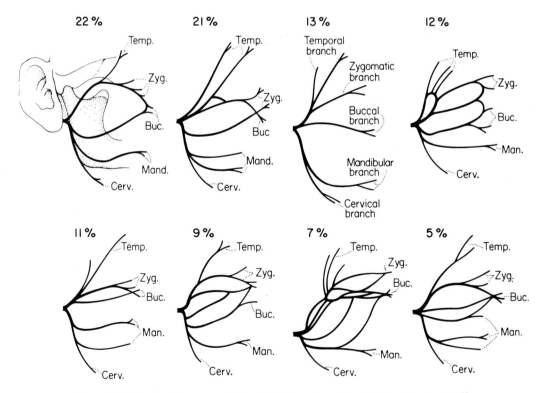

Figure 1.4. The facial nerve; variations in its branches. (Modified from Davis et al.[43])

volvement of a major portion of the gland; (3) malignancies of the deep lobe of the parotid gland; (4) malignant neoplasms having a clinical presentation of VIIth nerve paresis; (5) recurrent malignancy; and (6) certain benign tumors, principally the mixed tumor, which compromise the nerve. Work et al.[46] have reviewed the last of these indications. The facial nerve should be preserved if possible in the following instances: (1) all benign tumors and cysts; (2) *early* low-grade malignant neoplasms of the lateral lobe; and (3) recurrent benign mixed tumors. The last two may require segmental resection of the VIIth nerve and a total parotidectomy. In short, it is the relationship of the neoplasm to the nerve that dictates sacrifice or preservation of the nerve. This holds true for both benign and malignant neoplasms. If the nerve is compromised, a frozen section diagnosis of low-grade neoplasm does not alter the decision to resect.

Special note of two other nerves is necessary. These nerves are the great auricular nerve and the auriculotemporal nerve. The latter is small and branches from the posterior surface of the mandibular nerve. It is significant in its relation to Frey's syndrome. It ascends through or deep to the substance of the parotid gland and takes a vertical course just anterior to the external auditory meatus. The great auricular nerve, usually the largest branch of the cervical plexus, usually lies behind and tends to parallel the external jugular vein. In parotidectomy, the nerve or its anterior branches may be found below the tip of the mastoid process.

The frequency of injury to the facial nerve during surgery of the parotid gland is difficult to assess. Not only is it difficult to compare results in series, the definition of injury to the nerve differs according to the duration of follow-up of the patient and to the grade of paralysis, which is a subjective observation. Ward[47] has studied the circumstances during parotid gland surgery in which the facial nerve might be injured.

In his series, limited surgery carried as great a risk of injury to the nerve as during extended surgery. Extended surgery provided greater risk of injury to the facial nerve on secondary exploration (71%) than on primary exploration (6.5%). Two primary factors are responsible for the increased susceptibility of the facial nerve to injury during multiple operations on the gland: (1) ischemic anoxia of the nerve as a result of surgical interference with the vasa vasorum; and (2) adherent scar tissue.

To facilitate identification of the nerve and a demonstration of the macroscopic extent of tumor,

intravital staining of the parotid gland with 2.5% methylene blue solution may be used.[48] Staining is essentially restricted to normal salivary tissue; any tumor or lymph nodes within the gland are demonstrable by their failure to take up the blue dye.

Submandibular Gland

This salivary gland lies in the submandibular triangle and extends over the superficial surfaces of the anterior and posterior bellies of the digastric muscle.

The posterior border of this gland lies in close proximity to the lower portion of the parotid gland at the jaw, where the stylomandibular ligament separates them. The lymph nodes lie on the superficial upper border of the gland; other nodes lie anterior and posterior to the gland. Anteriorly, the submandibular gland lies directly against the mylohyoid muscle.

In surgical procedures it is best to remove the entire nodal and glandular contents of the submandibular compartment rather than perform partial excision of the gland.

Identification of nerves is less critical but required. The mandibular branch of the facial nerve is identified superficial to the facial vessels. The hypoglossal nerve and submandibular ganglion are identified from below upward and appear on the hyoglossus muscle.

Sublingual Glands

The sublingual gland is approximately one-half the size of the submandibular gland. These salivary glands lie in the floor of the mouth, below the mucosa and above the mylohyoid muscle. The glands relate laterally to the mandible, medially to the styloglossus muscle, posteriorly to the hyoglossus muscle and anteriorly to the genioglossus muscle. The two sublingual gland masses almost meet in the midline in front of the genioglossus muscle. There are about 20 excretory ducts from the sublingual gland that empty into the floor of the mouth, although an occasional duct may empty into the submandibular duct. The most frequent lesion for this site is the ranula. Malignancy is uncommon.

SALIVARY GLAND TUMORS

In terms of general incidence, tumors of the salivary glands comprise less than 3% of all neoplasms in the head and neck.[49] Between 75 and 85% are found in the parotid glands. This predominant involvement of the parotid gland is reflected in the instance of the mixed tumor, wherein the parotid gland is affected approximately 10 times as often as the submandibular gland.[50] The sublingual gland is almost never a primary site for this neoplasm.

Approximately 10 to 20% of all salivary gland tumors arise outside of the major salivary glands and occur in the lacrimal glands, mucous glands of the palate, lips, tongue, nasopharynx, accessory sinuses and larynx.[51] The palate is the most frequent site of minor salivary gland tumors (see Chapter 2). Benign tumors are much more common than malignant ones; they account for over four-fifths of parotid tumors but for less than half of the tumors of the other salivary glands. According to Eneroth,[51, 52] one of six tumors in the parotid gland, one of three in the submandibular gland and almost half of the tumors of the palate will be malignant. The prognosis for any given type of malignant tumor is most favorable when the primary site is in the palate region, less favorable when it is in the parotid gland and least favorable in the submandibular gland.

The over-all incidence of salivary gland tumors is essentially the same throughout the world. There is, however, a demonstrable influence of geography on the salivary gland distribution of the tumors. Mixed tumors seem to occur with the same frequency among the Caucasian populations anywhere in the world. African Negroes present more often with mixed tumors of the minor and lesser major salivary glands.[53] In Pretoria, the parotid gland was involved with mixed tumors four and one-half more times in the Caucasian population than in Negroes.[54] The latter population, however, manifested submandibular and minor salivary gland mixed tumors two to three times as often as the whites. Submandibular tumors occur with a relatively greater frequency among the Chinese in Malaya and in Ugandans and West Indians. There is no significant sex predilection among the whites of Europe and the United States. In the nonwhite United States population and in Africa, salivary gland tumors are more often found in women.

Several interesting and probably significant associations with the occurrence of salivary gland tumors have been made. One of these is the association of cancer of the salivary glands with carcinoma of the breast. Berg et al.[55] followed up 396 patients with carcinoma of a major salivary gland and found that the subsequent incidence of breast cancer was eight times the expected figure. This increase is somewhat greater than the known risk of second breast cancer developing in a patient who already has a mammary carcinoma.

These data have been challenged and supported.[56–59] There are strong statistical reasons to doubt the validity of the claim and the protagonists state either that there is no increased risks of a subsequent breast cancer in either black or white women or strong support for the validity of population-based surveys.[56, 57] Table 1.5 modified from Prior and Waterhouse[56] presents a simplified comparison of four surveys of the association of breast and salivary gland cancer. Prior and Waterhouse[56] further enhanced their findings by reversing the sequence. Taking the breast as the primary site, they found a significant statistical difference (P < 0.05) between observed and expected numbers.

The head and neck region has often been the area of predilection for the occurrence of radiation-implicated tumors. There is now convincing evidence for the relationship between thyroid cancer and prior irradiation. A growing body of information also points to a similar relationship with neoplasia of the salivary glands.[60–64]

The observations on the possible induction of salivary gland tumors in patients who have received radiation for benign conditions have not reached the level of statistical confidence obtained in studies of malignant thyroid tumors. Reports of small series or individual cases are the usual data currently available. Larger studies such as that of the Michael Reese Group[61] suffer from an absence of a matched control group. Despite a freedom from statistical uncertainty, however, important correlations have emerged:

Table 1.5
Association of Breast and Salivary Gland Tumors

Author	No. of Patients with Salivary Gland Tumors	Breast Tumors		P Value
		Expected	Observed	
Berg et al.[55]	396	0.9	7	<0.001
Moertel and Elveback[58]	297	4.0	4	—
Dunn et al.[59]	349	4.2	8	—
Prior and Waterhouse[56]	453	2.0	6	<0.05

1. The literature dealing with salivary gland tumors and radiation exposure nearly exclusively relates to irradiation administered accidently, for diagnostic purposes, or for the treatment of benign disorders.

2. Therapeutic irradiation for a malignancy in the anatomical region is not successfully implicated. It is presumed that high-dosage radiation may lead to a lower incidence of secondary malignancy compared to low- or medium-dosage exposure.

3. The latent periods for induced neoplasms of the salivary tissues and thyroid gland following postnatal therapeutic exposure in infancy or later are clearly longer than those following prenatal diagnostic irradiation.

4. The latent period has averaged 15 to 20 years or more for salivary gland tumors after irradiation. A similar latency is observed in bomb survivors in Japan.[64]

5. It is apparent that there is no general pattern of age and radiosensitivity to carcinogenesis of salivary tissue. The duration of risk has not been clearly defined. As Mole[65] has pointed out, while a 10-year survey is likely to provide a good guide to the total number of induced neoplasias after radiation exposure during fetal life, a 25-year or longer survey is required to assess total induction in patients who received radiation treatments in adult life.

6. The parotid gland is the salivary tissue site in nearly three-quarters of the reported cases.

7. The induced salivary gland tumors are more often of a benign type with the benign mixed tumor accounting for nearly 50% of the radiation-related tumors of salivary tissues. The mucoepidermoid carcinoma is the most common malignant salivary gland tumor following these forms of irradiation.

Radiographic procedures in reality play only an ancillary role in the preoperative definition of salivary gland neoplasms.[66, 67] In most cases, their use not only is not helpful, they are also not indicated. Plain film x-rays are essentially useful only if they demonstrate calculi. Most parotid gland calculi are radiolucent. As for sialography, its use may be summarized by quoting Quinn,[66] "sialography searches for stones, strictures and sialectasia." A "hot" salivary gland scan with Technitium 99 pertechnetate is virtually diagnostic of Warthin's tumor which preferentially absorbs and concentrates the radionucleide. Cervical ultrasound, utilizing the B-mode and gray scale is said to be useful in differentiating solid from cystic salivary gland lesions, if that indeed is a necessary preoperative requirement. Finally, computed tomographic scanning may prove useful in the assessment of neoplastic extension beyond the salivary gland into fascial spaces of the neck.

Unusual in children (vide infra), salivary gland tumors nevertheless may present over a wide range of years, extending from childhood to adults over the age of 80 years. At the time of primary treatment, the average patient is approximately 45 years old.

Because the parotid gland so dominates the statistics and since we will address the minor and lesser major salivary gland tumors in another chapter, further generalizations concerning the salivary gland tumors in this chapter will relate predominantly to the parotid glands.

Concerning the location of tumors in the parotid glands, the greatest number (about 80%) are found in the superficial and caudal parts of the gland, and most frequently the presenting symptom is a lump in the region of the ear. It is good clinical practice to consider every "lump," every tumor thus localized, as a probable tumor of the parotid gland.

Symptomatology is, on the whole, not very impressive. A considerable delay or time lag between clinical onset of the tumor and treatment is fairly characteristic of salivary gland tumors, regardless of whether they arise in the major or minor salivary glands. Rapid growth need not necessarily be caused by a malignant tumor. Infection of the glandular tissue and ducts can be caused by a malignant tumor and can very easily confuse the clinical picture. On the other hand, slow growth does not of necessity imply only a benign tumor. Inspection and palpation are obviously important. Pharyngeal extension can be inspected in the tonsillar region. Color changes are seen in hemangiomas. Pain need not point toward malignancy. A benign tumor located deep in the gland can sometimes cause a painful mastoid process.

Of the tumors in the deep parotid lobe, only a few attain the size to grow between the mandible and the mastoid process and fill the parapharyngeal space, causing the pharyngeal wall to bulge in medially (vide infra). In Eneroth's[51] study, less than 1% of the parotid tumors proved to be clinically parapharyngeal. Sometimes a tumor in the deep portion of the gland can increase to such an extent that the superficial part is compressed, and the tumor then is falsely considered to be superficial. Such a tumor will displace the facial nerve laterally, stretch it, and produce an abnormally descending trunk, which can easily be injured if the true situation is not realized.[49]

A benign parotid tumor usually presents as a freely mobile, nontender mass, which is located just in front of or below the auricle. There are no other associated physical findings.

Facial Nerve Paralysis

Facial nerve paralysis is unusual and seen in far-advanced cases. When noted, the process is almost always malignant.[68] It should be remembered that a malignant growth can circumvent a nerve branch without causing nerve signs or symptoms. Fixation of the mass and ulceration of the overlying skin are additional indications of malignancy.

As indicated above, neoplastic invasion of the facial nerve is an ominous preoperative clinical sign. The anatomical and therapeutic significance and consequences of this morbid event follow.

Nerve fibers are joined together in fascicles or funiculi. The *connective tissues* which bind the fibers together follow the course of the funiculi. Their terminology is confused and it is best, for the sake of clarity, to divide them into three compartments: *endoneurium* which represents all connective tissue structures within the funiculi; *perineurium* which forms a specialized sheath around each fascicle; and the *epineurium* which is the extrafascicular connective tissue.[69]

The *endoneurium* consists of predominently longitudinally oriented collagen fibers and fibroblasts condensed around each nerve fiber and more loosely arranged between the nerve fibers. A few septa separate each fascicle into several compartments and contain arterioles and venules. The spaces between the collagenous sheaths and septa contain fluid. This is separated from the blood stream by a "blood nerve barrier" (tight junction between endothelial cells) and from the epineurial lymphatics by the perineurium.

The *perineurium* begins at the level of the radicular nerve and consists of concentric layers of spindle cells separated by collagen and elastic laminae. The thickness of the perineurium varies within the same nerve. Its function is that of a diffusion barrier separating the endoneurial fluid from epineurial lymph. The elastic component of the perineurium likely provides tensile strength to nerve bundles.

The loose areolar tissue separating the fascicles and surrounded by a denser fibrous sheath is the *epineurium*. It contains the vasa vasorum and lymphatics which drain into regional lymph nodes.

From the above, it is clear that the only lymphatic spaces in the nerve coverings are in the epineurium. Experimental and necropsy studies have failed to demonstrate *any* perineurial or endoneurial lymphatics. On the other hand, epi-, peri-, and endoneurial extension of salivary gland malignancies are well recognized. For adenoid cystic carcinomas, regardless of their salivary tissue origin, invasion of nerve is so common as to be proverbial. In my experience, all adenoid cystic carcinomas larger than 1 cm will manifest extensions into at least the perineurial spaces. One should distinguish between perineural and perineurial growth. Perineural refers to growth around a nerve; perineurial means the more specific growth within the perineurium.

While it is well known that adenoid cystic carcinomas and other malignancies can propagate along neural routes, it is less appreciated that on rare occasions a neural spread of epithelial tissues is not a manifestation of malignancy.[70] Perineural and endoneurial growth may be found in sclerosing adenosis and papillomatosis of the breast and in an otherwise normal pancreas.

The little known organ of Chievitz (Chievitzen organ) has also been confused with perineural invasion in patients with oral carcinoma.[71, 72] These juxtaoral organs are not neoplastic but rather a normal persistence of included ectoderm (? neuroepithelial). The organ tissue is typically located in the spatium buccotemporale adjacent to the fascia buccotemporale and innervated by the buccal nerve. Lutman[72] points out the epithelium of the organ of Chievitz is not anaplastic and the nests are not actually in the perineural spaces, but instead lie between or adjacent to double or single axons or tiny nerves.

Neoplastic involvement of the facial nerve represents 5% of all lower motor neuron facial paralyses. Its preoperative presence in a patient with a malignant tumor of the parotid gland is a serious prognostic sign. It indicates an aggressive local invasion and a high potential for metastasis. The incidence of facial palsy in patients with malignant lesions has ranged from 8 to 33% in individual classes of parotid malignancy. Conley and Hamaker[73] record an over-all incidence of 12% in their series of 279 patients; Eneroth and Hamberger[74] record an incidence of 14%. The tumors associated with the facial palsy are those with the highest incidence of metastases and lowest cure rate, i.e., high-grade or undifferentiated carcinomas (Fig. 1.5). Upon analysis of the position of the tumors, Conley[73] indicates they are more often in the deep lobe or in combination with the superficial lobe and/or beyond the confines of the gland.

While spontaneous facial paralysis adds considerable doubt on a favorable outcome for the host

(100% mortality in the series of Eneroth and Hamberger[74]), it is not hopeless. The basic treatment is radical parotidectomy. This usually includes the platysma muscle and occasionally the skin, the masseter muscle anteriorly, the posterior belly of the digastric and stylohyoid muscles medially and inferiorly along with a deep jugular dissection, the tip of the mastoid, the conchal cartilage, and the cuff of sternocleidomastoid muscle posteriorly. The fallopian canal is opened to secure the proximal line of resection if the main trunk is involved. Conley[73] adds to the above a radical neck dissection if the neoplasm is a high-grade lesion. An extended radical procedure is advised by Conley[73] if the neoplasm goes beyond the above perimeters.

Parotid tumors should be explored and a histological diagnosis made. I do not recommend preliminary biopsy. The potential danger of cell spillage and implantation recurrence is always present. This is lessened by needle biopsy or aspiration (vide infra), but the specimen obtained is difficult to interpret. More important, the operation to be done depends greatly on the gross appearance of the tumor and the gland, especially whether or not the facial nerve is involved in tumor spread. Every parotid tumor operation is thus an exploratory procedure.

Clinical Staging

Staging of salivary gland neoplasms is of very recent origin and appears to have been initiated by Spiro et al.[75] Their proposed clinical staging for carcinoma of the parotid is presented in Table 1.6. The T1 designation is reserved for any lesion 3 cm or less in size that is solitary, freely movable and shows no evidence of VIIth nerve dysfunction. A T2 lesion is one between 3.1 and 6.0 cm, solitary, without ulceration or deep fixation and with a normally functioning VIIth nerve. A tumor in the T3 category is one with any one of the following: larger than 6.0 cm, multiple nodules, ulceration or deep fixation, or VIIth nerve palsy. Spiro et al.[73] indicate that "fixation" means *complete* immobility.

Division into three clinical stages follows application of the N0 and N1 designations. Providing that the neck is clinically negative (N0), patients with T1 and T2 lesions are placed into stage I and II respectively. Any patient with clinical evidence of metastases to lymph nodes (N1) or with T3 lesion is considered to be in stage III.

Following the correlation of the above clinical staging with histological findings, Spiro et al.[75] pointed out the following trends. Low-grade mucoepidermoid carcinomas, adenocarcinoma grade I and acinous cell carcinomas were least likely to metastasize to regional lymph nodes or distant sites. More than 70% of these patients presented with stage I disease. In contrast, about 50% of their remaining patients who had tumors that usually manifest a more aggressive behavior (carcinoma ex pleomorphic adenoma, adenoid cystic carcinoma, mucoepidermoid carcinomas other than grade I, squamous cell carcinomas, and higher grade adenocarcinomas) were in the stage III category when first seen.

At this writing, following the initiative of Spiro et al.[75] there is a retrospective study to expand the system and prepare a classification. The histolog-

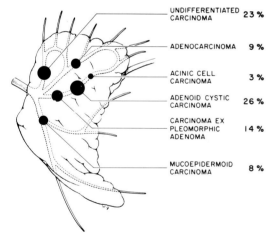

UNDIFFERENTIATED CARCINOMA	23 %
ADENOCARCINOMA	9 %
ACINIC CELL CARCINOMA	3 %
ADENOID CYSTIC CARCINOMA	26 %
CARCINOMA EX PLEOMORPHIC ADENOMA	14 %
MUCOEPIDERMOID CARCINOMA	8 %

Figure 1.5.   Carcinomas of parotid gland and facial paralysis.

Table 1.6
Clinical Staging, Parotid Gland*

T1	T2	T3
0–3 cm and solitary and freely mobile and CR VII intact	3.1–6 cm and solitary and freely mobile or skin fixation and CR VII intact	6 cm or multiple nodules or ulceration or deep fixation or CR VII dysfunction

* Modified from Spiro et al.[75]

ical classification is intended to be a modification of that proposed by the World Health Organization (W.H.O.).[76]

Radiotherapy

The indications for radiotherapy as a modality in the management of salivary gland neoplasms have evolved from ones of palliation to more precise definition. The indications are almost restricted to the treatment of carcinoma. Suggestions such as those by McEvedy and Ross[77] for the treatment of mixed parotid tumors by enucleation and radiotherapy, are, in my opinion, regressive. For recurrent mixed tumors (nonoperable for a variety of reasons), the effectiveness of irradiation is still undefined.

As a primary form of treatment, radiotherapy has been used for malignancies in patients with advanced lesions in which resection is not possible.

It is in the immediate postoperative period in cases where residual or microscopic foci of neoplasm is present or suspected that there has been considerable advocacy. Fletcher and Jesse[78] state that postoperative irradiation is not indicated for low-grade malignancies (low-grade mucoepidermoid carcinoma, well-differentiated adenocarcinoma and acinous cell carcinoma) unless there is disease at the place of excision. In that instance, the postoperative irradiation should be given to the tumor bed. These authors further indicate that for a high-grade neoplasm, not only the bed, but also the temporal bone and base of skull and neck should be irradiated. Five thousand rads should be given to the entire tumor bed if no gross tumor has been left behind. The dose is increased to 6,000 rads if there is suspected or definable residual tumor. In the M. D. Anderson series postoperative irradiation for high-grade malignancies reduced the local failure from 36 to 11%, but the follow-up periods were variable.[76]

The complications of irradiation are related to the primary tumor and whether it is possible to protect sensitive structures. In the case of the major salivary gland, the main complications are soreness and difficulty in swallowing secondary to radiation mucositis of the oral cavity and pharynx. Dryness of the mouth produces changes in the oral flora with rapid dental decay unless an appropriate dental prophylaxis is instituted. Trismus may develop because of radiation-induced fibrosis. Besides dental cavities and periodontal disease, osteoradionecrosis of the mandible is always a possibility. Moderately severe problems may present in the ear. Dryness, scaling and chondritis may be sequalae. Uncommonly a serous otitis externa or

media with pain and partial loss of hearing may occur. Fletcher and Jesse[78] point out that facial nerve graft takes may be reduced after irradiation.

Perhaps the most informed and least biased evaluation of the role of radiation therapy and salivary gland tumors has been presented by Chang.[79] He wisely points out that a salivary gland tumor is an excellent example of the proposition that whereas radiosensitivity may determine to some extent radiocurability, a higher level of radiosensitivity does not necessarily mean a higher rate of curability and vice versa. If there is a difference in radiosensitivity inherent in various histological types of salivary gland neoplasms, it does not seem to be a decisive factor in curability. The adenoid cystic carcinoma serves as a case in point. This tumor appears to be relatively more radiosensitive than other salivary malignancies. While there may be a dramatic response to irradiation, this response is temporary and local recurrence is frequent. Perhaps linear energy transfer radiation, combined with a lower oxygen enhancement ratio and a higher relative biological effectiveness will have a more decisive effect on this group of malignancies. The indications and contraindications for radiotherapy of salivary gland tumors as proposed by Chang[79] are presented in Table 1.7.

Neck Dissection

The place of neck dissection in the management of carcinomas of the parotid gland needs better clarification. This, to some degree, has been accomplished for American surgeons[75, 80] and appears to be in contrast to Scandinavian policy, at least as enunciated by Eneroth and Hamberger.[74] These authors advocate radical neck dissection for all tumors, even without suspect palpable lymph nodes in the neck, except for benign tumors and low-grade mucoepidermoid carcinomas.

Decision for neck dissection should be based on: (1) the presence or absence of clinically positive lymph nodes; (2) a clear appreciation that only the high-grade adenocarcinomas and mucoepidermoid carcinomas, squamous cell carcinomas, and carcinomas ex pleomorphic adenoma manifest a significant *lymphatic* spread; (3) an appreciation that adenoid cystic carcinomas and acinic cell carcinomas involve lymph nodes of the region by *contiguous* spread far more often than by the lymphatic route; (4) observations that there will be a high probability that neoplastic recurrence will occur with an equal frequency in the operated neck without regard to whether the removed lymph nodes were positive or negative; (5) needle

Table 1.7
Salivary Gland Tumors: Radiotherapy*

General Indications	Poor or Contraindications
1. Residual malignant tumor after surgery.	1. Benign tumors which can be treated by surgery.
2. Microscopic malignant tumor at resection margin.	2. Far advanced salivary gland malignancies.
3. Unresectable primary carcinoma.	3. Patient factors (medical contraindication).
4. Unresectable recurrent or incompletely resectable tumor.	
5. Malignant lymphoma.	
6. Metastatic salivary gland carcinoma. Metastasis to the salivary gland.	

* After Chang.[79]

biopsy or aspirate of suspicious lymph nodes will provide necessary preoperative information; and (6) the suggestion that a prophylactic neck dissection is likely never indicated.

Recurrence of Salivary Gland Tumors

The presence of a neoplasm in the submandibular gland requires at least a complete excision of that gland. This axiom of treatment accounts for the relatively low recurrence rate of benign tumors of that gland as compared to the parotid gland.

In the parotid gland, the absence of recurrence of a benign salivary gland tumor and an acceptable rate of recurrence from a malignant lesion is directly related to the experience and skill of the surgeon and the disavowment of enucleation in favor of at least a lateral lobectomy. The conversion to the latter form of management has reduced the benign mixed tumor recurrence from 8 to 2% at the Mayo Clinic[81] and to 0 in the series reported by Skolnik et al.[80]

The shift toward total parotidectomy and more radical excision has also reduced the recurrence of malignant neoplasms, but it still remains disconcertingly high. Solace should not be had in *only* 5-year follow-up periods since recurrences respect no time limit. This is especially true for adenoid cystic and acinous cell carcinomas. Spiro et al.[73] record an over-all local recurrence of 27% in their patients with carcinoma of the parotid gland. This is increased to 60% in patients with stage III tumors. Hodgkinson and Woods,[82] in an evaluation having follow-up periods of at least 5 years, record a 38% rate of local recurrence. Their study is of further interest since 64% of patients in the recurrence group had sacrifice of the VIIth nerve during their initial surgical procedure. Kagan et al.[83] report nearly 50% of the patients in their study had recurrences (as many as two per patient). As would be expected, the neoplasms manifesting the

greatest propensity for recurrent disease were adenoid cystic, high-grade mucoepidermoid, high-grade glandular and squamous cell carcinomas.

Distant Metastases

There is no question that disseminated disease from carcinomas of the parotid gland have been underestimated. This is evident in any series extended beyond a 5-year surveillance.[73–75, 84] The frequency of this event varies with the clinical stage of the disease and is highest with high-grade malignancies (high-grade adenocarcinomas and mucoepidermoid carcinomas and adenoid cystic carcinomas). Eneroth and Hamberger[74] observe there is a nearly 1:1 correlation with spontaneous facial palsy. Nearly one-third of the patients with these neoplasms, given time, will manifest distant metastases. Of these, Spiro et al.[75] point out that there is no evidence of a local treatment failure.

The experience reported from the University of Michigan substantiates the foregiving and, in addition, clearly indicates that if follow-up periods are long enough (15 to 40 years), not even carcinomas usually considered as low grade (with or without VIIth involvement) can be excluded. Our observations on acinous cell carcinoma are pertinent in that respect (see page 43).

The primary metastatic sites are the lungs, followed by bones and disseminated disease. While nearly all patients with distant metastases die within 24 months of their discovery, some are capable of leading a useful and prolonged life. Those patients with a solitary metastasis from an adenoid cystic carcinoma are such exceptions.

Benign Mixed Tumor

The mixed tumor is a slowly growing, usually well-demarcated, essentially benign tumor of salivary glands. It is most commonly found in the parotid gland (particularly the tail), where it makes

Table 1.8
Parotid Gland Tumors: Histological Diagnoses in Reported Series

Classification	Foote and Frazell[33] (776 cases)	Bardwill[171] (153 cases)	Eneroth[37] (802 cases)	Lambert[276] (83 cases)
Mixed tumors				
Benign	447 (58%)	36 (34%)	569 (70.9%)	44 (53%)
Malignant	46 (6%)	34 (22%)		1 (1%)
Warthin's tumor	50 (6.5%)	5 (3%)	41 (5.1%)	16 (19%)
Mucoepidermoid carcinoma				
Low-grade	45 (6%)	32 (21%)	34 (4.2%)	5 (6%)
High-grade	45 (6%)			
Adenoid cystic carcinoma	15 (2%)	13 (8%)	19 (2.4%)	2 (2%)
Acinous cell carcinoma	21 (3%)	8 (5%)	36 (4.5%)	3 (5%)
Adenocarcinoma (miscellaneous)	32 (4%)	16 (11%)	17 (2.1%)	
Oncocytic cell tumor	1 (0.1%)	1 (1%)	4 (0.5%)	1 (1%)
Squamous cell carcinoma	26 (3%)	8 (5%)	1 (0.1%)	1 (1%)
Miscellaneous				
Benign	3 (0.4%)			
Malignant	0		15 (1.8%)	5 (6%)
Unclassified				
Benign	4 (0.6%)			
Malignant	30 (4%)			2 (2%)

up approximately 65% of all neoplasms of that gland (Table 1.8). In the parotid gland, it is most often outside the facial nerve and behind the mandibular branch. Rauch,[89] in a review of 4,245 mixed tumors, found 92.5% in the major salivary glands (84% in the parotid and 8% in submandibular); 0.5% in the sublingual gland, and 6.5% in the minor salivary glands of the respiratory and digestive tracts. In another large series of over 6,000 cases, oral involvement accounted for 5.5% of all mixed tumor sites, whereas 2.5% were found in the nasopharyngeal tract. About 7% occur in the minor salivary glands and 4% arise in the hard and soft palate with an equal frequency.[90] The upper lip is more often the site than the lower lip and the oropharynx is involved 10 times as often as the epipharynx. Ectopic sites such as the mandible and choristomatous lesions in the ear account for a small number.

Mixed tumors present more often in women at all sites with the exception of the pharynx. No age is immune but the majority of patients are in the fifth decade of life. Minor salivary gland mixed tumors usually present in patients over 50 years old.

The usual history is that of a slow-growing or apparently stationary, painless mass. In some patients, there may be a history of recent rapid growth after a period of relatively long quiescence, or the converse may be true. The average interval between onset of signs and/or symptoms is almost 6 years.

The clinical examiner usually describes the tumor as being rather firm, smooth and movable. Size varies from a centimeter or less to large and disfiguring masses. Ulceration of the overlying skin or mucous membrane is unusual. Initially they are solitary; multiple nodulation is a manifestation of recurrent tumors (Figs. 1.6 and 1.7). Generally lobulated and globular, the tumor appears to be surrounded by a capsule of variable thickness, completeness and density. Compression of surrounding tissue produces the impression of invasion. This is more obvious in tumors of the submandibular gland than of the parotid. This "pseudopenetration" of the "capsule" has no adverse prognostic significance and should not be used as a criterion for "semimalignancy."[36, 37, 91] Regardless of the completeness of the capsule or its absence, the tumor is clearly demarcated.

Eneroth[91] has made detailed studies on the capsule and so-called satellitosis. The majority of apparently separate foci of tumor, outside of the capsule, are in reality outgrowths of the main mass. This can be demonstrated by serial sections.

Morphological diversity and complexity (Figs. 1.8 to 1.11) is the hallmark of mixed tumors, but, by definition, both epithelial and mesenchymal elements must be present for diagnosis. Without these elements the lesion cannot be regarded as a true mixed tumor. Two types of cells determine the pleomorphic structure of the tumor: an inner row of epithelial cells and an outer layer of myoepithelial cells. These may be arranged in a wide

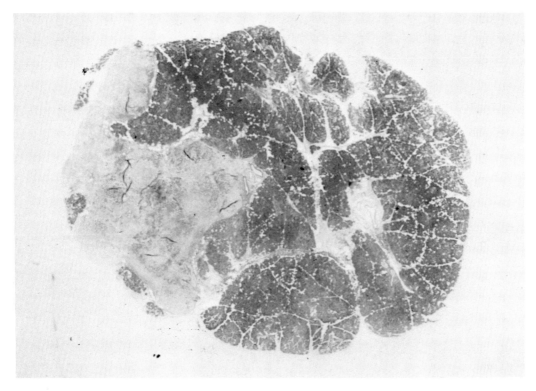

Figure 1.6. Lobulated benign mixed tumor of parotid gland. Primary excision.

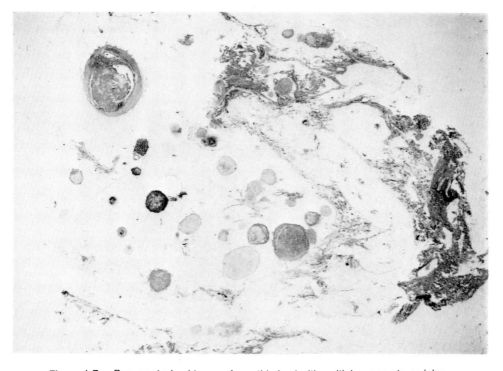

Figure 1.7. *Recurrent* mixed tumor of parotid gland with multiple, separate nodules.

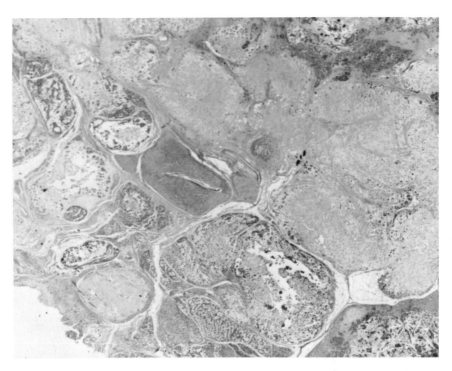

Figure 1.8. Recurrent, histologically benign mixed tumor of parotid gland. The nodules of tumor are composed predominantly of chondroid matrix. Note the severe compression of a branch of the VIIth nerve in the *center*.

number of patterns associated with a scant or abundant stroma, which, in turn, may be mucoid, fibroid, chondroid, vascular or myxochondroid. Calcification and ossification are unusual. Exuberant epithelial participation may suggest malignancy, but without destructive infiltration and the other findings discussed below, caution should be exercised. Approximately 36% of benign mixed tumors manifest an almost equal distribution of myxoid and cellular areas; 22% are predominantly cellular and 12% may be categorized as extremely cellular.[33] Tyrosine crystals (Fig. 1.12), found predominately in the nonepithelial areas of mixed tumors, are apparently unique to these tumors.[92] Their significance is unknown.

The clinical course of the biological behavior of mixed tumors is more dependent upon the type and adequacy of treatment than upon microscopic appearance. If one classifies mixed tumors, as did Foote and Frazell,[33] into (1) principally myxoid, (2) equally myxoid and cellular, (3) predominantly cellular and (4) extremely cellular, the recurrence rates of the cellular and extremely cellular variants tend to be highest. The fallacy in using these criteria for prognostication lies in the fact that 80% of these lesions fail to manifest expected recurrences. It is necessary then to look elsewhere. Authors have given recurrence rate figures ranging

from 5 to 50% of cases. This wide range reflects (1) inclusion of cases in the preparotidectomy era, i.e., enucleation, and (2) failure to maintain long-term observations, since recurrences may be long delayed.

The primary reason for recurrence, or probably more aptly persistence, is inadequate removal at the onset, i.e., enucleation versus removal of a margin of uninvolved gland. The tumors persist or recur because pseudopods or parts of the tumor are not removed at the time of operation due to neglect or fear of damaging the facial nerve. Rupture or seeding are other reasons. Adequate surgical removal, at least superficial parotidectomy, *must* be performed. Enucleation belongs to the past. For tumors deep to the facial nerve, the procedure of total conservative parotidectomy is completed by removal of that portion of the gland deep to the nerve with preservation of the nerve and all its branches. For tumors in the submandibular and minor salivary glands, total excision is recommended. Radiation has not been shown to be an effective form of treatment. Using this form of management, "recurrences" should be markedly reduced, and, if they occur, are also treated by meticulous resection. The vast majority of mixed tumors behave like benign neoplasms.

The recurrence rates of mixed tumors offered in

the literature vary widely. This variation in reported series would appear to be due to two factors: firstly, an inadequate follow-up period (many must therefore be considered as only interim reports); secondly, to histological confusion over the malignant potential of these tumors.[93] There are two probable causes of recurrence following operation: first, that tumor cells have been left behind; and second, that the recurrence is not in fact a recurrence but another tumor. We consider the latter as unusual and presume that patients who present with a recurrent parotid tumor do so because of inadequate surgical removal at the time of the initial operation.

A *primary multicentric* origin of mixed tumor does occur. It is of such low frequency, however, that it would not be used as rationalization for recurrence. In my personal experience, the incidence of multifocal origin of a mixed tumor is 0.5% of mixed tumors of the parotid gland. Warthin's tumor and acinous cell carcinoma are far more often multicentric. The finding of multiple foci of mixed tumor is, on the other hand, a nearly constant finding in recurrent tumors.

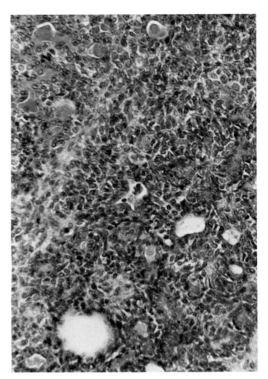

Figure 1.10

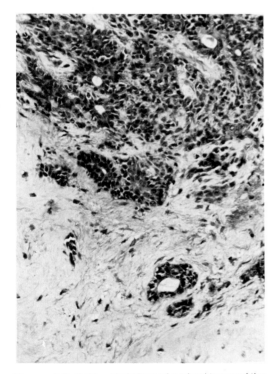

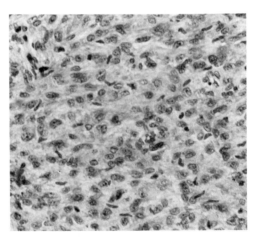

Figure 1.11

Figures 1.9–1.11. Variations of a mixed tumor of the parotid gland. These range from the parvicellular (chondroid) lesion in Figure 1.9 through the cellular lesions of Figures 1.10 and 1.11. Figure 1.11 demonstrates an unusual degree of myoepithelial proliferation.

Recurrence of a mixed tumor is very likely independent of the microscopic appearance of the lesion. The same may be said for completeness or incompleteness of the tumor's capsule. Epithelial hypercellularity of a mixed tumor is not associated with any more higher local recurrence rate than the usual essentially benign-appearing tumor. In fact, Vandenberg et al.[94] noticed that patients with benign mixed tumors had a more favorable prognosis when the tumor was of a purely or predom-

inantly epithelial type. In two relatively large series, the majority of the recurrent mixed tumors
were hypocellular with an abundant chondromyxoid or myxoid stroma.[95, 96]

Even though mixed tumors manifest a slow
growth, recurrences are associated with significant
morbidity.[97] These include compromise of the facial nerve, an accelerated rate of recidivous tumors
(Table 1.9) and the supervention of malignancy.

Total parotidectomy with dissection and preservation of the facial nerve is the preferred operative procedure for the first recurrence. If parotidectomy has been performed as the initial procedure, Fu et al.[97] advise excisional biopsy of the
recurrent nodule with a surrounding cuff of subcutaneous muscle and scar tissue with preservation
of the nerve. This may require the use of the
operating microscope. Certain highly selected patients with recurrent mixed tumors of the parotid
gland will require en bloc resections of the recurrent tumor with the facial nerve and immediate
grafting.[42, 46]

The role of radiation therapy is controversial
and to date, only limited in success.

The time required for recurrent mixed tumors
to be clinically manifest is extremely variable,
ranging from a few months to over three decades.
In general, the time interval is between 2 and 5
years between the observation of recurrence and
presentation for additional treatment.

"Malignant Mixed Tumor"

The terms "malignant mixed tumor" and carcinoma ex pleomorphic adenoma have been used
interchangeably.[101–104] While there is usually no
confusion in the minds of therapists, the designations actually signify two different histopathological entities.

Carcinoma ex pleomorphic adenoma or carcinoma arising in a mixed tumor refers to an epithelial malignancy in which remnants of a mixed
tumor matrix can be identified. Capable of assuming any epithelial subtype, the carcinoma is usually
a ductal carcinoma (Fig. 1.13). Metastases contain
only the carcinoma. This form of "malignant
mixed tumor" is overwhelmingly the most common form. Carcinoma ex pleomorphic adenoma
is furthermore increasingly being recognized.

The true malignant mixed tumor is considerably
less common. It exists in two histological forms:
one in which a histologically benign mixed tumor
inexplicably metastasizes without any signal alterations in histological character; and the other in
which both epithelial and stromal elements are
malignant and metastasize together. In effect, because of the heterologous malignancy, the latter

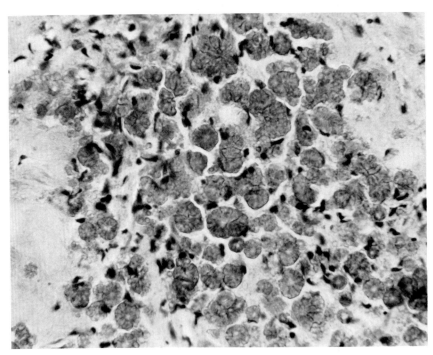

Figure 1.12.   A cluster of extracellular tyrosine crystals in a mixed tumor.

form is a carcinosarcoma (Fig. 1.14). Needless to say both forms of true malignant mixed tumor are nearly medical curiosities, especially the tumor whose biological behavior belies its benign histological appearance.[102, 105] The carcinosarcomatous form has been seen by me three times in 15 years. In each a chondrosarcoma co-existed with a ductal carcinoma. One was in the palate, the other two, in the submandibular gland.

Carcinoma ex pleomorphic adenoma presents in *two* basic clinical forms. The more common is that in a patient with a known benign mixed tumor for a considerable period of time, either because of no prior treatment or because of recurrences. In short, it appears the malignant change is a function of time, either in the recividous or in the primary tumor. A smaller number of patients present with carcinoma ex pleomorphic adenoma without the foregoing sequence. In this instance, the carcinoma is present at the first surgical removal in a patient whose clinical history is short, often less than 1 year. These patients tend to be one or three decades younger than the more common clinical type.

The majority of patients with carcinoma ex pleomorphic adenoma give an almost uniform history. Tumor has usually been present for some time (10 to 15 years), with or without recurrences, and suddenly manifests a rapid growth 3 to 6 months before admission. This may be accompanied by pain and paralysis of the facial nerve. Perineural invasion was found in nearly 50% of the patients studied by LiVolsi and Perzin.[104] The patients are generally a decade older than those with benign mixed tumor. The risk of malignant transformation of this type of tumor increases with the preoperative duration of the tumor. Judged by my experience and that of Spiro et al.,[101] nearly 50% of patients have had at least one surgical procedure before admission. The *number* of recurrences do not appear to be related. Similarly, there

Table 1.9
Recurrences: Primary and Recidivous Mixed Tumors

Author	Primary	Percentage of Recurrences	Recidivous	Percentage of Recurrences
Grage et al.[98]	48	10.0	21	29.0
Winsten and Ward[99]	60	30.0	17	35.3
Molnar et al.[100]	75	10.6	18	33.9

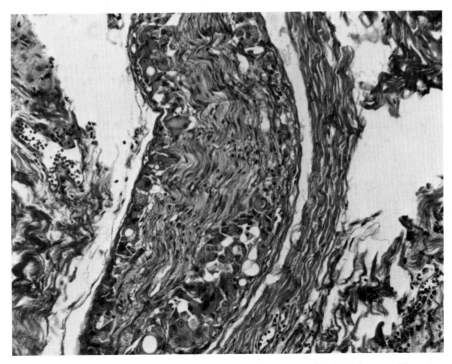

Figure 1.13. Ductal carcinoma ex pleomorphic adenoma manifesting intraneural invasion.

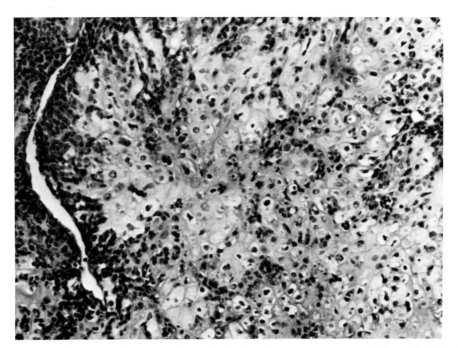

Figure 1.14. True malignant mixed tumor. Shown is the chondrosarcoma component. The epithelial part was of duct cell type.

is a lack of any significant morphological change or progression in the mixed tumor, regardless of the number of recurrences. This observation, however, may be due to a sampling error. Adding credence to the effect of time on the mixed tumor is the study by Eneroth and Zetterberg.[106] These workers have shown, by microspectrophotometric DNA analysis, a difference in the DNA content between morphologically benign mixed tumors of short duration and those with a long preoperative duration of tumor. The latter are characterized by the occurrence of a small fraction of tetraploid cells in the population.

Although historical and clinical features may lead one to suspect the malignancy of a mixed tumor, the diagnosis is a histopathological one. In large series with satisfactory follow-up, "malignant mixed tumors" (very likely all carcinomas ex pleomorphic adenoma) comprise from 2 to 5% of the entire mixed tumor category (Table 1.10). All of the salivary tissues may be the site of carcinoma ex pleomorphic adenoma. In descending order of incidence, the salivary sites are: parotid; submandibular gland and the minor salivary glands of the palate; lip; paranasal sinuses; nasopharynx; and tonsil. Tumors in the parotid gland have ranged from 0.5 to 12.0 cm in diameter. Those in the submandibular gland tend to be less than 6.0 cm

when discovered. A similar size is noted for tumors in the palate.

Formerly, all mixed tumors were considered to be malignant. This judgment was based upon a high recurrence rate (30 to 40%) after inadequate initial treatment, and the occasional appearance of an obviously malignant, rapidly growing and distantly spreading neoplasm after many years of quiescence. An additional handicap in the assessment of malignant mixed tumors is the "lumping" tendency of earlier pathologists. Most of the so-called malignant mixed tumors would now be diagnosed as adenoid cystic carcinomas. The presence of multiple, simultaneously occurring, benign mixed tumors, although rare, may be yet another explanation for the apparent "metastasis" of a mixed tumor.

In brief, the histological criteria for carcinoma ex pleomorphic adenoma are those given by Eneroth[37]: "the presence of mesenchymal (e.g., myxoid, chondroid or fibroid) tumor tissue in a malignant tumor also containing epithelial structures excludes it from other forms of carcinoma and makes it necessary to assign it to the group of carcinoma *in* pleomorphic adenoma."

The carcinoma ex pleomorphic adenoma has certain gross and microscopic features which assist in the diagnosis.

On gross examination these tumors usually appear encapsulated, but in some areas the capsule is disrupted or infiltrated by the malignant component. Some tumors are indeed poorly circumscribed. On cut-section, the surface may resemble a benign mixed tumor, but areas of necrosis and hemorrhage are prevalent. These findings along with advanced softness, cystic change and an irregular border should always alert the surgeon and pathologist to the possibility of a malignant lesion.

For confidence in the microscopic diagnosis, vestiges of the maternal mixed tumor should be identified.[107] In my experience and that of Spiro et al.[101] and LiVolsi and Perzin,[104] the class of epithelial malignancy most often encountered is the adenocarcinoma, usually of ductal type and of a varying differentiation.

It is important to appreciate that carcinoma ex pleomorphic adenoma may be focal, thus requiring multiple sections of the parotid tumor. It is distressing to receive consultation cases from which only two sections of a 5- to 10-cm mass have been taken when the same pathologist will elaborately dissect and sample a leiomyomatous uterus! Suspicious microscopic findings *requiring* further sections are: (1) micronecrosis (Fig. 1.15) and hemorrhage; (2) excessive hyalinization (Fig. 1.16) in a mixed tumor; (3) dystrophic calcification and ossification of stroma; (4) more than the usual bosselation; and (5) destructive infiltrative growth at the periphery of the tumor. According to Eneroth et al.,[108] infiltrative behavior is the single most reliable index. In my experience, this feature may be difficult not only to find, but also to define.

The cellular atypism of malignancy is usually present in the infiltrative masses, but it can also be found elsewhere in the tumor. I have also regarded solid or nearly solid, cellular areas of epithelial elements, usually in microductular form and pos-

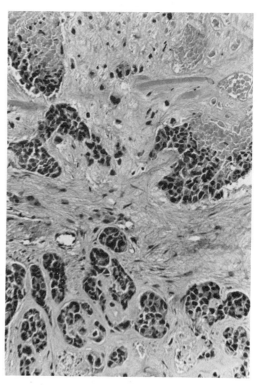

Figure 1.15. Focal areas of micronecrosis in a carcinoma ex pleomorphic adenoma.

Table 1.10
Frequency of "Malignant Mixed Tumors"

Except for the data from the study by Chaudhry et al.,[283] all other information is from a series dealing with the major salivary glands (predominantly the parotid gland).

Authors	No. of Salivary Gland Tumors	No. of "Malignant Mixed Tumors"	Percentage of "Malignant Mixed Tumors"
Foote and Frazell[33]	877	57	7
Eneroth[37]	802	16	2
Morgan and Mackenzie[277]	151	14	9.3
Moberger and Eneroth[278]	2,211	34	1.8
Skolnik et al.[279]	116	2	1.7
Brown et al.[280]	286	12	4.2
Mustard and Anderson[107]	287	16	5.5
Wheelock et al.[281]	209	15	5.3
Freeman et al.[282]	545	5	0.9
Chaudhry et al.[283]	1,414	29	2.0
Saksela et al.[103]	119	6	5.0
Spiro et al.[101]	2,743	146	5.4

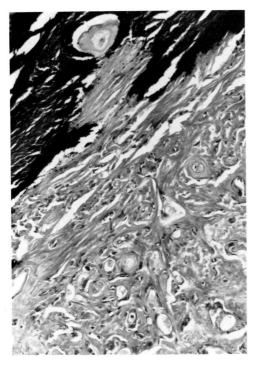

Figure 1.16. Excessive hyalinization and ossification in a carcinoma ex pleomorphic adenoma.

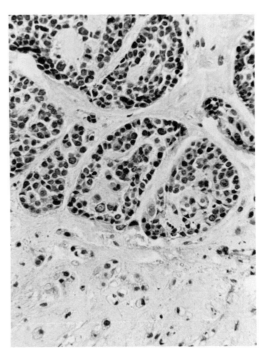

Figure 1.17. Carcinoma ex pleomorphic adenoma with carcinoma cells arranged in a lobular arrangement.

sessing glassy-looking nuclei and arranged in a pattern reminiscent of lobular carcinoma of the breast as pathognomonic (Fig. 1.17). If it can be shown that these cytomorphological alterations are *confined* to foci within an otherwise benign mixed tumor, the term "carcinoma in situ" may be used. Carcinoma in situ in a mixed tumor is a *histological* malignancy and has no clinical or biological corollary.[104]

The importance of recognizing carcinoma ex pleomorphic adenoma lies in its accelerated recurrence rate and high metastatic rate; it was 43% of the cases presented by Eneroth et al.[108] and 70% in the series reported by Gerughty et al.[102] Regional lymph nodes and lungs represented the favorite metastatic sites. In the Sloan-Kettering Memorial Cancer Center experience,[101] the incidence of cervical lymph node metastases was 25%. From the same study, the over-all incidence of distant metastasis was at least 32%. Distant sites were lungs, bone and brain. Nearly one-third of the patients with metastases manifested multiple site involvement. Death intervened within 1 year after the discovery of distant spread. The greater number of patients manifesting distant spread than regional lymph node involvement illustrates once again that carcinomas of major salivary glands, if

persistent, favor hematogenous over lymphogenous metastasis.

Compared with adenoid cystic carcinoma, mucoepidermoid tumor and acinic cell carcinoma, "carcinoma ex mixed tumor" or malignant mixed tumor has the poorest prognosis. Of 29 patients described by Foote and Frazell,[33] 12 were dead in less than 2 years; 21 died in less than 6 years and 2 were alive with inoperable recurrences. A 48.4% 5-year survival indicates the grave prognosis for this tumor. This is re-enforced by Spiro et al.[101] who present net or determinate "cure" rates at 5-, 10- and 15-year intervals of 40, 24 and 19% respectively.

Treatment for this neoplasm is a radical total parotidectomy. Whether or not radical dissection of the involved nodes should be done prophylactically is a moot point, but involved nodes should also be removed at the time of parotidectomy.

Adenoid Cystic Carcinoma

Adenoid cystic carcinoma (cylindroma, adenocystic carcinoma) is a malignant epithelial tumor which develops in major and minor salivary glands (for a discussion on adenoid cystic carcinoma of the minor salivary glands, see Chapter 2). The most likely sources of the neoplasm are the canaliculi and the intercalated ducts of the peripheral duct system of the salivary glands.

The role of the myoepithelial cell in the production of adenoid cystic carcinoma remains as controversial as it does in other salivary gland tumors. With only few exceptions, the cells have been identified in all adenoid cystic carcinomas examined with the electron microscope.[109] Whether or not it is capable of being recognized, I believe the myoepithelium plays a key modifying role in the architectural forms taken by the carcinoma.

Fortunately, the term adenoid cystic carcinoma is now in much more common use than the older "cylindroma." The latter is a diffuse conception, indicating several independent and nonrelated types of neoplasms and is best discarded from both clinical and pathological nomenclatures. Even "adenoid cystic carcinoma" is to some degree a misleading description, as cystic structures are not entirely typical in this type of tumor as they are in mucoepidermoid tumors or Warthin's tumors.

The neoplasm is uncommon in the major salivary glands, comprising about 4% of all tumors of those glands.[33] Incidence in the parotid gland lies between 2 and 5% of all tumors of the gland. A relative guide to its frequency in the parotid gland is that the mucoepidermoid tumor exceeds the occurrence of adenoid cystic carcinoma by a ratio of 2:1. On the other hand, the neoplasm develops with a far greater relative frequency in the minor and lesser major salivary glands (see Chapter 2). It is the most common malignant tumor of the submandibular gland. The tumor has also been recognized in a number of other glandular tissues including the lacrimal and ceruminous glands, esophagus, breast, Bartholin glands of vulva, uterine cervix and prostate gland.[110]

Both sexes are affected with about equal frequency. Presentation in childhood is unusual and the mean age at the time of clinical diagnosis is in the midforties. Pain and "spontaneous" paralysis of the facial nerve occur in nearly one-third of the patients.[111] The other clinical findings are those associated with a palpable resistance in the region of the parotid gland.

One of the most outstanding features of this neoplasm, regardless of its site of origin, is its marked tendency to invade nerves. It is this proclivity that accounts for the high frequency of pain and of paralysis of the facial nerve when the neoplasm arises in the parotid gland. In our own surgical experience, invasion of the nerves is an almost constant microscopic finding (Fig. 1.18). Although extension of neoplasm through nerves is not peculiar to the adenoid cystic carcinoma, this neoplasm certainly manifests this morbid finding more often than other epithelial neoplasms in the head and neck.[112] Blanck et al.[113] consider such an

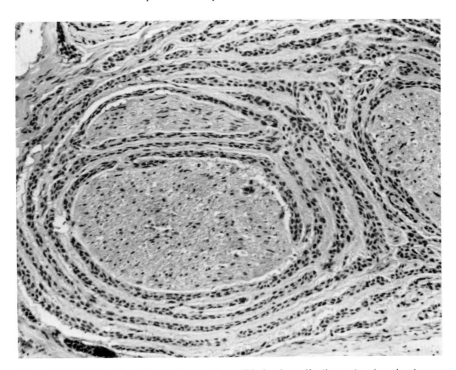

Figure 1.18.   Adenoid cystic carcinoma of parotid gland manifesting extension about nerves.

involvement occurring in association with adenoid cystic carcinomas of the parotid gland as implying a nearly hopeless prognosis. The same dim outlook also applies to the clinical appearance of facial nerve paralysis, a finding which is surprisingly constant in various studies of the neoplasm. According to Eneroth,[37] the majority of patients who suffer facial nerve invasion die within 8 years from the clinical onset of the neoplasm.

Primary adenoid cystic carcinomas of the major salivary glands are commonly monolobular and usually measure 2 to 4 cm at the time of operation. The neoplasms are unencapsulated but appear circumscribed. Like its counterpart in the upper respiratory tract and minor salivary glands, the apparent gross delimitation of the neoplasm belies the infiltration into adjacent apparently normal tissue. On cut section the neoplasm is moist and gray-pink in appearance.

Microscopically there is interplay between the stroma of the neoplasm and the neoplastic epithelial elements. The latter consists of usually rather uniform basaloid cells possessing little cytoplasm and regular nuclei (Fig. 1.19). The cells may be

arranged in anastomosing cords, festoons, solid nests or masses, or in gland-like spaces. It is important to recognize that the neoplasm is not always cribriform or adenoid cystic in appearance. There is an extreme variation in the amount and character of the interstitial stroma of adenoid cystic carcinomas. The stroma may vary from a hyaline eosinophilic material to a mucinous myxoid interstitium.

The relatively wide spectrum of histological appearances of adenoid cystic carcinomas can be imperfectly divided into four main patterns: cribriform or classic; tubuloglandular; solid cellular; and hyaline or cylindromatous. At the light microscopic level, the classic or cribriform adenoid cystic carcinoma appears to consist of anastomosing cords of cells, often surrounding acellular areas. The acellular spaces may contain variable amounts of mucin and what appears to be a hyalinized material. Even under the light microscope, these spaces lack a glandular orientation and electron microscopic evaluation has shown them to be pseudocysts.[114, 115] The pseudocysts constitute an extracellular compartment lined by highly repli-

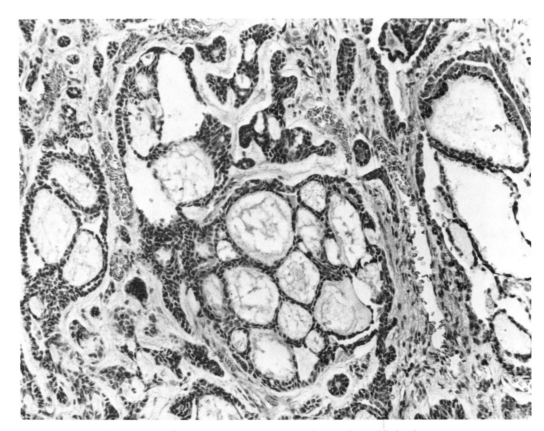

Figure 1.19.   Cribriform adenoid cystic carcinoma of parotid gland.

cated basement membranes which correspond to the hyaline material seen with routine microscopy and staining. True lumina are actually inconspicuous and sparsely distributed in the cellular areas. Aggregations of fine filaments are also common in the pseudocysts.[114, 115] The filaments resemble the microfibrils usually associated with both collagen and elastic fibers. Fine structure analysis has further demonstrated a continuity between the interstitium and the pseudocysts.[115] Elastic tissues have also been identified in the pseudocysts and adjacent to epithelial islands.[116]

The pronounced development of membrane material yields the microscopic picture found in the cylindromatous type of adenoid cystic carcinoma. Reasons for the abundant basement membrane material in the cylindromatous form are unclear. It is noteworthy that the dermal eccrine cylindroma and the presumably related membranous adenoma (see page 50) of salivary glands share this propensity.

The mucosubstances in adenoid cystic carcinomas have been rather intensely investigated. It is fully apparent that these substances abound in different sites in the tumors and they are produced by the various tumor cells. The mucins present in tumor ducts appear to be neutral glycoproteins and sialomucins, whereas those of the pseudocysts are mainly typical connective tissue mucopolysaccharides.[117] The staining characteristics of the pseudocysts of adenoid cystic carcinoma are essentially the same as those of the chondroid and myxoid areas of the mixed tumors. Furthermore the staining of the epithelial secretions are similar in both tumor types.

Histological grading of adenoid cystic carcinomas into high, low and intermediate grades has led some workers to consider grading has a prognostic implication.[118-121] Low-grade carcinomas are those lesions showing a predominance of a cribriform or cylindromatous pattern. High-grade carcinomas, or those with a solid pattern, are said to be associated with a worse prognosis. Nearly an equal number of investigators including myself have found no confirmation of such a relationship.[122-125] Location and clinical stage are determinant factors.

There should not be confusion with mixed tumors manifesting "cylindromatous" patterns. Evans and Cruickshank[36] point to the isomorphism of the adenoid cystic carcinoma: the presence of myxochondroid or fibroid components occurring in a lesion with a cylindromatous pattern is a clear indication that the growth is not an adenoid cystic carcinoma. These authors, in a masterpiece of

brevity, state: "Islets of chondromatous elements with a myxomatous change induced by the histolysis of tumor tissue in the common 'mixed tumor' are strange to the adenocystic carcinoma."[36] The highly invasive pattern and neural invasion further confirm the diagnosis of adenoid cystic carcinoma.

The long-term prognosis is grave and all studies clearly indicate that a much longer follow-up than 5 years is necessary to disclose a definite prognosis in adenoid cystic carcinoma. Foote and Frazell[33] indicate that only 25% of the patients are free of neoplasm 5 or more years after treatment. According to Blanck et al.,[113] the determinate survival rate after the first histological verification is near 75% for 5 years and only 13% for 20 years. Spiro et al.[122] point out that differences in cure rate are dependent upon the site of origin of the primary. When the parotid gland was involved, the 10-year determinate cure rate was 29% as compared with 23% in the mouth, 10% in the submandibular gland and 7% in the paranasal sinuses and larynx. Conley and Dingman[124] using standard life-table methods conclude the probability of being dead from adenoid cystic carcinoma of *all* sites in the head and neck is 31% and by the end of 15 years is 62%. For major salivary glands the figures are more favorable, 24% and 43% respectively. They are reduced in minor salivary gland primaries to 36% and 77% respectively. A comparison of survival rates as influenced by site of the neoplasm is presented in Table 1.11.

The fairly high recurrence rate may well be due to unsatisfactory primary surgical treatment and a failure to recognize the neural extension and insidious infiltration of adenoid cystic carcinomas. Because of the prolonged clinical course it is important to persist with treatment in spite of recurrences so that longer periods of freedom from symptoms may be achieved.

The prognostic significance of metastases is difficult to ascertain since this is usually a late find-

Table 1.11
Relation of Site of Primary to Survival Rates of Adenoid Cystic Carcinomas
Determination survivals are from the data presented by Eneroth et al.[284]

Follow-up Time (Years)	Percentage of Determinate Survival		
	Parotid Gland	Submandibular Gland	Palate
5	73	50	80
10	39	25	44
15	21	0	38
20	13	0	36

ing. Approximately 40% of the cases may manifest either regional or distant metastases or both. The lungs are frequent sites of distant metastases. Often multiple recurrences precede metastases. Because of the often slow growing course, I consider resection of solitary metastases to lung and selected bones as appropriate in selected cases.[126] Relatively prolonged survival may occur in patients with distant metastases, as occurred in 20% of the patients studied by Spiro et al.[122] Death supervened within 1 year of the appearance of these metastasis in one-third of the patients (Fig. 1.20). According to Spiro et al.,[122] the incidence of distant metastases in patients dying of the disease approaches 70%. Lymph node involvement by adenoid cystic carcinomas is of a relatively low order; approximately 15%.[122, 124, 127, 128] When it occurs it does *not* usually result from embolic lymph node metastasis. Rather, a direct invasion of the lymph nodes from tumor in the perinodal soft tissue occurs.[127, 128] This accounts for the often observed sparing of lymph nodes except in the vicinity of the primary, be it parotid gland or submandibular gland (Fig. 1.21).

As with tumors of any histological type, "cure" is achieved with the greatest frequency in patients with the smallest primary lesion. Surgery appears to offer the best chance for eradication of this disease, but the stubbornness and recurrent lesions

that are the hallmarks of adenoid cystic carcinoma have raised questions over the relative merits of any given surgical procedure. Failure of the primary procedure, however, usually means incurability, but not necessarily failure at good palliation.[124] It is possible that better results may be achieved in some cases by more aggressive, ablative surgery or by combinations of surgery and irradiation. The latter has been exploited after the advent of megavoltage treatment and emergence of the concept of the treatment of subclinical and microscopic disease immediately postoperatively. Conley and Dingman[124] outline the principal applications of irradiation: (1) treatment of nonresectable recurrences; (2) augment surgical management when residual disease is present; (3) palliation in the inoperable patient; (4) to gain temporary control in surgically inaccessible tumors; and (5) in the physiologically infirm. A review of the various roles played by radiation therapy is offered by Cummings.[129]

Mucoepidermoid Carcinoma

The descriptive cliche, "a distinctive group of neoplasms" is contained in the opening paragraphs of nearly all of the major reports dealing with the group of salivary gland tumors called mucoepidermoid tumors. The implication this cliche may convey is that both the microscopic

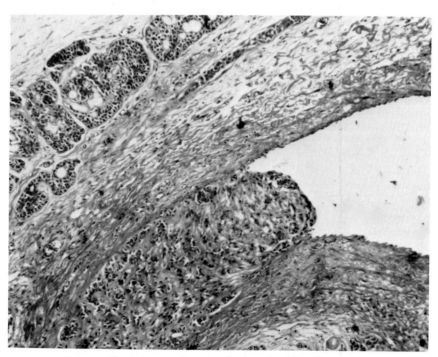

Figure 1.20.   Intravascular extension by adenoid cystic carcinoma.

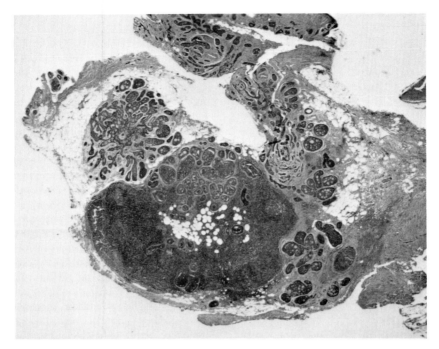

Figure 1.21. Paraparotid lymph node invaded by adenoid cystic carcinoma. The invasion is by contiguous extension and not by lymphatic spread. (Courtesy of M. S. Allen, Jr., M.D.)

appearance and the clinical behavior of the neoplasm are fairly stereotype. Nothing could be further from actual practice.

The name *mucoepidermoid* was given to these salivary gland lesions in 1945 by Stewart et al.[130] when they split the neoplasms off from the broader category of mixed tumors. They chose the designation to emphasize the two main histological features of these tumors, and the term is actually a contraction of "mixed epidermoid and mucus-secreting cell patterns." Clear cells and an abundant lymphoid stromal component are also relatively common.

Mucoepidermoid carcinomas comprise between 3 and 9% of all salivary gland tumors. The majority apparently arise from the epithelium of the large ducts of both major and minor salivary glands. The parotid gland is most commonly involved by the neoplasms. They constitute approximately 10% of all intraoral minor salivary gland tumors, and the palate is the most frequent site. Next to the parotid gland, the palate is the most common localization of a mucoepidermoid carcinoma.

The relative incidence of mucoepidermoid carcinomas is, however, higher in the glands of the palate than in the parotid and submandibular glands. Of the malignant salivary glands tumors of the palate, parotid gland and submandibular gland, the mucoepidermoid carcinoma makes up approximately 26, 21 and 10%, respectively.[132, 133] Mucoepidermoid carcinomas may occur at any age with the highest incidence in patients who are between their fourth and fifth decades of life. There is a slight female predominance.

Clinical presentation varies and, in so doing, relates to the histological composition of the neoplasm. Symptoms and signs are unusual apart from those which mimic mixed tumors. Some tumors may manifest a fixation to the surrounding tissues, pain, and, in some patients, a facial paralysis is also a possible morbid event associated with the neoplasm. The mean duration between the initial swelling and histological verification is quite long; Jakobsson et al.[134] indicate an average of 6.4 years. The more malignant variants have a mean time interval of about 1.5 years. The tumor may be either solid, cystic or semicystic. Cystic composition is unusual in the high-grade malignant carcinomas.

Mucoepidermoid carcinomas are composed of essentially three to six cell types[135]:

1. "Maternal" cells. These cells are small, approximately the size of a lymphocyte, round or oval in shape and have small, round nuclei. The cytoplasm is scanty, is basophilic and is not stained by mucicarmine, periodic acid-Schiff (PAS) or

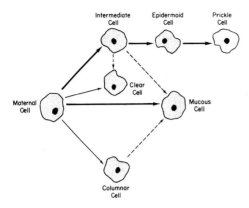

Figure 1.22. Scheme for the histogenesis of mucoepidermoid carcinomas. (Modified from Sikorowa.[135])

Sudan IV stains. These cells occur in the medium-sized or large ducts of the salivary glands. The maternal cell is the progenitor for all of the other cell types (Fig. 1.22).

2. Intermediate cells. This form of cell was designated by Foote and Frazell[33] as an "intermediate cell type." These cells are oval in shape and are a little larger than the maternal cells. They contain a small, darkly staining nucleus and a scanty, pale eosinophilic cytoplasm. The intermediate cells resemble the cells of the Malpighian layer of the squamous epithelium of the mucous membranes. Like the maternal cell, the intermediate cells do not contain either mucin or fat. PAS stains are also negative. Intermediate cells have a potential ability for further differentiation. They may differentiate both toward glandular forms and toward epidermoid, prickle and clear cells.

3. Epidermoid cells. These cells also fail to stain with mucicarmine or fat stains and give only a faint PAS reaction. When arranged in a pavement-like fashion, the epidermoid cells form solid areas and nests which closely resemble squamous cell carcinomas. More mature cells manifest a homogenous, hyaline cytoplasm with keratinization of individual cells and, on rare occasions, the formation of keratin pearls. The presence of intercellular bridges increases their resemblance to squamous cell epithelium.

4. Clear cells. These variably sized and shaped cells have distinct outlines and a hydropic, water-clear cytoplasm. Their nuclei, usually centrally placed, are small, vesicular or pyknotic. Mucicarmine and fat stains are negative, and the cells contain no glycogen.

5. Columnar cells. These cells resemble the cells found in the major secretory ducts of the salivary glands. They transform into mucous cells and in this transitional form, their cytoplasm acquires a slight tendency to stain with mucicarmine.

6. Mucous cells. Since mucous cells occur in the normal ductular epithelium of the salivary glands, their appearance in a mucoepidermoid tumor is expected. Usually large, sometimes swollen or balloon-shaped, these cells have distinct cell boundaries. Their small nuclei are usually compressed and located near the periphery of the cell. Their foamy or reticular cytoplasm is slightly basophilic and pale and gives a prominent positive reaction to mucicarmine and PAS stains. Metachromasia is also exhibited.

If a cell becomes engorged with the produced mucus, its cell membrane ruptures and the mucus is released into the stroma. Some of the cells disintegrate through the liberation of the mucus; others are desquamated into the lumen of mucus-containing cysts. Microcysts and macrocysts are lined with single or multiple layers of mucous cells. Sometimes, particularly in mucoepidermoid carcinomas of the hard palate, the mucous cells acquire a signet-ring appearance. Transition of maternal and intermediate-type cells into mucous cells can readily be seen in many tumors.

There is a wide variation in the cellular makeup of individual mucoepidermoid carcinomas. Specific appearances depend on the relative frequency of the six cell types. Virtually all authors writing on the subject of mucoepidermoid carcinomas have spent a major part of their reports defining or refining the inter-relationships of the cell types in an effort to present a histological classification possessing some prognostic portent.

The first such attempt was by the originators of the diagnostic term.[130] They divided the tumors into two groups, a "qualified" benign group and a "highly favorable" and "relatively favorable" group. The latter class, at the time of their report, had not been shown to be capable of metastasis. Malignant forms were those tumors with either the histological features found in an ordinary squamous cell carcinoma or those tumors with a "transitional-cell carcinoma" appearance. In the malignant tumors, there was a predominance of epidermoid and/or intermediate cell types. Mucous elements and columnar cells were not prominent.

Foote and Frazell[33] followed with their very significant contribution and confided that the strict separation into benign and malignant types was too sharp and too arbitrary, particularly so since, by the time of their study, it had been noted that some of the earlier lesions classified as benign had actually metastasized. These authors emphasized that all cell types were found in most of the tumors. In highly malignant tumors, mucous-containing cells were not numerous, and epidermoid and intermediate cells dominated the histological picture. They further reiterated that epidermoid cells were conspicuous in most low grade tumors. Because of the difficulty in dividing the carcinomas into categories of low-grade or high-grade malignancy and because there was so much overlapping of histological features, Foote and Frazell[33] suggested a more rational approach. They referred to the whole group of mucoepidermoid tumors as malignant and divided the lesions into three degrees of malignancy: high, intermediate and low.

Jakobsson et al.[134] have approached the problem differently. Acknowledging the work of others in dividing their cases into two or more groups according to morphology, they pointed out the difficulty in establishing definite histological criteria for these various divisions. They divide mucoepidermoid tumors into high- and low-grade malignancy with the sole criterion being the demonstration of invasion. In their study, other histological features gave no clear-cut indication of the prognosis, although cystic and well-differentiated adenomatous structures were more often seen in the low-grade tumors. Solid epithelial areas were more often found in high-grade tumors. Despite the fact that their paper is an outstanding one from the point of view of the biological activity of mucoepidermoid carcinomas, there is a glaring deficiency; their definition of "invasion" is never clarified except by a photomicrograph depicting perineural invasion. Certainly "invasion" by a neoplasm that is characteristically unencapsulated is difficult to define.

It is our opinion, after review of our own surgical material and of series presented in the literature, that many of the mucoepidermoid tumors described as benign or of "low-grade malignant potential" follow a clinical course not unlike that of a benign mixed tumor of the salivary glands.[134, 136, 137] This course is characterized by a slow growth, fairly frequent recurrences and a rare, histologically inexplicable, ability to metastasize. High-grade malignancies, on the other hand, run a much more aggressive course, with a high rate of recurrences and frequent local and distant metastases.

We are further convinced that because it is not possible by light microscopy to distinguish between a highly differentiated, yet metastasizing tumor and a histologically, hypothetically benign mucoepidermoid tumor, the patient and surgeon are best served by regarding all forms of mucoe-

pidermoid tumors as carcinomas. The study of Eneroth et al.[138] also presents good evidence to contradict the existence of a recognizable benign form. According to Jakobsson et al.,[134] the malignant types manifest their malignancy within the first 5 years of the follow-up period after primary treatment.

Healey et al.[139] and Foote and Frazell[33] separate mucoepidermoid carcinomas into three grades of malignancy: "low-grade," "high-grade" and "intermediate." The intermediate subgroup is made up of moderately well-differentiated mucoepidermoid carcinomas that behave much like the "low-grade" carcinomas, except they have a higher incidence of recurrences and occasionally manifest metastases.

Well-differentiated or low-grade carcinomas are those mucoepidermoid tumors in which there are well-formed glandular or cystic spaces (Fig. 1.23). These cysts are lined by a single layer of mucin-producing cells. Focal areas in the cysts are lined by flattened epidermoid cells and, in some areas, proliferations of intermediate cells infolded into the cyst lumens. The cells manifest no pleomorphism. Mitoses are extremely rare. According to Healey et al.,[139] this group of tumors manifests a variable degree of infiltration into adjacent structures.

Intermediate types of mucoepidermoid carcinomas have a greater tendency to form solid nests of cells and are more cellular than the low-grade carcinomas (Fig. 1.24). Epidermoid cells and in-

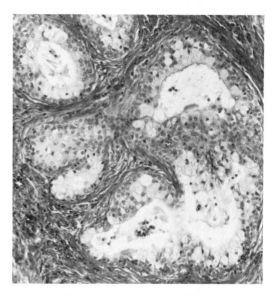

Figure 1.23. Low-grade or well-differentiated mucoepidermoid carcinoma.

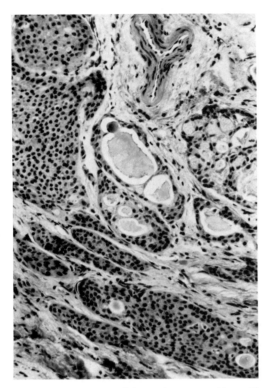

Figure 1.24. Intermediate-grade mucoepidermoid carcinoma.

termediate-type cells are more frequent, and cystic spaces are less prominent. The cells show a slight to moderate pleomorphism, and occasional mitoses are present. These carcinomas have a greater tendency to be locally invasive.

High-grade mucoepidermoid carcinomas manifest considerable anaplasia. According to Woolner et al.,[136] three main patterns are found. (1) The bulk of the lesion is squamous cell in character and resembles squamous cell carcinoma of other sites. Mucous cells are limited in number and often present only in focal areas. These cells may be so few in number that they may be missed unless sampling of the tumor is adequate (Fig. 1.25). (2) The carcinoma is composed of an abundance of cellular mucus and an equally prominent squamous cell distribution. The most striking anaplastic feature is the presence of small, hyperchromatic cells with a rather coarse chromatin pattern. Mitoses are numerous. (3) Carcinomas in which all cell lines and differentiation are present, but in the unusually prominent peripheral zone of basal cells or intermediate cells, there is anaplasia and frequent mitoses. These carcinomas exhibit considerable local aggressiveness and infiltrate adjacent

tissues with ease. From the foregoing, it can be seen that carcinomas showing marked cyst formation usually show little cellular anaplasia and a minimal local aggressiveness.

A modicum of assistance for prognostication may be achieved by assessing the DNA content of cells in smears obtained by asperation. Noninvasive tumors have been found to be associated with a diploid or near diploid DNA content, whereas invasive mucoepidermoid carcinomas are found to have a triploid or near-triploid DNA content.[140, 141]

Mucoepidermoid carcinomas are said to be prone to recurrences. Frazell[142] reported that 15% of the low-grade and 60% of the high-grade carcinomas recur. Stevenson and Hazard[143] reported that 75% of the carcinomas recur. Bhaskar and Bernier,[137] on the other hand, record a relatively low (15%) recurrence rate in their series. Our experience and that of Jakobsson et al.[134] would seem to indicate a recurrence rate intermediate between the foregoing extremes, i.e., 30%.

When recurrences appear, they usually do so during the first postoperative year. The histological appearance of the neoplasm does not change even with repeated recurrences.

The ability of mucoepidermoid carcinomas to metastasize also varies according to different studies. It has been stated that 66% of the high-grade mucoepidermoid carcinomas are associated with local lymph node metastases and in 33%, multiple cutaneous, osseous, pulmonary and cerebral metastases may occur.[33, 142]

Metastatic foci may contain only pure epidermoid forms, pure mucus-producing adenocarcinoma, or be mixed in character. This clonal pattern is taken to indicate or reflect a mosaic structure in the primary with subpopulations endowed with varying differentiative capacities. Both recurrences and metastases are usually associated with the more anaplastic forms of mucoepidermoid carcinomas, and both the local recurrences and the metastases contribute significantly to the death of the host.

Most authors consider the mucoepidermoid carcinoma to be of relatively low radiosensitivity. Complete regression as a result of radiation therapy is probably not achievable. Therefore, treatment is primary surgical removal, with the extent of surgery governed by the location of the tumor in the gland, the presence or absence of palpable regional lymph nodes and the histological appearance of the tumor.[144, 145] Jakobsson et al.[134] are of the opinion that parotidectomy should always be complemented by a radical neck dissection in high-grade mucoepidermoid carcinomas.

The 5-year survival of all patients with mucoepidermoid carcinoma is nearly 90%. Determinate survival rates of the whole group (both high- and low-grade carcinomas) shows that, as expected, the low-grade carcinomas have a definitely benign course. This can be judged with relatively great accuracy after only 5 year's observation, unlike that for adenoid cystic carcinomas and acinous cell carcinomas.[134]

Spiro et al.[75] record a 44% incidence of metastases to cervical lymph nodes for their parotid mucoepidermoid carcinomas other than low grade. Survival in their series of intermediate- and high-grade carcinomas appeared to be stage dependent in that when the carcinomas were analyzed according to stage, the 5-year cure rate varied from 100% to 65% to 10% in stages I, II and III respectively. A 5-year survival of 41.6% is given as the Mayo Clinic experience[144] with high-grade mucoepidermoid carcinomas and this survival is nearly matched by data provided by Jakobsson et al.[134]

For highly differentiated mucoepidermoid carcinomas of the palate, the 5-, 10-, 15- and 20-year determinate survival rate is 100%.[131] The 5- and 10-year determinate survival rates of poorly differentiated mucoepidermoid carcinomas of the palate are 17% and 0%, respectively.[131]

Elsewhere in this text, mucoepidermoid carcinomas of other less common sites are discussed. Despite the fact that the mucous glands of the larynx, trachea and bronchi are phylogenetically similar to those in the salivary glands, mucoepidermoid carcinomas of these glands are rare.[146-148] In the bronchi, the mucoepidermoid carcinomas are particularly viscious with all patients dead of their disease within approximately 1.5 years of the onset of symptoms, regardless of the type of treatment.[148]

The conjunctival mucoepidermoid carcinoma is also rare but there are suggestions that it is more locally aggressive than squamous cell carcinoma of the conjunctiva.[149]

Acinous Cell Carcinoma

Baden and Wallen[150] point out that the adjectival form of acinus is *acinous* and therefore neither acinous or acinic is grammatically correct as a name for this salivary gland tumor. The appropriate, although not widely used, designation is then "*acinous cell carcinoma.*"

Acinous cell neoplasms were not recognized as a specific class of salivary gland tumors until the early 1950s. Credit is given to Buxton et al.[151] for being the first to ascribe a "malignant ability" to these lesions. Since that time there has been an

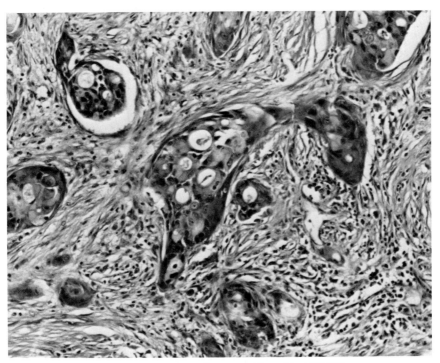

Figure 1.25. High-grade mucoepidermoid carcinoma.

Table 1.12
Incidence of Acinous Cell Carcinoma—Parotid Gland

Authors	Total No. of Parotid Tumors	No. of Acinous Cell Tumors	Percentage of all Parotid Tumors	Percentage of Malignant Parotid Tumors
Foote and Frazell[33]	766	21	2.7	
Beahrs et al.[167]	760	24	3.2	14.8
Grage et al.[164]	272	11	4.0	16.9
Bardwill[171]	153	8	5.2	7.2
Hanna and Gaisford[172]	300	7	2.3	9.1
Mustard and Anderson[107]	287	10	3.4	13.5
Vandenberg et al.[94]	145	4	2.1	19.0
Eneroth et al.[154]	2,102	63	2.9	

evolution by pathologists and surgeons to consider acinous cell neoplasms as carcinomas.[152–154] This trend has not been without its detractors. Evans and Cruickshank[36] hold firmly to the notion that there are only occasional "facultative malignant variants" of acinic cell tumors. Others assume a purely academic and post hoc stance and consider the neoplasms merely as *tumors*, dividing them into "benign" or "malignant" on the basis of their biological course in the host.[32, 155, 156] This type of reasoning has culminated in the rather grim outlook that some patients will have unnecessary radical surgery and some patients will have insufficient surgery for these lesions.[156] Disconcerting as that may sound, it is more disturbing that pathologists appear to be prisoners of their own nomenclature. The epitome of such semanticism appears to have been reached by Thackray and Sobin[32]: "There seems to be more necessity to change the name to carcinoma if a tumor happens to metastasize than there is justification for calling those that have not yet done so adenomas." Would that the patients who have died of their acinous cell carcinomas be so reassured!

Acinous cell carcinomas account for between 2.5 and 4% of all tumors of the parotid gland (Table 1.12). Their incidence in salivary tissues other than the parotid gland is of a low order (Table 1.13) and is dominated by an origin from minor salivary glands of the oral cavity.[157] The carcinoma ranks only behind Warthin's tumor in its frequency of bilateral parotid gland involvement which is approximately 3%.[157] Characteristically presenting in patients who are in their fifth decade of life, the acinous cell carcinoma also figures prominently in the malignancies of salivary glands in childhood.[158] Only the mucoepidermoid carcinomas are more common.

Acinous cell neoplasms, because of their unique position at the distal end of the salivary unit, are

Table 1.13
Acinous Cell Carcinoma: Incidence in Minor Salivary Glands

Author	Total No. of tumors	Percentage Malignant	No. of Acinous Cell Carcinomas
Fine et al.[168]	79	47	1
Spiro et al.[31]	492	88	2
Frable and Elzay[169]	73	42	0
Chaudhry et al.[170]	1,414	40	4

particularly well suited to test our hypothesis of pathogenesis (vide supra) which considers the development of salivary gland neoplasia as an epigenetic event superimposed upon the process of cell renewed by stem or reserve cells. For the acinous carcinoma, these cells are believed to reside in the intercalated duct or its embryonic precursor, the terminal epithelial cluster and tubule (Fig. 1.26). Since de-differentiation of a fully developed acinous cell carcinoma is not probable, the varying patterns of differentiation seen in acinous cell carcinomas are attributed to the attempts of the terminal tubule or intercalated duct reserve cells to approximate the neoplastic equivalent of the normal phenotypic expression of acinous lobules. The fullest expression of this process of neoplastic differentiation is the classically defined acinous cell carcinoma. Those acinous cell carcinomas with imperfect differentiation retain areas of tubular or solid epithelial masses.

Grossly, the neoplasms are usually solitary masses, often with well-defined margins. A thin capsule may be present. Most of the tumors measure up to 3.0 cm but may be larger than 5.0 cm at the time of their discovery. Multilobulation may be a conspicuous feature and while multinodularity is prominent in recurrent carcinomas, it may also be present in primary lesions. The latter is regarded by us as a multifocal origin. It is our belief that the acinous cell carcinoma ranks second

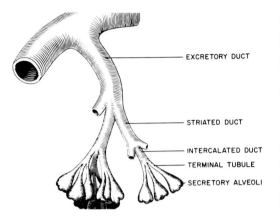

Figure 1.26. Schematic presentation of the salivary duct system. Acini and acinous cell carcinomas are believed to be derived from the terminal portions; the intercalated ducts and terminal tubules.

only to Warthin's tumor in frequency of multifocal origin and like Warthin's tumor, the acinous cell carcinoma may arise in ductal or acinar inclusions in paraparotid or intraparotid lymph nodes. On cross-section the tumor appears to be composed of brittle, gray-white solid or cystic tissue. The gross appearance of the tumor, in particular its cut surface, does not resemble the smooth, glistening surface typical of the mixed tumor of salivary glands.

The histological growth patterns of acinous cell carcinomas fall into one or a combination of the following: (1) acinar-lobular; (2) microcystic; (3) follicular; (4) papillary cystic; (5) medullary; (6) ductologlandular; and (7) primitive tubular. The last three patterns are those foci most closely resembling intercalated ducts and cells from the terminal tubules of the embryo and early postnatal parotid gland (Figs. 1.27 and 1.28). This is confirmed not only by their light-microscopic appearance but also by their ultrastructural features.[159–161] These patterns never comprise the entire tumor and more differentiated, recognizable acinous carcinoma is evident in most sections examined. The

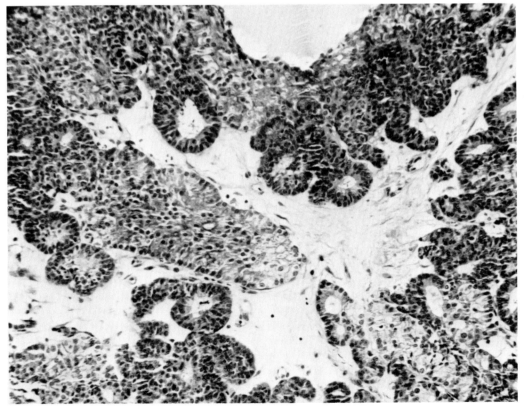

Figure 1.27. Differentiating acinous cell carcinoma. Note the tubular forms and solid foci. These correspond to the terminal tubules and buds of the embryonic salivary gland.

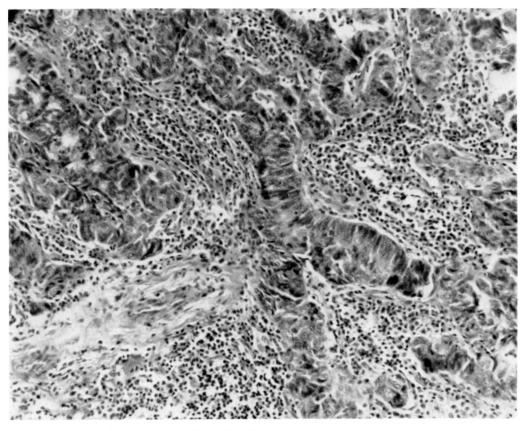

Figure 1.28. Undifferentiated focus in an acinous cell carcinoma.

primitive tubular patterns, however, manifest an infiltrative growth in contrast to the usual blunt, circumscribed growth of the more differentiated acinous cell carcinomas.

A conspicuous lymphoid infiltrate is often associated with the carcinoma. In some carcinomas, the character and circumscription of the lymphoid component is such to strongly suggest an origin within intraparotid aggregates or in small lymph nodes. Calcification may be prominent. Usually it takes the form of calcospherites but may also present in a dystrophic form within broad areas of collagenous tissue.

The acinous cell carcinoma in its classical form bears a rather marked resemblance to normal lobules of the parotid gland (Fig. 1.29). Granular (secretory-type) cells are either a prominent or an exclusive component. The cells are round or polygonal with eccentrically placed nuclei and inconspicuous nucleoli. The cytoplasm is usually finely or coursely granular, but may be focally clear in some areas. Occasionally, the clear cells may be diffuse. The tumor cells usually manifest a baso-

philic hue on routine hematoxylin and eosin stained histological sections. Mitotic figures are rare and when present are usually found in the less differentiated tubular cells.

The results of the application of special staining techniques have been discussed by Abrams et al.[162] The degree of reactivity is related to the level of differentiation of the cells. Only the PAS reaction is positive in all cell types in all growth patterns.

It is generally considered that there is not a good correlation between histological appearance of the acinous cell carcinoma and its biological course in the host. On the basis of the seven growth patterns mentioned above and other features, I have graded acinous cell carcinomas into high and low grades. High-grade carcinomas manifest intravascular extension, local finger-like invasion and have medullary, ductuloglandular or primitive tubular foci. Done in a retrospective fashion, such grading correlates fairly well with recurrences and metastases, but the fallibility of even such post hoc grading is evident by the occasional patient with a low-grade carcinoma who follows the same postoperative course as a patient with a high-grade carcinoma.[163] The grading system is unlikely to be adequate to serve as a complete intraoperative (frozen-section) guide to the surgeon because of sampling error. Whether or not preoperative DNA content assessment is practical is also conjectural. From the work of Eneroth et al.,[141, 154] it is suggested the DNA content of acinous cell carcinoma is equivalent to that of cells from a poorly differentiated adenocarcinoma. While this finding argues strongly against the existence of a totally benign variety of acinous cell tumor, there is further evidence that the DNA content correlates best with the invasiveness of the carcinoma.[141]

In the final analysis, while adverse histological features may be identified, it is the clinical extent of the primary tumor and the adequacy of primary removal which determine prognosis and survival.[152]

The observations on our patients with acinous cell carcinoma and that of others clearly indicate a patient with an acinous cell neoplasm is ill-served by considering the tumor as benign (Table 1.14). They should also dispel further ambiguity over the malignant potential of these neoplasms. Clinical experience certainly refutes statements such as: "The number of cases that ultimately become malignant and metastasize is so small that these tumors are not entitled to be grouped all together under the generic term acinic cell carcinomas. Neither are they to be regarded as semi-malignant growths."[36]

Ambiguity over the malignancy of acinic cell neoplasms has had its counterpart in the therapeutic philosophy applied to the management of these neoplasms. Eneroth et al.[154, 163] have recommended the most aggressive, and Godwin et al.,[155] the most conservative forms of treatment. The former advocate total parotidectomy *and* neck dissection. The latter suggest the "best" treatment is an excision of the tumor with a margin of parotid gland. Considering the tumors as essentially benign, Abrams et al.[162] recommend "lobectomy for lesions in the superficial lobe or tail of the parotid gland or total parotidectomy for those in deeper portions." The fate of the facial nerve in patients with these carcinomas has also been debated. Grage et al.[164] advise routine VIIth nerve resection.

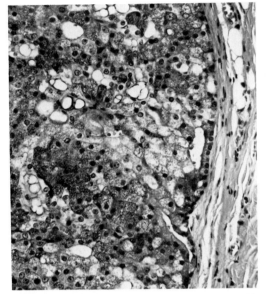

Figure 1.29. Acinous cell carcinoma of the parotid. Note the close resemblance to normal acinar structures of the salivary glands.

Table 1.14
Recurrence and Metastasis: Acinous Cell Carcinoma

Authors	No. of Patients	Local Recurrence	Metastasis*	Death Due to Neoplasm
Abrams et al.[162]	18	10	Indeterminate	3
Beahrs et al.[167]	12	1	4	4
Buxton et al.[151]	21	8	—	7
Eneroth et al.[163]	63	12	10	7
Foote and Frazell[33]	21	4	—	7
Fox et al.[165]	46	22	—	7
Godwin et al.[155]	27	16	4	3
Gorlin and Chaudhry[166]	10	2	5	—
Grage et al.[164]	8	5	4	1
Spiro et al.[152]	67	22	8	8
The University of Michigan	31	14	11	8

* Includes cervical lymph node and distant metastases.

Others sacrifice the nerve only when there is clinical or gross involvement.[152, 153]

The place of neck dissection is also controversial. Only Eneroth and his associates have recommended a routine radical neck dissection.[163] It is of interest that Fox et al.[165] advise against radical neck dissection even though that judgement was made after a study of a series in which the frequency of metastases to cervical lymph nodes (3/46 cases) was nearly equal to that occurring in Eneroth's series (4/47 cases).[163]

Based on our data and that provided by Chong et al.[153] and Abrams et al.,[162] enucleation and local excision of these carcinomas is to be condemned. An 85% recurrence rate in our series and a 67% rate in Chong's series[153] should underscore that opinion.

Recurrences are markedly reduced by total parotidectomy, but as is evident in our series and that of Chong et al.,[153] the capriciousness of the neoplasm, clearly enhanced by failure of primary management, mitigate statements concerning the ultimate prognosis in these patients. It is the clinical stage of the carcinoma which determines prognosis.

It would seem quite clear that the best opportunity for cure lies in complete surgical removal of the neoplasm at the time of initial treatment. For this, a total parotidectomy is the procedure of choice. This is predicated on the unpredictable invasiveness of the carcinoma, high-grade foci that occur in a significant number of the carcinomas, and a potential for multifocal origin of some of the tumors. A relatively low incidence of metastases to the cervical lymph nodes (approximately 10%) does not warrant *elective* neck dissection. The management of the facial nerve cannot be predicted on the basis of a retrospective analysis of the behavior of these carcinomas. That decision is best left to the surgeon who in each patient bases his decision on clinical and/or gross findings.

The full malignant potential of acinous cell carcinoma can only be realized in studies with long term follow-up. Given that, there is clear evidence that these neoplasms exhibit a higher degree of malignancy than is usually ascribed to them. It has also been demonstrated that both the recurrences and appearance of metastases may be very late.[152, 153, 164] Four of the 11 patients studied by Grage et al.[164] died of their disease. The average survival before death was 13 years. Eight of our 35 patients died of their disease after similar lengths of time. Eneroth et al.[154] record a determinate survival at 5 years of 90%, declining to 56% at 20 years. Of the 69 patients with acinous cell

carcinoma reported by Chong et al.,[153] 16 died of their disease. The influence of primary treatment on prognosis is quite clear in the latter study. All deaths occurred in patients who had local excision. Citing clinical extent of the tumors as most important for ultimate survival, Spiro et al.[152] record determinate "cure" rates of 76, 63 and 55% at 5, 10 and 15 years respectively.

Death may be caused by both local extension and hematogenous dissemination. The lungs and skeleton, particularly the spinal column, are the metastatic sites of predilection.

Experience with irradiation of acinous cell carcinoma is very limited. There is a suggestion of radiosensitivity and postoperative external irradiation is used in selected patients who have locally advanced disease.

Adenocarcinoma

In a way, these malignant neoplasms of the major salivary glands are those glandular malignancies that cannot be placed into other more definable classes such as carcinomas of the acinous cell, mucoepidermoid and adenoid cystic types. They have either been placed in the category of miscellaneous carcinomas or the term has been used in a generic sense. Foote and Frazell[173] included adenoid cystic carcinomas under the heading of adenocarcinoma, and a similar "lumping" has only been recently clarified for adenocarcinomas of minor salivary glands[174] (see Chapter 2). Some adenocarcinomas arise from mixed tumors of long standing (an occurrence we are becoming more to respect) and a few appear to have arisen from a pre-existing adenoid cystic carcinoma. Others seem to occur *ab initio*.

Because these neoplasms have been, in effect, "hidden" in most reports, their true incidence is difficult to establish. In a series of 1,678 tumors of the parotid gland studied by Blanck et al.,[175] 47 (2.8%) were considered to represent this type of neoplasm. These neoplasms made up 15.7% of the 299 malignant parotid neoplasms in their material. Earlier reports consider the incidence to be much lower. There is no apparent sex difference and patients have been reported who have been in the early second decade to the seventh decade of life. The mean interval between the first symptom and the first histological verification of the tumor in Blanck et al.'s[175] series was nearly 4 years. Symptoms and signs apart from a palpable mass are unusual.

At their discovery the neoplasms vary in size from less than 3 cm to more than 5 cm in diameter. The tumor is firm and hard and usually manifests some degree of attachment to adjacent tissues. Adenocarcinoma of the major salivary glands, like its counterparts in the upper respiratory tract and minor salivary glands, may be papillary or non-papillary and mucus-secreting or non-mucus-secreting.

In general, its microscopic appearance is similar to that of adenocarcinomas of the gastrointestinal tract, a feature already noted for adenocarcinomas of minor salivary gland origin. In the parotid, there is, however, a greater tendency to form cystic and papillary structures. A papillary growth was manifested in 42 of the 47 examples studied by Blanck et al.[175] These papillary structures are often found as projections from the walls of cystic lumina.

The cells of the neoplasm are cylindrical, of a variable height and often form papillary excrescences, acini or solid masses. In some examples, the cells may be signet ring in type. Mucus production, as determined by the mucicarmine stain, is present in most of the neoplasms. Blanck et al.[175] observed a rather marked lymphoid stroma in seven of their cases. It is to be noted that an abundant lymphoid tissue accompaniment in the adenocarcinoma is more common than in mucoepidermoid or acinous cell carcinomas. The principal differential diagnosis is mucoepidermoid carcinoma, and this rests on the demonstration of squamous cells differentiation.

Evans and Cruickshank[36] consider all adenocarcinomas as highly malignant neoplasms that metastasize to the regional lymph nodes and distant viscera. Blanck et al.,[175] however, after dividing their cases into invasive (high-grade malignant) and noninvasive (low-grade malignant), consider the high-grade adenocarcinomas to behave clinically like a low-grade mucoepidermoid carcinoma. It is important to recognize that this division into high- and low-grade malignancy is based on a histological *staging* (local destructive infiltration) and not on any histological *grading* characteristics.

Recurrences occur most often in high-grade adenocarcinomas and, in these patients, recurrence is a serious omen. Of 15 patients with local recurrence, 10 (nine high-grade and one low-grade), i.e., 67%, died from their neoplasms.[175] Metastases occur predominantly in the high-grade adenocarcinomas. The regional lymph nodes and distant metastases to the skeleton, lungs and other lymph node groups are the sites. In the series reported by Blanck et al.[175] all except 1 of their 13 patients with regional and/or distant metastases died from their neoplastic disease.

The determinate survival rate in Blanck et al.'s[175] series fell from 78% for the patients followed up for 5 years to 41% for the 20-year group. In the 28 patients with a high-grade tumor, the determinate survival rate fell from 70 to 20%. In the 19 patients with low-grade neoplasm, the corresponding drop was from 94 to 83%. The most effective treatment to date has been total excision.

Primary carcinomas arising from the major duct system of the salivary glands are a very small and unusual class of neoplasms. Substantiating the diagnosis of a Stensen's duct carcinoma is not an easy task since there is considerable difficulty in identifying these neoplasms as distinct from those arising in the gland proper or secondarily involving the gland from the buccal mucosa. Primary carcinomas of Stensen's duct may be mucoepidermoid, squamous cell or adenocarcinomatous in appearance. Benign tumors of the parotid duct are not as rare as cancers of the duct, and possibly represent ectopic salivary gland tissue which has become neoplastic.[176] A review of proved cancers of the parotid duct has been presented by Gaisford et al.[176] Treatment is surgical and it must be relatively radical.

An apparently related group of salivary duct carcinomas has been described by Kleinsasser et al.[177] and Evans and Cruickshank.[36] Many of the histological features of these neoplasms bear a strong resemblance to ductal lesions of the breast, i.e., intraductal papillary proliferation, mucoid variants, comedocarcinomas, intraductal cribriform patterns and, occasionally, lesions resembling adenosis of the breast. Fayemi and Toker[178] are further impressed with the resemblence to prostatic carcinoma. This group of salivary duct carcinomas occurs predominantly in men between the fifth and sixth decades and most frequently arises within the parotid gland. The clinical course of patients with this malignancy varies from a gradual progression to rapid growth associated with hematogenous and lymphatic dissemination.

Like mammary carcinomas, the salivary duct carcinomas also contain myoepithelial cells (Fig. 1.30).

Undifferentiated Carcinomas

These neoplasms are rare and are usually highly malignant carcinomas. Authorities such as Patey et al.[179] do not feel there is justification for removing these neoplasms or the trabecular carcinomas from the major generic classification of adenocarcinomas. The poor level of differentiation of these carcinomas certainly should indicate that, if generalizations about the prognosis for adenocarci-

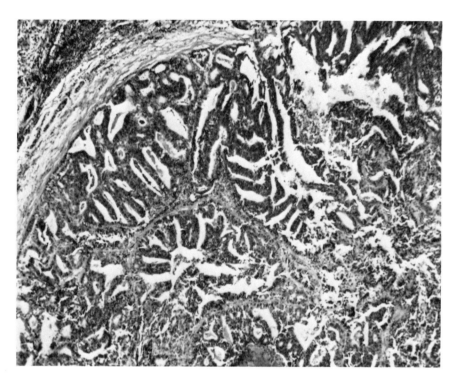

Figure 1.30.   Salivary duct carcinoma of parotid gland.

nomas are to be made, the undifferentiated malignancies should be separated.

Undifferentiated carcinomas make up not more than 3% of all tumors of the major salivary glands and from 1 to 4.5% of all malignat neoplasms of the parotid gland.[180] The seventh and eighth decades of life are the time periods of greatest occurrence, but undifferentiated carcinoma may arise at nearly any age. There is no sex difference. Over one-third of the reported cases appear to have been superimposed on a previously diagnosed mixed tumor, often one of long standing.[36, 179] When an undifferentiated carcinoma has developed within a pre-existing mixed tumor, there is histological evidence of the underlying tumor in the form of one or more of its components. Usually such residues consist of acellular hyaline masses. Areas with histological structures characteristic of poorly differentiated solid carcinoma may also occur in other types of malignant salivary tumors such as adenoid cystic carcinomas and high grade adenocarcinomas.

The undifferentiated and poorly differentiated carcinomas usually grow in solid or trabecular patterns and have been divided into spheroidal, spindle, round and small cell types. This simplistic cell typing is a throwback to the morbid anatomists and serves no known clinicopathological significance.

The small cell undifferentiated carcinoma of salivary gland origin merits special consideration, in that it has been likened, histologically, to the oat cell carcinoma of the lung. Koss et al.,[181] in their report of 14 cases of the anaplastic, small cell carcinoma of *minor* salivary glands, postulated a neuroectodermal origin (Kulchitsky-like cells). These lesions manifest a high frequency of metastasis to cervical lymph nodes (50%) and an overall poor prognosis. The inability of investigators to find characteristic neurosecretory granules in these tumors certainly jeopardizes a neuroectodermal progenitor cell theory and these small cell carcinomas may be only yet another variation of anaplastic carcinoma.[182]

Blanck et al.,[180] after a study of 75 cases of poorly differentiated carcinomas of the parotid gland, consider these malignancies to have a much worse prognosis than other carcinomas, apart from carcinoma ex pleomorphic adenoma. This is especially true for the 5-year determinate survival rate.[179]

Trabecular adenocarcinomas are extremely rare forms of undifferentiated carcinomas of the major salivary glands. In Eneroth's series,[37] they made up only 0.6% of all tumors.

The neoplasms are composed of closely packed polymorphous neoplastic cells arranged in rather characteristic cords or trabeculae. The trabeculae vary in width and are separated by thin connective tissue stromal elements. The cells are somewhat larger and more polygonal than those found in the solid undifferentiated carcinomas of the salivary glands.

In view of the few cases recorded, or at least recognized, opinions on the neoplasm's behavior cannot be definitely given. However, because of the incidence of recurrence and metastases, as well as the high mortality rate, trabecular adenocarcinomas appear to be highly malignant neoplasms of the parotid gland.

Clear Cell Carcinoma

The so-called nonmucinous "clear cells" which occur in neoplasms of a variety of tissues (kidneys, thyroid gland, uterus and sweat glands, including the major and minor salivary glands) continue to perplex investigators and elude a precise definition. In the instance of tumors of the salivary tissues, the clear cell is slowly emerging from its enigmatic status. This is attributed to the results of histochemical and/or ultrastructural analyses.[18, 38, 183-185] These studies have shown that the clear cell (nonmucinous) appearance is the light microscopic manifestation of three basic factors, depending upon the particular gland lesion being investigated.[186] First, clear cells may contain large amounts of cytoplasmic glycogen and a normal complement of subcellular organelles; second, they contain little or no demonstrable glycogen and a paucity of organelles; and third, the cells may appear clear because of a postremoval or fixation artefact. The latter phenomenon is seen in occasional oncocytic lesions and acinous cell carcinomas.

From the foregoing, then, one may simplistically classify the primary nonmucinous cell tumors of salivary tissue as glycogen-rich, nonglycogen containing, and produced by artefact.

This categorization of clear cells does not relate to the cell of origin and is nothing more than a structural (cell) descriptive interpretation.

Clear cells may predominate or be only a component of major and minor salivary gland tumors. When present in other definable tumors, artefact is the likely basis.

The cell of origin of the clear cell neoplasm remains problematical, not only because of its rarity, but also because of varying interpretations of electron and light microscopic findings. In some instances two cell types, epithelial and myoepithelial, are described. In others, only one or the other is said to be present. Additionally, not all of the tumors have contained glycogen. The conclusion

of Donath et al.[38] appears to be a scientifically based compromise. They have designated this group of lesions as *epithelial-myoepithelial carcinomas of intercalated ducts.* This term embraces those tumors previously described as adenomyoepithelioma, glycogen rich (myoepithelial or clear cell tumors), and tubular adenomas. The variable morphological presentation of these tumors may be explained by the participation of both epithelial and myoepithelial cells or by the two-sided nature of the myoepithelial cell itself. This two-sided character is expressed in part by the position of the cells (an epithelial interface and a stromal and basement membrane interaction). Also, the "epithelial" part of the myoepithelial cell situated toward the lumen is remarkably poor in cell organelles and hence looks pale under the light and electron microscopes. Pinocytotic vesicles and glycogen granules, on the other hand, are regularly present on the cell surface adjacent to the basement membrane.

The description of the two-sided, normal myoepithelial cell corresponds to the ultrastructural appearance of the biphasic form of the neoplasms as given by Donath et al.[38] The inner layer of cells in their tumors contained few organelles. The other cells were rich in organelles and glycogen and manifested myoepithelial characteristics.

Other forms of the clear cell tumor appear monophasic and composed of relatively large polygonal cells with a clear nonvacuolated cytoplasm arranged in compressed cords or tubules, or in cohesive masses.[186]

If glycogen is present within the clear cells there is a positive reaction to PAS and Best's carmine stain, which is soluble with diastase digestion. Glycogen is also demonstrable in electron micrographs. The type of glycogen present in the tumor cells is that of single particles (beta-type).

The clear cell tumors may be found in major and minor salivary tissues.[31, 187] In the latter they have been recorded in the nasal cavity, paranasal sinuses, oral cavity and larynx.

There is a strong probability that the majority, if not all, of the nonmucinous clear cell tumors in major and minor salivary glands are at least low-grade carcinomas. This is in concert with the interpretations applied to clear cell tumors of the thyroid gland.[188] The relative undifferentiation of the nonglycogen tumors indicates an immature cell similar to the reserve cell of salivary ducts. Clear cell tumors in the major salivary glands sometimes possess a capsule, while others, like the tumors in the minor salivary tissues manifest an irregular, noncircumscribed infiltrative growth pattern.

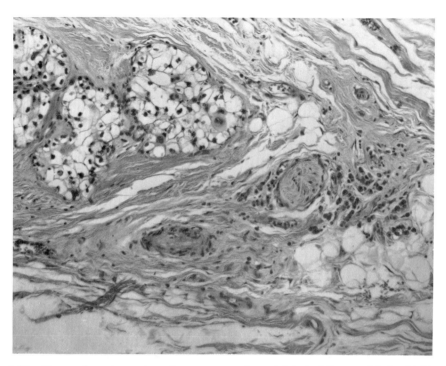

Figure 1.31. Clear cell carcinoma (nonglycogen or mucin containing) of the parotid gland infiltrating near nerve branches.

In my own experience of three cases, one patient manifested a local, destructive, infiltrative growth in the hard palate, another (with tumor in the parotid gland) demonstrated perineural invasion, and the third patient's lesion (parotid gland) eventually metastasized to regional lymph nodes after three recurrences. Because of this behavior and indications from the literature I consider all clear cell lesions as carcinomas with a biological behavior akin to the low-grade and intermediate-grade mucoepidermoid carcinoma (Fig. 1.31).

The true clear cell carcinoma must always be distinguished from a metastatic renal cell carcinoma to salivary tissue. Aside from subtle and inconstant histochemical differences, the only sure way to separate the lesions is by clinical exclusion of the primary. Differences in vascular patterns, organoid arrangement and cytoplasmic differentiation have failed to be conclusive criteria.

Primary Squamous Cell Carcinoma of the Parotid Gland

The frequency with which a *primary* squamous cell carcinoma occurs in the parotid gland is not easy to ascertain by a review of reports in the literature. Data are presented that indicate the incidence ranges from 0 to 3.4% of all parotid tumors.[39] The neoplasm, in reality, is perhaps one

Table 1.15
Primary Squamous Cell Carcinoma of the Parotid Gland

Author	No. of Parotid Tumors	No. of Primary squamous Cell Carcinomas
Foote and Frazell[33]	766	26 (3.4%)
Batsakis et al.[39]	580	2 (0.3%)
Eneroth[51]	2,158	7 (0.3%)
Eneroth[37]	802	1 (0.1%)
Woods et al.[81]	1,360	20 (1.5%)
Spiro et al.[75]	1,875	10 (0.5%)
Conley[42]	1,538	16 (1.0%)

of the most unusual of parotid neoplasms (Table 1.15). Eneroth[37] has cited an incidence of 0.1% and included primary squamous cell carcinoma of the parotid in a "miscellaneous" category along with primary melanoma and malignant supporting tissue neoplasms of that gland. Woods et al.[81] after studying 1,360 primary tumors of the parotid gland, gave an incidence of 1.5% for primary squamous cell carcinomas. These neoplasms made up nearly 10% of their *primary malignant* tumors of the parotid gland. In the study by Spiro et al.,[75] there were 10 cases of the neoplasm in a total of 1,875 parotid tumors (0.5%). These made up 3% of all primary malignant neoplasms of the parotid gland.

These statistics contrast with the 3.4% incidence given by Foote and Frazell[33] and this is due to refinements in histopathological diagnosis and classification since the publication of their paper. Before ascribing a primary origin of a squamous cell carcinoma in the parotid gland, one *must* exclude mucoepidermoid carcinoma and extension or metastases to the gland from an extraparotid source. Foote and Frazell[33] were cognizant of this axiom. With reference to mucoepidermoid carcinomas, this quotation from their paper is pertinent: "We have on a number of occasions classified certain salivary gland tumors as squamous and then later changed this classification to mucoepidermoid after more material from the primary, recurrent or metastatic tumors became available for study."[33]

It can be safely stated that if metastases and mucoepidermoid carcinomas are excluded, the frequency of primary squamous cell carcinoma is 1% or less of all parotid gland tumors. This figure is very near the 1.5% incidence given for metastases to the parotid gland from squamous cell skin cancer of the head and neck and only slightly less than primary squamous cell carcinomas of the submandibular gland.[51, 189]

The site of origin of the primary neoplasms is very likely salivary ducts, but in nearly all cases, the neoplasm has obliterated any identifiable point of origin.

To my knowledge, all or nearly all of the acceptable primary squamous cell carcinomas of the parotid gland have been well- or moderately well-differentiated carcinomas. There is no mucus production, and intracellular keratinization, intercellular bridges and keratin pearl formation are often noted.

Local recurrence and regional lymph node metastases are the usual outcome for patients with this malignancy. Spiro et al.[75] report seven of their 10 patients eventually manifested lymph node metastases. Ultimate survival appears to depend more on the clinical stage of the disease than on the histological appearance of the tumor. Distant metastases are not a prominent feature.

Lymphoma of the Parotid Gland

Cervical lymph node involvement is by far the most common primary presentation of lymphoma in the head and neck. Extranodal presentation is distinctly not commonplace and primary presentation in parotid tissues is especially not commonplace. In the collected data of Freeman et al.[190] from 1,467 cases of extranodal lymphomas, 69 presented in the salivary glands. Lymphocytic

Table 1.16
Primary Lymphomas of the Parotid Gland

Authors	No. of Parotid Neoplasms	No. of Lymphomas
Batsakis and Regezi[186]	580	2
Foote and Frazell[33]	776	0
Berdal et al.[68]	479	3
Leegaard and Lindeman[49]	100	0
Hugo et al.[193]	187	2
Eneroth[37]	802	0

lymphomas, followed by histiocytic lymphomas accounted for an aggregate of 64% of the lymphomas.

Exclusive of this Registry study, Nime et al.[191] found that only 14 of 43 possible cases recorded in the literature were sufficiently documented to warrant the diagnosis of primary lymphoma of the salivary glands. The same authors could find but one case in a total of 2,636 lymphomas. Table 1.16 is further testimony of the rarity of these lesions in salivary glands.

In order to qualify as a primary lymphoma of the salivary gland, the following criteria must be fulfilled: there must be no known extrasalivary lymphoma at the time of diagnosis; there must be histological proof that the lymphoma involves the salivary parenchyma and is not a secondary invader from paraparotid lymph nodes; and there must be architectural and cytological confirmation of the malignant nature of the lesion. Atypical (pseudolymphomatous) reaction must be ruled out.[186]

The parotid gland is involved much more frequently than the submandibular gland, and I know of no case reported from the sublingual glands. This predilection for site may be related to the normal presence of lymphoid tissues and lymph nodes in the parotid gland. Lymph nodes and encapsulated aggregates are absent in the embryonic and adult submandibular and sublingual glands.

It is very likely that most, if not all, primary lymphomas in the parotid gland arise in this intraglandular lymphoid tissue. Lymphomas which arise in association with a previously existing lymphoepithelial lesion (with or without Sjogren's syndrome) have a different histogenesis.[192] Patients with Sjogren's syndrome are known to have an increased incidence of intraglandular and extraglandular lymphoproliferative disorders. This is similar to an increased incidence of lymphomas associated with other presumed autoimmune disorders.

As far as prognosis is concerned, primary lymphomas of the salivary glands, whether arising as extranodal lymphomas or within intrasalivary gland lymph nodes, with or without associated benign lymphoepithelial lesions (in the absence of Sjogren's syndrome), appear to have a more favorable prognosis than do lymphomas in general.

Nime et al.[191] claim that 92% ($^{11}/_{12}$) of primary salivary gland lymphomas have shown no evidence of additional lymphoma 2 to 8 years after diagnosis. In effect these are stage I lymphomas. Lymphomas in patients with Sjogren's syndrome, on the other hand, are often rapidly fatal, and many patients survive less than 3 years after diagnosis. As a rule this group of patients manifests a generalized lymphoma.

Monomorphic Adenomas

Since publication of the first edition of this book, there has been a considerable advance in our knowledge of this group of salivary gland tumors beyond the original limited definition of basal cell adenoma. In the event, there has been a considerable widening of the histomorphological spectrum of the so-called salivary gland adenoma. The following characteristics now apply to these lesions: (1) they are essentially monomorphic in *cellular* composition, epithelial or, more rarely, myoepithelial; (2) the origin of the monomorphic epithelial tumor is most likely the intercalated duct or reserve cell; (3) many epithelial tumors are multicentric in a given salivary gland; (4) epithelial adenomas are most often reported as arising from minor salivary tissues, principally the lip, rarely the upper airway; (5) there is an undeniable microscopic and histogenetic similarity of the epithelial tumors to dermal appendage tumors (eccrine cylindroma and spiradenoma, trichoepithelioma); (6) left to their natural course, many monomorphic adenomas would likely evolve into mixed tumors (pleomorphic adenoma); (7) hybrid forms, intermediate to mixed tumors and occasionally adenoid cystic carcinoma can be identified; and (8) the biological activity of monomorphic adenomas is benign and not unlike the mixed tumor; whether a histogenetically related malignant tumor exists (malignant basaloid tumor) is conjectural.

It is now quite clear that the benign basaloid tumor (basal cell adenoma) described by Kleinsasser and Klein[194] and Batsakis[195] is but one histomorphological expression of a varied yet limited potential of the progenitor cells. The full potential is very likely expressed as a mixed tumor. In that regard, evidence that basal cell adenomas

do not contain myoepithelial cells and are something other than a variant of mixed tumor is inconclusive.

Electron microscopic studies have presented a varied summary of the cellular components of the monomorphic adenoma.[196–199] According to some investigators, the tumors are purely epithelial; to others, myoepithelial cells participate to a limited extent (Fig. 1.32). With little dissent, however, the intercalated duct cell is considered the primary cell of origin. The presence of secretory granules does not exclude the intercalated duct cell.

The original descriptions of the basal cell adenoma contained no reference to an intercellular secretion product and the absence was considered as a differential diagnostic feature. That this is no longer tenable is evidenced by the light and electron microscopic findings of a replicated basal lamina (basement membrane) in several of the described tumors.[198, 199] If this membrane material is abundant, there is a striking similarity of the salivary tumor to dermal-type cylindromas.[200] We have designated such salivary tumors as *membranous adenomas*.[200] To my knowledge membranous adenomas have occurred only in the parotid gland and like the majority of monomorphic epithelial lesions may in reality be hamartomas.[201]

From the foregoing, it can be seen that the only recently recognized monomorphic adenoma has many forms; basal cell adenoma, membranous adenoma, tumors intermediate to mixed tumor and adenoid cystic carcinoma (hybrid forms), and myoepithelioma (Fig. 1.33).

Basal cell and membranous adenoma. The primary distinction between these two forms is the presence of intercellular ground substance in the latter.[200] This material appears to be a replicated basal lamina. Modifying terms such as tubular, canalicular, papillary and solid refer to their architectural growth pattern. The basal cell adenoma pattern is most often seen in the minor salivary glands and in those of the upper lip particularly.[202] The clinical appearance of these minor salivary tumors is that of a circumscribed, nonulcerated nodule, that is usually solid. They have varied in size from 0.4 to 2.0 cm in greatest dimension. The tumors are painless and a mucocele is suggested. An awareness of gradual enlargement is often the only reason for medical consultation. There is no sex predilection and the median age of Nelson and Jacoway's[203] patients was 60 years (33 to 73 years). Preoperative duration has ranged from a few months to many years, usually the latter. The canalicular form is the most common type in the minor salivary glands. It manifests what has been

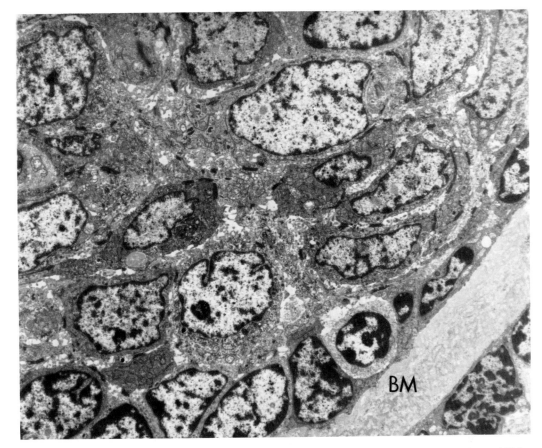

Figure 1.32. Monomorphic adenoma. Nests of cells surrounded by multilayered basement membrane (*BM*). The peripheral cells are anchored to the membrane by semidesmosomes and are interconnected by prominent desmosomal junctions. Only a few organelles are in the cytoplasm. (Courtesy of M. Klima, M.D.)

considered as a pathognomonic vascular pattern that serves to distinguish it from the adenoid cystic carcinoma, i.e., small capillaries and venules predominating in microcytic areas of the tumor.[204]

In contrast, the vascularity of the adenoid cystic carcinoma is indistinctly found in the supporting stroma and absent in microcytic spaces (Fig. 1.34). Epithelial induction of the stroma is absent in the classical form of basal adenoma. Mitoses are rare to absent. The tumors are benign and recurrence is rare.

To date, the parotid gland is the major salivary gland of predilection for both classic and membranous forms of the monomorphic adenoma. In this site, too, patients with the classic type are usually older than 50 years at the time of presentation with a mean age of 60 years in the cases reported. Membranous lesions tend to be found a decade earlier.[200, 201, 205] Both forms are usually less than 3.0 cm and have a tendency to lie superficial to

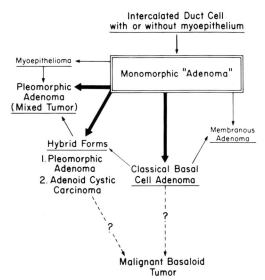

Figure 1.33. Proposed inter-relationship of monomorphic adenomas and other lesions.

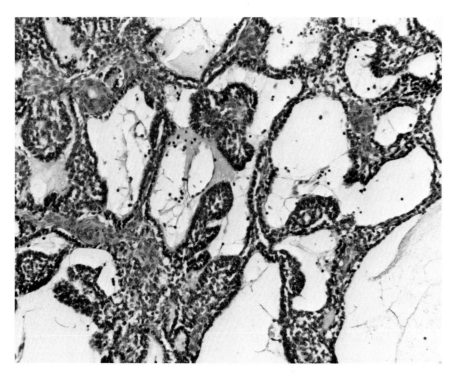

Figure 1.34. The distinctive vascular pattern of a canalicular basal cell adenoma.

the main body of the gland where they may be grossly mistaken for a hyperplastic lymph node because of their color and encapsulation. In the nonmembranous forms, the stroma is usually inconspicuous or may be lattice-like if a canalicular architecture predominates. The usual architecture is either a solid basaloid or trabecular. The tumors manifest a prominent capsule (Fig. 1.35). Basisquamous whorling in globular ends of epithelial islands resembling the terminal buds during embryogenesis may be a prominent histological feature. The combination of the basisquamous foci and a loose stroma may impart an ameloblastomatous appearance to selected fields of the tumor.

Lateral lobectomy is curative. Recurrences are seldom seen.

The homologous nature of salivary gland and epidermal tumors is nowhere so striking as it is with the membranous variant of monomorphic adenoma and sweat gland tumors such as eccrine spiradenoma and eccrine cylindroma.[200, 201, 205] Parotid basal cell adenomas certainly resemble benign cutaneous basaloid tumors. Both show ovoid club-shaped islands and focal areas of a whorling pattern comprised of central basal-type cells surrounded by a peripheral palisade of smaller basaloid cells. With the addition of intercellular ground-substance, the homology is nearly complete (Fig. 1.36). Both are multicentric in origin and are biologically benign. A rare diathesis of dermal type cylindromas of the parotid gland and tubular adenomas of the skin has been reported.[205]

Hybrid basal cell adenoma. Under this subclassification, I include those monomorphic tumors that possess histological features suggesting an evolution to either adenoid cystic carcinoma or benign mixed tumor. The latter is by far more common and my experience with the hybrid basal cell of adenoid cystic tumor is so limited that a prediction of its biological course is not possible.[204] The basal cell and membranous adenoma may be considered as either the benign homologues of adenoid cystic carcinoma or as the "non-pleomorphic" forms of mixed tumor.

The importance of recognizing the monomorphic epithelial adenomas lies in distinguishing them from adenoid cystic carcinoma. Little harm accrues to the patient in whom these lesions are "buried" under the diagnosis of mixed tumor, but for the patient whose lesion is misdiagnosed as an adenoid cystic carcinoma, the implications are evident.

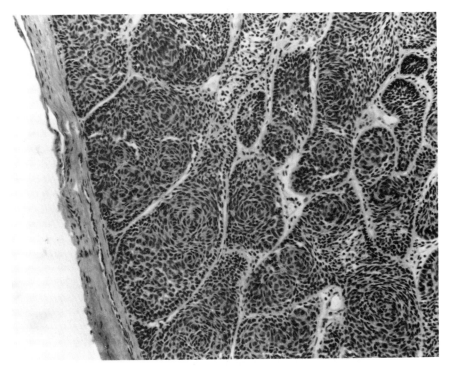

Figure 1.35. Encapsulated basal cell adenoma.

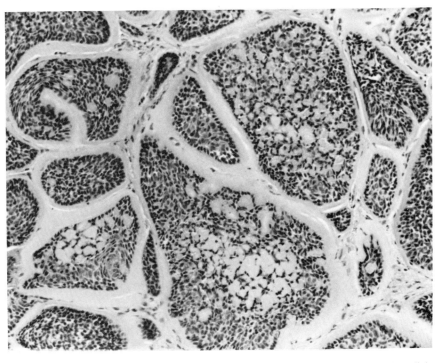

Figure 1.36. So-called membranous adenoma of parotid gland. Note the prominent extracellular hyaline material and the near identity with dermal eccrine cylindroma.

Myoepithelioma

This tumor is difficult to confirm by electron microscopic examination and nearly impossible by means of light microscopy. It is my opinion that the myoepithelioma is a one-sided (monomorphic) variant of mixed tumor and rarely exists in true monomorphic form (Fig. 1.37). Its incidence is less than the 1% of salivary gland mixed tumors which manifest a predominance of myoepithelial cells.

Adenosine triphosphatase and alkaline phosphatase histochemical reactions are not reliable as universal markers for salivary myoepithelial cells and definitive diagnosis rests on electron microscopic confirmation of the myoepithelium.[206, 207]

Two types of myoepithelial cell morphology exist: a slender elongated (stromal-like) cell and a more polyhedral, usually eosinophilic cell. The light microscopic manifestations of tumors composed of these cells are a tumor with bands and bundles of spindle cells and one having a plasmacytoid appearance.

Sciubba and Goldstein[206] have reviewed these tumors in the major and minor salivary glands. There is no sex preference and there is a tendency for those occurring in the palate to present in teenagers and young adults. Clinically, the tumors are indistinguishable from mixed tumors. The tumors are biologically benign and a definable ma-

lignant variant has not been defined. Histological and electron microscopic features helpful to distinguish the myoepithelioma from mesenchymal tumors are offered by Meriono and LiVolsi.[208]

Warthin's Tumor (Cystadenolymphoma, Papillary Cystadenoma Lymphomatosum)

It has been almost 50 years since Warthin[209] described and presented for the first time in the American literature the tumor, *papillary cystadenoma lymphomatosum*. Since not all of the tumors are papillomatous, the term *cystadenolymphoma* has also found wide use. Many times, however, either by form of tribute, or more likely, through facility, the neoplasm has been called Warthin's tumor.

Many of the reports that followed Warthin's were by pathologists who, perhaps piqued by the unusual association of lymphoid and epithelial tissue displayed by the tumor, presented a variety of histogenetic theories. Two studies stand out among the several hundred recorded in our literature: Thompson and Bryant's[210] elucidation of the phatogenesis of the lesion, and the review of the clinical features by Chaudhry and Gorlin.[211] Early reports include many hypotheses for the development of the Warthin tumor. The currently accepted theory is an origin from heterotopic sal-

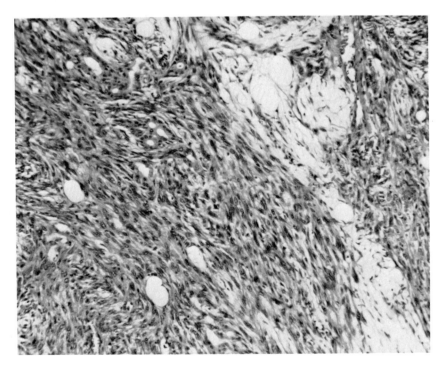

Figure 1.37. Prominent myoepithelial cell proliferation in a mixed tumor of parotid gland.

ivary gland tissue within lymph nodes external to or within the parotid gland.

Thompson and Bryant[210] studied the embryonic development of the salivary glands and found that, whereas the submaxillary and sublingual glands develop as compact entities, the parotid gland develops in a loose arrangement containing aggregates of lymphoid tissue, and encapsulation occurs late in ontogeny. Thus, lymph nodes become enclosed with the parotid gland, and salivary ducts and acini become included in these nodes, as well as in nodes outside of the definitive gland which were excluded by the formation of the capsule. It is from these ductal epithelial elements, incorporated in lymphoid tissue outside of and within the parotid capsule, that the tumors arise. The finding of ductal inclusions in lymph nodes in or near the parotid, the occasional multicentricity of Warthin's tumor in several apparently uninvolved lymph nodes and the relatively undisturbed lymph nodal architecture seen about tumors removed at an early stage of their formation are features supporting this thesis. The cause of the oxyphilic alteration in the epithelial elements is not known.

Although Warthin's tumor has been reported as occurring in a wide age span (2.5 to 92 years), 82% are found in patients between 41 and 70 years of age (average 55.6 years). There is a decided (5:1) male predominance,[211] and a rare case has been reported in a Negro.

The tumor is asymptomatic. Only 10% of patients present with complaints other than a symptomless mass, those complaints being pain, pressure sensations or rapid increase in size of the tumor. Facial nerve weakness has been reported only once. The lack of discomfort accounts for the relatively long duration before diagnosis. The average duration is 3 years, and reports give a range of 2 weeks to 30 years.

Despite reports of the tumor occurring in sites other than the parotid gland or its environs, Warthin's tumor is best considered as a lesion of the parotid gland, where it represents 6 to 10%[212, 213] of all parotid gland tumors, second in frequency of benign tumors only to the mixed tumors. It occurs most often in the lower pole of the gland next to the angle of the mandible. Because of the pathogenetic relationship described above, the tumor may arise in lymph nodes superficial or medial to the parotid gland. In a number of instances, the tumors have been bilateral.[213] Because of the intimate relationship of the tail of the parotid gland with the submaxillary gland, we doubt the validity of the latter being reported as a primary site. A few unquestionable Warthin tumors have

been noted in the lower lip and the palate, but doubts exist about the credibility of reported tumors in the oropharynx, hypopharynx, posterior nasal space, larynx and thyroid gland.[213]

The tumor is well defined, soft or fluctuant or, if deep within the gland, firm to palpation. The average size is given as 3.6 cm with a range of 1 to 8.5 cm at the time of surgical removal.

Aspiration biopsy and staining of the air-dried smears of the aspirates with May-Grunwald-Giesma stain may permit a correct diagnosis in up to 83% of the cases,[214] but repeated biopsy may be required, and, in most cases, the patient will come to surgery anyway.

The tumor is encapsulated and round or oval with a smooth or lobulated surface. It is usually cystic or semisolid and compressible. A fluid of variable character but usually mucoid and brown-tinged, exudes from the cut surface. On section, multiple irregular cystic spaces with papillary projections are seen. Solid areas are gray and may manifest many small white nodules representing lymphoid follicles. The cut section may present a pseudotuberculous appearance.

Microscopically, an epithelium having a tubulopapillary-cystic pattern is within lymphoid tissue or a lymph node. The latter has sinuses, lymph follicles and, usually an embracing connective tissue capsule. Lymph node architecture may be so compressed and distorted by the epithelial components that sinuses may not be readily evident, but follicles are usually seen.

The epithelium is a double layer of oxyphilic, finely granular cells, an inner layer of round, cuboidal or polygonal cells, and an outer zone of nonciliated, tall columnar or clavate cells (Fig. 1.38). The nuclei of the inner cells are vesicular, while those of the outer layer are usually pyknotic and situated uniformly toward the luminal surface. Not all of the cells have the same intensity of staining with eosin; some are pale and distinctly granular, whereas others are intensely red and homogeneous. Mucus or goblet cells may be interspersed in the epithelial layer. A piling up of epithelium or focal areas of squamous metaplasia may occasionally be seen. Sebaceous elements may be prominent. A fine basement membrane separates the epithelium from the lymphoid tissue. The fluid within the cystic spaces of the tumor and into which papillae project has a homogeneous or finely granular eosinophilic appearance.

Phosphotungstic acid-hematoxylin stains on paraffin-embedded tumors demonstrate numerous fine, blue-black granules (mitochondria) in the cytoplasm of both cell types in the epithelial layer.

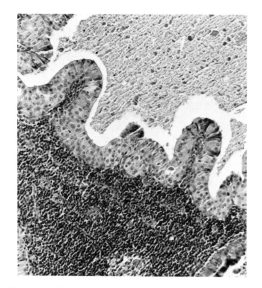

Figure 1.38. Classical appearance of a Warthin's tumor.

Positive histochemical reactions for phosphatases, esterase and various mitochondrial enzymes are demonstrable, but not in significantly greater degree than in normal parotid gland ducts, although certain qualitative differences exist.

Ultrastructural examination of the epithelial cell cytoplasm finds it packed with mitochondria in both apical and basal areas.[215, 216] Many are in groups, are enlarged and manifest increased numbers of cristae. The staining variation noted under the light microscope correlates with the numbers of mitochondria in the cells.

The Warthin tumor is particularly amenable to surgical removal. It is usually superficially placed, and the facial nerve is rarely involved by the tumor. While well-defined, the tumor does not usually shell out easily, and this factor, with the desire not to spill the cyst contents, requires removal of adjacent gland. Radiation may decrease the size of the lesion but does not effect its regression and is not a substitute for surgical removal.

Recurrence rates are difficult to compute from reports because of insufficient follow-up. Six of 49 tumors encountered at Memorial Hospital (New York City) manifested recurrence.[33] Incomplete excision, operative spillage of tumor contents or, more likely, growth from a new focus are held responsible. Multicentricity at first excision has been repeatedly noted.

Earlier reports of malignant Warthin's tumor has been refuted by many authors.[33, 213] Two case reports[217, 218] are more convincing. The patients, in both instances, had received irradiation to the neck

8 and 13 years earlier. In view of the fact that these two cases, of almost 600 cases of Warthin's tumor reported in the literature, are the only reasonably acceptable examples of malignancy certainly speaks for a spontaneous malignant propensity of such low order as to be practically nonexistent.[219] Involvement by lymphoma is reported. The lymphoid component of Warthin's tumor has been shown to be composed predominantly of complement receptor B-lymphocytes.[220]

Sialadenoma Papilliferum

The relationship, or at least histological similarity between some epidermal appendage tumors and some salivary gland tumors, is again highlighted by this rarely recognized tumor of major and minor salivary tissues. Described for the first time in 1969,[221] an acceptable documentation of the lesion has occurred only six additional times by 1978.[222] In a relatively rich experience in salivary gland tumors, this author has never seen such a lesion, or perhaps, at best, never recognized it. Only the first examples have been reported in the parotid gland; the remainder are in the oral cavity with a preference for the palate. The tumor has always occurred in late adulthood, is circumscribed and biologically benign after excision. Wherever it has occurred the tumor is described as a painless, papillary, exophytic growth. Microscopically the lesion consists of numerous papillary folds of epithelium and tortuous, widely dilated salivary ducts. Supporting connective tissue cores are well vascularized. Oxyphilic, mucous and squamous cells line the papillae. If the accompanying lymphoid infiltrate is marked, a Warthin's tumor is suggested. In every report, the similarity to syringoadenoma papilliferum of sweat gland origin is mentioned.

Sebaceous Cell Lesions

Ectopia of sebaceous glands is a well-recognized phenomenon in the head and neck, particularly in such locations as the mucocutaneous junctions, the buccal mucosa (Fordyce's condition) and within the parotid gland. An estimated 33% of the adult population is said to possess atypical sebaceous structures, some even with holocrine scretion, in their parotid glands.[223] Their presence in other salivary glands is considerably less frequent. Table 1.17 presents the conditions in which sebaceous gland components may be found in the parotid gland. Exclusive of their presence in normal glands, they are most often found in association with recognizable salivary gland tumors, i.e., mixed tumors, mucoepidermoid carcinomas and Warthin's tumors.

The origin of sebaceous elements in the major salivary glands is unknown. None of the proposed theories (metaplasia, developmental inclusions, pluripotential duct cell) satisfy all contingencies. It is likely all play a variable role. An ectodermal derivation of the parotid gland explains their being found most often in that gland, but does not explain the less frequent occurrence in the submandibular gland. As far as neoplasia is concerned, the least attractive hypothesis is the metaplastic proposal.

True neoplastic lesions are unusual and are to be distinguished from normal foci and hyperplasias. In order of decreasing frequency, the neoplasms are sebaceous lymphadenoma, sebaceous carcinoma and sebaceous adenoma.

The sebaceous lymphadenoma is a distinct clinicopathological entity in the region of the parotid gland. Less than 12 examples had been reported by 1976,[224] but this is an underestimation of the incidence. The tumor is composed of sebaceous glands in a matrix of benign lymphoid tissue. Terminal tubule buds and keratinization may be found. In some instances, the circumscription of the tumors, compression of adjacent parotid tissue and an absence of sebaceous elements in the uninvolved gland raised the likely possibility of origin in para- or intraparotid lymph nodes. This is identical to the proposed origin of Warthin's tumor. An extraparotid origin also holds true for most of the so-called sebaceous carcinomas of the parotid region. One must carefully exclude adnexal origin before the acceptance of an intraparotid primary origin.[223, 225]

Sebaceous carcinoma of the parotid gland may simulate either a mucoepidermoid carcinoma or a squamous cell carcinoma. All have similar growth patterns with poorly defined margins and a finger-like as well as blunt invasion. Necrosis is a common finding and focal areas of keratinization is usually evident. Once diagnosis is established, an aggressive surgical management is required to reduce recurrences and metastases.[226]

Since carcinomas of the sebaceous elements in the parotid exist, a benign form (adenoma) likely exists. I have never seen one.

Neoplasms arising from sebaceous elements in minor salivary gland-bearing tissues are even more unusual despite their known distributions.[227, 228] The presence of sebaceous glands in oral (Fordyce's spots) or paraoral sites may almost be considered within the physiological norm. Sebaceous glands on the lips, frenum, retromolar region of the palate and tongue are said to occur in over 80% of the population. In these sites, they are noticed chiefly in middle-aged and elderly subjects. They have not been found in infants less than 4 months of age and rarely in children under 3 years.

The sebaceous elements are single or grouped pin-head sized granules which are symmetrically located chiefly on the upper lip, lateral portion of the lower lip, and the buccal mucosa at the angle of the mouth. They may be scattered over the buccal mucosa but are especially prominent on the mucosa lateral to the anterior pillar of the fauces and retromolar gingiva. The upper lip contains from 10 to 100 foci with the upper 2 mm of the vermillion border essentially devoid of the glands.

There are no reported carcinomas from the sebaceous components in these areas and only unconvincing examples of benign neoplasia. A rare example of sebaceous glands surrounding a malignancy of the anterior commissure of the larynx has been recorded.

Oncocytic Lesions

So named because of their size and oxyphilic cytoplasm, oncocytic cells may be best considered as somatic mutants. The cells are not of a new or specific cell lineage, but rather they represent parenchymal elements of acini or intralobular ducts of normal or abnormal salivary tissue which have undergone cytoplasmic changes induced by unknown influences. Table 1.18 outlines the surgical-pathological presentations of the oncocyte in salivary gland tissues. In the majority of instances, the cells appear as isolated findings, or in groups within an aging salivary gland (predominantly parotid). Clinically tumorous lesions (oncocytosis versus oncocytoma) make up less than 1% of all salivary gland tumors (Table 1.19). Warthin's tumor, while manifesting typical oncocytes, is not appropriately regarded as an oncocytoma since its

Table 1.17
Sebaceous Gland Elements in the Parotid Gland

Condition	Estimated Frequency
"Normal variant"	33% of adult population
Histological accompaniment of salivary gland tumors (in or adjacent to tumor)	20% of salivary gland tumors
Sebaceous lymphadenoma	12 cases reported
Sebaceous carcinoma (unaccompanied by other tumors)	6 cases reported
Sebaceous adenoma	Doubtful existence

Table 1.18
Surgical-Pathological Manifestations of the Oncocyte in Salivary Glands

Type of Presentation	Approximate Frequency
1. Occurring singly or in small groups as an accompaniment of age	Rarely before 50 years; nearly 100% after 70 years
2. As above, but in association with definable salivary gland tumors; i.e., adenoid cystic carcinomas, adenocarcinomas, etc.	Less than 10%
3. Benign hyperplasias or neoplasia A. Diffuse multi-nodular (oncocytosis) B. Solitary tumor (oncocytoma) C. Bilateral diffuse or solitary	Less than 1% of all salivary gland tumors
4. Warthin's tumor	
5. Malignant oncocytic or oncocytoid tumor	

Table 1.19
Incidence of Oncocytomas of Salivary Glands

Author	No. of Parotid tumors	No. of Oncocytomas	Percentage
Buxton et al.[151]	280	3	1.0
Foote and Frazell[33]	877	1	0.1
Kirklin et al.[239]	909	4	0.4
Blanck et al.[235]	1,678	13	0.8
Tandler et al.[234]	1,578	12	0.7
Johns et al.[233]	580	4	0.7

diagnosis requires the additional feature of a lymphoid component.

Results obtained by electron microscopy suggest that oncocytic transformation of epithelial cells is certainly not a degenerative process.[229-231] The transformation should be regarded as a re-differentiation of the epithelial cells which develop an increased but unbalanced metabolism. Unlike normal mitochondria, oncocyte mitochondria produce only very small quantities of high-energy phosphate (ATP). The conditions prevailing are much the same as those in brown adipose tissue, which also contain a large number of mitochondria and serves for chemical thermoregulation. The functional defect of the oncocyte mitochondria thus takes the form of a mitochondriopathy (Fig. 1.39). Apparently, the oncocytes try to compensate for this functional defect by an increased number of mitochondria and increasing the surface area of the mitochondrial membrane.[232] Mitochondria are the major component of the cell for which the establishment of some degree of continuity with other membrane elements exist. Oncocytic transformation must then be considered as a consequence of an acquired disturbance of the mitochondrial enzyme organization. Since oncocytes are able to divide, this abnormal metabolic activity is passed on to their offspring.

The electron microscopic appearance of the oncocyte is one of a cell filled by an excessive accumulation of mitochondria (to which it owes its oxyphilic staining). The cristae are stacked closely together in the center, or with longitudinal mitochondria having transverse tubular cristae. Occasionally, the mitochondria are often larger than normal ones and there may be a considerable number of bizarre forms. Organelles other than mitochondria are sparse. A variable degree of mitochondrial division may be present.

The definition of an oncocyte, solely by light microscopic examination of hematoxylin and eosin-stained sections, is not precise. Fine structural studies have demonstrated that many different intracytoplasmic structures may be responsible for the same light microscopic appearances.[229] An eosinophilic and granular cytoplasm may be imparted by (1) mitochondrial hyperplasia, (2) smooth endoplasmic reticulum, (3) dense lysosomal-like bodies, (4) secretory granules and (5) other cell organelles.

To qualify for the designation of oncocyte (Table 1.20) a cell should meet the following standards. (1) The cell in question makes its appearance sometime after the organ in which it occurs has reached histological maturity. (2) The cell should manifest a high level of oxidative activity. (3) The cell must possess an unusually large number of mitochondria (many, or all may be hypertrophoid and abnormal in appearance). (4) Special cytoarchitectural features such as basal infolding, brush borders, etc. should be in a state of regression or absent. Histochemical demonstration of the mitochondria-rich cytoplasm is the minimal additional step toward documentation. Failing this, the surgical pathologist must report to the descriptive adjective "oncocytoid" for a presumptive lesion.

It must be appreciated that histochemical demonstration of mitochondria is not infallible.[223] Negative histochemical reactions may be had in lesions where electron microscopy clearly demonstrates excess numbers of mitochondria. The most likely explanation for this phenomenon is delay in fixation from the time of separation of the tumor from its blood supply to its being placed in fixative with a resulting loss of necessary enzyme radicals needed for a positive stain. The histochemical stains are not of value in excluding the diagnosis when negative. In order to rule out a suspected diagnosis of oncocytic neoplasm, the tissue must be examined by the electron microscope.

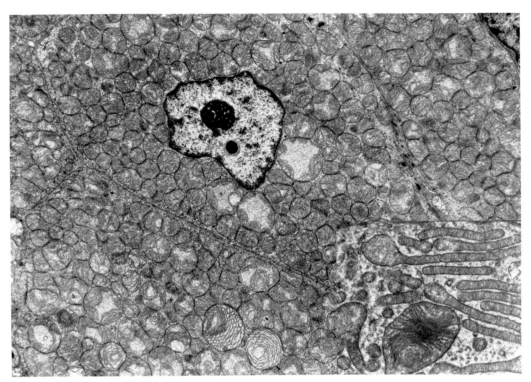

Figure 1.39. Electron micrograph of mitochondria-filled cytoplasm of an oncocytoma. *Inset* shows the often grotesque shape of the mitochondria.

Table 1.20
Cellular Characteristics of the Salivary Gland Oncocyte

Hematoxylin and Eosin Appearance	Histochemical Reactions	Electron Microscopic Appearance
1. Cellular enlargement (10 to 15 μm)	1. PTAH* and BAAF stains demonstrate numerous mitochondria	1. Two oncocytic cells: epithelial and myoepithelial
2. Cytoplasm variably filled with acidophilic granules	2. High levels of various, predominantly *mitochondrial enzymes*	2. Marked hyperplasia of mitochondria—often many bizarre and swollen forms
3. Coalescence of granules may produce a pale, dark or homogeneous (colloid) cytoplasm.	3. Relatively high levels of enzymes usually associated with microsomes or other cytoplasmic fractions	3. Beta-type glycogen in cytoplasmic matrix and in granular deposits in mitochondria
4. Nucleoli not prominent	4. Variable and weak stains with Sudan stains	4. Relative paucity of other cell organelles (lysosomal bodies and secretory granules)
	5. Strong luxol fast blue reaction	5. Desmosomal attachment between oncocytes
	6. Metachromasia with thionin and cresyl violet	
	7. Variable PAS reaction	

* PTAH, phosphotungstic acid hematoxylin; BAAF, Bensley's acid analine fuchsin; PAS, periodic acid-Schiff.

The neoplastic versus hyperplastic basis for many of the oncocytic lesions has not been settled.[234] It is our contention that the majority of tumors are the result of oxyphilic metaplasia and hyperplasia. Nevertheless, both benign and malignant oncocytomas occur.

It is difficult, if not impossible, especially with isolated cases, to clearly separate lesions that are hyperplastic from those that are neoplastic (Fig. 1.40). In general, the hyperplastic lesion contains cells with a nearly normal nuclear-cytoplasmic ratio, inconspicuous nucleoli and a normal polarity of the long axis of the cells to the basal membrane and to other cells. In contrast, oncocytomas usually consist of cells with larger nuclei, increased nuclear-cytoplasmic ratio (generally with a prominent nucleolus) and often with an altered polarity. A true oncocytoma contains no lymphoid tissue. The diagnostic term should be reserved for tumors composed solely or mainly of oncocytes. Solid oncocytomas consist of lobes and lobules of the typical swollen, eosinophilic cells. The cells are arranged in solid sheets or cords and occasionally in a tubular or acinar fashion (Fig. 1.41). Papillary oncocytomas are not substantially different from papillary cystadenoma or carcinomas except for their distinctive cytoplasmic characteristics. Mi-

toses are sparse to absent in both benign and malignant oncocytomas.

The parotid gland is the most common site of oncocytomas in the salivary glands and in the entire head and neck region. The submandibular gland is only rarely involved.[235] The tumors are generally noncystic and are encapsulated. Often lobulated, they rarely exceed 5.0 cm in diameter. Bilaterality and multinodularity have been conspicuous features in some series. In accordance with the age at which oncocytes make their appearance, most patients are in their sixth decade.[231]

The growth rate of an oncocytoma is typically slow and the mass in the parotid gland has usually been present for several years before removal. Recurrences after an apparently complete removal of a benign oncocytoma are unusual. If a recurrence presents, it usually does so within the first 5 postoperative years.

Oncocytomas arising in the minor salivary glands are even more unusual than those of the major glands. Most of the oncocytic lesions of the oral mucous glands and the mucosa and submucosal ducts of the upper respiratory tract are oncocytic hyperplasia rather than neoplasm.[236] Cohen and Batsakis[237] have recorded 20 papillary, cystic oncocytic "cystadenomas" from such diverse

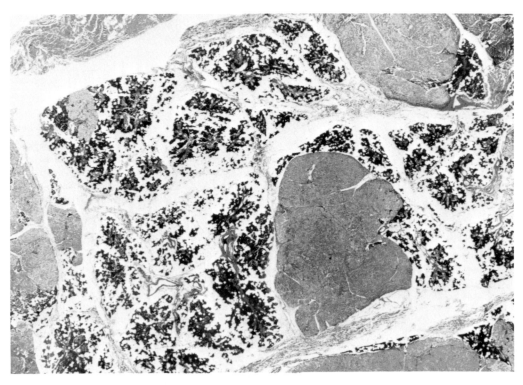

Figure 1.40. Nodular, diffuse oncocytosis.

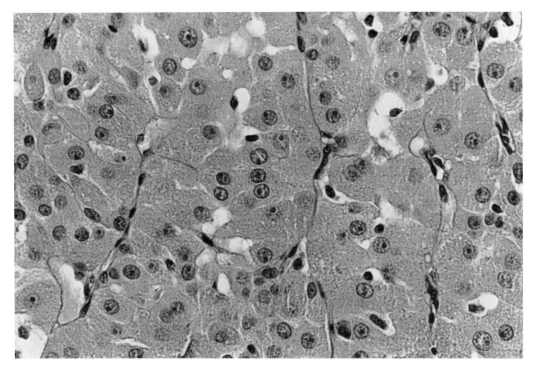

Figure 1.41.   Oncocytoma. (Contributed by J. L. Cornog, Jr., M.D.)

sites as the accessory tear glands, buccal mucosa, palate, nasopharynx and larynx. It is to be noted that most of the extrasalivary gland oncocytomas are cystic and papillary rather than solid in configuration. Most of the laryngeal and upper airway oncocytic lesions are asymptomatic. When symptoms present, they are the result of a polypoid, space-occupying tumor.

Malignant tumors composed of oncocytes are unusual (Fig. 1.42). Johns et al.[233] accepted only 11 cases in the world literature in 1977. The malignant oncocytoma does not have sufficient histological differences from benign oncocytomas to permit its ready recognition. The gross appearance, i.e., solid rather than cystic, and the anatomical location do, however, appear to be significant. In this regard, we consider solid oncocytomas of the nose, paranasal sinuses and larynx to be grade I carcinomas.

The biological course of the oncocytic carcinoma is one of multiple aggressive recurrences with bony involvement (sinuses) or regional lymph node metastases.[238] Seven of the 11 patients reviewed by Johns et al.[233] manifested regional lymph metastases at some time during their disease process. Short-term follow-up of these patients suggests a good survival rate. Since the prognosis is not affected by the oncocytic character of the

cells alone, the long-term prognosis is very likely that of adenocarcinoma and acinous cell carcinoma. If that be the case, it would suggest that the 20-year survival may not share the short-term statistics.

Metastases to the Parotid Gland and Regional Metastases to Parotid Lymph Nodes

The majority of the metastatic involvements of the parotid gland are of a regional nature and are related to the anatomy of the parotid lymphatic system. Conley and Arena[240] found that the secondary involvements are usually the result not of direct contiguous involvement, but more often of metastases into intra- or paraparotid lymph nodes. Hematogenous spread is usually minimal.

Lymph nodes associated with the parotid gland drain lymph from the scalp, face and the external ear. These lymph nodes also drain the eyelids, external nose and the lacrimal glands, as well as the sinonasal, nasopharyngeal or oropharyngeal cavities (Fig. 1.43).

Conley and Arena[240] state that the parotid gland contains 20 to 30 "follicles" and lymph nodes with a rich network of interconnecting lymph vessels. Paraparotid lymph nodes are found around the external surface of the gland and are particularly numerous in the pretragal and supratragal areas.

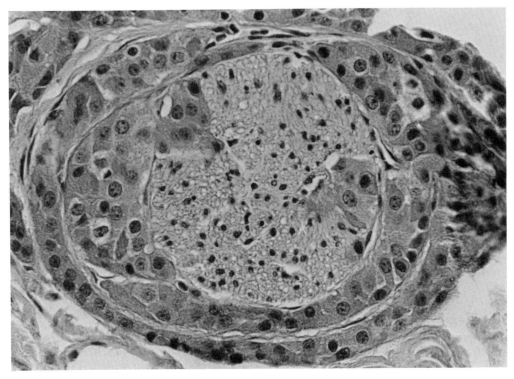

Figure 1.42.   Oncocytic carcinoma invading nerve. (Contributed by J. L. Cornog, Jr., M.D.)

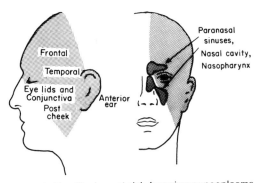

Figure 1.43.   Regions at risk for primary neoplasms capable of metastasizing to parotid lymph nodes.

Intraglandular and paraglandular lymph nodes communicate freely with each other and drain into the cervical lymphatic network. According to Graham[241] almost all of the parotid lymph nodes lie lateral to the posterior facial vein as it courses through the gland. These observations seem to be borne out clinically in that metastatic involvement of parotid lymph nodes is usually lateral to the vascular bundle.[242]

Exclusive of the hematogenous route, four modes of entrance exist for neoplasms to secondarily involve the parotid gland: (1) direct, with involvement of paraglandular lymph nodes; (2) secondary disposition from a paraglandular lymph node; (3) retrograde extension through lymphatics from lymph node involvement in the neck; and (4) a contiguous direct extension with lymph node involvement.

Because of the richness of the lymphatics, the pre- and supratragal lymph nodes are favorite repositories for metastases from the temple, scalp and ear. Next in frequency of involvement are the lymph nodes in association with the lateral, posterior, deep and inferior portions of the gland. The anterior portion of the gland is only rarely involved by a metastasis.[240]

The high risk patients for metastases to the parotid are those with deeply invasive melanoma or large, poorly differentiated squamous cell carcinomas of the skin of the ipsilateral eyelid and conjuctiva, frontal, temporal, posterior cheek and anterior ear. Over one-half of the patients with neoplasms of those areas will manifest parotid gland metastases during the course of their disease. Occult metastases from this group of cancers may be as high as 25% and nearly one-third of the patients may have the parotid metastasis of the first manifestation of metastatic disease.[243]

Malignant melanomas and squamous cell carcinomas dominate the tabular classifications of types of neoplasms producing regional metastases to the parotid nodes. Each share equally in making up about 80% of the total number.[242] A wide diversity of epithelial and soft tissue neoplasms make up the remainder. Contiguous involvement is most often by neoplasms of the supporting tissues. Melanoma of the temporal scalp is the single most frequent cause of regional metastases to the parotid lymph nodes and has a proclivity to the paraparotid lymph nodes. Melanomas in this area manifest an 80% incidence of metastasis to the parotid lymph nodes. Primary melanomas from other areas about the head and neck tend to metastasize to the parotid nodes in less than 50% of the cases.[242] Melanomas of the face may metastasize to the parotid region before they are discernible in the neck.

In all cases of lymphatic spread to the parotid gland, the metastatic foci are in the lymphoid tissue (Fig. 1.44). This may be obscured by an over-run of the lymph nodes of the metastasis giving an appearance of intraparenchymal localization.

Metastases from squamous cell primaries are predominantly intraglandular. The offending carcinoma may have its primary site in the mucosal lining of the oral cavity, sinuses or pharynx, or in the ear. In my experience, metastatic squamous cell carcinomas to the parotid gland are not well differentiated, many appearing as nonkeratinizing.

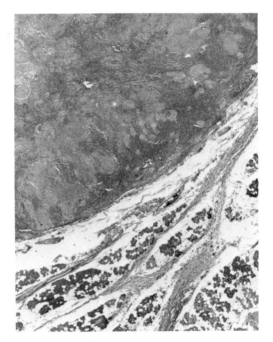

Figure 1.44. Metastatic lymphoepithelioma to intraparotid lymph node.

The rare primary squamous cell carcinoma of the parotid gland, on the other hand, is a well-differentiated, usually keratinizing neoplasm.

In the majority of patients manifesting regional parotid or parotid gland metastases, there is also evidence of metastases in the neck and/or disseminated disease. The prognosis, therefore, for all varieties (para- or intraglandular) and by any histological type of neoplasm is grave. Over-all survival is 12.5% for 5 years. Conley and Arena[240] record 5-year determinate survivals of 14.3% for parenchymal parotid gland involvement, 9.4% for intraglandular lymph node involvement, and 14.3% for paraglandular lymph node metastatic disease. Treatment, whenever feasible, is composite resection of the primary neoplasm, parotid gland and neck dissection.

Infraclavicular sites for primaries with metastases to the parotid region are led by the lungs, followed by breast, kidney and gastrointestinal tract.[244] Metastases to the submandibular gland follow the same site preferences.

The foregoing has dealt with carcinomatous metastases. Involvement of the salivary glands by a contiguous spread of a malignant tumor is usually due to a sarcoma of adjacent structures. The involvement of intraglandular lymphoid tissue or the salivary gland proper by lymphomas has been stated to be surprisingly rare except for the salivary gland lesions in Burkitt's lymphoma.[245] This may be due to sampling artefact since the data presented by Freeman et al.[190] are contradictory.

Tumors of the Deep Lobe of the Parotid Gland with Parapharyngeal Growth of Parotid Tumors

Most tumors of the parotid gland are found superficial to the facial nerve. Two-thirds of the mixed tumors, for example, are located in the superficial lobe, where most have an infra-auricular position. Preauricular locations are less common. In a few cases, the tumors are situated relatively far forward on the cheek and these lesions are thought to have arisen from accessory salivary gland tissue in the region of the anterior part of the excretory duct system.[246] Parapharyngeal extension of salivary gland tumors and tumors of the deep lobe of the parotid gland is unusual, yet when they occur they present diagnostic difficulties.

The wedge-shaped parotid gland has its base facing laterally and its medial border is close to the lateral pharyngeal wall in front of the anterior pillar of the tonsil. The deep lobe of the parotid gland comprises only a small part of the total gland substance. It lies deep to the facial nerve and is in continuity with the rest of the gland by a narrow triangular aperture. The boundaries of this aperture are: above, the base of the skull; anteriorly, the medial pterygoid muscle and the ascending ramus of the mandible; posteriorly, the styloid process, its muscles and the stylomandibular ligament. The deeper portion of the gland, where it is in relation to the anterior pillar of the fauces, is also related to the superior constrictor muscle. In effect, the deep lobe of the parotid gland is sandwiched between the ramus of the mandible and the mastoid process.

The largest single experience with these tumors is that of the Sloan-Kettering Memorial Cancer Center who reported 130 deep lobe tumors of a population of 1217 previously untreated patients (11%).[247] This coincides closely with the data presented by Hanna et al.[248] who dealth with 35 definite cases, or a 12% incidence.

The rarity of these lesions not only may lead to diagnostic difficulties, surgical management of deep lobe tumors may be difficult or even hazardous. This is occasioned because the deep lobe lies beneath the branches of the facial nerve and is often behind the ramus of the mandible.

Because of the anatomical restrictions outlined above, a tumor developing in the deep parotid tissues finds its most unencumbered growth projection medially. Clinical features also reflect this mode of presentation. Growth into the "stylomandibular canal or tunnel" is facilitated in some measure because the part of the gland extending toward the tunnel is covered by a thin fascia, in contrast to a fibrous capsule over the lateral aspects of the parotid gland.[249] Clinical presentation is often in the mouth or the pharynx. The narrow stylomandibular tunnel often fixes and draws the tumors at this point and gives them an hourglass appearance or "dumbbell tumor." There is a bulge in the mouth in the affected side of the palate. This mass is usually asymptomatic but dysphagia, sore throat, earache, aural "stuffiness," an inability to retain dentures or a feeling of something sticking in the throat may bring the patient in for evaluation. The patients of Hanna et al.[248] presented most often with a swelling in the region of the parotid gland in front of the ear.

Among a total of 481 cases of parotid gland tumors admitted to the Ear, Nose and Throat Department of Rikshospitalet, Oslo, 21 tumors of the dumbbell type were found, a relatively high frequency of parotid lesions bulging into the pharynx.[250] Fifteen of them could be seen both parapharyngeally and in the retromandibular fossa. In six cases, the tumor was only seen parapharyngeally. A much lower incidence of parapharyngeal extension has been reported from the Karolinska

Sjukhuset. Only nine (1%) of 1,108 cases of parotid gland tumors proved to be clinically parapharyngeal at that institution.[250] Partial explanation for this statistical difference is perhaps related to the shorter preoperative duration of the tumors from Karolinska Sjukhuset.[250]

The relative ratio of benign to malignant salivary gland tumors in the superficial portion of the parotid gland holds true also for tumors arising in the deep lobe of the gland. The majority of the tumors are benign mixed tumors. Hanna et al.[248] give a 23% malignant tumor incidence. Mucoepidermoid and acinous cell carcinomas appear to be the most common malignant histological types. Hanna et al.[248] contend that there is an excellent chance of cure in spite of the technical diffculties attendant to the removal of thes tumors. This is confirmed by Nigro and Spiro[247] who contend that most deep lobe tumors can be excised through a conventional parotidectomy excision, sparing the facial nerve. They record only two recurrences in patients with benign tumors. In patients with malignant deep lobe tumors, 5-, 10- and 15-year determinate "cures" were 61, 52 and 48% respectively, almost identical with those reported for all patients with carcinoma of the parotid gland. Of their patients, 19% manifested cervical lymph node metastases during the course of their disease.

Multiple Tumors of the Major Salivary Glands

The development of tumors in two or more salivary glands is an unusual phenomenon. Only 27 (1.3%) of 2,072 patients with major salivary gland tumors who presented at Memorial Hospital, New York City, had involvement of more than one gland.[251] In a total of 1,678 patients observed during a follow-up period from 10 to 50 years, a salivary gland tumor developed in both glands in only 11 cases.[252] Bilateral simultaneous or synchronous tumors are even more unusual.[253] A nonpost-operative multifocal involvement of a single gland is also unusual.

Warthin's tumor is the most common salivary gland tumor to be bilateral, multifocal in the same gland, and associated synchronously with other neoplastic salivary gland lesions. The oncocytic tumors and the benign mixed tumor follow distantly in all three categories. It is my subjective impression that of the malignant lesions, it is the acinous cell carcinoma which is most often bilateral.

SALIVARY GLAND TUMORS IN CHILDREN

The over-all incidence of noninflammatory tumors of the salivary glands in children is quite low, accounting for less than 5% of all salivary gland tumors in all age groups.[254, 255]

With few dissentors, malignant neoplasms have been estimated as representing 25% of the childhood salivary gland tumors, and this correlates well with the expected rate of malignancy in adult salivary gland tumors. The malignant variants are dominated by the mucoepidermoid carcinomas (the most common) and adenocarcinomas. Among the latter, acinous cell carcinomas are most often reported. Almost all other histological variations of tumor encountered in adults have been reported in children. The benign mixed tumor (pleomorphic adenoma) is the most common form of benign epithelial tumor.[158, 256]

A considerable number of benign tumors of salivary glands in children are vascular in origin. If this large proportion of nonepithelial salivary gland tumors is excluded from a statistical review, a disproportionately high percentage (approximately 50%) of salivary gland tumors in children behave in a malignant fashion.[257, 258] Table 1.21 from Schuller and McCabe[256] confirms this. Mixed tumors are definitely unusual in infancy and early childhood and most examples are recorded as presenting in adolescence or late childhood. In Kauffman and Stout's[254] series, no tumor was known to have been present before the age of 7 years. Despite their biological benignancy, mixed tumors in children have manifested a relatively high recurrence rate. This finding may only reflect a more conservative surgical approach in the small child.

As far as the biological activity of the malignant forms of epithelial tumors is concerned, there is little evidence to indicate a different course from their counterparts in adults. While the mucoepidermoid carcinoma spans the entire age period, adenoid cystic carcinomas, acinous cell carcinomas and adenocarcinomas are almost exclusively diseases of the older child or adolescent. The undifferentiated carcinomas of the major salivary glands are seen primarily in infants and young children with a secondary peak in frequency in adolescence. Rapid growth, local fixation or inoperability at the time of initial examination, and widespread metastases, all characterize the undifferentiated carcinoma.

Vascular tumors are the most common neoplasms or neoplastic-like proliferations occurring in the salivary glands during infancy and childhood. Of the tumors making their clinical appearance during the first year of life, the capillary hemangioma is the predominant lesion, making up well over one-half of the total number of salivary gland tumors.[259] The parotid gland is by far the favorite site for the vascular tumors, with only a few examples being reported from the other salivary glands. There is a rather striking sex dominance, in that almost all series present a prominent female population.[260]

The diagnosis of a hemangioma of the parotid gland can usually be made with reasonable accuracy without a tissue examination. The fact that this lesion is the principal cause of parotid gland swellings in infants is certainly significant for establishing a presumptive diagnosis. A concomitant hemangioma or a telangiectasia in the overlying skin is also fairly common. Even without the overlying cutaneous changes, a bluish discoloration of the skin is characteristic. Crying may produce an increase in the size of the facial mass. The tume-

Table 1.21
Salivary Gland Tumors in Children*

Nonvascular Benign			Malignant Epithelial		
Classification	No.	Percentage of all Benign	Classification	No.	Percentage of all Malignant
Mixed tumor	94	85.6	Mucoepidermoid carcinoma	73	48.9
Lymphoepithelial lesion	3	2.7	Acinous cell carcinoma	18	12.2
Cystadenoma	3	2.7	Undifferentiated	14	9.4
Warthin's tumor	3	2.7	Adenocarcinoma	11	7.5
			Carcinoma ex pleomorphic adenoma	9	6.0
			Adenoid cystic carcinoma	6	4.0
			Squamous cell carcinoma	3	2.0

* Modified from Schuller and McCabe.[256]

faction is soft, may have a "cystic feel" or even be compressible. The tumors are located at the angle of the jaw and often extend anteriorly over the ramus of the mandible. The lobe of the ear may be displaced by the mass. Most characteristically, the salivary gland enlargement is noted during the first 6 months of life, with a period of maximum growth between the fourth and sixth months.

Resected specimens lack a distinctly demarcated mass in the salivary gland. Rather, the appearance is one of a hypertrophied gland with variation in size from two to five times that of the normal infant's parotid gland. The enlargement appears to be due to an increase in size of individual lobules of the gland. These are purple-red and spongy, and impart a distinctly congested appearance. The microscopic appearance is characteristic and variations are minimal. The lobular architecture of the gland is preserved and accentuated. Vasoformative elements replace the parenchyma and surround isolated acini and ducts. (Fig. 1.45). Endothelial proliferation with vascular differentiation, unaccompanied by other tissues, is the hallmark of this tumor.

The multifocal nature of the hemangiomatous process is indicated by the finding of vasoformative foci within juxtaparotid musculofascial tissues and in the interlobular septae. Nuclear pleomor-

phism and atypism are absent, but there may be a high mitotic index.

The controversy over whether these lesions are true neoplasms or vascular malformations has not been resolved. The cavernous form, seen in older children and adults, is best considered either as a malformation or as a consequence of trauma. The appropriate treatment for these lesions is controversial, but nonsurgical modalities, such as external or interstitial irradiation or the injection of sclerosing agents, are not advised. A watchful expectancy for spontaneous regression is often thwarted by parental pressures, but there is a high percentage of involution.[261] Recurrences after excision are unusual and are more prone to occur when the patient is less than 4 months old.[262]

In contrast to the hemangiomas, the glandular parenchyma associated with *lymphangiomatous* involvement is not replaced or atrophic but intact. Microscopically, islands and lobules of normal-appearing glandular tissue are separated by thin-walled lymph-containing spaces. In later stages a considerable fibrous connective tissue thickening of the walls of the dilated lymph channels may occur.

Two examples of an extremely rare form of congenital epithelial tumor of the parotid gland have been reported by Vawter and Tefft.[263] They were diagnosed in newborns and had developed during fetal life. Designated by their describers as "embryomas," the tumors manifested repeated local recurrences.

ASPIRATION BIOPSY AND PAROTID GLAND TUMORS

Studies on aspiration biopsy were performed as early as the 1930's, but as a diagnostic tool, the technique has not gained wide acceptance among head and neck surgeons and pathologists. The Scandinavian workers have had the greatest depth in study.[264-266]

The possibility of risk of tumor dissemination or implantation is an important issue. No matter how fine the needles used for aspiration, the procedure will inevitably produce microtrauma in its passage through the tissues, with the consequent risk of local neoplastic spread along the needle tract or distantly through punctured blood or lymphatic vessels. The risk of local tumor implantation due to aspiration biopsy has been investigated in mixed tumors. Follow-up of 141 patients for at least 5 years after aspiration biopsy has shown no local recurrence after surgical removal of the benign mixed tumor.[267] Robbins et al.[268] and Berg

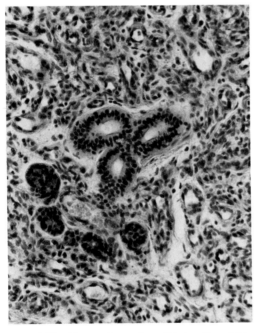

Figure 1.45. Hemangioma of parotid gland in a child. Note replacement of the acinar parenchyma.

Table 1.22
Salivary Gland Tumors—Thin Needle Aspiration*

	No. of Cases	Percentage of Correct Diagnosis	Percentage of False Positives	Percentage of False Negatives
Benign mixed tumor	215	93	4	3
Warthin's tumor	45	80	0	20
Adenoid cystic carcinoma	45	66	0	33
Acinous cell carcinoma	34	65	0	35
Mucoepidermoid carcinoma	18	62	0	38
Carcinoma ex pleomorphic adenoma	7	100	0	0
Oncocytoma	4	100	0	0

* Modified from Frable and Frable.[270]

and Robbins[269] after study of the technique in patients with breast carcinoma, concluded that aspiration biopsy is not detrimental to the patient and that "clinically no reason can be found not to use aspiration biopsy when it is indicated."[269]

Aspiration biopsy of salivary gland tumors with a fine needle (22 gauge) yields adequate material for cytological analysis. Benign neoplasms in these sites, such as the oncocytic tumors (Warthin's tumor and oncocytoma) and mixed tumors, can, in most instances, be recognized from a study of aspiration biopsy material.[266] Zajicek and Eneroth,[266] after studying 100 consecutive cases of salivary gland carcinomas, have also presented histocytological features which may be helpful in the differentiation between various types of salivary gland carcinoma—adenoid cystic, acinous cell, adenopapillary, mucoepidermoid adenocarcinoma, trabecular and undifferentiated.

Koivuniemi et al.,[265] dealing with other tumors in the head and neck as well as salivary gland lesions, report a 2.3% false-positive diagnostic rate and a 5.5% false-negative rate with cytological aspiration biopsy. These workers describe a Millipore filter technique that has distinct advantages over the ordinary smear preparations.

Table 1.22 from Frable and Frable[270] summarizes the results of thin-needle aspiration biopsy as presented in several series. Lindberg and Akerman[271] report on a retrospective study of the primary cytological reports correlated with the final diagnosis in 461 patients. Exact aggrement was achieved in 63% of the cases, "good" and not misleading agreement in a further 18%, false reports in 8%, and an unsatisfactory specimen in 11% of patients. The greatest reliability was present with a mixed tumor (93.5% accurate diagnoses). The most difficult tumor groups for successful correlation were malignant cystic tumors and mucoepidermoid carcinomas.

Spiro et al.[75] relate the following statistics from 125 patients who had 144 aspiration biopsies of salivary gland tumors: diagnostic in 62%, nondiagnostic in 21%, and an erroneous benign diagnosis in 17%.

While diagnostic accuracy can be improved by a needle-core biopsy, I agree with Spiro et al.[75] that the form of *primary* treatment will be altered in relatively few instances even if a diagnosis of cancer is obtained preoperatively. The same cannot be categorically said, however, for recurrent carcinomas and lymph node metastases.

Electron Microscopy in the Diagnosis of Salivary Gland and Other Neoplasia of the Head and Neck

While a case may be argued for wider use of electron microscopy as an aid to histological diagnosis in problem cases such as tumors of uncertain histogenesis, it must be emphasized that in the end, a diagnosis is reached by looking at the patient, the hematoxylin and eosin sections and the electron micrograph, in that order.[272]

Pathologists, consciously or subconsciously categorize tumors by recognizing the histological and cytological similarities between neoplastic cells and their normal counterparts. As dedifferentiation of the cells increases, the recognition of these similarities by light microscopy becomes increasingly difficult to the point where the origin and nature of certain neoplasms cannot be ascertained with certainty. This leads then to the differential diagnosis of poorly differentiated carcinoma, melanoma or lymphoma, a triumverate all too familiar to the head and neck surgeon. In these instances, the elucidation of fine structure is of considerable assistance. There is a point, however, where the differentiation is so low that ultrastructural diagnostic features are difficult to recognize. Furthermore, the area under inspection by electron microscopy is small and sampling error plays a role. Finally, in some poorly differentiated tumors, there may not be a single ultrastructural feature by which the origin of the neoplastic cell can be recognized. In these instances, tentative conclusions can be reached by analysis of the cytoplasmic membranes, organelles, cytoplasmic inclusions, and the topographical relationships of the neoplastic cells.[273]

In order that the head and neck surgeon appreciates the limitations of electron microscopy as a diagnostic tool, he should be moderately conversant with what the microscopist looks for when he deals with a difficult histological lesion. The following and Table 1.23 present a partial listing.

1. Filaments. These may be seen to some degree in many cells. They appear in abundance in muscle and epithelial neoplasms. When seen in epithelium, tonofilaments are usually arranged in bundles and are often associated with desmosomes. Myofilaments tend to be randomly distributed throughout tumor cells. A parallel alignment with suggestions of cross-banding is indicative of muscle tumors. Actin-like fibrils and characteristic dark bodies characterize smooth muscle lesions. Rhabdomyosarcomas possess thick and thin filaments, even when cross-striations are absent on light microscopy. Differentiation between tonofilaments and myofilaments is difficult. Filaments in muscle tumors are primarily actin (60 Å), which is close to the diameter of tonofilaments (40 to 50 Å).

2. Desmosomes. Epithelial cells often (if not always) and mesenchymal cells, rarely, have desmosomes. Attached bundles of tonofilaments in squamous cell carcinoma are particularly abundant. Since myoepithelial cells normally have desmosomes, their neoplastic counterparts will also be expected to possess them.

3. Secretory Granules and Other Inclusions. These include melanosomes, APUD granules, mucus, lipid and glycogen. Neurosecretory granules (dense core granules) are found in neuroectodermal lesions such as paragangliomas, esthesioneuroblastomas, etc. Homogenous secretory granules are typical in acinous cell carcinomas. Granular secretory granules are found in mucoepidermoid carcinomas. Autophagic vacuoles are seen in granular cell tumors. Lipid droplets and glycogen granules are nonspecific, but their presence or absence assists in differential diagnosis. Premelanosomes with their characteristic lattice work signifies melanic-producing tumors. The Langerhans granules of Histiocytosis X are distinctive.

4. Lysosomes. This organelle is not indicative of any specific tumor. Numerous lysosomes of char-

acteristic structure occur in cells of macrophage lineage.

5. Mitochondria. Pleomorphic and hyperplastic mitochondria are indicative of oncocytes. In themselves, however, the number, size and shape assist only in differential diagnosis.

6. Endoplasmic Reticulum. Protein secreting cells tend to rough endoplasmic reticulum; steroid cells to smooth.

7. Pinocytotic Vesicles. These are found in neurogenous and smooth muscle tumors, but not in other mesenchymal tumors.

8. Microvilli. Prominent relatively straight and intracellular clusters of microvilli are characteristic of epithelial cells.

9. Intercellular (Matrix) Fibrils. These are looked for in supporting tissue neoplasms such as fibrogenic lesions are in epithelial lesions producing abundant replicated basement membrane material such as the adenoid cystic carcinoma.

10. Basement Membrane and Cell Relationship Arrangements. Epithelial cells often cluster in a single basket of basement membrane. Mesenchymal cells tend to lie independently, often without an identifiable basement membrane.

Utilizing the aforementioned features of neoplastic cells, Regezi and Batsakis[274] found that electron microscopy provided a final definitive diagnosis in 5% of 161 head and neck tumors. They further suggest this percentage can be substantially increased if ultrastructural examination is reserved for equivocal tumors by light microscopy. It should be understood that subcellular analysis, by itself, cannot define malignancy. There is, however, a tendency toward more hyperplasia of organelles and cytoplasmic disarray in histologically malignant tumors. The light microscope remains the better tool for evaluation of malignancy.

Satisfactory preservation of the cytoarchitecture of tissue is a prerequisite for the identification of specific ultrastructural features essential for diagnosis. The quality of tissue preservation bears an important relationship to the time interval between tissue removal and immersion of the tissue into the fixative. Prolonged fixation is also disadvantageous for ultrastructural study. The selection of fixatives is important and varies with authors. McDowell and Trump[275] have compared the merits of formaldehyde, formaldehyde-glutaraldehyde combinations and gluteraldehyde in phosphate buffers. They recommend a combination of 4% commercial formaldehyde and 1% glutaraldehyde in a buffer of 176 mOsm/liter. This fixative is stable for at least 3 months if stored at 4°C. Alcohol must be avoided because of the severe

Table 1.23
Subcellular Structures Important for Ultrastructural Diagnosis

Subcellular structures	Cells	Neoplasms
Filaments		
Tonofilaments	Epithelium	Squamous, salivary gland, and odontogenic tumors
Desmosomes	Epithelium	Squamous, salivary gland, and odontogenic tumors
	Endothelium	Endothelioma
	Myoepithelium	Myoepithelioma
	Rarely connective tissue cells	Rarely connective tissue tumors
Myofilaments	Myoepithelium	Myoepithelioma
	Smooth muscle cells	Smooth muscle tumors
	Striated muscle cells	Striated muscle tumors, pericytoma?
Organelles		
Mitochondria	Oncocytes	Warthin's tumor, some pleomorphic adenomas and oncocytomas
Autophagic vacuoles		Granular cell myoblastoma, congenital epulis of newborn, and granular cell ameloblastoma
Pinocytotic vesicles	Myoepithelium	Myoepithelioma and some pleomorphic adenomas?
	Schwann cells	Neurogenous tumors
	Endothelium	Endothelioma?
	Smooth muscle cells	Smooth muscle tumors
Melanosomes and premelanosomes	Melanocytes and nevus cells	Nevi, melanomas, and neuroectodermal tumor of infancy
Secretory granules	Acinar cells	Acinic cell carcinoma, mucoepidermoid carcinoma
Neurosecretory (catecholamine) granules	Sympathetic (adrenergic) nerve cell endings, paraganglion cells, and Merkel cells	Neuroblastomas, pheochromocytomas, and paragangliomas
Langerhans granules	Langerhans cells	Histiocytosis X
Deposits		
Lipid (in abundance)	Fat cells	Lipomatous tumors, xanthomas and renal cell carcinoma
Glycogen (150–300 Å) (in abundance)	Skeletal muscle cells and clear cells	Striated muscle tumors, Ewing's tumor, mesenchymal chondrosarcoma, clear cell tumors, and renal cell carcinoma
Other		
Basement lamina	Epithelium, endothelium, myoepithelium, Schwann's cells, and smooth muscle cells	Epithelial tumors, endothelioma, myoepithelioma, neurogenous tumors, and smooth muscle tumors
Microvilli	Grandular epithelium	Glandular tumors

cytoplasmic damage it produces. Retrieval of tissues from paraffin embedded material for electron microscopy is generally fruitless. With few exceptions, there are considerable morphological changes.

REFERENCES

1. McFarland, J.: Tumors of the parotid region. Surg. Gynecol. Obstet. 57:104, 1933.
2. McFarland, J.: The histopathologic prognosis of salivary gland mixed tumors. Am. J. Med. Sci. 203:502, 1942.
3. Seifert, G., and Donath, K.: Die Morphologic der Speicheldrusenerkrankungen. Arch. Otorhinolaryngol. 213: 111, 1976.
4. Ackerman, L. V., and del Regato, J. A.: Cancer—Diagnosis, Treatment and Prognosis. 3rd Ed., St. Louis, C. V. Mosby Co., 1962.
5. Redman, R. S., and Sreabny, L. M.: The prenatal phase of the morphosis of the rat parotid gland. Anat. Record 168: 127, 1971.
6. Cutler, L. S., and Chaudhry, A. P.: Cytodifferentiation of the acinar cells of the rat submandibular gland. Dev. Biol. 41:31, 1974.
7. Jacoby, F., and Leeson, C. R.: The post-natal development of the rat submaxillary gland. J. Anat. 93:201, 1959.

8. Chang, W. W. L.: Changes in the cell population of rat submandibular gland during postnatal growth. Anat. Rec. 175:289, 1973.

9. Leeb, I. J.: Ethionine induced degeneration and regeneration in the rat parotid gland: an electron microscope study. Am. J. Anat. 142:29, 1975.

10. Hanks, C. T., and Chaudhry, A. P.: Regeneration of rat submandibular gland following partial extirpation. A light and electron microscopic study. Am. J. Anat. 130:195, 1971.

11. Bressler, R. S.: Fine structure of the differentiating acini in submandibular glands of isoproterenol-treated rats. Am. J. Anat. 138:431, 1973.

12. Yamashina, S., and Barka, T.: Localization of peroxidase activity in the developing submandibular gland of normal and isoproterenol-treated rats. J. Histochem. Cytochem. 20:855, 1972.

13. Slaukin, H. C., and Bauetta, L. A.: Developmental Aspects of Oral Biology. Academic Press, New York, 1972.

14. Fleischmajer, R., and Billingham, R. E.: Epithelial-Mesenchymal Interactions. W. W. Bolt, New York, 1968.

15. Regezi, J. A., and Batsakis, J. G.: Histogenesis of salivary gland neoplasms. Otolaryngol. Clin. N. Amer. 10:297, 1977.

16. Eversole, L. R.: Histogenic classification of salivary tumors. Arch. Pathol. 92:433, 1971.

17. Toner, P. G., Carr, K. E., and Wyburn, G. M.: The Digestive System—An Ultrastructural Atlas and Review. Butterworths, London, 1971.

18. Hamperl, H.: The myoepithelia (myoepithelial cells)—Normal state, regressive changes, hyperplasia; tumors. Curr. Top. Pathol. 53:161, 1970.

19. Chisholm, D. M., Waterhouse, J. P., Kraucunas, E., and Sciubba, J. J.: A quantitative ultrastructural study of the pleomorphic adenoma (mixed tumor) of human minor salivary glands. Cancer 34:1631, 1974.

20. Tandler, B., Denning, C. R., Mandel, I. D., and Kutscher, A. H.: Ultrastructure of human labial salivary glands. III. Myoepithelium and ducts. J. Morphol. 130:227, 1970.

21. Archer, F. L., and Kno, V. C. Y.: Immunohistochemical identification of actyomysin in myoepithelium of human tissues. Lab. Invest. 18:669, 1968.

22. Puchtler, H., Waldrop, F. S., Carter, M. G., and Valentine, L. S.: Investigation of staining, polarization and fluorescence microscopic properties of myoepithelial cells. Histochemie 40:281, 1974.

23. Hubner, G., Klein, H. J., Kleinsasser, O., and Schiefer, H. G.: Role of myoepithelial cells in the development of salivary gland tumors. Cancer 27:1255, 1971.

24. Mylius, E. A.: The identification and the role of the myoepithelial cell in salivary gland tumors. Acta Pathol. Microbiol. Scand. 50 Suppl. 139, 1960.

25. Azzopardi, J. G., and Smith, O. D.: Salivary gland tumours and their mucins. J. Pathol. Bacteriol. 77:131, 1959.

26. Doyle, L. E., Lynn, J. A., Panopio, I. T., and Crass, G.: Ultrastructure of the chondroid regions—benign mixed tumor of salivary gland. Cancer 22:225, 1968.

27. Welsh, R. A., and Meyer, A. T.: Mixed tumors of human salivary gland. Arch. Pathol. 85:433, 1968.

28. Hoshino, M., and Yamamato, I.: Ultrastructure of adenoid cystic carcinoma. Cancer 25:186, 1970.

29. Tandler, B.: Ultrastructure of adenoid cystic carcinoma of salivary gland origin. Lab. Invest. 24:504, 1971.

30. Pierce, G. B.: Neoplasms, differentiations and mutations. Am. J. Pathol. 77:103, 1974.

31. Spiro, R. H., Koss, L. G., Hajdu, S. E., and Strong, E. W.: Tumors of minor salivary origin—a clinicopathologic study of 492 cases. Cancer 31:117, 1973.

32. Thackray, A. C., and Sobin, L. H.: Histological Typing of Salivary Gland Tumors. Geneva, W.H.O., 1972.

33. Foote, F. W., Jr., and Frazell, E. L.: Tumors of the major salivary glands. Cancer 6:1065, 1953.

34. Glaser, A.: Die Geschwulste der Kopfspeicheldrussen. Volk und Gesundheit, Berlin, 1967.

35. Seifert, G.: Die Mundspeicheldrusen. In Spezielle Patholo-

gische Anatomie, Vol. I, edited by W. Doerr and E. Vehlinger, Julius Springer, Berlin, 1966.

36. Evans, R. W., and Cruickshank, A. H.: Epithelial Tumours of the Salivary Glands. W. B. Saunders Company, Philadelphia, 1970.

37. Eneroth, C. M.: Histological and clinical aspects of parotid tumors. Acta Otolaryngol. Suppl. 191:1, 1964.

38. Donath, K., Seifert, G., and Schmitz, R.: Zur Diagnose and Ultrastruktur des tubularen Speichelgangcarcinoms; epithelial-myoepitheliales Schaltstuckcarcinom. Virchows Arch. (Path. Anat.) 356:16, 1972.

39. Batsakis, J. G., McClatchey, K. D., Johns, M. E., and Regazi, J.: Primary squamous cell carcinoma of the parotid gland. Arch. Otolaryngol. 102:355, 1976.

40. Frommer, J.: The human accessory parotid gland: its incidence, nature, and significance. Oral Surg. 43:671, 1977.

41. Beahrs, O. H.: The surgical anatomy and technique of parotidectomy. Surg. Clin. N. Am. 57:477, 1977.

42. Conley, J.: Salivary Glands and the Facial Nerve. Grune & Stratton, New York, 1975.

43. Davis, R. A., Anson, B. J., Budinger, J. M., and Kurth, L. E.: Surgical anatomy of the facial nerve and parotid gland based upon a study of 350 cervicofacial halves. Surg. Gynec. Obstet. 102:385, 1956.

44. Beahrs, O. H., and Adson, M. A.: The surgical anatomy and technic of parotidectomy. Am. J. Surg. 95:885, 1958.

45. Cocke, W. M., and Finley, J. M.: Management of the facial nerve. Clin. Plast. Surg. 3:389, 1976.

46. Work, W. P., Batsakis, J. G., and Bailey, D. G.: Recurrent benign mixed tumor and the facial nerve. Arch. Otolaryngol. 102:15, 1976.

47. Ward, C. M.: Injury of the facial nerve during surgery of the parotid gland. Br. J. Surg. 62:401, 1975.

48. Cheesman, A. D.: Intra-vital staining as an aid to parotid gland surgery. Clin. Otolaryngol. 2:17, 1977.

49. Leegaard, T., and Lindeman, H.: Salivary gland tumors: clinical picture and treatment. Acta Otolaryngol. 263:155, 1970.

50. Leading Article: Salivary gland tumours. Lancet 1:655, 1969.

51. Eneroth, C. M.: Salivary gland tumors in the parotid gland, submandibular gland, and the palate region. Cancer 27:1415, 1971.

52. Eneroth, C. -M.: Incidence and prognosis of salivary-gland tumours at different sites. A study of parotid, submandibular and palatal tumours in 2632 patients. Acta Otolaryngol. 263:174, 1970.

53. Edington, G. M., and Sheiham, A.: Salivary gland tumours and tumours of the oral cavity in Western Nigeria. Br. J. Cancer 20:20, 1966.

54. Schulenburg, C. A. R.: Salivary gland tumours; report of 105 cases. S. Afr. Med. J. 28:910, 1954.

55. Berg, J. W., Hutter, R. V. P., and Foote, F. W., Jr.: The unique association between salivary gland cancer and breast cancer. J.A.M.A. 204:771, 1968.

56. Prior, P., and Waterhouse, J. A. H.: Second primary cancer in patients with tumours of the salivary glands. Br. J. Cancer 36:362, 1977.

57. Newell, G. R., Krementz, E. T., and Roberts, J. D.: Multiple primary neoplasms in blacks compared to whites. Further cancers in patients with cancer of the buccal cavity and pharynx. J. Natl. Cancer Inst. 52:639, 1974.

58. Moertel, C. G., and Elveck, L. R.: The association between salivary gland cancer and breast cancer. J.A.M.A. 210:306, 1969.

59. Dunn, J. E., Bragg, K., Sautter, C., and Gardipec, C.: Breast cancer risk following a major salivary gland carcinoma. Cancer 29:1343, 1972.

60. Rice, D. H., Batsakis, J. G., and McClatchey, K. D.: Postirradiation malignant salivary gland tumor. Arch. Otolaryngol. 102:699, 1976.

61. Schneider, A. B., Favus, M. J., Stachura, M. E., Arnold, M. J., and Frohman, L. A.: Salivary gland neoplasms as a late consequence of head and neck irradiation. Ann. Int. Med. 87:160, 1977.

62. Southwick, H. W.: Radiation-associated head and neck tumors. Am. J. Surg. 134:438, 1977.

63. Belsky, J. L., Takeichi, N., Yamamoto, T., Cihak, R. W., Hirose, F., Ezaki, H., Inove, S., and Blot, W. J.: Salivary gland neoplasms following atomic radiation: additional cases and reanalysis of combined data in a fixed population, 1957–1970. Cancer 35:555, 1975.

64. Takeichi, N., Hirose, F., and Yamamoto, H.: Salivary gland tumors in atomic bomb survivors, Hiroshima, Japan. I. Epidemiologic observations. Cancer 38:2462, 1976.

65. Mole, R. H.: Late effects of radiation in carcinogenesis. Br. Med. Bull. 29:78, 1973.

66. Quinn, H. J., Jr.: Symposium: Management of tumors of the parotid gland. II. Diagnosis of parotid gland swelling. Laryngoscope 86:22, 1976.

67. Noyek, A. M., Zizmor, J., Musumeci, R., Sanders, D. E., and Renouf, J. H. P.: The radiologic diagnosis of malignant tumors of the salivary glands. J. Otolaryngol. 6:38, 1977.

68. Berdal, P., Gronas, H. E., and Mylius, E. A.: Parotid tumors: clinical and histological aspects. Acta Otolaryngol. 263:160, 1970.

69. Blackwood, W., and Corsellis, J. A. H.: Greenfield's Neuropathology, 3rd Ed., pp. 693–694, Year Book Medical Publishers, Chicago, 1976.

70. Endes, P., and Adler, P.: Non-malignant perineural spread of epithelial tissue in the orofacial region. Virchows Arch. (Pathol. Anat.) 374:81, 1977.

71. Krammer, E. B., and Zenker, W.: Letter to the Editor. Am. J. Clin. Pathol. 62:371, 1974.

72. Lutman, G. B.: Epithelial nests in intraoral sensory nerve endings simulating perineural invasion in patients with oral carcinoma. Am. J. Clin. Pathol. 61:275, 1974.

73. Conley, J., and Hamaker, R. C.: Prognosis of malignant tumors of the parotid gland with facial paralysis. Arch. Otolaryngol. 101:39, 1975.

74. Eneroth, C. -M., and Hamberger, C. -A.: Principles of treatment of different types of parotid tumors. Laryngoscope. 84:1732, 1974.

75. Spiro, R. H., Huvos, A. G., and Strong, E. W.: Cancer of the parotid gland. A clinicopathologic study of 288 primary cases. Am. J. Surg. 130:452, 1975.

76. American Joint Committee for Cancer Staging and Final-Result Reporting: Manual for staging of cancer, 1977. Chicago, Ill., 1977.

77. McEvedy, B. V., and Ross, W. M.: The treatment of mixed parotid tumours by enucleation and radiotherapy. Br. J. Surg. 63:341, 1976.

78. Fletcher, G. H., and Jesse, R. H.: The place of irradiation in the management of the primary lesion in head and neck cancers. Cancer 39:862, 1977.

79. Chang, C. H.: Radiation therapy. In Diseases of the Salivary Glands, edited by R. R. Rankow and I. M. Polayes, pp. 343–355. W. B. Saunders Co., Philadelphia, 1976.

80. Skolnik, E. M., Friedman, M., Becker, S., Sisson, G. A., and Keyes, G. R.: Tumors of the major salivary glands. Laryngoscope 87:843, 1977.

81. Woods, J. E., Chong, G. C., and Beahrs, O. H.: Experience with 1,360 primary parotid tumors. Am. J. Surg. 130:460, 1975.

82. Hodgkinson, D. J., and Woods, J. E.: The influence of facial-nerve sacrifice in surgery of malignant parotid tumors. J. Surg. Oncol. 8:425, 1976.

83. Kagan, A. R., Nussbaum, H., Handler, S., Shapiro, R., Gilbert, H. A., Jacobs, M., Miles, J. W., Chan, P. Y. M., and Calcaterra, T.: Recurrences from malignant parotid salivary gland tumors. Cancer 37:2600, 1976.

84. Rafla, S.: Malignant parotid tumors: natural history and treatment. Cancer 40:136, 1977.

85. Chisholm, D. M., Waterhouse, J. P., Kraucunas, E., and Scuibba, J. J.: A quantitative ultrastructural study of the pleomorphic adenoma (mixed tumor) of human minor salivary glands. Cancer 34:1631, 1974.

86. Takeuchi, J., Sobue, M., Yoshida, M., Esaki, T., and Katoh, Y.: Pleomorphic adenoma of the salivary gland. With special reference to histochemical and electron microscopic studies and biochemical analysis of glycosaminoglycans in vivo and in vitro. Cancer 36:1771, 1975.

87. Quintarelli, G., and Robinson, L.: The glycosaminoglycans of salivary gland tumors. Am. J. Pathol. 51:19, 1957.

88. Willis, R. A.: Pathology of Tumours, 4th Ed. Butterworths, London, 1967.

89. Rauch, S.: Die Speicheldrusen des menschen. G. Thieme, Stuttgart, 1959.

90. Rauch, S., Seifert, G., and Gorlin, R. J.: Disease of the salivary glands: tumors. In Thoma's Oral Pathology, edited by R. J. Gorlin and H. M. Goldman, 6th Ed., p. 1013. C. V. Mosby Co., St. Louis, 1970.

91. Eneroth, C. -M.: Mixed tumors of major salivary glands: prognostic role of capsular structure. Ann. Otol. Rhinol. Laryngol. 74:944, 1965.

92. Nochomovitz, L. E., and Kahn, L. B.: Tyrosine crystals in pleomorphic adenomas of the salivary gland. Arch. Pathol. 97:141, 1974.

93. Mallet, K. J., and Harrison, M. S.: The recurrences of salivary gland tumours. J. Laryngol. Otol. 85:439, 1971.

94. Vandenberg, H. J., Kambouris, A., and Pryzbylski, T.: Salivary tumors: Clinicopathologic review of 190 patients. Am. J. Surg. 108:480, 1964.

95. Naeim, F., Forsberg, M. I., Waisman, J., and Coulson, W. F.: Mixed tumors of the salivary glands: Growth pattern and recurrence. Arch. Pathol. Lab. Med. 100:271, 1976.

96. Krolls, S. O., and Boyers, R. C.: Mixed tumors of salivary glands. Long-term follow-up. Cancer 30:276, 1972.

97. Fee, W. E., Jr., Goffinet, D. R., and Calcaterra, T. C.: Recurrent mixed tumors of the parotid gland—results of surgical therapy. Laryngoscope 88:265, 1978.

98. Grage, T. B., Lober, P. H., and Shanon, D. B.: Benign tumors of the major salivary glands. Surgery 50:625, 1961.

99. Winsten, J., and Ward, G. E.: Mixed tumors of the parotid gland. Surgery 42:1029, 1957.

100. Molnar, L., Ronay, P., and Dobrossy, L.: Mixed tumours of the parotid gland. Oncology 25:143, 1971.

101. Sprio, R. H., Huvos, A. G., and Strong, E. W.: Malignant mixed tumor of salivary origin. A clinicopathologic study of 146 cases. Cancer 39:388–396, 1977.

102. Gerughty, R. M., Scofield, H. H., Brown, F. M., and Hennigar, G. R.: Malignant mixed tumors of salivary gland origin. Cancer 24:471–486, 1969.

103. Saksela, E., Tarkkanen, J., and Kohonen, A.: The malignancy of mixed tumors of the parotid gland. A clinicopathological analysis of 70 cases. Acta Otolaryngol. 70:62–70, 1970.

104. LiVolsi, V. A., and Perzin, K. H.: Malignant mixed tumors arising in salivary glands. I. Carcinomas arising in benign mixed tumors: A clinicopathologic study. Cancer 39:2209–2230, 1977.

105. Youngs, G. R., and Scheuer, P. J.: Histologically benign mixed parotid tumour with hepatic metastasis. J. Pathol. 109:171–172, 1973.

106. Eneroth, C.-M., and Zetterberg, A.: Malignancy in pleomorphic adenoma. A clinical and microspectrophotometric study. Acta Otolaryngol. 77:426–432, 1974.

107. Mustard, R.A., and Anderson, W.: Malignant tumors of the parotid gland. Ann. Surg. 159:291, 1964.

108. Eneroth, C. -M., Blanck, C., and Jakobsson, R. A.: Carcinoma in pleomorphic adenoma of the parotid gland. Acta Otolaryngol. 66:477–492, 1968.

109. Nochomovitz, L. E., and Kahn, L. B.: Adenoid cystic carcinoma of the salivary gland and its histologic variants. A clinicopathologic study of thirty cases. Oral Surg. 44:394, 1977.

110. Headington, J. T., Teears, R., Niederhuber, J. E., and Slinger, R. P.: Primary adenoid cystic carcinoma of skin. Arch. Dermatol. 114:421, 1978.

111. Berdal, P., deBesche, A., and Mylius, E.: Cylindroma of salivary glands: report of 80 cases. Acta Otolaryngol. 263:170, 1970.

112. Ballantyne, A. J., McCarten, A. B., and Ibanez, M. L.: The

extension of cancer of the head and neck through peripheral nerves. Am. J. Surg. 106:651, 1963.

113. Blanck, C., Eneroth, C. -M., Jakobsson, F., and Jakobsson,
P. A.: Adenoid cystic carcinoma of the parotid gland.
Acta Radiol. Scand. 6:177, 1967.

114. Tandler, B.: Ultrastructure of adenoid cystic carcinoma of
salivary gland origin. Lab. Invest. 24:504, 1971.

115. Hoshino, M., and Yamamoto, I.: Ultrastructure of adenoid
cystic carcinoma. Cancer 25:186, 1970.

116. Adkins, K. F., and Daley, T. J.: Elastic tissues in adenoid
cystic carcinomas. Oral Surg. 33:562, 1974.

117. Bloom, G. D., Carlsoo, B., Gustafsson, H., and Henriksson,
R.: Distribution of mucosubstances in adenoid cystic
carcinoma. A light and electron microscopic study. Virchows Arch. (Pathol. Anat.) 375:1, 1977.

118. Byers, R. M., Jesse, R. H., Guillamondegui, O. M., and
Luna, M. A.: Malignant tumors of the submaxillary
gland. Am. J. Surg. 126:458, 1976.

119. Eneroth, C. -M., Hjertman, L., and Moberger, G.: Malignant tumors of the submandibular gland. Acta Otolaryngol. 64:514, 1967.

120. Eby, L. S., Johnson, D. S., and Baker, H. W.: Adenoid
cystic carcinoma of the head and neck. Cancer 29:1160,
1972.

121. Grahne, B., Lauren, C., and Holsti, L. R.: Clinical and
histological malignancy of adenoid cystic carcinoma. J.
Laryngol. 91:743, 1977.

122. Sprio, R. H., Huvos, A. G., and Strong, E. W.: Adenoid
cystic carcinoma of salivary origin. A clinicopathologic
study of 242 cases. Am. J. Surg. 128:512, 1974.

123. Osborn, D. A.: Morphology and the natural history of
cribriform adenocarcinoma (adenoid cystic carcinoma).
J. Clin. Pathol. 30:195, 1977.

124. Conley, J., and Dingman, D. L.: Adenoid cystic carcinoma
in the head and neck (cylindroma). Arch. Otolaryngol.
100:81, 1974.

125. Fu, K. K., and Leibel, S. A., Levine, M. L., Friedlander, L.
M., Boles, R., and Philips, T. L.: Carcinoma of the major
and minor salivary glands. Analysis of treatment results
and sites and causes of failures. Cancer 40:2882, 1977.

126. Mountain, C. F., Khalil, K. G., Hermes, K. E., and Frazier,
O. H.: The contributions of surgery to the management
of carcinomatous pulmonary metastases. Cancer 41:833,
1978.

127. Allen, M. S., Jr., and Marsh, W. L., Jr.: Lymph node
involvement by direct extension in adenoid cystic carcinoma. Absence of classic embolic lymph node metastasis.
Cancer 38:2017, 1976.

128. Ganzer, U.: Behandlung und Prognose des adenoidzys-
tischen Karzinoms. Laryng. Rhinol. 53:901, 1974.

129. Cummings, C. W.: Adenoid cystic carcinoma (cylindroma)
of the parotid gland. Ann. Otol. 86:280, 1977.

130. Stewart, F. W., Foote, F. W., Jr., and Becker, W. F.:
Mucoepidermoid tumors of salivary glands. Ann. Surg.
122:820, 1945.

131. Eneroth, C. -M., Hjertman, L., and Moberger, G.: Mucoepidermoid carcinoma of the palate. Acta Otolaryngol. 70:
408, 1970.

132. Eneroth, C. -M., and Hjertman, L.: Benign tumours of the
submandibular gland. Pract. Otorhinolaryngol. 29:166,
1967.

133. Eneroth, C. -M., Hjertman, L., and Moberger, G.: Malignant tumours of the submandibular gland. Acta Otolaryngol. 64:514, 1967.

134. Jakobsson, P. A., Blanck, C., and Eneroth, C. -M.: Mucoepidermoid carcinoma of the parotid gland. Cancer 22:
111, 1968.

135. Sikorowa, L.: Mucoepidermoid tumors of salivary glands.
Pol. Med. J. 3:1345, 1964.

136. Woolner, L. B., Pettet, J. R., and Kirklin, J. W.: Mucoepidermoid tumors of the major salivary glands. Am. J.
Clin. Pathol. 24:1350, 1954.

137. Bhaskar, S. N., and Bernier, J. L.: Mucoepidermoid tumors
of major and minor salivary glands. Cancer 15:801, 1962.

138. Eneroth, C. -M., Hjertman, L., Moberger, G., and Soder-

berg, G.: Mucoepidermoid carcinomas of the salivary
glands. With special reference to the possible existence of
a benign variety. Acta Otolaryngol. 73:68, 1972.

139. Healey, W. V., Perzin, K. H., and Smith, L.: Mucoepidermoid carcinoma of salivary gland origin: classification,
clinical-pathologic correlation, and results of treatment.
Cancer 26:368, 1970.

140. Eneroth, C. -M., and Zetterberg, A.: The relationship between the nuclear DNA content in smears of aspirates
and prognosis of mucoepidermoid carcinoma. Acta Otolaryngol. 80:429, 1975.

141. Eneroth, C. -M., and Zetterberg, A.: A cytochemical method
of grading the malignancy of salivary gland tumours
preoperatively. Acta Otolaryngol. 81:489, 1976.

142. Frazell, E. L.: Clinical aspects of tumors of the major
salivary glands. Cancer 7:637, 1954.

143. Stevenson, G. F., and Hazard, J. B.: Mucoepidermoid carcinoma of salivary gland origin. Cleve. Clin. Q. 20:445,
1953.

144. Thorvaldsson, S. E., Beahrs, O. H., Woolner, L. B., and
Simons, J. N.: Mucoepidermoid tumors of the major
salivary glands. Am. J. Surg. 120:432, 1970.

145. Eversole, L. R.: Mucoepidermoid carcinoma: review of 815
reported cases. J. Oral Surg. 28:490, 1970.

146. Thomas, K.: Mucoepidermoid carcinoma of the larynx. J.
Laryngol. Otol. 85:261, 1971.

147. Larson, R. E., Woolner, L. B., and Payne, S. W.: Mucoepidermoid tumors of the trachea. J. Thorac. Cardiovasc.
Surg. 50:131, 1965.

148. Turnbull, A. D., Huvos, A. G., Goodner, J. T., and Foote,
F. W., Jr.: Mucoepidermoid tumors of bronchial glands.
Cancer 28:539, 1971.

149. Rao, N. A., and Font, R. L.: Mucoepidermoid carcinoma
of the conjunctiva. A clinicopathologic study of five cases.
Cancer 38:1699, 1976.

150. Baden, E., and Wallen, N. G.: Acinous cell tumor of the
floor of the mouth. J. Oral Surg. 23:163, 1965.

151. Buxton, R. W., Maxwell, J. H., and French, A. J.: Surgical
treatment of epithelial tumors of the parotid gland. Surg.
Gynecol. Obstet. 97:401, 1953.

152. Spiro, R. H., Huvos, A. G., and Strong, E. W.: Acinic cell
carcinoma of salivary origin. A clinicopathologic study
of 67 cases. Cancer 41:924, 1978.

153. Chong, G. C., Beahrs, O. H., and Woolner, L. B.: Surgical
management of acinic cell carcinoma of the parotid
gland. Surg. Gynec. Obstet. 138:65, 1974.

154. Eneroth, C. -M., Jakobsson, P. A., and Blanck, C.: Acinic
cell carcinomas of the parotid gland. Cancer 19:1761,
1966.

155. Godwin, J. T., Foote, F. W., and Frazell, E. L.: Acinic cell
adenocarcinoma of the parotid gland. Am. J. Pathol. 30:
465, 1954.

156. Sharkey, F. E.: Systematic evaluation of the World Health
Organization Classification of salivary gland tumors: a
clinicopathologic study of 366 cases. Am. J. Clin. Pathol.
67:272, 1977.

157. Levin, J. M., Robinson, D. W., and Lin, F.: Acinic cell
carcinoma: collective review, including bilateral cases.
Arch. Surg. 110:64, 1975.

158. Krolls, S. O., Trodahl, J. N., and Boyers, R. C.: Salivary
gland lesions in children: A survey of 430 cases. Cancer
30:459, 1972.

159. Erlandson, R. A., and Tandler, B.: Ultrastructure of acinic
cell carcinoma of the parotid gland. Arch. Pathol. 93:130,
1972.

160. Batsakis, J. G., Wozniak, K. D., and Regezi, J. A.: Acinic
cell carcinoma: a histogenetic hypothesis. J. Oral Surg.
35:904, 1977.

161. Bloom, G. D., and Henriksson, R.: Some ultrastructural
features of acinic cell carcinoma. J. Laryngol. 91:947,
1977.

162. Abrams, A. M., Cornyn, J., Scofield, H. H., and Hansen, L.
S. L.: Acinic cell adenocarcinoma of the major salivary
glands: Clinicopathologic study of 77 cases. Cancer 18:
1145, 1965.

163. Eneroth, C. -M., Hamberger, C. A., and Jakobsson, P. A.: Malignancy of acinic cell carcinoma. Ann. Otol. 75:780, 1966.

164. Grage, T. B., Lober, P. H., and Arhelger, S. W.: Acinic cell carcinoma of the parotid gland. Am. J. Surg. 102:765, 1961.

165. Fox, N. M., ReMine, W. H., and Woolner, L. B.: Acinic cell carcinoma of the major salivary glands. Am. J. Surg. 106:860, 1963.

166. Gorlin, R. J., and Chaudhry, A.: Acinic cell tumor of the major and minor salivary glands. J. Oral Surg. 15:304, 1957.

167. Beahrs, O. H., Woolner, L. B., Carveth, S. W., and Devine, K. D.: Surgical management of parotid lesions. Arch. Surg. 90:890, 1960.

168. Fine, G., Marshall, R. B., and Horn, R. C.: Tumors of the minor salivary glands. Cancer 12:653, 1960.

169. Frable, W. J., and Elzay, R. P.: Tumors of minor salivary glands. Cancer 25:932, 1970.

170. Chaudhry, A. P., Vickers, R. A., and Gorlin, R. J.: Intraoral minor salivary gland tumors. Oral Surg., 14:1194, 1961.

171. Bardwill, J. M.: Tumors of the parotid gland. Am. J. Surg. 114:498, 1967.

172. Hanna, D. C., and Gaisford, J. C.: Parotid gland tumors, diagnosis and treatment. Am. J. Surg. 104:737, 1962.

173. Foote, F. W., Jr., and Frazell, E. L.: Tumors of the major salivary glands. Atlas of Tumor Pathology, Section IV, Fascicle II. Armed Forces Institute of Pathology, Washington, D. C., 1954.

174. Batsakis, J. G., Holtz, F., and Sueper, R. H.: Adenocarcinoma of nasal and paranasal cavities. Arch. Otolaryngol. 77:625, 1963.

175. Blanck, C., Eneroth, C. -M., and Jakobsson, P. A.: Mucusproducing adenopapillary (non-epidermoid) carcinoma of the parotid gland. Cancer 28:676, 1971.

176. Gaisford, J. C., Hanna, D. C., and Sotereanos, G. C.: Primary cancer of Stensen's duct. Arch. Otolaryngol. 82: 45, 1965.

177. Kleinsasser, O., Klein, H. J., and Hubner, G.: Speichelgangcarcinome. Arch. Klin. Exp. Ohren. Nasen. Kehlkopfheilkd. 192:100, 1968.

178. Fayemi, A. O., and Toker, C.: Salivary duct carcinoma. Arch. Otolaryngol. 99:366, 1974.

179. Patey, D. H., Thackray, A. C., and Keeling, D. H.: Malignant disease of the parotid. Br. J. Cancer 19:712, 1965.

180. Blanck, C., Backstrom, A., Eneroth, C. -M., and Jakobsson, P. A.: Poorly differentiated solid parotid carcinoma. Acta Radiol. 13:17, 1974.

181. Koss, L. G., Spiro, R. H., and Hajdu, S.: Small cell (oat cell) carcinoma of minor salivary gland origin. Cancer 30:737, 1972.

182. Wirman, J. A., and Battifora, H. A.: Small cell undifferentiated carcinoma of salivary gland origin: an ultrastructural study. Cancer 37:1840, 1976.

183. Echevarria, R. A.: Ultrastructure of the acinic cell carcinoma and clear cell carcinoma of the parotid gland. Cancer 20:563–571, 1967.

184. Mohamed, A. H., and Cherrick, H. M.: Glycogen-rich adenocarcinoma of minor salivary glands. A light and electron microscopic study. Cancer 36:1057–1066, 1975.

185. Goldman, R. L., and Klein, H. Z.: Glycogen-rich adenoma of the parotid gland. An uncommon benign clear-cell tumor resembling certain clear-cell carcinomas of salivary origin. Cancer 30:749–754, 1972.

186. Batsakis, J. G., and Regezi, J. A.: Selected controversial lesions of salivary tissues. Otolaryngol. Clin. N. Am. 10: 309–328, 1977.

187. Ferlito, A.: Histological classification of larynx and hypopharynx cancers and their clinical implications. Acta Otolaryngol. Suppl. 342, 1976.

188. Stoll, W., and Lietz, H.: Zur Kenntnis und Problematik des hellzelligen Adenomes in des Schilddruse. Virchows Arch. (Pathol. Anat.) 361:163–173, 1973.

189. Ridenhour, C. E., and Pratt, J. S., Jr.: Epidermoid carcinoma of the skin involving the parotid gland. Am. J. Surg. 112:504, 1966.

190. Freeman, C., Berg, J. W., and Cutler, S. J.: Occurrence and prognosis of extranodal lymphomas. Cancer 29:252–260, 1972.

191. Nime, F. A., Cooper, H. S., and Eggleston, J. C.: Primary malignant lymphomas of the salivary glands. Cancer 37: 906, 1976.

192. Batsakis, J. G., Bernacki, E. G., Rice, D. H., and Stebler, M. E.: Malignancy and the benign lymphoepithelial lesion. Laryngoscope 85:389, 1975.

193. Hugo, E., McKinney, P., and Griffith, B. H.: Management of tumors of the parotid gland. Surg. Clin. N. Am. 53: 105, 1973.

194. Kleinsasser, O., and Klein, H. J.: Basalze iladenome der Speicheldrusen. Arch. Klin. Exp. Ohren. Nasen Kehlkopfheilkd. 189:302, 1967.

195. Batsakis, J. G.: Basal cell adenoma of the parotid gland. Cancer 29:226, 1972.

196. Luna, M. A., and Mackay, B.: Basal cell adenoma of the parotid gland. Case report with ultrastructural observations. Cancer 37:1615, 1976.

197. Jao, W., Keh, P., and Swerdlow, M. A.: Ultrastructure of the basal cell adenoma of the parotid gland. Cancer 37: 1322, 1976.

198. Min, B. H., Miller, A. S., Leifer, C., and Putong, P. B.: Basal cell adenoma of the parotid gland. Arch. Otolaryngol. 99:88, 1974.

199. Klima, M., Wolfe, S. K., and Johnson, P. E.: Basal cell tumors of the parotid gland. Arch. Otolaryngol. 104:111, 1978.

200. Headington, J. T., Batsakis, J. G., Beals, T. F., Campbell, T. E., Simmons, J. L., and Stone, W. D.: Membranous basal cell adenoma of parotid gland, dermal cylindromas, and trichoepitheliomas. Comparative histochemistry and ultrastructure. Cancer 39:2460, 1977.

201. Reingold, I. M., Keasbey, L. E., and Graham, J. H.: Multicentric dermal-type cylindromas of the parotid glands in a patient with florid turban tumor. Cancer 40:1702, 1977.

202. Christ, T. F., and Crocker, D.: Basal cell adenoma of minor salivary gland origin. Cancer 20:214, 1972.

203. Nelson, J. F., and Jacoway, J. R.: Monomorphic adenoma (canalicular type): Report of 29 cases. Cancer 31:1511, 1973.

204. Bernacki, E. G., Batsakis, J. G., and Johns, M. E.: Basal cell adenoma. Distinctive tumor of salivary glands. Arch. Otolaryngol. 99:84, 1974.

205. Crumpler, C., Scharfenberg, J. C., and Reed, R. J.: Monomorphic adenoma of salivary glands. Trabecular-tubular, canalicular and basaloid variants. Cancer 38:193, 1976.

206. Sciubba, J. J., and Goldstein, B. H.: Myoepithelioma: Review of the literature and report of a case with ultrastructural confirmation. Oral Surg. 42:328, 1976.

207. Garnett, J. R., and Harrison, J. D.: Alkaline-phosphatase and adenosine triphosphatase histochemical reactions in the salivary glands of cat, dog and man with particular reference to the myoepithelial cells. Histochemie 24:214, 1970.

208. Meriono, M. J., and LiVolsi, V. A.: Pleomorphic adenomas of the parotid gland resembling mesenchymal tumors. Oral Surg. 44:405, 1977.

209. Warthin, A. D.: Papillary cystadenoma lymphomatosum. J. Cancer Res., 13:116, 1929.

210. Thompson, A. S., and Bryant, H. C., Jr.: Histogenesis of papillary cystadenoma lymphomatosum (Warthin's tumor) of the parotid salivary gland. Am. J. Pathol. 26:807, 1950.

211. Chaudhry, A. P., and Gorlin, R. J.: Papillary cystadenoma lymphomatosum (adenolymphoma): a review of the literature. Am. J. Surg. 95:923, 1958.

212. McGurk, F. M., Main, J. H. P., and Orr, J. A.: Adenolymphoma of the parotid gland. Br. J. Surg. 57:321, 1970.

213. Cohen, M. A., and Batsakis, J. G.: Warthin's tumor revisited. Mich. Med. 67:1341, 1968.

214. Eneroth, C.-M., and Zajicek, J.: Aspiration biopsy of sali-

vary gland tumors. II. Morphological studies on smears and histologic sections from oncocytic tumors (45 cases of papillary cystadenoma lymphomatosum and 4 cases of oncocytoma). Acta Cytol. 9:355, 1965.

215. Tandler, B., and Shipkey, F. H.: Ultrastructure of Warthin's tumor. I Mitochondria. J. Ultrastruct. Res. 11:292, 1964.

216. McGavran, M. H.: The ultrastructure of papillary cystadenoma lymphomatosum of the parotid gland. Virchows Arch. (Pathol. Anat.) 338:195, 1964.

217. Little, J. W., and Rickles, N. H.: Malignant papillary cystadenoma lymphomatosum: report of a case with a review of the literature. Cancer 18:1851, 1965.

218. DeLa Pava, S., Knutson, G. H., Mukhtar, F., and Pickren, J. W.: Squamous cell carcinoma arising in Warthin's tumor of the parotid gland: first case report. Cancer 18: 790, 1965.

219. Seifert, G., Heckmayr, M., and Donath, K.: Carcinome in Papillaren Cystadenomolymphomen der Parotis Definition und Differentialdiagnose. Z. Krebsforsch. 90:25, 1977.

220. Cossman, J., Deegan, M. J., and Batsakis, J. G.: Warthin tumor: β-lymphocytes within the lymphoid infiltrate. Arch. Pathol. Lab. Med. 101:354, 1977.

221. Abrams, A. M., and Finck, F. M.: Sialadenoma papillferum. A previously unreported salivary gland tumor. Cancer 24:1057, 1969.

222. Freedman, P. D., and Lumerman, H.: Sialadenoma papilliferum. Oral Surg. 45:88, 1978.

223. Batsakis, J. G., Littler, E. R., and Leahy, M. S.: Sebaceous cell lesions of the head and neck. Arch. Otolaryngol. 95: 151, 1972.

224. Baratz, M., Loewenthal, M., and Rozin, M.: Sebaceous lumphadenoma of the parotid gland. Arch. Pathol. Lab. Med. 100:269, 1976.

225. MacFarlane, J. K., Viloria, J. B., and Palmer, J. E.: Sebaceous cell carcinoma of the parotid gland. Am. J. Surg. 130:499, 1975.

226. Shulman, J., Waisman, J., and Morledge, D.: Sebaceous carcinoma of the parotid gland. Arch. Otolaryngol. 98: 417, 1973.

227. Guiducci, A. A., and Hyman, A. B.: Ectopic sebaceous glands: a review of the literature regarding their occurrence, histology and enbryonic relationships. Dermatologica 125:44, 1962.

228. Epker, B. N., and Henney, F. A.: Intraoral sebaceous gland adenoma. Cancer 27:987, 1971.

229. Askew, J. B., Jr., Fechner, R. E., Bentinck, D. C., and Jenson, A. B.: Epithelial and myoepithelial oncocytes: ultrastructural study of a salivary gland oncocytoma. Arch. Otolaryngol. 93:46, 1971.

230. Tandler, B.: Fine structure of oncocytes in human salivary glands. Virchows Arch. (Pathol. Anat.) 341:317, 1966.

231. Hamperl, H.: Oncocytem and oncocytome. Virchows Arch. (Pathol. Anat.) 335:452, 1962.

232. Schulz, H.: Electron microscopy of oncocytomas and carcinoid tumors. Results Cancer Res. 44:63, 1974.

233. Johns, M. E., Regezi, J. A., and Batsakis, J. G.: Oncocytic neoplasms of salivary glands: an ultrastructural study. Laryngoscope 87:862, 1977.

234. Tandler, B., Hutter, R. V. P., and Erlandson, R. A.: Ultrastructure of oncocytoma of the parotid gland. Lab Invest. 23:567, 1970.

235. Blanck, C., Eneroth, C. M., and Jakobsson, P. A.: Oncocytoma of the parotid gland: neoplasm or nodular hyperplasia. Cancer 25:919, 1970.

236. Gallagher, J. C., and Puzon, B. Q.: Oncocytic lesions of the larynx. Ann. Otol. Rhinol. Laryngol. 78:307, 1969.

237. Cohen, M. A., and Batsakis, J. G.: Oncocytic tumors (oncocytomas) of minor salivary glands. Arch. Otolaryngol. 88:71, 1968.

238. Gray, S. R., Cornog, J. L., Jr., and Seo, I. S.: Oncocytic neoplasms of salivary glands. A report of fifteen cases including two malignant oncocytomas. Cancer 38:1306, 1976.

239. Kirklin, J. W.: Parotid tumors: Histopathology, clinical

behavior, and end results. Surg. Gynec. Obstet. 92:721, 1951.

240. Conley, J., and Arena, S.: Parotid gland as a focus of metastasis. Arch. Surg. 87:757, 1963.

241. Graham, J. W.: Metastatic cancer in the parotid lymph nodes. Med. J. Aust. 2:8, 1965.

242. Pope, T. H., Jr., and Lehmann, W. B.: Parotid metastasis to parotid nodes. Arch. Otolaryngol. 86:673, 1967.

243. Storm, F. K., Eilber, F. R., Sparks, F. C., and Morton, D. L.: A prospective study of parotid metastases from head and neck cancer. Am. J. Surg. 134:115, 1977.

244. Parkin, J. L., and Stevens, M. H.: Unusual parotid tumors. Laryngoscope 87:317, 1977.

245. Wright, D. H.: Burkitt's tumour. A postmortem study of 50 cases. Br. J. Surg. 51:245, 1964.

246. Eneroth, C. M., Fluur, E., and Moberger, G.: Unusual localization of mixed tumors in the parotid region. Pract. Otorhino Laryngol. 28:108, 1966.

247. Nigro, M. F., and Spiro, R. H.: Deep lobe parotid tumors. Am. J. Surg. 134:523, 1977.

248. Hanna, D. C., Gaisford, J. C., Richardson, G. S., and Bindra, R. N.: Tumors of the deep lobe of the parotid gland. Am. J. Surg. 116:524, 1968.

249. Berdal, P., and Hall, J. G.: Parapharyngeal growth of parotid tumors. Acta Otolaryngol. 263:164, 1970.

250. Eneroth, C. M.: Discussion of paper by Berdal et al. (reference 68).

251. Turnbull, A. D., and Frazell, E. L.: Multiple tumors of the major salivary glands. Am. J. Surg. 118:787, 1969.

252. Carlsoo, B., and Ekstrand, T.: Unilateral multiple mixed tumours of the parotid gland. J. Laryngol. 91:629, 1977.

253. Brill, A. H., and Fitzhugh, G. S.: Bilateral synchronous mixed tumors of the parotid gland. Arch. Otolaryngol. 101:751, 1975.

254. Kauffman, S. L., and Stout, A. P.: Tumors of the major salivary glands in children. Cancer 16:1317, 1963.

255. Castro, E. B., Huvos, A. G. Strong, E. W., and Foote, F. W., Jr.: Tumors of the major salivary glands in children Cancer 29:312, 1972.

256. Schuller, D. E., and McCabe, B. F.: The firm salivary mass in children. Laryngoscope 87:189, 1977.

257. Marlow, J. F., and Hora, J. F.: Parotid mucoepidermoid carcinoma in children. Laryngoscope 78:68, 1968.

258. Bhaskar, S. M., and Lilly, G. E.: Salivary gland tumors of infancy: report of 27 cases. J. Oral Surg. 21:305, 1963.

259. Nussbaum, M., Tan, S., and Som, M. L.: Hemangiomas of salivary glands. Laryngoscope 86:1015, 1976.

260. Goldman, R. L., and Perzik, S. L.: Infantile hemangiomas of the parotid gland: a clinicopathological study of 15 cases. Arch. Otolaryngol. 90:605, 1969.

261. Koop, C. E.: Surgical pros and cons. Surg. Gynec. Obstet. 135:274, 1972.

262. Wawro, N. W., Frederickson, R. W., and Tennant, R.: Hemangioma of the parotid gland in the newborn and in infancy. Cancer 8:595, 1955.

263. Vawter, G. F., and Tefft, M.: Congenital tumors of the parotid gland. Arch. Pathol. 82:242, 1966.

264. Soderstrom, N.: Fine Needle Aspiration Biopsy, Used As a Direct Adjunct in Clinical Diagnostic Work. Almquist and Wiksell, Stockholm, 1966.

265. Koivuniemi, A., Sadsela, E., and Holopainen, E.: Cytological aspiration biopsy in otorhinolaryngological practice: a preliminary report with special reference to method. Acta Otolaryngol. 263:189, 1970.

266. Zajicek, J., and Eneroth, C. M.: Cytological diagnosis of salivary-gland carcinomata from aspiration biopsy smears. Acta Otolaryngol. 263:183, 1970.

267. Zajicek, J.: Discussion of salivary gland tumours: clinical picture and treatment. Acta Otolaryngol. 263:155, 1970.

268. Robbins, G. F., Brothers, J. H., Eberhart, W. F., and Quan, S.: Is aspiration biopsy of breast cancer dangerous to the patient? Cancer 7:774, 1954.

269. Berg, J. W., and Robbins, G. F.: A late look at the safety of aspiration biopsy. Cancer 15:826, 1962.

270. Frable, W. J., and Frable, M. A.: Thin-needle aspiration

biopsy in the diagnosis of head and neck tumors. Laryngoscope 84:1069, 1974.

271. Lindberg, L. G., and Akerman, M.: Aspiration cytology of salivary gland tumors: diagnostic experience from six years of routine laboratory work. Laryngoscope 86:584, 1976.

272. Carr, I., and Toner, P. G.: Rapid electron microscopy in oncology. J. Clin. Pathol. 30:13, 1977.

273. Gyorkey, F., Min, K. -W., Krisko, I., and Gyorkey, P.: The usefulness of electron microscopy in the diagnosis of human tumors. Human Pathol. 6:421, 1975.

274. Regezi, J. A., and Batsakis, J. G.: Diagnostic electron microscopy of head and neck tumors. Arch. Pathol. Lab. Med. 102:8, 1978.

275. McDowell, E. M., and Trump, B. F.: Histologic fixations suitable for diagnostic light and electron microscopy. Arch. Pathol. Lab. Med. 100:405, 1976.

276. Lambert, J. A.: Parotid gland tumors. Milit. Med. 136:484, 1971.

277. Morgan, M. N., and Mackenzie, D. H.: Tumours of salivary glands: a review of 204 cases with five year follow-up. Brit. J. Surg. 55:284, 1968.

278. Moberger, J. H., and Eneroth, C. -M.: Malignant mixed tumors of the major salivary glands: special reference to the histologic structure in metastases. Cancer 21:1198, 1968.

279. Skolnik, E. M., Meyers, R. M., Tardy, E., Roos, J. C., and Saberman, M. N.: Malignancies of the parotid gland. Arch. Otolaryngol. 93:256, 1971.

280. Brown, J. B., Fryer, M. P., and Zografkis, G.: The treatment of primary malignant tumors of the parotid gland. Surg. Gynecol. Obstet. 129:40, 1969.

281. Wheelock, M. D., Putong, P., and Trota, J.: Pathologic features of neoplasms of the salivary glands. Am. J. Surg. 98:907, 1959.

282. Freeman, F. M., Beahrs, O. H., and Woolner, L. B.: Surgical treatment of malignant tumors of the parotid gland. Am. J. Surg. 110:527, 1965.

283. Chaudhry, A. P., Vickers, R. A. and Gorlin, R. J.: Intraoral minor salivary gland tumors. Oral Surg. 14:1194, 1961.

284. Eneroth, C. -M., Hjertman, L., and Moberger, G.: Adenoid cystic carcinoma of the palate. Acta Otolaryngol. 66:248, 1968.

CHAPTER 2

Neoplasms of the Minor and "Lesser" Major Salivary Glands

Neoplasms of the two "other" major salivary glands (submandibular and sublingual) and especially of the minor salivary glands have increasingly attracted the attention of surgeons and pathologists over the past decade. The formulation and general acceptance of sound histological classifications, an enhanced clinicopathological awareness and improved surgical techniques have been largely responsible for this surge of interest. While their over-all incidence is relatively low when compared to primary neoplasms of the parotid gland or to the vastly more numerous squamous cell carcinomas of the head and neck, their importance should not be underestimated. Virtually complete transference of classifications applied to neoplasms of the parotid gland can be made, certainly to the tumors of the submandibular and sublingual glands, and to the majority of neoplasms arising from the minor salivary glands and the glandular mucosa of the upper respiratory tract and mouth.

The frequency of occurrence and the biological behavior of these neoplasms are, however, often distinctly different from their counterparts in the parotid gland. These differences are largely due to the peculiar anatomical relationships of their sites of origin, the nature of the tumor bed and, perhaps most importantly, the delay between the onset of signs and symptoms and the seeking of medical advice. Delay may be occasioned by an undue complacency or inadequate treatment on the part of the primary physician or by the lulling of the patient into a false sense of security because of seemingly minor or innocuous symptoms.

Both of these serve as deterrants to successful surgical management. The surgical axiom of complete excision by the initial operator is probably even more important for these tumors than for those presenting in the parotid gland. In several regions of the head and neck (viz, submandibular gland, sublingual gland and areas within the oral cavity) this complete form of removal is facilitated by the absence of structures such as the facial nerve that have served as "obstacles" to the surgeon treating tumors of the parotid gland. Failure to achieve complete removal of several classes of minor salivary gland and lesser salivary gland tumors virtually assures "recurrences" through persistent growth. The general lack of radiocurability of these lesions offers little else to the patients besides repeated surgical excisions that may be disfiguring or a lingering, painful, clinical progression of the disease. Unfortunately, many patients, especially those with glandular neoplasms of the sinonasal tract, larynx and trachea, do not present themselves in time for a complete and effective removal of their neoplasm. The end result is much like that of the patient who has been mismanaged at the onset.

Although the location of the neoplasm and the time factor are more important, the fact that the incidence of malignant salivary gland tumors is considerably higher in minor or lesser salivary glands than in the parotid certainly is additive to the ultimate outcome of patients. It appears that the smaller the salivary gland, the greater the probability it will harbor a malignant neoplasm (Table 2.1). This inverse relationship holds true for almost all classes of salivary gland neoplasms. In this regard, benign mixed tumors of the upper respiratory tract are unusual, not numerous in the oral cavity and most numerous in the parotid and submandibular glands. Adenoid cystic carcinomas, on the other hand, are the most common malignant neoplasms of the minor and lesser salivary glands. This neoplasm so dominates the statistics that it has been suggested that the high rate of malignancy in minor salivary gland tumors is directly attributable to this neoplasm (Table 2.2).

Whether the relative incidence of malignancy in these glands is related to their cellular composition is conjectural. The parotid gland is composed of an almost exclusive *serous* cell population, whereas the lesser glands and the minor salivary glands are all or nearly all mucous in type.

TUMORS OF THE MINOR SALIVARY GLANDS

For the purposes of this presentation, neoplasms to be considered take their origin from the mucous membranes, minor salivary glands and other glands of similar general structure, wherever situated or whatever their secretion, in the head and neck.[1] The distribution and frequency of these glands in the oral and upper respiratory tracts have been outlined by Ranger et al.[2] Intraoral minor salivary glands number 450 to 750. They may be found in the mucosa of the lips and cheeks, hard and soft palate, uvula, floor of the mouth, posterior tongue, retromolar area and peritonsillar region. Additional glandular elements histologically identical to the intraoral glands are found in the nasopharynx, larynx, lacrimal glands, paranasal sinuses, trachea, skin and breast. The ratio between tumors of the major salivary glands, including the submandibular and sublingual glands, and those of the minor salivary glands is of the order of 5:1. Among the latter tumors, the majority

occur in the oral cavity, the palate being the site in somewhat over one-half of the cases.[3]

The incidence of benign versus malignant *minor* salivary gland tumors varies with the type of reporting institution and ranges from a high of 82% malignant rate from the M. D. Anderson Hospital (Houston, Texas)[4] to a low of 7% reported by Bergman.[5] My own assessment, after a review of 20 reports, totaling 945 neoplasms, is that 52.3% of minor salivary gland tumors fall into a malignant classification.

A handicap in all but recent assessments of minor salivary gland tumors has been the use of the term *adenocarcinoma* in a generic sense and in apparent synonymity to designate tumors of rather wise histological appearance. These have included adenoid cystic carcinoma, mixed tumors, mucoepidermoid tumors and true adenocarcinomas. True adenocarcinomas are justifiably gaining acceptance and recent reports are separating this distinctive lesion from its equally distinctive cousin—adenoid cystic carcinoma. In terms of sheer numbers, tumors of the intraoral regions far exceed those of other anatomical regions of the head and neck. For this reason, I have elected to consider neoplasms of the upper respiratory tract and the oral cavity separately.

Nose and Paranasal Sinus

Malignant neoplasms of the mucosal lining of the nasal and paranasal cavities make up less than 1% of all malignancies and approximately 15% of all neoplasms of the upper respiratory tract.[6] In all reported series, squamous cell carcinomas are by far the most plentiful (80 to 90%). Tumors of minor salivary gland origin and other glandular neoplasms comprise between 4 and 8% of sinonasal malignancies.[7] In order of greatest incidence, the major types of mucous gland neoplasms are as follows: adenoid cystic carcinoma, adenocarcinoma, pleomorphic adenoma (mixed tumor), mucoepidermoid carcinoma and undifferentiated carcinoma. Acinous cell carcinoma, carcinoma ex

Table 2.1
Incidence of Malignant Minor Salivary Gland Tumors

Author	No. of Cases	Percent Malignant
Reynolds et al.[104]	49	69
Brown et al.[105]	38	63
Chaudhry et al.[60]	1,414	54
Smith[106]	38	37
Edwards[107]	23	31
Stuteville and Corley[71]	80	91
Bardwil et al.[4]	100	87
Shumrick[74]	54	93
Potdar and Paymaster[108]	110	50

Table 2.2
Adenoid Cystic Carcinoma. Anatomical Site in Head and Neck*

	Anatomical Site								
	Oropharynx				Nose and Sinuses	Naso-pharynx	Larynx	Trachea	Lacrimal Gland
	Palate	Mouth	Tongue	Tonsil					
Number of adenoid cystic carcinomas	210	106	124	34	113	48	22	11	20
Percent of all mucosal gland tumors at site	29	24	54	26	37	54	32	82	50

* After Osborn[8]

pleomorphic adenoma and true neoplasms of oncocytic type are unusual.

For practical purposes, all minor salivary gland neoplasms of the sinonasal tract, regardless of their histological composition, behave in an aggressive manner. Cohen and Batsakis[1] have commented on the locally infiltrative character of the usually benign-acting oncocytoma when it occurs in this region (Fig. 2.1). Masquerading as "polyps" with variable degrees of nasal obstruction, carcinomas of the minor salivary glands often are unrecognized until the disease is beyond control. The neoplasms have most aptly been likened to a "fire which smolders unnoticed within the walls of a house."[7] When clinical and pathological diagnosis (regardless of histological subtype) is finally made, the disease may be beyond control.

Adenoid Cystic Carcinoma. There is definite agreement that this carcinoma is the most common malignant derivative of minor salivary tissues (Fig. 2.2). In all major series the adenoid cystic carcinomas make up approximately 35% of all minor salivary gland carcinomas. Table 2.2, after Osborn[8] presents the anatomical distribution of 557 adenoid cystic carcinomas in the mucosal surfaces of the head and neck. Figure 2.3, based on combined cases from four other investigators, presents a similar distribution.[9–12]

Adenoid cystic carcinomas, except those associated with invasion of nerves, do not present distinctive clinical findings. Those carcinomas presenting in the antrum are associated with facial pain and swelling and the duration of these symptoms may range from months to several years. Nearly half of the patients will give a history of 1 year or more. Lesions involving the nasal cavity and nasopharynx have nasal obstruction, deafness and diplopia as common clinical findings—clear evidence of local extension.

The age range for adenoid cystic carcinomas is quite broad but there are peaks in the fourth and fifth decades. Males predominate.

There are no distinguishing gross features. The most important aspect is the difficulty in surgically demarcating the tumor because of its insidious infiltrative growth. Spiro et al.[10] report some degree of fixation or extension to contiguous structures in 39 of 49 patients having their primary lesions in the paranasal sinuses, nasal cavity and pharynx. In these sites, the neoplasm is rarely less than 2 cm when histological diagnosis is made.

For tumors in the paranasal sinuses, the radiographic findings consist of a soft-tissue mass, usually extending beyond the confines of the sinus, erosion and destruction of the wall of the sinus, and invasion of surrounding structures. For radiographic demonstration of perineural spread by the neoplasm, tomography is imperative.[13] Perineural spread is usually along the maxillary and mandib-

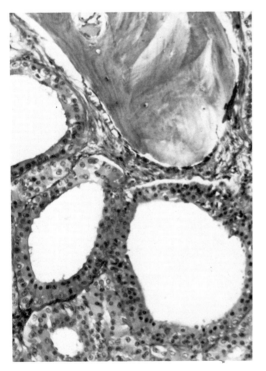

Figure 2.1 Oncocytoma of minor salivary gland invading wall of maxillary sinus.

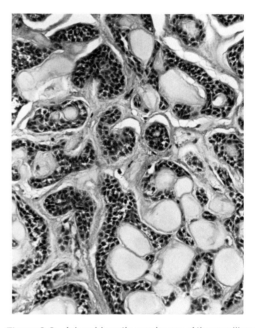

Figure 2.2. Adenoid cystic carcinoma of the maxillary sinus.

ADENOID CYSTIC CARCINOMA

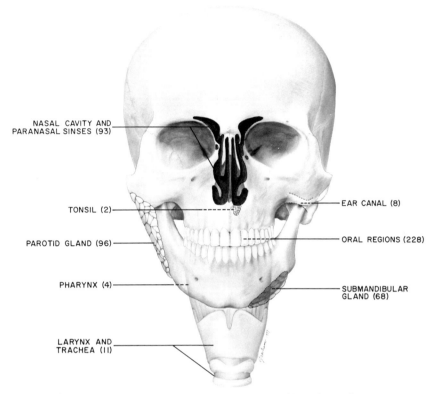

Figure 2.3. Distribution of head and neck adenoid cystic carcinomas.

ular divisions of the trigeminal nerve. The foramen ovale and foramen rotundum may be involved by extension of the neoplasm to the Gasserian ganglion.

The biological course of these carcinomas in the upper airway is one of relentless progression, local invasion, persistence of neoplasm after attempted surgical removal, and death. Spiro et al.[10] relate a 10-year determinate cure rate of only 7% for adenoid cystic carcinomas in the nasal cavity, antrum and larynx. This is to be compared to 29% for these carcinomas in the parotid gland, 23% for oral carcinomas and 10% for submandibular gland primaries.

Five-year follow-up periods are clearly inadequate and even 10-year survival data may not adequately convey the ultimate lethality of the adenoid cystic carcinomas since many of the survivors have persistent neoplasms.

Lymphogenous spread of adenoid cystic carcinomas of minor salivary gland origin, plays a relatively modest role, not unlike similar observations in major salivary gland adenoid cystic carcinomas.[8, 10] Spiro et al.[10] found 14% of their mucosal adenoid cystic carcinomas metastasized to regional lymph nodes, the lowest incidence of

lymphatic spread of all types of malignant tumor in their series. Conley and Dingman,[9] in their study of all head and neck adenoid cystic carcinomas, record a 16% metastatic spread to lymph nodes.

This low lymph node involvement contrasts sharply with a high blood-vascular dissemination. Systemic involvement is usually correlated with unequivocal evidence of uncontrolled disease at the primary site or in the neck. Spiro et al.[10] report a remote spread of the carcinoma in nearly 40% of 174 patients. These workers further note that adenoid cystic carcinomas accounted for 62% of distant metastases from all varieties of mucosal gland tumors. The lungs, bones and brain are the secondary foci of note and greatest incidence. Distant metastases are, however, accountable for but 10% of the deaths due to the neoplasm. Extensive local growth is the usual cause of death.

Adenocarcinoma. These neoplasms arise from both the surface epithelium and the minor salivary tissues. Batsakis et al.[14, 15] have pointed to the tendency of the adenocarcinoma to arise high in the nasal cavity and the ethmoid sinuses as compared to the adenoid cystic carcinoma. They have divided the adenocarcinomas into three basic clinicopathological forms: papillary, sessile and alveo-lar-mucoid. Included in this subclassification are those carcinomas that closely simulate colonic carcinomas. The latter are almost exclusively in the nasal cavity and are postulated to arise from nasal tissue possessing a common origin with that of the gastrointestinal tract.[16] Argentaffin cells may be present in the tumors. This carcinoma and very likely most of the adenocarcinomas arise from the pseudostratified columnar epithelium lining the airway. Others may be of seromucinous origin.

There are few benign papillary *neoplasms* in the upper respiratory tract; such lesions represent a focal papillary *hyperplasia* of mucosal or glandular elements or, as in the case of the cylindrial cell papilloma, a variant of nasal papilloma.

The papillary adenocarcinoma retains its cytological identity with the mucosal epithelium and may be mucinous or only sparsely so. It is of interest that the mucinous papillary adenocarcinoma is the form most often associated with woodworking.[17]

The sessile adenocarcinomas cover a broader expanse of the surface, retain little similarity to their cells of origin and manifest a worse prognosis than do the papillary, non-colonic-like type adenocarcinomas. The alveolar-mucoid variant shares this poorer prognosis. It may be polypoid or sessile. Its appearance has been likened to the colloid carcinomas of the breast or colon.

Figure 2.4 presents the anatomical localization of 95 adenocarcinomas of the nasal cavity, paranasal sinuses and nasopharynx as recorded in five series.[14, 16, 18–20] As with adenoid cystic carcinomas, there is a distinct male predominance and the neoplasms present most often in the fifth decade of life.

In the present decade, it has been pointed out that workers in the footwear repairing, wood and furniture industries have increased risks of developing nasal and paranasal adenocarcinomas.[21, 22]

In 1965, a clinical study suggested a relation between furniture making and nasal and paranasal adenocarcinomas in England.[23] This association has been confirmed by epidemiological studies in several areas of the world (Denmark, France, Belgium and Australia) as well as the United States.[24] Among furniture workers in England, the annual incidence for nasal and paranasal adenocarcinoma was 60/100,000, which approximates the rate for cancer of the bronchus in the general male population.

Brinton et al.[24] confirming earlier work[25] showed in their North Carolina study that a matched triplet analysis resulted in an odds ratio of 4.4 for employment as furniture workers and 1.5 for other woodworking occupations. The excess risk among furniture workers was apparent below and above age 65. Twenty-four of the 37 deaths from nasal cancer in their study were said to be due to max-

ADENOCARCINOMA

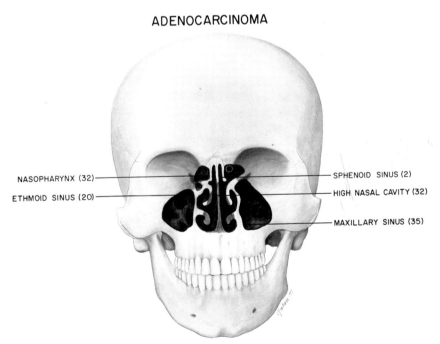

NASOPHARYNX (32)
ETHMOID SINUS (20)
SPHENOID SINUS (2)
HIGH NASAL CAVITY (32)
MAXILLARY SINUS (35)

Figure 2.4. Distribution of head and neck adenocarcinomas of minor salivary gland origin.

illary sinus primaries. Where the classification of the neoplasm was noted 4 of the 13 cases were adenocarcinoma.

Hadfield[22] is to be credited with the most comprehensive study of the relationship of adenocarcinoma of the paranasal sinuses and woodworkers in the furniture industry. He studied 92 cases (34 squamous cell carcinomas, 35 adenocarcinomas and 23 anaplastic carcinomas). For adenocarcinoma the male-to-female ratio was 10:1. In *all* 35 patients with adenocarcinoma the tumor appeared to originate in the ethmoid sinuses. In no patient with adenocarcinoma was there evidence of cervical lymph node metastases. Hematogenous spread was occasionally noted. Death was invariably due to intracranial extension of neoplasm. The carcinogen remains undetected.

The over-all biological behavior of adenocarcinoma is not unlike that of adenoid cystic carcinomas. Cervical lymph node metastases are variable. The data from the study by Spiro et al.[18] present the highest incidence of any series, 28%. Distant metastases, however, are far less than those recorded for adenoid cystic carcinoma.

Local uncontrolled growth accounts for the death of the patient. Again the 5-year survival estimates are not adequate for a considerable attrition occurs when observation periods are extended to 10 and 15 years. Papillary carcinomas

have little tendency to metastasize and the survival rate of this type of adenocarcinoma exceeds that of the other subtypes.

Depending on whether or not a papillary component dominates, the neoplasms vary from a soft, polypoid and friable granular mass to a poorly demarcated sessile tumor with a nodular gray surface that may be cystic, gelationous or hemorrhagic (Fig. 2.5).

The papillary carcinoma arises from the surface epithelium and retains cytological identification with this epithelium. Deviation from papillary hyperplasia, as seen in association with some forms of chronic sinusitis, is present in a higher mitotic index, nuclear and cytoplasmic pleomorphism and piling up of epithelium on papillae (Fig. 2.6). The papillae have less stroma than inflammatory papillation, and microinvasion may be found at the base. There is only a scant amount of mucicarminophilic material, and goblet cells are rare. In contrast to the other two forms, the papillary carcinoma is rather sharply localized with relatively normal sinus epithelium adjacent to the papillary process.

Sessile adenocarcinomas cover a broader expanse of surface and retain little similarity to either surface epithelium or glands. We consider *sessile* an appropriate designation, despite papillation, because of the gross configuration and because the

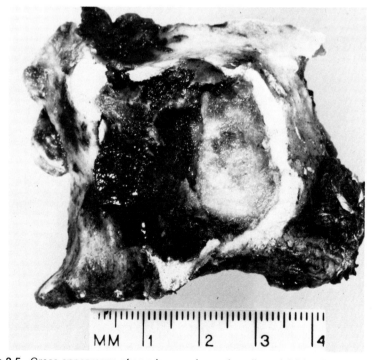

Figure 2.5. Gross appearance of an adenocarcinoma (sessile variety) involving the maxilla.

"papillae" here arise as a result of extension and confluence of ducts and through a crypt-like proliferation of the surface epithelium. There is a similarity to adenocarcinoma of the colon. The cells are nonciliated, columnar and have variable pseudostratification of nuclei. Nuclei are basally located and there is more hyperchromatism than in the papillary forms. Mucin and goblet cells, although greater in amount and number than in the papillary carcinoma, are not prominent. Necrosis, other than that from surface ulceration, is not conspicuous (Figure 2.7).

The mucoid adenocarcinoma, as the designation implies, is characterized by abundant mucus and usually retains little basic alveolar structure. Its localization within the lamina propria suggests origin from the seromucinous glands rather than from the surface epithelium. The neoplasm may be appropriately likened to the "colloid" carcinoma of the gastrointestinal tract and the breast and has little structural difference from these neoplasms. Goblet cells are plentiful, and extracellular mucin separates aggregates of carcinoma cells or interdigitates with the connective tissue stroma in the form of "mucoid" lakes. Signet ring cells may be present in the stroma or in medullary sheets (Fig. 2.8).

Of the three histological types, the papillary is least variable in morphology. Although there is some admixture of patterns in the sessile and alveolar mucoid variants, a dominant pattern prevails.

In patients with either adenoid cystic carcinoma or adenocarcinoma, death is due to uncontrolled and persistent disease at the primary site.[6, 26] It is ushered in by hemorrhage, infection, pansinusitis, meningitis and brain abscesses. The proximity of the ethmoid and sphenoid sinuses to the cranial

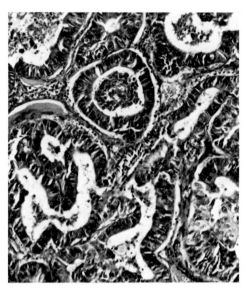

Figure 2.7. Sessile adenocarcinoma of the nose and paranasal sinuses.

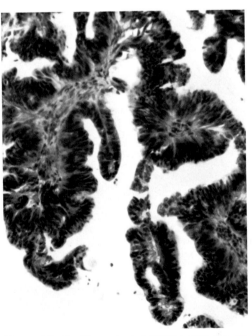

Figure 2.6. Papillary adenocarcinoma from the ethmoid sinus.

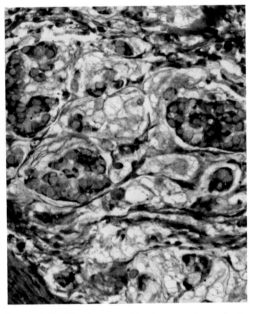

Figure 2.8. Alveolar-mucoid adenocarcinomas. The resemblence to so-called "colloid carcinomas" of the gastrointestinal tract and breast is striking.

cavity decrees to neoplasms of these sites a prognosis worse than that for neoplasms arising from the antrum or nasal cavity. These neoplasms are, at the most, only moderately radiosensitive, and their response to radiotherapy is one of incomplete regression. The extent of surgery required is debatable with some authors recommending a radical approach as the best chance for "cure." Rafla's[19] data indicate that perhaps the best results are obtained after a combined surgical and radiotherapeutic attack on the lesions.

My experience, combined with that of others, would indicate that regardless of the mode of treatment the over-all results are disappointing.[27]

A variety of factors influence survival of patients with neoplasms of the minor salivary glands. A major surgical ablation is the treatment of choice in potentially resectable primary and recurrent tumors.[18] Failure at this stage usually means incurability, but not necessarily failure at good palliation. For nearly all forms, irradiation will prove to be an effective and indispensable adjunct in the management of a majority of these patients.[28]

Other factors influencing survival have been selected by Spiro et al.[18] Their data suggest a more favorable outlook in women who are under 50 years of age. The effects of histological subtype are clearly seen in their statistics. Patients with carcinoma ex pleomorphic adenoma and anaplastic small cell carcinomas are seldom salvaged (11 to 17%). The outlook in subjects with adenoid cystic carcinomas and solid adenocarcinomas is somewhat better (20 to 30%), but this salvage falls off rapidly when surveillance is extended to 15 years. Within the adenocarcinoma group, survival is improved in patients who have papillary, papillocystic, or clear cell subtypes. Grading adenoid cystic carcinomas into high and low grades, however, is an academic exercise without a correlation to survival or response to treatment. Spiro et al.[18] record an over-all 10-year determinate cure rate for patients with mucoepidermoid carcinomas of 69.4% (range 78.6% to 50% in Grade I and Grade III carcinomas).

As expected the anatomical site of the primary lesion, bears heavily on survival. Forty-one percent of patients with minor salivary gland tumors in the oral cavity or oropharynx were salvaged in the Sloan-Kettering Memorial Cancer Center series.[18] Only 15.6% with patients with carcinomas of the sinuses or nasal cavity were salvaged. In patients whose primary lesion was 2 cm or less a survival of 55.6% was achieved. This dropped to 23% when the lesion exceeded 4 cm. Involvement of contiguous structures reduces the cure rate from 50% to 17% or less (Fig. 2.9).

Cervical node metastases seriously affect prognosis. They are particularly ominous if present at the first examination since less than 10% of such patients are salvaged. Spiro et al.[18] record a "cure" rate of 18.8% in patients who developed node involvement subsequent to initial treatment. This is to be compared to a 38.7% rate in patients who never manifested metastases to cervical lymph nodes. The carcinomas most likely to show metastasis to nodes are the poorly differentiated carcinomas, carcinoma ex pleomorphic adenoma and mucoepidermoid carcinomas. Distant metastases are seen in nearly all forms of minor salivary gland malignancy (Table 2.3) but occur most often in patients with adenoid cystic carcinoma (40%). Because of the possibility of additional survival following this event, Spiro et al.[18] recommend excision of the primary lesion whenever feasible, even if pulmonary metastases are present on admission. Additionally, I support resection of metastases, where feasible, if local control of the primary lesion has been achieved.

Based on determinate cases, the "cure" rate in the Sloan-Kettering Memorial Cancer Center series at 5, 10 and 15 years after treatment was 44.5, 32.6 and 21.4%, respectively.[18] This data is based on 311 patients having all forms of minor salivary gland malignancy.

Pleomorphic Adenoma. In contrast to its fre-

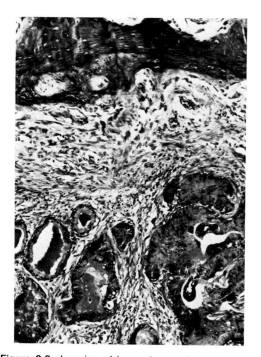

Figure 2.9. Invasion of bony sinus walls by adenocarcinoma.

Table 2.3
Carcinomas of Minor Salivary Glands: Distant Metastases*

	Total Patients	At Primary Treatment	After Primary Treatment	Percent with Metastases
Anatomical Site				
Oral cavity and oropharynx	292	13	67	27.4
Paranasal sinuses and nasal cavity	127	3	20	18.1
Larynx	15	3	5	46.7
Histological Classification				
Adenoid cystic	174	13	56	39.7
Mucoepidermoid	76	—	8	10.5
Adenocarcinoma				
Solid duct	106	2	15	16.0
Other	37	1	8	24.3
Carcinoma ex pleomorphic adenoma and malignant mixed tumor	13	—	1	7.7
Acinic cell	2	—	—	0.0
Oat cell	14	1	2	21.4
Colonic type	12	1	2	25.0
	434	18	92	25.3

* Modified from Spiro et al.[18]

quency in the major salivary glands, the mixed tumor (pleomorphic adenoma) is unusual in the upper respiratory tract. Judging from the scattered reports, the nasal cavity is the favored site of origin, followed distantly by the maxillary sinus and nasopharynx (Fig. 2.10).

Between 1949 and 1974, 40 cases in the nasal cavity were recorded in the Division of Otolaryngic Pathology of the Armed Forces Institute of Pathology (A.F.I.P.).[29] In the nasal cavity these lesions most often arise from the bony or cartilaginous parts of the nasal septum. One-fifth of cases arise from the lateral wall and usually involve a turbinate. Their initial lack of aggressiveness is indicated by an only infrequent extension into the adjacent sinuses.

Males and females are affected almost equally and the age of presentation is broad, 3 to 82 years. The chief complaints are nasal obstruction and less so, epistaxis. The patients usually seek medical attention within one year of the onset of these symptoms.

The size of the tumors are clinically deceptive in that they often are much larger than anticipated. In the A.F.I.P. series, the size of the tumors ranged from 0.7 to 7.0 cm.[29]

Typically the mixed tumor is a homogeneous, lobular mass, occasionally bosselated or cystic, but more often polypoid and translucent. Deviation from the usual gray-white appearance is most often due to hemorrhage.

Compagno and Wong[29] have pointed out that the intranasal mixed tumor differs from its counterparts in the major salivary glands by a greater cellularity. Epithelial elements rather than stromal elements predominate. At times the tumors may be composed almost entirely of epithelial cells with little or no stroma.

Local or total wide surgical excision usually excludes recurrences. In 31 of the 34 patients followed by Compagno and Wong[29] there were no recurrences. The distinctly uncommon myxoid stroma in intranasal mixed tumors has been cited as a histological reason for the low recurrence rate. In the 10% of patients experiencing recurrences, the lesion may extend into paranasal sinuses. It is to be noted that recurrence may be delayed so that it appears after the traditional 5-year period.

The monomorphic (basal cell) adenoma, while relatively frequent in the minor salivary glands of the oral cavity is an infrequent lesion of the upper airway. Here it may exist as such or present in a hybrid form, i.e., adenoid cystic carcinoma or, in evolution toward pleomorphic adenoma.

Carcinoma ex Pleomorphic Adenoma. Carcinoma ex pleomorphic adenoma arising from the mucous glands of the respiratory tract must be considered as unusual and hence considerably less than those arising in the oral cavity and major salivary glands. For the diagnosis there must be clear evidence of benign mixed tumor associated with a malignant, usually carcinomatous compo-

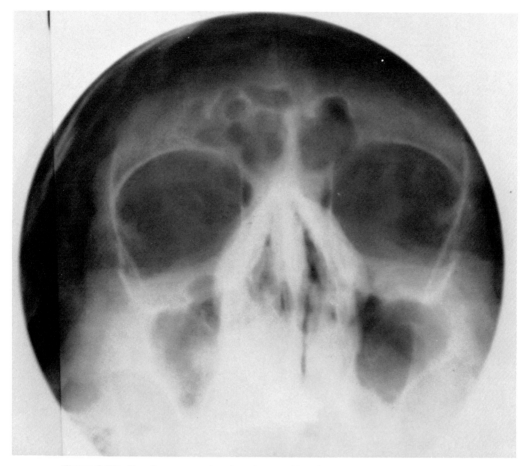

Figure 2.10. Roentgenogram showing pleomorphic adenoma (mixed tumor) of antrum.

nent. The maxillary antrum has been cited most often as the primary site in the upper airway. It appears to be more aggressive and lethal than either the adenoid cystic carcinoma or adenocarcinoma.[18]

Mucoepidermoid Carcinoma. Mucoepidermoid carcinomas rank third, behind adenoid cystic carcinomas and adenocarcinomas in their frequency in the respiratory tract. In the upper airway, they involve the antrum and nasal cavity most often but as it is with other mucous gland tumors, these neoplasms are not confined to a single group of air cells.

I ascribe to the histological grading of mucoepidermoid carcinomas into three arbitrary classes: low grade, intermediate grade and high grade. It is of interest, in this respect, that Foote and Frazell[30] placed none of their tumors of minor salivary gland origin in the low malignancy group.

The biological behavior of the intermediate-grade and high-grade mucoepidermoid carcinomas is like that of adenocarcinoma: recurrences, local extension and metastasis to lymph nodes and remote sites during the course of a prolonged illness.

Other Forms of Gland Cell Carcinoma. Acinous cell carcinoma, clear cell carcinoma, true oncocytomas, and anaplastic adenocarcinomas are all unusual in minor salivary glands and mucous glands. Each probably represent 0.5 to 1.0% of all mucous gland tumors.

Clear cell carcinomas are composed of relatively large cells with a clear cytoplasm which is negative for mucin stains (Fig. 2.11). They may or may not contain glycogen and may be papillary. All are locally infiltrative and very likely their biological behavior is akin to the intermediate-grade mucoepidermoid carcinoma.[31] It is to be noted here that "clear cells" may be present in varying degrees in other salivary gland neoplasms, particularly the acinous cell carcinomas and oncocytic lesions. Such cells are largely due to artefacts in the processing of tissue.

Lesions composed of oncocytes in the entire

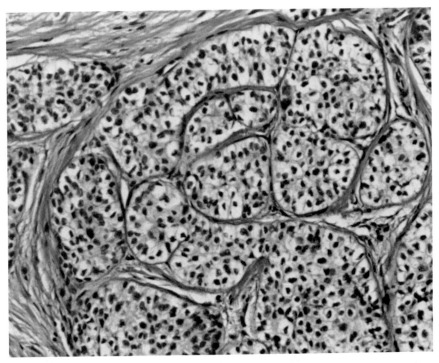

Figure 2.11. Clear cell carcinoma of minor salivary gland origin composed of nonmucin and nonglycogen containing duct cells.

upper respiratory tract are, with few exceptions, reactive or hyperplastic ones. Most are papillary or cystic in character. Solid, tumor-forming oncocytic lesions, oncocytomas, are rare in the airway and are the only oncocytic lesions warranting the designation of neoplasm.[1] The few examples reported have manifested an irregular, unencapsulated growth pattern and tend to invade locally. Very rarely a metastasis may occur.

The oncocyte, wherever it occurs, possesses the same histological and ultrastructural characteristics: acidophilic, granular cytoplasm and numerous, often tightly packed mitochondria.[32]

Undifferentiated adenocarcinomas or anaplastic forms of adenocarcinoma of the nasal cavity and paranasal sinuses are distinctly not common. Koss et al.[33] reported 14 examples of anaplastic, small cell carcinomas of the minor salivary glands and remarked on their histological similarity to oat cell carcinoma of the bronchus. Five of their cases were in the upper airway (nasal cavity, paranasal sinuses and epiglottis); the remainder were oral lesions.

All of the neoplasms were located beneath histologically normal surface epithelium whenever the latter was not ulcerated. Remnants of mucous salivary glands were identifiable in every one of the primary tumors.

The neoplasms are composed of elongated small cells with very scant cytoplasm and intensely hyperchromatic nuclei. The cells may be arrayed in sheets, in some instances having the general configuration of ducts; in other instances the cells infiltrate the stroma in a haphazard manner. Necrosis in the neoplasms is common. A hyaline stroma surrounding tumor cells may be prominent (Fig. 2.12). The cellular presentation is most often a monotonous one. Koss et al.[33] observed spindle and giant cell forms in one case and keratinization in another.

The anaplastic carcinomas manifest frequent cervical lymph node metastases (50% of Koss[33] series). Four of the 14 patients studied by Koss et al.[33] survived 5 years or longer.

Mucous Gland Tumors of the Larynx

Any form of malignant glandular neoplasm in the larynx must be considered unusual. Nearly all estimates place their frequency as less than 1% of all laryngeal cancer.[34–37] The neoplasms arise from the seromucinous glands and minor salivary tissue found in the mucosa. In the larynx, the greatest concentration of these structures is found in the false cords and just inferior to the anterior commissure. Lesser numbers are found in the aryepiglottic fold and the free portion of the glottis. The

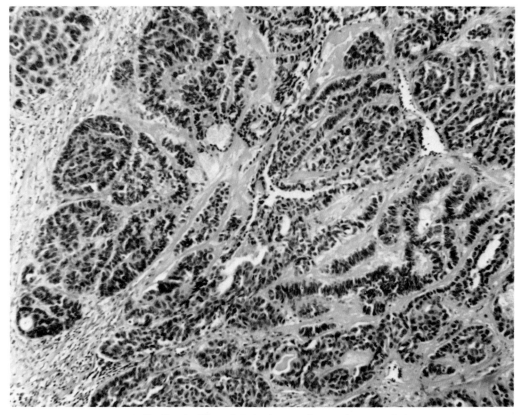

Figure 2.12. Poorly differentiated adenocarcinoma of paranasal sinus.

squamous lined portion of the vocal cord is said to be normally devoid of glands.

With minor exception, glandular neoplasms of the larynx are histologically indistinguishable from their counterparts in the major salivary glands and minor salivary tissues of the oral cavity and paranasal sinuses. Adenoid cystic carcinomas and adenocarcinomas comprise most of the histologic types.[38] Adenoid cystic carcinoma is the most common. Less commonly encountered are mucoepidermoid carcinomas, oncocytic carcinomas, mixed tumors and metastatic adenocarcinomas.

The age range of presentation of the neoplasms is wide but laryngeal adenoid cystic carcinomas have been primarily seen in patients in their sixth decade of life.[36, 38] Most of the adenocarcinomas have occurred in patients beyond the age of 60 years. There appears to be a conspicuous male predominance in adenocarcinomas of the larynx as opposed to a nearly equal sex involvement of adenoid cystic carcinomas.

Adenocarcinomas, in contrast to adenoid cystic carcinomas, are rarely subglottic. Supraglottic and transglottic involvement are about equal. Adenoid cystic carcinomas involve the supra- and subglottic

regions[37, 38] with approximately two-thirds of cases in subglottic structures.

Signs and symptoms are not unique to the glandular tumors. Neoplasms arising in the subglottis, regardless of histological type, usually are advanced when diagnosed and present with airway obstruction. Neoplasms in the supraglottic area tend to present later in the course of the disease, but are usually associated with sore throat, huskiness of voice and dysphagia. Pain is often a prominent symptom in adenoid cystic carcinomas, and may be attributed to their propensity to spread along nerves.

In gross configuration, adenocarcinomas usually form large, nonulcerated masses (Fig. 2.13). Adenoid cystic carcinomas manifest a lesser tendency to this large size.

Adenocarcinoma in situ has been described by Ferlito[38] among others. It is rarely observed and probably of multicentric origin.

Both adenoid cystic carcinomas and adenocarcinomas of the larynx are lethal diseases, with a subjective impression that adenocarcinoma is a more rapid killer. Almost all patients with adenocarcinomas are dead within 2 years of diagnosis.[36]

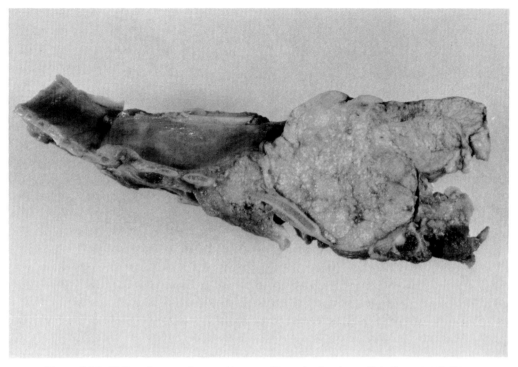

Figure 2.13. Bulky adenocarcinoma of larynx with predominant growth in the supraglottis.

Widespread pulmonary and hepatic metastases are related to the outcome. Approximately one-third of the patients with adenoid cystic carcinomas eventually manifest pulmonary metastases.[37] The clinical course is, however, more torpid with local recurrences and regional lymph node involvement. Follow-up of 3 or 5 years is inadequate. Recurrences are frequently delayed until 3 or 5 years, and there is an inverse proportion between survivors and nonsurvivors at 5-, 10- and 15-year intervals.[39] Primary radical surgery for adenocarcinomas and adenoid cystic carcinomas in no way appears to decrease recurrence rate or prolong survival.

Considerably less frequent carcinomas are the adenosquamous carcinoma (mixed adenosquamous), clear cell carcinoma, giant cell carcinoma (anaplastic giant cell adenocarcinoma), acinous cell carcinoma, mucoepidermoid carcinoma, carcinoma ex pleomorphic adenoma, anaplastic carcinoma (oat cell) and carcinosarcoma.[40–44]

The adenosquamous carcinoma is an admixture of adenocarcinoma with squamous cell carcinoma. Mingled in this pattern are areas of undifferentiated carcinoma (so-called "basaloid" carcinoma). The tumor seems to originate from glandular and ductal epithelium, regardless of whether they are squamous, basaloid or undifferentiated type and are arranged so as to form tubular, alveolar or ductal configurations.

A characteristic, albeit not constant finding, is the presence of large nests and solid masses composed of "glassy" cells bounded by fibrous tissue. Their cytoplasm is clear and periodic acid-Schiff (PAS)-negative. The surface epithelium may appear intact or neoplastic, but infiltration always originates from glandular epithelia.[40] This lesion appears distinct from mucoepidermoid carcinomas.

The clear cell carcinoma is extremely rare in the larynx. It shows the same morphological features as the clear cell carcinoma of the lung and major and minor salivary glands.

Giant cell carcinomas are also exceptional in the larynx.[42] This tumor is composed of numerous pleomorphic multinucleated giant cells, often with starry acidophilic and vacuolated cytoplasm supported by a delicate fibrovascular stroma. The tumor cells may resemble pleomorphic sarcomatous giant cells. Numerous atypical mitoses can be found. The cells may be isolated, in clusters, or around alveolar-like spaces. PAS-positive granules are present in the cytoplasm of some cells and some appear phagocytic. Necrosis and hemorrhage are inconspicuous. The relationship of the giant cell adenocarcinoma to other malignant giant cell tumors of the larynx is unclear.

Acinous cell carcinomas are nearly exclusively neoplasms of the major salivary glands and this relates to their extreme rarity in the larynx. Ferlito cites but two cases.[38]

Mucoepidermoid carcinomas have a predilection for the supraglottic larynx. Fechner[36] records nine possible examples from the literature.

A few acceptable cases of carcinoma ex pleomorphic adenoma of the larynx have been reported.[38] All exhibited an accelerated malignancy.

Undifferentiated and anaplastic small cell carcinomas are uncommon but by no means rare lesions in the larynx. The undifferentiated carcinoma is usually a surface lesion and possesses a basaloid appearance. The neoplasm is a highly malignant lesion. At this point it is pertinent to point out that basaloid variants of the adenoid cystic carcinoma may simulate this neoplasm and that there is a decided tendency for adenocarcinomas of the larynx to be poorly differentiated (Fig. 2.14).

Carcinosarcoma is perhaps the most rare of laryngeal neoplasms, if it exists at all. I agree with Ferlito[38] in considering almost all reported cases as collision tumors.

Metastases of glandular neoplasms must always be considered in the differential diagnosis of these tumors. On rare occasions, the laryngeal symptoms due to metastasis have been the presenting complaint. Renal cell carcinoma has been the most frequent secondary adenocarcinoma of the larynx, followed by melanoma, and primary lesions in breast, lung, prostrate gland and gastrointestinal tract. Levine and Applebaum,[45] in a recent review, record 38 cases. The lesions were evenly distributed in glottis, supraglottis and subglottis.

Benign, true neoplasms of the glandular elements of the larynx are even more unusual than the malignant variants; at least as attested by the literature.[46] The majority of pleomorphic adenomas occur in the subglottic region. The single acceptable case from the epiglottis was reported by Cotelingham et al.[46]

The vast majority of oncocytic lesions of the larynx, in our experience, are benign hyperplasias and not true neoplasms.[47-49] Nearly all of the clinically significant lesions have been cystic and correspond to their smaller counterparts seen at necropsy. The ventricle and false cord are the sites of predilection. In most instances the oncocytic cysts are retention cysts, formed by ectactic excretory ducts. The reported mean age of patients with oncocytic cysts of the larynx has been 64 years

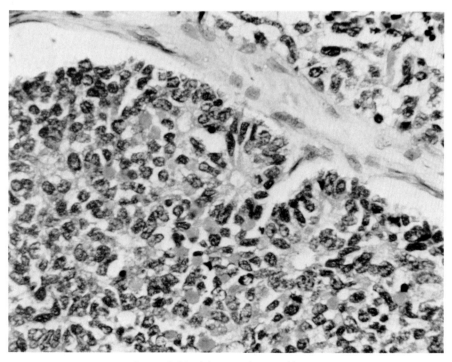

Figure 2.14. Adenocarcinoma of larynx.

with an age range of 48 to 88 years. This is analogous to the oncocytic tumors of major salivary tissue. There is a slight female predominance. On occasion there may be an intense inflammatory reaction about the cyst. This has misled authors into considering them as Warthin's tumors. This is inaccurate and very likely Warthin's tumor is a lesion restricted to the parotid gland. No unqualified example of a malignant oncocytic lesion in the larynx has been recorded.[49]

Despite the fact the larynx and lungs share a common embrological origin from primitive foregut, oat cell carcinomas are rarely described as arising in the larynx. Kyriakos et al.[50] could find only four cases in the literature and added three personal examples. Since not all tumors with the histological pattern and cytological characteristics of an oat cell carcinoma are of neuroectodermal derivation, the diagnostic term should be reserved for those lesions demonstrating ultrastructural evidence of neurosecretory granules. The prognosis of patients with laryngeal oat cell carcinomas is as grim as that for patients with pulmonary oat cell malignancies.

Trachea

Primary malignant disease of the trachea is infrequent, but probably not as rare as the literature supports. Gilbert et al.[51] reviewed 546 cases of primary tracheal *tumors* in adults and children. Five hundred and nine were in adults, and 49.1% of these were malignant. Of the malignant neoplasms, 79% were carcinomas. Salm[52] indicates that approximately 40 new cases are added to the literature each decade.

In terms of general incidence, one tracheal carcinoma occurs for every 180 bronchogenic or 75 laryngeal carcinomas. To date over 400 cases of primary carcinoma of trachea have been reported, and of these squamous cell carcinomas account for nearly 50% of the total.[53] There is an apparent correlation of tracheal squamous cell carcinoma and smoking. No such relationship exists for the malignant glandular neoplasms.

Of the glandular and minor salivary gland tumors, the adenoid cystic carcinoma dominates the statistics, exceeding adenocarcinomas by a ratio of almost 2:1. Adenoid cystic carcinomas make up from 20 to 35% of all primary tracheal malignancies. Other forms, such as the mixed tumor and mucoepidermoid tumor, are rarely identified in the trachea. There is no sex dominance, and the age peak is similar to that observed for carcinoma of the larynx and nasal sinuses. Malignant epithelial neoplasms in children are, however, very unusual.

There does not seem to be any significant difference in ultimate prognosis between squamous cell and glandular carcinomas. This is due to the insidious nature of tracheal neoplasms which may remain silent for long periods of time. Hoarseness, dyspnea and cough, in that order, are the principal complaints.[54]

X-ray examinations, while of value in determining the location and extent of the neoplasm, are of no great value in detection. Cytological examination is also not helpful in the early discovery of glandular malignancy. This is in contrast to a reported 75% positive rate for squamous cell carcinomas of that structure. Endoscopic examination and biopsy remain the one most reliable means of establishing the diagnosis.

Adenoid cystic carcinomas and adenocarcinomas appear to have a predilection for the upper one-third of the trachea in contrast to a distal localization for other epithelial neoplasms. Over 60% are on the posterior or lateral wall. Size, location and duration play a more important role in prognosis than does histological type. Adenocarcinomas are the most bulky, and at the same time, manifest deep penetration into the tracheal wall and adjacent mediastinum. Patients with neoplasms at the cervical end of the trachea have a better survival because these lesions are usually more amenable to radical resection.

Of the two more common tracheal tumors (squamous cell and adenoid cystic carcinoma), extension beyond the trachea occurs three times more frequently with the adenoid cystic carcinoma (58%) than with squamous cell carcinoma. Nevertheless, because of the duration of the lesion before diagnosis, all three types are characterized by extensive local invasion. If there is a tendency to intraluminal polypoid configuration among the three neoplasms, it is manifested most often by adenoid cystic carcinoma. Regardless of histological type, the patient with a small lesion has a better chance of 5-year survival.

Briefly, primary epithelial malignancy of the trachea can be said usually to follow an insidious course. It almost always recurs and is capable of producing both local and distant metastases. The neoplasms, particularly those of glandular derivation kill by local extension and involvement of vital structures, often over a period of many years. The deadliest of all three are the adenocarcinomas, which rapidly cause death after diagnosis. In terms of general survival (with recurrences), the adenoid cystic carcinoma is a poor leader. Squamous cell carcinomas are intermediate.

No primary carcinoma of the trachea can be said to offer a good prognosis. McCafferty et al.[55]

found only 51 of 392 patients (13%) survived to 3 years. Most patients with adenocarcinomas are dead within 6 months of diagnosis. Adenoid cystic carcinomas manifest a more protracted course, marred by recurrences, local invasion and metastases to lymph nodes. The predisposition to perineural invasion is obvious in this region also.

All three, squamous cell carcinomas, adenoid cystic carcinomas and adenocarcinomas, share the ability to metastasize locally to regional lymph nodes and to distant sites (lungs, liver, bone) via hematogenous routes. Death is due to uncontrolled local disease. Adenoid cystic carcinomas may delay their lethality for some time. Hadju et al.[53] found that three of their seven patients died of their disease 1, 12 and 13 years after diagnosis.

Radiotherapy is an effective form of treatment in only a small proportion of cases, the mainstay, if indeed there is such, being surgical removal. Endoscopic removal, while effecting significant periods of remission for adenoid cystic carcinomas, is usually associated with late local recurrences and a protracted, incapacitating terminal illness. For the unlikely localized lesions, sleeve resection and an end-to-end anastomosis are recommended.[55] Unfortunately, local extension and bulk often contradict this approach. Irradiation is probably not helpful in the palliation of any form of tracheal carcinoma, and there is always the risk of inducing tracheomediastinal fistulae.[56]

A final caution concerning tracheal carcinomas: patients (20%) may manifest synchronous or metachronous occurrences of a second carcinoma.

Intraoral Salivary Gland Tumors

All reports indicate a common pattern for sites of predilection of intraoral minor salivary gland tumors. The most common site for either benign or malignant neoplasms is the palate. This single site includes more than 50% of all tumors. Frable and Elzay[3] found that this held true for both benign and malignant variants in a review of 955 cases. This frequency coincides with the number of independent glandular aggregates found: 250 in the hard palate, 100 in the soft palate and 12 in the uvula.[57, 58] Tumors of the salivary glands of the palate occur almost as frequently as squamous cell carcinomas. Benign tumors have a particular affinity for the soft palate and the posterior one-third of the hard palate.

For involvement by benign tumors, the palate is followed by the upper lip and the buccal mucosa. The tongue, however, far exceeds the upper lip as the second most common site of primary malignant minor salivary gland tumors. The lower lip and the base of the tongue are unusual sites of

origin for benign mixed tumors.[59] The lower alveolus is more often affected than the upper alveolus. Tumors presenting in the cheek are more often benign than malignant.

A peculiarity of tumors of the minor salivary glands is that they practically never arise exactly in the midline, being found to one or the other side of the midline. This distribution is due to the distribution and arrangement of the minor salivary tissues of the palate.[58] Organized in an orderly manner and packed into irregular spaces created by dense fibrous bands in the submucosa, the minor salivary glands seldom extend anterior to a line drawn between the first molars. Anterior to this line, the spaces are filled with fibroadipose tissue. The glands also do not occur either in the midline of the hard palate or in the gingiva laterally. Both benign and malignant lesions characteristically occur as asymptomatic swellings that have been present for many months before diagnosis. Pain is inconstant and ulceration is unusual, even with malignant forms. If it is present, it is small in comparison with the total bulk of the tumor. This is in contrast to squamous cell carcinomas of the oral regions where ulceration is practically always a feature. Except for those presenting on the hard palate, the tumors are usually mobile.

Only reasonably accurate estimations of the frequency of the various histological types can be made. Of 1,320 tumors reviewed by Chaudhry et al.,[60] 800 were benign and 520 were malignant (this included all mucoepidermoid carcinomas). Benign mixed tumors were the most common, constituting nearly 56% of all intraoral minor salivary gland tumors. In the same series, adenoid cystic carcinomas were the most frequent malignant tumor, but they made up only 16% of all intraoral tumors. Other authors, reporting smaller series, place the incidence of the adenoid cystic carcinoma considerably higher. Of 1,106 cases of intraoral minor salivary gland tumors reported from 1945 to 1960, 10% were mucoepidermoid carcinomas.[60] Adenocarcinomas, adenopapillary lesions and adenomas are less often seen, and squamous cell carcinomas of the minor salivary glands and Warthin's tumor are rarely seen.[61] The distinctive acinous cell carcinoma is very rare in the minor salivary glands.

Salivary gland adenomas (pleomorphic and monomorphic) in the oral cavity are said to manifest a low recurrence rate. For both tumors, however, a lack of encapsulation is a common feature. This is not to be considered as a histological sign of malignancy. Because of the absence of a well-defined fibrous capsule, a risk of recurrence after surgical removal is enhanced. The frequency of local recurrence of both forms of adenoma, however, is surprisingly low. In a report from the Karolinska Sjukhuset, a series of 88 patients with palatal adenomas, there were only seven recurrences, equally distributed between pleomorphic and monomorphic adenomas.[62] As has been pointed out earlier (Chapter 1), the cellularity of the tumor does not correlate with incidence of recurrence. This observation is in agreement with the DNA values found in the nuclei of monomorphic adenomas. Eneroth and Zetterberg[63] have found that the DNA values (cytophotometric) of nuclei of these adenomas were identical with normal control cells. Highly differentiated mucoepidermoid carcinomas of the oral cavity, on the other hand, exhibit higher values which are comparable with those of malignant cells. Management of the intraoral adenomas is discussed by Worthington[64] ad Coates et al.[58] Radiological aspects are presented by Pinto et al.[65]

The relative incidence of mucoepidermoid carcinomas in the intraoral regions (10%) is higher than that reported for the major salivary glands (5%).[60, 61] Approximately 40% occur in the palate, more than 20% in the jaws (chiefly in the retromolar and tuberosity regions) and 20% in the floor of the mouth. The low-grade variety usually has signs and symptoms similar to benign mixed tumors, whereas the high-grade mucoepidermoid carcinomas behave not unlike squamous cell carcinomas that arise in the oral cavity.

On the basis of follow-up studies, low-grade mucoepidermoid carcinomas may be adequately treated by local excision without adverse results, particularly recurrences. High-grade carcinomas require radical surgery because of their high recurrence rate (20 to 50%) and the propensity for regional lymph node metastases.

Like their counterparts in the upper respiratory tract, *adenocarcinomas* have a sinister and lethal behavior. The incidence of adenocarcinoma in the mouth is difficult to establish, but recent reports point to a rate as high as 25%.[61] The palate, buccal mucosa, tongue, floor of mouth and the lips, in that order, are sites of predilection. Of lingual tumors, 21% are adenocarcinomas.[66]

The histological subclassification proposed by Batsakis et al.[6, 14] has some bearing on the prognosis (vide supra), with the papillary form less aggressive but nevertheless as prone to recurrence as the other histological variants.[67] Recurrences are the hallmark of this neoplasm and occur so often that, of all intraoral minor salivary gland tumors, "it offers the poorest prognosis, irrespec-

tive of the mode of treatment."[60] Ranger et al.[2] arrived at a similar conclusion after a study of 80 mucous gland tumors. Others report a less pessimistic appraisal. The variability of therapeutic results is due to: (1) misdiagnosis or misclassification; and (2) lack of aggressiveness or thoroughness during the primary attack on the lesion. Fifteen of 17 patients with intraoral adenocarcinomas reported by Chaudhry et al.[60] manifested one or more recurrences and four patients died of lymph node or pulmonary metastases.

In the lip the most common salivary gland tumors are benign: mixed tumor and monomorphic adenoma. Malignant salivary gland tumors of this site are rare. Adenoid cystic carcinomas and adenocarcinomas are the two malignant subtypes most often encountered.[68, 69] Table 2.4 presents the frequency of adenocarcinoma of the lip.

The prognostic outcome for patients with adenoid cystic carcinoma is somewhat better than for adenocarcinoma, with occasional reports indicating as high as 58% 5-year survival.[71] A near 30% 3-year survival and 10% 5-year survival is more nearly the consensus of most workers.[73] Shumrick[74] states the case succinctly in saying that the tumor "may give a respectable 3-year survival but drops sharply at 5 years and is disastrous at 6 to 8 years."

Recurrence rates are as high as for adenocarcinomas (50 to 60%), and this fact coupled with the tumor's locally destructive action and proneness to follow the routes of cranial nerves, does not lead to a happy outlook for the patient. Local excision is almost invariably associated with recurrences. Approximately 30% manifest distant metastases, primarily to the lungs (90%).[74] The role of radiotherapy is controversial and probably, at this time, best used only as an adjunct to primary surgical excision.[71]

Necrotizing Sialometaplasia. This benign lesion

Table 2.4
Adenocarcinoma of the Lips

Author	Total No. Minor Salivary Gland Tumors	Total No. Adenocarcinomas	No. in Lips
Chaudhry et al.[60]	94	17	2
Epker and Henny[61]	90	16	1
Soskolne et al.[72]	64	7	1
Crocker et al.[70]	38	1	0
Stuteville and Corley[71]	80	2	0
Frable and Elzay[3]	73	1	0

of salivary tissue occurs in two manners of presentation: (1) a spontaneous and often startling mucosal ulcer of the palate and (2) as a reaction to injury (usually iatrogenic) in minor salivary tissue of the oral cavity, nasal cavity and larynx, and the major salivary glands.[75-77]

The importance of this reparative process lies in two areas: the lesion is unfamiliar to the general surgical pathologist, and it may be mistaken by the uninformed for a squamous cell carcinoma or mucoepidermoid carcinoma.

Most of the reports in the literature have dealt with the lesion as it presents as an ulcer of the hard palate and surrounding tissues. The lesion in this site occurs predominantly in men with an observed age range of 23 to 66 years. The cause of the process is unknown and the disorder is self-healing (Fig. 2.15).

Abrams et al.[75] were the first to describe the microscopic appearance of necrotizing sialometaplasia. It includes: mucosal ulceration of the palate with pseudoepitheliomatous hyperplasia; ischemic lobular necrosis of the salivary glands; dissolution of acinar walls and release of mucous with a subsequent inflammatory and granulation tissue response; extensive squamous metaplasia of salivary acini and ducts, found almost invariably in multiple lobules; and a relatively intact salivary

lobular architecture despite extensive necrosis and inflammation (Figs. 2.16 and 2.17).

The lesion in the salivary tissues appears to be a unique response to injury. The degree of squamous metaplasia may be pronounced and the lobular infarct-like necrosis is a histopathological feature apparently unique to this lesion.

A definite diagnosis of the palate lesion is established only by microscopic examination of the lesion. Confirming the diagnosis eliminates the need for unnecessary surgery since *all* of the re-

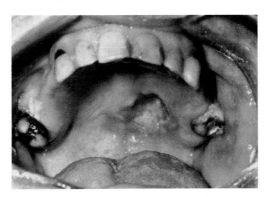

Figure 2.15. Intraoral appearance of necrotizing sialometaplasia of the palate. (Contributed by E. N. Myers, M.D.)

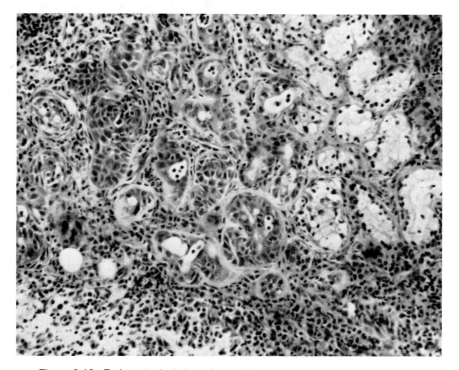

Figure 2.16. Early metaplasia in an intraoral area of necrotizing sialometaplasia.

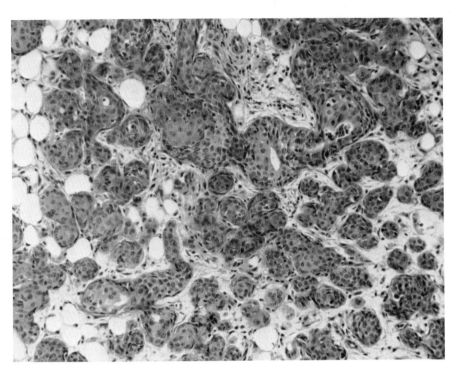

Figure 2.17. Late necrotizing sialometaplasia of palate.

ported patients have healed completely regardless of the mode of therapy: complete excision, incomplete excision, or no surgical treatment.

In the minor salivary tissues of the upper airway and larynx and in the major salivary glands, the lesion appears as the consequence of focal lobular sialadenitis or in specimens removed after prior surgical intervention. Thackray and Lucas[78] term the process in major salivary glands a "lobular regeneration." Except for the ulceration, so prominent in the palate lesions, the histological architecture and cytological changes are exactly those described in the palate.

SUBMANDIBULAR GLAND

The submandibular gland occupies most of the submandibular triangle and extends over the anterior and posterior bellies of the digastric muscles. Superiorly, the gland courses along its duct above the mylohyoid muscle where it relates to the posterior one-third of the tongue. The level of the hyoid bone is reached by the inferior aspect of the gland. The deep portion of the submandibular gland, which lies along its duct, is in direct relation to the sublingual gland. Only the sphenomandibular and stylomandibular ligaments separate the parotid gland from the posterior border of the submandibular gland.

There are two routes of lymphatic drainage. The most constant route ends in the jugulodigastric and upper deep cervical nodes after draining the posterior portion of the gland. The other route has efferents draining mainly the surface and lateral aspects of the gland and ending in the upper cervical and jugulodigastric nodes; many also go to the middle cervical nodes.

Only about 10% of all salivary gland neoplasms occur in the submandibular gland, but compared to the parotid gland, a considerably larger percentage are malignant. This observation holds even more abundantly true for the sublingual gland and minor salivary gland tumors.

Apart from benign mixed tumors and inflammatory lesions, other benign neoplasms of the submandibular gland are rare. It is estimated that approximately 40% of all tumors of the submandibular gland are benign mixed tumors. Eneroth and Hjertman,[79] after a study of 187 patients with submandibular gland tumors, treated between 1909 and 1965, classified 95 as benign mixed tumors. They occurred nearly four times as often as benign inflammatory tumors. Female patients exceed males by a ratio of 2:1.

Because there is a relative absence of pain and rather minor cosmetic disturbances, the preoperative duration of benign mixed tumors of the gland is relatively long—5 or more years in nearly one-half of the patients presented in various series. Malignancy in a mixed tumor (based on local destructive infiltration) of the submandibular gland is very unusual. Only 3 of 98 mixed tumors qualified in the series reported by Eneroth and Hjertsman.[79]

The importance of local accessibility and complete primary excision of any salivary gland tumors is amply in evidence in the statistics concerning benign mixed tumors of the submandibular gland. Less than 5.5% recur, and these are invariably in those patients who have had an apparently inadequate primary resection and present with a persistence of the tumor.[79] The usual treatment of a benign mixed tumor in this region is total excision of the gland. The operative field is devoid of a major nerve, but care must be exercised to avoid the cervical branch of the facial nerve.[80, 81]

Of 230 submandibular tumors studied by Rafla,[81] 116 were malignant. Hanna and Clairmont[82] reviewed reports entailing 632 submandibular salivary gland tumors. The benign versus malignant ratio was nearly equal: 52% benign and 48% malignant tumors. Table 2.5 presents a comparison of the frequency of the different types of salivary gland malignancy affecting the submandibular gland.

The percentage of lesions that manifest involvement of nerves is less than that expressed for parotid gland malignancies; 11 versus 18%. This is to be expected because of the more intimate relationship of the parotid gland to the facial nerve. Few patients manifest motor nerve paralysis, and this is probably attributable to the deeper location of the hypoglossal nerve in the submandibular triangle.

Anatomical relations of the gland also influence local spread of the malignant neoplasms, viz., invasion of the parapharyngeal space and related structures, the posterior one-third of the tongue and the anterior faucial pillars. Involvement of the soft palate and the palatal arches is also more common than seen with parotid gland malignancies. There is a particularly high rate of local recurrence in the submandibular area with adenoid cystic carcinomas. Extension along the lingual, alveolar, and hypoglossal nerves and invasion of the mandible are held accountable.

The above features and the relatively long interval before patients seek treatment accounts in considerable measure, for the rather disappointing results of treatment for malignancies of the submandibular gland. Adenoid cystic carcinomas in this location behave aggressively and manifest the same clinical course as they do in other salivary glands. Eight of 12 patients studied by Rafla[81] died with disease within 5 years, and 10 of 18 suffered from recurrent disease. Only one of 18 patients was alive and without disease at a 5-year follow-up.

Most of the mucoepidermoid carcinomas behave more aggressively and have a much lower survival rate than their counterparts in the parotid gland. Conley et al.[83] found that a significant number of the histologically low-grade mucoepidermoid carcinomas in the submandibular gland were ultimately fatal.

Accelerated death rates are seen with the other varieties of salivary gland malignancy.

Contemporary surgical thinking is toward more radical excision.[84] It seems reasonable to expect an improvement in results if en bloc or composite resections are performed in patients with less advanced disease. Intensive postoperative irradiation in selected cases is also warranted.

The submandibular gland as a site of a metastasis from a distant primary is a surgical curiosity.[85] This is considered to be due to an absence of intraglandular lymph nodes in contrast to the rich, intraglandular lymph node containing parotid glands. Involvement of contiguity from extensive primary lesions or metastases to the submandibular lymph nodes is regularly observed.

SUBLINGUAL GLANDS

Smallest of the major salivary glands, the sublingual glands are in close relationship to the duct

Table 2.5
Submandibular Gland Malignancy

Author	Benign	Malignant	Adenoid Cystic Carcinoma	Mucoepidermoid Carcinoma	Adenocarcinoma	Undifferentiated Carcinoma	Carcinoma ex pleomorphic Adenoma
Eneroth et al.[86] (157 cases)	95 (60%)	62 (40%)	25 (40%)	6 (10%)	0	15 (24%)	3 (5%)
Conley et al.[83] (115 cases)	61 (53%)	54 (47%)	17 (31%)	17 (31%)	8 (15%)	4 (7%)	4 (7%)
Spiro et al.[84] (217 cases)	96 (44%)	121 (56%)	42 (35%)	23 (19%)	14 (12%)	3 (2%)	23 (19%)

of the submandibular gland, lingual vessels and nerve, the hypoglossal nerve and the mucous membrane of the floor of the mouth. Secretions reach the floor of the mouth via 20 or more small excretory ducts.

The jugulodigastric and mid-deep jugular nodes are the major lymph nodes draining the gland area. Drainage from the anterior portion of the gland passes to the submandibular lymph nodes and intraglandular nodes and then to the mid-deep jugular node. These nodes are also in the course of drainage from the lip, floor of mouth and a portion of the tongue.

The importance of recognizing primary salivary gland tumors of this gland is that there is a striking predominance of malignant types. A review to 1969 indicates that only 46 examples of primary neoplasia of the sublingual gland have been reported.[87] Of these, 37 have been classified as malignant. Depending on the series, the total incidence of malignancy stands in contrast to that observed in the ⋅ other two major salivary glands—34% for the parotid gland and 50% in the submandibular gland.

There is a constancy in clinical presentation. All patients present with a mass under the tongue causing some discomfort. As with all tumors of the minor or lesser major salivary glands, there is delay (at least several months) between the onset of symptoms and the initial medical observation. This delay, however, is never as long as for the tumors of the minor salivary glands and partly accounts for the better prognosis manifested by patients with sublingual malignancies. Certainly an additional factor is the management by total excision of the gland, avoiding biopsy or local partial excision. The experience at the Columbia-Presbyterian Medical Center (New York City) is representative of this principle of primary management.[87] Since total gland excision was instituted in 1956, there have been no instances of local recurrence and only one instance of cervical lymph node metastasis.[87]

Adenoid cystic carcinomas and mucoepidermoid carcinomas are the types of neoplasms most often encountered, each representing approximately 40% of the lesions. Contrast with the parotid gland and submandibular gland is again noteworthy. Foote and Frazell[88] report only a 6% incidence of adenoid cystic carcinoma in the parotid and a 23% incidence in the submandibular. This re-emphasizes the apparent truth that the smaller the salivary gland the higher the incidence of adenoid cystic carcinoma.

ABERRANT SALIVARY GLAND TISSUE AND TUMORS

Aberrant salivary tissue is usually discovered by chance during surgical procedures for other lesions. Only rarely do neoplasms arise from these aberrant foci.

Since the foregut is abundantly supplied with a submucosal lymphoid component, it is not unusual to find aberrant tissue within the lymph nodes of the head and neck. Up to 1% of tonsils are said to contain ectopic salivary gland tissue. The body of the mandible, lower neck, hypopharynx, middle ear, sternoclavicular joint and along the thyroglossal duct are other noteworthy sites. Pesavento and Ferlito[89] updated earlier reviews in 1976. Salivary gland ectopias in the pituitary gland are quite common and may be readily found if sections of the pituitary are adequate in number. Schochet et al.[90] consider it probable that some pituitary tumors manifesting oncocytes are derived from these salivary nests.

Youngs and Scofield[91] have presented cogent reasons for concluding that heterotopic salivary gland tissue in the lower neck develops within the remnants of the precervical sinus of His by heteroplasia. The constant association of the salivary gland elements with sinuses, cysts or branchial cartilages along the lower anterior border of the sternocleidomastoid muscle certainly suggests an association with the branchial apparatus.

A variety of morphological types of salivary gland tumors has been reported to arise from the tonsil; only one such lesion (mixed tumor) has been recorded as arising from ectopic salivary glandular tissue in the middle ear.[92]

Salivary gland choristomas of the middle ear, while also rare, have been more often reported (eight cases).[93] Most of the patients initially manifest conductive losses and the salivary tissue is associated with ossicular abnormalities. In several cases, there has been an inextricable involvement of the salivary tissue with the facial nerve.

Salivary gland lesions of the jaws, particularly of the mandible, on the other hand, have a relatively high proportion of malignant neoplasms. The so-called static (developmental, latent, Stafne's bone cyst) is a benign rare affliction of the mandible that produces a circumscribed radiolucency anterior to the angle of the mandible and is usually located below the inferior dental canal.[94, 95] The lesion is not a true cyst, but rather an asymmetrical developmental defect in the mandible at or near the groove made by the facial artery where it crosses bone. Since the size of the defect (1 to 2 cm) does not change with time, the lesion has acquired the designation static. Most lesions, if not all, are due to ectopic submaxillary gland tissue. In most cases, exploration reveals a cup-shaped depression on the lingual aspect of the mandible which contains a portion of submaxillary gland tissue. In some instances the cavities may be empty at the time of surgery. The defects occur predominantly in women between the ages of 33 and 72 years and may be bilateral. There are no authenticated examples of neoplasms arising from this ectopic tissue.

Judging from the literature, *central* salivary gland *tumors* of the jaw bones are unusual but not rare.[96-99] For inclusion in this category and for confirmation of their central origin, the following criteria are necessary: (1) presence of intact cortical plates; (2) radiographic evidence of bone destruction; (3) an intact mucous membrane overlying the lesion; (4) another salivary gland primary or odontogenic tumor must be eliminated; and (5) histological examination of the tissue. The elimination of nonqualifying mandibular lesions is easier than for those located in the maxilla. It is perhaps for this reason that central tumors of the mandible exceed those of the maxilla by rates of 2 to 8:1.

Mucoepidermoid carcinomas are the most common histological type; adenoid cystic carcinomas are a distant second, followed by adenocarcinomas. Mixed tumors are very rarely found in a central osseous position. The majority of the mucoepidermoid carcinomas are mandibular; adenoid cystic carcinomas have a slight inclination toward a maxillary localization. Freeman et al.[100] have reported a rare carcinoma ex pleomorphic adenoma in the mandible.

In the maxilla, ectopic minor salivary gland tissue is probably the generating tissue. Origin in the mandible is most likely from mucous glandular inclusions in the retromolar area. Bhaskar[96] dismisses easily the possibility that these central tumors are from the lining of odontogenic cysts and further claims that the so-called "malignant ameloblastomas" of the mandible are in reality malignant salivary gland tumors in the jaws. A thorough review of aberrant salivary gland tissue and neoplasms has been presented by Miller and Winnick[101] and a comprehensive review of central mucoepidermoid carcinomas of the jaws has been provided by Browand and Waldron.[102]

Radiographs of the mucoepidermoid carcinomas of the jaws consistently show a destruction of bone, usually described as a multilocular or cystic radiolucency. Preoperative diagnoses are ameloblastoma and/or dentigerous cysts. As their designations indicate, all are malignant neoplasms. The adenoid cystic variety behaves not unlike its counterparts elsewhere. The central mucoepidermoid carcinoma has a rapid clinical onset, usually producing pain and a mass in less than 1 year. It is locally aggressive but does not metastasize readily. Metastatic lesions from mucoepidermoid carcinoma are usually limited to the regional lymph nodes. Microscopically, the metastatic lesions within the lymph nodes reflect the variable structure of the primary neoplasm.

Complete surgical excision of the tumors is the preferred treatment, with radiation therapy used to manage stubborn recurrences or inoperable lesions.

A tumor to be distinguished from an intraosseous mucoepidermoid carcinoma is that designated by W.H.O. as "malignant primary intraosseous carcinoma."[103] This lesion is independent of the gingival mucosa or any pre-existing odontogenic cyst. It presumably takes its origin from epithelial rests of Malassez or from the fusion of the facial embryonic buds. The tumor is mucin negative and is characterized by an alveolar or plexiform pattern of squamous differentiated cells. A basal palisading layer may suggest odontogenic origin.

The primary epidermoid intra-alveolar carcinoma may appear in childhood, but is primarily a disease of the sixth or seventh decades. Two-thirds of the patients are males. The mandible is more frequently affected than the maxilla (6:1). Clinical signs and symptoms are nonspecific. The tumor inhibits normal repair after dental extraction and will grow in the alveolus. Radiographs demonstrate a poorly defined, lytic area. Metastases are not very frequent, but when present, they are usually found in the regional lymph nodes (nearly one-third of cases). The prognosis appears to be independent of the form of treatment and is evaluated at 30 to 40% at 5 years.

REFERENCES

1. Cohen, M. A., and Batsakis, J. G.: Oncocytic tumors (oncocytomas) of minor salivary glands. Arch. Otolaryngol. 88:71, 1968.
2. Ranger, D., Thackray, A. C., and Lucas, R. B.: Mucous gland tumours. Br. J. Cancer 10:1, 1956.
3. Frable, W. J., and Elzay, R. P.: Tumors of minor salivary glands: a report of 73 cases. Cancer 25:932, 1970.
4. Bardwil, J. M., Reynold, C. T., Ibanez, M. I., and Luna, M. A.: Report of one hundred tumors of the minor salivary glands. Am. J. Surg. 112:493, 1966.
5. Bergman, F.: Tumors of the minor salivary glands. Cancer 33:538, 1966.

6. Batsakis, J. G.: Mucous gland tumors of the nose and paranasal sinuses. Ann. Otol. Rhinol. Laryngol. 79:557, 1970.

7. Mesara, B. W., and Batsakis, J. G.: Glandular tumors of the upper respiratory tract. Arch. Surg. 92:872, 1966.

8. Osborn, D. A.: Morphology and the natural history of cribriform adenocarcinomas (adenoid cystic carcinoma). J. Clin. Pathol. 30:195, 1977.

9. Conley, J., and Dingman, D. L.: Adenoid cystic carcinoma in the head and neck (cylindroma). Arch. Otolaryngol. 100:81, 1974.

10. Spiro, R. H., Huvos, A. G., and Strong, E. W.: Adenoid cystic carcinoma of salivary origin. A clinicopathologic study of 242 cases. Am. J. Surg. 128:512, 1974.

11. Eby, L. S., Johnson, D. S., and Baker, H. W.: Adenoid cystic carcinomas of the head and neck. Cancer 29:1160, 1972.

12. Lefstedt, S. W., Gaeta, J. F., Sako, K., Marchetta, F. C., and Shedd, D. P.: Adenoid cystic carcinoma of major and minor salivary glands. Am. J. Surg. 122:756, 1971.

13. Dodd, G. D., and Jing, B. S.: Radiographic findings in adenoid cystic carcinoma of the head and neck. Ann. Otol. 81:591, 1972.

14. Batsakis, J. G., Holtz, F., and Sueper, R. H.: Adenocarcinoma of nasal and paranasal cavities. Arch. Otolaryngol. 77:625, 1963.

15. Batsakis, J. G.: Mucous gland tumors of the nose and paranasal sinuses. Ann. Otolaryngol. 79:557, 1970.

16. Sanchez-Casis, G., Devine, K. D., and Weiland, L. H.: Nasal adenocarcinomas that closely simulate colonic carcinomas. Cancer. 28:714, 1971.

17. Michaels, L., and Hyams, V. J.: Objectivity in the classification of tumors of the nasal epithelium. Postgrad. Med. J. 51:695, 1975.

18. Spiro, R. H., Koss, L. G., Hajdu, S. I., and Strong, E. W.: Tumors of minor salivary origin. A clinicopathologic study of 492 cases. Cancer 31:117, 1973.

19. Rafla, S.: Mucous gland tumors of paranasal sinuses. Cancer. 24:683, 1969.

20. Gamez-Araujo, J. J., Ayala, A. G., and Guillnmondegui, O.: Mucinous adenocarcinomas of nose and paranasal sinuses. Cancer 36:1100, 1975.

21. Acheson, E. D., Cowdell, R. H., and Rang, E.: Adenocarcinoma of the nasal cavity and sinuses in England and Wales. Br. J. Ind. Med. 29:21, 1972.

22. Hadfield, E. S.: A study of adenocarcinoma of the paranasal sinuses in woodworkers in the furniture industry. Ann. R. Coll. Surg. Engl. 46:301, 1969.

23. MacBeth, R.: Malignant disease of the paranasal sinuses. J. Laryngol. 79:593, 1965.

24. Brinton, L. A., Blot, W. J., Stone, B. J., and Fraumeni, J. F., Jr.: A death certificate analysis of nasal cancer among furniture workers in North Carolina. Cancer Res. 37: 3473, 1977.

25. Brinton, L. A., Stone, B. J., Blot, W. J., and Fraumeni, J. F., Jr.: Nasal cancer in U.S. furniture industry counties. Lancet 2:628, 1976.

26. Tauxe, W. N., McDonald, J. R., and Devine, K. D.: A century of cylindromas. Arch. Otolaryngol. 75:364, 1962.

27. McDonald, J. R., and Havens, F. Z.: A study of malignant tumors of glandular nature found in the nose, throat and mouth. Surg. Clin. North Am. 28:1087, 1948.

28. Rounthwaite, F. J., Frei, J. V., Wallace, A. C., and Watson, T. A.: The effect of radiotherapy in the treatment of adenoid cystic carcinoma of the head and neck arising in minor salivary glands. J. Otolaryngol. 6:297, 1977.

29. Compagno, J., and Wong, R. T.: Intranasal mixed tumors (pleomorphic adenomas). A clinicopathologic study of 40 cases. Am. J. Clin. Pathol. 68:213, 1977.

30. Foote, F. W., and Frazell, E. L.: Tumors of minor salivary glands. Cancer 6:1065, 1973.

31. Batsakis, J. G., and Regezi, J. A.: Selected controversial lesions of salivary tissues. Otolaryngol. Clin. N. Am. 10: 309, 1977.

32. Johns, M. E., Regezi, J. A., and Batsakis, J. G.: Oncocytic neoplasms of salivary glands. An ultrastructural study. Laryngoscope 87:862, 1977.

33. Koss, L. G., Sprio, R. H., and Hajdu, S.: Small cell (oat cell) carcinoma of minor salivary gland origin. Cancer 30:737, 1972.

34. Houle, J. A., Joseph, P., and Batsakis, J. G.: Primary adenocarcinomas of the larynx. J. Laryngol. 90:1159, 1976.

35. Whicker, J. H., Weiland, L. H., Neel, H. B., III, and Devine, K. D.: Adenocarcinoma of the larynx. Ann. Otol. 83:487, 1974.

36. Fechner, R. E.: Adenocarcinoma of the larynx. Canad. J. Otolaryngol. 4:284, 1975.

37. Olofsson, J., and VanNostrand, A. W. P.: Adenoid cystic carcinoma of the larynx. A report of four cases and a review of the literature. Cancer 40:1307, 1977.

38. Ferlito, A.: Histological classification of larynx and hypopharynx cancers and their clinical implications. Acta Otolaryngol. Suppl. 342, 1976.

39. Sessions, D. G., Murray, J. P., Bauer, W. C., and Ogura, J. H.: Adenocarcinoma of the larynx. Canad. J. Otolaryngol. 4:293, 1975.

40. Ferlito, A.: Adenosquamous carcinoma of the larynx. A clinical and pathologic study. Report of four cases and review of the literature. Acta Otolaryngol. Belg. 30:390, 1976.

41. Frilito, A.: Primary anaplastic giant cell adenocarcinoma of the larynx. J. Laryngol. 90:1053, 1976.

42. Ribari, O., Elemer, G., and Balint, A.: Laryngeal giant cell tumors. J. Laryngol. 89:857, 1975.

43. Olofsson, J., and VanNostrand, A. W. P.: Anaplastic small cell carcinoma of larynx. Ann. Otol. 81:284, 1972.

44. Crissman, J. D., and Rosenblatt, A.: Acinous cell carcinoma of the larynx. Arch. Pathol. Lab. Med. 102:233, 1978.

45. Levine, H. L., and Applebaum, E. L.: Metastatic adenocarcinomas to the larynx: report of a case. Trans. Acad. Ophth. Otol. 82:536, 1976.

46. Cotelingham, J. D., Barnes, L., and Nixon, V. B.: Pleomorphic adenoma of the epiglottis. Arch. Otolaryngol. 103:245, 1977.

47. Thawley, S. E., Berlin, B. P., and Berkowitz, W. P.: Oncocytic hyperplasia of the larynx. J. Laryngol. 91:619, 1977.

48. Holms-Jensen, S., Jacobsen, M., Thommesen, N., and Ferreira, O.: Oncocytic cysts of the larynx. Arch. Otolaryngol. 83:366, 1977.

49. Johns, M. E., Batsakis, J. G., and Short, C. D.: Oncocyte and oncocytoid tumors of the salivary glands. Laryngoscope 83:1940, 1973.

50. Kyriakos, M., Berlin, B. P., and Kecskemeti, K. D.: Oatcell carcinoma of the larynx. Arch. Otolaryngol. 104:168, 1978.

51. Gilbert, J. G., Mazzarella, L. A., and Feit, L. J.: Primary tracheal tumors in the infant and adult. Arch. Otolaryngol. 58:1, 1953.

52. Salm, R.: Primary carcinoma of the trachea: a review. Br. J. Dis. Chest 58:61, 1964.

53. Hadju, S. I., Huvos, A. G., Goodner, J. T., Foote, F. W., Jr., and Beattie, E. J., Jr.: Carcinoma of the trachea: clinicopathologic study of 41 cases. Cancer 25:1448, 1970.

54. Weber, A. L., and Grillo, H. C.: Tracheal tumors: radiological, clinical and pathological considerations. Adv. Otorhinolaryngol. 24:170, 1978.

55. McCafferty, G. J., Parker, L. S., and Suggit, S. C.: Primary malignant disease of the trachea. J. Laryngol. Otol. 78: 331, 1964.

56. Birt, B. D.: The Management of malignant tracheal neoplasms. J. Laryngol. Otol. 84:723, 1970.

57. Hjertman, L., and Eneroth, C.-M.: Tumours of the palate. Acta Otolaryngol. Suppl. 263:179, 1970.

58. Coates, H. L. C., Devine, K. D., Desanto, L. W., and Weiland, L. H.: Glandular tumors of the palate. Surg. Gynec. Obstet. 140:589, 1975.

59. Goepfert, H., Giraldo, A. A., Byers, R. M., and Luna, M. A.: Salivary gland tumors of the base of the tongue. Arch. Otolaryngol. 102:391, 1976.

60. Chaudhry, A. P., Vickers, R. A., and Gorlin, R. J.: Intraoral minor salivary gland tumors: an analysis of 1,414 cases. Oral Surg. 14:1194, 1961.

61. Epker, B. N., and Henny, F. A.: Clinical, histopathologic, and surgical aspects of intraoral minor salivary gland tumors: review of 90 cases. J. Oral Surg. 27:792, 1970.

62. Eneroth, C.-M., Hjertman, L., and Moberger, G.: Salivary gland adenomas of the palate. Acta Otolaryngol. 73:305, 1972.

63. Eneroth, C.-M., and Zetterberg, A.: Nuclear DNA content as a criterion of malignancy in salivary gland tumours of the oral cavity. Acta Otolaryngol. 75:296, 1973.

64. Worthington, P.: The management of the palatal pleomorphic adenoma. Br. J. Oral Surg. 12:132, 1974.

65. Pinto, R. S., Kelly, D. S., and George, A. E.: Radiologic features of benign pleomorphic adenoma of the hard palate. Oral Surg. 39:976, 1975.

66. Burbank, P. M., Dockerty, M. B., and Devine, K. P.: A clinicopathologic study of 43 cases of glandular tumors of the tongue. Surg. Gynecol. Obstet. 109:573, 1959.

67. Allen, M. S., Jr., Fitz-Hugh, G. S., and Marsh, W. L., Jr.: Low-grade papillary adenocarcinoma of the palate. Cancer 33:153, 1974.

68. Heidelberger, K. P., McClatchey, K. D., Batsakis, J. G., and Van Wieren, C. R.: Primary adenocarcinoma of the lip. J. Oral Surg. 35:68, 1977.

69. Byers, R. M., Boddie, A., and Luna, M. A.: Malignant salivary gland neoplasms of the lip. Am. J. Surg. 134:528, 1977.

70. Crocker, D. J., Calalaris, C. J., and Finch, R.: Intraoral minor salivary gland tumors: report of 38 cases. Oral Surg. 29:60, 1970.

71. Stuteville, O. H., and Corley, R. D.: Surgical management of tumors of the intraoral minor salivary glands; report of 80 cases. Cancer 20:1578, 1967.

72. Soskolne, A., Sela, J., Ben-Amar, A., and Ulmansky, M.: Minor salivary gland tumors: a survey of 64 cases. J. Oral Surg. 31:528, 1973.

73. Adams, G. L., and Duvall, A. J.: Adenocarcinoma of the head and neck. Arch. Otolaryngol. 93:261, 1971.

74. Shumrick, D. A.: Treatment of malignant tumors of minor salivary glands. Arch. Otolaryngol. 88:74, 1968.

75. Abrams, A. M., Melrose, R. J., and Howell, F. V.: Necrotizing sialometaplasia. A disease simulating malignancy. Cancer 32:130, 1973.

76. Maisel, R. H., Johnston, W. H., Anderson, H. A., and Cantrell, R. W.: Necrotizing sialometaplasia involving the nasal cavity. Laryngoscope 87:429, 1977.

77. Fechner, R. E.: Necrotizing sialometaplasia. A source of confusion with carcinoma of the palate. Am. J. Clin. Pathol. 67:315, 1977.

78. Thackray, A. C., and Lucas, R. B.: Tumors of the major salivary glands. Atlas of Tumor Pathology, Fascicle 10, Washington, D. C., Armed Forces Institute of Pathology, 1974.

79. Eneroth, C.-M., and Hjertman, L.: Benign tumors of the submandibular gland. Pract. Otorhinolaryngol. 29:166, 1967.

80. Frable, M. A. S.: Submaxillary gland excision. Surg. Gynecol. Obstet. 131:1155, 1970.

81. Rafla, S.: Submaxillary gland tumors. Cancer 26:821, 1970.

82. Hanna, D. C., and Clairmont, A. A.: Submandibular gland tumors. Plast. Reconstr. Surg. 61:198, 1978.

83. Conley, J., Myers, E., and Cole, R.: Analysis of 115 patients with tumors of the submandibular gland. Ann. Otol. 8: 323, 1972.

84. Spiro, R. H., Hajdu, S. I., and Strong, E. W.: Tumors of the submaxillary gland. Am. J. Surg. 132:463, 1976.

85. Abramson, A. L.: The submaxillary gland as a site of distant metastases. Laryngoscope 81:793, 1971.

86. Eneroth, C.-M., Hjertman, L., and Moberger, C.: Malignant tumors of the submandibular gland. Acta Otolaryngol. 64:514, 1967.

87. Rankow, R. M., and Mignogna, F.: Cancer of the sublingual salivary gland. Am. J. Surg. 118:790, 1969.

88. Foote, F. W., Jr., and Frazell, E. L.: Tumors of the major salivary glands. Cancer 6:1065, 1953.

89. Pesavento, G., and Ferlito, A.: Benign mixed tumour of heterotopic salivary gland tissue in upper neck. Report of a case with a review of the literature on heterotopic salivary gland tissue. J. Laryngol. 90:577, 1976.

90. Schochet, S. S., McCormick, W. F., and Halmi, N. S.: Salivary gland rests in the human pituitary. Light and electron microscopical study. Arch. Pathol. 98:193, 1974.

91. Youngs, L. A., and Scofield, H. H.: Heterotopic salivary gland tissue in the lower neck. Arch. Pathol. 83:550, 1967.

92. Saeed, Y. M., and Bassis, M. L.: Mixed tumor of the middle ear: a case report. Arch. Otolaryngol. 93:433, 1971.

93. Mischke, R. E., Brackman, D. E., and Gruskin, P.: Salivary gland choristoma of the middle ear. Arch. Otolaryngol. 103:432, 1977.

94. Choukas, N. C., and Toto, P. D.: Etiology of static bone defects of mandible. J. Oral Surg. 18:16, 1960.

95. Uemura, S., Fujishita, M., and Fuchihata, H.: Radiographic interpretation of so-called developmental defect of mandible. Oral Surg. 41:120, 1976.

96. Bhaskar, S. N.: Central mucoepidermoid tumors of the mandible. Cancer 16:721, 1963.

97. Dhawan, I. K., Bhargava, S., Nayak, N. C., and Gupta, R. K.: Central salivary gland tumors of jaws. Cancer 26:211, 1970.

98. Silverglade, L. B., Olvares, O. F., and Olech, E.: Central mucoepidermoid tumors of the jaws: review of the literature and case report. Cancer 22:650, 1968.

99. Smith, R. L., Dahlin, D. C., and Waite, D. E.: Mucoepidermoid carcinoma of the jawbone. J. Oral Surg. 26:387, 1968.

100. Freeman, S. I., Van de Velde, R. L., Kagan, A. R., and Perzik, S. L.: Primary malignant mixed tumor of the mandible. Cancer 30:167, 1972.

101. Miller, A. S., and Winnick, M.: Salivary gland inclusion in the anterior mandible. Oral Surg. 31:79, 1971.

102. Browand, B. C., and Waldron, C. A.: Central mucoepidermoid tumors of the jaws. Report of nine cases and review of the literature. Oral Surg. 40:631, 1975.

103. Lathower, C. and Verhest, A.: Malignant primary intraosseous carcinoma of the mandible. Oral Surg. 37:77, 1974.

104. Reynolds, C. T., McAuley, R. L., and Rogers, W. P., Jr.: Experience with tumors of minor salivary glands. Am. J. Surg. 111:168, 1966.

105. Brown, R. L., Bishop, E. L., and Giradeau, H. S.: Tumors of the minor salivary glands. Cancer 12:40, 1959.

106. Smith, J. F.: Tumors of minor salivary glands. Oral Surg. 15:594, 1962.

107. Edwards, E. G.: Tumors of minor salivary glands. Am. J. Clin. Pathol. 34:455, 1960.

108. Potdar, G. G., and Paymaster, J. C.: Tumors of minor salivary glands. Oral Surg. 28:310, 1969.

CHAPTER 3

Non-neoplastic Diseases of the Salivary Glands

There has been an increasing emphasis on benign, non-neoplastic disorders of the salivary glands over the past decade. Attention is drawn to this heterogenous group of disorders not only because they may, at times, simulate neoplasms, but also because of the imperfections in the many modes of treatment, uncertainty in pathogenesis and histogenesis and because immunochemical techniques have opened new vistas of relationships between recurrent parotid diseases and autoimmune disorders.

Table 3.1 presents a classification of some of these disorders. While it is convenient to consider each type separately and in apparent isolation, this is too often artificial and academic. The clinician and the surgical pathologist labor under the proverbial "chicken and egg complex," particularly so in the categories of chronic recurrent parotitis, "sialectasis" and sialolithiasis. There is always uncertainty as to whether these disorders are due to a primary infection with secondary obstruction or primary obstruction with secondary infection. The limited tissue response repetoire manifested by the salivary glands and the similarities of sialographic appearances leads one to consider that he is dealing with different conditions, the principal differences being ones of degree and distribution. Care must be exercised, however, as with any "spectrum-appearing" disease state, that oversimplification of pathogenesis does not deter the search for specifics.

In the following discussion, we present a contemporary clinicopathological review of nonmalignant sialoadenopathies. The disorders range from those with known causal agents, i.e., specific infections, to salivary gland enlargements manifesting either complex or obscure pathogenesis.

VIRAL INFECTIONS

Mumps is by far the most common cause of parotid gland swelling. Although submandibular gland involvement may be present, the principal gland affected is the parotid. The disease has not been recognized in patients below the age of 1 year and is most common in, yet not limited to, the 4- to 5-year-old age group. Many cases are subclinical and account for misdiagnosis leading to referral for parotid gland enlargement.

The *clinical* diagnosis of mumps is reliable only during epidemics. Diagnosis is made by measuring serum antibodies to the mumps S and V antigens. A titer of more than 1:192 indicates recent infection. The virus may also be isolated from the urine from 6 days before to 13 days after salivary gland manifestations.

Other viral agents may also produce a parotitis and account for some of the inexplicable serological negatives in "mumps." Coxsackie, parainfluenza (type 1 and 3), the virus of lymphocytic choriomeningitis, herpes, echo virus, and influenza type A have all been incriminated as causal agents.[1]

A virus, usually latent within the salivary glands, can cause "salivary gland virus disease" affecting multiple organ systems in usually debilitated hosts. Diagnosis is made by finding characteristic intracellular inclusions.

INFLAMMATORY DISEASE

Acute Pyogenic or Suppurative Parotitis. Occurring throughout a very wide range of life, the clinical onset of acute parotitis is marked by a sudden onset of swelling of the gland and soft tissues in the periparotid region and is associated with a purulent discharge from Stensen's duct. The swelling is diffuse and involves the whole gland or the entire side of the face. The area is firm, tender, smooth and warm to palpation. There is a low-grade fever and a modest leukocytosis.

Pathogenesis is incompletely understood but a number of *predisposing* factors are known. Most prominent among these is the association with the postoperative period. So-called "surgical parotitis" accounts for approximately 30 to 40% of the cases of acute inflammatory parotitis and has been estimated to occur in 1:1,000 and 1:2,000 postoperative patients.[2, 3] Bilateral presentation occurs in 20% of this group and terminal neoplasms are the factors in the nonsurgical patient. The disease can occur ab initio in infants and in the elderly who are otherwise in good health. The provocative name, *nosocomial* parotitis may be applied to this form of parotitis in order to stress that the illness appears in hospitalized patients if their salivary secretions are impaired and oral and environmental hygiene is neglected.[4]

Retrograde infection is very likely the precipitating cause in acute parotitis. There is a known precipitous increase in oral bacteria during the

Table 3.1
Non-neoplastic Enlargements of the Salivary Glands

  I. Inflammatory
   A. Acute (specific)
     1. Viral (mumps, Coxsackie A, ECHO, and lymphocytic choriomeningitis)
     2. Bacterial (staphylococcal, streptococcal, pneumococcal, gram-negative)
       a. Acute suppurative of infancy
       b. Postsurgical
       c. Terminal debilitation
   B. Chronic (specific)
     1. Tuberculosis
     2. Actinomycosis, etc.
     3. ? Sarcoidosis
   C. "Recurrent subacute" and chronic recurrent
     1. Self-limited
     2. Progressive
     3. Lymphoepithelial lesion and Sjögren's syndrome
 II. Systemic and secondary metabolic
   A. Obesity, hypertension, diabetes mellitus
   B. Malnutrition and associated deficiencies (protein, vitamins)
   C. Alcoholism and alcoholic liver disease
III. "Hypersensitivity" and drug idiosyncrasy
 IV. Local (salivary gland) disturbances
   A. Sialolithiasis
   B. Sialoangiectasis
   C. Trauma, foreign body, fistula
   D. Parotid lymphadenopathy
   E. Cysts, mucocele and ranula
   F. Local duct obstructions (mucous plugs, congenital)
  V. Miscellaneous
   A. Pneumoparotitis
   B. Psychogenic
   C. Functional overactivity
   D. Idiopathic
   E. Irradiation sialoadenitis

postoperative period, and increased coagulase *Staphylococcus aureus* has been found in all subjects with dry mouth. In the newborn and aged with acute parotitis, *S. aureus* is the principal pathogen. During the middle ages, *Streptococcus viridans* accounts for approximately two-thirds of the cultures, the pneumococcus accounts for a little less than a quarter and the remainder reflect the dominant oral flora.

In children and nonsurgical cases, the disease may be recurrent. The course in these instances is variable and, while the disease often begins as a unilateral affliction, it later becomes bilateral. Occasionally both sides are simultaneously involved.[5]

In the majority of patients there is resolution after adequate antibiotic therapy. It is also noteworthy that hormonal factors play a role since, by the age of 15 years, most children have ceased to have recurrences. It has been suggested that the natural outcome of parotid gland infection caused by pyogenic organisms other than *S. aureus* is related to the resumption of function of the gland and that, with spontaneous salivation, the parotitis subsides. This may be partially true but gram-negative parotitis has been fatal in the very young and in the moribund (leukemic) patient.

Microscopically there is evidence of erosion of ducts with penetration of the exudate into the parenchyma. The lobular architecture of the parotid gland with its multiple septae prevents an early confluence of the small necrotic foci and leads to multiple small abscesses (Fig. 3.1).

Sialadenitis in childhood has been divided by Kaban et al.[6] into four separate classes (Table 3.2). Management of the disorders in this age group can be found in the reports of Kaban et al.[6] and Casterline and Jaques.[7]

SPECIFIC GRANULOMATOUS DISEASES

Hyperplasia of the intraparotid gland and periparotid lymph nodes may simulate localized tumors of the gland. On occasion, also, these lymph nodes with or without other lymphadenopathy may be the site of specific chronic infective granulomas. The granulomatous disease may be limited to the lymph nodes or may also involve the salivary gland itself. Any number of granulomatous diseases may secondarily involve the salivary glands, including actinomycosis and atypical mycobacterial infection, brucellosis, etc. Tuberculosis, animal scratch disease and the polyglot disorder, sarcoidosis, are singled out for special consideration.

Mycobacterium Tuberculosis. In the past, tuberculous lymphadenitis of the cervical lymph nodes was a fairly common disease, most frequently caused by ingestion of the bovine tubercle bacillus. At present, the frequency is considerably lower and infection is due more often to the human strain.

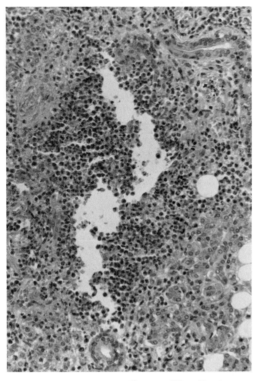

Figure 3.1. Acute suppurative parotitis with abscess formation.

In 1961 Donohue and Bolden[8] presented a collective review of 79 cases of presumed "primary" tuberculosis of the salivary gland. In 75% of the cases there was no family or personal history of tuberculosis.

The parotid gland is most often involved, and bilaterality is unusual. Tuberculous infection of the sublingual gland is rare, and the submandibular gland is intermediate in frequency of involvement. One-third of the cases present in the second and third decades of life. While considered "primary" the salivary gland lesions most likely arise from a focus in the tonsils or less often from around teeth. Ascent to the glands and regional lymph nodes is via the duct system, lymphatics or the facial nerve trunk. True secondary involvement of the salivary glands in generalized tuberculosis is quite variable, and in these instances the submaxillary and sublingual glands are far more often involved than the parotid glands.

Gross manifestations assume two rather distinct forms: (1) an acute inflammatory infection with diffuse gland involvement; and (2) a chronic, "encapsulated" tumorous type which may be asymptomatic for many years. Pain is a late manifestation and facial paralysis is rare.

At the present time concurrent pulmonary and salivary gland tuberculosis has become less prevalent, and has been replaced by involvement of the salivary glands and their associated lymph nodes with *atypical* mycobacterial infection.[9, 10] The salivary gland or cervical adenopathy generally appears acutely as a painless mass, which after

Table 3.2
Sialadenitis in Children

Type	Etiology	Predominent Organisms	Treatment	Outcome
Acute sialadenitis of submandibular gland	Obstruction: calculi, stenosis, stricture	Flora of mouth	Antibiotics, removal of stone, excision	No recurrence
Acute suppurative parotitis	Predisposition in prematures, systemic disease, or immunosuppression. Increased viscosity and decreased secretion	*Staphylococcus aureus*	Antibiotics	Usually one episode
Recurrent acute parotitis	No single factor. Reduced secretion	Mixed culture with alpha streptococcus	Antibiotics, possible parotidectomy	Multiple episodes. May be self-limited at puberty
Chronic parotitis	Varied (obstruction, autoimmune, heredity). Reduced secretion	No predominent organisms	Local (heat, massage) and sialogogues	Low grade; responsive to local treatment

a period of rapid growth, remains stationary in size. Systemic symptoms are usually not present. Occasional fistulae may be formed.

Animal Scratch Disease. This entity is also referred to as cat-scratch disease, but the feline is not the only offender. The disease appears to be increasing in frequency as the number and variety of pets increase in households. The disease is a necrotizing granulomatous affliction that may involve the parotid lymph nodes and simulate parotid salivary gland disease. Involvement of salivary parenchyma is by contiguous extension. It is not possible to completely separate animal scratch disease from other so-called viral granulomatous infections by histological study alone.

Sarcoidosis. This is a diagnosis made principally after exclusion of other possible granulomatous disorders. Association, if not synonymity, with Heerfordt's disease is now clear, but the basic alteration is uncertain. Parotid gland and/or parotid lymph node involvement is estimated to occur in approximately 6% of all cases. In the rare series where documentation by histological means has been done, the incidence is higher (one-third of cases).[11] Much like tuberculosis, the sarcoidal granulomas primarily involve the lymphoid tissue and not the parenchyma (Fig. 3.2). In passing, it is important to remember that, while caseous necrosis is not seen in sarcoidosis, the granulomas may manifest a noncaseating, usually fibrinoid, central necrosis.

CHRONIC RECURRENT SIALADENITIS

This poorly understood group of lesions affects the parotid gland more frequently than the submandibular. This is probably due, at least in part, to the anatomical differences of the two glands. The relatively long and narrow parotid duct makes it more prone to abnormalities in the character of the secretions than the submandibular gland with its shorter and wider duct. Clinically, there are recurrent attacks of parotid swelling associated with discomfort or pain. One or both glands may be involved and the process affects both children and adults. There is some tendency for the disease to terminate spontaneously at puberty, but some cases persist into adulthood.[12] Spontaneous recovery in those patients manifesting an adult clinical onset is not common.

Of the various predisposing factors which produce chronic recurrent inflammatory disease, three are fairly constant[13]: (1) a decreased secretion rate and flow; (2) stasis of secretions; and (3) alteration in the character of the secretion. Maynard[13] has

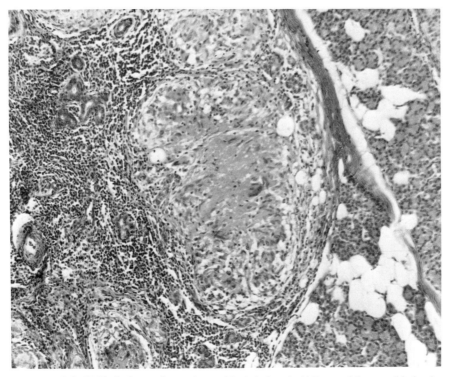

Figure 3.2. Epitheliod granuloma of sarcoidosis in lymphoid tissue of the parotid gland.

measured saliva secretion rates in these patients and has found a statistically significant reduction. This was true even on the unaffected side in patients with unilateral disease and in patients manifesting a spontaneous cure. The sequence of events may be as follows: a decrease in parotid secretion rate → retrograde infection → low-grade ductal infection → metaplastic ductal epithelium → obstruction (mucous plugs, stricture, calculus) → recurrent parotitis.

Reduction in the secretion rate may be initiated by a variety of causes, i.e., following viral infection, developmental, etc. Repeated ascending infections intervene and cultures have shown that the majority of organisms are similar to those of the normal flora of the mouth, indicating an opportunistic infection. Once established, this low-grade infection, if prolonged, induces mucous metaplasia in the ductal lining cells. Normally the parotid gland produces only small amounts of mucus. In recurrent parotid gland enlargement, excessive amounts are produced, yielding a flocculent secretion. This more "solid" material serves as a potential source for recurrent obstruction and as the nidus for calculi.

Some indirect support for the primary role of the ducts and ductal secretions has been provided by Tandler[14] in an elegant study of the chronically inflamed human submandibular gland. This craftsman points out that many of the ultrastructural changes in salivary glands previously attributed to autoimmune disease also occur in patients who are free of these disorders but whose salivary glands have undergone intermittent obstruction or infection. He further reaffirms that, in the absence of an escape route, secretions accumulate in the duct lumina, and when they reach some threshold concentration, precipitate (amorphous, tubular structure, crystalloids or any combinations). An associated increase in lysosomes may be responsible for the lytic events allowing the ductal contents and other debris to be liberated into the salivary parenchyma. The host response is uniformly one of polymorphonuclear leukocytes, followed by chronic inflammatory cells.

A peculiar inflammatory disease of the submandibular gland characterized by a progressive plasmacellular ductitis and known as Küttner's tumor needs special mention. This chronic, nonspecific and sclerosing sialoadenitis of the submandibular gland is well known in the European literature[15, 16] but is rarely commented on by American authors. This disorder is unilateral and affects men and women equally. Histogenetically the lesion appears to be a progressive (from interlobular to intercalated ducts) ductitis.[15] A plasma cell and lymphocytic infiltrate about the ducts eventually yields to an encasement of ducts in thick fibrous trabeculae. The present author has seen a similar process in the parotid gland, where in the end-stage, the term fibrosing (sclerosing) parotitis has been used.

Recurrent sialadenitis in adults is most often due to obstructive causes or concurrent systemic disease (calculi, mucus plugs, strictures, extraductal causes). On the other hand, a complete examination of the child with sialadenitis usually fails to disclose any concurrent local or systemic etiological factors. It has been reported that recurrent parotitis in children is histologically different from that in adults in that children have a *synsialitis,* inflammation of the supporting connective tissue of the gland, whereas adults have involvement of ducts and parenchyma.[9]

Chronicity of the recurrent attacks affects ultimate prognosis. The best prognosis is in men over the age of 40 years with less than 1-year histories of symptoms of unilateral, short-lived, parotid swelling. The worst prognosis is manifested by women over 40 years of age with *long* histories of infrequent bouts of painful, long-lasting swellings affecting *both* parotid glands.

From the pathological viewpoint, there are three significant changes in the glands: (1) ductal changes; (2) acinar alterations; and (3) lymphocytic infiltration of the glands. All three have their radiographic counterparts encompassed in the term "sialectasis."[17] In the recurrent "parotitis" group of patients, the sialogram demonstrates the architectural changes that have occurred during the progress of the disease. Maynard[13] demonstrated a progressive sequence of sialographic changes in his series of patients. These ranged from near normal in appearance to complete disruption of the gland. Intermediate findings are those of branch duct changes to "sialectasis," and eventually main duct changes of various degrees. The sialogram, according to Maynard,[13] reflects merely the degree of damage sustained by the glands after repeated attacks of obstruction and low-grade infection. He further cautions that many of the "sialectatic" changes shown are artefacts due to extravasated dye through weakened intralobular ducts. Nonetheless, he offers a classification based on sialographic appearances. Sialangiectasis, in itself, has been considered important as a forerunner for a spectrum of disorders.[18, 19]

As far as the importance of ductal epithelial changes versus acinar epithelial changes is concerned, both are equally significant. We have already stated the importance of the ductal metaplasia and increased mucus production. In relation to the acini, Furstenburg and Blatt say, "The mechanism which resists retrograde infection of salivary parenchyma by mouth organisms can operate successfully in the face of increased pressure gradients ... as long as the normal complement of acinar tissue is available and sufficiently productive to wash the organisms out of the duct."[20]

The lymphocytic infiltrate observed in the glands removed for recurrent parotitis is a response to ductal and acinar damage. Waterhouse[21] has shown that focal "lymphocytic adenitis" occurs in a high proportion of clinically normal salivary glands with loss of functional secretory gland acini and that the incidence increased with age. To be creditable as focal "lymphocytic adenitis" there must be an aggregate of 50 or more lymphocytes and histiocytes with a scattering of plasma cells adjacent to or replacing gland acini.[22] Such foci are commonly found in relation to small veins or at the edge of intralobular ducts.

During the progressive stages of recurrent parotid swelling there is also a progressive accumulation of lymphoid tissue around intralobular ducts and, subsequently, lymphoid replacement of the secreting glandular elements. There is also an accompanying hyperplasia of the intraparotid lymph nodes.

Chisholm et al.[22] have correlated, in the postmortem subject, the degree of lymphocytic infiltration in major and minor salivary glands. It has been shown that the changes observed in the submandibular gland accurately reflect the degree of focal lymphocytic adenitis present in the parotid and lacrimal glands. Furthermore, there has been shown a strong association of focal lymphocytic sialadenitis and rheumatoid arthritis in the postmortem subject. Finally, and of importance to the biopsy surgeon, there has been a significant degree of correlation between lymphocytic infiltrates in the labial salivary glands and focal lymphocytic submandibular adenitis (hence also the parotids). There is more than a suggestion also that the presence of lymphocytic foci in the labial glands in Sjögren's syndrome in fact reflects salivary gland involvement as a whole and that the lymphocytic foci found in one gland are related to others. The microscopist is cautioned however, to recall that chronic trauma (lip biting, etc.) to the lips may also produce a similar histological appearance in the labial glands.[23]

The association of focal lymphocytic adenitis and Sjögren's syndrome permits us entree to a discussion of this complex disorder. In a sense Sjögren's syndrome is the "stalking horse" for chronic parotitis studies and is to the parotid gland what Hashimoto's disease is to the study of thyroiditis. It is now generally agreed that the syndrome is a systemic disorder that also involves the salivary glands. It occurs mainly in women (90%) near their menopause and is associated with parotid, lacrimal and other salivary gland enlargement (predominantly parotid).

Mikulicz's Disease and Syndrome Sjögren's Syndrome and Benign Lymphoepithelial Lesion

Ever since Mikulicz[24] described in 1882 and published in 1892 his *single* unique case of a 42-year-old man with bilateral lacrimal, parotid and submaxillary swellings, his name has been associated with parotid disease. This association has been accompanied by confusion. What his patient actually had cannot be determined with certainty, but a heterogenous group of parotid lesions have been included under the eponymic designation "Mikulicz's disease."

The definition of Mikulicz's disease has been made so vague by papers published since his death that the diagnosis is almost meaningless, and we see no justification for using it other than in a historical context. If one wishes to honor this venerable investigator by retaining an eponymic designation, Mikulicz's syndrome *may* be appropriate, if it is used in a nonspecific *clinical* and not morphological context to refer to a bilateral enlargement of the lacrimal and salivary glands caused by a variety of diseases: leukemia, lymphoma, tuberculosis, sarcoid, etc.

With this preamble, one can now relate in a somewhat unencumbered manner to Sjögren's syndrome and benign lymphoepithelial lesion of the salivary gland.

The diagnostic terms lymphoepithelial lesion, chronic recurrent (punctate) parotitis or sialadenitis, sicca syndrome and Sjögren's syndrome share nearly common histopathological changes in the salivary tissues—a lymphoreticular cell proliferation, usually associated with atrophy of the acinar parenchyma, and a variety of ductal changes ending in the so-called "epimyoepithelial island."[13, 18, 25, 26]

The histopathological (and often the clinical) picture is one of a chronic inflammation (sialadenitis) with architectural variations (focal, punctate, nodular or diffuse) being related to severity and chronicity. The histological similarity, if not identity, combined with a uniform sialectasis and cases presenting pathological features intermediate in type between the extremes of focal and diffuse changes, clearly indicate an evolutionary spectrum perhaps beginning with an undefined duct injury. An analogous lesion may well be the follicular damage in thyroiditis.

It is my contention that the classically defined lymphoepithelial lesion[27, 28] is, in effect, an *end-stage* epithelial alteration with characteristic lymphocytic infiltration of the salivary parenchyma. In evolution to that stage, the lesion has passed through successive chronic inflammatory phases. Histopathological criteria to circumscribe the diagnosis are then most difficult to define except for the end-stage disease. The author reserves the diagnostic term—lymphoepithelial lesion—for a gland or part of a gland that is totally or nearly totally replaced by a chronic inflammatory infiltrate and in which only islands of metaplastic ducts are identified. For lesions falling short of this advanced change, I use the terms, chronic lymphoepithelial sialadenitis, chronic punctate parotitis[26] or chronic nonspecific sialadenitis.

The lymphoepithelial lesion is usually localized in a tumor-simulating fashion, but may be diffuse in the involved gland (Fig. 3.3). Lymphoid and epithelial components are present in every instance. In some examples, the lymphoid infiltrate may so dominate the histological picture that multiple sections will be required to find the islands of epithelium. The islands are the most characteristic structures as far as diagnosis is concerned and are formed by a metaplastic proliferation of altered ductal epithelium accompanied by myoepithelial cells (Fig. 3.4). The pathologist cannot help but be impressed by the developmental stages leading to the formation of the epimyoepithelial island. Beginning as a form of salivary duct (intercalated and striated) injury with periductal inflammation, the salivary changes progress through at least four histological stages. Each is characterized by nearly concomitant and progressive duct injury and

metaplasia with atrophy of acinar parenchyma and replacement by the ever-widening periductal inflammation. With disappearance of the duct lumina, myoepithelial prominence occurs so that the island is a mixture of these cells, altered duct cells, all permeated by lymphocytes of variable quantities. An extracellular, eosinophilic, hyaline-like material is often prominent in and about the islands. Similar strands or masses of this proteinaceous material may be present in the lymphocyte-replaced parenchyma. The cellular infiltrate may indeed be composed of mature lymphocytes, or be a mixed lymphocyte, histiocyte and plasma cell reaction. The pattern may be diffuse or follicular.

I am convinced, as are Seifert and Donath,[16] that myoepithelial cells are integral components of the islands of the lymphoepithelial lesion. Surprisingly, however, they are elusive to the electron microscopist.[29, 30]

The epithelial islands may be present in variable numbers in the punctate and chronic inflammatory stages. In the former, however, the histological appearance is dominated by dilated ducts with periductal chronic inflammation which is often coalescent.

The histopathological appearances of the salivary glands in the various stages of lymphoepithelial lesion and the glands from patients with Sjögren's syndrome are *identical*. Evidence that the benign lymphoepithelial lesion is a less highly developed form of Sjögren's syndrome is at present limited and debatable. If, as certain morphological evidence indicates, there is a histogenetic and pathogenetic relationship between chronic recurrent parotitis or punctate parotitis, the benign lymphoepithelial lesion and Sjögren's syndrome, this relationship is certainly not common. It is very clear that the pathological process in the salivary glands can be present in at least two different clinical forms: one, a disease which may occur in

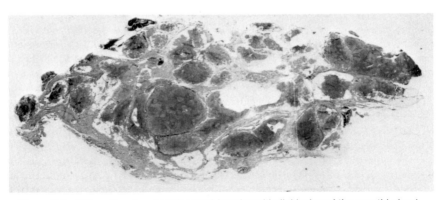

Figure 3.3. Diffuse (focal and coalescent) lymphoepithelial lesion of the parotid gland.

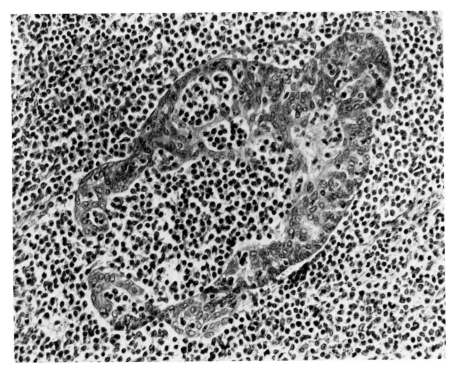

Figure 3.4. Over-all lobular architecture of the salivary gland is preserved in the benign lymphoepithelial lesion of the salivary gland. There is, however, atrophy of the glandular parenchyma with replacement by a dense lymphocytic infiltration. A hallmark of the disorder is the presence of islands of epithelial and myoepithelial cells. They are of ductal origin.

males and females; and the other, associated with systemic disease and is almost always seen in women.

Clinically, Sjögren's syndrome consists of three major components: (1) keratoconjunctivitis sicca, initiated by lesions in the lacrimal gland; (2) xerostomia with or without salivary gland enlargement resulting from damage to the salivary glands and the mucous glands of the oral cavity; and (3) connective tissue disease, usually rheumatoid arthritis. It is generally recognized that the diagnosis of the syndrome can be made when only two of the three features are present. This oversimplification does not convey the multifaceted and often systemic character of the disease (Fig. 3.5).

Other collagen diseases, such as lupus erythematosus, scleroderma or periarteritis nodosa may substitute for rheumatoid arthritis in the syndrome. The term "sicca syndrome" or "complex" may be applied when xerostomia and keratoconjunctivitis sicca occur in the absence of an associated collagen disease.

The sicca complex is the most common variant of the syndrome. The patient presents with xerophthalmia, xerostomia and painless parotid gland enlargement. From this, the syndrome can progress to one with a widely diversified range of clinical signs and symptoms characteristic of systemic involvement or remain as the "sicca syndrome."

Numerically, the greatest number of patients presenting with histological findings of lymphoepithelial lesions suffer only from chronic parotitis without ever developing more serious consequences of their disease; a small number evolve into a clinically recognizable form of Sjögren's syndrome or its variants. An even smaller number of patients, *with or without evidence of autoimmunity,* develop aggressive lesions of either the lymphoreticular or epithelial components of the lymphoepithelial lesion[25, 31, 32] (Fig. 3.5).

The development of lymphoreticular abnormalities in patients with Sjögren's syndrome is preceeded by a lymphocytic infiltrate that progresses to an intrasalivary gland lymphoreticular hyperplasia, increased numbers of plasma cells and the production of circulating antibodies. The development of serious autoimmune disease follows the loss of specific target autoimmunity (in the salivary gland) and results in generalized autoimmune dis-

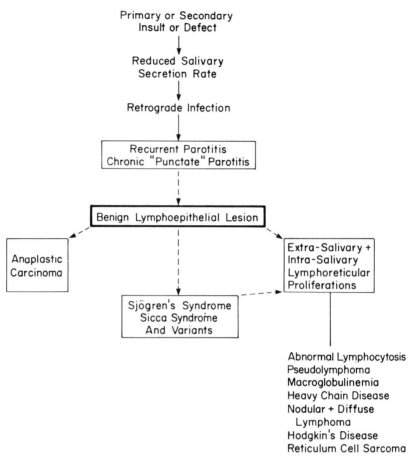

Figure 3.5. Salivary gland alterations leading to the benign lymphoepithelial lesion and hence to the development of malignancy. Neoplasia may arise from either the epithelial or the lymphoreticular components of the primary lesion.

ease. The loss of specific target autoimmunity in a few of these patients also leads to the development of abnormal or atypical lymphoreticular proliferations: pseudolymphomas, macroglobulinemias and hyperglobulinemias, malignant lymphoma. The pseudolymphomatous reaction is the most common and may be a precursor form to lymphoma.[25, 33]

Patients with Sjögren's syndrome and a malignant lymphoreticular disorder may first be seen in such a state, may develop the disorder from the classic benign condition, or may proceed through the pseudolymphomatous state.

To date, the majority of malignant lymphomas complicating the course of Sjögren's syndrome have been extrasalivary and have been classified as histiocytic lymphoma, lymphocytic lymphoma, Hodgkin's disease, macroglobulinemia and heavy chain disease.[34] There is, however, increasing documentation of a primary origin of the lymphomas

in the salivary glands themselves (See Chapter 1). It can also be categorically denied that the finding of islands eliminates the diagnosis of lymphoma.

It is important to appreciate that the advent of a lymphoma in a patient with lymphoepithelial lesions of the salivary tissues need not be associated with clinical or laboratory evidence of a systemic autoimmune disease. Furthermore, a progressive decline in globulin abnormalities and various antibody titers may presage the development of a histiocytic lymphoma in patients with Sjögren's syndrome.

The association of Waldenstrom's macroglobulinemia and Sjögren's syndrome is a particularly interesting one. Patients with the benign, uncomplicated form of Sjögren's syndrome usually have little or no increase in their serum IgM levels. However, as they develop extraglandular infiltrates, the IgM concentration can become quite increased. At this point, investigations may indicate the IgM is monoclonal (single light chain type) in nature. This may be essential in characterizing these patients as having Waldenstrom's macroglobulinemia because the histopathological appearance of this disorder is quite similar to or identical with the pseudolymphoma phase of atypical hyperplasia.

Unlike the lymphomas arising in relation to a pre-existing lymphoepithelial lesion, the development of carcinomas from the metaplastic epithelial islands has not been associated with clinical evidence of a systemic autoimmune disorder. Nor would it be expected. Carcinomatous transformation is a very unusual occurrence, with many of the reported cases manifesting a geographic or racial disposition (Eskimos and Indians).[25, 35] The carcinomas appear as nonkeratinizing carcinomas and often present as malignant caricatures of the epithelial islands. Intraparotid metastases from a primary lesion of the upper airway must always be excluded.

Of the many extrasalivary manifestations of disease found in patients with Sjögren's syndrome, disorders of the lymphoreticular system are prominent. These may be nodal or extranodal. Of the latter, the lungs, kidneys, gastrointestinal tract and spleen are most often involved. It is of further interest that clinical aspects of the syndrome may be absent with only the lymphoepithelial lesion of salivary glands serving as a pathogenetic link.[25]

The unusual pleural and pulmonary complications of Sjögren's syndrome are similar to those seen in rheumatoid arthritis. Similar pulmonary lesions are also found in patients in whom there is no coexistent rheumatic disease; indeed, it is in the sicca complex alone that the pulmonary lesions are most frequently encountered.[25] These lesions are, for the most part, entirely nonspecific (bronchitis, pulmonary infections and pneumonia and bronchiectasis). The findings of lymphomatoid granulomatosis of the lung or lymphoid interstitial pneumonia, are more directly related.[36, 37] According to Sutinen et al.,[36] more than one-quarter of all published cases of lymphoid interstitial pneumonia have been diagnosed in patients with Sjögren's syndrome. The pulmonary disorders are thought to be counterparts to the salivary gland lesion.

A focal lymphocytic minor sialadenitis (labial) has been demonstrated in approximately 70% of patients manifesting Sjögren's syndrome (Fig. 3.6).[38–40] Twenty percent of the patients with rheumatoid arthritis alone will manifest similar findings. Greenspan et al.[40] performed a quantitative study of the inflammatory reactions in lip biopsy specimens. They found the size of the perivascular foci of lymphocytes was directly related to the number of such foci in specimens. The *number* of foci further has served as a valuable index of the severity of major salivary gland involvement and has correlated well with the findings of reduced stimulated parotid flow rate, decreased pertechnetate uptake and beta$_2$-microglobulin concentration in saliva.[41] Patients with a marked lymphocytic infiltration of labial tissues also exhibit (90%) a markedly decreased or absent tear lysozyme concentration.[42]

Biopsy of other mucous gland areas such as the palate and nasal mucous membrane should reveal findings similar to those in labial biopsy specimens, but offers no diagnostic advantage.

It is of interest that epithelial islands are rarely found in labial biopsy material.

The labial biopsy findings in patients with Sjögren's syndrome and progressive systemic sclerosis (scleroderma) have presented a somewhat different pattern (Fig. 3.7). Cipoletti et al.,[43] observing that there is a 17% association between the syndrome and scleroderma, categorized the morphological alterations in the minor salivary glands of the lip as (1) fibrosis with lymphocytes, (2) fibrosis without lymphocytes, and (3) normal. A moderate to marked fibrosis, in the absence of a significant mononuclear cell infiltrate correlated with many severe visceral features of progressive systemic sclerosis. The intralobular fibrosis of the labial salivary glands strongly resembles the changes seen in Brunner's glands of the duodenum. The fibrosis may indeed reflect features of systemic sclerosis rather than being a manifestation of Sjögren's syndrome. In addition, the aggressive fibrosis is consistent with the hypothesis that the scleroderma fibroblast eventually becomes autonomous in its oversynthesis of collagen.

As indicated, the etiology and pathogenesis of Sjögren's syndrome remain obscure. Intensive immunological investigations, however, have led to significant clues. From these studies it is clear that genetic, viral and immunological factors are intermingled and form a changing background on which various immunopathological disorders develop. Investigations in the homologous leukocytic antibody (HLA) system suggest an involvement of the immune-response gene in the pathogenesis. Sjögren's syndrome is primarily involved with HLA-DW^3 and only secondarily with HLA-B8, which is itself strongly associated with DW^3 owing to a linking disequilibrium.[44] The correlation with DW^3/B8 may account for the relationship between Sjögren's disorder and other B8 associated dis-

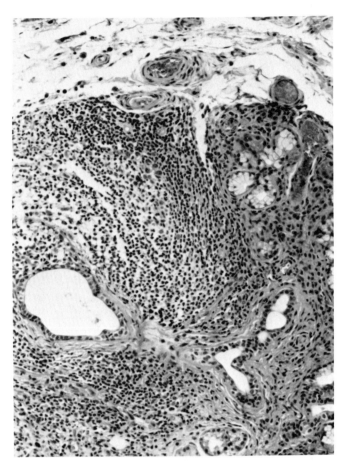

Figure 3.6. Biopsy specimen of the lip from a patient with Sjogren's syndrome. Minor salivary gland acini are replaced by mononuclear (lymphocyte) and plasma cell infiltrate.

eases. The genetic component is further highlighted when one studies the various disorders resulting from the mating of New Zealand (NZB) black mice with other strains.[45] The NZB mouse spontaneously develops an autoimmune disorder with several features like those present in human autoimmune disorders.[46] Mating the NZB mouse to a number of normal mouse strains will result in a complete masking of the autoimmune phenomena. In the human subject any genetic predisposition to Sjögren's syndrome is probably polygenic in nature and difficult to confirm.[47]

Deegan,[45] among others,[48] has reviewed the clinical laboratory findings in Sjögren's syndrome. The hypergammaglobulinemia seen in the majority of patients is usually broad based and polyclonal, with the IgG fraction particularly increased. IgM and IgA levels may also be increased, but not as notably as IgG. Because of intermediate-sized complexes or aggregates of the increased

immunoglobulins a hyperviscosity syndrome may be added to the system complex.[49]

The incidence of rheumatoid factor in Sjögren's syndrome is significantly increased. The variation in frequency in different series is due to the sensitivity of testing measures. Patients with either the sicca complex or the syndrome have rheumatoid factor in their sera. However, the antigenic determinants on the IgG molecule that the factors are directed against differ for the two groups.[45] Lymphocytes obtained from labial biopsies in patients with Sjögren's syndrome actively synthesize rheumatoid factor.[50]

Antinuclear antibodies are quite common in patients with Sjögren's syndrome.[48] Most investigators report their presence in more than 50% of the patients. The patterns are variable. Approximately 10% of patients manifest a positive lupus erythematosus cell (LE) preparation. These patients almost exclusively are those with rheuma-

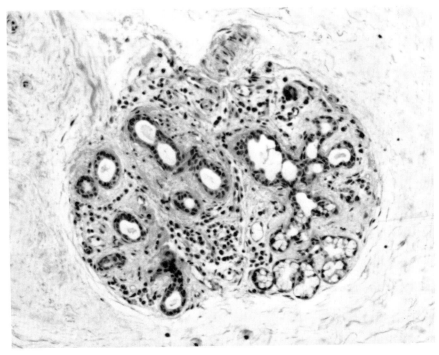

Figure 3.7. Biopsy specimen of the lip from a patient with systemic sclerosis (scleroderma). Note the atrophy of acini produced by collagen and the encasement of the lobule by connective tissue.

toid arthritis. Anti-DNA antibodies are occasionally present in those patients with systemic LE in association with the syndrome. These patients should be observed for the development of systemic LE.

Anti-DNA antibodies are heterogeneous with specifities to distinct antigenic sites on the DNA molecule. Antibodies to native or double-stranded DNA (DS-DNA) and to single-stranded or denatured DNA (SS-DNA) are found in the sera of many subjects with connective tissue diseases. Low levels of DS-DNA antibodies are usually found in Sjögren's syndrome, rheumatoid arthritis, scleroderma, and mixed connective tissue disease. High levels are often associated with systemic LE.

When patients with Sjögren's syndrome are studied for ANA by immunofluorescence, 48 to 68% are positive on tissue substrates but no characteristic pattern of immunofluorescent staining is observed.[48]

Complement fixing and precipitating antibodies to a variety of organ and tissue extracts have been repeatedly demonstrated in patients with Sjögren's syndrome. Antisalivary duct antibodies are present in the sera of about two-thirds of the patients with the syndrome and concomitant rheumatoid arthritis, but are present in less than 20% of the patients with the sicca complex alone.[51] This antibody ap-

pears to be more closely related to the presence of rheumatoid arthritis than Sjögren's syndrome. There is little correlation between its presence and the lymphocytic sialadenitis.

Autoantibodies in Sjögren's syndrome identified by precipitin test with sonicated extract of human tissue culture have been characterized as (1) precipitin SS-A, (2) SS-B, and (3) rheumatoid arthritis precipitin (RAP). Studies have shown that precipitins SS-A and SS-B are present in high frequency in sera from patients with Sjögren's syndrome without associated rheumatoid arthritis and are absent or present in low frequency in many other connective tissue diseases.[48] On the other hand, patients with Sjögren's syndrome and clinical features consistent with rheumatoid arthritis (SS-RA) usually do not have SS-A and SS-B but have RAP. Table 3.3 shows the incidence of specific ANA in Sjögren's sicca syndrome and Sjögren's syndrome with rheumatoid arthritis.

Other autoantibodies detected include those to gastric parietal cells, mitochondria and thyroid gland. There is also an increased incidence of antimitochondrial, antithyroglobulin and antimicrosomal antibodies.[52]

Studies of the cell mediated immune aspects of Sjögren's syndrome indicate an impairment of these mechanisms. Patients with disease limited to

Table 3.3
Frequency of Antibodies to Precipitins SS-A, SS-B and RAP* in Sjögren's Syndrome

Disorder	Percentage of Patients with Positive Test		
	SS-A	SS-B	RAP
SS-Sicca syndrome	70	48	5
SS-Rheumatoid arthritis	9	3	76

* RAP, rheumatoid arthritis precipitin.

the salivary glands are not as impaired as those with rheumatoid arthritis or extrasalivary lymphoid infiltrates. Berry et al.[53] have claimed that 93% of patients with Sjögren's syndrome are reactive to an extracted parotid antigen in a leukocyte migration assay. These same workers also demonstrated a positive correlation between reactivity in the assay system and the extent of lymphoid infiltrate in labial biopsy specimens.

A corollary of the wide variety of antibodies and cell-mediated immune defects can be found also in the NZB mouse.[45] Decreased levels of thymosin are present as early as 2 months of age. This is followed by a loss of suppressor T-cell activity and precedes the emergence of autoantibodies. There further may be a direct correlation between loss of suppressor cell activity and the onset of antibody producing clones of B-cells. The decrease in cell mediated immunity may also impair the animal's immunological surveillance system and lead to the development of malignant lymphoma noted in a large number of older NZB mice. The similarity of many of these features to Sjögren's syndrome, while apparent, requires additional studies.

A viral etiology for Sjögren's syndrome has received considerable support. Virus-like particles have been identified during electron microscopic examination of salivary and other tissues from patients with the syndrome.[54] Antigammaglobulin antibodies, similar to rheumatoid factor, are involved in the neutralization of certain virus-antibody complexes and studies have shown that there is a considerable amount of immunoglobulin and rheumatoid factor synthesis in labial biopsy specimens.[45]

There is little agreement over the proper management of these diseases. From the otolaryngologist's standpoint, there is less controversy. A localized parotid or other salivary gland lesion cannot be accurately diagnosed by clinical methods, and they all should be removed by subtotal parotidectomy. Symptoms of the benign lymphoepithelial lesion are often mild, and no further treatment may be necessary once the diagnosis is established. Often the swelling subsides spontaneously. Recurrences may be treated by further surgery.

The management of Sjögren's syndrome usually requires a joint otolaryngological and medical attack. Treatment is mainly symptomatic. All patients in whom disease is suspected should have a sialogram and biopsy of the parotid, whether or not the gland is enlarged. X-ray therapy would seem to be contraindicated, as it would tend to destroy any remaining functional salivary tissue in the oral cavity and pharynx. A conservative parotidectomy may be required if secondary bacterial infection becomes severe.

SALIVARY GLAND ENLARGEMENT IN SYSTEMIC OR "METABOLIC" DISORDERS

Sialography has permitted an assessment of the normal variation in size of the parotid gland. While there exists considerable interindividual variation in normals, the differences between right and left glands is minimal. In general, there is a reduction in parotid gland mass with increasing age. This is seen chiefly in men.[55] Women in menopause *may* manifest an enlargement.

There is a definite association between asymptomatic parotid gland enlargement and various metabolic diseases or related disorders. Lack of local heat, induration and tenderness differentiate these disorders from an inflammatory parotitis.

The parotid glands are usually the only major salivary glands involved, or their enlargement at least dominates the clinical picture. In many of the enlargements, the etiology and pathogenesis is obscure despite definite relationship to diseases such as obesity, chronic alcoholism and portal cirrhosis. Dietary deficiency (lack or excess) undoubtedly plays a role in many cases, but many patients do not manifest such findings. The occasional patient with *unilateral* involvement, rather than the much more common bilateral and symmetrical enlargement, indicates that local factors may also be implicated. Psychic stimuli to salivary gland secretion also play a role.

Ill-defined acute and chronic phases exist and appear to be in relation to excessive or prolonged stimuli. In the early stages, histological evidence points to this in the relative absence of resting acini and hypertrophy of glandular tissue. The so-called chronic phase may manifest a replacement by fat. The hypertrophy and fatty replacement probably represent various stages of the same process.

Identifiable metabolic disorders such as diabetes mellitus, hypertension, hyperlipidemias and obesity are often so intermixed that the singling out of one as the underlying cause is impossible.

MALNUTRITION

All conditions of starvation or malnutrition predispose the victims to swelling of the parotid gland and, in some communities where malnutrition represents a way of life, swelling of the parotid glands is so widespread that an epidemic is simulated. The term "nutritional mumps" has been applied to these conditions.[56, 57]

Kenaway,[58] studying a large group of natives with asymptomatic parotid gland swelling in the Upper Nile River Valley, found an associated pellagra in 65%, cirrhosis in 31%, diabetes or latent diabetes mellitus in 10% and beriberi in 2% of the study population. Kwashiorkor and a deficiency of vitamin A have also been related to the disorder. Some few reports comment on a higher incidence of parotid gland tumors in patients with chronic enlargement of the gland due to malnutrition, but there are no convincing data.

The parotid enlargement is bilateral or symmetrically diffuse. It is due to an increase in acinar size, where individual cells are enlarged up to 50% of their normal dimension and are distended with secreting granules. If fatty replacement has not occurred, the glands revert to their normal size if adequate nourishment is provided. Replacement of acinar parenchyma of the major salivary glands by fibroadipose tissue is an age-related event. It furthermore is independent of general adiposity. Approximately one-quarter of the parenchymal cell volume is normally lost between childhood and old age.

ASYMPTOMATIC PAROTID GLAND SWELLING AND ALCOHOLIC CIRRHOSIS

This relationship is now well recognized and fully documented. A history of alcoholism and/or an alcoholic-related cirrhosis is diagnostically important. The association of parotid gland enlargement with nonalcoholic cirrhosis is so rare that it can be used as a differential diagnostic feature.[59] The parotid gland swelling may focus attention to an underlying liver disease, sometimes, even in the precirrhotic stage. Decreases or increases in glandular size seem to correlate with improvement or decompensation of the cirrhotic process.

The incidence of asymptomatic parotid gland swelling in association with alcoholism-alcholoic cirrhosis varies from 30 to 80%, with the discrep-

ancies largely due to an overlooking of the glandular disorder in the cirrhotic patient. Sex distribution and age spread parallels that of cirrhosis.

Current evidence suggests that the swellings are more related to a relative or absolute protein deficiency than to an endocrine abnormality associated with the cirrhotic state. There is, however, an often associated gynecomastia. The histological changes are similar to, if indistinguishable from, the affected glands in malnourished patients.

Regardless of the etiological factors, the appearance of the face is fairly characteristic. The parotid gland enlargement is usually bilateral and symmetrical although, on occasion, one gland may show predominance. Normally the parotid glands are not palpable. In this disorder they become easily palpable in the preauricular region and between the ascending ramus of the mandible and the anterior border of the upper part of the sternocleidomastoid muscle. If the enlargement is pronounced, the face assumes a trapezoid configuration with the ears almost hidden in the frontal view.[60] This should not be confused with a similar appearance presenting in patients with hypertrophy of the masseter muscles. In this disorder, there is a "flattening" out effect to the jaw, especially at the angle of the mandible.

Stensen's duct is permeable and the oral orifice is normal. The resting salivary output is within normal limits, but with a periodicity. The amylase activity of the saliva is increased up to threefold over normal. Because of this and because of the histological appearance, Bonnin et al.[61] advocate the use of the term "parotidosis" to signify their belief that the glandular enlargement is an adaption to increased salivary functions.

Sialograms manifest a "leafless winter-tree" appearance because of the lack of normal arborization. This is the result of displacement of the ducts farther from each other and, to a lesser extent, from the compression of the smaller interlobular canaliculi due to acinar hypertrophy. Biopsy specimens have manifested the following histological features in order of decreasing frequency: (1) an increased size of the acini due to increased size of individual acinar cells, which in turn, is due to an increased number of secreting granules; (2) fatty infiltration; and (3) mild to moderate fibrosis, confined to the interlobular septae and without chronic inflammatory cells. The ductal epithelium is seemingly unaffected. The aforementioned findings are not constant and may occur in varying combinations. It is considered that the acinar hypertrophy and increased zymogen granules occur predominantly in early stages, while fatty atrophy and fibrosis dominate the later stages.

The association of parotid gland enlargement and diabetes mellitus is not striking or as convincing as that of cirrhosis and malnutrition. Levine et al.,[62] studying Pima Indians, found that glandular swelling was no more frequent in diabetics than in nondiabetics. Age and obesity were more important in predicting parotid size than the blood sugar concentration. Other metabolic phenomena occurring in diabetics have not been sufficiently excluded, viz., hyperlipoproteinemia. Nonetheless, it has been claimed that the bilateral parotid gland enlargement may be an early warning sign of latent diabetes. There is, however, no evidence that the salivary gland enlargement is due to a compensatory swelling following impairment of the insulogenic functions of the pancreas.

The occasional biopsy specimen has manifested a marked fatty infiltration and some increase of zymogen granules in the acinar epithelium. These are nonspecific and may indeed be related to the fact that most of the subjects are obese.

HYPERSENSITIVITY AND REACTION TO DRUGS

Drug effects on the salivary glands, predominantly the parotid glands, are of two types: (1) idiosyncratic; and (2) direct (iodine and heavy metal) and not on an allergic basis.[12, 63, 64] Allergy has, however, been implicated for some cases of recurrent "parotitis." An inflammatory (clinical) swelling of salivary glands can occur after the injection of certain heavy metals such as mercury and bismuth. The glands are enlarged, edematous and tender.

Iodine "mumps," a diffuse and tender swelling of the salivary glands and surrounding tissues, sometimes occurs 2 or 3 days after the injection of iodide-containing compounds. The swellings persist for 4 to 6 days and then subside. In many instances the submaxillary glands are more affected. Salivary flow is increased and the saliva is clear, much like that in heavy metal-induced enlargement.

Salivary gland enlargement has also been recorded as an idiosyncratic side-effect of a small number of widely differing drugs. In view of the widespread use of medications, this adverse reaction must be considered comparatively rare. Atropine with its know drying effect produces enlargement of the glands due to the inability of the more viscid, thick saliva to exit from the gland and the ducts.

In a like manner, any drug causing xerostomia predisposes to an ascending parotitis. Phenylbutazone, capable of producing "dry-mouths" in nearly 20% of patients taking the drug, may have the rare complication of parotid enlargement. Oxyphenbutazone has also been incriminated. Recurrent salivary gland enlargement can, however, occur without evidence of an ascending infection. This is described in patients receiving phenothiazine derivatives, all of which exert an atropine-like action. Isoproterenol has a sialadenotropic action in rats and has been associated with salivary gland enlargement in man.[65] Methimazole, thiocyanates and thiourea drugs may have salivary gland enlargement as a side effect.

SIALOLITHIASIS AND OTHER OCCLUSIVE DISEASES OF SALIVARY GLANDS

In contrast to tumors which have their greatest frequency in the parotid gland, between 80 and 90% of all salivary gland calculi occur in the submandibular gland.[66, 67] Less than 20% are found in the parotid gland and only 1% in the sublingual gland. The calculi in the minor salivary glands are located in the mucosa of the anterior part of the oral cavity, usually in proximity to the labial commissure, and are generally small, firm, nontender movable nodules usually covered by a normal mucosa.

Calculi are present in nearly two-thirds of patients with chronic sialadenitis. A single calculus is present in approximately 75% of cases, and involvement of more than one salivary gland is seen in less than 3% of cases. Sialolithiasis is a disease of middle age, affecting men slightly more often than women. Calculi in the salivary gland of children are rare entities and occur most often in the submandibular gland.

The calculi are predominantly composed of calcium phosphate in the form of hydroxyapatite with small amounts of magnesium, carbonate and ammonium. The organic matrix is made of various carbohydrates and amino acids. Signs and symptoms vary somewhat, depending on the glands involved and the position of the calculus in the gland. Minor salivary gland calculi appear as asymptomatic, usually freely movable, submucosal nodules, no greater than 0.5 cm. Sialoliths within the glandular parenchyma are associated with less severe symptoms than those producing duct obstruction.

The characteristic signs and symptoms of sialolithiasis of the major glands in the early stages are recurrent episodes of pain and swelling, usually associated with eating, lasting 2 to 3 hours, and then gradually subsiding. Subsequently, if obstruction is not relieved, and this is particularly true for parotid duct calculi, there is an associated infection (*Streptococcus viridans* most often) and symptoms increase in severity, swellings do not subside and relationship to meals is not as clearly defined.

Associated signs and symptoms in patients with submandibular gland obstruction are: (1) unilateral sore throat or swelling which is unrelated to a pharyngitis and is not responsive to the usual form of treatment; (2) palpable submandibular lymph nodes, especially within the gland itself; (3) a palpable or visible concretion within Wharton's duct, and/or similar palpable masses within the gland proper; and (4) expression of a purulent exudate.

Calculi of the parotid gland (Fig. 3.8) and Stensen's duct are smaller than those of the submandibular gland and, in contrast to the symptoms of calculi produced in the latter, may be seemingly unrelated to food intake and often prolonged for several days. This has been related to the greater ease of secondary infection and also because the patient has neglected the early signs and symptoms, usually seeking medical attention after the condition has been present for 2 or more years.

The diagnosis of sialolithiasis is made through a combination of the clinical history, palpation and radiography. The smaller size of parotid calculi has already been noted. In addition to this they tend to crumble more easily than those of the submandibular gland. They are not often palpable because of the deeper anatomical location of Sten-

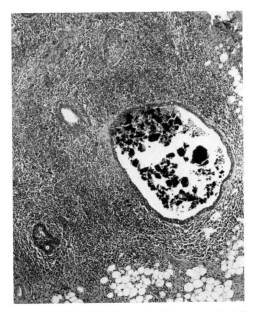

Figure 3.8. Parotid gland sialolith surrounded by heavy chromic inflammatory infiltrate. There is marked metaplasia of the duct linings.

sen's duct. Radiographic examination may not be helpful since, again in contrast to the submandibular gland, the majority of parotid calculi are radiolucent. In the radiographic investigation of parotid gland calculi, intraoral films are essential. In other projections they may be obscured by the teeth or bone and show only as a negative shadow in a sialogram. For submandibular calculi, occlusal radiographs will reveal the location, size and number of calculi in nearly 90 to 95% of cases. Sialography and probing of the ducts for diagnostic purposes are probably contraindicated, not only because of the lack of significant additional information gained, but also because the hazards of infection are too great.

Treatment varies with the duration and severity of the symptoms and with the location and number of calculi. For the rare minor salivary gland stone, excisional biopsy is recommended. Elsewhere, where feasible, the offending stone should be removed, with the foreknowledge that this procedure may not be curative and that recurrences, especially in the parotid gland, will manifest themselves. The most satisfactory way to treat calculi of the submandibular gland is by total removal of the gland. Parotidectomy is indicated for those patients with secondary chronic and recurrent sialadenitis and sialolithiasis of that gland.

Hamartomatous or acquired vascular lesions about the parotid gland may clinically mimic a primary parotid lesion. Because calcification of an intravascular thrombus (phlebolith) may also present radiographically as a salivary calculus, a differential diagnosis may be difficult. Table 3.4 from O'Riordan[68] lists some of the radiological features of phleboliths and salivary calculi.

Other, considerably rarer causes for obstructive sialoadenopathy are edematous stenosis of the ducts, strictures, congenital atresia of ducts, indi-

Table 3.4
Radiological Features of Salivary Calculi and Phleboliths

Calculus	Phlebolith
Uniformly opaque; may be laminated, if large, especially in the submandibular gland	Usually laminated with opaque centers, uniformly opaque, if small
Usually shaped by duct and, therefore, elongated	Usually circular
One or two*	Multiple
Sialography, filling defect at site	Sialography, outside of duct system

* Salivary calculi are rarely multiple, whereas phleboliths are usually multiple.

rect main duct obstruction from diseases of an accessory lobule and trauma to the parotid papilla caused by cheek biting, ill-fitting dentures and pericoronitis.

Stricture obstruction of Stensen's and Wharton's ducts have been divided into (1) papillary obstruction, which may be either acute ulcerative obstruction or chronic fibrotic stenosis, and (2) duct obstruction. This differential is important since it dictates management. Acute ulcerative papillary obstruction is usually caused by acute trauma to the papilla and is treated conservatively with saline rinses and massage. In the chronic form, scarring is present and if the gland is normal, papillotomy and ductoplasty is carried out.[9]

CYSTS, PSEUDOCYSTS, FISTULAE AND SIALECTASIS OF THE SALIVARY GLANDS

Cystic lesions, as a group, comprise approximately 5% of all salivary gland tumors, but, if neoplasms are excluded, this number is reduced considerably. Their importance, however, lies in the fact that the majority are unilateral and, in almost one-half of the cases, they have simulated a mixed tumor, necessitating surgical removal and histopathological examination.

True cysts are unusual and occur most often in the parotid gland. They manifest considerable variation in their linings, cuboidal duct-like or tall mucus-secreting cells with occasional zones of squamous metaplasia to the rare epidermoid cyst or keratoma. Mucoceles, are most often not true cysts (vide infra). The simple cysts, keratomas, and occasionally mucoceles must be distinguished from mucoepidermoid tumors. Rarer cysts are the branchial cysts. Those originating from the second branchial cleft may present in the lower pole of the parotid gland, while the first branchial cleft occurs in the preauricular position of the gland. Bilateral cystic disease may occasionally be found in the salivary glands of children with fibrocystic disease of the pancreas and may rarely be manifested as congenital bilateral polycystic parotid glands.[69]

Cystic lesions of the branchial apparatus are discussed more fully in Chapter 26. It is pertinent, however, to present here the infrequently reported *lymphoepithelial cyst* of the parotid gland and immediate environs. Bhaskar and Bernier[70, 71] avoid calling these lesions "branchial cysts" since this would imply a specific embryological origin for these cysts. They consider the terms, "benign lymphoepithelial cyst" or "benign cystic lymph nodes" as more appropriate. It is highly probable, how-

ever, that these lesions arise from remnants of the branchial apparatus. By 1973 only 20 cases had been reported in the literature,[72] a clear underrepresentation.[73] All of the lesions have been unilateral and most have been diagnosed in patients who have been in their fifth decade of life. Their size has varied from 1.0 to 7.0 cm. Besides an integral lymphoid component, the cysts manifest a lining of squamous, cuboidal, columnar, or any combination of these cells. Although most authors do not make the distinction, Bhaskar and Bernier[70] reported that over four-fifths of the lesions contained medullary sinusoids within the lymphoid tissue. The contents of the cysts vary from a thinwatery fluid to a thick, opaque and gelatinous material. While these lesions are clearly lymphoepithelial in their composition, they have not had any relationship to the lymphoepithelial lesion of chronic sialadenitis or any immune disorders.

Salivary gland fistulae are mainly characterized by a unilateral swelling in the area of the duct or by the flow of saliva into the skin surface. Rarely does a fistulae open to the oral mucous membrane. Because of their susceptibility to trauma, the parotid gland ducts are most commonly involved. The disorder is almost always the result of traumatic severance of the duct.

Mucous plugs may well be more prevalent than calculi as a cause for parotid gland obstruction. In contrast to parotid gland calculi that are usually located in Stensen's duct, mucous plugs are generally found within major ducts of the gland itself. They also manifest a greater tendency for recurrences.

Mucous retention cysts, mucoceles and ranulas constitute a related group of lesions capable of producing salivary gland enlargement.

The mucosa of the oral cavity abounds with small mucous glands. Retention of the secretions from these glands leads to mucous retention cysts *or* mucoceles.[74] They are most frequently located on the mucosal aspects of the lips, cheeks and ventral surfaces of the tongue.[75] They occasionally may present on the dorsal surface of the tongue or palate. Within the oral cavity these lesions are painless, soft tissue swellings which are fluctuant. As they enlarge and approach the surface they manifest a typical bluish-white "frog-belly" appearance. Their protrusion into the oral cavity makes them susceptible to trauma.

For many years it has been considered that stenosis or obstruction of the excretory ducts of salivary glands was responsible for mucoceles and mucous retention cysts. Since the investigation of Bhaskar et al.,[76] and surgical pathological confirmation that most mucoceles are devoid of an epithelial lining, pathological distinction must be made between mucous retention cysts and mucocele. The latter, while it may evolve from a mucous retention cyst, does not represent true cystic formation of an obstructive origin. In the majority of reported series, mucoceles do not possess an epithelial lining. Rather they represent an extravasation of mucus into the surrounding tissues. Epithelial-lined mucous cysts (mucous glands or metaplastic squamous cells) result from intermittent duct obstruction. Complete block of an excretory duct leads to atrophy (a sclerosing sialadenitis) rather than the formation of a mucocele.[77] The theory that mucoceles represent extravasation of mucus is substantiated by findings after severance of the submaxillary ducts in rats, where escape of mucus into the surrounding tissue forms a mucocele comparable to the human type, whereas direct ligation produces acinar atrophy.

Treatment for mucoceles-mucous retention cysts is surgical excision, either partial by marsupialization, or complete. Shira[74] has outlined techniques. Escape of the contents of a mucous retention cyst during trauma or surgical removal will lead to recurrence in the form of a mucocele. For both lesions it is frequently difficult to determine exactly the extent and margins of the lesions.

The ranula is usually a retention phenomena in the floor of the mouth and results from obstruction of the duct of the major salivary glands, usually the sublingual gland. Some represent remnants of the cervical sinuses.

Two varieties of ranula may be defined. Each has a different clinical behavior and appearance, and each requires different methods of treatment. These two varieties have been called simple ranulas and plunging ranulas. The simple ranula is a true retention cyst of the numerous salivary glands that lie in the submucosal layers of the lining of the oral cavity. It is epithelially lined and results from obstruction of ducts. The plunging ranula extends beyond the mucous membranes into the floor of the mouth and into the fascial planes of the neck. The extent of the plunging ranula is considered to be a function of time and they are almost always the result of mucous extravasation. Therefore, they are more correctly pseudocysts. These pseudocysts may appear either as the classical sublingual ranula or as a submandibular mass without visible intraoral connection. The simple ranula is usually unilateral, painless and of a translucent bluish appearance. If large, they can cause deviation of the tongue and cross the midline submucosally. They may rupture spontaneously.

Treatment of the smaller ranulas in the floor of the mouth is performed primarily by excision or marsupialization of the cyst wall. Plunging ranulas provide a greater challenge. According to Quick and Lowell,[78] the accepted technique consists of meticulous dissection of the pseudocyst and an excision in continuity with the sublingual gland of origin.

MISCELLANEOUS CAUSES

Bilateral and symmetrical enlargement of the parotid glands has been seen in association with chronic relapsing pancreatitis. Sialographic examination and the few tissue specimens examined are indistinguishable from the parotid enlargement associated with cirrhosis and malnutrition.

Uremia may be a rare cause of salivary gland (parotid and submaxillary) enlargement. The glands may remain enlarged for long periods of time and manifest a decreased salivary flow and sluggish responses to stimuli. High local concentration of ammonia may be important in the genesis.

Blatt[79] has described a parotid-masseter hypertrophy—traumatic occlusion syndrome. The syndrome ranges from simple glandular swelling and associated pain to a recurring obstructive sialodochitis. The salivary gland swelling is apparently caused when the buccomasseteric portion of Stensen's duct is compressed by traumatic occlusion or masseteric hypertrophy.

Pneumoparotitis results in certain patients who produce a high intrabuccal pressure. The clinical state is usually complicated by infection of the gland and probably by an underlying congenital predisposition. Partially related to the foregoing are the subparotid and submandibular gland swellings that occur rarely during endoscopy (approximately 1:1,000 endoscopic examinations).[80] These are usually bilateral and completely painless. The swellings are of two etiological types: (1) those due to direct temporary duct occlusion during endoscopy; and (2) those due to filling of cervical air sacs representing blind branchial cleft remnants. The former decompresses spontaneously in 2 to 12 hours; the latter can be deflated by local pressure.

Intubation is also responsible for rather striking enlargement of all salivary glands during induction of anesthesia. In this instance, however, it is postulated that an overactive pharyngeal reflex is triggered by the instrumentation, and this produces a vasodilation and hyperemia of the salivary glands.[81]

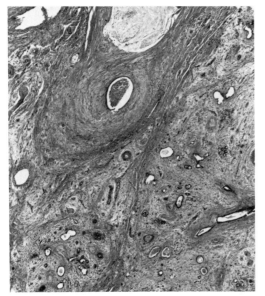

Figure 3.9. Postirradiation sialadenitis (chronic). Only ductal elements persist in a matrix of connective tissue.

Unusual and not clear-cut causes are parotid swelling related to "school phobia," where alpha-adrenergic stimulation is cited as the cause,[82] and excessive corn starch ingestion over a prolonged period of time.[83]

IRRADIATION SIALADENITIS

Acute, tender and painful swelling of the major salivary glands has long been recognized as a sequel to irradiation to the head and neck regions. Early and constantly following acute radiation damage to the salivary glands there is an elevation of serum and urinary amylase, a qualitative and quantitative alteration of the saliva leading to an invariable dryness of the mouth between 2 and 6 hours after irradiation and certain dental lesions which do not occur when only teeth are irradiated.[84]

The histological changes observed in the glands are in harmony with the clinical features and hyperamylasemia. The acute reaction varies with the serous-mucous composition of the salivary glands. Serous glands and acini are far more susceptible to injury. Marked degranulation, disruption of serous cells and pools of zymogen granules appear in acini and are directly related to the dose or level of radiation. In many parotid glands, acinar arrangement may be indiscernible, and the serous cells become vacuolated and appear near rupture. In contrast, the epithelial lining of inter-

calated and interlobular ducts remains intact and the larger secreting ducts are only moderately dilated. Mucous portions of salivary glands manifest little, if any, histological changes. An acute inflammatory reaction accompanies these cellular changes and is manifested by purulent exudate in ducts, suppurative foci along the septae and cell infiltrates in the serous acini.

In spite of these microscopic findings of severe acute tissue damage, systemic abnormalities are uncommon and the reaction subsides rather quickly without specific therapy. The acute alterations progress to a chronic stage where the glands have few, if any, acini left and consist of a ductal framework with interlobular and periductal fibrosis and chronic inflammatory cells.[85] Subsequently atrophy of the gland occurs (Fig. 3.9).

REFERENCES

1. Brill, S. J., and Gilfillan, R. F.: Acute parotitis associated with influenza type A.: A report of twelve cases. New Engl. J. Med. 296:1391, 1977.
2. Schwartz, A. W., Devine, K. N., and Beahrs, O. H.: Acute postoperative parotitis ("surgical mumps"). Plast. Reconstr. Surg. 25:51, 1966.
3. Beahrs, O. H., and Woolner, L. B.: Surgical treatment of disease of salivary glands. J. Oral Surg. 27:119, 1969.
4. Lundgren, A., Kylen, P., and Odkvist, L. M.: Nosocomial parotitis. Acta Otolaryngol. 82:275, 1976.
5. Leake, D. L., Krakowiak, F. J., and Leake, K. C.: Suppurative parotitis in children. Oral Surg. 31:174, 1971.
6. Kaban, L. B., Mulliken, J. B., and Murray, J. E.: Sialadenitis in childhood. Am. J. Surg. 135:570, 1978.
7. Casterline, P. F., and Jaques, D. A.: The surgical management of recurrent parotitis. Surg. Gynec. Obstet. 146:419, 1978.
8. Donohue, W. B., and Bolden, T. E.: Tuberculosis of the salivary glands: a collective review. Oral Surg. 14:576, 1961.
9. Epker, B. N.: Obstructive inflammatory disease of the major salivary glands. Oral Surg. 33:2, 1972.
10. Wong, M. L., and Jafek, B. W.: Cervical mycobacterial disease. Tr. Am. Acad. Ophth. Otol. 78:75, 1974.
11. Hammer, J. E., and Scofield, H. H.: Cervical lymphadenopathy and parotid gland swelling in sarcoidosis: a study of 31 cases. J. Am. Dent. Assoc. 74:1224, 1967.
12. Banks, P.: Non-neoplastic parotid swelling: a review. Oral Surg. 25:732, 1968.
13. Maynard, J. D.: Recurrent parotid enlargement. Br. J. Surg. 52:784, 1965.
14. Tandler, B.: Ultrastructure of chronically inflamed human submandibular gland. Arch. Pathol. Lab. Med. 101:425, 1977.
15. Räsänen, O., Jokinen, K., and Dammert, K.: Sclerosing inflammation of the submandibular salivary gland (Kuttner tumour). Acta Otolaryngol. 74:297, 1972.
16. Seifert, G., and Donath, K.: Die Morphologie der Speicheldrüsenerkrankungen. Arch. Otorhinolaryngol. 213:111, 1976.
17. Patey, D. H., and Thackray, A. C.: Chronic "sialectatic" parotitis in the light of pathological studies on parotidectomy material. Br. J. Surg. 43:43, 1955.
18. Bark, C. J., and Perzik, S. L.: Mikulicz's disease, sialoangiectasis, and autoimmunity based upon a study of parotid lesions. Am. J. Clin. Pathol. 49:683, 1968.
19. Blatt, I. M.: On sialectasis and benign lymphosialadenopathy. Laryngoscope 74:1684, 1964.
20. Furstenberg, A. C., and Blatt, I. M.: Intermittent parotid

swelling due to ill-fitting dentures—an entity, its diagnosis and treatment. Laryngoscope 68:1165, 1958.

21. Waterhouse, J. P.: Inflammation in the salivary glands. Br. J. Oral Surg. 3:161, 1966.

22. Chisholm, D. M., Waterhouse, J. P., and Mason, D. K.: Lymphocytic sialadenitis in the major and minor glands: a correlation in postmortem subjects. J. Clin. Pathol. 23: 690, 1970.

23. Kerr, D.: Personal communication.

24. von Mikulicz, J.: Concerning a peculiar symmetrical disease of the lacrimal and salivary glands. Med. Class. 2:165, 1937.

25. Batsakis, J. G., Bernacki, E. G., Rice, D. H., and Stebler, M. E.: Malignancy and the benign lymphoepithelial lesion. Laryngoscope 85:389, 1975.

26. Hemenway, W. G.: Chronic punctate parotitis. Laryngoscope 61:485, 1971.

27. Godwin, J. T.: Benign lymphoepithelial lesion of the parotid gland (adenolymphoma, chronic inflammation, lymphoepithelioma, lymphocytic tumor, Mikulicz disease): report of eleven cases. Cancer 5:1089, 1952.

28. Morgan, W. S., and Castleman, B.: A clinicopathologic study of Mikulicz's disease. Am. J. Pathol. 29:471, 1953.

29. Boquist, L., Kumilien, A., and Ostberg, Y.: Ultrastructural findings in a case of benign lymphoepithelial lesion (Sjogren's syndrome). Acta Otolaryngol. 70:216, 1970.

30. Yarington, C. T., and Zagibe, F. T.: The ultrasturcture of the benign lympho-epithelial lesion. J. Laryngol. 83:361, 1969.

31. Hyman, G. A., and Wolff, M.: Malignant lymphomas of the salivary glands: review of the literature and report of 33 new cases, including four cases associated with the lymphoepithelial lesion. Am. J. Clin. Pathol. 65:421, 1976.

32. Thomas, P.: Sjogren's syndrome disimmunoglobulinemia and malignant disease. Post. Med. J. 49:349, 1973.

33. Causey, J. Q.: The benign lymphoepithelial lesion—a harbinger of neoplasia. S. Med. J. 69:60, 1976.

34. Azzopardi, J. G., and Evans, D. J.: Malignant lymphoma of parotid associated with Mikulicz disease (benign lymphoepithelial lesion). J. Clin. Pathol. 24:744, 1971.

35. Arthaud, J. B.: Anaplastic parotid carcinoma. ("Malignant lymphoepithelial lesion") in seven Alaskan natives. Am. J. Clin. Pathol. 57:275, 1972.

36. Sutinen, S., Sutinen, S., and Huhti, E.: Ultrastructure of lymphoid interstitial pneumonia. Virus-like particles in bronchiolar epithelium of a patient with Sjogren's syndrome. Am. J. Clin. Pathol. 67:328, 1977.

37. Weisbrot, I. M.: Lymphomatoid granulomatosis of the lung, associated with a long history of benign lymphoepithelial lesions of the salivary glands and lymphoid interstitial pneumonitis. Report of a case. Am. J. Clin. Pathol. 66: 1792, 1976.

38. Chisholm, D. M., and Mason, D.: Labial salivary gland biopsy in Sjogren's disease. J. Clin. Pathol. 21:656, 1968.

39. Berry, H., Bacon, P. A., and Davis, J. D.: Cell-mediated immunity in Sjogren's syndrome. Ann. Rheum. Dis. 31: 298, 1972.

40. Greenspan, J. S., Daniels, T. E., Talal, N., and Sylvester, R. A.: The histopathology of Sjogren's syndrome in labial salivary gland biopsies. Oral Surg. 32:217, 1974.

41. Michalski, J. P., Daniels, T. E., Talal, N., and Grey, H. M.: Beta$_2$ microglobulin and lymphocytic infiltration in Sjogren's syndrome. New Engl. J. Med. 293:1228, 1975.

42. Tabbara, K. F., Ostler, H. B., Daniels, T. E., Sylvester, R. A., Greenspan, J. S., and Talal, N.: Sjogren's syndrome: a correlation between ocular findings and labial salivary gland histology. Trans. Am. Acad. Ophth. Otolaryngol. 78:467, 1974.

43. Cipoletti, J. F., Buckingham, R. B., Barnes, E. L., Peel, R. L., Mahmood, K., Cignetti, F. E., Pierce, J. M., Rabin, B. S., and Rodnan, G. P.: Sjogren's syndrome in progressive systemic sclerosis. Ann. Int. Med. 87:535, 1977.

44. Chused, T. M., Kassan, S. S., Opelz, G., Moutsopoulos, H. M., and Terasaki, P. I.: Sjogren's syndrome associated with HLA-Dw3. New Engl. J. Med. 296, 1977.

45. Deegan, M. J.: Immunologic diseases of the salivary glands. Otolaryngol. Clin. N. Am. 10:351, 1977.

46. Carlsoo, B., and Ostberg, Y.: Ultrastructural observations on the parotitis autoimmunica in the NZB/NZW hybrid mice. Acta Otolaryngol. 85:298, 1978.

47. Shearn, M. A.: Sjogren's Syndrome. Philadelphia, W. B. Saunders Co., 1971.

48. Nakamura, R. M., and Tan, E. M.: Recent progress in the study of autoantibodies to nuclear antigens. Hum. Pathol. 9:85, 1978.

49. Blaylock, W. M., Waller, M., and Normansell, D. E.: Sjogren's syndrome: hyperviscosity and intermediate complexes. Ann. Int. Med. 80:27, 1974.

50. Anderson, L. G., Cummings, N. A., Asofsky, R., Hylton, M. B., Tarpley, T. M., Tomasi, T. B., Wolf, R. O., Schall, G. L., and Talal, N.: Salivary immunoglobulin and rheumatoid factor synthesis in Sjogren's syndrome. Am. J. Med. 53:456, 1972.

51. Whaley, K., Webb, J., McAvoy, B. A., Hughes, G. R. V., Lee, P., MacSween, R. N. M., and Buchanan, W. W.: Sjogren's syndrome. II. Clinical associations and immunological phenomena. Quart. J. Med. 42:513, 1973.

52. Anderson, L. G., Tarpley, T. M., Talal, N., Cummings, N. A., Wolf, R. O., and Schall, G. G.: Cellular-versus-humoral autoimmune responses to salivary gland in Sjogren's syndrome. Clin. Exp. Immunol. 13:335, 1973.

53. Berry, H., Bacon, P. A., and Davis, J. D.: Cell-mediated immunity in Sjogren's syndrome. Ann. Rheum. Dis. 31: 298, 1972.

54. Shearn, M. A., Tu, W. H., Stephen, B. G., and Lee, J. C.: Virus-like structures in Sjogren's syndrome. Lancet 1:568, 1970.

55. Ericson, S.: The normal variation of the parotid size. Acta Otolaryngol. 70:294, 1970.

56. DuPlessis, D. J.: Parotid enlargement in malnutrition. S. Afr. Med. J. 30:700, 1956.

57. Nash, L., and Morrison, L. F.: Asymptomatic chronic enlargement of the parotid glands: review and report of a case. Ann. Otol. Rhinol. Laryngol. 58:646, 1949.

58. Kenaway, R. M.: Endemic enlargement of the parotid gland in Egypt. Trans. R. Soc. Trop. Med. Hyg. 31:339, 1937.

59. Borsanyi, S. J., and Blanchard, C. L.: Asymptomatic enlargement of the parotid glands in alcoholic cirrhosis. South. Med. J. 54:678, 1961.

60. Borsanyi, S., and Blanchard, C. L.: Asymptomatic enlargement of the parotid glands: its diagnostic significance and particular relation to Laennec's cirrhosis. J. A. M. A. 174: 20, 1960.

61. Bonnin, H., Moretti, G., and Geyer, A.: Les grosses parotides des cirrhoses alcoliques. Presse Med. 62:1449, 1954.

62. Levine, S. B., Sampliner, R. E., Bennett, P. H., Rushforth, N. B., Burch, T. A., and Miller, M.: Asymptomatic parotid enlargement in Pima Indians: Relationship to age, obesity, and diabetes mellitus. Ann. Intern. Med. 73:571, 1970.

63. Banks, P.: Hypersensitivity and drug reactions involving the parotid gland. Br. J. Oral Surg. 5:60, 1967.

64. Sprinkle, P. M.: Recurrent salivary gland disease. Laryngoscope 78:654, 1968.

65. Borsanyi, S. J.: Chronic asymptomatic enlargement of the parotid glands. Ann. Otol. Rhinol. Laryngol. 71:857, 1962.

66. Blatt, I. M.: Studies in sialolithiasis. III. Pathogenesis, diagnosis and treatment. South Med. J. 57:723, 1964.

67. Holst, E.: Sialolithiasis of minor salivary glands: report of 3 cases. J. Oral Surg. 26:354, 1968.

68. O'Riordan, B.: Phleboliths and salivary calculi. Br. J. Oral Surg. 12:119, 1974.

69. Mihalyka, E. E.: Congenital bilateral polycystic parotid glands. J. A. M. A. 181:634, 1962.

70. Bhaskar, S. N., and Bernier, J. L.: Histogenesis of branchial cysts. Am. J. Pathol. 35:407, 1959.

71. Bernier, J. L., and Bhaskar, S. N.: Lymphoepithelial lesions of salivary glands. Cancer 11:1156, 1958.

72. Weitzner, S.: Lymphoepithelial (branchial) cyst of parotid gland. Oral Surg. 35:85, 1973.

73. Richardson, G. S., Clairmont, A. A., and Erickson, E. R.:

Cystic lesions of the parotid gland. Plast. Reconstr. Surg. 61:364, 1978.

74. Shira, R.: Simplified technic for the management of mucoceles and ranulas. J. Oral Surg. 20:374, 1962.

75. Cataldo, E., and Mosadomi, A.: Mucoceles of the oral mucous membrane. Arch. Otolaryngal. 91:360, 1970.

76. Bhaskar, S. M., Bolden, T. E., and Weinnmann, J. P.: Pathogenesis of mucoceles. J. Dent. Res. 35:863, 1956.

77. Sela, J., and Ulmansky, M.: Mucous retention cyst of salivary glands. J. Oral Surg. 27:619, 1969.

78. Quick, C. A., and Lowell, S. H.: Ranula and the sublingual salivary glands. Arch. Otolaryngol. 103:397, 1977.

79. Blatt, I. M.: The parotid-masseter hypertrophy—traumatic occlusion syndrome. Laryngoscope 79:624, 1969.

80. Slaughter, R. L., and Boyce, H. W., Jr.: Submaxillary salivary gland swelling developing during peroral endoscopy. Gastroenterology 57:83, 1969.

81. Bonchek, L. I.: Salivary gland enlargement during induction of anesthesia. J. A. M. A. 209:1716, 1969.

82. Rosefsky, J. B.: Parotid swelling and school phobia. Arch. Otolaryingol. 92:390, 1970.

83. Jastak, R.: An unusual cause of parotid enlargement. Henry Ford Hosp. Med. J. 15:259, 1967.

84. Kashima, H. K., Kirham, W. R., and Andrews, J. R.: Postirradiation sialadenitis: a study of the clinical features, histopathologic changes and serum enzyme variation following irradiation of human salivary glands. Am. J. Roentgenol. Radium Ther. Nucl. Med. 94:271, 1965.

85. Seifert, G., and Geier, W.: Zur Pathologie der Strahlen-Sialadenitis. Z. Laryng. Rhinol. 50:385, 1971.

CHAPTER 4

"Leukoplakia," "Keratosis" and Intraepithelial Squamous Cell Carcinoma of the Head and Neck

The histopathological diagnoses of lesions arising from the two "biologically cheap" tissues of the human body—squamous epithelium and fibrous connective tissue—are made more often than the pathologist would like to admit by subjective rather than objective analysis. For borderline squamous lesions, particularly of the oral regions, upper respiratory tract, and the uterine cervix, institutions and individual pathologists may be categorized as conservative or aggressive in their diagnoses, each according to their subjective training. This subjectivity has spawned a number of imprecise and often indefinable criteria and diagnostic terms. "Premalignant," atypical hyperplasia, leukoplakia, keratosis, pachyderma, etc., are examples of the latter in common usage. One should be chary in his use of the adjective "premalignant." According to current nomenclature, the term implies a condition which may either be reversible *or* may eventually result in recognizable malignancy.

There have been only isolated studies showing an evolution from a benign lesion to a malignant one. McGavran et al.,[1] studying laryngeal keratosis, put the situation in proper perspective: "In our opinion the premalignant nature of keratosis and the metamorphosis of keratosis to cancer are based in the main upon repetition of previously reported cases with an increment each time of a few more clinical cases. These studies certainly raise the question of a premalignant state, but they hardly serve to provide the requisite clinical proof."[1]

The circumstantial evidence is admittedly strong, especially when in situ carcinoma or severe dysplasia is adjacent to areas of infiltrating squamous carcinoma. In the very broadest of contexts, these lesions may then be considered "premalig-nant." But if we extend the concept further, chronic inflammation in the mouth and larynx secondary to local irritation may also be considered premalignant, and the very breadth of the concept reduces its value to an academic rather than clinical usefulness.

Benign squamous cell hyperplasias should not be confused with squamous cell carcinomas in the upper aerodigestive tracts. Most often the lesions are epithelial responses to injury. Some may present as clinical leukoplakia or clinical keratosis (vide infra), while others are localized papillomatous lesions. In the oral cavity, the squamous cell hyperplasias occur in a wide range of clinical presentations.

Papillary hyperplasia is often restricted to the hard palate, and with few exceptions to patients with ill-fitting dentures. It has been estimated that 2 to 11% of denture patients will manifest this form of hyperplasia. The principal cause is frictional irritation. Removal or correction of the ill-fitting denture may be followed by regression or disappearance of the lesions. The distribution of the lesions often conforms to the relief area of the denture and may spread up the lingual slope of the alveolar ridge and rarely to the buccal mucosa.

Microscopically there are seen multiple polygonal projections of epithelium arising in a broad base and surrounding or surmounting a vascular, often inflamed connective tissue core. Epithelial hyperplasia may be marked and dyskeratosis may be present. The lesion is exophytic and the surrounding tissue is normal. There have been no documented cases of squamous cell carcinoma arising from this lesion as a precursor.

Pseudoepitheliomatous hyperplasia representing an exaggerated epithelial response to a stimulus or injury is not infrequent in the oral epithelium (Fig. 4.1). The lesion overlies or is at the margin of an inflammatory lesion. It also frequently occurs over the so-called granular cell myoblastoma. The importance of the lesion is in the danger it may be considered a squamous cell carcinoma. A form of primary pseudoepitheliomatous hyperplasia is the keratoacanthoma that occurs singly or occasionally in multiple forms in the oral mucosa, especially the lip.

Two distinctive forms of hyperplasia have attracted considerable attention in the oral surgery literature: white sponge nevus[2-4] and Heck's disease (focal epithelial hyperplasia).[5, 6] White sponge nevus has acquired numerous synonyms since its original description. It is a rare familial ectodermal disorder affecting both sexes equally. The practical significance of the disorder is that it would appear to be entirely benign and usually requires no treatment other than the important step of reassuring the patient. The epithelium is thickened and parakeratotic, with the superficial cells manifesting a "washed out" appearance and pyknotic nuclei. Vacuolation of the cells is prominent. Chronic inflammatory cell reaction in the corium is minimal or absent.

Clinically the disorder presents as a diffuse,

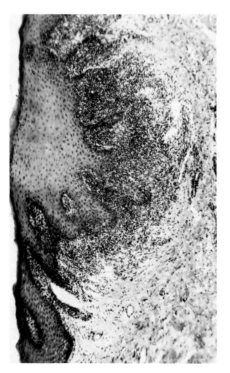

Figure 4.1. Localized hyperplasia in nicotinic stomatitis.

grayish-white lesion appearing as a spongy, soft and asymptomatic change in the mucosa. The entire oral mucosa tends to be involved, with the most obvious lesions on the buccal mucosa, floor of mouth and ventral surface of the tongue. Lesions of a similar character may also be present in the vagina, or the labia and rectum. The disorder may appear at birth, infancy or in childhood and reaches its maximum severity at puberty

The focal epithelial hyperplasia first described by Heck[5, 6] is characterized by an unusual hyperplastic response of the buccal, labial and lingual mucosae in the mouths of a small percentage of American Indian children. Except for isolated single reports in other races, the disorder is strikingly confined to the American Indian ancestry. It has never been observed in an adult. Causal factors are unknown, but the frequent familial occurrence suggests a genetically determined disease. The possibility of a viral origin has not been eliminated. Oral examination reveals multiple, soft, sessile papules which are both discrete and confluent. They may be normal or pale in color. The lower lip is most prominently affected. Microscopic findings consist essentially of acanthosis and parakeratosis of the squamous epithelium without evidence of dyskeratosis.

Oral lichen planus must also be singled out as a source of histopathological difficulty. Lichen planus is a complex chronic mucocutaneous disease which appears in different forms. Because of the variable clinical features and unknown cause, recognition of the disorder is sometimes difficult. As Silverman and Griffith[7] point out, there are reasons for concern regarding the diagnosis, since many patients have symptoms requiring treatment and a tenuous relationship between oral lichen planus and carcinoma has been reported. In the oral cavity lichen planus most often presents in the following forms: *reticular*, a lace-like and/or punctate keratosis overlying a normal-appearing mucosa; *erosive*, an erythematous mucosa with erosion and pseudomembrane formation, associated with a reticular keratotic pattern; *plaque*, a light and homogeneous keratosis. The erosive form is by far the most common. Lichen planus can occur on any oral mucosal site and is usually present in more than one area. The buccal mucosa is involved in over three-quarters of the patients. The occurrence of oral lichen planus in the general population is less than 1%. Even though there appears to be an increased prevalence of squamous cell carcinoma in patients with oral lichen planus, there is no good evidence that the disorder is "premalignant".

Other lesions of the oral mucous membranes besides the foregoing that may appear white on clinical examination are those associated with lupus erythematosus (discoid or systemic) and moniliasis, and, except for the latter (which may be scraped off), these may qualify for the *clinical* designation of leukoplakia. This emphasizes the wide variety of microscopic features that may be found in clinical leukoplakia.

"LEUKOPLAKIA"

The literal meaning of "leukoplakia" is nothing more than white *plaque*, and the term has been used by clinicians and pathologists alike for any mucosal lesion that could be described in this way. Traditionally the term has also carried a "premalignant" connotation. Such a generalization is not warranted, since there are a number of white mucosal lesions in the oral and upper respiratory tract that are either benign or only exceptionally associated with the subsequent appearance of malignancy. A mucosal white patch, however, cannot be dismissed too lightly for, as Hartwell[8] has put it, "If a painless, unobtrusive, or even unnoticed white patch in the mouth had no more significance than a callus on a laborer's hands, then there would be no problem to discuss." The danger is, particularly in intraoral leukoplakia, that the lesion may either be associated with precursor changes of malignancy or actually mask a carcinoma.

As a counter-reaction to the indiscriminate use of the term, many workers in recent years, particularly morphological pathologists, have reserved the term for lesions considered to show *histological* evidence of "premalignancy." This approach is illogical since "premalignancy" is even more elusive than leukoplakia. Furthermore, just as not all white lesions are potentially malignant, so not all potentially malignant lesions appear as white patches. Indeed, the latter often appear erythematous rather than white. Mashberg et al.,[9] in a study of 144 early asymptomatic oral squamous cell carcinomas, found that 98% were erythroplasias or had an erythroplastic component. By contrast only 5% of the lesions were white and without a red component.

The term "leukoplakia," in my opinion, should *never* be used by the pathologist. It is a clinical diagnosis, the histological counterpart of which may range widely and for which no standards or uniformity have or can be applied.[10] Descriptive terms such as hyperplasia, hyperplasia with graded atypism, and "borderline lesions" adequately convey the pathologist's subjective impression of the lesions and are intellectually honest.

To most oral surgeons and head and neck surgeons, the term "leukoplakia" means just what it was originally intended, i.e., a white patch.[11, 12] The occurrence of a white area, flat or raised, in the mucous membranes depends heavily on the presence of a cornified opaque zone on the surface. In healthy oral mucosa, there is an orderly progression of epithelial cells toward the surface, and a continuous desquamation takes place without keratin accumulation. The underlying changes in the squamous epithelium may range from a harmless hyperplasia to invasive carcinoma.

The usual leukoplakic lesion falls into three basic categories: (1) a simple keratosis as a response to a mild irritant or stimulus. The width of the stratum corneum is increased and there may also be an accentuation of the stratum granulosum with acanthosis. Some extension of the rete ridges may be apparent, particularly in the mucosa of the tongue and alveolar mucosa. Chronic inflammation is usually minimal or absent; (2) various combinations of hyperkeratosis, parakeratosis and acanthosis with inflammatory reaction beneath the epithelium; (3) a mucosal lesion which, while probably manifesting hyperkeratosis, is, however, dominated by dyskeratosis or variable degrees of abnormal orientation and proliferation of epithelial cells. In this form, the width of the stratum corneum may be very great or minimal. If the atypicality is severe, differentiation from intramucosal carcinoma (carcinoma in situ) may be difficult. In these borderline lesions, subjectivity plays its greatest role in the interpretation by the pathologist.

Clinical oral leukoplakia is not uncommon and is found most often in men over the age of 40 years (90%). As indicated, there is little correlation between the clinical appearance of the leukoplakic lesions and their histological features. Waldron and Shafer[13] reviewed 3,256 tissue specimens clinically diagnosed as leukoplakia ("keratosis," "white patch"). Microscopic study showed that 80% were varying combinations of hyperorthokeratosis, hyperparakeratosis, and acanthosis without evidence of epithelial dysplasia. Mild to moderate dysplasia was noted in 12% of specimens and severe epithelial dysplasia or carcinoma in situ was found in 4.5%. Infiltrating squamous cell carcinoma was diagnosed in 3% of the specimens. The region at greatest risk for "leukoplakic cancer" is the floor of the mouth.

The buccal mucosa is the site of greatest occurrence in the mouth, followed by the alveolar mucosa, tongue, lip, palate, floor of mouth and gingiva, in that order. In the buccal mucosa, the lesions are particularly common at the occlusal line, where irritation from malocclusion or bad occlusal habits are most likely to be manifested. The mucosa of the lower lip is an area of predeliction in pipe smokers and the hard palate is a common site in both the pipe and cigarette smoker.

The number of cases of leukoplakia that may progress to carcinoma can not be assessed with clarity, but there is a significant association of all varieties of leukoplakia adjacent to surgically removed oral cancer. Predictions of the development of "leukoplakia" into carcinoma have ranged from 2 to 70% and reflect the variable criteria for histological diagnosis. Excellent reviews concerning this association have been provided.[14, 15]

"ERYTHROPLAKIA"

The term "erythroplakia" has been used to describe the *clinical* appearance of a red patch of the mucous membrane which does not represent some specific or nonspecific inflammatory lesions.[16] Thus, like leukoplakia, the term carries no histopathological connotation. However, once the more innocuous inflammatory lesions are eliminated, most and probably all cases of true clinical erythroplakia represent some epithelial dysplasia ranging from mild forms to invasive carcinoma. The red appearance of the lesions is explained when the lesions are examined microscopically. An orthokeratin or parakeratin surface is absent and the connective tissue papillae with engorged capillaries between the rete ridges lie close to the surface. In the dysplastic epithelium, there is generally a failure of the cells to show any significant maturation. Individual cell keratinization, pearl formation, and surface keratinization are negligible until actual invasion begins, at which time cellular maturation may commence. In the examples studied by Shafer and Waldron,[16] erythroplakia manifested no sex preference and was most frequently seen in the sixth and seventh decades. The most common site in females was the mandibular alveolar mucosa-mandibular gingiva-mandibular sulcus. In men, the floor of the mouth and retromolar areas were the sites of predelection. The most significant finding in their study was that 91% of the tissue specimens studied manifested invasive carcinoma, carcinoma in situ, or severe epithelial dysplasia.

SIGNIFICANCE OF LARYNGEAL KERATOSIS

The normal epithelial covering of the larynx is a nonkeratinizing squamous epithelium except for the lining of the laryngeal ventricle and the subglottic areas where pseudostratified, ciliated, columnar epithelium exists. Much like leukoplakia, the term clinical *keratosis* does not denote a definite or specific entity, for its microscopic appearances are extremely variable. The use of the term implies a whitish plaque which may be raised above the surface or any similar exudate on the top of a vocal cord. It may be localized to a small portion of the vocal cord or may extend widely to involve practically the entire larynx. The lesion is not necessarily accompanied by an inflammatory reaction in the surrounding tissue (Fig. 4.2). Putney[17] considers the irregular, papillary type of keratoses as more ominous than the flat variety with no sharp line of demarcation between the keratosis and normal mucosa.

After surveying the reports in the literature, it is obvious that one man's premalignant keratosis is another's benign hyperkeratinization. In addition, through clinical and pathological use, many terms have gained acceptance as synonyms for keratosis. Such terms include hyperkeratosis, leukoplakia, chronic hypertrophic laryngitis and pachyderma laryngis. Many authors, without describing their histological criteria, imply, nevertheless, various degrees of atypism and consider the lesions as precancerous regardless of the histological appearance. In defining laryngeal keratosis, Norris and Peale[18] require a keratinizing cell layer present in the mucosa. This is a generally agreed upon basic change. In addition to keratin production, other changes in the epithelium that may be encountered

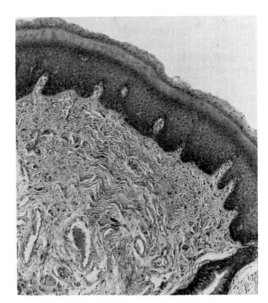

Figure 4.2. Laryngeal "keratosis" associated with basal cell hyperplasia. Histologically benign.

are acanthosis, parakeratosis, presence of a granular cell layer and various dyskeratotic changes.

There is certainly justification for distinguishing between simple (histological) keratosis (keratin production) with a normal cellular cytology and keratin production in a lesion manifesting cellular atypism.[19] Although both are benign lesions, the latter has a statistically poorer prognosis with respect to the association of a later developing carcinoma.

Clinical keratosis is typically found in middle-aged white men. In a study of 116 cases, Norris and Peale[18] found an 82% incidence among males whose average age was 51 years. McGavran et al.[1] record an almost identical average age in 74 of 84 cases of keratosis. Keratosis has long been associated with the smoking of cigarettes and voice abuse, and in certain instances manifests a persistent tendency to recur after local removal. The tendency to recur is greater in those lesions showing the greatest degree of associated cellular atypism.

The malignant potential of "keratosis" of the larynx is difficult to assess since few papers define the histopathological abnormality considered under the term. Of Norris and Peale's[18] 116 cases, 86 were classified as "leukoplakia" (here defined as keratosis with atypia) and 30 as keratosis (without atypia). Eleven of 86 examples of "leukoplakia" later gave rise to carcinoma (4 in situ), whereas only one of the 30 keratoses was followed by the development of carcinoma. In the study by McGavran et al.,[1] only three of 84 cases of keratosis studied were subsequently found to have carcinoma. Thirty percent, however, manifested recurrent keratoses following excisional biopsy. A further statistical study by Putney and O'Keefe[20] indicated that 27 of 67 cases of laryngeal keratosis were later found to have squamous cell carcinoma (six of the seven examples were diagnosed within 6 months of the original biopsy).

At the present time, all that may be concluded concerning keratosis is: (1) keratosis without associated cellular atypia is a benign lesion and is reversible with little inclination to progress further to atypical change or carcinoma. (2) While there is by no means an obligatory progression from keratosis, with or without atypia, to cancer, the risk is small yet significant.

The treatment of keratosis should be conservative surgical excision. Lederman[21] considers irradiation to be indicated only rarely. He writes that such treatment is too radical for a benign disorder and, should keratosis or carcinoma recur or occur after the primary irradiation, its prior use would preclude further similar therapy. Putney and

O'Keefe[20] recommend the use of vocal cord stripping as treatment for keratosis. This is to be done in conjunction with the exclusion or removal of known laryngeal irritants (cigarette smoke and alcohol). If carcinoma in situ is present in association with a keratosis, irradiation is considered by some as the treatment of choice.

CARCINOMA IN SITU

Carcinoma in situ, or intraepithelial carcinoma, is essentially a microscopic diagnosis and is more appropriately considered a histopathological entity rather than a clinical entity. It may be defined as a proliferative disorder of the epithelium in which all of the generally accepted cytological criteria of malignancy are manifested except one—invasive qualities. It is a carcinoma confined to the epithelial layer. A fine diagnostic line separates severe epithelial dysplasia from carcinoma in situ. The crossing of this line by a pathologist depends on his training, experience, location of the lesion in question and subjectivity (Figs. 4.3 to 4.6).

In general, squamous cell carcinomas in situ of the mucous membranes of the body are similar in their histological appearance. The behavior of intraoral and laryngeal lesions, however, cannot be equated with that of the more commonly occurring and far more extensively studied carcinoma in situ of the cervix. Before 1952 there were few studies relating to this lesion as it occurred in the larynx. In the instance of the larynx, it appears that less rigorous criteria for the diagnosis have been applied than for carcinoma in situ of the cervix.[22]

The usual microscopic criteria upon which a diagnosis is made include the following, as described by Evans.[23]

1. There is a proliferation of rather small (variable) cells with basophilic cytoplasm and a disproportionately large nucleus. These cells are crowded together and their nuclear axes often lie perpendicular to the surface of the mucosa. Although the cells not infrequently appear uniform, most lesions manifest varying degrees of cellular pleomorphism.

2. The prickle cell layer is replaced by the atypical and immature cells. Only infrequently is there evidence of isolated cell keratinization. The normal flat squames are not usually found in the surface layers. Exceptionally there is a very attenuated superficial layer of mature squamous cells.

3. There is a disorganization and loss of the normal cellular stratification of the mucosal cells with a replacement of the entire thickness of the epithelium by abnormal cells. The transition from

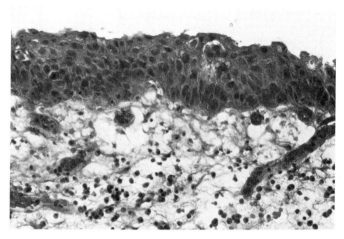

Figure 4.3. A "borderline" lesion from the vocal cord.

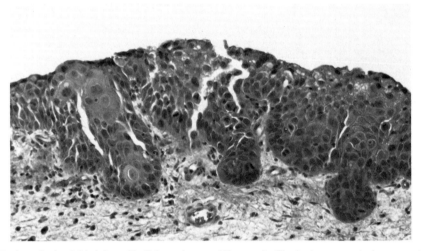

Figure 4.4. A nonleukoplakic intraepithelial carcinoma of the mouth. The lesion presented as an erythroplasia.

normal stratified epithelium to carcinoma in situ may be gradual, but often it is sudden and so abrupt as to leave an easily recognized demarcation line. The affected area stains more deeply than, and therefore contrasts sharply with, the adjacent and paler normal epithelium. There may be extension of the intraepithelial process into underlying or adjacent mucous glands, replacing the whole or part of the epithelium of one or more glands and their excretory ducts.

4. There must be a sharp and distinct line of demarcation between the intraepithelial proliferation and the underlying stroma (formerly considered an intact basement membrane). When the atypical epithelial elements appear to reach out beyond the confining limits of the epithelium, the lesion is no longer in situ and is now considered

invasive. The invasion may be superficial and limited and considered as "microinvasion." This lesion carries the same prognosis as the in situ parent.

Personal experience also indicates that while the over-all thickness of the mucosa may be increased, nearly equal numbers of lesions show a thinning or no significant change in thickness. The most consistent finding is the loss of normal architectural arrangement of the cells in the mucous membrane; mitoses and cellular pleomorphism are too variable to be of significant assistance. It is also to be remembered that individual cell keratinization or "pearl" formation are very uncommon in carcinoma in situ of the mucosa. In fact, these microscopic findings are much more consistent with a transformation of the lesion into a superficially

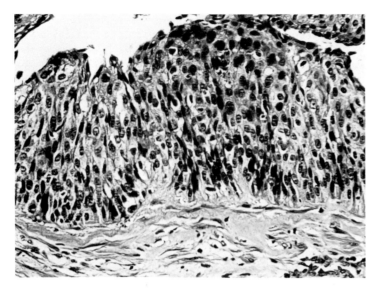

Figure 4.5. Carcinoma in situ of larynx. This field lay adjacent to invasive squamous cell carcinoma.

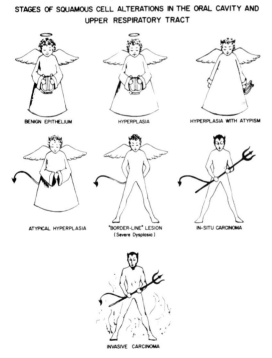

STAGES OF SQUAMOUS CELL ALTERATIONS IN THE ORAL CAVITY AND UPPER RESPIRATORY TRACT

BENIGN EPITHELIUM   HYPERPLASIA   HYPERPLASIA WITH ATYPISM

ATYPICAL HYPERPLASIA   "BORDER-LINE" LESION (Severe Dysplasia)   IN-SITU CARCINOMA

INVASIVE CARCINOMA

Figure 4.6. This fanciful presentation of epithelial alterations (with apologies to Dr. Hugh Grady) serves more to highlight the pathologist's impressions than to imply a progression of the lesions through the various stages.

invasive carcinoma. According to Shafer,[24] either of these two findings mandate a search for evidence of invasion.

The above criteria are by no means absolute or uniformly conformed to in microscopic diagnosis. This is reflected in the diverse opinions that may be rendered by several pathologists on the same lesions. The prevalent opinion is that if the in situ lesions are left untreated, there is a transmutation to invasive carcinoma. The frequency of this change is not known, nor are there good data on the time required for this change to occur. The majority of evidence is circumstantial rather than obtained through a documented chain of events.

While carcinoma in situ of the mouth may present as a form of clinical leukoplakia, the usual clinical manifestation of the lesion is described as an "erythroplasia," signifying a velvety red hyperplastic change in the mucosa.[25] These are harmless looking and consequently dismissed because they resemble an area of inflammation. They are of particular concern if found along the floor of the mouth or on a faucial arch. Several eponymic designations used to describe intraepithelial carcinoma of other sites have also been applied to the intraoral lesions, viz., erythroplasia of Queyrat and Bowen's disease. This usage is not condoned and may serve to confuse the surgeon. Rupert Willis,[26] in typical fashion, stated, "For the pathologist, ... there is only one entity, intraepithelial carcinoma, the structural variants of which do not call for distinctive names."

The peak age incidence for oral carcinoma in situ (fifth through seventh decades) coincides almost exactly with the age of the occurrence of invasive squamous cell carcinoma. Observations of the biological course of these lesions, like those elsewhere in the upper aerodigestive tract are limited. All that can be said at this time is that some are cured surgically, some may recur after removal, they may increase in size or severity or may regress or disappear without surgical management, and they may remain static or may undergo malignant transformation.[15, 24, 27, 28]

A significant number of intraoral in situ carcinomas also have invasive carcinoma in the adjacent areas. This association is so high, in fact, that I advise thorough clinical and pathological examination, to find a coexistent carcinoma. The investigations of Slaughter et al.[29] confirm this high index of suspicion. While the prognosis for a localized lesion of carcinoma in situ is relatively good, the patient must be considered at high risk and should not be lost to follow-up study.

In the larynx, carcinoma in situ is also often associated with a nearby invasive squamous cell carcinoma.[30] The lesion can present on or involve any part of the larynx, although it is most commonly found in the vocal cords. The lesions appear as circumscribed or more diffuse, grayish-white or more reddish thickenings of the vocal cords with either a smooth or granular surface. The anterior part of the cord is usually involved; on occasion the lesion is found in the middle third. In some instances the neoplastic thickening is more diffuse and may involve the entire cord or extend into the subglottic space. Sometimes the apparent origin is near the anterior commissure. In these instances, there is not infrequent extension across the commissure into the other cord or downward into the subglottic region. The mobility of the cord is unimpaired in most instances.

The main pathological difficulties relate to (1)

clinical and histopathological similarities to chronic laryngitic changes which often accompany or precede the in situ lesion, and (2) the microscopic changes are, in many cases, more extensive than the clinically visible changes.

Stout[31] and Stout et al.[32] have reported on the association of size of the clinically recognized lesion and coexistent invasive carcinoma. The noninvasive lesions (limited to in situ carcinoma) are, as a rule, smaller than those with limited invasion. Those with marked invasion were the ones covering the most extensive area. Stout[31] concluded that the size of the lesions at the time of the onset of infiltration is not so much a question of the length of duration as of the growth activity of the tumor tissue. This may, in part, explain the fact that the average age of patients with squamous cell carcinoma in situ of the larynx is not significantly lower than that of invasive carcinomas.

Table 4.1 and the following text summarize the principal points of this chapter:

1. There is insufficient, *documented* evidence to consider a histologically benign lesion of the larynx as "precancerous." This is not to deny, however, that certain clinical and pathological lesions are commonly found in association with either carcinoma in situ and invasive carcinoma. These range from the larynx of the leutic and the alcohol and tobacco abuser to those designated as bearing "keratosis" and/or "leukoplakia." These represent laryngeal reaction to injury and do not differ from similar lesions in other mucosal regions, where a *premalignant* connotation has not applied.

2. The term *leukoplakia* should be abandoned as a *definitive* clinical, and by all means, patholog-

Table 4.1
Squamous Cell Lesions of the Upper Aerodigestive Tract

1. Squamous cell hyperplasia with or without keratosis. }	Histologically benign; also called "keratosis."
2. Squamous cell hyperplasia with or without keratosis, plus atypia or dysplasia; may be graded into mild, moderate, severe.* }	Histologically benign; also called "keratosis" with atypia. The more severe the atypia, the greater the statistical association with carcinoma. This association does not imply a histogenetic progression.
3. Carcinoma in situ.	Histologically an intraepithelial carcinoma. Insufficient evidence to conclude it is inevitably biologically malignant.
4. Carcinoma with microinvasion or superficial stromal invasion }	Biologically malignant.
5. Carcinoma, invasive.	

* Atypia and dysplasia have been used interchangeably. The differences are moot. Atypia usually refers to cellular (cytological) abnormalities while dysplasia usually relates to tissue and/or architectural changes. Atypia allows a greater latitude in description.

ical diagnostic term. It is a *descriptive* term, that by both clinical and pathological misunderstanding has degenerated into a dangerous (for the patient) form of terminology. Additionally, emphasis on the white patch detracts from the more typical appearance of carcinoma (nonkeratinizing) which is erythematous and granular. Leukoplakia is imparted by keratin; carcinoma in situ is typically nonkeratinizing.

3. Much like leukoplakia, the term *keratosis* does not denote a definite or specific entity, for its microscopic appearances are very variable. Distinction should be made between simple (histological) keratosis (keratin production) with normal cellular cytology and architecture and keratin production in a lesion manifesting cellular atypia (dysplasia). Although both are benign, the latter has a statistically poorer prognosis with respect to being associated with a later developing carcinoma.

4. *Carcinoma in situ* may be defined as an abnormal proliferative disorder of an epithelium whose architectural disorganization and cytological atypia exceeds that associated with dysplasia. Because of its association with definable invasive carcinoma, it *may* be considered as an intraepithelial carcinoma.

5. The terms *microinvasive carcinoma* and *carcinoma with superficial invasion* refer to lesions with shallow and biologically early stromal invasion by either a lesion possessing histological features of an in situ carcinoma or one that manifests no evidence of a phase of in situ carcinoma. Carcinoma in situ and microinvasive carcinoma appear to behave in a similar biological manner and if coexisting invasive carcinoma can be eliminated, the two lesions may be treated alike.

REFERENCES

1. McGavran, M. H., Bauer, W. C., and Ogura, J. H.: Isolated laryngeal keratosis. Its relation to carcinoma of the larynx based on a clinicopathologic study of 87 consecutive cases with long-term follow-up. Laryngoscope 70:932, 1960.
2. Cohen, L., and Young, A. H.: The white sponge naevus. Br. J. Oral Surg. 5:206, 1968.
3. Young, W. F.: Familial white folded dysplasia of the oral mucous membranes. Oral Surg. 5:93, 1967.
4. McGinnis, J. P., and Turner, J. E.: Ultrastructure of white sponge nevus. Oral Surg. 40:644, 1975.
5. Witkop, C. J., and Niswander, J. D.: Focal epithelial hyperplasia in Central and South American Indians and Ladinos. Oral Surg. 20:213, 1965.
6. Hettwer, K. J., and Rogers, M. S.: Focal epithelial hyperplasia (Heck's disease) in a Polynesian. Oral Surg. 22:466, 1966.
7. Silverman, S., Jr., and Griffith, M.: Studies on oral lichen planus. II. Follow-up on 200 patients, clinical characteristics and associated malignancy. Oral Surg. 34:705, 1974.
8. Hartwell, S. W., Jr.: Intraoral "leukoplakia." Cleve. Clin. Q. 34:127, 1967.
9. Mashberg, A., Morrissey, J. B., and Garfinfel, L.: A study of the appearance of early asymptomatic oral squamous cell carcinoma. Cancer 32:1436, 1973.
10. Sprague, W. F.: A survey of the use of the term "leukoplakia" by oral pathologists. Oral Surg. 16:1067, 1963.
11. Hellinger, M. J., Karpas, C. M., and Sellers, W., Jr.: A clinicopathologic correlation of oral white lesions: study of forty-five cases. Oral Surg. 16:1365, 1963.
12. King, O. H., Jr.: Intraoral leukoplakia? Cancer 17:131, 1964.
13. Waldron, C. A., and Shafer, W. G.: Leukoplakia revisited. A clinicopathologic study of 3256 oral leukoplakias. Cancer 36:1386, 1975.
14. Cawson, R. A.: Premalignant lesions in the mouth. Br. Med. Bull. 31:164, 1975.
15. Pindborg, J. J., Deftary, D. K., and Mehta, F. S.: A follow-up study of sixty-one oral dysplastic precancerous lesions in Indian villagers. Oral Surg. 43:383, 1977.
16. Shafer, W. G., and Waldron, C. A.: Erythroplakia of the oral cavity. Cancer 36:1021, 1975.
17. Putney, F. J.: Borderline malignant lesions of the larynx. Arch. Otolaryngol. 61:381, 1955.
18. Norris, C. M., and Peale, A. R.: Keratosis of the larynx. J. Laryngol. Otol. 77:635, 1963.
19. Fechner, R. E.: Laryngeal keratosis and atypia. Canad. J. Otolaryngol. 3:516, 1974.
20. Putney, F. J., and O'Keefe, J. J.: The clinical significance of keratosis of the larynx as a premalignant lesion. Ann. Otol. Rhinol. Laryngol. 62:348, 1953.
21. Lederman, M.: Keratosis of the larynx. J. Laryngol. Otol. 77: 651, 1963.
22. McNelis, F. L., and Esparza, A. R.: Carcinoma in situ of the larynx. Laryngoscope. 81:924, 1971.
23. Evans, R. W.: Histopathological Appearances of Tumors with a Consideration of Their Histogenesis and Certain Aspects of Their Clinical Features and Behavior, 2nd Ed., Williams & Wilkins Co., Baltimore, 1966.
24. Shafer, W. G.: Oral carcinoma in situ. Oral Surg. 39:227, 1975.
25. Shedd, D. P.: Clinical characteristics of early oral cancer. J.A.M.A. 215:955, 1971.
26. Willis, R. A.: Pathology of Tumours, 3rd Ed., p. 289. Butterworths, London, 1960.
27. Mincer, H. H., Coleman, S. A., and Hopkins, K. P.: Observations on the clinical characteristics of oral lesions showing histologic epithelial hyperplasia. Oral Surg. 33:389, 1972.
28. Hamperl, H.: Preinvasive carcinoma. Recent Results Cancer Res. 44:53, 1974.
29. Slaughter, D. P., Southwick, H. W., and Smejkal, W.: "Field cancerization" in oral stratified squamous epithelium: clinical implications of multicentric origin. Cancer 6:963, 1953.
30. Bauer, W. C.: Concomitant carcinoma in situ and invasive carcinoma of the larynx. Canad. J. Otolaryngol. 3:533, 1974.
31. Stout, A. P.: Intramucosal epithelioma of the larynx. Am. J. Roentgenol. Radium Ther. Nucl. Med. 69:1, 1953.
32. Altmann, F., Ginsberg, I., and Stout, A. P.: Intraepithelial carcinoma (cancer in situ) of the larynx. Arch. Otolaryngol. 56:121, 1952.

CHAPTER 5

Squamous Cell "Papillomas" of the Oral Cavity, Sinonasal Tract and Larynx

Squamous cell tumors, whether true neoplasms or epithelial reactivities to tissue injury, are the most common tumors of the oral cavity and the upper respiratory tract. The very broad and loosely defined category of squamous cell lesions called "papillomas" is important not only for the possibility for diagnostic error it may present, but also because many of the so-called "papillomas" of the sinonasal tract and larynx are refractory or at least very stubborn in their response to treatment. I seriously doubt that a precise definition of a true *neoplastic* papilloma can be made. It is my contention that the majority do not represent neoplasms in the usual sense. "Papillomatous," in my usage, refers to the low power and/or gross architecture of the lesion and does not necessarily imply a neoplastic basis for the origin of the lesion.

In the following discussion, I present a clinico-pathological appraisal of squamous papillomas of the head and neck mucous membranes. Since a florid type of papillomatosis occurs only infrequently in the oral cavity, and since most oral "papillomas" are most likely a response to injury, their significance is considerably less than those of the nasal and paranasal cavities and the larynx.

SQUAMOUS CELL PAPILLOMAS OF THE ORAL CAVITY

In the oral cavity, as elsewhere, the term papilloma is often indiscriminately applied to any elevated soft tissue growth. The usual example of this is a fibroepithelial polyp. The hard and soft palate and the uvula are the most common sites of origin for squamous papillomas in the oral cavity. They may occur at all ages, but appear predominantly between the ages of 20 and 50 years. The palate, gingiva, tongue, cheek and lip account for over 90% of the lesions.[1, 2] The lesions most often occur singly, but multiple papillomas sometimes occur in the oral mucosa. They are usually small, the patient often being unaware of their presence. They may be broad-based or pedunculated. Non-keratinized papillomas are generally soft, whereas those manifesting considerable keratinization are firmer in consistency.

The typical oral papilloma may be either keratinizing or nonkeratinized and is a pedunculated lesion with a cauliflower-like structure.[3] Histologically there is a proliferation of benign squamous cells in an arborescent growth and thin connective tissue cores. The oral papilloma is not premalignant, and recurrences seldom appear after excision. Statements concerning the precancerous nature of the lesions may be due to confusion of this benign lesion with verrucous carcinoma. Multiple papillomas have been associated with ichthyosis hystrix and the focal dermal hypoplasia syndrome.

Intraoral condyloma acuminatum may present as a gingival hyperplasia but can also be multiple or single pedunculated or cauliflower-like lesions indistinguishable from their counterparts in the vaginal and perianal regions.[4]

PAPILLOMAS OF THE SINONASAL TRACT

Numerous designations have been given to epithelial papillomas of the nasal cavity and the paranasal sinuses. Hyams[5] has counted at least 20 synonyms. Commonly used terms have been: inverted, Schneiderian, transitional cell, cylindrical, hard, soft and true papilloma. The word "papilloma" has also been inappropriately applied to the considerably more common allergic or inflammatory polyp, to hyperplastic sinusitis with or without squamous metaplasia, to polypoid or papillary squamous cell carcinoma and to localized benign hyperkeratosis.

Several other factors contribute to the confusion related to these lesions and make the extraction of information from the literature under the categorical heading of *papilloma* nearly impossible. Whether or not the papillomas of the upper respiratory tract are true neoplasms or pronounced responses to tissue injury is debatable and cannot be answered at this time. It is fairly certain, however, that allergy does not play a role in the genesis of nasal, paranasal sinus and upper respiratory tract *papillomas*.

For the pathologist seeking to define the biological behavior of these lesions, the descriptive adjective "transitional" used to describe a class of nasal and paranasal sinus papillomas is probably the most disconcerting. Osborn,[6–8] in his several articles concerning benign and malignant epithelial lesions of the upper respiratory tract, has his own application, but he never fully describes its meaning. He stresses "relative persistence of basement membrane" and infolding as indispensable to the diagnosis. The following, taken from one of Osborn's more recent papers, is representative of his justification for using the terms transitional papilloma and carcinoma: "It will be clear that my definition of transitional cell carcinoma in the upper respiratory tract differs fundamentally from that of the earlier writers, the concept being based on the morphology of an organized epithelium instead of a single cell. Transitional cell papilloma and carcinoma of the urinary tract are so-called because they arise from, and tend to, reproduce transitional epithelium. The application of the term to tumors of similar morphology in the upper respiratory tract would seem to be a logical extension of its use."[6] I take a contrary opinion and would restrict "transitional" to the urothelium of the lower genitourinary tract and pelves and ureters. There is only a vague resemblance of the nasal papilloma and the true transitional cell epithelium found in the urinary tract. Furthermore, while some authors claim there is a "striking resemblance" of the inverted papillomas of the urinary bladder to the nasal papillomas, I am singularly not of that persuasion, and refer the reader to the papers by Henderson et al.[9] and DeMeester et al.[10] for comparison. There is also a distinct difference in behavior since no inverted papilloma of the bladder has manifested recurrence.

A similar condemnation applies to the use of the term "transitional" to refer to the normal epithelium from which arises a highly radiosensi-

tive variant of squamous cell carcinoma of the nasopharynx, tonsils and base of tongue (lymphoepithelioma). If one must use the designation, it should be used in the context offered by Ringertz,[11] who stated that the epithelium appeared to represent a *transition between* squamous and glandular epithelium. Earlier, Nicholson[12] had recognized transitional epithelium as an incompletely differentiated squamous type of epithelium.

The majority of the papillomas are nonkeratinizing, squamous cell in type (either wholly or partially so) and represent benign extensions of squamous metaplasia, whereas the squamous cell carcinoma represents the malignant variant. Figure 5.1, modified after Müller et al.,[13] depicts the proposed origin of the epithelial papilloma by a proliferation of the replacement or reserve cells of the mucosa.

Despite the histological similarities between papillomas of the nose and sinuses and papillomas of the laryngotracheal tree, there does not seem to be a pathogenetic relationship. The virtual *absence* of epithelial papillomas of the sinonasal tract in the preadolescent patient is in sharp distinction to the relatively high incidence of laryngeal papillomas in prepubertal children. This divergence is, in part, attributed to the uniqueness of the "Schneiderian membrane" or epithelium that forms the mucosa of the nasal and paranasal cavities, with the exception of the specialized olfactory area of the superior part of the nasal cavity. The Schneiderian epithelium is considered ectodermal in origin, whereas the remainder of the respiratory tract derives its mucosa from the entoderm.

The following discussion, concerning squamous

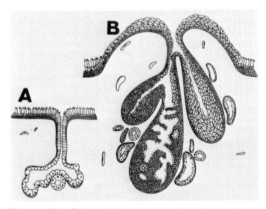

Figure 5.1. Schematic representation of the histogenesis of the inverted papilloma. *A*, normal nasal mucosa and gland are depicted. *B*, pronounced basal cell hyperplasia and epidermoid metaplasia replaces the respiratory epithelium and proliferates inward into an edematous stroma.

papillomas of the nasal cavity and paranasal sinuses, is derived from several solid, well-documented papers and from my own surgical pathological experience.[5,14-16] The collective incidence of papillomas of the sinonasal tract in relation to the inflammatory or allergic polyps is 2.7%. The *over-all* frequency is low and has ranged from 0.01 to 4.7% of "neoplastic" lesions in the sinuses and nasal cavity.[5]

Three and possibly four histomorphological types of papilloma have been categorized, primarily on an anatomical basis. These are: (1) the keratotic lesions arising from the stratified squamous epithelium lining the vestibule of the nose; (2) inverted papilloma, originating primarily from the lateral nasal walls; (3) fungiform or septal papilloma; and (4) cylindrical cell papilloma.

The papilloma of the vestibule actually represents a collection of clinicopathological lesions ranging from a localized, papillomatous keratosis on a fibroepithelial *polyp*, in which the squamous epithelium is merely a passive participant, to a keratinizing squamous papilloma exactly like those found on the surfaces of the body (Fig. 5.2). The clinicopathological course of these lesions is identical to the expected benign behavior of their counterparts elsewhere on the skin.

Within the two principal remaining types, inverted papilloma and fungiform papilloma, there are many similarities. There is a male dominance in incidence, with the fourth and fifth decades of life being the time of greatest frequency. There is a tendency for the fungiform variety to occur earlier in life. Both types are composed of hyperplastic squamous or stratified columnar epithelium, with most of the histological features of one being common to the other. Both types are subject to multiple recurrences (persistences).

Without historical evidence of location and gross intranasal involvement it may be impossible to distinguish the two types of epithelial papilloma. The third variant, cylindrical cell papilloma, (Fig. 5.3), is the least common and because of its rarity is often confused with a glandular malignancy or adenoma. As one gains experience with these lesions, it is clear that cylindrial cell areas occur in nearly all forms of nasal epithelial papillomas and that exclusiveness of that type of epithelium is likely time-related before reserve cell replacement. In the following discussion, I have addressed the three types separately, but in practice have referred to the group as *epithelial papillomas*.

Inverted Papilloma

Norris,[16, 17] acknowledging our lack of scientific basis for considering nasal papillomas as neoplasms, suggests a possible alternative term for this lesion: "inverting epithelial hyperplasia." Certainly the rare papillary sinusitis may be difficult to distinguish from the inverted papilloma and indeed some authors consider both diseases to be the same. The principal reason for the retention of the term *inverted papilloma* is its distinctiveness and familiarity. To do otherwise would be to introduce another source of confusion.

The highly descriptive term "inverting" is derived from the histological appreciation that the neoplastic (or hyperplastic) epithelium *inverts* into the underlying stroma and the lesion is endophytic rather than exophytic from a microscopic viewpoint (Fig. 5.4).

The inverted papilloma is almost exclusively a lateral nasal wall lesion. A common site is at the junction of the antrum and ethmoid sinus. In Hyams[5] large series no inverted papilloma originated primarily from the nasal septal surface. Unilaterality and nonmultiple involvement is also characteristic of this type of papilloma. In this respect, primary origin (not secondary involvement) from the roof or floor of the nasal cavity is very unusual.

The gross appearance of the inverted papilloma is one of fairly large size, often bulky, deep red to gray in color and with a variable (friable to firm) consistency. Marked vascularity and edema of the stroma with gross translucency are conspicuous features (Fig. 5.5).

There is a male predominance, and available statistics indicate the inverted papilloma is uncommon in Negroes. Clinical symptoms are domi-

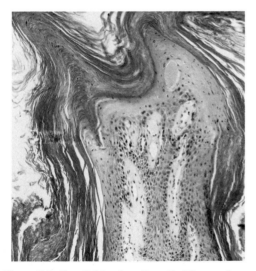

Figure 5.2. Keratinizing "papilloma" of the nasal vestibule.

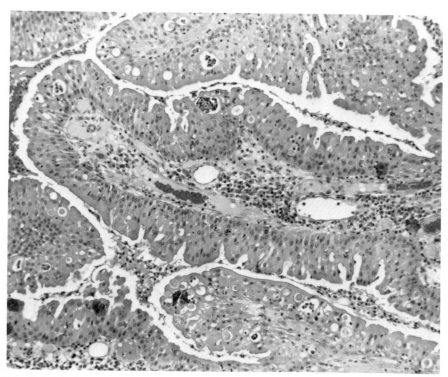

Figure 5.3. Cylindrical cell papilloma. This variant of epithelial papilloma of the nasal cavity is often mistaken for a papillary adenocarcinoma. The photomicrograph represents an area of a lesion composed entirely of cylindrical cells. Cylindrical cell foci, however, may be found in many predominantly squamous epithelial papillomas of the nose.

nated, as expected, by unilateral obstruction and nasal "stuffiness."[18] A few patients manifest epistaxis, postnasal drip and sinus headaches. Patients may allow the lesions to reach considerable bulk through neglect of the seemingly innocuous symptoms. There is a distinctive absence of allergic history in patients with lateral wall (inverted) papillomas.

From a histological standpoint, the designation *inverted* is appropriately descriptive. The epithelium of the lesion inverts into the underlying stroma instead of an exophytic proliferation as is characteristic of papillomas in general. The majority of inverted papillomas manifest an epidermoid or squamous cell pattern, but, in addition to this prominent cellular component, the surface frequently may be lined by a uniform single layer of typical, often ciliated, columnar epithelium of the respiratory type (Fig. 5.6). Surface keratin with a distinct underlying granular cell layer was noted in approximately 10% of Hyam's[5] cases. Desquamation of surface epithelium is common on the exposed surfaces.

Individual cells are uniform and retain a polarity with adjoining cells. Some cells are rich in glycogen, and this is seen in routine sections as intracytoplasmic vacuoles, pushing the cell nucleus to one side. Intercellular bridges can easily be seen in all layers and especially in the layers adjacent to the basement membrane. Nuclear uniformity (size and chromogenicity) are consistent features. Occasional mitosis may be present.

A distinctive feature is the consistent finding of microscopic mucous cysts interspersed throughout the epithelium of the papilloma (Fig. 5.7). The demonstration of these cysts may require the use of mucin stains.[5] A distinct and intact basement membrane separates and defines the epithelial component from the underlying connective tissue stroma.

The stromal density varies from a loose edematous matrix to one of more compact and fibrous nature. The degree of associated stromal inflammation is also variable, varying from insignificant to moderate. Eosinophils are not a prominent cell, but plasma cells may, on occasion, dominate the infiltrate.

Fungiform Papilloma

An exophytic or mushroom-shaped lesion with a thin central core of connective tissue, the fungiform papilloma of the nasal cavity is most consist-

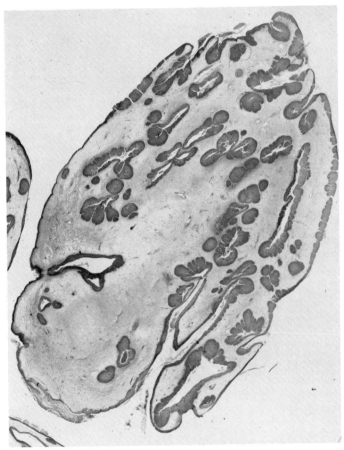

Figure 5.4. Inverted papilloma of the lateral nasal wall. Polypoid in gross configuration, the epithelium of the lesion inverts into the stroma.

ent with the common concept of a papilloma. In contrast to the lateral wall localization of the inverted papilloma, fungiform papillomas arise almost exclusively from the surface of the nasal septum. Grossly, the lesion is a raised verrucous or cauliflower-like excrescence with a firm, often rubbery consistency. It lacks the translucency of the inverted papilloma, is gray to pink, and is attached to the mucous membrane by a broad base. The clinical symptoms and age of patients are similar to those with lateral wall papillomas. Because of superficial excoriation, epistaxis may be more common.

Dominantly squamous or epidermoid in character, the fungiform variety of intranasal papilloma may also manifest a single layer of respiratory-type epithelium on its surface. This finding, however, is less often seen than in the inverted papilloma. In short, the histological features are similar to those found in inverted papillomas, even to the presence of mucous cysts within the epithelium. Superficial excoriation is common. The sup-

porting tissue core is usually delicate, usually devoid of seromucinous glands and only sparsely vascular. An accompanying inflammatory exudate is unusual (Fig. 5.8).

Cylindrical Cell Papilloma

Admittedly rare, this form of papilloma is depicted as a ragged, beefy and papillary growth found in the maxillary sinus or in conjunction with lesions of the adjacent lateral nasal wall or ethmoid sinus.

The lesion is characterized by Hyams[5] as a "proliferation of multi-layered columnar cells" with eosinophilic cytoplasm, round to oval uniform and dark nuclei and occasionally ciliated. Squamous or epidermoid elements are either absent or inconspicuous (Fig. 5.3).

CLINICAL BEHAVIOR

Until recently, confusion existed concerning the clinicobiological behavior of the entire class of

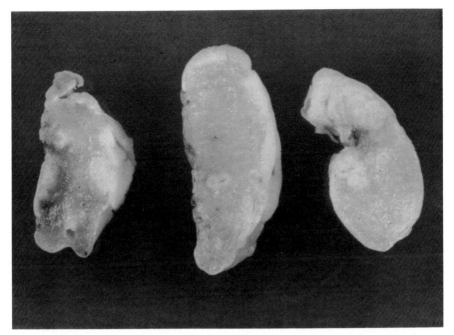

Figure 5.5. Sectioned polypoid masses from an inverted (lateral wall) papilloma. The more opaque epithelial proliferation may be seen inverting into the moist and edematous stroma.

papillomas of the upper respiratory tract. Some authors have considered these lesions as uniformly malignant, some as premalignant and others as perfectly benign. Certainly the question of whether these lesions are precancerous is not any easy one to answer. This is due partly to their rarity and partly because there often has been inadequate follow-up over a long period of time.

The major clinical problem is that of recurrences. This more appropriately is an expression of persistence after inadequate removal. From 25 to 75% of all nasal and paranasal papillomas will recur at least once, regardless of the histological type.[19, 20] Prediction of those which will recur cannot be made by microscopic examination. In any given series, there is a greater tendency for the inverted papillomas to be recurrent.

Apparent multicentricity of the inverted papillomas is probably a misconception and is more likely the extension of the disease via metaplasia of adjacent mucosa.[5] Removal of a lateral wall inverted papilloma *must* always be accompanied by inspection of the adjacent sinus to rule out metaplastic extension. While both the nasal cavity and adjacent sinuses are often involved by the papillomatous process, the disease may be limited to only one or the other. The confinement of a papilloma to the lateral nasal wall is relatively low in occurrence.

The literature concerning inverted papillomas includes frequent references to an eventual malignant "transformation" in a pre-existing papilloma. Marcial-Rojas[21] believes that this occurs more often than the literature indicates and likens the diagnostic problem to that associated with villous papillomas of the rectum. Hyams[5] assumes a conservative stance and desires to discourage the use of the term "premalignant" in describing an inverted papilloma in order to reduce over-treatment.

Our own experience, like that of Brown[22] and Norris[16] is contrary to that of Marcial-Rojas.[21] Marked atypia, short of carcinoma, can be expected in approximately 10% of inverted papillomas. Unlike a Mayo Clinic series,[23] we have not been impressed with a higher or more rapid rate of recurrence in such atypical inverted papillomas. In that respect, a prediction of the biological activity of any inverted papilloma cannot be made solely on the basis of histological appearance.

Malignant transformation of an inverted papilloma, if it occurs, must be of a low order. Osborn[6] considers it to be less than 2% of cases. On the other hand, an invasive squamous cell carcinoma *arising* in the same anatomical area as the inverted papilloma (an *associated* carcinoma) is not unusual (13% in Hyam's series).[5] This finding certainly underscores Marcial-Rojas' admonition to obtain multiple sections of the often bulky resected specimens.[21]

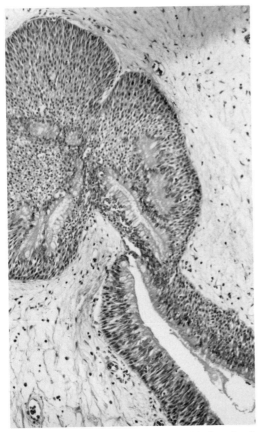

Figure 5.6. Ciliated and respiratory epithelium lies in a single layer over squamous epithelium in an inverted papilloma.

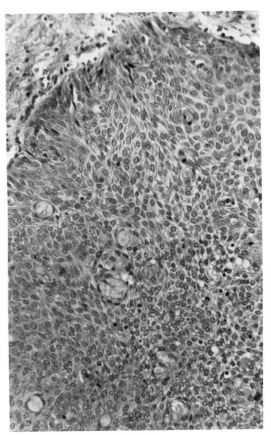

Figure 5.7. Microscopic mucous cysts in an inverted papilloma.

Combined lesions of papilloma and carcinoma (most often squamous cell) fall into three histological categories. In one group the carcinoma and the inverted papilloma occupy the same anatomical region but there is no evidence the papilloma has given rise to the cancer. Papillomas with a focus of invasive carcinoma confined within make up the second group. The third category is represented by the patients who after treatment for an inverted papilloma, develop invasive cancer without again exhibiting further evidence of papillomas. Lasser et al.[20] found 16 such cases in the literature. In 15 cases that I studied, all the carcinomas were squamous cell and fell into categories 1 and 2 nearly equally. Fechner and Sessions[24] and Schoub et al.[25] record what they consider to be metastases from a typical papilloma. Their documentation, particularly that of Schoub's[25] is not satisfactory and this author categorically denies the possibility of such an event.

The septal or fungiform papillomas present no problem concerning their premalignant state or malignant potential. They are either benign (the vast majority) or represent a papilloma-like squamous cell carcinoma. Hyam's[5] data again are representative. He found no associated malignancies with septal papillomas. This is perhaps related to the extreme rarity of squamous cell carcinomas per se on the nasal septum.

The treatment of nasal and paranasal cavity papillomas may be a frustrating experience for the head and neck surgeon. In general, experiences with radiotherapy have led to the conclusion that it is ineffectual and always raises the specter of inducing malignancy. Because of the propensity for extension by contiguity, the lesions should be excised widely. In patients with tumor isolated to the septum or the inferior turbinate, a limited surgical resection may prove to be adequate therapy, and, in these instances, early adequate surgical removal usually effects a cure. For large and bulky and recurrent papillomas in any location, all of the problems of the treatment of neoplasms in this anatomical area are encountered. The tu-

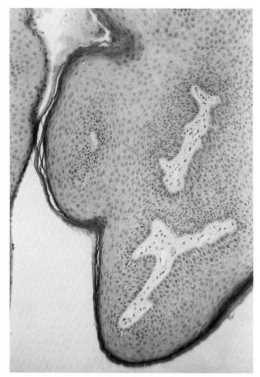

Figure 5.8. Papilloma of the nasal septum; it is called fungiform to distinguish it from the inverted papilloma.

mor should be widely and deeply excised—widely because of the metaplasia in adjacent areas and the possibility of coexistent carcinoma near the main tumor, and deeply to remove downward proliferations.

Unrestricted growth of even the histologically benign inverted lesions may produce death by extension through eroded bones into vital structures. The benign proliferation, although often recurrent and locally aggressive, does not invade adjacent bony confines but produces a pressure atrophy. De novo malignancy or associated squamous cell carcinomas destroy bone by invasion, and, in these instances, the danger of direct extension into the cranial cavity is the greatest. The relatively low-grade malignancy of the associated carcinomas is evidenced by only rare examples of cervical lymph node metastases and systemic dissemination. Nevertheless, this should not be used to underestimate the considerable morbidity and local aggressiveness leading to death.

PAPILLOMAS OF THE LARYNX

The two most common tumors of the larynx in infancy and young children are papillomas (squamous cell) and subglottic hemangiomas. Of all the benign growths of the larynx, the squamous cell papilloma is the one most frequently encountered at any age and it is the most common of all laryngeal tumors in childhood.

The above said, I also hasten to add that "papillomas" of the larynx, much like those of the nasal and paranasal cavities, are frustrating clinical and pathological lesions. A considerable measure of confusion arises from the indiscriminate use of the term "papilloma" as a label for a variety of lesions that do not qualify; viz., inflammatory polyps, pseudoepitheliomatous hyperplasia, speakers nodules, etc. Fortunately this practice is on the wane. Another source of difficulty is the histological similarity, if not identity, of the papillomas occurring in childhood and those presenting in the adult patient. This feature, coupled with the fact that there is a considerable temporal overlap into adulthood for some of the so-called childhood variety of papilloma, has led to "fuzzy concepts" over the biological activity of laryngeal papillomas. Clinical pronouncements have consequently ranged from "a benign, self-limited disease" to "a premalignant state."

There are sufficient biological behavioral differences to consider that (at least) two forms of laryngeal papillomas exist: a "juvenile" type and a papilloma of adults, inappropriately called "senile."[26–31] The juvenile papilloma may occur at any age, but is much more often a lesion of childhood. Spontaneous involution is a characteristic of the juvenile type of papilloma, and this too may occur at any age, but appears most often at the time of puberty. An occasional individual may continue to develop new lesions or recurrences throughout life. Andrews[32] cites an 85-year-old man with laryngeal papillomatosis since early childhood. In contrast to adult papillomas, where single papillomas dominate the statistics, multiple papillomatosis is the rule in the child with laryngeal involvement (80 to 90% of series).

The juvenile papillomas may occur anywhere in the larynx, chiefly on the true and false cords and in the anterior commissure. They frequently extend subglottically and on occasion involve the trachea, bronchi or epiglottis. Tracheal and bronchial spread of papillomas is almost always preceded by a tracheotomy. Only 1% of laryngeal papillomas are associated with tracheal papillomas, while 36% of the tracheal lesions have been associated with concurrent or previous laryngeal papillomas.[33] The pharynx and soft palate are less often sites of the lesion and these papillomas are almost never encountered in the esophagus below the level of cricopharyngeus.[34]

The pathogenesis of the juvenile papilloma, while very likely distinct from the solitary laryngeal papilloma of the adult, is still not completely settled. Juvenile papillomas have been transmitted by a filterable agent to both skin and mucous membrane, and they are currently thought to be a response to a viral agent. Electron microscopic studies, while failing to clearly identify a virus in these lesions, have provided sufficient ancillary findings that a viral etiology is little doubted.[35–37] The papilloma virus is most likely a tumorogenic virus belonging to a group collectively called papova viruses. Papova is an acronynm of papilloma, polyoma and vacuolating.

The juvenile papillomas are not neoplastic lesions but represent an abnormal tissue response to an initiating factor (viral). The development of squamous cell carcinoma in a previously benign papilloma is a rare event, almost always associated with prior irradiation.[38] It is of further interest that in even those instances the malignancy is in the subglottic larynx or in the trachea.[39, 40] Similarly, invasive papillomatosis, that unusual lesion without cytological evidence of malignancy, shows a predisposition for the tracheobronchial tree rather than the larynx. By contrast, however, there is not the relation of radiation to invasive bronchial or tracheal papillomatosis.[39]

There is, however, considerable morbidity with these lesions. They cannot be eradicated completely; recurrences and persistence of lesions may lead to multiple surgical excisions, and acute respiratory obstruction may often require tracheostomy. On the other hand, spontaneous disappearance may supervene. With respect to the recurrences, trauma to the upper respiratory tract's mucous membranes, whether surgical or infectious, appears to play a decisive role.

There does not appear to be a sex difference and whites and blacks are equally affected. The age of clinical onset varies from the newborn to adulthood. Respiratory obstruction can be insidious and progressive or sudden in character. In the young patient a change in phonetics, beginning with hoarseness, that may progress to complete aphonia is the usual presenting sign. The juvenile lesions appear as white to pinkish-red glistening mulberry-like nodules. They are usually friable and may reach the size of a cherry before removal. Ease of bleeding is a constant feature.

Microscopically, the structures are sessile or papillary and composed of a vascular connective tissue core covered by stratified squamous epithelium (Fig. 5.9). Multiple (secondary or tertiary) branches are present. Mitoses may be easy to find,

but these are never atypical and the cells are mature and well differentiated. There is no tendency to invade stroma or submucosal tissues except for the rare so-called invasive papillomatosis.[39]

There are no distinctive histological differences between the juvenile and adult papillomas. Holinger et al.[41] feel there are, however, clinical differences. The adult papilloma is more friable, leaving a cleaner surface after forceps removal, whereas in children the lesions appear to be more "deep-seated" and have a tougher consistency. The adult papilloma is usually a solitary formation. After the age of 40 years, virtually all laryngeal papillomas are single and not multiple.

The otolaryngologist is faced with four problems in dealing with laryngeal papillomatosis: (1) the obstructive location of the lesions; (2) their multiplicity; (3) high recurrence rate; and (4) the ability of the papillomas to seed previously uninvolved mucosa. Untreated or uncontrolled, the papillomas can reduce the patient to a respiratory cripple and require numerous hospital admissions for treatment.[42–44]

Because of a general lack of success in eradicating the lesions from the respiratory tract, there is no single widely accepted form of management. Antibiotics, hormones, electrocoagulation, ultrasound, cryotherapy, radiation, transfer factor, sur-

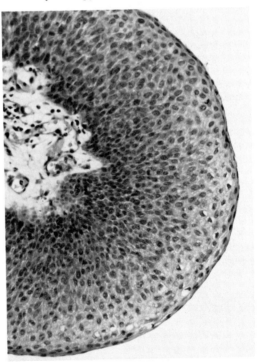

Figure 5.9. So-called juvenile papilloma of the larynx. This lesion occurred in a 4-year-old boy.

gical excision, carbon dioxide laser beams and autogenous vaccines have all been used with varying degrees of success. The laryngeal destruction, arrested development, chronic cicatricial stenosis and induction of malignancy seen as late sequellae to radiotherapy have led to its abandonment as a form of treatment.

At times, only one or two forceps removals are necessary to arrest the development of the disease; in others, removals over a protracted time are required. In one extreme case, 166 procedures were performed over a 4-year period. Approximately 30% of the patients require tracheostomy to alleviate airway obstruction.

The philosophy of management for the multiple recurring papillomas of childhood should be one of conservatism.[44] The more aggressive the treatment, the more certain complications will develop. A 12 to 14% mortality rate has been expressed for the disease, and this relatively high rate for an inherently benign disease is chiefly the result of complications of treatment.

At the time of this writing, there is no doubt that endoscopic excision of papillomas, possibly by microsurgical methods, remains the most effective procedure and the principal means of therapy.[45, 46] Tracheotomy favors the spread of the disease around the site of the tracheostoma and into the tracheobronchial tree. Even in children with advanced papillomatosis, it may be possible to avoid tracheotomy by endoscopic excision of the obstructing growths.

It is difficult to find any reliable data that are helpful in determining the incidence of benign versus malignant papillomas of the larynx in *adults*. The controversy may be likened to that surrounding adenomatous polyps of the colon in some respects. Simply stated, there are two anatomically distinct squamous cell papillomas of the adult laryngeal mucosa. The least common is a "florid type" that is related to, if not the same as, the juvenile papilloma.[47] These are multiple, confluent and tend to recur often after simple extirpation. They are essentially benign and the diagnosis warrants conservation in treatment. Foci of anaplasia or atypia may be present but are confined to the cells of the basal portion of the growth.

The most common adult lesion is the *solitary* squamous cell papilloma. This lesion is unrelated to the juvenile lesions. Most examples of this type do not recur after simple surgical excision. They usually manifest no significant degree of atypia in the papillary pattern of squamous cells overlying fibrous stalks.

The diagnosis of *malignancy* in a papillomatous tumor is often especially difficult. It is further doubted that "malignant degeneration" occurs in papillomas, all papillary carcinomas having been malignant from the onset and not having evolved through a period of benign growth. Two studies by Altmann et al.[48, 49] underline the difficulty the pathologist encounters. These workers published an important study dealing with the incidence of intraepithelial anaplasia in carcinoma of the larynx.[48] Papillary tumors were purposely omitted from this study of intraepithelial carcinoma because the authors (including A. P. Stout) were uncertain whether intraepithelial changes in these lesions should or could be considered a sign of true malignancy. Undaunted, however, Altmann and Stout with Basek[49] later published a report dealing with intraepithelial anaplastic changes in papillomas of the adult larynx. They recommended that, whenever anaplasia is observed in papillary growths, repeated biopsies are essential along with a close follow-up. They, however, observed that anaplastic changes in the epithelium of papillomas seem less significant than those developing in nonpapillomatous laryngeal epithelium.

This summation of their investigations should not be viewed as begging the issue, because there is no clear-cut line of separation between the benign laryngeal papilloma and the "malignified" papilloma. Some solace may be had, however, by recognizing that the solitary and isolated malignant papilloma with complete or transepithelial atypia (not isolated or focal anaplasia) is rare. As a consequence, conservatism (simple excision) is the treatment of choice. The rate of recurrence with such treatment has been estimated at 20%.

The histological criteria for malignancy in a papilloma should not be different from that used for in situ carcinoma elsewhere in the mucous membranes of the head and neck. Hyperkeratosis, regarded by some as a "threatening sign" of malignancy, is not.

The true papillary squamous cell carcinoma, in my experience, is found almost exclusively in the area of the upper aerodigestive tract from the base of the tongue to the true cords. In this region the tumor is solitary, usually in the oro- or hypopharynx and occurs in young adults of both sexes. Unless induced by irradiation or other means, the papillary squamous cell carcinoma does not pass through a benign papilloma phase.

NASAL POLYPS

The relatively commonplace and to some, mundane, nasal and sinus polyp has little or no relationship to the squamous papilloma. Its importance lies in its elusive pathogenesis, the often gross similarity to the much more morbid papilloma, relationship to systemic diseases and hypersensitivity, and an occasional departure from the stereotyped histological appearance that may be alarming to a pathologist.

Nasal polypi are rarely seen before the age of 5 years. Even children with asthma and rhinitis (mean age of 6 years) are not prone to the development of polyps. Only one (0.1%) of the 1,501 pediatric patients studied by Settipane and Chafee[50] had nasal polyps. The same investigators indicate the frequency in the general population of adults to be 4.2%; the adult asthmatic population manifested an incidence of 6.7%. It is of further interest that asthmatics with negative results of allergy skin tests to inhalant allergens have significantly more nasal polyps than asthmatics with positive skin test results. Of a total of 211 patients with nasal polyps, 71% had asthma and 29%, rhinitis only.[50] The frequency of nasal polyps increases with advancing years.

The pathogenesis of nasal polypi (polypoid rhinosinusitis) is as yet unknown. They often recur, sometimes repeatedly and occasionally with surprising rapidity. The widespread belief that the condition is a consequence of a topic hypersensitivity is not supported in many cases.[51] Evidence of local IgE formation has been found in some nasal polypi, but this is not constant. Other suggested causes include bacterial, enzymatic deficiencies and increased osmotic pressure in the submucosa, secondary to short chain mucopolysaccharides. Ultimately the immediate genesis rests with congestion of the local vascular system and an associated myxomatous change in connective tissue.

Some pathologists and clinicians have attempted to divide the nasal polypi into allergic and inflammatory types. Often it is the eosinophil concentration that is said to favor the former over the latter. I have not been successful in that ability. The percentage of eosinophils varies with the stage and the intensity of the reaction by the mucosa.

Nasal polyps represent a focal reactive prominence of the lamina propria mucosae. In these projections, there is: (1) a variable, often pronounced edema; (2) variable proliferation of connective tissue fibroblasts; and (3) an inflammatory infiltrate that ranges from acute to lymphofollicular.

The components of nasal polyps are then, the epithelium, stroma, cellular infiltrate and the vascular system (Fig. 5.10).

Mucous glands may be found in all polyps and the density of occurrence varies from polyp to polyp in the same patient. The density of the glands is reduced from that of the normal mucosa and the majority are found in the distal half of a

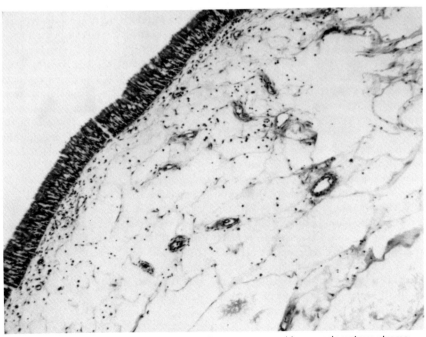

Figure 5.10. Nasal polyp with intact surface mucosa and loose, edematous stroma.

polyp.[52] The mucus-producing ability of a polyp is also reduced and slight as compared with the normal nasal mucosa.[52] The glands in a polyp are tubular and differ from those in the nose and are formed from the surface epithelium after a polyp has attained a certain size.[53] The glands are not occlusion glands—all have a duct leading to the surface of the polyp and presumably have been formed by a downgrowth of epithelium, secondary canalization and then dichotomous division of tubules. Degeneration and cystic change occurs in the glands and may or may not be accompanied by a similar change in the stroma. Ultrastructural studies of polyps indicate an increased amount of transudated fluid in the epithelial layer resulting in distended intercellular spaces, deformity of cell contour and looseness of epithelial cells and vacuolation of epithelial cell cytoplasms. There is also an increase in goblet cell population. Eosinophils, mast cells, and plasma cells have shown subcellular characteristics of antigen-antibody phenomena in some cases.[54] In several studies there has been a significant relation between local IgE production and the density of eosinophilic infiltration of the polypi.[55]

Secondary changes in polyps include increasing collagenization, infarct, surface ulceration and formation of a pyogenic granuloma reaction, mucoid liquefaction, metaplasia of surface epithelium, the rare development of carcinoma in this metaplastic epithelium, and stromal cell atypia. Repeated neovascularization accompanied by fibrosis may yield a polypoid lesion that microscopically will simulate an angiofibroma. Unsuspecting pathologists will also be perturbed by the occasional polyp with atypical change in the stromal fibroblasts. This phenomenon has occurred most often in the choanal or posterior polypi in the author's experience.

The importance of polyposis with stromal atypia lies in their similarity to malignant sarcoma cells and the catastrophic effects of the misinterpretation of such lesions as malignant (Fig. 5.11). Proliferation of stromal fibroblasts and mesenchymal cells is a response to an excess of intercellular fluid. The stromal cells attempt to check this expansion by an increase in collagen synthesis.[56] According to Klenhoff and Goodman,[57] all "inflammatory" polyps of the nasal cavity contain mesenchymal cells of varying degrees of atypicality. These are usually focal and may be in a palisade configuration. These rarely suggest malignancy. The lesions depicted by Smith et al.[58] and Compagno et al.,[59] however, exceed this minimal atypism. The former restricted their study to the antrochoanal polyp; the latter to all polyps. The antrochoanal polyp originates from the maxillary antrum and often extrudes into the nasal fossa

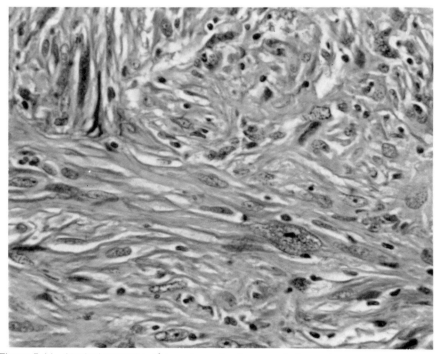

Figure 5.11. Atypical stromal cells in a choanal polyp; so-called pseudosarcomatous change.

through an abnormally enlarged accessory ostium. They comprise between 3.5 to 6.5% of all polyps and occur primarily in the teen-ager and young adult. Although the lesions usually appear as a unilateral and solitary lesion, other polyps have been found in approximately 7.5% of the patients. A significant number of the hosts also manifest bilateral maxillary sinus disease. Because of their position, the clinical presentations of the choanal polyp differ somewhat from the other forms of polypi but it is uniformly agreed that it possesses no unique structural features except for a paucity of mucous glands and eosinophils. Recognition of the reactive, albeit atypical, nature of the cells (fibroblasts and histiocytes) is their presence in a histological structure indistinguishable from the usual nasal polyp and the absence of other sarcomatous features.

Nasal polypi occurring in two generalized disorders merit discussion. The first is the syndrome of recurrent nasal polypi, occurring with asthma and an idiosyncrasy to analgesics, particularly aspirin. While nasal polyposis is much more common in men (60%), the syndrome is manifested nearly twice as often in women than men.[51] Atopy is no more prevalent than in the general population. The syndrome's sequence appears to be the appearance of nasal polyps, followed by asthma and then an aspirin idiosyncrasy. Other analgesics are also capable of producing reactions in these patients. A current hypothesis has the syndrome a result of an abnormality of prostaglandin production or a response to prostaglandins.[51]

The second systemic disorder is cystic fibrosis. As indicated above, nasal polyposis is almost exclusively a disease of adults and is in fact so unusual in children that the finding of a polyp should occasion a search for cystic fibrosis. While the majority of cases occur in already documented cases, there are reports where nasal polypi preceeded the diagnosis by up to 12 years. Nasal polypi in patients with cystic fibrosis have an overall incidence of 6 to 25% and the majority are detected in children between the ages of 4 to 13 years.[60] Sinus radiographs invariably reveal opacity of the maxillary and ethmoid sinuses. This is due both to the accumulation of viscid mucopurulent material in the sinuses and polypoid thickening of the sinus lamina propria. The appearance on rhinoscopy in patients with established involvement depends on the severity of symptoms and ranges from a mild congestion to bulky, multiple and most often bilateral polypi. Microscopically there are no specific features to permit an unequivocal diagnosis related to cystic fibrosis. Even eosinophils may be abundant. There is, however, a tendency for inspissation of secretions in the microcystic spaces of the polyp and a coexisting hyperplasia of the mucus-producing elements of the epithelium and lamina.

The rhinolith is not usually considered in the differential diagnosis of "polyps" of the nasal cavity but it may present in a somewhat similar manner. Rhinoliths are calcareous bodies infrequently found within the nasal cavity and the maxillary antrum. They are formed as a result of complete or partial encrustation of a foreign body, usually of endogenous, but occasionally of exogenous origin. In the former, the nidus is composed of purulent exudate, blood products and cellular debris. Around the nidus, mineral salts, especially calcium phosphate and carbonate, are deposited to form a rough surface. Rhinoliths are usually unilateral, associated with some nasal or sinus disease or anatomical abnormality and are found principally in adult females. The size of rhinoliths varies considerably but nearly all rhinoliths are symptom-producing. Nasal obstruction, malodorous nasal discharge with local pain, epistaxis and fever are not uncommon. Rhinoliths are most often located in the nasal cavity around the inferior choncha. In some cases, they may be entirely intrasinusoidal, or because of pressure necrosis of the wall of the maxillary sinus, project into that airspace.

REFERENCES

1. Waldron, C. A.: Oral epithelial tumors. In Oral Pathology, edited by R. J. Gorlin and H. M. Goldman, pp. 801–803. C. V. Mosby, Co., St. Louis, 1970.
2. Lucas, C. M.: Pathology of Tumors of the Oral Tissues. Little, Brown and Co., Boston, 1964.
3. Greer, R. O., and Goldman, H. M.: Oral papillomas. Clinicopathologic evaluation and retrospective examination for dyskeratosis in 110 lesions. Oral Surg. 38:435, 1974.
4. Summers, L., and Booth, D. R.: Intraoral condyloma acuminatum. Oral Surg. 38:273, 1974.
5. Hyams, V. J.: Papillomas of the nasal cavity and paranasal sinuses. Ann. Otol. Rhinol. Laryngeal. 80:192, 1971.
6. Osborn, D. A.: Nature and behavior of transitional tumors in the upper respiratory tract. Cancer 25:50, 1970.
7. Osborn, D. A.: Transitional cell growths of the upper respiratory tract. J. Laryngol. Otol. 70:574, 1956.
8. Osborn, D. A., and Winstron, P.: Carcinoma of the paranasal sinuses. J. Laryngol. Otol. 76:387, 1961.
9. Henderson, D. W., Allen, P. W., and Bourne, A. J.: Inverted urinary papillomas. Report of five cases and review of the literature. Virchows Arch. (Pathol. Anat.) 366:177, 1975.
10. DeMeester, L. J., Farrow, G. M., and Utz, D. C.: Inverted papillomas of the urinary bladder. Cancer 36:505, 1975.
11. Ringertz, N.: Pathology of malignant tumors arising in the nasal and paranasal cavities. Acta Otol Laryngol. (suppl.) 27:31, 1938.
12. Nicholson, G. W.: The heteromorphoses of the human body. Guys Hosp. Rep. 72:75, 1922.
13. Müller, R., Bechtelsheimer, H., and Tolsdorff, P.: Zur formalen Genese des sog. invertierten Papillom (invertiertes

Epitheliom). Z. Laryng. Rhinol. 52:300, 1973.

14. Suh, K. W., Facer, G. W., Devine, K. D., Weiland, L. H., and Zujko, R. D.: Inverting papilloma of the nose and paranasal sinuses. Laryngoscope 85:35, 1977.

15. Vrabec, D. P.: The inverted Schneiderian papilloma. A clinical and pathological study. Laryngoscope 85:180, 1975.

16. Norris, H. J.: Papillary lesions of the nasal cavity and paranasal sinuses. Part I. Exophytic (squamous) papillomas. A study of 28 cases. Laryngoscope 72:1784, 1962.

17. Norris, H. J.: Papillary lesions of the nasal cavity and paranasal sinuses. Part II. Inverting papillomas. A study of 29 cases. Laryngoscope 73:1, 1963.

18. Skolnik, E. M., Loewy, A., and Friedman, J. E.: Inverted papilloma of the nasal cavity. Arch. Otolaryngol. 84:61, 1966.

19. Ridolfi, R. L., Lieberman, P. H., Erlandson, R. A., and Moore, O. S.: Schneiderian papillomas: a clinicopathologic study of 30 cases. Am. J. Surg. Pathol. 1:43, 1977.

20. Lasser, A., Rothfield, P. R., and Shapiro, R. S.: Epithelial papilloma and squamous cell carcinoma of the nasal cavity and paranasal sinuses. Cancer 38:2503, 1976.

21. Marcial-Rojas, R. A., and Delleon, E.: Epithelial papilloma of nose and accessory sinuses. Arch. Otolaryngol. 77:634, 1963.

22. Brown, B.: The papillomatous tumours of the nose. J. Laryngol. Otol. 78:889, 1964.

23. Mabrey, T. E., Devine, K. D., and Harrison, E. G., Jr.: The problem of malignant transformation in a nasal papilloma. Arch. Otolaryngol. 82:296, 1964.

24. Fechner, R. E., and Sessions, R. B.: Inverted papilloma of the lacrimal sac, the paranasal sinuses and the cervical region. Cancer 40:2303, 1977.

25. Schoub, L., Timme, A. H., and Uyss, C. J.: A well differentiated inverted papilloma of the nasal space associated with lymph node metastases. S. Afr. Med. J. 47:1663, 1973.

26. Majoros, M., Parkhill, E. M., and Devine, K. D.: Papilloma of the larynx in children: a clinicopathologic study. Am. J. Surg. 108:470, 1964.

27. Björk, H., and Weber, C.: Papilloma of the larynx. Acta Otolaryngol. 46:499, 1956.

28. Björk, H., and Teir, H.: Benign and malignant papillomas of the larynx in adults. A comparative clinical and histological study. Acta Otolaryngol. 47:95, 1957.

29. Klos, J.: Clinical causes of laryngeal papillomatosis in children. Ann. Otol. Rhinol. Laryngol. 79:1132, 1970.

30. Szpunar, J.: Laryngeal papillomatosis. Acta Otolaryngol. 63: 74, 1967.

31. Holinger, P. H., Schild, J. A., and Maurizi, D. G.: Laryngeal papilloma: review of etiology and therapy. Laryngoscope 78:1462, 1968.

32. Andrews, A. H., Jr.: Surgery of benign tumors of the larynx. Otolaryngol. Clin. North Am. 3:517, 1970.

33. Lynn, R. B., and Takita, H.: Tracheal papilloma. Canad. Med. Assoc. J. 97:1354, 1967.

34. Nuwayhid, N. S., Ballard, E. T., and Cotton, R.: Esophageal papillomatosis. Case report. Ann. Otol. 86:623, 1977.

35. Boyle, W. F., Riggs, J. L., Oshiro, L. S., and Lennette, E. H.: Electron microscopic identification of papova virus in laryngeal papilloma. Laryngoscope 80:1102, 1973.

36. Lundquist, P. G., Frithiof, L., and Wersall, J.: Ultrastructural features of human juvenile laryngeal papillomas. Acta

Otolaryngol. 80:137, 1975.

37. Spoendlin, H., and Kistler, G.: Papova-virus in human laryngeal papillomas. Arch. Otorhinolaryngol. 218:289, 1978.

38. Rabbett, W. F.: Juvenile laryngeal papillomatosis: the relation of irradiation to malignant degeneration in this disease. Ann. Otol. Rhinol. Laryngol. 74:1149, 1965.

39. Fechner, R. E., Goepfert, H., and Alford, B. R.: Invasive laryngeal papillomatosis. Arch. Otolaryngol. 99:147, 1974.

40. Zehnder, P. R., and Lyons, G. D.: Carcinoma and juvenile papillomatosis. Ann. Otol. 84:614, 1975.

41. Holinger, P. H., Johnston, K. C., and Anison, G. C.: Papillomas of the larynx: a review of 109 cases with a preliminary report of aureomycin therapy. Ann. Otol. Rhinol. Laryngol. 59:547, 1950.

42. Bone, R. C., Feren, A. P., Nahum, A. M., and Winkelhake, B. G.: Laryngeal papillomatosis: immunologic and viral basis for therapy. Laryngoscope 86:341, 1976.

43. Gross, C. W., and Crocker, T. R.: Current management of juvenile laryngeal papillomata. Laryngoscope 80:532, 1970.

44. Holinger, P. H., Schild, J. A., and Weprin, L.: Pediatric laryngology. Otolaryngol. Clin. North Am. 3:625, 1970.

45. Szpunar, J.: Juvenile laryngeal papillomatosis. Otolaryngol. Clin. N. Am. 10:67, 1977.

46. Fearon, B., and MacRae, D.: Laryngeal papillomatosis in children. J. Otolaryngol. 5:493, 1976.

47. Rock, J. A., and Fisher, E. R.: Florid papillomatosis of the oral cavity and larynx. Arch. Otolaryngol. 72:593, 1960.

48. Altmann, F., Ginsberg, I., and Stout, A. P.: Intraepithelial carcinoma (cancer in-situ) of the larynx. Arch. Otolaryngol. 56:121, 1952.

49. Altmann, F., Basek, M., and Stout, A. P.: Papilloma of the larynx with intraepithelial anaplastic changes. Arch. Otolaryngol. 62:478, 1955.

50. Settipane, G. A., and Chafee, F. H.: Nasal polyps in asthma and rhinitis. J. Allergy Clin. Immunol. 59:17, 1977.

51. Wilson, J. A.: Nasal polypi. Clin. Otolaryngol. 1:3, 1976.

52. Tos, M., and Mogensen, C.: Mucous glands in nasal polyps. Arch. Otolaryngol. 103:407, 1977.

53. Tos, M.: Mucous glands in the developing human rhinopharynx. Laryngoscope 87:987, 1977.

54. Toppozada, H. H., and Talaat, M. A.: Human nasal epithelium and cellular elements in chronic allergic rhinitis. Otorinolaringologie 37:333, 1975.

55. Chandra, R. K., and Abrol, B. M.: Immunopathology of nasal polypi. J. Laryngol. 88:1019, 1974.

56. Busuttil, A., More, I.A.R., and McSeveney, D.: Ultrastructure of the stroma of nasal polyps. Cilia in stromal fibroblasts. Arch. Otolaryngol. 102:589, 1976.

57. Klenhoff, B. H., and Goodman, M. L.: Mesenchymal cell atypicality in inflammatory polyps. J. Laryngol. 91:751, 1977.

58. Smith, C. J., Echevarria, R., and McLelland, C. A.: Pseudosarcomatous changes in antrochoanal polyps. Arch. Otolaryngol. 99:228, 1974.

59. Compagno, J., Hyams, V. J., and Lepore, M. L.: Nasal polyposis with stromal atypia. Review and follow-up study of 14 cases. Arch. Otolaryngol. 100:224, 1976.

60. Berman, J. M., and Colman, B. H.: Nasal aspects of cystic fibrosis in children. J. Laryngol. 91:133, 1977.

CHAPTER 6

Squamous Cell Carcinomas of the Oral Cavity and the Oropharynx

Oral and oropharyngeal cancers may seem trivial statistically, but they remain obstinate clinical problems. Oral cancer (primarily squamous cell carcinomas) accounts for approximately 5% of all malignant tumors in the population of the United States. In 1962 approximately 6,000 deaths in the United States were attributed to oral cancer. In 1967, the number had risen to 7,000 deaths.[1] According to the 1975 projections by the American Cancer Society, more than 23,000 United States citizens will have cancer of the oral cavity during the year, with about 8,200 of them dying despite treatment.[2] In England and Wales, one of every 100 cancer deaths is attributed to this group of neoplasms.[3] It has been postulated that one of every three persons who develop an *intraoral* cancer will die within a 5-year period after the diagnosis.

Paradoxically, in view of the foregoing, the mouth is readily accessible for inspection, biopsy, and radiotherapy—yet the outstanding feature of these neoplasms, "is the poor prognosis of a form of cancer which presents exceptionally good opportunities for early treatment."[3] The major implication is that early diagnosis is not being made. Approximately 60% of oral carcinomas are well advanced at the time of their diagnosis. Several factors are at play to occasion the delay in diagnosis. First, approximately three-quarters of all cases of oral cancer occur in patients over the age of 60 years. A related statistic is that between two-thirds and three-quarters of these patients are edentulous. If the patient wears satisfactorily functioning dentures or he does not have dentures, he assumes that no examination of his dentures or his mouth is necessary.[4] A second factor must lie in the general unawareness of the oral cancer prob-

lem by the practitioner. Sixty-nine of 100 oral cancers referred to the Royal Marsden Hospital had *not* been recognized by a dental surgeon.[3] A third factor is the over-all failure of "screening techniques" to significantly contribute to earlier diagnosis.[5]

Oral cytological examinations, in a manner similar to the cytological examinations for uterine cancer, have been proposed as a major tool to assist in early diagnosis. The American Dental Association has editorially stated that "oral cytology should be a part of every oral examination in which the dentist detects even the least suspicious lesion."[6] Despite this recommendation and the numerous studies of oral exfoliative cytology reported in the past two decades, the application and the reliability of the procedures are still controversial. There is, however, general agreement on several points[1]:

1. Oral cytology is *not* a substitute for biopsy.

2. Oral cytology has a *potential* for early detection of malignant lesions.

3. Oral cytology is *useful* as an adjunct for more precise categorization of visible mucosal lesions not warranting biopsy.

4. The value of oral cytology is *limited* if cancer is *clinically suspected.*

5. Oral cytology *may* be useful for repeated follow-up examinations to indicate an appropriate site for biopsy of diffuse or multicentric lesions.

The issue of whether oral cytology is applicable to mass population screening is unsettled, although the majority opinion seems to be that it is not practical at this time.

Let us examine some of the above points in greater detail. A negative cytology report precludes neither malignancy nor other disease. The false-negative frequency in reported series has been quite high. The false-negative rate for oral cytological examination determined in the study by Folsom et al.[1] was 31%. This represented 46 lesions proved malignant by biopsy and contrasts to only six instances of a false-positive cytology. The latter are considered to be of far less consequence since biopsy proved the lesions benign and the patients were not subjected to unnecessary surgery. Folsom[1] warns, however, that the false-negative rate of cytological examinations derived from his study may approximate that to be expected in general dental practice today.

The reliability rate of oral cytological examination appears to vary, depending upon the specific oral site being examined. The vermillion surface of the lip and the attached gingiva have a poor degree of reliable cytological examination with a significantly high false-negative rate. For other areas, the reliability is somewhat better. In Folsom's[1] study the reliability (proven by biopsy) was as follows: 27% for the attached gingiva, 38% for lip lesions, 56% for the oral pharynx, 60% for buccal mucosa, 71% for the tongue, 73% for the palate, and 89% for the floor of the mouth. These statistics reflect the opinions of other workers that the more densely keratinized areas or hyperkeratotic lesions are the least amenable to correct cytological interpretation. Cytological examination is furthermore applicable primarily to epithelial lesions. It is seldom useful in the evaluation of nonepithelial malignant or benign conditions.

SQUAMOUS CELL CARCINOMAS OF THE ORAL REGIONS

Squamous cell carcinomas are the most common malignant tumors of the oral cavity, representing a little over 90% of all oral malignancies. In the United States, this form of neoplasm accounts for 7 to 8% of all malignancies. Bhaskar[7] considers that in the United States, more than 20,000 new cases of oral cancer occur each year and that about one-half of this number die of or with this disease annually. In Britain, 2,400 new cases are registered each year and the number of deaths annually is half the number of new cases.[8]

Oral squamous cell carcinoma is predominantly a disease of men, and, while carcinomas of the lips occur more often than their intraoral counterparts, significant geographic distributions prevail (vide infra). Further extensions of this geographic influence are the observations that in certain countries of the East and Far East, oral and pharyngeal carcinomas account for almost half of all malig-

nant neoplasms. On the lips and in the oral cavity there is a regional incidence that, along with features of histological classification, stage of disease, and form of treatment, plays an important role in prognosis for patients and biological activity of the neoplasm itself.[9-12]

In the following discussion, squamous cell carcinomas of the oral regions are presented according to their presumed site of origin, and each is considered separately. From a pathogenetic basis and from an over-all incidence basis (only slightly more than 0.5% of all lesions biopsied by dentists are squamous cell carcinomas), this may be an artificial strategy; it does stress, we hope, the value of *thorough* oral examination.

Before this exercise, however, let us consider some features of oral cancer at large. Early asymptomatic oral squamous cell carcinomas are primarily located in three areas: the floor of the mouth, ventral or lateral tongue and the soft palate complex.[13, 14] These lesions are more often *erythroplastic* than white and the invasive carcinomas cannot be distinguished from in situ lesions by color alone. Induration is not a feature of the early and asymptomatic carcinoma, nor does minimal size (less than 1 cm) preclude the existence of invasion.

The cause of oral cancer remains elusive despite some known direct relationships such as tobacco chewing and the use of betel nut. The risk of mouth cancer in the heavy smoker and drinker may be as much as 15 times greater than in those who neither smoke nor drink. More than 70% of mouth cancers occur in the dependent parts most exposed to food and saliva. Surveillance and biopsy of snuff-dippers mucosae, however, have led some investigators to conclusions that snuff, per se, or chewing tobacco do not act as carcinogens.[15]

A variety of different tumor-node-metastasis (TNM) classifications have been proposed for carcinoma of the oral cavity but none have gained a universal acceptance. A classification with considerable merit is that proposed by Rapidis et al.[16] wherein they take into consideration site (S) and pathology (P) in addition to the conventional tumor (T), node (N) and metastasis (M) in common use. These five variables have been compared favorably to the traditional TNM classification. Table 6.1 presents this STNMP classification for intraoral carcinomas.

Cervical lymph node metastases from oral carcinomas certainly define a high risk category of patients and this has been well documented.[17-20] The adverse effect of cervical lymph node metastases is clearly evident by the presentation of

Table 6.1
STNMP Classification for Intraoral Carcinomas (Rapidis et al.)[16]

S (Site)		T (Tumor)		N (Node)	
S1	Lip, skin	T1	Tumor less than 20 mm in diameter	N0	No palpable nodes
S2	Lip, mucous membrane	T2	Tumor between 20 mm and 40 mm in diameter	N1	Equivocal node enlargement
S3	Tongue	T3	Tumor between 40 mm and 60 mm in diameter	N2	Clinically palpable homolateral regional node(s) not fixed.
S4	Cheek		and/or extending beyond the primary region		
S5	Palate		and/or through adjacent periosteum	N3	As N2 but fixed
S6	Floor of mouth		and/or through the capsule	N4	Clinically palpable contralateral or bilateral node(s) not fixed.
S7	Alveolar process	T4	Any tumor greater than 60 mm in diameter	N5	As N4 but fixed.
S8	Antrum		and/or extending to involve adjacent structures		
S9	Central carcinoma of bone				

M (Metastasis)		P (Pathology)	
M0	No distant metastasis	P0	Hyperkeratotic lesion showing atypia
M1	Clinical evidence of distant metastases without definite histological and/or radiographic confirmation.	P1	Carcinoma in situ
		P2	Basal cell carcinoma
		P3a	Verrucous carcinoma
M2	Proven evidence of metastases beyond the regional nodes.	P3b	Well-differentiated squamous cell carcinoma
		P3c	Moderately differentiated squamous cell carcinoma
		P3d	Poorly differentiated squamous cell carcinoma

Table 6.2
Carcinoma of the Oral Regions: Admission Lymph Node Status, Memorial Cancer Hospital[17]

Anatomical Site	No. of Patients	No. with Involved Node (%)
Floor of mouth	804	315 (39%)
Tonsil	650	395 (61%)
Tongue		
Base	136	103 (76%)
Oral	314	98 (31%)
Palate		
Hard	123	16 (13%)
Soft	299	110 (37%)
Buccal mucosa	248	93 (36%)
Gingiva	179	62 (35%)
	2,753	1,192 (43%)

data in Tables 6.2 and 6.3.[17, 18, 20] Not only the number of lymph nodes but also of evidence, fixation and size are directly correlated to survival. The levels of cervical lymph node involvement are those used at Memorial Cancer Center, New York, and are depicted in Figure 6.1. Level I refers to those lymph nodes within the submandibular and submental triangles. The chain of nodes along the upper, middle and lower third of the jugular vein are levels II, III and IV respectively. Level V describes the nodes along the accessory nerve and in the posterior cervical triangle. Spiro et al.[18] indicate the incidence of *multiple* node involvement increases as the metastatic disease from the intraoral carcinoma becomes clinically apparent at the lower levels in the neck.

Contralateral spread of metastases is thought to occur in three ways: by crossing efferent lymphatics; by actual spread over the midline via efferent lymphatics after regional nodes have been involved, producing collateral lymph flow; or as in certain anatomical areas where there is no definite midline and the superficial lymphatics form a network with the capacity to direct flow to either side. Contralateral metastases from the gums and buccal mucosa are unusual, but they are significant from the tongue and floor of mouth. The incidence in tongue lesions varies from 4% for the mobile portion to 25% for those at the base. Spread of the carcinoma from the floor of the mouth most frequently involves the homolateral submandibular nodes with the upper and middle jugular nodes following very closely in frequency. When contralateral involvement is present (17%), however, the prevalent pathway is by way of the upper jugular nodes with the submandibular nodes involved two-thirds as frequently.[19]

Although a significant reduction in local and regional failure rates in oral cancer has been achieved, their magnitude is still unacceptable to most head and neck surgeons. An ideal dose and delivery of preoperative radiation has yet to be defined. The results of multiple drug chemotherapy are somewhat encouraging but require further clinical trials. Shah et al.[21] state that in more than half of their patients with carcinoma of the oral cavity (total of 758 patients), initial treatment failed to control the carcinoma before 5 years. Recurrent disease manifested itself either at the primary site, the neck, or both. Seventy-three percent of these patients eventually died of their disease. Factors for this lack of control were: (1) sex; females seemed to have an over-all poor prognosis compared with males; (2) stage of disease; recurrent disease increased as the stage advanced; (3) depth of invasion; (4) neoplasm at resection margins; and (5) clinically positive lymph nodes; if microscopically confirmed, the failure rate was significantly increased.

With respect to "adequate" surgical margins, it is evident that a pathologist's report of adequate excision is most dependable if no irradiation has been used previously in the management of the patient. Lee[22] has pointed out that inadequate tumor margins are most often reported back to the surgeon who has operated on an intraoral lesion— an incidence of 15%, compared with the hypopharynx, 3%, and larynx, 4%.

Until recently radical neck dissection was not questioned as the treatment for clinically apparent metastases within the neck from head and neck squamous cell carcinomas. Support has been clearly evident by observations that as the extent of lymph node involvement increases from solitary to multiple ipsilateral and bilateral lymph nodes, cure rates progressively decline. Modification from the classic en bloc radical neck are largely dependent on location of the cancer, stage and clinical judgment on the presence or absence of metastases.

The apparent plateauing of survival and recurrences within the dissected neck has led to advocacy of combined or integrated management of the neck.[23-25]

Surgery and radiation therapy can be integrated in the following ways: (1) surgical resection of the primary lesion and cervical node metastases with radiation used for recurrences; (2) surgery followed by radiation therapy for both primary site and the entire neck; (3) curative radical irradiation for the primary lesion and planned preoperative radiation and neck dissection; (4) planned preoperative irradiation to the primary lesion alone and/or to the neck. Surgical excision is mandatory in this instance, while in (3) surgical excision of the primary is used only for recurrences.

Pros and cons can be given for pre- or postoperative irradiation, but control of the cancer within the neck appears to be the same whether the irradiation is delivered before or after surgery.[26] The sequence in which radiation therapy and surgery are administered to the neck depends primarily on the decision regarding the treatment of the primary lesion. In a patient with clinically

Table 6.3
Influence of Histologically Positive Lymph Nodes on Survival

Lymph Nodes	5-Year "Cure" Rate	
	Roswell Park[20] (N = 256)	Memorial[18] (N = 557)
Histologically positive		
1. Single	39%	30%
2. Two	25%	—
3. Three or more	11%	24%
4. Contralateral	—	25%
5. Bilateral	—	5%
Histologically negative	60%	60%
	(N = 160)	(N = 194)

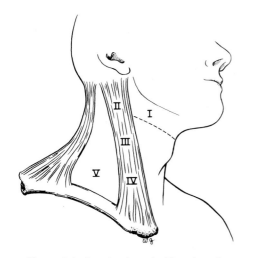

Figure 6.1. Levels of cervical lymph nodes.

positive nodes and the primary treated by radiation therapy, 5,000 rads in 5 weeks is delivered to the neck and the appropriate surgical procedure follows in 3 to 4 weeks.[26] If the initial treatment of the primary lesion is by surgery, the appropriate surgical procedure within the neck is done simultaneously and radiation therapy, 5,500 rads in 5½ weeks, is delivered three weeks later.[26]

Subclinical disease (N0) in the neck cannot be ignored. Jesse[26] indicates that 32% of patients N0 with oral cavity and faucial arch primary cancers will develop cancer in the neck if not electively treated. He further relates treatment to the neck *after* a node develops is successful in 75% of patients whose primary cancer remains controlled. The case for prophylactic elective neck dissection has been reviewed by Nahum et al.[27] Nearly all of the arguments for neck dissection can apply also to elective radiotherapy to the neck. However, the effectiveness of surgical resection is clearly shown by Manfredi and Jacobelli.[28] A significant reduction in survival occurs with the onset of clinical cervical disease. A comparison of 5 years' results in a group of patients who underwent a therapeutic or prophylactic dissection showed a survival rate of 24.7% and 57.6%, respectively.[28]

Million[29] has indicated that 4,500 to 5,000 rads in 4½ to 5 weeks has prevented metastasis from patients staged N0 whose primary tumor is controlled. Fletcher[30] considers that the same dose eradicates in excess of 90% of subclinical disease, whereas 3,000 rads in 3 weeks to 4,000 rads in 4 weeks eradicates only 60 to 70%.

At present, elective neck dissection and elective irradiation appear equally beneficial in removing nodes containing subclinical metastases. Planned integrated therapy of carcinomas of the oral cavity and faucial arch, supraglottic larynx, hypopharynx and nasopharynx is outlined by Jesse.[26]

In the foregoing we have discussed two of three therapeutic modalities for the treatment of epidermoid cancer in the neck. The third, *chemotherapy*, can be of value in selected cases.[31, 32] The goal of this modality, as it is for any cancer therapy, is to eliminate all cancer cells in the host with as little adverse effect as possible. To accomplish this goal, the ideal agent should be able to destroy a relatively large mass of tumor with as little damage to normal cells as possible. Additionally, it must exhibit systemicity—the ability to destroy neoplastic cells in a discriminative fashion wherever they may be in the body.[33–36] No such chemotherapeutic agent exists at the present time. Like surgery and radiotherapy, chemotherapy lacks specificity and systemicity. Chemotherapy also shares

with experimental immunotherapy and hormonal therapy the problem that resistant variants may arise and become predominant through selective inhibition of sensitive cell populations.

Perhaps one of the most important concepts to grasp in the chemotherapy of cancer is that neoplastic cells are not rapidly dividing cells. In a steady state, cell renewal equals cell loss; but in cancer, cell loss equals only 95 to 97% of cell renewal. Thus squamous cell carcinomas have the same, or even slower, cell growth rates, and a slightly decreased rate of cell loss. Cancer, then, may be regarded as a disease of cell accumulation rather than proliferation.

Therapy with chemotherapeutic agents is selected with the foregoing in mind and the agents are best classified by their mode of action. Class I drugs (e.g., nitrogen mustard and gamma irradiation) are equally toxic for both proliferating and resting cells. The margin of safety for therapeutic use is then minimal.

Phase-specific drugs (vincristine, vinblastine, methotrexate) act on a specific part of the cell cycle. Methotrexate and 6-mercaptopurine interfere with DNA synthesis; vinblastine interferes with the postmitotic phase; vincristine acts in two places and also perhaps during mitosis, when it interferes with spindle formation and subsequent chromosome separation. Normal cells are unaffected by brief exposure to phase-specific drugs, but this is a short-lived.

Cycle-specific agents (fluorouracil, cyclophosphamide) destroy both proliferating cells and resting cells, but cells in the cycle are far more sensitive.

It is becoming apparent that there is not often much to be gained from the use of anticancer drugs as a form of "last-resort" treatment after failure to control by conventional surgical and radiotherapeutic measures. The most likely anticipated result of such treatment is some temporary systematic relief with occasionally some objective evidence, again usually temporary, of tumor regression, all gained at the risk of increased morbidity and mortality. There is, however, evidence that a planned adjunctive use of chemotherapeutic agents with irradiation or surgery or both may offer substantial hope for tumor irradication or control.[37]

A number of currently available drugs such as methotrexate and bleomycin have a definite activity against squamous cell carcinoma of the head and neck; to a lesser extent, this holds true for 5-fluorouracil in relation to adenocarcinoma. To date, however, responses are generally short and accompanied by substantial toxicity.[38] De Vita et al.[37] considers squamous cell cancers of the head and neck in a category "responsive to drugs for which clinically useful improvement in survival of responders has not been clearly demonstrated."

Methotrexate, bleomycin and cis-diamminedi-chloroplatinum (II) (cis-DDP) are the three agents most actively investigated at this writing. DDP has been demonstrated to be at least as active as the other two drugs in epidermoid carcinomas of the head and neck. DDP is one of several platinum compounds which strongly inhibits cellular replication by action on DNA. Its toxic effects strike the hematopoietic, auditory, gastrointestinal and renal system. Effects on the kidney may be reduced by induced and vigorous diuresis.[38]

The final role, either single, in combination, or combined with other modalities of drug treatment of squamous cell carcinoma of the head and neck awaits definition by carefully controlled, non-biased clinical trials. Histological evaluations of the effect on tumor are available.[39, 40] For methotrexate, 5-fluorouracil and bleomycin, the light and electron microscopic changes are similar and these, in turn, are similar to the changes wrought by irradiation. In short, the changes are those of an increase in differentiation of the squamous cell carcinoma, with the end result of solid and necrotic keratin balls. The appearance of residual differentiated (keratinized) cells is likely the result of elimination of undifferentiated cells rather than a direct stimulation of differentiation of primitive neoplastic cells.

Immunotherapy (manipulations that augment the ability of a tumor-rejection immune response to inhibit growth or spread of an existing tumor) has not been successfully applied to epidermoid carcinomas of the head and neck. The theoretical potential of a systemic treatment with a high degree of specificity and low toxicity has yet to be fulfilled. If that cannot be provided immunotherapy offers no advantage over simpler, conventional treatment methods. Another major limitations of tumor inhibition via tumor-rejection immunity is the relative weakness of the response. At present, it appears that immunotherapy should be reserved for those situations which involve a minimal tumor bulk, such as that which remains after optimum conventional treatment.[41]

Carcinomas of the Lips. Carcinomas of the mucous membrane or the vermillion area of the lips are the most common malignant neoplasms of the oral mucous membranes. They make up between 25 and 30% of all carcinomas of the oral regions. The lower lip is the primary site in over 95% of the cases. Despite the relatively high frequency for this anatomical region, carcinomas of the lower lip constitute only 0.6% of all cancer in man.[42]

The disease, as it presents in the United States, has a pronounced male predominance (95%). Elsewhere, particularly in Scandinavia, women manifest a significant number of carcinomas of the lip as opposed to their American sisters.[43] Women also have a greater tendency to develop carcinomas of the upper lip. The greatest number of cases present in patients 50 to 70 years old, but the disease is not limited to that period. Bernier and Clark,[44] studying a select population (service personnel), found a substantial number of patients who were younger than 40 years of age.

There is considerable agreement over the rather striking association of carcinoma of the lip and complexion and occupation. The disease is rare in Negroes and is most frequently observed in subjects with a fair or ruddy complexion, particularly in those who are outdoor workers and who have considerable exposure to sunlight. Tobacco users, particularly pipe smokers, are said to manifest a predilection. Additional observations concerning the demographic and geographic incidence of carcinoma of lip in the United States may be found in the report by Szpak et al.[45] and Ju.[46] It is to be noted that squamous cell carcinoma of the lip and skin comprise a significant proportion of the malignant neoplasms in renal and homograft recipients.[47]

On the lower lip, the carcinomas are most often found originating on the exposed vermillion border, outside the line of contact with the upper lip. While the middle one-third of the lip and the buccal commissures may be the site of origin, most carcinomas (85%) of the lower lip arise at a point about halfway between the midline and the commissure. The upper lip is an uncommon site for carcinoma to develop, but, when it is primary there, the neoplasm is frequently near the midline.

Surprisingly, in view of its exposed position, carcinoma of the lip is not often diagnosed early. Many patients relate a delay of up to 2 years before seeking medical attention. Nearly half of a series of 190 patients had carcinomas of the lip measuring more than 1.5 cm in diameter at the time of initial examinations.[48]

Squamous cell carcinomas are by far the dominant histological type of neoplasm. Occasionally a basal cell carcinoma from the skin of the upper lip will extend onto the labial surface. The remainder of the epithelial lesions are of minor salivary gland origin and have been presented elsewhere (see Chapter 2). Approximately 85% of the squamous cell carcinomas are well differentiated and would fall into Broder's I and II classifications.[49] Spindle cell variants are rare but nevertheless important to recognize because they may be confused with supporting tissue neoplasm (Figs. 6.2 and 6.3). Multifactoral microscopic grading of the primary tumors in a TNM classified series of squamous cell carcinoma of the lip has indicated a significant correlation between the histopatholog-ical grade and recurrences, frequency of metastases and mortality.[50]

The uncommon variant of squamous cell carcinoma, the adenoid squamous cell carcinoma, with few exceptions occurs on the skin of the head and neck and may be an oral lesion as well. For those on the lips, a relatively high percentage occur on the upper lip.[51, 52] In accordance with its general tendency, those on the lips manifest a decreased

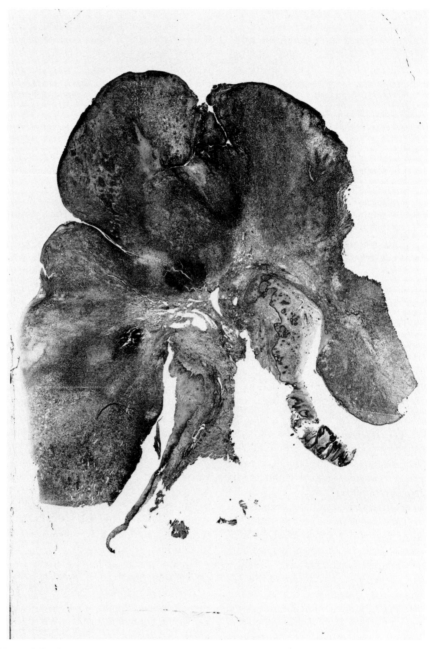

Figure 6.2. Polypoid pleomorphic carcinoma. (Courtesy of A. Someren, M.D.) See Chapter 9.

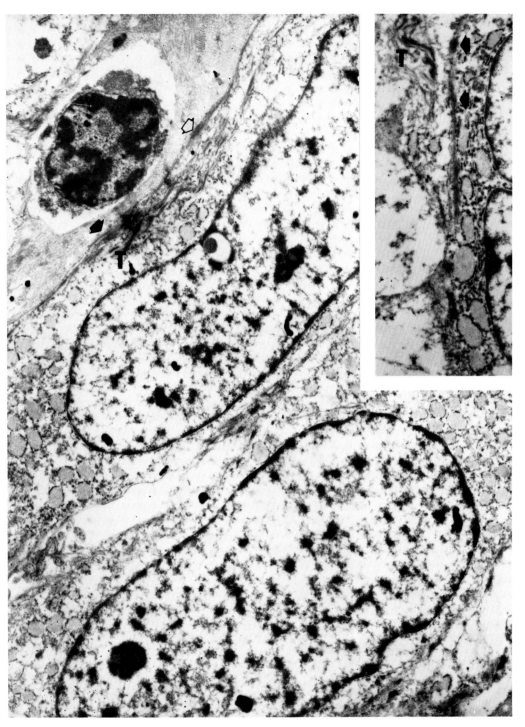

Figure 6.3. Ultrastructural appearance of the carcinoma in Figure 6.2. Tumor cell exhibits poorly defined desmosomes (*arrows*) and tonofilaments (T). Magnification, ×10,000; inset, ×6,400. (Courtesy of A. Someren, M.D.)

tendency to metastasize and have manifested a high cure rate.

Keratoacanthomas should be distinguished, if possible, from well-differentiated carcinomas of the lip. Nearly three-quarters of the keratoacanthomas occur in the head and neck and of these nearly 10% are localized on the lips, where they are equally distributed between upper and lower lips.[53] Most have been at the mucocutaneous junction; others have occurred on the vermillion.

Even more rare is a basal cell carcinoma apparently confined to the mucosal surface.[52]

Three morphological types of squamous cell carcinoma are seen: exophytic, ulcerative and verrucous. The exophytic type is only slightly more common than the ulcerative form. The typical *verrucous squamous cell carcinoma* only rarely occurs on the lips. Many of the labial carcinomas arise in areas of clinical leukoplakia and may present as nodular, warty outgrowths (exophytic) or begin as small ulcers. Both of these gross forms may begin as a seemingly stubborn blister or "cold sore." Both the ulcerative and exophytic carcinomas may reach considerable size because of their relatively indolent course. The ulcerative carcinoma manifests a relatively more rapid infiltration and invasion and is usually of a higher histological grade than the exophytic carcinoma. As a general rule, carcinomas of the upper lip are also more rapidly growing than those of the lower lip.

Carcinomas of the lip tend to have an indolent and often protracted clinical evolution. There is a greater tendency to lateral and peripheral spread than for deep invasion. Metastases to lymph nodes are late and relatively infrequent when one compares these carcinomas with others in the oral regions.[42] In common, however, with other oral carcinomas, the potential for metastasis increases with increasing size of the lesion and the duration present before treatment. Metastasis is also closely related to the degree of differentiation in the carcinoma, and the location on the lip influences the proclivity for metastasis.[50, 54] Carcinomas of the commissures are more likely to manifest this adverse finding than carcinomas of other sites on the lip. Involvement of the commissure also adversely affects recurrence rates. With either upper or lower lip primaries, the recurrence rate is double when the lesion involves the commissure.[55]

Statistics concerning metastases vary according to the reporting institution and whether or not the patient has received any prior treatment before institution of "definitive" management. Metastases to lymph nodes may be expected to occur in 5 to 10% of the patients at some time during the

biological course of their disease.[56] Unusually, node involvement is said to be present on initial examination. Most metastases present within 2 years after discovery of the primary lesion. The submandibular lymph nodes are the chief secondary deposit sites. Neoplasms near the midline may involve the submental group of lymph nodes. Distant metastases are unusual.

At the risk of overstatement, treating carcinoma of the lip by either surgical excision or radiotherapy produces remarkably similar results. The prognosis is excellent.[55] A recent statistical mortality rate for carcinoma of the lips has been expressed as 0.1 per 100,000 population.[42] Even these few deaths have been attributed to inadequate treatment or mismanagement.

An 80 to 90% 5-year cure rate has been expressed for carcinomas of the lower lip. All workers agree that the upper lip neoplasms are more virulent in their clinical behavior and in their ability to metastasize. Martin et al.[57] reported 21 patients and found metastases in nearly half the group. Their 5-year survival for patients with lesions of the upper lip was only 41% as compared with a greater than 70% survival rate for patients with carcinomas of the lower lip. Regardless of the site of origin, the presence of metastases has a profound affect on survival, reducing the near 90% survival rate (lower lip) to a 50% 5-year salvage.[58–60]

Table 6.4, presenting comparative data from the studies by Krause et al.[59] and Wurman et al.,[60] clearly indicates the significance of size of the labial carcinoma to the frequency of regional lymph node metastases. Table 6.5, modified from Lund et al.,[50] also points out the morbidity for metastases in persistent and recurrent carcinomas. Lip cancer kills primarily in two ways: (1) spread into the pterygoid fossa and middle cranial fossa, possibly along the inferior dental nerve; (2) extensive neck disease localized to the anterior and upper neck.[61]

Carcinoma of the Buccal Mucosa. Buccal carcinomas, in contrast to carcinomas of the lip, are

Table 6.4
Frequency of Regional Lymph Node Metastases*

Site	T1 (<2 cm)	T2 (2–4 cm)	T3 (>4 cm)
Lip	5%	52%	73%
Oral tongue	42%	43%	72%
Floor of mouth	38%	65%	71%

* From data presented by Krause et al.[59] and Wurman et al.[60]

Table 6.5
Carcinoma of Lip: Relationship of Recurrence to Metastasis*

	Patients without Recurrence	Incidence of Metastases (%)	Patients with Persistent and Recurrent Carcinoma	Incidence of Metastases (%)
T1	207	2	14	7
T2	143	2	20	20
T3	31	16	13	46
Total	381	3	47	23

* Modified from Lund et al.[50]

prone to the running of an aggressive course. The cheek forms the lateral wall of the oral cavity and is made up of the buccinator muscle, external fibroadipose tissue and skin. The mucosal surface connected with the cheek extends from the upper to the lower gingivo-buccal gutters, where the mucosa reflects itself to cover the upper and lower alveolar ridges and forms the commissures of the lips and the related ramus of the mandible. The neoplasms are encountered at the commissure of the mouth, along the occlusal plane of the teeth or at the retromolar areas.

Buccal carcinomas present in patients of a more advanced age than other oral carcinomas. O'Brien and Catlin[62] and others[63, 64] record a mean age in the seventh decade. Exclusive of rather striking geographic differences, the disease is one of men with a ratio dominance of 4 to 10:1. Women in the southeastern United States bear buccal carcinomas with almost the same incidence as men. Geographic variation of both the sex dominance and numerical frequency is intimately related to oral hygiene and the chronic use of local irritants. Tobacco chewing, in particular, appears to play an important role in the pathogenesis of buccal squamous cell carcinomas. Khanolkar[65] reports that 415 of 576 oral cancers in Indians arose from the buccal mucosa. This preponderance more than implies local factors of major importance. In India and the Far East, the chewing of betel nut has been the "whipping boy." Its significance cannot be denied, but it is not possible to implicate this habit alone. The chewing of the nut is probably additive and supplements poor oral hygiene. "Snuff-dipping" by Southern women in the United States is held responsible for the marked incidence in that sex in the rural areas of this part of the nation.

Buccal carcinomas are usually insidious in their clinical behavior. Trismus produced by neoplastic infiltration or submaxillary adenopathy may be the first clinical evidence of their presence. Pain is usually intense only in ulcerating carcinomas.

Virtually all authors agree that there are three distinctive clinicopathological types of buccal carcinoma: (1) exophytic, (2) ulceroinfiltrative and (3) verrucous. The exophytic is most common, and the verrucous type is the least common. The latter is a rather distinctive clinicopathological entity and is found most often on the buccal mucosa in contrast to other areas of the body. All three varieties are well to moderately well differentiated and arise often in association with areas of clinical leukoplakia. Ackerman and del Regato[42] claim that except for carcinoma of the tongue, no other lesion is so often associated with a leukoplakic patch. The majority of the neoplasms arise on the part of the mucosa lying against the lower third molars. Very often the expansiveness of the neoplastic growth obscures the definite site of origin.

Exophytic carcinomas are found most commonly at the level of the buccal commissure and present as a soft white outgrowth in an area of leukoplakia. Early on they may appear benign from both gross and clinical aspects. They do not often ulcerate and may be asymptomatic unless there is secondary infection. Ulceroinfiltrative carcinomas involve the buccinator muscle early and often present as a deep excavating ulcer with diffuse peripheral extensions. Untreated, both exophytic and ulceroinfiltrative carcinomas are extensively destructive, particularly the latter type. They invade deeply, may ulcerate through the skin and invade the adjacent bones. Extension to the pharyngomaxillary fossa may occur easily from posteriorly situated lesions. Invasion of the anterior pillars of the soft palate, alveolar ridges or pterygoid fossa makes "curative" therapy nearly impossible.

The verrucous carcinoma is a "low-grade" squamous cell carcinoma, most commonly found in the mandibular buccal sulcus and the alveolar mucosa of the mandibular ridge. A smaller number are found on the maxillary alveolar mucosa and occasionally they may be found on the tip of the tongue. This type of carcinoma is not limited to the oral cavity. Similar lesions occur on the hand, scrotum and the mucosa of the penis, vulva, larynx and nasal fossa. Kraus and Perez-Mesa[66] studied 105 cases and described 77 in the oral cavity. Fifty of the 77 intraoral carcinomas presented on the buccal mucosa. Duckworth[67] estimates that verrucous carcinomas represent less than 5% of all oral cancers (Table 6.6).[66, 68] The neoplasm usually evolves in an indolent fashion in areas of leukoplakia. There is a striking correlation with the chewing of tobacco and the use of snuff.

Recognition of verrucous carcinoma is important for two reasons: (1) it is often underdiagnosed as a benign hyperplasia; and (2) it carries the most favorable prognosis of all forms of buccal carcinoma.[66, 69] The clinical appearance of the verrucous carcinoma is that of a piled-up growth or large papillary mass with a micronodular or mammilated surface. It is relatively soft when compared to the other forms of carcinoma unless there has been a superimposed infection. The degree of keratinization (often considerable) determines the color of the lesion, white or reddish-white.

Verrucous carcinomas may grow to considerable size with a conspicuous lateral or surface spread (Fig. 6.4). Deep extension, however, should never be minimized in the surgical planning for treatment. Downgrowth penetrates the buccal soft tissues, invades the maxilla or mandible and may even extend through the cheek to present onto the surface of the skin. This local aggressiveness belies its relatively innocuous appearance, and no matter how wide or deep the neoplasm extends, it maintains its well differentiated appearance. The microscopist may be deceived in considering the lesion as benign, even after repeated biopsy specimens.

Microscopically, the verrucous carcinoma is characterized by a thick layer of proliferating squamous epithelium whose individual cells are not cytologically malignant (Figure 6.5). The advancing margin consists of either bulbous masses of neoplasm or long, finger-like extensions of well-differentiated epithelium. Epithelial pearls and small cysts are often seen, but cellular atypism or mitoses are rare. The basement membrane is intact and there are no groups or nests of squamous cells breaking through to invade in the usual sense of microscopic invasion (Figure 6.6). A heavy inflam-

Table 6.6
Verrucous Carcinoma: Distribution of Lesions*

Site	No. of Cases
Oral Cavity	77
Buccal mucosa	50
Gingiva	21
Tongue	3
Palate	2
Tonsillar pillar	1
Nasal Cavity	4
Larynx	15
Total	96

* As reported by Kraus and Perez-Mesa[66] and Biller et al.[68]

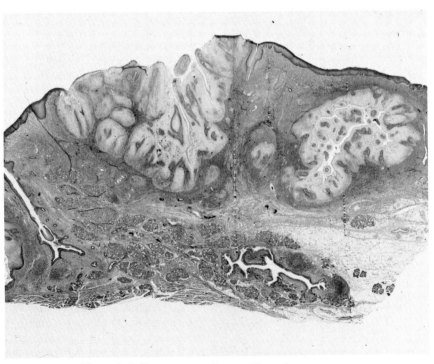

Figure 6.4. Verrucous carcinoma of buccal mucosa.

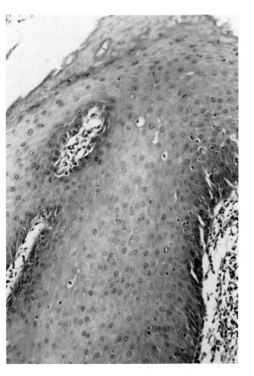

Figure 6.5. Verrucous carcinoma of buccal mucosa. The regularity of the cells is deceptive.

matory reaction in the adjacent stroma is also characteristic.

Keratoacanthomas, squamous papillomas and pseudoepitheliomatous hyperplasias are the three principal lesions that require differentiation. The former is very rare in the oral cavity. The central stromal core of the papilloma with its rich vascularity is distinctly different from the connective tissue matrix of the verrucous carcinoma where it is very inconspicuous. Reactive hyperplasia is never as coarsely papillated or verrucoid, and its anastomosing epithelial nests are slender and pointed.

The recurrence rate for all types of buccal carcinoma is high. Waldron[43] considers this to be due to multicentric foci in a widely "conditioned" area of mucosa. It is not uncommon, particularly with the verrucous carcinomas, to have the patients manifest several other oral primary carcinomas. Goethals et al.[70] recorded that 31% of his patients developed a second oral carcinoma. The prognosis of buccal carcinomas is dependent upon the clinicopathological type, how early the lesions are detected, their anteroposterior location and mode of therapy.

Until recently, survival figures had not been established with consideration of the usually ex-

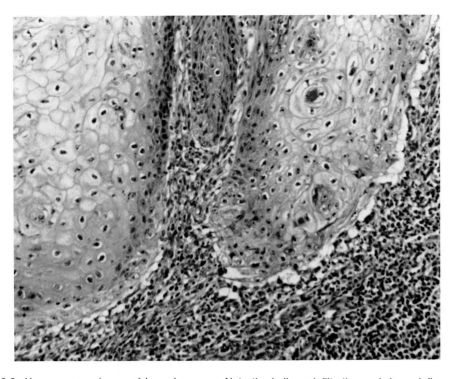

Figure 6.6. Verrucous carcinoma of buccal mucosa. Note the bulbous infiltration and dense inflammatory reaction.

cellent outcome associated with the verrucous carcinoma. If the buccal carcinoma is detected in its early stages, good results are obtainable by either radiotherapy or simple excision. Preparatory roentgen therapy is often used but, except for localized lesions, is probably not curative when used as the sole therapeutic measure. Peroral radiotherapy is practical only in limited lesions of the posterior half of the buccal mucosa and in particular for those carcinomas that have invaded the anterior pillar of the soft palate. A combination of external and internal (peroral) irradiation may control, but not cure, the carcinoma.

Exophytic carcinomas are said to be particularly suitable for curietherapy. This form of management should not be applied to lesions that have already invaded the alveolar ridges and the anterior pillar of the soft palate.

Kraus and Perez-Mesa[66] claim that verrucous carcinomas manifest a poor response to irradiation. Their data strongly suggest that this form of primary treatment is contraindicated for this type of buccal carcinoma. Four of 17 patients so treated developed a highly malignant carcinoma with anaplasia, metastases and a rapid progressive death (Tables 6.7 and 6.8).

Table 6.7
Verrucous Carcinoma and Radiation Therapy

Author	No. Treated by Radiation Alone	No. with Recurrence
Oral		
Ackerman[201]	7	7
Perez et al.[202]	17	17
Goethals et al.[70]	1	1
Fonts et al.[69]	4	2
Demian et al.[203]	2	2
Kraus and Perez-Mesa[66]	13	13
Laryngeal		
Ryan et al.[204]	3	3
Burns et al.[205]	8	1
Biller and Bergman[206]	4	2

Table 6.8
Verrucous Carcinoma: Metastases

Author	No. of Cases	Metastasis
Ackerman[201]	31	1
Kraus and Perez-Mesa[66]	105	4*
Goethals et al.[70]	55	0
Ryan et al.[204]	20	0

* All occurred following failure of radiation therapy and all were anaplastic carcinomas.

In general, the prognosis of ulceroinfiltrative carcinoma is the poorest of the group. When either this form or the exophytic carcinoma have invaded the soft palate, upper alveolar ridge or the pterygoid fossa, even the most radical management is very likely doomed to failure. In this respect, the biological expectations for an exophytic carcinoma are heavily dependent on the stage of development when first treated.

Posterior one-third buccal carcinomas have a poor outlook because of their tendency to invade the anterior faucial pillars and the soft palate. Carcinomas in a localized retrocommissural location have the best prognosis.

The lymphatics of the buccal area drain into the submental, submandibular, lateral pharyngeal, and superficial and deep parotid lymph nodes before proceeding to the deep jugular nodes. Lymphatic spread of advanced cancer of the buccal mucosa is most frequent to the ipsilateral submandibular nodes. Involvement of the deep cervical lymph nodes is not common.[71]

As indicated above, the lesions are seldom small when first noted. Radiation therapy of small nonverrucous carcinomas may be used with acceptable results. If the carcinoma invades bone or infiltrates soft tissues, surgical intervention is indicated, the extent of which will be dictated by the boundaries of the disease. Table 6.9 from Dhawan et al.[72] lists the sites of spread from advanced buccal carcinoma.

Metastases, most often to the regional lymph nodes, will occur in about 50% of cases of buccal carcinoma. This statistic applies almost exclusively to carcinomas of the exophytic and ulceroinfiltrative types. Metastasis from verrucous carcinomas are seldom noted. The metastatic harbinger is first noted in the submaxillary lymph nodes. Distant metastases occur with somewhat less frequency than in other oral carcinomas.

Death in all forms of buccal carcinoma is usually due to the results of local, uncontrolled disease and is related to over-all debilitation. As expected, the 5-year survival for treated verrucous carcinomas is the highest of the three clinicopathological types and ranges from 60 to 75%. Goethals et al.[70] report a 75% 5-year survival in 55 patients treated by diathermy excision. The over-all survival, however, is considerably lower (30% 5-year) and reflects the interplay of location, histological type and therapy. O'Brien and Catlin[62] found that 64% (160 of 240 patients) had extension of their carcinomas past the buccal mucosa and/or metastases at the time of admission to their center. Regional lymph nodes were involved in 37% of this group.

Table 6.9
Carcinoma of the Buccal Mucosa Infiltrative and Metastatic Patterns*

Local Infiltration	Percent	Lymph Nodes	Percent
Infratemporal fossa	70	Submandibular (ipsilateral)	58
Skin	58	Upper-deep cervical	10
Alveolus	52	Submandibular (contralateral)	4
Anterior pillar	12	Submental	4
Palate	6	Negative nodes	38
Tongue	4		
X-ray evidence of invasion of mandible	42		

* From data presented by Dhawan et al.[72]

Paymaster,[63] reviewing 467 cases of buccal carcinoma treated by a variety of means, expressed an over-all survival of 43% for 5 years. Lampe[73] reported on 30 cases of buccal carcinoma treated by radiation therapy and claimed a 50% 5-year survival. An interesting group of statistics has been offered by O'Brien and Catlin,[62] who reported a 52% determinate survival (5 years) in 248 patients. These authors noted that earlier series from their own institution (225 patients) manifested a 28% 5-year survival. The increased survival in the more contemporary series was attributed to the use of surgical resection rather than radiation.

Surgical removal thus appears to have more favorable survival data associated with it, but this may only reflect selection criteria. Nevertheless, radical removal of a verrucous carcinoma, regardless of the extent of bone invasion, should not be contraindicated since it may be life-expanding for the patients. Similar radical removal for advanced ulceroinfiltrative and exophytic carcinomas is ill-advised.

Carcinoma of the Gums (Gingiva and the Alveolar Mucosa). Squamous cell carcinomas of the gingiva and alveolar mucosa are less common than those of the lips and tongue and comprise approximately 10% of all oral malignant neoplasms.[74] The two anatomical areas are herein considered together, acknowledging, at the same time, that some authors and institutions subdivide the region into gingiva and alveolar mucosa.

Carcinomas of the gums generally occur in the premolar and molar regions with the lower jaw affected more often than the upper.[75] As with other squamous cell carcinomas in the oral regions, there is a male predominance, generally in a ratio of 4:1 over women. Oral habits peculiar to the geographic locales influence the sex distributions and, much like buccal carcinomas, there is an increased frequency of carcinoma of the gums in rural

women of the Southeastern United States.[76] Patients are usually in their sixties at the time of diagnosis. In the lower gums, carcinomas usually arise in the molar area or the posterior third of the dental arch. They rarely take origin in the anterior third. A similar preference is manifested for carcinomas of the upper gums.

The clinical diagnosis may be difficult, since the signs and symptoms may be confused with benign inflammatory or reactive lesions so common in these areas. Thoma[77] considered this group of carcinomas as the most misdiagnosed of any form of carcinoma in the oral cavity. Carcinomas of the maxillary antrum may infiltrate the upper gingiva and produce an intraoral ulceration. In some of these instances it may be impossible to establish a gingival or antral origin.

The carcinomas may be superimposed upon an area of severe periodontal disease or areas of "leukoplakia." Many of the carcinomas appear to arise at the free gingival margin close to the surface of a tooth. Alveolar ridge carcinomas occur most often in edentulous areas. Interference with mastication or the fitting of a denture is usually the first clinical sign. Ackerman and del Regato[42] state that there is often a history of extraction of teeth and surgical treatment for a suspected alveolar abscess before a correct diagnosis is made.

Gingival carcinomas may be nodular and plaque-like, ulcerating or papillary and exophytic. Carcinomas of the alveolar mucosa of the edentulous patient are usually papillary and fungating in character. All forms have a significant spreading tendency that carries them over the mucosal surface. A high level of differentiation characterizes the majority of the carcinomas. Willen et al.[78] have shown that histological grading, mode and stage of invasion, and cellular response can be scored so as to be prognostically helpful.

Invasion of the underlying bone occurs in nearly

50% of carcinomas of the gums.[79, 80] This occurs relatively early in the ulcerating type. It is this invasion that is responsible for the often observed loosening of teeth associated with the carcinomas. Resected specimens have demonstrated that osseous invasion occurs more often than is suspected.[79, 80] It is frequently present even though the dental x-rays are negative for bone involvement.

Metastases from both maxillary and mandibular carcinomas are first to the submandibular nodes. Mandibular carcinomas manifest this tendency to a greater degree than do the maxillary carcinomas. There is approximately a 25% clinical error rate in the clinical evaluation of palpable lymph nodes associated with carcinoma of the gums.[81] Fine-needle biopsy of the lymph nodes reduces this error.[82] As a general rule, the metastases prove to be less differentiated than the primary tumor. The metastatic rate averages approximately 30% but has been reported to be as high as 88%.[83, 84]

Treatment of these carcinomas is primarily surgical, and bone involvement is an important determinant. The role of radiotherapy, either alone or in combination therapy is outlined by Nathanson et al.[85] and Love et al.[86] En bloc dissection of the primary lesion, the mandible and lymph nodes, with or without postoperative irradiation, appears to be the method of choice for mandibular carcinoma.[84, 87, 88] A similar radical approach is taken for maxillary gum carcinomas. Given an adequate therapy, the prognosis for the patient with carcinoma of the gum is better than that associated with carcinoma of the tongue. There is no real difference in 5-year survival between upper and lower jaw carcinomas, and several authors have reported as high as 50% 5-year survival.[75, 81] If metastases are present at the time of primary treatment the prognosis is considerably worse. Backstrom et al.[82] record a 5-year determinate survival of 7% compared with 41% for patients with carcinoma of the gums without cervical metastases.

Left to their own devices, carcinoma of the upper and lower gums becomes widely expansive. In the upper gum, lateral extension results in infiltration of the gingivobuccal gutter and soft tissues of the cheek; medially the palate is invaded and bone invasion results in penetration of the antrum.

Nonepidermoid cancers of the gum are far outnumbered by the epidermoid cancers. In a 20-year survey at Memorial Hospital in New York, 606 cases of epidermoid and 26 cases of nonepidermoid cancer were inventoried.[89] Nineteen of the nonepidermoid cancers were of minor salivary gland origin and four were melanomas. It is estimated that about 6% of minor salivary gland cancers arise in the gum. Mucoepidermoid carcinomas and adenoid cystic carcinomas appear equally prevalent and their behavior is similar to those found in the major salivary glands.

Carcinoma of the Tongue. Carcinoma of the tongue is only slightly less common in total incidence than carcinoma of the lip and exceeds or closely approximates the total incidence of all other intraoral primary sites combined.[90] Squamous cell carcinomas make up approximately 97% of all malignant lesions of the tongue. Glandular malignancy and supportive tissue tumors account for the remainder (see appropriate sections). An estimated 1,625 persons will have died from cancer of the tongue in the United States in 1970, with approximately 2,700 new cases being diagnosed.[91]

Carcinoma of the tongue is predominately a disease of men and one of middle life. Frazell and Lucas[92] found that four-fifths of their patients were in their sixth to eighth decades. The disease, however, is also seen in the young[93] (vide infra). Because of the association with pre-existing Plummer-Vinson syndrome, Scandinavian women have a higher incidence than American women.

Poor oral hygiene and habits, the use of tobacco and alcohol and the coincidence of syphilis are all important underlying or predisposing factors. Trieger et al.[93] found that 18% of their series also had a diagnosis of syphilis. Three-fourths of their series were heavy drinkers, with 50% manifesting unequivocal evidence of hepatic cirrhosis, and 90% smoked excessively. The squamous cell carcinomas of the tongue in tobacco and alcohol users are also noted to be more aggressive. More of this group die due to their carcinoma or a second primary lesion than do nonusers. This difference is not explained by a difference in tumor stagings, patient's ages or type of treatment received.[94] As with other forms of oral and paroral cancer, there is a geographical variation, which is probably related to oral habits. In India for example, there is a disproportionately high occurrence of carcinoma of the tongue.[95] Location in the tongue differs in the Indian, however, with the base of the tongue affected three times more frequently than the anterior or mobile portion of the tongue.

The symptoms, clinical findings and biological behavior of carcinoma of the tongue vary considerably with the location of the neoplasm. In some institutions, cancer of the tongue refers to neoplasms arising in the oral or mobile portion; tumors of the base of the tongue, i.e., posterior to the line of the circumvallate papillae, are included in the anatomical region of the oropharynx.

Frazell and Lucas[92] suggested the following anatomical subdivisions of the tongue in regard to the location of carcinoma: (1) posterior third—lesions arising posterior to the circumvallate papillae and the glossopalatine fold; (2) anterior two-thirds—further subdivided into an anterior third and middle third including the lateral border and ventral surface of the tongue; and (3) dorsum of the tongue—the part of the tongue anterior to the circumvallate papillae, but excluding the lateral border.

Although there is some individual series variation, carcinoma of the tongue is most often found on the lateral border of the middle third. In the large series reported by Frazell and Lucas,[92] 45% were located in this area, 20% in the anterior third, and only 4% on the dorsum of the tongue. When all series are considered, it may be said that approximately three-fourths of the cancers occur in the oral portion of the tongue. In this location, the squamous cell carcinomas tend to be more histologically mature. The growth pattern is usually infiltrative, ulcerative and exophytic. According to Conley[96] the lesions are already more than 2 cm in diameter at the time of first clinical examination. The dorsum of the tongue, the tip and the ventral surface are the least common sites for the primary lesion. The neoplasms arising from the ventral surface extend directly toward the floor of the mouth, and, in many instances, it is difficult or impossible to determine the exact site of origin.

A tabulation of the presenting symptoms of patients with squamous cell carcinoma of the tongue is presented in Figure 6.7. Local pain, often simulating a sore throat, is an important symptom of carcinoma of the posterior third of the tongue.

There is often too long a delay in seeking medical attention after the symptoms are noted. An average time lapse of at least 4.6 months has been recorded.[97] Carcinomas of the posterior third of the tongue tend to be clinically silent until they have become extensive. They are, of course, difficult to visualize and tend to be deeply infiltrative, taking the path of least resistance, which is the intrinsic lingual musculature. An area of induration noted on deep palpation is the most common finding. Small areas of ulceration are usually present.

Carcinomas arising in the vallecular area often present in the pre-epiglottic space after extension anteriorly. Those originating on the glossopalatine sulcus, early in their course, invade the superficial and deep zones of the tongue and extend up to the lateral pharynx. Because of their infiltrative character and difficult visualization, they often extend into the oral tongue or have clinical lymph node metastases before diagnosis is made. Neoplastic involvement of the lingual nerve is responsible for the pain in the ear on the affected side in patients with advanced or moderately differentiated carcinoma of the tongue or floor of the mouth.[98]

In the anterior two-thirds of the tongue there are two primary growth patterns with all intermediate grades: infiltrative and exophytic. Early on they usually present as a nondescript area of focal thickening or roughness or as clinical leukoplakia. Other forms of presentation are as a painless, superficial ulceration or desquamation. The deeply infiltrative types may manifest little or no surface ulceration until late in the course of the disease. Other forms are exophytic or ulcerating, fungating masses. The predominatly exophytic varieties have less tendency to infiltrate deeply.

Squamous cell carcinoma of the tongue may

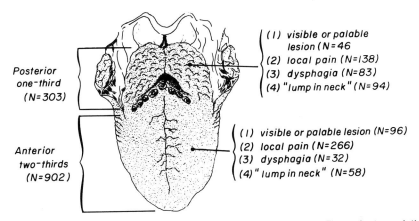

Figure 6.7. Presenting symptoms in carcinoma of the tongue (1,205 patients). The patient population on which this illustration is based is that studied by Frazell and Lucas.[92]

arise in apparently normal epithelium, in areas of clinical leukoplakia or on a pre-existing chronic glossitis. In the latter instances, multiple and separate primary carcinomas should always be sought. Squamous cell carcinomas of the tongue are usually moderately well differentiated. The exception to this is the group of carcinomas arising from the base of the tongue. These carcinomas are distinctly less well differentiated as a group. Lund and associates,[99] using a multifactorial microscopic grading system achieved a high correlation with scoring and predictability of lymph node metastases. Others have found similar relationships with stromal reactions (round cell infiltrate and stromal acid mucosubstances).[100]

Metastasis to the cervical lymph nodes is said to occur more frequently from carcinomas of the tongue than from any other intraoral primary neoplasm. Early metastasis is also a detrimental feature and occurs with sufficient frequency that it must be assumed even if palpable lymph nodes are not present. Any treatment of the patient must be directed with this factor in mind. Frazell and Lucas[92] found that 40% of their 1,554 patients had lymph node involvement on admission, and over 20% manifested bilateral involvement. Contralateral involvement was present in 3% of the cases studied. Lymphatic drainage of the organ favors involvement of homolateral side lymph nodes. The propensity for metastases from carcinomas of the base of the tongue is even greater. Approximately 70% of patients have unilateral or bilateral metastases upon first examination.[96] Metastases invariably develop first in the subdigastric node and spread downward along the jugular chain to involve, in untreated cases, the entire supraclavicular region.[98] Distant metastasis from carcinoma of the tongue is also not uncommon. The lungs and liver are most often the site of deposits.

Carcinomas of the middle third are so situated that the neoplasm gains ready access to the anterior tonsillar pillars, the tonsil, retromolar area and floor of mouth, and may diffusely involve the entire tongue. The frequency of metastasis is high from this site. Metastases from carcinomas arising from the anterior third are slightly less frequent in occurrence than from carcinoma on the middle third. Carcinomas from the tip and dorsum of the tongue are unusual and are more indolent in their behavior. The size of the primary lesion does not necessarily correlate with the presence or likelihood of metastases. Carcinoma of the base of the tongue exhibits a high frequency of metastases to cervical lymph nodes (uni- and bilateral). According to Sessions et al.,[101] 34% of patients with occult

ipsilateral metastases go on to develop contralateral metastases.

The prognosis for patients with carcinoma of the tongue is influenced significantly by a number of factors.[92] Obviously early diagnosis and management of the primary lesion before extension is the key to a successful outcome. The anteroposterior location of the primary neoplasm is important in this respect. There is a marked decrease in 5-year survival as the primary site moves to the posterior third of the tongue. The size and degree of spread of the primary lesion adversely affect prognosis. Lesions greater than 2 cm have a more lethal effect. Finally, the incidence of histologically proven metastases certainly mars 5-year survivorship.

The prognostic significance of palpable lymph nodes has been well documented. Their presence nearly halves 5-year survival figures.[102] Histologically proved metastases in the palpable lymph nodes reduces survivorship for an additional quarter. Frazell and Lucas[92] reported a 5-year cure rate of 67% in patients who did not develop metastases in lymph nodes during the course of their treatment. In patients with involved nodes on admission, the cure rate was only 17%. Small neoplasms of the anterior third of the tongue without involvement of adjacent structures are associated with the highest cure rate, i.e., 80% or better for 5 years. The middle third carcinomas, unless detected early have a much reduced survival rate (i.e., 30%) because of extension into the floor of the mouth, mandible and posteriorly into the tonsillar area.

Posterior third carcinomas are detected late, reach a large size, are less differentiated, have a higher metastatic rate and extend widely into the surrounding structures. For these reasons, despite apparently adequate extirpation, they have a survival rate of less than 15% for 5 years. The histological appearance of the neoplasms is of less importance than the location, size and presence of metastasis, but there is some correlation between the level of differentiation and aggressive behavior.

Therapy of lingual cancer, because of the character of the primary and the early metastases, tends to be radical. Several approaches are used at different centers.[102–109] Lampe and Fayos,[105] treating squamous cell carcinoma of the oral part (anterior two-thirds), primarily by radiotherapy of the lingual tumor and reserving surgery for neck gland dissection and for "salvage after radiotherapeutic failures," report results as good as, if not better than those reported for solely surgical management. Despite this, surgical removal is the therapy most widely used and tends to be radical in extent. Hemiglossectomy, unilateral resection of the mandible and radical neck dissection are the usual surgical approaches.

The combined use of irradiation and surgery is necessary for extensive involvement. MacComb et al.[98] claim that radiation therapy is not tolerated well by patients who are alcoholics and heavy smokers and recommend surgical intervention only in this class of patient. The debate between radiotherapist and surgeon over the role of their methods of treating squamous cell carcinoma continues.[110] Frazell[108] has presented an excellent review of both sides of the issue as it relates to the mobile portion of the tongue. As long as the widely divergent viewpoints persist, it seems unlikely that any one form of treatment will receive unanimous endorsement.

It should be recognized that depending on the facilities at hand and the experience and skill of the therapist, small lesions (3.0 cm or less) may be treated successfully by either local surgery or irradiation (anterior two-thirds of the tongue). Chances of disease control diminish with increasing size of the lesion and with increasing incidence of cervical metastases, regardless of the mode of treatment (Table 6.10).

The recurrence rate for carcinoma of the tongue is relatively high, even for those lesions in the anterior third. Skolnik and Saberman[102] indicate nearly 40% of anterior third tumors recur at the primary site. A cumulative recurrence rate of 90% by 2 years has been recorded for carcinoma of the tongue base.[111] Persistence, recurrence and uncontrolled primary disease is responsible for the death of patients. The immediate causes of death are pneumonia, extension into vital structures, obstruction and cachexia.

Squamous Cell Carcinoma of the Floor of the Mouth. Some institutions do not separate the floor of the mouth from the tongue or gums in their statistical reporting of intraoral carcinomas. Where subdivision has been made to isolate floor

of the mouth carcinomas (the U-shaped area between the lower gum and the tongue), the frequency of carcinoma approaches that for the tongue and accounts for approximately 10 to 15% of all oral carcinomas.[112, 113] It is at least the second most common site for squamous cell carcinomas in the oral cavity[114] and is the most common intraoral site in Negroes.[115] Approximately 500 people in the United States die each year from carcinoma of the floor of the mouth.[116]

The most frequent site of origin is in the anterior segment of the floor of the mouth at the midline and lateral to or involving the frenulum. At its onset the lesion may be deceptively small, but with progression of time the characteristic exophytic or papillary appearance is obtained. The lesion rarely begins as an ulcer.

Unhappily, a high proportion of the carcinomas arising in this area are advanced when first seen (Table 6.11). Their infiltration is deceptive but may extend to reach the gums, tongue and genioglossus muscle. Spread along the periosteum is common once the mandible is reached by the infiltrative growth. Invasion of the root of the tongue is an ominous prognostic event. In some respects, these neoplasms are harder to control than those from the buccal mucosa and the tongue. This is due to the loose submucosal tissues of the submental and submandibular spaces which facilitate extension.

The disease is one of males predominantly, and the men are usually in their fifth to seventh decades of life. Most are heavy users of tobacco and alcohol.

Metastases to cervical lymph nodes may be an early occurrence but are usually a later manifestation than that observed in carcinoma of the tongue (Fig. 6.8). Submental lymph nodes are rarely involved, and metastasis to distant sites is rare and often occurs after the primary and/or

Table 6.10
Cancer of the Anterior Tongue: Comparison of Methods of Primary Control*

Primary Lesion	Radiation Therapy (%)	Surgical Therapy (%)
T1	86	86
T2	93	79
T3	63	50
T4	50	34

* From the report by Frazell.[108]

Table 6.11
Cancer of the Floor of the Mouth: Stage of Disease (TNM) on Admission to the Head and Neck Service, Memorial Cancer Center, N. Y.*

Stage of Neoplasm	1935–1949 (285 Cases)	1950–1963 (349 Cases)
	% of total	
Stage I	20	23
Stage II	34	32
Stage III	34	35
Stage IV	12	10

* Data are from Harrold.[118] The failure to achieve early diagnosis is clearly evident in the nearly identical percentage of patients in each stage for the years studied.

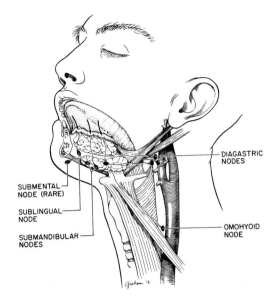

Figure 6.8. Lymphatic routes: carcinoma, floor of mouth.

regional metastases have been apparently controlled. Some contradiction to the latter is found in patients who undergo necropsy. Kolson et al.[117] found distant metastasis in 12 of 27 patients who had a postmortem examination.

The carcinomas are usually well differentiated and prognosis is considerably more affected by size and extent of the disease than by the microscopic appearance.[118] Multifocal carcinomas should be looked for, and there is a surprisingly high (20.3%) incidence of primary carcinomas in other sites.[117] More than half of these occur in the head and neck area.

The importance of a thorough routine oral screening examination is borne out by the study of Kolson et al.,[117] who found that 50% of their 108 patients had their carcinomas confined to the floor of the mouth when first seen. Usually the carcinomas are large or lymph node metastases are present before patients seek medical advice. The incidence of lymph node metastases during the course of the disease ranges from 35 to 70%. As with all areas in the head and neck, a palpable neck mass does not mean metastases to lymph nodes. Examination of Kolson et al.'s[117] 46 radical neck dissection specimens indicated no microscopic neoplasm in 30% of patients who had palpable nodes.

Therapeutic guidelines may be found in a number of reports.[116–120] The most favorable lesions appear to be adequately treated by excision or irradiation with equal success. Figure 6.9, after

Harrold,[118] gives the relation of survival to the status of the nodes. Ipsilateral lymph node involvement markedly reduces the salvage rate (25%) and pre-operative irradiation does not appear to influence the outcome significantly.[117]

Squamous Cell Carcinoma of the Palate. I have elected to separate anatomically the hard and soft palates in the discussion of squamous cell carcinomas. The uvula and soft palate form a clinico-oncological unit and are considered as part of the oropharynx (the palatine arch). Neoplasms of this region are discussed later. An additional justification for this seemingly artificial separation is the fact that the large proportions of neoplasms arising in the hard palate are of mucous or salivary gland origin. Ackerman and del Regato[42] estimate that for every squamous cell carcinoma of the hard palate, there are three or four glandular tumors. This applies principally to an American population. There are significant geographic differences; viz., in India, where local irritants play such a conspicuous etiological role, the frequency of squamous cell carcinomas of the hard palate is very much increased. In an Indian study (17-year) of tumors of the hard palate, Ramulu et al.[121] found only six benign tumors and 1,100 malignant lesions, most of which were squamous cell carcinomas. This extraordinary incidence is largely due to the peculiar habit of smoking *chuttas* with the burning end inside the mouth.

Squamous cell carcinomas may arise in the midline or to one side or the other of the hard palate close to the upper gingiva. They are usually ulcerated but at times may be verrucous. The neoplasm is only rarely sharply localized and is

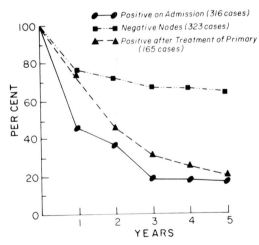

Figure 6.9. Influence of lymph node metastases on survival: carcinoma of the floor of the mouth. Data presented are from Harrold's study.[118]

often surrounded by areas of clinical leukoplakia. Eneroth et al.[122, 123] have found that nearly three-fourths of the squamous cell carcinomas of the palate are well differentiated and have devised a histological host response grading system that may be additive to other factors for prognosis.

An excellent study of squamous cell carcinoma of the palate (hard *and* soft) has been presented by Ratzer et al.[124] Their report concerned 422 patients with squamous cell carcinoma of the palate seen at Memorial Hospital (New York City) over a 22-year period. This number actually represented a "mixed bag" of cases, including *all* patients (early lesions, late lesions, treated and not treated). Two hundred ninety-nine cases were from the soft palate and 123 originated from the hard palate.

Carcinoma of the palate is a disease of elderly men and is usually detected in the seventh decade of life. From a prognostic standpoint, the size of the tumor, rather than anatomical site, appears to have the greater influence. In the Memorial Hospital series, the cure rate was slightly better, but not significantly so, for patients with tumors of the *hard* palate.[124] Lesions greater than 3.0 cm have a marked decrease in 5-year cure rates, i.e., 54% versus 16%.[124] Enlargement of the neoplasm to the extent of invading adjacent structures also reduces the prognosis. When the palatal carcinoma is confined to the primary site of origin, the cure rate is nearly twice that of neoplasms that have involved adjacent structures such as the gingiva, tongue and buccal mucosa. Over-all results are *much worse* with hard palate tumors manifesting local extension than for those of the soft palate.

The most striking decline in survival is seen in those patients who present with cervical lymph node metastases compared to those with carcinoma confined to the oral cavity (Table 6.12). Cure rate at the Memorial Hospital was only 8% when nodes were present on admission.[124] When cervical metastases developed subsequent to control of the primary tumor, the 5-year cure rate was 15%. Distant metastases are *said* to be unusual.

Squamous cell carcinomas of the palate may be treated successfully by either radiation therapy or surgery. Most current workers favor the latter mode. For both hard and soft palate tumors, the choice of treatment is based on a number of factors: (1) site of origin; (2) size of the neoplasm; (3) stage of the disease; and (4) previous therapy, if any. In general, surgery is preferred for almost all squamous cell carcinomas of the hard palate.[124] Some early and well-confined cancers of the soft palate are amenable to surgical excision with sub-

Table 6.12
Carcinoma of the Palate: Stage of Disease on Initial Examination

Stage of Disease	Hard Palate	Soft Palate	Percentage
	No. of cases		
In situ	0	14	3
Localized	60	85	34
Invasion of adjacent structures	40	85	30
Metastases to regional or cervical lymph nodes	16	110	30
Distant metastases	1	3	1

* Data are derived from the report by Ratzer et al.[124]

sequent functional disability. More diffuse lesions are best treated by radiation therapy. Cervical lymph node metastases are best treated by radical neck dissection. Advanced local lesions with local regional lymph node involvement are probably best managed by combined radiation and surgical therapy. Death of patients who have carcinomas of the palate is due to uncontrolled disease with extension into adjacent structures, including bone.

Basal cell carcinoma rarely occurs on the oral mucosa. Liroff and Zeff[125] have reported such a lesion of the palatal mucosa and reviewed the four other oral basal cell carcinomas in the literature.

Oral Carcinomas in Children. Benign tumors occur far more often than malignant tumors in the oral cavities of children. Jones,[126] basing his conclusions on a study of subjects from Northern Ireland, estimates that 1 person in 1,500 develops a tumor in the mouth before the age of 16. In his Belfast group of subjects, he discovered only two carcinomas (one of the lip and the other from the alveolus) in a 14-year period. He also concluded that 7.5% of the oral soft tissue lesions were malignant.

Although rare, a pattern has emerged from the various and isolated cases of oral carcinomas in childhood.[127] The duration of symptoms averages a period of weeks rather than months. The neoplastic growth rate is rapid because the neoplasm has arisen on already growing tissues. Metastases occur early to regional lymph nodes. No obvious etiological factors are usually demonstrable, but it has been reckoned that congenital disorders of the skin such as chronic ichthyosis or other ectodermal defects may predispose the child to the development of intraoral carcinoma.[128]

In the oral cavity, the junction of the anterior two-thirds and posterior one-third of the tongue is said to be a common site of involvement. Pichler et al.[129] have reviewed the literature and could cull but 11 cases of documented squamous cell carcinoma of the tongue in the first two decades of life. The youngest patient was a newborn.

Distant Metastases from Oral Cancer. It has been taught and perpetuated in texts that oral epithelial malignancies rarely spread below the level of the clavicles. Topazian[130] has traced the origin of this traditional viewpoint back to 1906, when Hitchings found that less than 1% of head and neck cancers were associated with distant metastases. Castigliano and Rominger[131] and others[132, 133] are beginning to lay this myth to rest. In their reviews, the former authors demonstrated a progressive increase in the number of distant metastases from oral malignancies, from a figure of 2% in 1943 to 15% in 1957. Hoye et al.[132] concluded that, if *sought for,* a high number of patients will manifest distant metastases. These workers further demonstrated that *all* histological grade IV lesions produced distant metastases. Their study, however, was not restricted to the neoplasms of the oral cavity. The lung is the favorite site for metastases.

The most likely reason for the increasing recognition of remote secondary lesions from oral cancers is the increasing life span after treatment in the present and recent decades. Certainly the number of necropsies performed affects the number and the reliability of the statistics.

EFFECT OF LYMPH NODE METASTASIS ON SURVIVAL IN ORAL CANCER

The very significant and detrimental influence upon prognosis of cervical lymph node metastases from carcinomas of the oral region has been emphasized in the preceding pages. Table 6.13 (from Blady's[134] study) re-emphasizes these facts. From this information it can safely be stated that the clinical staging of the neoplasm is far more important for defining prognosis than is the histological classification of the particular carcinoma.

According to MacComb and Fletcher,[135] more patients die from recurrent or uncontrolled regional neck lymph node cancer than from localized primary disease. It is the attack on these metastatic sites that has generated the controversy. Whether a primary surgical treatment or a primary radiotherapeutic management is superior or even equally effective is at the center of the controversy. An important ancillary argument is the matter of *prophylactic treatment,* regardless of the form of the treatment.

Neoplasms of specific index sites in the oral cavity, oropharynx and laryngopharynx usually manifest characteristic metastatic patterns to the cervical lymph nodes. The distribution of clinically positive lymph nodes from these sites has been well described by Lindberg.[136] Since there is no evidence (experimental or clinical) that the presence or absence of regional lymph nodes has a demonstrable effect on the development of tumor immunity, their treatment is integral in the management of the disease.[137]

Southwick[138] rightfully points out that even individuals with a special training and interest in the treatment of head and neck cancer have difficulty in accurately assessing whether an enlarged lymph node contains metastatic neoplasm. The incidence of microscopic disease in neck dissection specimens considered clinically negative at the time of their removal ranges from a low of 25% to a high of 60% (Table 6.14). This is too great an inaccuracy to be reliable.

Accuracy of clinical assessment of nodal metastases has been nicely studied by Spiro et al.[18] In 732 patients with squamous cell carcinoma of the oral cavity and oropharynx, and with pathological verification of the presence or absence of lymph node metastases in the ipsilated neck dissection, these workers record a 15% false negative assessment and a 10% false positive evaluation. In the

Table 6.13
Incidence of Cervical Metastases: Primary Examination

Site of Neoplasm	Incidence (%)	5-Year Survival (%)
Anterior two-thirds of tongue	45.0	16.2
Base of tongue	70.0	24.0
Floor of mouth	41.0	19.0
Cheek	37.0	23.0
Soft palate	47.0	17.0
Tonsil	66.0	21.0
Nasopharynx	71.0	15.0

* Data are from the report by Blady.[134]

Table 6.14
Incidence of Clinically Occult Cervical Metastases
The general unreliability of clinical palpation is evidenced from the variable incidence reported by these workers.

Author(s)	Incidence (%)
Lyall and Shetlin[207]	60
Kremen[208]	50
Southwick et al.[209]	40
Sako et al.[210]	27.6
Ward et al.[211]	25
Spiro et al.[18]	15

same series, clinical assessment was more accurate in 70 patients who underwent bilateral neck dissection. A correct preoperative clinical diagnosis was made in 130 of 140 neck specimens (93%).

Questions can also be asked about the accuracy of *pathological* examination, sectioning and microscopic evaluation of the resected lymph nodes. In regional lymph nodes draining cancer from some regions of the body, the commonly employed methods of sectioning the lymph nodes can account for an approximately 30% false pathological interpretation.[139] The failure to identify a metastasis wthin a lymph node depends upon the number of sections examined and the location of the metastasis within the node. Increase in the percentage probabilities of identifying various sized lesions in different sized nodes can be had by using the methods described by Wilkinson and Hause.[139] The characteristics of epidermoid carcinoma metastatic from the mucosa of the head and neck are such that the high false negative rate given above very likely does not apply to those metastases.

Since it is not the purpose of this book to detail surgical or radiotherapeutic management, the reader is referred to several excellent sources for critical assessments of one form of treatment over another and for guidelines on whether to electively treat the neck in patients with squamous cell carcinomas of the oral cavity and faucial arch.[135, 138, 140–144]

THE OROPHARYNX

There is no unanimity among surgeons, therapists and pathologists on what structures should be included in the anatomical area designated as oropharynx. The M. D. Anderson Hospital (Houston, Texas) approach is a very logical and clinically useful one.[145] These workers divide the oropharynx into two main structures: the palatine arch and the orpharynx proper (Fig. 6.10). The palatine arch is composed of the anterior faucial pillars and the soft palate. While these structures share characteristics of the oral cavity and the oropharynx, tumors from the region are treated, both surgically and radiotherapeutically, in a manner that parallels the management of oropharyngeal neoplasms.

The oropharynx proper, in the above schema, is composed of the following: (1) soft palate, including the uvula; (2) anterior faucial pillars, retromolar trigones; (3) glossopalatine sulci (glossotonsillar or palatoglossal); (4) tonsillar beds; (5) posterior faucial pillars; (6) base of tongue; (7) valleculae;

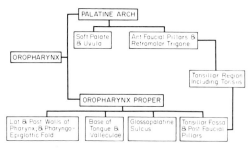

Figure 6.10. This schematic presentation of anatomical regions of the oropharynx is based on the M. D. Anderson Hospital (Houston, Texas) concept of the oropharynx.[145]

(8) lateral and posterior oropharyngeal walls from the level of the soft palate to the level of the hyoid bone; (9) pharyngoepiglottic fold. The anterior faucial pillars are considered by some authors as oral structures, and the neoplasms from these sites do indeed behave like oral carcinomas. In our opinion, this is too academic a splintering, especially since overgrowth of the neoplasms may obscure precise sites of origin. The tonsillar region includes the tonsils, the tonsillar bed and both (anterior and posterior) faucial pillars. This site is the second most common site for cancer in the upper air passages, but except for very early lesions, involvement of a single site in the region is unusual. In most cases, the site of origin is *ascribed* to the anterior faucial pillar or to the tonsillar bed. Only exceptionally can the posterior faucial pillar be pinpointed as the site of origin.

The designation "retromolar trigone" refers to the anterior aspects of the anterior pillar and is a common site for squamous cell carcinoma. The soft palate region begins at the junction of the anterior and posterior faucial pillars and includes the uvula for the purposes of this presentation. The base of the tongue lesions have been considered in the section concerning squamous cell carcinomas of the tongue. The base of the tongue blends laterally with the glossopharyngeal sulci and posteriorly with the valleculae. Lesions of this area are considered as a unit. Neoplasms arising from the pharyngeal walls from the level of the soft palate to the level of the hyoid are also considered as oropharyngeal. Neoplasms originating on the pharyngoepiglottic folds are also assigned to the oropharynx as they manifest more of the clinicopathological characteristics of neoplasms from that region than of neoplasms of the aryepiglottic folds.[145]

The malignant gradient increases as the origin of carcinomas moves posteriorly in the oral cavity and reaches the oropharynx. Thus, carcinomas of the base of the tongue tend to be more extensive (60 to 70% are T3 and T4) and more biologically aggressive than carcinomas of the tonsillar region as compared to those of the buccal mucosa or the alveolar ridge.[146] From the standpoint of histological differentiation, carcinomas in the oropharynx are more often undifferentiated and anaplastic, in contrast to the more differentiated carcinomas of the mouth (Fig. 6.11).

The most striking feature of the oropharyngeal carcinomas, however, is their high proclivity for metastases. For carcinomas of the soft palate there is an incidence of metastases of 40%, somewhat over 50% for carcinomas of the tonsillar pillars, retromolar area, tonsillar fossa and pharynx, and up to 70% for carcinomas at the base of the tongue.[147]

Bilateral and contralateral metastases are increased in oropharyngeal primaries because of the richer network of lymphatics. The primary lymphatic connections of oropharyngeal lesions drain into the superior deep jugular lymph nodes and the subdigastric lymph nodes. There are lesser direct connections with the superior spinal accessory and mid-deep jugular lymph nodes. The retropharyngeal lymph node area is the closest and most direct drainage site, but, curiously enough, these nodes are not as frequently involved as the superior deep jugular nodes. The prognosis, however, is grave when the retropharyngeal lymph nodes are involved.

All of the factors noted above are deterrents to

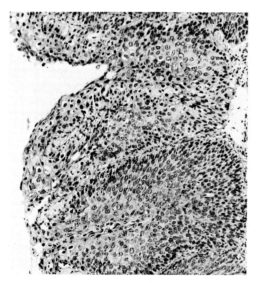

Figure 6.11. Squamous cell carcinoma of oropharynx.

an effective therapeutic control. The majority of oropharyngeal carcinomas are graded as T2, T3, N1 and N2 when first seen. Primary carcinomas of the soft palate are more superficial and tend to remain localized for a longer period of time. As they extend, they involve the tonsillar pillars, pterygoid plate and the nasopharynx. Primary carcinomas of the tonsillar fossa, tonsillar pillars and the retromolar areas advance toward the pharyngeal wall, base of the tongue, the mandible and internal pterygoid muscle. Carcinomas of the pharyngeal wall spread readily along the pharynx in a longitudinal fashion. Laterally, these carcinomas invade the tonsil, the tonsillar fossa and the base of the tongue.

Cure rates for oropharyngeal carcinomas are very poor when one considers the more common incidence of the disease in older age groups (essentially males in their sixth decades of life), coupled with those who tend toward increased consumption of tobacco and chronic alcoholism, and the high risk for second primaries.

The principal attack on oropharyngeal cancer is by means of supervoltage irradiation.[146-148] The results of a combined radiotherapeutic and surgical approach, however, remain the yardstick and the mark that any single modality must achieve for carcinomas in this area.[148] Conley[147] has expressed the current sentiments: "Perhaps the greatest deficiency in the application of irradiation is the failure to recognize that it is neither a cure nor can it effect a cure if applied in a persistent program, especially if the cancer is radioresistant, and, more particularly, if there has been failure to ascertain the presence of local or occult recurrences and early distant dissemination."

After a re-evaluation of an individual neoplasm's radioresistance, a composite surgical resection of the primary lesion with its regional lymphatic bed offers the best hope for "cure" in the instance of an irradiation failure. This approach, obviously, depends upon whether the patient qualifies for this aggressive management.

Supervoltage irradiation, the primary modality used for these neoplasms, is augmented by surgery in instances where[147]: (1) irradiation has little chance for complete success in large and radioresistant carcinomas; (2) carcinomas have recurred after an initial disappearance; (3) metastases are present in the cervical lymph nodes; (4) the patient cannot tolerate the debilitating effects of intensive irradiation; (5) there are postirradiation complications such as radionecrosis. In the treatment of oropharyngeal carcinomas, therefore, surgery plays an important supporting role. It is also recognized that when irradiation controls, nothing else matches it in excellence.[147]

In the past decade, there has been a significant advance in survival figures for oropharyngeal cancer. These have ranged from 15 to 25% and 30 to 50% depending on the site in the oropharynx and the stage of the primary and lymph nodes at the time of presentation of the patient. Cancers of the soft palate are usually stage I at the time of discovery. These neoplasms also have a lower incidence of metastases to lymph nodes. The cure rate is near 50%. Carcinomas in the region of the tonsil, tonsillar pillars and the retromolar areas are usually more advanced at the time of their discovery and are more anaplastic. They also have a higher incidence of metastases. The cure rate is approximately 35%. Carcinomas of the pharynx are the most difficult to control locally. They are usually advanced, manifest a high incidence of metastases, including spread to the retropharyngeal lymph nodes, have a relatively higher rate of recurrence and a high rate of postsurgical complications. The cure rate is approximately 25%. Failure to eradicate the cancer at the primary site remains the single most important reason for a patient's death, but as aggressive management for these lesions becomes more successful, greater numbers of patients survive only to succumb to distant metastases and second primary lesions.[149]

Carcinomas of the Palatine Arch. The palatine arch is literally a junctional area between the oral cavity and the laryngopharynx. The majority of the mucosal malignancies are squamous cell carcinomas. The squamous cell carcinomas of the soft palate and the uvula are usually well differentiated and are reportedly easier to control than the less well differentiated carcinomas of the anterior pillars and the retromolar trigone. In turn, carcinomas of the pharyngeal wall are usually even less differentiated and resistant to management.

Carcinomas of the palatine arch are predominantly diseases of elderly males (60 to 70 years old) who are heavy users of tobacco and maintain a heavy alcoholic intake. Pain is an important symptom. Trismus usually indicates the neoplasm has already deeply infiltrated. Since early metastasis is not characteristic, palpable adenopathy at the time of admission is usually not present. The propensity to metastasize is increased as the neoplasm increases in size or biologically ages.

Left to themselves, the neoplasms invade the buccal mucosa and the hard palate and eventually present cervical lymph node metastases. It is reasonable to expect contralateral node metastases from a carcinoma of a midline structure such as the palatine arch which is so richly endowed with lymphatics. Fletcher and Lindberg[150] have reported an incidence of 24% of contralateral nodes in 88 cases of carcinoma of the soft palate and tonsil fossa, whereas Rider[151] has reported an incidence of 4% in cases of carcinoma of the tonsillar area.

In the management of carcinomas of the oropharynx, it must be recalled that neoplasms of this area are a part of a regional diathesis of carcinoma of the upper aerodigestive tract. Strong et al.[152] report a "field cancerization" in 11 of 73 patients with carcinomas of the palatine arch. This corresponds to the generally quoted 10 to 20% incidence of an associated carcinoma(s) of the upper aerodigestive tract.

Difficulty in defining the gross margins of the lesions makes mere "local" excision unsatisfactory. In this respect, even the initial recognition of the carcinoma is difficult. An ulcerative and infiltrative character is more often seen than a papillary or exophytic pattern of growth. In fact, many of the T1 tumors are very inconspicuous, being little more than areas of erosion.

Rider[151] has emphasized the sinister significance of a palatine arch tumor to the base of the tongue and the frequency with which this is the area of residual disease after radiation and the cause of failure (30 to 40%). Ackerman and del Regato[42] state: "in general, carcinomas of the soft palate presenting trismus and deep infiltration are not curable by radiation therapy." Fletcher et al.[153] prefer combined radical radiotherapy and radical surgery approach.

The prognosis for patients with carcinomas in this region is difficult to ascertain with certainty because of the inclusion, in statistics, of carcinomas of the tonsils or hard palate and buccal carcinomas, as well as lower gum carcinomas that have infiltrated the retromolar trigone area. A 27% 5-year survival has been quoted by Perussia.[154] Strong et al.[152] report that the combined 3-year survival rate of 60 patients with a determinate carcinoma was 24 of 60, or 40%.

Russ et al.[155] have discussed squamous cell carcinoma of the *soft palate* in their personal experience with 38 examples. Radiation therapy to the primary tumor and neck is the preferred modality of initial treatment. Because the soft palate is rich in lymphatics, these tumors tend to be infiltrative locally and invasive of adjacent areas when first detected. If surgery is chosen, the resection must encompass wide margins and can result in severe handicaps of deglutition and phonation not readily corrected by a prosthesis or reconstruction.

Russ et al.[155] record a 5-year survival of 33% and indicate attempts at salvage after recurrence are usually unsuccessful.

Carcinomas of the Tonsils and Tonsillar Region. Carcinomas from this region of the oropharynx account for 1.5 to 3% of all cancers and are second in frequency only to carcinoma of the larynx among the malignancies of the upper respiratory tract.[156, 157] Approximately 12,000 new cases of carcinoma from this region are diagnosed each year.[158] Men are affected more often than women, and the neoplasm is one of older patients, being most commonly seen in the seventh decade in men and in the sixth decade in women. Squamous cell carcinoma of the tonsil is rare in people under 40 years of age. Only 11 cases had been treated at the M. D. Anderson Hospital from 1944 to 1976.[59] Their 5-year survival is considerably less than adults.

In comparison to adjoining area, the tonsil is relatively insensitive from a clinical point of view; this accounts for the paucity of symptoms in an early cancer of the tonsil. A sore throat may be the only symptom, and the first indication of the neoplasm may be a metastasis in the neck. A little over 90% of the epithelial malignancies of the tonsillar area are squamous cell carcinomas of varying levels of histodifferentiation. They tend to be undifferentiated and to metastasize early in their biological course. In a Roswell Park[160] series of 123 cases, 32% were well differentiated squamous cell carcinomas; 40%, moderately well differentiated; 28%, poorly differentiated; 5%, anaplastic carcinomas. Three percent were classified as lymphoepitheliomas.

The diagnostic terms "transitional cell carcinoma" and "lymphoepithelioma," formerly of considerable currency in the literature and in clinical practice, are now being used less often to define neoplasms in this region and upper respiratory tract. It is now generally accepted that these two lesions are not entities unto themselves, arising from specific epithelia, but, rather, are squamous cell carcinomas of low differentiation, albeit often with distinctive clinical and histopathological features. A more detailed consideration of these two terms will be found in the sections concerned with the sinonasal tract and the nasopharynx. If the carcinomas of the tonsillar area are classified according to schemes that still consider the lymphoepithelioma and transitional cell carcinoma as separate tumors, their frequencies are 15 and 13%, respectively.

The gross features of carcinoma of the tonsillar area, and particularly of the tonsil, have been well described by Ackerman and del Regato.[42] Tonsil carcinomas, in their early stages, are usually found arising near the upper pole of the tonsil. The better the differentiation of the neoplasm, the more likely it will be exophytic. The less differentiated carcinomas (lymphoepithelioma and transitional cell carcinoma) do not infiltrate deeply and tend to spread in a superficial manner. Ulceration is more common in the nonexophytic types. Extension of tonsillar carcinomas to the soft palate, the glossopharyngeal sulcus and the base of the tongue is common and occurs early in the course of the disease. Scanlon et al.[161] have reported that 50% of patients with carcinoma of the tonsil have metastases in the cervical lymph nodes at first presentation. Not only is there a high incidence of subclinical lymph node metastases, a small number of occult tonsillar carcinomas are first manifested by cervical lymph node metastasis.[162]

The stage of the disease, like that for other oral and oropharyngeal carcinomas, is the determinant for prognosis and response to treatment. Extension of the carcinoma into the base of the tongue is of prime local importance. One-third of carcinomas of the tonsil region manifesting invasion of the base of the tongue will recur.[163] Tonsillar cancers do not respect the anatomical divisions of the tonsillar region (beds pillars) but rather behave like cancers of the lymphatic field of the oropharynx.

Irradiation is the primary mode of treatment for carcinomas in this area, although radical primary surgery, once considered as a less suitable alternative, is also used with encouraging results.[156] Calamel and Hoffmeister,[164] compared surgical and irradiation therapy results and have presented optimistic figures for survival after surgery. TNM stage III lesions treated surgically had a 67% 3-year survival and a 0% survival if treated by irradiation. Stage IV 3-year survivals were 43% with surgical treatment and 0% with irradiation. Whicker et al.[157] record an over-all 5-year survival of 48% in patients undergoing surgical procedures designed to cure.

Teloh[165] has reported an over-all 5-year survival of 7.5%, a 15% 5-year survival for stage III carcinomas and a 0% survival for stage IV carcinomas. Similarly poor over-all survivals have been reported by Martin and Sugarbaker[166] and Walker and Schulz.[167] Seda and Snow[156] report an over-all 3-year survival (for all stages) of 20%. Treatment in their study was a combined radiotherapy and surgical approach.

Guidelines for radiotherapy of neoplasms in this region may be found in the reports by Dalley[168] and others.[169-171]

HYPOPHARYNX

The hypopharynx is defined as the anatomical area extending from the superior margin of the epiglottis to the inferior border of the cricoid. Three subdivisions are recognized: the *posterolateral wall*, the *pyriform sinus* and the *postcricoid area*.

Symptomatically the hypopharynx is a "semi-silent" area of the gullet which is drained by a rich network of lymphatics, superiorly in the retropharyngeal chain to the node of Rouviere near the base of the skull, laterally to the jugular chain and anteriorly through the thyrohyoid membrane. If early diagnosis of hypopharyngeal lesions is to be made, attention must be paid to seemingly minor complaints.[172] The possibility of neoplasm should be suspected in patients with persistent sore throat or pain on ingestion of hot foods or liquids. Late symptoms such as dysphagia, huskiness of voice, cervical adenopathy, difficulty in handling saliva and weight loss all herald an advanced stage of the disease. Referred ear pain is evidence of the neoplasm's invasion of the superior laryngeal nerve. History of Plummer-Vinson syndrome and an excessive use of alcohol and tobacco are also important in suspecting the possibility of carcinoma in the hypopharynx.

Ahlbom[173] has pointed out the frequency with which carcinoma of the oral cavity, pharynx or the esophagus in women is accompanied by the Plummer-Vinson syndrome. This syndrome is a true precancerous syndrome and is characterized clinically by sideropenic anemia, achlorhydria and generalized atrophy of the mucous membranes of the mouth, pharynx and esophagus. In Jacobsson's series of 322 patients treated in Stockholm,[174] 60% were women (203) and 90% gave evidence of the syndrome.

The *pyriform* sinus is more frequently involved than the other sites in the hypopharynx. In a series of 230 patients, 61% of the neoplasms were primary in the pyriform sinus, 24% in the postcricoid area and 15% in the posterolateral walls of the pharynx.[175] The great majority of carcinomas of the hypopharynx are squamous cell and are rather undifferentiated. In general, they are less differentiated than carcinomas of the endolarynx. Most of the neoplasms also share the tendency, sooner or later, to invade the larynx and metastasize to the cervical lymph nodes. The neoplasms of the pyriform sinus manifest the greatest frequency of cervical lymph node involvement.

The lymphoepithelioma is an extremely rare cancer in the laryngohypopharyngeal regions. Ferlito[176] has reported one case in the pyriform sinus and despite searching was able to find only one other example.

Invasion of the jugular vein may also result in distant visceral metastasis. Willis[177] found 29 of 64 cases at necropsy to manifest extension to the jugular vein. Twenty-four of these 29 had metastases to the lungs, liver and bones. Coutard[178] cites similar statistics. Table 6.15 relates the influence of metastases on survival in hypopharyngeal carcinomas. Over 5-year survivorship in major series is low: Sloan-Kettering Memorial Cancer Center, 25%[172]; Mayo Clinic, 47%[179]; Roswell Park, 28%[180]; and the University of Toronto, 20%.[181] These data include all forms of primary and secondary treatment.

Carcinomas of the Pyriform Sinus. Cancers of the pyriform sinus include those of the aryepiglottic fold, arytenoid, medial and lateral walls of the pyriform sinus. The pyriform sinus per se is defined as extending from the pharyngoepiglottic fold superiorly to the cricopharyngeal fold inferiorly and from the inner aspect of the thyroid ala laterally to the aryepiglottic fold and the posterior lateral boundary of the larynx medially.

There appears to be no prognostic significance in dividing the carcinomas according to their position on the upper and lower portions of the sinus.

Table 6.15
Influence of Metastases on Survival: Hypopharyngeal Carcinomas*

A. Hypopharynx—General		
Metastases	No. of Patients	Absolute 5-Year Survivals
None	16/74	2/16 (12%)
Regional	52/74	4/52 (8%)
Distant	2/74	0/2
Unknown	4/74	

B. Hypopharynx—According to Site		
Site	Patients with Cervical Node Metastases	5-Year Survival
	%	%
Pyriform sinus	70	9.1
Postcricoid area	40	20.0
Postpharyngeal wall	50	20.6

* Data presented are derived from the reports by Bryce[175] and Truluck and Putney.[107]

This exercise is also clinically misleading since the majority of the carcinomas cross the arbitrary dividing line at the level of the internal laryngeal nerve.

Local extension from the primary site is medially along the inner border of the thyroid ala to encroach upon the endolarynx, onto and over the aryepiglottic fold into the supraglottic portions of the larynx, onto the posteriocricoid mucosa and anteriorly into the soft tissues of the neck. A considerable number of patients will manifest metastases during the course of this disease. Of 52 patients studied by McGavran et al.,[182] 43 had histologically proved ipsilateral cervical lymph node metastases, predominantly in the upper jugular chain. This finding leaves little room for academic rhetoric regarding the necessity of including the cervical lymph nodes in primary therapy regardless of the clinical evaluation. Contralateral node metastasis are also a problem in approximately 10% of the patients. Second primaries occur in the head and neck in about 12% of cases.[182]

Death is due to persistence of disease in the area or in the neck. Distant metastasis are found in about 10 to 20% at necropsy.[182] The 3- and 5-year cure rates expressed by McGavran et al.[182] were 50 and 41%, respectively. Their patients were treated primarily by radical surgery. Radiotherapeutic measures are potentially curative in only a few patients with localized disease and in whom cervical lymph node metastases are absent.[182-185] Irradiation alone has yielded low 5-year survivorship (6 to 8%).[185]

Eisbach and Krause[186] reviewed their experience with 104 patients with squamous cell carcinoma of the pyriform sinus and reported 3-year determinate survival rates as follows: radiation therapy, 10%; surgery, 56%; and combined therapy, 40%. Evaluation of their local recurrence rate yielded the following: radiation therapy, 58%; surgery, 5%; and combined therapy, 28%. These data were interpreted to suggest that preoperative irradiation hampered the assessment of adequate resection margins during the surgical procedure. These workers[186] also observed that radiation therapy is quite effective in controlling subclinical lymph node metastases.

Postcricoid Carcinomas. Carcinomas from this region of the hypopharynx are biologically the worst of the lot. The causes of failure to "cure" the carcinoma in this region are: (1) presentation of a patient at a relatively late stage of disease; and (2) recurrent or residual disease. The over-all salvage rate for postcricoid carcinoma does not exceed 20 to 25%.[187, 188] Despite this low survival rate, the surgical management has become more radical.[188, 189] Som and Nussbaum[188] state that the surgical procedure of choice for postcricoid carcinoma must solve three problems.

1. The need for wide resection because: (a) most patients manifest a carcinoma at an advanced stage on primary examination; (b) there is a high incidence of "skip" areas of "multiple primaries" in the pharynx and cervical esophagus.

2. The frequent involvement of the mediastinal lymph nodes and the consequent need for resection of lymph node-bearing tissue in the tracheoesophageal angle below the level of the manubrium as well as the need for a routine neck dissection where feasible.

3. Reconstructive surgery after elimination of the neoplasm.

Som[190] has commented on the significance of metastases in the lymph nodes at the tracheoesophageal angle and superior mediastium. What often has been referred to as "recurrence at the lower suture line" often proves to be the result of direct extension from lower cervical lymph nodes and the involved nodes in the mediastinum. Experience with the primary or even secondary lesion and the combined use of radiation therapy has not been good. There has been no enhancement of survival, and its use has seemingly complicated the reconstructive procedures.

Ogura[187] has concurred in the use of surgical means for the treatment of this group of neoplasms. Future surgical management and its direction is expressed by Som and Nussbaum[188]: "It may well be that wide excision of larynx, pharynx and entire esophagus with resection of the manubrium and excision of mediastinal lymph nodes is the ultimate procedure of choice in the surgical treatment of carcinoma of the hypopharynx and cervical esophagus".

Carcinoma of the Pharyngeal Wall. The pharyngeal wall includes the posterior and lateral mucosal walls of the pharynx extending from the nasopharynx superiorly to the cricopharyngeus aperture and pyriform fossa below and to the posterior edge of the pharyngeal tonsils laterally. Carcinomas from this region are particularly vicious and are considered far more lethal than laryngeal carcinomas or carcinomas of the anterior part of the tongue. Pharyngeal wall carcinomas also have a much poorer prognosis than do carcinomas of the pyriform sinus or the extrinsic larynx (two areas in which carcinomas of the wall are often included for survival statistics). Carcinomas of the pyriform sinus are more common.

In accordance with the majority of squamous cell carcinomas of the mucosal surfaces of the head and neck, this carcinoma is also one of advancing age and of males. The peak age incidence is between 60 and 70 years. Clinical symptoms, sore throat and dysphagia are innocuous. A few patients experience "foreign-body" sensations in the throat, hemoptysis and aural pain.

Nearly all the carcinomas are squamous cell carcinomas and many are large and fungating. Most are situated in the midposterior pharyngeal wall and occasionally can be seen by depressing the base of the tongue. In a large series, 78% were larger than 5 cm in diameter when first discovered.[191] In testimony to the insidious progress of the disease, almost one-quarter of the patients will manifest cervical metastases as their first symptom or sign.

Carcinomas of the posterior wall of the pharynx are capable of prevertebral spread to the posterior tonsillar pillar and fauces and in advanced lesions there may be involvement of the soft palate and the nasopharynx. Inferior and lateral growth involves the mouth of the esophagus, the lateral wall of the pharynx and the pyriform sinus. Regional lymph node involvement is common. Over half the patients will manifest involved lymph nodes at the time therapy is instituted and two-thirds will eventually show lymph node metastases.[191-192] The ominous "field effect" seen elsewhere in the oral cavity and upper respiratory tract is also significantly associated with pharyngeal wall carcinomas. Excluding cancer of the skin, 28 of 164 patients studied by Cunningham and Catlin[191] had a second neoplasm, the most frequent area of involvement being the head and neck region.

Although small, localized cancers of the pharyngeal walls can be "cured" by irradiation, surgery plays a more important role in the management of these neoplasms. Combinations of surgery and radiotherapy may salvage a few patients not controlled by either method alone. Regardless of the therapy, the stage of the disease thwarts the physician.[193] The gross 5-year cure rate is 19% with a net determinate cure rate of 21%.[191] This compares poorly with other squamous cell carcinomas of the head and neck—anterior two-thirds of tongue (43%), larynx (47%) and cheek mucosa (42%). The rate is similar to that expressed for the base of the tongue (21%) and higher than that for the cervical esophagus (5%).[194]

Retropharyngeal Lymph Nodes and Carcinomas of the Pharyngeal Walls. The retropharyngeal lymph nodes play an important role in the total management of carcinomas of the nasopharynx and the orohypopharynx. Much credit is due to Ballantyne[195] in re-emphasizing their significance, particularly in reference to carcinomas of the pharyngeal walls.

The lymph nodes are found in the areolar tissue behind the musculature of the pharynx and are divided into medial and lateral groups. The lateral retropharyngeal lymph nodes lie close to the internal carotid arteries and superiorly lie near the base of the skull. More accessible, the medial group of lymph nodes are more closely applied to the musculature of the pharynx. Draining the nasopharynx and the wall of the pharynx, the lymph nodes' efferent pathways are variable but tend to course to the lymph nodes in the deep lobe of the parotid gland, to the nodes beneath the superior end of the sternocleidomastoid muscle and to those in the posterior triangle of the neck.

Neoplastic or inflammatory involvement of the retropharyngeal lymph nodes may produce a pain complex or syndrome. This is a characterized by pain and stiffness in the neck on the same side as the lesion. The pain frequently radiates to the eye and forehead on the ipsilateral side.

In a series of 34 patients with cancer of the pharyngeal walls treated surgically at the M. D. Anderson Hospital, positive retropharyngeal nodes were found in 44%.[195] An enhancement of survival may be had by the removal of these positive lymph nodes.

MULTIPLE MALIGNANCIES IN PATIENTS WITH CANCER OF THE HEAD AND NECK

The occurrence of separate primary malignancies occurring in patients was formerly considered as rare and unusual. The recent literature (already cited in the preceding pages), and especially the investigations by Moertel et al.,[196] gives ample proof that this is not the case. With improved cancer therapy and palliation, this phenomenon is expected to increase and the possibility of a second primary lesion should always be kept in mind in the management of patients with head and neck neoplasms. The survival after the removal of a second primary lesion may greatly exceed that of a nonoperative management of a lesion considered to be a recurrence or a metastasis.[197] Whenever a patient with a primary carcinoma of the oral cavity and upper respiratory tract is suspected of having either a late or an "unusual" metastasis, a new primary carcinoma must be considered.

The criteria generally accepted, yet at times difficult to fulfill, for multiple primary lesions are those proposed by Warren and Gates[198]: (1) the neoplasms must be clearly malignant; (2) each neoplasm must be geographically separate and distinct; (3) the possibility that one of the cancers is a metastasis from the other(s) must be excluded.

The literature strongly suggests that the existence of a malignant neoplasm implies an increased susceptibility to the development of a second malignancy and further that a malignant neoplasm in one organ may be associated with an increased susceptibility in another organ of the same or associated system. Moertel et al.[196] do not concur. Their evidence indicates that the specific type of second cancers is probably largely determined by the age of the patient and his expected longevity.

While the foregoing may be true, in general, for visceral or parenchymatous organs, we take issue for its pertinence in the mouth and upper respiratory tract. Local predisposing factors, whether environmental, habitual or familial, seem to play a governing role. Chronic irritation from smoking or poor dental hygiene and the Plummer-Vinson syndrome predisposes, not local areas, but an entire "field" in the head and neck.

Bachulis and Williams[197] found in their male population that three-fourths had an initial primary neoplasm in the skin, colon, pharynx, larynx, bladder or prostate gland. Sixty percent of this patient group developed subsequent (separate) carcinomas in the *same* anatomical sites.

In a series of 1,919 patients admitted to the Head and Neck Service of the Roswell Park Memorial Hospital (Buffalo, N. Y.) with primary malignant tumors of the head and neck, more than one primary lesion was diagnosed in 144 (7.5%).[199] In 44% of this group, the second head and neck cancer developed within 24 months of the first cancer. Time intervals between the two cancers may extend to many years. Another primary head and neck malignancy was observed in 18% of patients with multiple malignancies as compared to 3.3% of all malignant lesions reported for the general population.

The Mayo Clinic's experience is also informative.[196] Of 732 patients with proved squamous cell carcinomas of the oral cavity, 64 (8.7%) were found to have two or more discrete oral cancers. Clinical leukoplakia was found in 75% of these patients. An additional 55 patients with oral cancer had independent carcinomas of the lips, pharynx or esophagus, thus increasing the over-all occurrence of multicentric lesions to 16.3%.

The lips are also frequent sites for multicentric cancers. Six percent of 1,300 patients with cancer of the lips had multicentric neoplasms.[196] Over one-half of these were simultaneous. Both multiple and single lesions showed a strong predilection for the lower lip. Forty-five of the 1,300 patients also had carcinomas of the oral cavity, pharynx, larynx or esophagus, an occurrence rate of 3.5%.

As evidenced by the Mayo Clinic experience, the larynx presents similar statistics.[196] Of 1,100 patients with squamous cell carcinomas of the larynx proved at operation during a 10-year period, a total of 18 (1.6%) were found to have two discrete carcinomas. Eleven of these neoplasms were simultaneous, and seven were interval lesions. In addition, 22 patients had an associated squamous cell carcinoma of the lips, oral cavity, pharynx or esophagus.

Related statistics are offered by Ju[200] in an excellent study to determine the behavior of cancer of the head and neck during its late or terminal phases. His material came from 2,700 autopsies in the Francis Delafield Hospital (New York City). Three hundred forty patients had primary malignancies in the head and neck area. A high incidence of second or third primary cancers was found in this group of patients in comparison with an over-all incidence of 6% multiple primary lesions in the general necropsy group. Excluding carcinoma of the prostate gland as a second primary lesion, the rate was still a high 15.5%.

REFERENCES

1. Folsom, T. C., White, C. P., Bromer, L., Canby, H. F., and Garrington, G. E.: Oral exfoliative study: reviews of the literature and report of a three-year study. J. Oral Surg. 33:61, 1972.
2. Silverberg, E., and Holleb, A. I.: Major trends in cancer, 25-year survey. Cancer 25:2, 1975.
3. Leading Article: Oral cancer: a stubborn problem. Lancet 1:299, 1972.
4. Storer, R.: Oral cancer, letter to the editor. Lancet 1:430, 1972.
5. Selbach, G. J., and von Haam, E.: The clinical value of oral cytology. Acta Cytol. 7:337, 1963.
6. Editorial: Oral cytology. J. Am. Dent. Assoc. 74:899, 1967.
7. Bhaskar, S. N.: Synopsis of Oral Pathology, 3rd Ed. C. V. Mosby, St. Louis, 1969.
8. Binnie, W. H.: Epidemiology and etiology of oral cancer in Britain. Proc. Roy. Soc. Med. 69:737, 1976.
9. Easson, E. C., and Palmer, M. K.: Prognostic factors in oral cancer. Clin. Oncol. 2:191, 1976.
10. Bruun, J. P.: Time lapse by diagnosis of oral cancer. Oral Surg. 42:139, 1976.
11. Malawalla, A. M., Silverman, S., Mani, N. J., Bilimoria, K. F., and Smith, L. W.: Oral cancer in 57,518 industrial workers of Gujarat, India. A prevalence and followup study. Cancer 37:1882, 1976.
12. Mendelson, B. C., Hodgkinson, D. J., and Woods, J. E.: Cancer of the oral cavity. Surg. Clin. N. Am. 57:585, 1977.
13. Mashberg, A., Morrissey, J. B., and Garfinkel, L.: A study of the appearance of early asymptomatic oral squamous cell carcinoma. Cancer 32:1436, 1973.
14. Mashberg, A., and Meyers, H.: Anatomical site and size of

222 early asymptomatic oral squamous cell carcinomas. A continuing prospective study of oral cancer. II. Cancer 37:2149, 1976.

15. Smith, J. F.: Snuff-dippers lesions. A ten-year followup. Arch. Otolaryngol. 101:276, 1975.

16. Rapidis, A. D., Langdon, J. D., Patel, M. F., and Harvey, P. W.: STNMP. A new system for the clinicopathological classification and identification of intra-oral carcinomata. Cancer 39:204, 1977.

17. Spiro, R. H., and Strong, E. W.: Mouth cancer, a surgical perspective. Clin. Bull. 6:3, 1976.

18. Spiro, R. H., Alfonso, A. E., Farr, H. W., and Strong, E. W.: Cervical node metastasis from epidermoid carcinoma of the oral cavity and oropharynx. A critical assessment of current staging. Am. J. Surg. 128:562, 1974.

19. DiTroia, J. F.: Nodal metastases and prognosis in carcinoma of the oral cavity. Otolaryngol. Clin. N. Am. 5:333, 1972.

20. Kalnins, I. K., Leonard, A. G., Sako, K., Razack, M. S., and Shedd, D. P.: Correlation between prognosis and degree of lymph node involvement in carcinoma of the oral cavity. Am. J. Surg. 134:450, 1977.

21. Shah, J. P., Cendon, R. A., Farr, H. W., and Strong, E. W.: Carcinoma of the oral cavity. Factors affecting treatment failure at the primary site and neck. Am. J. Surg. 132:504, 1976.

22. Lee, J. G.: Detection of residual carcinoma of the oral cavity, oropharynx, hypopharynx and larynx: a study of surgical margins. Tr. Am. Acad. Ophth. Otol. 78:49, 1974.

23. Lingeman, R. E., Helmus, C., Stephens, R., and Ulm, J.: Neck dissection: radical or conservative. Ann. Otol. 86:737, 1977.

24. Strong, E. W.: Preoperative radiation and radical neck dissection. Surg. Clin. N. Am. 49:271, 1969.

25. Beahrs, O. H., and Barber, K. W., Jr.: The value of radical dissection of structures of the neck in the management of carcinoma of the lip, mouth and larynx. Arch. Surg. 85:49, 1962.

26. Jesse, R. H.: The philosophy of treatment of neck nodes. Ear, Nose, Throat J. 56:58, 1977.

27. Nahum, A. M., Bone, R. C., and Davidson, T. M.: The case for elective prophylactic neck dissection. Laryngoscope 87:588, 1977.

28. Manfredi, D., and Jacobelli, G.: Neck dissection in the treatment of head and neck cancer: results in 1162 cases. In Cancer of the Head and Neck, edited by R. G. Chambers, A. M. P. deLimpens, D. A. Jaques, and R. T. Routledge, pp. 221–224, Excerpta Medica, Amsterdam, 1975.

29. Million, R. R.: Elective neck irradiation for TxNo squamous carcinoma of the oral tongue and floor of mouth. Cancer 34:149, 1974.

30. Fletcher, G. H.: Elective irradiation of subclinical disease in cancers of the head and neck. Cancer 29:1450, 1972.

31. Nahum, A. M.: Overview of chemotherapy of cancer of the larynx. Canad. J. Otolaryngol. 4:4, 1975.

32. DeWys, W. D.: Current concepts of chemotherapy combined with other modalities for head and neck cancer. Canad. J. Otolaryngol. 4:195, 1975.

33. Schenken, L. L.: Proliferative character and growth modes of neoplastic disease as determinants of chemotherapeutic efficacy. Cancer Treat. Rep. 60:1761, 1976.

34. Skipper, H. E.: Kinetic behavior versus response to chemotherapy. Prediction of response to chemotherapy. Natl. Cancer Inst. Monogr. 34:2, 1971.

35. Valeriote, F., and von Putten, L.: Proliferative-dependent cytotoxicity of anticancer agents: a review. Cancer Res. 35:2619, 1975.

36. Donegan, W. L., and Harris, P.: Regional chemotherapy with combined drugs in cancer of the head and neck. Cancer 38:1479, 1976.

37. DeVita, V. T., Jr., Young, R. C., and Canellos, G. P.: Combination versus single agent chemotherapy: a review of the basis for selection of drug treatment of cancer. Cancer 35:98, 1975.

38. Wittes, R. E., Cvitkovic, E., Shah, J., Gerold, F. P., and Strong, E. W.: cis-Dichlorodiammine-platinum (II) in the treatment of epidermoid carcinoma of the head and neck. Cancer Treat. Rep. 61:359, 1977.

39. Hattowska, H., and Borowicz, K.: Histologic evaluation of treatment of epidermoid carcinoma in the oral cavity with methotrexate and 5-fluorouracil. J. Oral Surg. 32:508, 1974.

40. Michaels, L.: Differentiation of squamous carcinoma of the larynx as a determinant of prognosis. Canad. J. Otolaryngol. 4:873, 1975.

41. Bartlett, G. L., Kreider, J. W., and Purnell, D. M.: Immunotherapy of cancer in animals: models or muddles. J. Natl. Cancer Inst. 56:207, 1976.

42. Ackerman, L. V., and del Regato, J. A.: Cancer: Diagnosis, Treatment and Prognosis, 4th Ed. C. V. Mosby, St. Louis, 1970.

43. Waldron, C. A.: Oral epithelial tumors. In Thoma's Oral Pathology, edited by R. J. Gorlin and H. M. Goldman, p. 820. C. V. Mosby, St. Louis, 1970.

44. Bernier, J. L., and Clark, M. L.: Squamous cell carcinoma of the lip. Milit. Surg. 109:379, 1951.

45. Szpak, C. A., Stone, J. J., and Frenkel, E. P.: Some observations concerning the demographic and geographic incidence of carcinoma of the lip and buccal cavity. Cancer 40:343, 1977.

46. Ju, D. M. C.: On the etiology of cancer of the lower lip. Plast. Reconstr. Surg. 52:1511, 1973.

47. Mullen, D. L., Silverberg, S. G., Penn, I., and Hammond, W. S.: Squamous cell carcinoma of the skin and lip in renal homograft recipients. Cancer 37:729, 1976.

48. Sharp, G. S.: Cancer of the lip. Oral Surg. 6:516, 1948.

49. Judd, E. S., and Beahrs, O. H.: Epithelioma of the lower lip. Arch. Surg. 59:422, 1949.

50. Lund, C., Sogaard, H., Elbrond, O., Jorgensen, K., and Andersen, A. P.: Epidermoid carcinoma of the lip. Histologic grading in the clinical evaluation. Acta Radiol. 14:465, 1975.

51. Johnson, W. C., and Helwig, E. B.: Adenoid squamous cell carcinoma (adenocanthoma): A clinicopathologic study of 155 patients. Cancer 19:639, 1966.

52. Weitzner, S.: Adenoid squamous cell carcinoma of the vermillion mucosa of lower lip. Oral Surg. 37:589, 1974.

53. Kohn, M. W., and Eversole, L. R.: Keratoacanthoma of the lower lip: report of cases. J. Oral Surg. 30:522, 1972.

54. del Regato, J. A.: Roentgen therapy of carcinoma of the lower lip. Radiology 51:499, 1948.

55. Bailey, B. J.: Management of carcinoma of the lip. Laryngoscope. 87:250, 1977.

56. Jorgensen, K., Elbrond, O., and Andersen, A. R.: Carcinoma of the lip. A series of 869 patients. Acta Otolaryngol. 75:312, 1973.

57. Martin, H., MacComb, W. S., and Blady, J. V.: Cancer of the lip. Ann. Surg. 114:226, 1941.

58. Hendricks, J. L., Mendelson, B. C., and Woods, J. E.: Invasive carcinoma of the lower lip. Surg. Clin. N. Am. 57:837, 1977.

59. Krause, C. J., Lee, J. G., and McCabe, B. F.: Carcinoma of the oral cavity. Arch. Otolaryngol. 97:354, 1973.

60. Wurman, L. H., Adams, G. L., and Meyerhoff, W. L.: Carcinoma of the lip. Am. J. Surg. 130:470, 1975.

61. Brown, R. G., Poole, M. D., Calamel, P. M., and Bakamjian, V. Y.: Advanced recurrent squamous carcinoma of the lower lip. Am. J. Surg. 132:492, 1976.

62. O'Brien, P. H., and Catlin, D.: Cancer of the cheek (mucosa). Cancer 18:1392, 1965.

63. Paymaster, J. C.: Cancer of the buccal mucosa: a clinical study of 650 cases in Indian patients. Cancer 9:431, 1956.

64. Martin, H. E., and Pfleuger, O. H.: Cancer of the cheek (buccal mucosa). Arch. Surg. 30:721, 1935.

65. Khanolkar, V. R.: Oral cancer in India. Acta Unio Int. Contra Cancrum 15:67, 1959.

66. Kraus, F. T., and Perez-Mesa, C.: Verrucous carcinoma. Cancer 19:26, 1966.

67. Duckworth, R.: Verrucous carcinoma presenting as mandibular osteomyelitis. Br. J. Surg. 49:332, 1961.

68. Biller, H. F., Ogura, J. G., and Bauer, W. C.: Verrucous carcinoma of the larynx. Laryngoscope 81:1323, 1971.

69. Fonts, E. A., Greenlaw, R. H., Rush, B. F., and Rovin, S.: Verrucous squamous cell carcinoma of the oral cavity. Cancer 23:152, 1969.

70. Goethals, P. L., Harrison, E. G., Jr., and Devine, K. D.: Verrucous squamous carcinoma of the oral cavity. Am. J. Surg. 106:845, 1963.

71. Skolnick, E. M., Campbell, J. M., and Meyers, R. M.: Carcinoma of the buccal mucosa and retromolar area. Otolaryngol. Clin. N. Am. 5:327, 1972.

72. Dhawan, I. K., Agarwal, S. B., Madan, N. C. and Sharma, U.: The extent of surgical resection for advanced cancer of the buccal mucosa. Surg. Gynec. Obstet. 137:31, 1973.

73. Lampe, I.: Radiation therapy of cancer of the buccal mucosa and lower gingiva. Am. J. Roentgenol. Radium Ther. Nucl. Med. 73:628, 1955.

74. McCarthy, P. L., and Shklar, G.: Diseases of the Oral Mucosa, p. 318. McGraw-Hill, New York, 1964.

75. Cady, B., and Catlin, D.: Epidermoid carcinoma of the gum. Cancer 23:551, 1969.

76. Rosenfeld, L., and Callaway, J.: Snuff dippers cancer. Am. J. Surg. 106:840, 1963.

77. Thoma, K. H.: Development and dissemination of oral cancer. N.Y. State Dent. J. 16:366, 1950.

78. Willen, R., Nathanson, A., Moberger, G., and Anneroth, G.: Squamous cell carcinoma of the gingiva. Histological classification and grading of malignancy. Acta Otolaryngol. 79:146, 1975.

79. Whitehouse, G. H.: Radiological bone changes produced by intraoral squamous carcinomata involving the lower alveolus. Clin. Otolaryngol. 1:45, 1976.

80. Byars, L. T.: Extent of mandibular resection required for treatment of oral cancer. Arch. Surg. 70:914, 1955.

81. Erich, J. B., and Kragh, L. V.: Results of treatment of squamous cell carcinoma arising in mandibular gingiva. Arch. Surg. 79:100, 1959.

82. Backstrom, A., Jakobsson, P. A., Nathanson, A., and Wersall, J.: Prognosis of squamous cell carcinoma of the gums with cytologically verified cervical lymph node metastases. J. Laryngol. 89:391, 1975.

83. Krishnamurthi, S., and Shanta, V.: Evaluation of treatment of advanced primary and secondary gingival carcinoma. Br. Med. J. 2:1261, 1963.

84. Martin, H. E.: Cancer of the gums. Am. J. Surg. 54:765, 1941.

85. Nathanson, A., Jakobsson, P. A., and Wersall, J.: Prognosis of squamous-cell carcinoma of the gums. Acta Otolaryngol. 75:301, 1973.

86. Love, R., Stewart, I. F., and Coy, P.: Upper alveolar carcinoma—a 30 year survey. J. Otolaryngol. 6:393, 1977.

87. Brown, R. L., Suh, J. M., Scarborough, J. E., Wilkins, S. A., and Smith, R. R.: Snuff dippers' intra-oral cancer: clinical characteristics and response to therapy. Cancer 18:2, 1965.

88. Simons, J. N., Masson, J. K., and Beahrs, O. H.: Results of radical treatment for intra-oral cancer. Am. J. Surg. 106:819, 1963.

89. Cady, B., and Hutter, R. V. P.: Nonepidermoid cancer of the gum. Cancer 23:1318, 1969.

90. Tiecke, R. W., and Bernier, J. L.: Statistical and morphological analysis of four hundred and one cases of intraoral squamous cell carcinoma. J. Am. Dent. Assoc. 49:684, 1954.

91. Silverberg, E., and Grant, R. N.: Cancer Statistics, 1970. CA. 20:11, 1970.

92. Frazell, E. L., and Lucas, J. C.: Cancer of the tongue: report of the management of 1,554 patients. Cancer 15:1085, 1962.

93. Trieger, N., Ship, I. I., Taylor, G. W., and Weisberger, D.: Cirrhosis and other predisposing factors in carcinoma of the tongue. Cancer 11:357, 1958.

94. Johnston, W. D., and Ballantyne, A. J.: Prognostic effect of tobacco and alcohol use in patients with oral tongue cancer. Am. J. Surg. 134:444, 1977.

95. Khanolkar, V. R.: Oral cancer in Bombay, India: a review of 1,000 consecutive cases. Cancer Res. 4:313, 1944.

96. Conley, J.: Cancer of the tongue. In Cancer of the Head and Neck, edited by J. Conley, pp. 270–277. Butterworths, Washington, D.C., 1967.

97. Flamant, R., Hayem, M., Lazar, P., and Denoix, P.: Cancer of the tongue: study of 904 cases. Cancer 17:377, 1964.

98. MacComb, W. S., Fletcher, G. H., and Healey, J., Jr.: Intraoral cavity. In Cancer of the Head and Neck, edited by E. W. MacComb and G. H. Fletcher, pp. 89–151. Williams & Wilkins Co., Baltimore, 1967.

99. Lund, C., Sogaard, H., Elbrond, O., Jorgensen, K., and Andersen, A. P.: Epidermoid carcinoma of the tongue. Histologic grading in the clinical evaluation. Acta Radiol. Therap. Phys. Biol. 14:513, 1975.

100. Paavolainen, M., Tarkkanen, J., and Saksela, E.: Stromal reactions as prognostic factors in epidermoid carcinoma of the tongue. Acta Otolaryngol. 75:316, 1973.

101. Sessions, D. G., Stallings, J. O., Brownson, R. J., and Ogura, J. H.: Total glossectomy for advanced carcinoma of the base of the tongue. Laryngoscope 83:39, 1973.

102. Skolnik, E. M., and Saberman, M. N.: Cancer of the tongue. Otolaryngol. Clin. North Am. 2:603, 1969.

103. Spiro, R. H., and Strong, E. W.: Surgical treatment of cancer of the tongue. Surg. Clin. N. Am. 54:759, 1974.

104. Whitehurst, J. O., and Droulias, C. A.: Surgical treatment of squamous cell carcinoma of the oral tongue. Arch. Otolaryngol. 103:212, 1977.

105. Lampe, I., and Fayos, J. V.: Radiotherapeutic experience with squamous cell carcinoma of the oral part of the tongue. J. Univ. Mich. Med. Ctr. 33:215, 1967.

106. Horiuchi, J., and Adachi, T.: Some considerations on radiation therapy of tongue cancer. Cancer 28:335, 1971.

107. Truluck, C. H., Jr., and Putney, F. J.: Survival rates in cancer of the tongue, tonsil and hypopharynx. Arch. Otolaryngol. 93:271, 1971.

108. Frazell, E. L.: A review of the treatment of cancer of the mobile portion of the tongue. Cancer 28:1178, 1971.

109. Maddox, W. A., Sherlock, E. C., and Eva.   . B.: Cancer of the tongue: review of thirteen-year experience, 1955–1968. Am. Surg. 37:642, 1971.

110. Vermund, H., and Golin, F. F.: Role of radiotherapy in the treatment of cancer of the tongue. A retrospective analysis on TNM-staged tumors treated between 1958 and 1968. Cancer 32:333, 1973.

111. Spanos, W. J., Shokovsky, L. J., and Fletcher, G. H.: Time, dose and tumor volume relationships in irradiation of squamous cell carcinomas of the base of the tongue. Cancer 37:259, 1976.

112. Shaw, H. J., and Hardingham, M.: Cancer of the floor of the mouth: surgical management. J. Laryngol. 91:467, 1977.

113. Bertholsen, A., Hansen, H. S., and Rygard, J.: Radiation therapy of squamous carcinoma of the floor of mouth and the lower alveolar ridge. J. Laryngol. 91:489, 1977.

114. Correa, J. N., Bosch, A., and Marcial, V. A.: Carcinoma of the floor of the mouth: review of clinical factors and results of treatment. Am. J. Roentgenol. Radium Ther. Nucl. Med. 99:302, 1967.

115. Leffall, L. D., and White, J. E.: Cancer of the oral cavity in Negroes. Surg. Gynecol. Obstet. 71:347, 1965.

116. Barton, R. T.: Surgical treatment of carcinoma of the floor of the mouth. Am. J. Surg. 133:971, 1971.

117. Kolson, H., Spiro, R. H., Rosewit, B., and Lawson, W.: Epidermoid carcinoma of the floor of the mouth. Arch. Otolaryngol. 93:280, 1971.

118. Harrold, C. C., Jr.: Management of cancer of the floor of the mouth. Am. J. Surg. 122:487, 1971.

119. Erich, J. B., and Kragh, L. V.: Treatment of squamous cell carcinoma of the floor of the mouth. Arch. Surg. 79:94, 1959.

120. Hardingham, M., Dalley, V. M., and Shaw, H. J.: Cancer of the floor of the mouth: clinical features and results of management. Clin. Oncol. 3:227, 1977.

121. Ramulu, C., Prasad, C. S. V., Krishnamurthy, K., and

Reddy, C. R. R. M.: Benign tumors of the hard palate. Indian J. Surg. 36:113, 1974.

122. Eneroth, C.-M., Hjertman, L., and Moberger, G.: Squamous cell carcinoma of the palate. Acta Otolaryngol. 73:418, 1972.

123. Eneroth, C.-M., and Moberger, G.: Histological malignancy grading of squamous cell carcinoma of the palate. Acta. Otolaryngol. 75:293, 1973.

124. Ratzer, E. R., Schweitzer, R. J., and Frazell, E. L.: Epidermoid carcinoma of the palate. Am. J. Surg. 119:294, 1970.

125. Liroff, K. P., and Zeff, S.: Basal cell carcinoma of the palatal mucosa. J. Oral Surg. 30:730, 1972.

126. Jones, J. H.: Non-odontogenic oral tumors in children. Br. Dent. J. 119:439, 1965.

127. Jones, B. J.: Oral carcinoma in the young patient with a report of two cases. Br. J. Oral Surg. 8:159, 1970.

128. Lancaster, L., and Fournet, L. F.: Carcinoma of the tongue in a child. J. Oral. Surg. 27:269, 1969.

129. Pichler, A. G., Williams, J. R., and Moore, J. A.: Carcinoma of the tongue in childhood and adolescence: report of a case and review of the literature. Arch. Otolaryngol. 95:178, 1972.

130. Topazian, D. S.: Distant metastasis of oral carcinoma. Oral Surg. 14:705, 1961.

131. Castigliano, S. G., and Rominger, C.: Distant metastases from carcinoma of the oral cavity. Am. J. Roentgenol. Radium Ther. Nucl. Med. 71:997, 1954.

132. Hoye, R. C., Herrold, K. McD., Smith, R. C., and Thomas, L. B.: A clinicopathological study of epidermoid carcinoma of the head and neck. Cancer 15:741, 1962.

133. Schneider, M.: Epidermoid carcinomas of the oral cavity: a review. Am. J. Med. 244:628, 1962.

134. Blady, J. V.: The present status of treatment of cervical metastases from carcinoma arising in the head and neck region. Am. J. Surg. 111:56, 1971.

135. MacComb, W. S.: Radical neck dissection. In Cancer of the Head and Neck, edited by W. S. MacComb and G. H. Fletcher, pp. 488–506. Williams & Wilkins Co., Baltimore, 1967.

136. Lindberg, R. D.: Distribution of cervical lymph node metastases from squamous cell carcinoma of upper respiratory and digestive tracts. Cancer 29:1446, 1972.

137. Hammond, W. G., and Rolley, R. T.: Retained regional lymph nodes: Effect on metastases and recurrence after tumor removal. Cancer 25:368, 1970.

138. Southwick, H. W.: Elective neck dissection for intraoral cancer. J.A.M.A. 217:454, 1971.

139. Wilkinson, E. J., and Hause, L.: Probability in lymph node sectioning. Cancer 33:1269, 1974.

140. Jesse, R. H., and Lindberg, R. D.: Evaluation of clinically negative neck: squamous cell carcinoma of oral cavity and faucial arch. J.A.M.A. 217:453, 1971.

141. Cody, B.: Carcinoma of the oral cavity—evaluation and management. Surg. Clin. North Am. 51:537, 1971.

142. Northrop, M., Fletcher, G. H., Jesse, R. H., and Lindberg, R. D.: Evolution of neck disease in patients with primary squamous cell carcinoma of the oral tongue, floor of mouth, and palatine arch, and clinically positive neck nodes either fixed or bilateral. Cancer 29:23, 1972.

143. Scanlon, P. W., Soule, E. H., Devine, K. D., and McBean, J. B.: Cancer of base of tongue. Am. J. Roentgenol. Radium Ther. Nucl. Med. 105:26, 1969.

144. Rouviere, H.: Anatomy of the Human Lymphatic System. Edwards Brothers, Inc., Ann Arbor, Mich., 1938.

145. Fletcher, G. H., and MacComb, W. S.: Radiation Therapy in the Management of Cancers of the Oral Cavity and Oropharynx. Charles C Thomas, Springfield, Ill., 1962.

146. Rubin, P.: Cancer of the head and neck: oropharynx. J.A.M.A. 217:940, 1971.

147. Conley, J.: Concepts in Head and Neck Surgery. Georg Thieme Verlag, Stuttgart, 1970.

148. Fletcher, G. H., Jesse, R. H., Healey, J. E., Jr., and Thoma, G. W.: Oropharynx. In Cancer of the Head and Neck, edited by W. S. MacComb and G. H. Fletcher, pp. 179–212. Williams & Wilkins Co., Baltimore, 1967.

149. Jesse, R. H., and Sugarbaker, E. U.: Squamous cell carcinoma of the cropharynx: Why we fail. Am. J. Surg. 132:435, 1976.

150. Fletcher, G. H., and Lindberg, R. D.: Squamous cell carcinomas of the tonsillar area and palatine arch. Am. J. Roentgenol. Radium Ther. Nucl. Med. 96:574, 1977.

151. Rider, W. D.: Epithelial cancer of the tonsillar area. Radiology 78:760, 1962.

152. Strong, M. S., DiTroia, J. F., and Vaughan, C. W.: Carcinoma of the palatine Arch: a review of 73 patients. Trans. Am. Acad. Ophtholmol. Otolaryngol. 75:957, 1971.

153. Fletcher, G. H., MacComb, W. S., Chau, P. M., and Farnsley, W. G.: Comparison of medium voltage and supervoltage roentgen therapy in the treatment of oropharynx cancers. Am. J. Roentgenol. Radium Ther. Nucl. Med. 81:375, 1959.

154. Perussia, A.: Cited by Ackerman, L. V., and del Regato, J.: Cancer Diagnosis, Treatment and Prognosis, 4th ed, p. 279. C. V. Mosby, St. Louis, 1970.

155. Russ, J. E., Applebaum, E. L., and Sisson, C. A.: Squamous cell carcinomas of the soft palate. Laryngoscope 87:1151, 1977.

156. Seda, H. J., and Snow, J. B., Jr.: Carcinoma of the tonsil. Arch. Otolaryngol. 89:756, 1969.

157. Whicker, J. H., DeSanto, L. W., and Devine, K. D.: Surgical treatment of squamous cell carcinoma of the tonsil. Laryngoscope 84:90, 1974.

158. Rolander, T. L., Everts, E. C., and Shumrick, D. A.: Carcinoma of the tonsil: a planned combined therapy approach. Laryngoscope 81:1199, 1971.

159. Johnston, W. D., and Byers, R. M.: Squamous cell carcinoma of the tonsil in young adults. Cancer 39:632, 1977.

160. Chen, T. Y., Johnson, R., and Sako, K.: Carcinoma of the tonsillar fossa. In Cancer of the Head and Neck, edited by R. G. Chambers, A. M. P. Janssen deLimpens, D. A. Jaques, and R. T. Routledge, pp. 190–198. Excerpta Medica, Elsevier, New York, 1975.

161. Scanlon, P. W., Gee, V. R., Erich, J. B., Williams, H. L., and Woolner, L. B.: Carcinoma of the palatine tonsil. Am. J. Radium Ther. Nucl. Med. Roentgenol. 80:781, 1958.

162. Micheau, C., Cachin, Y., and Caillou, B.: Cystic metastases in the neck revealing occult carcinoma of the tonsil. A report of six cases. Cancer 33:228, 1974.

163. Rider, W. D.: Epithelial cancer of the tonsillar area. Radiology 78:760, 1962.

164. Calamel, P. M., and Hoffmeister, F. S.: Carcinoma of the tonsil: comparison of surgical and radiation therapy. Am. J. Surg. 114:4, 1967.

165. Teloh, H. A.: Cancer of the tonsil. Arch. Surg. 65:693, 1952.

166. Martin, H., and Sugarbaker, E.: Cancer of the tonsil. Am. J. Surg. 52:158, 1941.

167. Walker, J. H., and Schulz, M. D.: Carcinoma of the tonsil. Radiology 49:162, 1947.

168. Dalley, V. M.: The place of radiotherapy in the treatment of tumors of the base of the tongue. Am. J. Roentgenol. Radium Ther. Nucl. Med. 105:26, 1969.

169. Scanlon, P. W., Soule, E. H., Devine, K. D., and McBean, J. B.: Cancer of the base of the tongue. Am. J. Roentgenol. Radium Ther. Nucl. Med. 105:26, 1969.

170. Fleming, P. M., Matz, G. J., Powell, W. J., and Chen, J. Z. W.: Carcinoma of the tonsil. Surg. Clin. N. Am. 56:125, 1976.

171. Concannon, J. P.: Radiotherapy as the initial form of treatment for epidermoid carcinoma of the tonsil and the base of the tongue. J.A.M.A. 217:940, 1971.

172. Shah, J. P., Shaha, A. R., Spiro, R. H., and Strong, E. W.: Carcinoma of the hypopharynx. Am. J. Surg. 132:439, 1976.

173. Ahlbom, H. E.: Simple achlorhydric anaemia, Plummer-Vinson syndrome, and carcinoma of the mouth, pharynx, and esophagus in women. Br. Med. J. 2:331, 1936.

174. Jacobsson, F.: Carcinoma of the hypopharynx: a clinical study of 322 cases, treated at radium-hemmet, from 1939 to 1947. Acta Radiol. 35:1, 1951.

175. Bryce, D. P.: Pharyngectomy in the treatment of carcinoma of the hypopharynx. In Cancer of the Head and Neck, edited by J. Conley, pp. 341–346, Butterworths, Washington, D.C., 1967.

176. Ferlito, A.: Primary lymphoepithelial carcinoma of the hypopharynx. J. Laryngol. 91:361, 1977.

177. Willis, R. A.: The Spread of Tumours in the Human Body. J. & A. Churchill, Ltd., London, 1934.

178. Coutard, H.: De la roentgen therapic des cancers du pharynx. Radiophys. Radiother. 3:203, 1934.

179. Carpenter, R. J., DeSanto, L. W., Devine, K. D., and Taylor, W. F.: Cancer of the hypopharynx. Analysis of treatment and results in 162 patients. Arch. Otolaryngol. 102:716, 1976.

180. Razack, M. S., Sako, K., Marchetta, F. C., Calamel, P., Bakamjian, V., and Shedd, D. P.: Carcinoma of the hypopharynx: success and failure. Am. J. Surg. 134:489, 1977.

181. Briant, T. D. R., Bryce, D. P., and Smith, T. J.: Carcinoma of the hypopharynx—a five year follow-up. J. Laryngol. 6:353, 1977.

182. McGavran, M. H., Bauer, W. C., Spjut, H. J., and Ogura, J. H.: Carcinoma of the pyriform sinus: the results of radical surgery. Arch. Otolaryngol. 78:826, 1963.

183. Lederman, M.: Cancer of the pharyngo-laryngeal groove with special reference to the sinus pyriformis. J. Laryngol. 67:641, 1953.

184. Sherlock, E. C., and Cain, A. S.: Tumors of the hypopharynx. South. Med. J. 64:641, 1953.

185. Andre, P., and Pinel, J.: Exercise chirurgicale associce a la radiotherapie dans le traitment des cancers du sinus pyriforme. Ann. Otolaryngol. 79:6, 1962.

186. Eisback, K. J., and Krause, C. J.: Carcinoma of the pyriform sinus. A comparison of treatment modalities. Laryngoscope 87:1904, 1977.

187. Ogura, J. H.: Cancer of the hypopharynx and larynx. Am. J. Med. Sci. 244:501, 1962.

188. Som, M. L., and Nussbaum, M.: Surgical therapy of carcinoma of the hypopharynx and cervical esophagus. Otolaryngol. Clin. North Am. 2:631, 1969.

189. Harrison, D. F. N.: Surgical management of cancer of the hypopharynx and cervical esophagus. Br. J. Surg. 56:95, 1969.

190. Som, M. L.: Surgical treatment of carcinoma of post-cricoid region. N.Y. State J. Med. 61:2567, 1961.

191. Cunningham, M. P., and Catlin, D.: Cancer of the pharyngeal wall. Cancer 20:1859, 1967.

192. Wang, C. C.: Radiotherapeutic management of carcinoma of the posterior pharyngeal wall. Cancer 27:894, 1971.

193. Lederman, M.: Cancer of the pharynx. J. Laryngol. 81:151, 1967.

194. Goodman, J.: End results in cancer of cervical esophagus.

Personal communication, 1966, cited by Cunningham and Catlin.[191]

195. Ballantyne, A. J.: Significance of retropharyngeal nodes in cancer of the head and neck. Am. J. Surg. 108:500, 1964.

196. Moertel, C. G., Dockerty, M. B., and Baggenstoss, A. H.: Multiple primary malignant neoplasms. I, II, and III. Cancer 14:221; 231; 238, 1961.

197. Bachulis, B. L., and Williams, R. D.: Multiple primary malignancies. Arch. Surg. 92:537, 1966.

198. Warren, S., and Gates, O.: Multiple primary malignant tumors: survey of the literature and statistical study. Am. J. Cancer 16:1358, 1932.

199. Marchetta, F. C., Sako, K., and Camp, E.: Multiple malignancies in patients with head and neck cancer. Am. J. Surg. 110:537, 1965.

200. Ju, D. M. C.: A study of the behavior of cancer of the head and neck during its late and terminal phases. Am. J. Surg. 108:552, 1964.

201. Ackerman, L. V.: Verrucous carcinoma of the oral cavity. Surgery 23: 670, 1948.

202. Perez, C. A., Kraus, F. T., Evans, J. C., and Powers, W. E.: Anaplastic transformation in verrucous carcinoma of the oral cavity after radiation therapy. Radiology 86:108, 1966.

203. Demian, S. D. E., Bushkin, F. L., and Echevarria, R. A.: Perineural invasion and anaplastic transformation of verrucous carcinoma. Cancer 32:395, 1973.

204. Ryan, R. E., Jr., DeSanto, L. W., Devine, K. D., and Weiland, L. H.: Verrucous carcinoma of larynx. Laryngoscope 87:1989, 1977.

205. Burns, H. P., van Nostrand, A. W. P., and Bryce, D. P.: Verrucous carcinoma of the larynx. Management by radiotherapy and surgery. Ann. Otol. 85:538, 1976.

206. Biller, H. F., and Bergman, J. A.: Verrucous carcinoma of the larynx. Laryngoscope 85:1698, 1975.

207. Lyall, D., and Shetlin, C. F.: Cancer of the tongue. Ann. Surg. 135: 489, 1952.

208. Kremen, A. J.: The case for elective (prophylactic) neck dissection. In Cancer of the Head and Neck, edited by J. Conley, pp. 183–185. Butterworths, Washington, D.C., 1967.

209. Southwick, H. W., Slaughter, D. P., and Trevino, E. T.: Elective neck dissection for intraoral cancer. Arch. Surg. 80:905, 1960.

210. Sako, K., Pradier, R. N., Marchetta, F. C., and Pickren, J. W.: Fallibility of palpation in the diagnosis of metastasis to cervical nodes. Surg. Gynecol. Obstet. 118:989, 1964.

211. Ward, G. E., Edgerton, M. T., Chambers, R. G., and McKee, D. M.: Cancer of the oral cavity and pharynx and results of treatment by means of the composite operation (in continuity with radical neck dissection). Ann. Surg. 150:202, 1959.

CHAPTER 7

Cancer of the Nasal Cavity and the Paranasal Sinuses

Malignant neoplasms of the nasal cavity and the paranasal sinuses comprise between 0.2 and 0.8% of all malignancies and 3% of cancers involving the upper respiratory tract and the upper alimentary tract.[1] Carcinoma of the maxillary antrum is a typical example with less than one case per 200,000 people per annum.[2] Perhaps more so than other neoplasms in the head and neck, cancers of the nose and paranasal sinuses present more unresolved problems for both surgeons and radiotherapists. The fate of patients with this disease is highly dependent upon the fullest cooperation between these two groups of physicians.[3]

A variety of factors are responsible for the poor prognosis associated with cancer in these anatomical regions. These include: (1) the advanced stage of the disease at the time of diagnosis; (2) the complex anatomy of the region involved; and (3) the reluctance of many surgeons to pursue an aggressive form of treatment. Because malignancy of the nasal chambers and paranasal sinuses so often masquerades as a chronic inflammatory condition, the patient and the physician are very often deluded into procrastination. Patients with cancer of the antrum or ethmoid sinuses rarely seek medical help until their neoplasms are advanced, the average delay between the onset of the first symptoms and final diagnosis being 6 months.[4]

As Rubin[5] points out: "Before cancer of the nose and paranasal sinuses can be cured, one must think of its possible existence." A good chance for control may be had if diagnosis can be made in the early to moderately advanced stages. Rubin[5] has divided the insidious progression of cancer in these anatomical regions into four clinical phases. In phase I, the neoplasm is obscured by symptoms of a sinusitis, and diagnosis requires drainage, access to the cavities and biopsy. In phase II, it is the radiologist who bears the greatest diagnostic

burden. In this phase, a dull ache may appear as the neoplasm erodes the walls of the nose and sinuses. Any area of bone destruction or assymmetrical sclerosis in a sinus demands immediate clarification.[5] Phase III is characterized by fairly obvious signs of malignancy. Radiographic evidence of bone destruction is now no longer subtle, and hypesthesias and deep pain herald nerve invasion. In phase IV, there is gross and distant spread of the neoplasm with major deformity. The diagnosis is obvious and the chances for cure are virtually nil.

The intimate inter-relationships and unity between the nasal passages and sinuses are largely responsible for the ease with which malignant tumors spread from one sinus to another. Although the maxillary sinus is involved in at least 80% of all cases, the disease is limited to this cavity in only 25% of patients.[4] Even this figure, depressing though it is, probably represents an overoptimistic viewpoint.[4] Discernible bone destruction is found in from 70 to 80% of cases.[6] The cancers may extend through the innumerable foramina and fissures of the bones making up the sinus complex. In addition, there are perineural, vascular and lymphatic extension into adjacent structures. Conley[6] reports that in 45% of his patients there was direct positive invasion of the orbit and that 80% manifested invasion of the nerves. Ten percent of his patients had extension of their neoplasms to the pterygoid plates.

It is manifestly clear that approximately three-quarters of patients with paranasal sinus cancer die of their disease. The natural history of the neoplasia is also clear; patients present late and die slowly. Harrison[7] comes directly to the point when he says of these patients, "There is little hope of any worthwhile improvement except to ensure that those who are potentially curable are cured." Eschewing classification, he considers patients having a "possibility" of cure as being divisible into three groups; early, late, and intermediate. Early neoplasms are small, localized, treatable and uncommon. Survival for patients with such lesions approximates 75% for 5 years. Survival for patients with late or advanced cases is reduced to approximately 7%. Patients who present with carcinomas in the intermediate group may be expected to have an over 50% 5-year survival depending on the response to therapy.

CLASSIFICATION

There is no generally accepted classification for tumors of the nasal fossa or the paranasal sinuses. Because of their grouping about the nose, the neoplasms have been simply classified as "nasal tumors." This form of classification should be abandoned. Tumors of the postnasal chambers with their special problems require a separate identity; similarly, classifications should separate tumors of the anterior nose and each of the sinuses.

Lederman[3] and Rubin[5] present the historical development of tumor classifications for this anatomical region. As with all such classifications, probably none is suitable for a universal adoption without modifications. The intrinsic deficiencies of any system of classification are that all classifications are dependent upon clinical and radiological evaluation of tumor extent. Nowhere is this more difficult than in the deep recesses of the nasal sinuses.[4] Table 7.1 presents Rubin's[5] attempt to classify paranasal sinus cancer and is based on modifications of early efforts of Ohngren,[8] Dodd et al.[9] and Sisson et al.[10] Lederman's[3] suggested classification has considerable merit and divides the region and sites into: (1) superior region (suprastructure); (2) middle region (mesostructure); and (3) inferior region (infrastructure). A schematic representation (after Lederman[3]) of the subdivisions of the upper jaw is seen in Figure 7.1. The tumor-node-metastases (TNM) classification based on this scheme is presented in Table 7.2.

In Lederman's[3] classification, primary emphasis is on the mesostructure and suprastructure since the infrastructure, or buccal part of the upper jaw, is outside the nasal and sinus cavities. Tumors arising from the infrastructure usually have their origins in the alveolar ridge, hard palate or about the teeth. It is also possible for neoplasms to invade the buccal cavity from the floors of the nose or the antrum. Because of the two-way invasion possibilities, Lederman[3] regards these neoplasms as legitimately belonging to the infrastructure of the up-

Table 7.1
Classification of Paranasal Sinus Cancer*

T (Tumor)
  T1. Infrastructure site of neoplasm in anterior and inferior compartment without bone destruction.
  T2. Suprastructure location of neoplasm in posterior and superior compartment without bone destruction; both compartments are involved.
  T3. Radiographic evidence of bone destruction. Invasion of nares or cheek muscles; enlargement of infraorbital foramina or orbital destruction. No soft tissue invasion of the orbit or eye. No involvement of oral cavity.
  T4. Invasion of skin of cheek; fistula may be present, orbital and eye invasions, invasion of oral cavity with fistula and extension to ethmoid, sphenoid or frontal sinuses.

N (Lymph nodes)
  N0. No involvement of primary station lymph nodes (includes retropharyngeal, jugulodigastric and the submandibular and parotid lymph nodes).
  N1. Palpable, movable, involved nodes.
  N2. Contralateral or bilateral nodes.
  N3. Fixed neck nodes.
  N4. Nodes in mediastinum or beyond primary station levels.

M (Metastasis)
  M0. No metastasis
  M1. Distant metastasis

* After Rubin.[5]

per jaw. The mesostructure or nasal portion of the jaw includes the antrum and the respiratory part of the nasal fossa (including the inferior turbinate, the whole of the nasal septum and the vestibule of the external nose). Since the bony components of the mesostructure offer only a weak barrier to the spread of cancer in the region, tumors arising here spread rapidly and render precise determination of origin difficult or impossible.

Tumors of the nasal fossa may extend backward to involve the nasopharynx and the base of the skull. Posterior penetration by an antral tumor may produce invasion of the pterygoid region. The cranial part (suprastructure) of the upper jaw is largely made up of the ethmoid and its turbinates and the olfactory part of the nasal fossa. Tumors of the frontal and sphenoid sinuses are included, for classification purposes, in the suprastructure. In 273 of the 610 previously untreated patients studied by Lederman,[3] there was involvement of both supra- and mesostructures.

The histological type of neoplasm also influences therapeutic considerations.[11, 12] Over 50% of the cancers of the nasal cavity and paranasal sinuses are squamous cell carcinomas of varying differentiation. Frazell and Lewis[11] found that 81% (337 of 416 cases) of the carcinomas were squamous cell in type. In this chapter emphasis is placed on squamous cell malignancies and on over-all survivals. The other categories of malignancy affecting the nose and paranasal sinuses may be found in other chapters in this text.

Lederman[3] has succinctly presented the principles of treatment for carcinomas in the upper jaw

Table 7.2
Tumor-Node-Metastases (TNM) Classification of Tumors of the Upper Jaw*

I. Region and sites
  A. Superior (suprastructure)
    1. Ethmoidal labyrinth
    2. Frontal sinus
    3. Sphenoid sinus (without nasopharyngeal involvement)
    4. Olfactory part of nasal fossa (above the middle turbinate)
  B. Middle (mesostructure)
    1. Maxillary sinus
    2. Respiratory part of nasal fossa: vestibule and septum
    3. Lateral wall, inferior turbinate
  C. Inferior (infrastructure)
    1. Floor of maxillary sinus
    2. Floor of nose
    3. Dental (odontogenic) tumors
    4. Tumors manifesting a simultaneous involvement of the antrum and hard palate, or the palate and the floor of the nasal fossa
II. Primary neoplasm (T).
  A. T1. Tumor limited to one sinus or a tissue of origin, e.g., turbinate, septum or nasal vestibule
  B. T2. Limited horizontal spread to same region or two adjacent or vertically related regions.
  C. T3.
    1. Tumor involving three regions (with or without orbital involvement)
    2. Extension of the tumor beyond the upper jaw, e.g., nasopharynx, cranial cavity, skin, buccal cavity or pterygopalatine fossa
III. Regional lymph nodes (N)
  A. N0. No palpable lymph nodes
  B. N1. Mobile homolateral lymph nodes
  C. N2. Mobile contralateral or bilateral lymph nodes
  D. N3. Fixed homolateral or bilateral lymph nodes
IV. Distant metastases (M).
  A. M0. No evidence of distant metastases
  B. M1. Distant metastases

* Reproduced from Lederman[3] by permission.

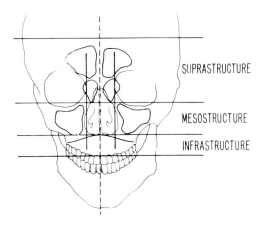

Figure 7.1. Subdivisions of the upper jaw (after Lederman[3]). Division into supra-, meso- and infrastructures is accomplished by drawing two parallel lines across the frontal section of the skull—one line passing through the floor of the orbits, the other through the floor of the antra. The two vertical lines serve to separate the ethmoid and nasal fossa from the maxillary sinus. The nasal septum separates the ethmoid and nasal fossa into right and left sides.

and has pointed out the limitations of both radical surgery and radiotherapy. Because of these limitations, the most appropriate form of management is a combination of the two. The combination that seems to be best is radiation followed by surgery. He cites one important contradiction to preoperative radiation for carcinoma of the upper jaw—involvement of the malar bone.[3]

In the following discussion, I present a clinicopathological assessment of carcinomas of the nasal cavity and the paranasal sinuses. An *attempt* has been made to consider carcinoma arising from specific areas. This has been done with the full realization that seeming confinement of a neoplasm to a single region is not usually found. Table 7.3 presents the relative frequency with which cancer affects the sinuses and nasal cavity.

CARCINOMAS OF SPECIFIC REGIONS

Carcinoma of the Nasal Cavity. The nasal cavity opens externally through the anterior nares and communicates posteriorly with the nasopharynx via the choanae. A midline nasal bony septum divides the cavity into right and left nasal fossae. The roof of the nasal cavity is formed by the nasal cartilage, nasal bone, nasal process of the frontal bone and the body of the sphenoid bone. The floor is composed of the hard palate (palatine process of the maxilla and the horizontal processes of the palatine bone). The inferior, middle and

Table 7.3
Cancer of the Nasal Cavity and the Paranasal Sinuses

Author	Anatomical Site of Origin				
	Maxillary Antrum	Nasal Cavity	Ethmoid Sinus	Sphenoid Sinus	Frontal Sinus
Ireland and Bryce[13]	124	22	33	4	
Osborn and Winston[14]	63		31		
Frazell and Lewis[11]	261	113	40	1	1
Tabah[15]	36		14	1	1
Conley[6]	60	15	15	2	3
Lederman[3]	356	154	172		4
Lewis and Castro[48]	451	237	75	3	6
Larsson and Martensson[29]	346	14	19	—	—
Boone et al.[47]	70	28	20	2	1

superior conchae or turbinates project into the nasal cavity from each lateral nasal wall. The turbinates incompletely divide the fossae into meatuses. These are inferior and lateral to their respective turbinates. The sphenoethmoidal recess lies immediately above and behind the superior meatus. Each nasal fossa has further been divided (physiologically and clinically) into a lower, or respiratory, portion and an upper, or olfactory, portion. The upper, or olfactory, portion of the nasal fossa lies above a line passing at the level of the free border of the middle turbinate.

Primary malignant tumors of the nasal cavity are relatively rare lesions, yet this region may be the site of a variety of histological types of neoplasms, both benign and malignant. Our concern here is with the malignant epithelial neoplasms (primarily squamous cell carcinomas).

Carcinoma of the nasal cavity is primarily a disease of males. Three-fourths of the patients are over 50 years of age, and the mean age at the time of diagnosis is the mid-fifties. Unilateral nasal obstruction with or without epistaxis is the most common presenting symptom. Chronic sinusitis or nasal polyps precede or are associated with the carcinomas in approximately 15% of the cases.[16] Smoking from early age is a noticeable habit among these patients. There is a modest tendency for the carcinomas to be in the right side of the nasal cavity; approximately 5% are bilateral.[16]

The lateral walls of the nasal cavity are the most frequently involved sites; approximately 50% arise on the turbinates. Other sites, in order of decreasing frequency, are septum, vestibule, posterior choanae and the floor of the nasal cavity. The majority of the carcinomas are polypoid or papillary (67%); one-third are ulcerated. Nearly 85% of the carcinomas are squamous cell type, varying in their histological differentiation from well differentiated to anaplastic. Invasion of adjacent bone

occurs in over one-third of the carcinomas.[16] Regional lymph node metastases are not frequent. In the series of Bosch et al.,[17] only 12% of the patients presented nodes on admission; another 5% developed metastatic nodes during the follow-up.

Radiotherapy, alone, or in combination with surgery has been the primary mode of treatment for cancer of the nasal cavity. Bosch et al.[17] report an over-all 5-year survival of 56%, of which 49% was achieved by radiation therapy alone, plus an additional 5% salvage after surgical failure. Early T1N0 lesions have a very good prognosis, with a 5-year survival of 91%. As Bosch et al.[17] point out, series which analyze the results of tumors of the paranasal sinuses and nasal cavity separately show that the results obtained in cancer of the latter are better (Table 7.4).

Carcinomas of the nasal vestibule and the nasal septum often present diagnostic problems because of their rarity. The nasal vestibule may be defined as that recess or slight dilation immediately within the aperture of the nostril which is bounded by the medial and lateral crus of the alar cartilages, extends to the apex of the nose, is lined by skin containing hair and sebaceous glands and is contiguous with the lateral margins of the columella and septum. Inasmuch as neoplasms of the vestibule extend to adjacent structures and the septum and lateral nasal walls are usually involved, the term "anterior intranasal carcinoma" may be more appropriate.[18]

The neoplasms are usually low-grade squamous cell carcinomas and almost never metastasize.[19] When metastasis does occur, however, it is generally to the prevascular lymph node associated with the facial artery at the notch of the mandible or to the supraparotid lymph nodes.[19] Surgical removal of the lesions with wide margins has accomplished eradication of the carcinomas. Similar results are obtained with radiation therapy.[18, 19]

Primary squamous cell carcinomas of the nasal septum usually arise on the anterior septum or near the mucocutaneous junction. Carcinomas arising at the mucocutaneous junction of the septum tend to infiltrate along the lines of cleavage into the nasal labial fold and deeply into the nostril.[20]

The signs and symptoms of a septal carcinoma are largely innocuous and a malignancy may be easily overlooked in its early stages. An anterior lesion often causes a sore area inside the nostril. Examination will reveal a nodular, wart-like lesion or a small, raised ulcerated area. Persistent crusting in the nostril may be present for several months before the diagnosis is made and then only after perforation of the septum has occurred. Septal carcinomas are more serious than the carcinomas of the vestibule and they should be vigorously treated even though some form of previous therapy has been carried out.

Deutsch[20] has reviewed the pertinent literature and favors surgical excision as the primary treatment, but also acknowledges the good results obtainable by radiotherapy.[21] In the 27 cases of septal carcinoma reviewed by Deutsch,[20] 45% were living from 2 weeks to 9 years after treatment. Twelve patients had combined therapy, six were treated with radiotherapy alone and five by surgery alone. There were definite metastases in 32% of the cases reviewed. Twelve of 14 patients with cancer of the nasal septum treated at the M. D. Anderson Hospital (Houston, Texas) were alive and well after 4 years.[19] Seven patients were treated solely by surgery, six received radiotherapy and one patient was treated by combined therapy.

A study of 14 personal cases of septal carcinomas has led me[22] to conclude the following: (1) The prognosis of a patient with carcinoma of the nasal septum correlates inversely with the *size* of tumor at diagnosis and the presence of metastasis. (2) Regional metastases may present early or relatively late during the course of the disease. They occur in approximately 10% of reported cases. (3) Because of the midline position of the tumor, metastases may occur in either side of the neck.

(4) Prophylactic neck dissection is not warranted. (5) Regardless of the mode of treatment or combination of techniques, metastatic disease almost excludes a successful outcome.

Carcinomas of the Frontal and Sphenoid Sinuses. The sphenoid sinus lies deep in the head and is bounded by many neurovascular structures. There are two landmarks for locating the sphenoid sinus—the nasal septum and the sinus ostium. The septum marks the midline and the sphenoidal sinuses lie at each side of it. The sphenoidal sinus ostium lies in the upper one-third of the anterior wall of the sinus. It lies posterior and lateral to the middle and superior turbinates in the sphenoethmoidal recess. The recess, in turn, is located in the posterosuperior portion of the lateral nasal wall. Anteriorly, the sinus is related to the nasal cavity. Inferiorly, it is related to the nasopharynx and the nasal cavity. Two vital structures are adjacent to the thin walls of the sinus. These are the pituitary gland and the internal carotid artery. The optic chiasm and nerve, frontal lobe of the brain and the cavernous sinus lie in close proximity to the sinus.

If the frontal sinuses develop as evaginations from the frontal recesses of the middle meatuses, they have no duct, but drain directly into the nose. A nasofrontal duct of variable lengths occurs *only* when the sinuses develop from anterior ethmoidal cells. Because of their developmental peculiarities, asymmetry, absence or multiple sinuses may occur. The posteroinferior walls of some frontal sinuses contain bulging domes of frontal cells. These are really anterior ethmoidal sinuses that have become crowded into the frontal bone. Pneumatization of ethmoidal cavities may spread across the top of the orbits, creating supraorbital cells.

Most of the neoplastic involvements of these sinuses are secondary to carcinomas from the ethmoid sinus or the nasopharynx. The diagnosis of a primary neoplasm of the frontal or sphenoid sinuses poses three problems: (1) to localize the lesions to these sinuses from the presenting symptom-sign complex; (2) to determine whether the disease is primary in the sinuses or secondary from

Table 7.4
Comparison of Survival: Carcinoma of the Nasal Cavity versus Paranasal Sinuses

Study	No. of Patients		5-Year Survival (%)	
	Antrum	Nasal Cavity	Antrum	Nasal Cavity
Lewis and Castro[48]	453	237	23	40
Lederman[3]	248	97	25	38
Badib et al.[16]	268	45	13	56
Boone et al.[47]	70	28	35	63

neighboring structures; (3) to separate neoplastic lesions from inflammatory disease. There have been over 100 cases of reputed primary carcinomas of the frontal sinuses reported in the literature.[4, 23] Many of these had ethmoid region involvement also, and a proof of origin in the frontal sinus was lacking. The vast majority of the neoplasms has been squamous cell carcinomas.

The presenting symptoms of a carcinoma of the frontal sinus are those of acute frontal sinusitis with pain and swelling over the affected sinuses. Erosion of bone occurs rapidly and few patients survive more than 2 years. Carcinomas of the sphenoid sinus are more difficult to diagnose since they present as either nasopharyngeal or sphenoethmoidal tumors. In addition, signs and symptoms are often referred to the neurovascular structures about the sinus rather than the sinus itself.[24]

Carcinomas of the Maxillary and Ethmoid Sinuses. Largest of the paranasal sinuses, the maxillary sinuses (antrum of Highmore) occupy the center of the superior maxillary bone. Each sinus is roughly pyramidal in shape. The summit of the pyramid is toward the malar region. The base or the medial wall of the sinus is toward the nasal fossa. The anterior wall corresponds to the cheek and the canine fossa and extends up to the border of the floor of the orbit. The infratemporal space lies posterolaterally and the pterygopalatine fossa lies posteromedially.

The floor of the orbit forms the roof of the sinus, and the alveolar process of the maxilla forms the floor of the antrum. The thin wall forming the base of the sinus pyramid is divided in two by the insertion of the inferior turbinate. The maxillary ostium or communication between the sinus and the nasal fossa is located in the upper one-half of the lateral nasal wall. Under normal conditions the maxillary sinuses are lined by a ciliated columnar epithelium.

The ethmoid sinuses are insinuated between the orbit, brain, nasal chamber and the maxillary sinus. Besides the main body of the labyrinth itself, there are three other parts of the sinus: the perpendicular plate, the crista galli, and the cribriform plate. The ethmoid labyrinth contains approximately 10 air cells and is located between the orbit and the upper portion of the nasal cavity on either side. According to their site of drainage, the air cells are divided into an anterior and posterior group. The anterior group drains into the middle meatus, and the posterior into the superior meatus. The anterior cells are more numerous and also smaller than the posterior cells. They cause two swellings in the middle meatus—the bulla ethmoidalis and the aggar nasi. The surgical anatomy of this region is elegantly presented by Pearson.[25]

Carcinoma of the Maxillary Antrum. The majority of carcinomas in the paranasal sinuses start in the mucosa of the maxillary antrum and the ethmoid labyrinth. Approximately 80% of the cancers of the paranasal sinuses arise in the antrum.[26] There is, as yet, no known cause of antral carcinomas, but an important etiological association appears to be chronic sinusitis. Long-standing chronic sinusitis leads to a metaplasia of the normal respiratory epithelium lining the maxillary sinus and it is this metaplastic epithelium that is probably the origin of most antral carcinomas.[27] There are also on record cases in which cancer has developed in long-standing antro-oral fistulas.

Squamous cell carcinomas are the most frequent histological type of carcinomas occurring in the antrum and usually constitute nearly 80% of the neoplasms from that paranasal sinus.[28, 29] Carcinoma of the antrum is approximately twice as common in men, and it is disease of relatively advanced age. Nearly 95% of patients are over 40 years of age.

At the beginning of this section, I alluded to the evolution of classifications for paranasal sinus carcinomas and the deficiencies associated with them. This is especially true for those adopted for use in carcinomas of the maxillary sinus. They suffer from both intrinsic inaccuracies and an apparent failure to relate T (extent of primary tumor) categories to clinical experience of the spread of these neoplasms. Harrison[30] has taken a critical look at classifications in this light and suggests the following T grouping:

T1. Tumor limited to the antral mucosa with no evidence of bone erosion.

T2. Bony erosion without evidence of involvement of skin, orbit, pterygopalatine fossa or ethmoidal labyrinth.

T3. Bony erosion with involvement of the foregoing structures.

T4. Tumor extension to the nasopharynx, sphenoidal sinus, cribriform plate or the pterygopalatine fossa.

Chaudhry et al.[26] have divided the most important signs and symptoms of carcinoma of the maxillary antrum into five major groups. *Group I* includes oral signs and symptoms. According to Larsson and Martensson,[29] oral subjective symptoms occurred in 26% of their cases and represented the first symptoms observed by the patient in 15%. The oral signs and symptoms appear when the neoplasm arises on the floor of the antrum and is followed by a downward extension. An unexpected localized or referred pain in the upper premolar or molar teeth may be the first, subtle evidence. This may be due to pressure or to actual involvement of the posterior superior dental nerve by the neoplasm. A loosening of teeth or an alteration in their alignment is the next most common oral sign. Other symptoms referable to the oral cavity may be a swelling of the palate, the alveolar ridge or the gingivobuccal sulcus. Following extraction of loose or aching teeth, there may be failure of the sockets to heal or the development of an antro-oral fistula. Trigmus may result from neoplastic extensions into the pterygoid fossa through the infratemporal surface of the antrum.

Group II is comprised of nasal symptoms and is due to medial extension of the neoplasm. In order of their frequency, the symptoms are: unilateral nasal stuffiness, unilateral nasal discharge (ranging from clear and watery to purulent and blood-tinged) and chronic epistaxis. Protrusion of the neoplasm into the nasal cavity may often be seen.

Group III is composed of ocular signs and symptoms, and these arise from extension upward through the floor of the orbit. Dislocation of the eye and diplopia may occur. Sometimes the neoplasms extend anteriorly through the lower orbital margin and may be seen or palpated behind the lower lid. Ocular symptoms occurred in 23% of Larsson and Martensson's[29] patients—in about 5% as the initial symptoms.

Group IV includes facial symptoms arising from the neoplastic involvement of the anterior wall of the antrum. Extension through the anterolateral wall gives a bulging of the cheek, often first observed as a filling of the nasolabial fold. Facial asymmetry and disfigurement follow, and, in advanced cases, the skin becomes infiltrated or even ulcerated. Due to invasion of the infraorbital nerve, numbness or paresthesia of the skin of the cheek is not an uncommon symptom.

Group V includes all forms of neurological symptoms except those presenting in the other four groups. The majority of the symptoms are due to neoplastic involvement of the seventh and eighth nerves and the meninges. As a consequence of this involvement, there may be unilateral deafness, unilateral facial paralysis and even hemiplegia. Chaudhry et al.[26] also included generalized headache and referred pain in this group.

The medial, anterior and downward extensions of antral carcinomas produce the classical clinical symptoms of this form of cancer, i.e., asymmetry of the face, a tumor bulge palpable or visible from the oral cavity and tumor in the nasal cavity visible by anterior rhinoscopy. Each of these symptoms is present in 40 to 60% of all cases, and one or more of them is present in nearly 90% of the cases.[27]

The roentgenographic findings consist of a soft tissue shadow in the antrum region and, in at least 90% of the cases, signs of bone destruction in the walls of the antrum and the adjacent bony structures.[27, 29] It certainly must be regarded as an expression of rather late discovery that about 90% of the cases *on admission* have clinical and roentgenological evidence of bone destruction. Ordinary roentgen films should be complemented by tomography for additional evidence of bone destruction. The only sure way to get an early diagnosis of antral cancer seems to be exploratory surgery. The most widely accepted technique is the incisional biopsy through a Caldwell-Luc approach or through the nasal cavity.

The salvage rate for cancer in this location is quite low. The experience of Marchetta et al.[31] is fairly typical. These workers treated 119 patients with squamous cell carcinoma of the maxillary antrum at Roswell Park Memorial Institute. In every patient, the neoplasm had extended beyond the antral cavity to invade the cheek, nose, palate or orbit. In no patient was the diagnosis made when the tumor was still confined to the antrum. One of the aforementioned sites was grossly involved in 22% of the patients, two sites in 50%, three sites in 26% and all four areas in 1%.

Despite the local invasiveness of this malignancy, palpable lymph nodes suggesting metastatic disease are infrequent at the time of admission. The lymphatics of the maxillary sinus end in the retropharyngeal, submandibular and jugular nodes, but positive involvement occurs far less than with carcinomas of the oral cavity. Between 10 and 18% of patients manifest cervical lymph node metastases at the time of admission.[27, 31] Cervical metastases, however, increase during the period of observation so that between 25 and 35% of patients eventually have spread of their disease to the regional lymph nodes.[27, 32] Approximately 10% will terminally manifest generalized metastases.[26, 32]

Larsson and Martensson[29] have pointed to the pronounced correlation between the degree of cervical lymph node involvement and invasion of the oral cavity by the antral malignancy. There is an almost twofold increase in lymph node metastases when this form of invasion has occurred. A paranasal cancer, therefore, behaves like an oral carcinoma when it enters the oral cavity, at least with regard to its propensity for metastatic spread.

If a significant advance in prognosis is to be made for this relatively lethal neoplasm, it will be obtained by an optimal cooperation between surgery and radiotherapy.[33] Even then, however, the 5-year cure rate, in unselected series, will barely exceed 25%.[27] If the lesion is diagnosed early and is confined to the nasoantral area of the maxillary sinus, radical surgical excision appears to provide the most satisfactory results.[34] In unselected series, however, usually only 35 to 45% of the cases can be regarded as operable (considering the probability of removal of the neoplasm and toleration of the mutilating defects).[27] Destruction of the base of the skull or of the pterygoid process, infiltration of the mucous membrane in the nasopharynx, or inoperable lymph node metastases are usually considered as contraindications to surgery. A block resection of the upper jaw from a facial incision often supplemented by a piecemeal removal of surrounding tissue and/or removal of the orbital contents or excision of parts of the cheek is the preferred surgical approach. Obviously this requires extensive prosthetic or surgical reconstruction.

Because the majority of patients with carcinoma of the antrum are diagnosed only when their disease is at an advanced stage, cure by radiotherapy or surgery alone is unlikely. In recent years, a policy of combined therapy has been promulgated as the most effective means of improving cure rates. There is a wide range of opinions regarding the best way to combine surgery and radiotherapy in operable cases. Radiotherapy should in most cases *precede* surgery since, theoretically, the risk of subsequent surgery should be reduced by preoperative radiotherapy.

In most therapy centers, a telecobalt unit or 4 mcv linear accelerator is used to produce a curative dose of external irradiation.[4] After about 2 months, when there has been subsidence of the radiation reaction, radical resection is performed in cases considered operable. In series of *unselected* cases, the above combined therapy has yielded an absolute 5-year cure rate of about 25% and a cure rate, in the operated cases, of nearly 45%.[2] In patients with advanced and inoperable disease, radiation therapy has produced cure rates of 12 to 19%.[29, 35] Reversing the therapy sequence in operable cases or relying primarily upon radiation treatment of the neoplasm has not produced cure rates superior to those obtained by combined therapy (preoperative radiation and surgical resection). Cervical lymph node metastases are best treated by an en bloc dissection with or without pre- or postoperative radiation therapy.[27, 34, 36]

The forsaking of maxillectomy (except for irradiation failure) in favor of combination chemotherapy and irradiation has been advocated by Sakai et al.[37] They regard the best mode of treatment to be a combination Co-60 gamma irradiation and continuous intra-arterial infusion of 5-fluorouracil. Table 7.5 presents a synopsis of their results with these modalities as compared to other forms of management in their patients.

Cancer of the Ethmoid Sinuses. Primary cancer of the collection of air cells making up the ethmoid sinus is relatively rare. Neoplasms in this area are more usually part of a regional disease. Larsson and Martensson[29] found 19 (5.6%) of 334 cases of cancer of the sinuses arising from the ethmoid. Hara[38] found that in 5 of 92 cases (5.5%) the ethmoid air cells alone were involved. Fitz-Hugh and Gorman[39] found 5 of 77 cases involving the ethmoid only. A larger percentage is reported by Lederman et al.[40]—25% (176 of 715 tumors of the upper jaw).

The dominant type of cancer involving the sinus is the squamous cell carcinoma. Sarcomas are much less common and adenocarcinoma and adenoid cystic carcinomas are relatively rare[14, 41] (see Chapter 2). Weaver[42] quotes an incidence of 7.2% for "adenocarcinomas" in 1,176 cases of paranasal sinus cancer, but adds that it is his impression that primary adenocarcinomas of the ethmoid sinus are being seen with an increasing frequency.

There is a slight male preponderance, and, although the peak incidence is in the mid-fifties, there is a wide range. Nasal obstruction, which may be associated with a bloody discharge, is the most frequent symptom and is more common than

Table 7.5

Maxillary Sinus Carcinoma: Results of Treatment, Osaka Medical School*

Treatment and Years of Study	No. of Patients	5-Year Survival (%)
Combination irradiation and surgery (1957–1966)	114	36.9
Irradiation only (1957–1966)	168	12.7
Irradiation with intra-arterial 5-fluorouracil (1967–1969)	25	36.1
Irradiation with intra-arterial infusion (1967–69) of other agents	35	35.7
Irradiation only (1967–1969)	45	35.2
Linac x-ray irradiation (1970–1971)	61	15.9
Irradiation with 5-fluorouracil infusion (1972–1973)	80	39.3†

* Modified from Sakai et al.[37]

† Three-year relative survival rate.

in antral carcinomas. Advanced cases may present with visible bone expansion, producing a characteristic broadening of the nasal region. A unilateral anosmia may follow neoplastic extension through the cribriform plate. Destruction of the bony walls, opacification and a trabecular pattern of the air cells are seen on radiological examination. Diagnosis is made by examination of biopsy specimens obtained via a Caldwell-Luc approach or through the nose.

The lymphatic drainage of the ethmoid sinus is to the lateral retropharyngeal nodes and thence to the upper deep cervical chain.[43] The incidence of nodal metastases is, however, low. This has been attributed, at least in part, to a poor lymphatic drainage or to a clinical inaccessibility of primary nodes. Distant metastases have been considered uncommon.[3]

Because synchronous involvement of the antrum and ethmoid sinus is common, the general principles of treatment for ethmoidal cancers are similar to those for carcinomas of the antrum. However, radical surgical excision is made difficult because of the proximity of the ethmoid sinuses to the base of the skull and the often advanced stage of the disease at the time of diagnosis.

Jesse et al.[19] have reviewed the pros and cons for the various methods of radical treatment (sur-

gical and radiotherapeutic). Many workers favor preoperative radiation with the full knowledge that this requires extreme care to avoid or minimize postoperative complications.[43] Mobile metastases to the cervical nodes are probably best treated by radical neck dissection. Fixed lymph nodes are an indication for palliative irradiation.[43] The results of treatment vary considerably and are partially dependent on the histological types (i.e., adenocarcinomas, adenoid cystic carcinomas or supporting tissue malignancies). Crude over-all 5-year survivals of 20 to 25% are to be expected.[3, 44]

In Table 7.6, the 5-year survival data of carcinomas of the paranasal sinuses are presented. These figures have been culled from 15 reports published between 1950 and 1971. The neoplasms represented are all carcinomas and the series contains selected as well as unselected patients. The near 25% survival average indicates that failure to establish early diagnosis thwarts an effective management.

Lymphomas of the Paranasal Sinuses. Malignant lymphoma involving the paranasal sinuses is an unusual occurrence and it is usually localized to this extranodal site when discovered.[45, 46] The incidence in reported series varies, but it is unusual to record as high a frequency as reported from the Massachusetts Eye and Ear Infirmary. Between

Table 7.6
Carcinoma of the Paranasal Sinuses: Results of Treatment—5-Year Survivals

Author	Form of Treatment	Location of Tumor	No. of Cases	5-Year Survival
				%
Capps[49] (1950)	Irradiation before surgery	Nose and sinuses	52	27.0
Schall[50] (1951)	Predominantly surgery	Nose and sinuses	202	26.5
Mattick and Streuter[51] (1954)	Irradiation before surgery	Antrum	68	10.0
Larsson and Martensson[29] (1954)	Irradiation before surgery	Nose and sinuses	294	23.0
Struben[52] (1957)	Surgery before irradiation	Sinuses	76	13.0
Snelling[53] (1957)	Irradiation before surgery	Antrum and ethmoids	115	28.0
Dalley[54] (1957)	Various combinations of surgery and irradiation	Antrum and ethmoids	215	28.5
Tabb[55] (1959)	Radical surgery following irradiation	Antrum	60	10.0
Baclesse et al[56] (1960)	Irradiation	Antrum	94	20.0
Frazell and Lewis[11] (1963)	Radical surgery	Antrum	163	29.0
Zange and Scholtz[57] (1963)	All methods	Antrum	116	25.0
Spratt and Mercado[2] (1965)	Primary irradiation	Antrum	69	15.0
Pointon[12] (1969)	Megavoltage only	Antrum and ethmoids	105	25.0
Pointon[12] (1969)	Intracavitary radium	Antrum and ethmoids	146	28.0
Tabb and Barranco[34] (1971)	Various combinations including chemotherapy	Antrum	102	27.0

1946 and 1970, 8% of their paranasal sinus malignancies were classified as some form of lymphoma.[45]

Some features of these lesions are presented in Chapter 23. Others are presented here. Patients with this form of malignancy are usually in their sixth decade of life and present with nasal obstruction and/or swelling of the cheek. In most patients, symptoms are insidious and of relatively long duration. The antral-ethmoidal complex is the most common area involved, but the tumor is not usually confined to the sinuses. Regardless of site, the disease has spread to other sinuses or adjacent soft tissue by the time of diagnosis. Concurrent generalized lymphoma is unusual. The most common histological form is histiocytic lymphoma.

Treatment has been nearly restricted to irradiation of the involved sites. Prophylactic treatment of regional lymph nodes has also been advocated but this is debated since most patients have negative results upon examination of their necks at the time of presentation to a physician. There are indications, however, that the presence of adenopathy with extranodal lymphoma of the head and neck halves the 5-year survival rate. A poor prognosis is also suggested when the primary lesion fails to respond to radiation therapy. Following irradiation, the 5-year survival rates have ranged from 50 to 70%.

REFERENCES

1. Grant, R. N., and Silverberg, E.: Cancer Statistics: 1970, pp. 8, 14. American Cancer Society, Inc., New York, 1970.
2. Spratt, J. S., Jr., and Mercado, R., Jr.: Therapy and staging in advanced cancer of the maxillary antrum. Am. J. Surg. 110:502, 1965.
3. Lederman, M.: Cancer of the upper jaw and nasal chambers. Proc. R. Soc. Med. 62:55, 1969.
4. Harrison, D. F. N.: The management of malignant tumors of the nasal sinuses. Otolaryngol. Clin. North Am. 4:159, 1971.
5. Rubin, P.: Cancer of the head and neck: nose, paranasal sinuses. J.A.M.A. 219:336, 1972.
6. Conley, J.: Concepts in head and neck surgery, p. 57. Georg Thieme Verlag, Stuttgart, 1970.
7. Harrison, D. F. N.: Problems in surgical management of neoplasms arising in the paranasal sinuses. J. Laryngol. 90:69, 1976.
8. Ohngren, L. G.: Malignant tumours of the maxillo-ethmoidal region: a clinical study with special reference to the treatment with electrosurgery and irradiation. Acta Otolaryng. (suppl.) 19:1, 1933.
9. Dodd, G. D., Collins, L. C., Egan, R. L., and Herrera, J. R.: The systemic use of tomography in the diagnosis of carcinoma of the paranasal sinuses. Radiology 72:379, 1959.
10. Sisson, G. A., Johnson, N. E., and Amiri, C. S.: Cancer of the maxillary sinus: clinical classification and management. Ann. Otol. Rhinol. Laryngol. 72:1050, 1963.
11. Frazell, E. L., and Lewis, J. S.: Cancer of the nasal cavity and accessory sinuses: a report of the management of 416 patients. Cancer 16:1293, 1963.
12. Pointon, R. C. S.: Neoplasia of the nose and sinuses. J. Laryngol. 83:407, 1969.
13. Ireland, P. E., and Bryce, D. P.: Carcinoma of the accessory nasal sinuses. Ann. Otol. Rhinol. Laryngol. 75:698, 1966.
14. Osborn, D. A., and Winston, P.: Carcinoma of the paranasal sinuses. J. Laryngol. 75:387, 1961.
15. Tabah, E. J.: Cancer of the paranasal sinuses: a study of the results of various methods of treatment in fifty-four patients. Am. J. Surg. 104:741, 1962.
16. Badib, A. O., Kurohara, S. S., Webster, J. H., and Shedd, D. P.: Treatment of cancer of the nasal cavity. Am. J. Roentgenol. Radium Ther. Nucl. Med. 106:824, 1969.
17. Bosch, A., Vallecillo, L., and Frias, Z.: Cancer of the nasal cavity. Cancer 37:1458, 1976.
18. Des Prez, J. D., and Kiehn, C. L.: Carcinoma of the nasal vestibule. Am. J. Surg. 114:587, 1967.
19. Jesse, R. H., Butler, J. J., Healey, J. E., Jr., Fletcher, G. H., and Chau, P. M.: Paranasal sinuses and nasal cavity. In Cancer of the Head and Neck, edited by W. S. McComb and G. H. Fletcher, Williams & Wilkins Co., Baltimore, 1967.
20. Deutsch, H. J.: Carcinoma of the nasal septum: report of a case and review of the literature. Ann. Otol. Rhinol. Laryngol. 75:1049, 1966.
21. Wang, C. C.: Treatment of carcinoma of the nasal vestibule by irradiation. Cancer 38:100, 1976.
22. Weimert, T. A., Batsakis, J. G., and Rice, D. H.: Carcinomas of the nasal septum. J. Laryngol. 92:209, 1978.
23. Brownson, R. J., and Ogura, J. H.: Primary carcinoma of the frontal sinuses. Laryngoscope 81:71, 1971.
24. Alexander, F. W.: Primary tumors of the sphenoid sinus. Laryngoscope 73:537, 1963.
25. Pearson, B. W.: The surgical anatomy of maxillectomy. Surg. Clin. N. Am. 57:701, 1977.
26. Chaudhry, A. P., Gorlin, R. J., and Mosser, D. G.: Carcinoma of the antrum: a clinical and histopathologic study. Oral Surg. 13:269, 1960.
27. Larsson, L. G., and Martensson, G.: Maxillary antral cancers. J.A.M.A. 219:342, 1972.
28. Cantril, S. T., Parker, R. G., and Lund, P. K.: Malignant tumors of the maxillary sinus: correlating study of clinical, anatomical and pathologic aspects of supervoltage roentgen therapy. Acta Radiol. 58:105, 1962.
29. Larsson, L. G., and Martensson, G.: Carcinoma of the paranasal sinuses and the nasal cavities. Acta Radiol. 42:149, 1954.
30. Harrison, D. F. N.: Critical look at the classification of maxillary sinus carcinomata. Ann. Otol. 87:3, 1978.
31. Marchetta, F. C., Sako, K., Mattick, W. L., and Stinziano, G. D.: Squamous cell carcinoma of the maxillary antrum. Am. J. Surg. 118:805, 1969.
32. Windeyer, B. W.: Malignant tumors of the upper jaw. Br. J. Radiol. 16:362, 1943.
33. Cheng, V. S. T., and Wang, C. C.: Carcinomas of the paranasal sinuses. A study of sixty-six cases. Cancer 40:3038, 1977.
34. Tabb, H. G., and Barranco, S. J.: Cancer of the maxillary sinus. Laryngoscope 81:818, 1971.
35. Hamberger, C. A., Martensson, G., and Sjögren, H. A.: Treatment of malignant tumors of the paranasal sinuses, cancer of the head and neck. In International Workshop on Cancer of the Head and Neck, pp. 224–229. Butterworth, Washington, D.C., 1967.
36. Kurchara, S. S., Webster, J. H., Ellis, F., Fitzgerald, J. P., Shedd, D. P., and Badib, A. O.: Role of radiation therapy and of surgery in the management of localized epidermoid carcinoma of the maxillary sinus. Am. J. Roentgenol. Radium Ther. Nucl. Med. 114:35, 1972.
37. Sakai, S., Fuchihata, H., and Hamasaki, Y.: Treatment policy for maxillary sinus carcinoma. Arch. Otolaryngol. 82:172, 1976.
38. Hara, J. H.: Malignant tumors of the paranasal sinuses. West. J. Surg. 63:348, 1955.
39. Fitz-Hugh, G. S., and Gorman, J. B.: Cancer of the nasal accessory sinuses. South. Med. J. 53:155, 1960.
40. Lederman, M., Busby, E. R., and Mould, R. F.: The treat-

ment of tumors of the upper jaw. Br. J. Radiol. 42:561, 1969.

41. Weaver, D. F.: Low grade cancer of the ethmoid sinus. Laryngoscope 69:284, 1959.

42. Weaver, D. F.: Cancer of the ethmoid sinuses. Arch. Otolaryngol. 74:333, 1961.

43. Bleehen, N. M.: Ethmoid sinus cancer. J.A.M.A. 219:346, 1972.

44. Murphy, W. T.: Radiation Therapy, 2nd Ed., pp. 308–310. W. B. Saunders Co., Philadelphia, 1967.

45. Sofferman, R. A., and Cummings, C. W.: Malignant lymphoma of the paranasal sinuses. Arch. Otolaryngol. 101: 287, 1975.

46. Lehrer, S., and Roswit, B.: Primary malignant lymphoma of the paranasal sinuses. Ann. Otol. 87:81, 1978.

47. Boone, M. L., Harle, T. S., Higholt, H. W. and Fletcher, G. H.: Malignant disease of the paranasal sinuses and nasal cavity. Am. J. Roentgenol. 102:625, 1968.

48. Lewis, J. S., and Castro, E. B.: Cancer of the nasal cavity and paranasal sinuses. J. Laryngol. 86:255, 1972.

49. Capps, F. C. W.: Discussion on malignant disease of the nasal cavity and sinuses. Proc. R. Soc. Med. 43:665, 1950.

50. Schall, L. A.: Malignant neoplasms of the nose, paranasal sinuses and nasopharynx. Trans. Am. Acad. Ophthalmol. Otolaryngol. 55:209, 1951.

51. Mattick, W. L., and Streuter, M. A.: Carcinoma of the maxillary antrum. Surgery 35:236, 1954.

52. Struben, W. H.: Malignant tumors of paranasal sinuses, treatment and results. Ann. Otol. Rhinol. Laryngol. 66: 754, 1957.

53. Snelling, M. D.: Discussion on the radiation treatment of cancer of the antrum and ethmoid. Proc. R. Soc. Med. 50: 529, 1957.

54. Dalley, V. M.: Discussion on the radiation treatment of cancer of the antrum and ethmoid. Proc. R. Soc. Med. 50: 533, 1957.

55. Tabb, H. G.: Maxillectomy in carcinoma of the antrum. Laryngoscope 69:119, 1959.

56. Baclesse, F., Ennuyer, A., and Calle, R.: Les epitheliomes du sinus maxillaire traites par roentgentherapie transcutane seule. J. Radiol. Electrol. Med. Nucl. 41:368, 1960.

57. Zange, J., and Scholtz, H. J.: 25 Jahe Behandlung bosartiger Geschwulste der Nase und Nebenholen in Jena und ihr Ergebniss. Z. Laryngol. Rhinol. Otol. 42:614, 1963.

CHAPTER 8

Carcinomas of the Nasopharynx

Because of the relatively unyielding nature of the bony limits of the nasopharynx, neoplasms from this area manifest a tendency for early extension and proliferation into the nasal cavities and the oropharynx. In addition to this local infiltration, metastatic spread to the cervical lymph nodes is common to nearly all types of nasopharyngeal carcinomas. The pharyngeal fascia, because of its anatomical relationships, is easily transgressed by neoplasms, and extension along the pharyngeal space is thereby facilitated.

GROSS AND MICROSCOPIC ANATOMY

The nasopharynx is in the most cephalad portion of the pharynx.[1] Its vaulted roof is occupied by the pharyngeal tonsil (a usually atrophic collection of lymphoid tissue in the adult) and lies primarily beneath the body of the sphenoid. A small recess, the pharyngeal bursa, lies in the midline in relation to the posterior aspect of the pharyngeal tonsil and extends up the back in the wall of the pharynx. The posterior wall of the nasopharynx, with which the roof gradually merges, is related to the first two cervical vertebrae. Its mucosa contains scattered lymphoid patches.

The openings of the Eustachian tubes occupy most of the lateral walls of the pharynx. Roughly triangular in shape, these tubes have their apices superiorly. Their anterior margins merge with the soft palate posteriorly. The posterior margin forms the torus tubarius, which corresponds to the internal extension of the cartilagenous part of the Eustachian tube. The fossa of Rosenmuller, the lateral recess of the pharynx, contains lymphoid tissue and lies behind the posterior margins of the tubal openings and between them and the posterior wall of the nasopharynx. The floor of the nasopharynx is formed by the upper surface of the soft palate and is the most mobile of all the parts of the region.

There are few published works on the regional distribution of squamous and ciliated epithelia of the nasopharynx. In stillborn and newborn infants, the nasopharynx is covered solely by a pseudo-stratified columnar epithelium.[2] Although there are exceptions, most authors state that, with advancing age, the ciliated epithelium is replaced by a stratified epithelium over rather large areas. Ali,[3] however, found no significant variation in the amount of squamous epithelium in subjects whose ages ranged between 10 and 80 years. From these observations, Ali[3] assumed that an epithelial transformation to squamous cell type takes place primarily during the first decade of life. Yeh[2] disagrees and considers the squamous epithelium as always being metaplastic.

Regardless of the initiating stimulus to change, the distribution and frequency of occurrence of stratified squamous epithelium have been mapped and outlined by Ali.[3] In the various age groups studied, about 80% of the posterior wall is covered by squamous epithelium, except for the part of the mucosa overlying the pharyngeal tonsil. The lining of the anterior and lateral walls is almost evenly shared between squamous and ciliated epithelia. Alternating patches of these two epithelia characterize the mucosa of the lateral walls. Under "normal" conditions, approximately 60% of the total mucosal surface of the nasopharynx is stratified squamous epithelium after the subject has passed 10 years of life.

There are variations in the appearance of the squamous epithelium with increasing age. Between the ages of 10 and 50 years, there is little keratinization except that found in deep crypts. After 50 years, acanthosis and keratinization may usually be seen in the exposed portions of the posterior and lateral walls of the nasopharynx. The anterior wall, normally, does not exhibit keratinization. Ciliated epithelium covers approximately 40% of the area of the anterior wall, but only 15 to 20% of the posterior walls. According to Ali,[3] half of the area of the lateral walls is lined by ciliated epithelium, but it appears only in irregular patches.

A third epithelium is present in the nasopharynx. The cells of this epithelium, although histologically separable from those of squamous epithelium, contain keratohyalin granules. The similarity of this epithelium to urothelium has prompted the designation "transitional," a term that has been misused so often (see Chapter 5) that it should be abandoned in favor of *intermediate*. The intermediate epithelium has five or six cell layers and no cilia. The deepest layer of cells has a cuboidal or even columnar shape. This is followed by layers of polyhedral cells, and finally all is surmounted by a row of rounded cells.

The distribution of the intermediate epithelium is almost always between patches of squamous and ciliated epithelium and is present in a region proximal to the oropharyngeal isthmus where it separates the nasopharynx from the oropharynx. The lining of the pharyngeal tonsil and that of the lateral walls show the greatest amount of the intermediate epithelium. Here it separates the alternating patches of squamous and ciliated epithelium.

Mucus-secreting glands in the tunica propria of the mucosa of the posterior wall of the nasopharynx are located close to the basement membrane. Elsewhere, the glands (mixed mucous and serous secreting) are below the level of the tunica propria and occasionally may be seen between muscle bundles. Melanin pigmentation may be found in the basal cells of all three types of epithelia. Ali[3] found a high incidence of pigmentation in the epithelia of Indians and Malays.

ETIOLOGICAL FACTORS

Every medical student's lode of answers for examiners contains the fact that nasopharyngeal tumors are among the most common of cancers in the Chinese. This is undeniable. There is a particularly high density among the population of South China, especially in the Kwantung Province.[4] In Hong Kong, cancer of the nasopharynx represents 18% of *all* malignant neoplasms,[5] as compared to 0.25% in a worldwide (white) survey[6]; 2.0% in New York[7]; and about 8% of all malignant neoplasms seen in specialized ear, nose and throat clinics.[8] Martin and Irean[4] have further investigated the racial susceptibility to nasopharyngeal cancer and consider that such a susceptibility exists not only in Chinese, but also to some extent in all Oriental races except the Japanese. Table 8.1 after Prasad[9] outlines the geographic variation of cancer of the nasopharynx.

The racial predisposition for nasopharyngeal carcinomas is present among Chinese whether

Table 8.1
Geographic Distribution of Nasopharyngeal Cancer

Nation	Percent of Head and Neck Malignancy	Percent of All Malignancy
U.S.A.	2.0	0.3
Canada	—	0.3
United Kingdom	2.0	1.3
Scandinavia	—	0.4
India	—	0.5
Japan	—	0.1
Kenya	25.5	—
Malaysia and Singapore	—	13.2
Indonesia	—	13.9
Hong Kong	—	18.0
China (Canton)	56.9	—
Taiwan	—	21.0

they are in their native country or have been "transplanted" to other lands. This has given rise to the statement that if one passes, in the street, a cross-eyed Chinese with a swelling in his neck, the diagnosis of carcinoma of the nasopharynx can practically be made in passing.

Buell[10] has carried out a noteworthy study in the Chinese population of California. Chinese who were born in the United States have about a 20-fold greater mortality from cancer of the nasopharynx than the Caucasoid population of California. Immigrants from China have 30 to 40 times greater mortality. While Buell's[10] evidence does not prove a genetic inheritance, it does show that conditions for selection are present and may be held accountable for the statistically different mortality rate.

Smoke and nasal nasopharyngeal cancer have had many correlations. Their most interesting ramifications have been present in Africa. Whatever the primary factors, be they genetic or environmental, cancer of the nasopharynx seems to be common in people with the following characteristics: male; a low nasal index; a high frequency of severe nonallergic vasomotor rhinitis; poor nutritional habits associated with an excess of carbohydrates, often with deficiencies in vitamins A and B; and scanty masculine body hair.

Evidence for the oncogenic potential of the Epstein-Barr herpes virus (EBV) has accumulated rapidly.[11-14] Although a causal relationship has not yet been firmly established, there is considerable indirect evidence to support the hypothesis that EBV is at least partially responsible for the production of certain forms of human cancer. This evidence is based on serological data, immunofluorescence studies, animal models and electron microscopic studies of tissue from human malignant neoplasms. Employment of DNA hybridization and immunofluorescence have consistently shown a "fingerprint" of the EBV in biopsy material of Burkitt's lymphoma and carcinoma of the nasopharynx. Additionally, the injection of EBV or EBV-infected cells can induce malignancy in animals.

Consistently high titers of EBV-related antigens occur in nasopharyngeal carcinoma but are usually not found in other squamous cell carcinomas of the upper respiratory tract, mouth or pharynx. In the nasopharynx, antibodies against EBV (early antigen and capsid antigen) are found only in association with two histological types: poorly differentiated carcinomas and the lymphoepithelial carcinoma.[15] Titers are roughly proportional to the stage of the disease with high levels in advanced or relapsing disease and low levels during remission and in long-term survivors. No major serological differences are apparent among Chinese and white patients with carcinoma. There is, however, a suggestion of a reduced serological response among whites.[16]

The viral genomes are not carried by the tumor-infiltrating lymphocytes of the carcinoma (largely T-cells) but by the carcinoma cells themselves. They also express the EBV-specific nuclear antigen. It is also quite likely that the nasopharyngeal carcinoma-associated genome is slightly different from the Burkitt's lymphoma-associated genome.

No matter the strength of the circumstantial evidence, doubts can be raised over the specificity of the association between nasopharyngeal carcinoma and EBV. The virus infects the majority of all adult human populations in all countries. Its seroepidemiology resembles other horizontally transmitted viruses with the regular presence of passively transmitted antibody in the newborn and subsequent decline and reappearance of activity induced antibody after infection. Timing and extent of seroconversion are closely related to socioeconomic status. After a primary infection the virus is very likely a permanent resident of the nasopharynx in most individuals. Because of the ubiquitous presence of EBV in adults and because of the long duration between childhood infection and the adult development of nasopharyngeal carcinoma, an answer to the question of whether EBV is an etiological cofactor or *passenger* in neoplastic tissues will be extremely difficult to obtain.[17] Where the virus ranks with inhaled carcinogens, host-cell genetics, cellular enzyme systems, and nutritional status is still unclear.

HISTOPATHOLOGY OF NASOPHARYNGEAL CANCER

In order to put the following discussion in proper perspective, this quotation from Scanlon et al.[18] seems appropriate: "there is probably no other single group of cancers of the respiratory system about which there is less agreement in the world literature with regard to the correct and proper pathological classification," as tumors of the nasopharynx. Because of this lack of uniformity in pathological classification, statistics relating to the frequency of types of neoplasm and survival are often nontransferable from one institution to another. An acceptable classification of malignant nasopharyngeal neoplasm is therefore essential in efforts to determine prognosis and/or effectiveness of treatment. Perez et al.[19] have presented just such a workable classification.

Our primary concern in this chapter, however, is to deal with the most common malignant epithelial neoplasm of the nasopharynx, the squamous cell carcinoma and its confusing and misrepresented variants. Discussions of the other neoplasms (i.e., tumors of the reticuloendothelial system, including plasma cell tumors, melanomas, minor salivary gland and other glandular neoplasms, and supporting tissue neoplasms) are presented elsewhere in this text.

Two basic forms of squamous cell carcinoma present in the nasopharynx: keratinizing and nonkeratinizing. Pathologically, the former present no problem, nor have they spawned any controversy. This is not true for the nonkeratinizing variants. Pathological disagreement in the literature has involved only the group of neoplasms which lack obvious squamous or glandular differentiation by light microscopy and to which a wide variety of names have been applied—lymphoepithelioma, transitional cell carcinoma, transitional cell epidermoid carcinoma, anaplastic carcinoma, embryonal cell carcinoma, basocellularis carcinoma, spinocellularis carcinoma, squamous cell carcinoma and epidermoid carcinoma. These are all synonyms for the nonkeratinizing (nonglandular) carcinomas.

Nonkeratinizing neoplasms by ordinary light microscopy are recognized by their large polyhedral cells usually forming a characteristic plexiform pattern, often stratified, and sometimes manifesting intercellular bridges. Neither mucin or keratin is formed by the cells, and glandular differentiation is not present. Many of the neoplasms histologically correspond to what have been called "transitional cell" carcinomas.

An important variant of the nonkeratinizing squamous cell carcinoma is the so-called *"lymphoepithelioma."* In the past, the undifferentiated character of the neoplasm and the intermingling of the neoplastic cells with lymphocytes obscured its true nature. There is no reason to deny that the lymphoepithelioma is a squamous cell carcinoma, albeit nonkeratinizing and apparently undifferentiated. By electron microscopy, keratin formation and desmosomes are present. The homogenous character of the keratinizing and nonkeratinizing tumors has been illustrated by the electron microscopic findings of Svoboda et al.,[29] who demonstrated squamous cell characteristics in undifferentiated neoplasms presenting no evidence of squamous differentiation by light microscopy. The light and electron microscopic studies of Michaels and Hyams[21] clearly indicate that tumor cells take origin from squamous epithelium, but are of an extreme degree of dedifferentiation.

While I can see no justification in retaining the descriptive term "transitional" to describe neoplasms of the upper respiratory tract, the same is not true for the term "lymphoepithelioma." If it is recognized that a lymphoepithelioma is an undifferentiated squamous cell carcinoma with a distinctive microscopic appearance and a favorable response to radiation therapy, it is worthwhile to retain the term as a diagnostic appellation. Histogenetically it has been shown that both the classical squamous and the undifferentiated carcinomas can arise from *any* of the epithelia normally present in the nasopharyngeal cavity, i.e., respiratory, squamous or intermediate types.[22]

Lymphoepithelioma. It has already been considered that the diagnostic term lymphoepthelioma be retained. Its use, however, is conditioned by recognizing that the lesion it denotes is an undifferentiated squamous cell carcinoma with an accompanying lymphocytic component. It is no more than a nonkeratinizing squamous cell carcinoma infiltrating the lymphoid stroma of the nasopharynx or a neoplasm with a reactive accumulation of lymphocytes among the tumor cells.

The term *lymphoepithelioma* was first used as a diagnosis by Regaud[23] and Schmincke[24] independently in 1921 to designate certain highly radiosensitive neoplasms of the nasopharynx and tonsils. Schmincke's[24] original description has not been improved upon during the ensuing half-century; if anything, other attempts have only confused the clinicopathological issues concerning these neoplasms. Schmincke[24] described the lesion as "a cellular, diffusely infiltrating, growth whose uniqueness rests in the syncytial structure which is permeated by lymphocytes. The cells are large, with rounded or oval and vesicular nuclei showing nuclear atypism, numerous mitoses, and varying amounts of chromatin with one or two prominent nucleoli. They occur in anastomosing cords of trabeculae and in nests, or islands. Occasionally they break away in areas and resemble sarcoma."

Subdivision of lymphoepitheliomas has been made into a *Regaud type* of tumor and a *Schmincke type* of tumor. In a Regard tumor one can see nests of nonkeratinizing squamous cells embedded in a lymphoid stroma; in a Schmincke tumor, one sees isolated transitional cells scattered in the lymphoid tissue. Such a distinction is meaningless because it has no bearing on prognosis and merely depends on the size of the epithelial nests.

In addition to his description, Schmincke[24] precisely categorized the neoplasm when he stated that the epithelial nature of the tumor was evident from the cellular and nuclear structure. He emphasized that the neoplasms were carcinomas and that the lymphocytes did not actively participate in the genesis of the lesion. The passive participation of the lymphoid component in lymphoepitheliomas has finally been accepted by the majority of authorities in head and neck oncology, but not without a struggle.

Part of the doubts as to the epithelial *versus* mesenchymal origin of the neoplasm relates to the normal histology of the nasopharynx, and, in particular, to the evolution and involution of the lymphoid tissues of the area and the transformation of the ciliated epithelium to squamous epithelium. The lymphoid tissue of the nasopharynx undergoes physiological involution with advancing age, but it does not completely disappear, even at old age. Furthermore, the amount of lymphoid tissue is quite variable from person to person and reflects each subject's own responses to injury and their host-defense mechanisms.

Quick and Cutler[25] recognized the neoplasms for what they are—undifferentiated epithelial tumors. Ewing,[26] however, impressed by some of the variants, observed "the tumor seems to spring directly from the lymphoid reticulum." It was, no doubt, this appearance that led some authors to believe "lymphoepitheliomas," or, at least, some so-called, were primary lymphoid tumors.[27, 28]

The important points to be garnered from the above discussion are: (1) there is no specific "lymphoepithelium" from which these neoplasms arise; (2) the lymphocytes present are incidental and not neoplastic ingredients; (3) "lymphoepitheliomas" manifest a considerable range of variation in their microscopic appearances.

Teoh,[29] after examining hepatic metastases, confirmed the incidental character of the lymphocytic component by finding only epithelial elements in the metastatic foci. The lymphocytes are not restricted to this neoplasm, and, in the metastases, may or may not be associated with epithelium. Even in metastases, lymphocytes are associated with other forms of epithelial malignancy.

The variable spectrum of histological appearances has been a source of inadvertent confusion. Cappell[30] recognized this spectrum, but became too rigid in his subdivision into two subgroups— *Regaud* and *Schmincke* types (vide supra). The former is recognizable as a carcinoma; the latter is less obviously so and resembles a sarcoma. There are no prognostic differences between the two lesions, and the designation of a variant resembling a sarcoma, particularly reticulum cell sarcoma, by an eponynm does little to aid a surgical pathologist in the often difficult task of distinguishing between a lymphoepithelioma and a lymphoma.

The histological criteria for diagnosis are: (1) syncytial bands or strands of nonkeratinizing squamous cells; (2) penetration of the neoplastic mosaic by lymphocytes; (3) no significant fibrous connective tissue stroma. The epithelial cells are generally pale and most often have indistinct cell borders so as to make the aggregates of cells appear syncytial. Discontinuity of plasma membranes may account for this appearance. Mitoses are usually conspicuous and the round or reniform nuclei often contain one or two large nucleoli. Lymphocytes infiltrate the stroma separating the cells or nests and may lie in intimate association with the epithelial cells (Fig. 8.1).

Between the obviously epithelial "lymphoepitheliomas" and the variant in which the epithelial character of the neoplasm is not so readily apparent lies a group of lesions varying not only in their epithelial/lymphoid proportions, but also in the size, shape and geographic arrangement of the tumor cells. Sometimes there is a mixture of polyhedral, "transitional" and fusiform cells in varying proportions which are arranged in a sarcoma-like pattern. At other times, the haphazard masses of fairly nondescript and large, round cells closely resemble reticulum cells and reticulum cell sarcoma (Fig. 8.2). Even an experienced and skilled pathologist will, on occasion, find it difficult to distinguish between reticulum cell sarcoma (or other lymphomas) and undifferentiated carcinomas.

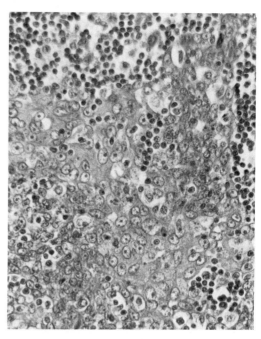

Figure 8.1. Lymphoepithelioma of the nasopharynx. Note the undifferentiated, pale epithelial cells with indistinct cell borders. The syncytial nests of epithelial cells in this example lie in an intimate relationship to lymphocytes.

Neither lymphosarcoma nor reticulum cell sarcoma is particularly common in other than the cervical lymph nodes in the head and neck region. It is rare for reticulum cell sarcoma to present initially in the mucosa or submucosa of the head and neck, but it occasionally occurs in Waldeyer's ring or in the sinuses. Only six cases of reticulum cell sarcoma occurred among 1,000 cases of cancer of the nasopharynx in the series reported by Yeh.[2] Higher, yet still variable, percentages have been cited by other authors. These are reviewed by Larsen et al.[31]

Larsen et al.[31] elaborate further on the diagnostic problems related to punch biopsy specimens. These specimens are often a source of dilemma for the surgical pathologists. This is especially true if the specimen is small or if it comes from nonlymphoid tissue. Often the specimen is distorted and squeezed. The delicate lymphoid and reticulum cells suffer much more than do the hardier connective tissue or squamous cells. As a result of the artefactual distortion, the reticuloendothelial cells resemble the cells of undifferentiated squamous cell carcinomas. In the absence of a recognizable epithelial structure, the diagnosis of lymphoepithelioma may have to rest upon the absence of cytoplasmic pyroninophilia and the presence of

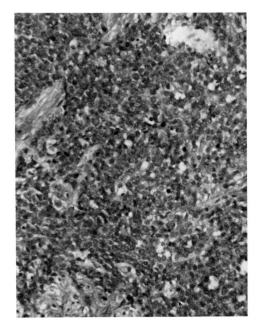

Figure 8.2. Lymphoepithelioma. The haphazard arrangement of the cells in this example renders the neoplasm difficult to distinguish from a reticulum cell sarcoma (histiocytic lymphoma).

desmosome-tonofilament complexes demonstrated by electron microscopy.[32]

In paraphrase of Ewing,[26] Larsen et al.[31] and Al-Saleem et al.,[33] the wisest course for a pathologist to follow is to recognize his diagnostic limitations and to request and utilize clinical data, other laboratory information, and consultation with the surgeon. The surgeon, in turn, should consider performing lymph node biopsy or rebiopsy with a scalpel.

Carcinomas of the nasopharynx make up nearly 98% of all cancers of the region. Nearly four-fifths of the carcinomas are classified as "epidermoid type," of which there are two basic types: keratinizing and nonkeratinizing squamous cell carcinomas. Both types exhibit various degrees of differentiation and can be subdivided into well, moderately well and poorly differentiated carcinomas. Most of the squamous cell carcinomas of the nasopharynx are of the nonkeratinizing variety, and even the keratinizing squamous cell neoplasms have a tendency to be poorly differentiated. These carcinomas can present in spindle-cell forms, clear-cell forms and combined cell populations in the same neoplasm.

Two other major subdivisions of nasopharyngeal carcinomas exist. These are the uncommon adenocarcinomas and a variably-sized group of carcinomas best regarded as "unclassified." The size of this unclassified category of carcinomas does not necessarily depend upon the experience of the surgical pathologist, since, as Yeh[34] has pointed out, a great proportion of this group has arisen from defects in the biopsy-obtained specimen. Crushing artefact and fragility of the neoplastic cells make accurate classifications difficult. Yeh[34] placed 11% of 1,437 cancers of the nasopharynx into this category. Adenocarcinomas, whether mucus-secreting or not, and with or without an adenoid cystic pattern, can arise from the surface ciliated epithelium, the duct epithelium or the minor salivary glands of the region. Yeh's[34] experience with carcinoma in situ of the nasopharynx is exactly like my own, i.e., an apparent *absence* of intraepithelial carcinomas other than in relation to an established invasive carcinoma.

The relative frequency of the histological types of carcinoma, especially of the keratinizing and nonkeratinizing squamous cell carcinomas, cannot be ascertained with any degree of certainty since it is entirely dependent on the individual author's training and subjective opinion. Therefore, Yeh,[34] who dislikes the term lymphoepithelioma and favors "transitional," found only 3.0% of the former and 16% of the latter among 1,437 cases. Perez et al.,[19] considering only the keratinizing and nonkeratinizing squamous cell carcinomas, classified 20 of 66 cases as keratinizing and 12 of the remaining 46 cases as lymphoepithelioma. The remainder of the nonkeratinizing carcinomas in their series would presumably fit into the category of "transitional" carcinoma. Perez et al.[19] placed only one neoplasm of the 79 they examined into the "unclassified" category.

CLINICOPATHOLOGICAL CORRELATION

The incidence of nasopharyngeal cancer is different among the races. In Caucasian populations this cancer usually comprises 0.25 to 0.50% of all malignant tumors.[35, 36] A male predominance is commonly reported in this disease; this is especially evident among the Chinese. Cancer of the nasopharynx tends to appear at an earlier age than most other forms of adult cancer; the mean age is in the late forties. Because of their location, nasopharyngeal neoplasms remain asymptomatic for an undesirable length of time or produce only trivial symptoms that are usually overlooked. The result is a delay in diagnosis and the start of treatment, both of which decrease the opportunities for cure.

Laing[37] has described two early stages in the

course of nasopharyngeal carcinomas. The "silent stage" is the period when only the symptoms of irritation are present. In the majority of patients this takes the form of a postnasal irritation requiring repeated attempts to "clear the throat." The "stage of superficial ulceration" follows by a few weeks or longer. Interference with the ciliary function of the mucosa by the neoplasm results in a stagnation and decomposition of secretions and halitosis. Repeated and forceful attempts at aspiration traumatize the friable surface of the ulcerated neoplasm and produce recurrent bleeding from the nasopharynx. *Considerable* epistaxis and nasal obstruction are not early signs. They usually indicate a massive space-occupying lesion, with pressure necrosis and fungation. Definite presenting signs and symptoms may be due to: (1) obstruction produced by the tumor; (2) local invasion of either the cranial or orbital cavities, i.e., cranial nerve paralyses or proptosis; and (3) swelling in the neck due to metastasis in a lymph node.

Since local extension plays a determining role in the production of signs and symptoms, it will be wise to consider, at this point, the manner of growth of nasopharyngeal carcinomas. Lederman[38] has pointed out that neoplasms of the nasopharynx extend not so much by *expansive* spread into contiguous natural cavities, as by *infiltration* into neighboring regions such as the cranial cavity, orbit and parapharyngeal space. It is this type of local aggressiveness that leads to a variety of cliniconeurological, ophthalomological and otolaryngological syndromes.

Lederman[38] further reports significant differences in the frequency with which the various areas of the nasopharynx are primarily involved by neoplasm. His estimations, by his own admission, are only approximate, since a precise origin is difficult and often impossible. The lateral wall, including the fossa of Rosenmüller is the most common site; the floor is only occasionally involved. Primary neoplasms of the nasopharyngeal roof are second in number only to those of the lateral walls. Posterior wall lesions are approximately one half the number from the roof and lateral walls.

Carcinomas taking their origins from the lateral walls and the fossa of Rosenmüller may spread in several directions[38]: (1) *medially*, to the lumen of the nasopharynx and forward across the ostia of the tubes toward the nasal fossa. Intraluminal (Eustachian tube) spread into the middle ear is unusual; (2) *inferiorly*, to the oropharynx and soft palate; (3) *anteriorly*, after breaching the fascial space around the levator palati muscle. Once

through this not very substantial barrier, neoplastic extension may occur throughout the length of the fascial space from the apex of the petrous temporal bone to the soft palate.

The parapharyngeal space is very vulnerable to neoplastic extension. It may be conveniently divided into three compartments by the styloid process and its muscles and the fascial extensions from the carotid sheath, which bridge the area between the posterolateral wall of the pharynx and the prevertebral fascia.[38] Convergence of the fascial spaces take place just below the apex of the fossa of Rosenmüller, and here neoplastic penetration into all compartments of the parapharyngeal space can readily occur.

The three compartments of the parapharyngeal space are: 1. *Prestyloid compartment.* Here lies the internal maxillary artery and the inferior dental, lingual and auriculotemporal nerves. The upper part of this space is in relation to the lateral nasopharyngeal wall and the fossa of Rosenmüller. At a lower level it relates to the tonsillar bed. Access into the prestyloid compartment by a neoplasm may permit spread to (a) the base of the skull, foramen ovale, foramen spinosum and the greater wing of the sphenoid; (b) submaxillary gland; and (c) the parotid gland.

2. *Retrostyloid compartment.* The carotid vessels and the carotid sheath, the last four cranial nerves, the cervical sympathetic nerves and lymph nodes occupy this compartment of the parapharyngeal space.

3. *Retropharyngeal compartment.* Median in position, this compartment separates the nasopharynx from the prevertebral muscles and contains the lateral retropharyngeal node of Rouviere along with other lymph nodes. Metastatic involvement of these nodes, in particular the retropharyngeal node of Rouviere, may lead to secondary invasion and compression of the carotid sheath and contents. Destruction of the lateral portion of the atlas may also occur.

The roof of the fossa of Rosenmüller is related to both the foramen lacerum medium and to the floor of the canal formed for the internal carotid artery as it lies in the petrous temporal bone. A neoplasm of the fossa of Rosenmüller finds its most ready entry into the cranial cavity by extension along the canal for the internal artery. While it is maintained that tumors growing from the roof and from the fossa of Rosenmüller are more inclined to grow into the cranial base, the neoplasms of the posterior and lateral walls are just as inclined for such an intracranial extension.

The rich lymphatic network servicing the nasopharynx makes cervical node involvement from neoplasms in the area frequent (Fig. 8.3). These may be bilateral, not only from lesions in the midline, but also because of a lymphatic crossover. In the 150 cases described by Lederman,[38] the frequency of metastases to the cervical lymph nodes was as follows: jugulo-digastric node, 70%; the upper deep cervical nodes, 66%; the jugulo-omohyoid node, 34%; the spinal accessory node, 28%; the inferior cervical node, 20%.

Lymph drainage from the roof and the posterior wall of the nasopharynx takes place mainly to the lymph nodes lying behind the pharynx in the vicinity of the jugular foramen. Metastases to these nodes can compress the ninth up to and including the twelfth cranial nerves *and* the upper portion of the sympathetic trunk. As a result of this involvement, the so-called foramen jugulare syndrome may appear. The syndrome consists of paralysis of the trapezius and sternocleidomastoid muscle, the palate, pharynx and recurrent nerve.

Lymphatics in the lateral wall drain partly into the retropharyngeal nodes and less often into the submandibular glands behind and below the angle of the mandible and into the deeper lymph nodes in the neck along the internal jugular vein. Despite the richness of lymphatics and the relatively high total incidence of metastases, lymph node groups regularly involved are few in number. This has been attributed to the limited territory of the primary in the nasopharynx.

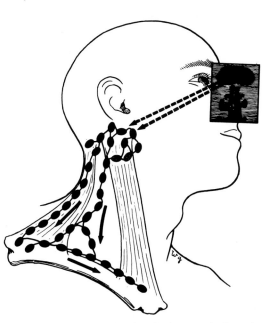

Figure 8.3. Pathways for lymphatic spread of carcinoma of the nasopharynx.

Since the majority of the carcinomas arise in the lateral or posterosuperior walls, it is not common to see metastases in the lymph nodes in the anterior triangle of the neck, except for the jugulodigastric lymph node. Spread of the carcinomas locally into the oropharynx, parapharyngeal space or the floor or the nasopharynx increases the involvement of nodes to include even the submandibular lymph nodes.[38] Retropharyngeal lymph node involvement may be "deduced or assumed" when neoplastic involvement of the last four cranial nerves is clinically present.

From the foregoing, it may be seen that a neoplasm taking origin in the fossa of Rosenmüller and the lateral wall of the nasopharynx may produce significant and characteristic symptoms referrable to the middle ear cleft in addition to symptoms originating from the nasopharynx. These "tubal occlusive" symptoms combined with the nasopharyngeal symptoms constitute a significant, yet moderately early, clinical picture of nasopharyngeal carcinomas. They are the most common manifestations of malignant neoplasm in the nasopharynx. In Laing's[37] experience this syndrome was demonstrated in the great majority of his patients *before* the appearance of regional metastases or neuro-opothalmic signs. Lederman[38] records that 55% of his patients presented with an obstruction of the Eustachian tubes or the nasal passages.

Local invasion by the neoplasms invariably brings about involvement of the cranial nerves, most commonly the motor nerves of the eye, the trigeminal and the last four bulbar cranial nerves. Because the foramen lacerum, the apex of the petrous temporal bone and the adjacent cavernous sinus, where the nerve trunks of the third to sixth cranial nerves and the internal carotid artery are situated, lie above the fossa of Rosenmüller, these structures are frequently involved by an upward infiltration of the neoplasm arising from this most frequent site of origin. The fifth cranial nerve is the earliest and most commonly involved; the second and third divisions are first, causing numbness and tactile anesthesia and, later, neurological pain along their distribution. The next most commonly involved nerve is the abducens, with a resultant paralysis of the lateral rectus muscle and diplopia.

A mass in the neck due to a metastasis in the cervical lymph nodes is the initial symptom or sign of a squamous cell carcinoma (with or without an associated lymphoid stroma) in the nasopharynx in approximately 50% of all cases.[39, 40] A study from Glasgow illustrates this point.[41] Half of the

24 patients in the series presented with a metastasis in the neck, and 21 of the patients manifested metastases by the time a definite diagnosis was made. The average time between onset and a definite diagnosis of carcinoma of the nasopharynx was nearly 10 months. In well over half of the cases, the nasopharynx was not at first suspected as the primary site.

Loke's[42] experience at Kuala Lumpur is also instructive. Of 134 cases of primary lymphoepithelioma of the nasopharynx, 110 presented first with enlarged cervical lymph nodes without *any* symptoms referable to the nasopharynx. Only after repeated examination was a tumor found in that location. Loke[42] also found that 268 of 430 cases of cervical lymph node showing a "lymphoepithelioma" pattern did not have a detectable primary growth at the time the patient presented for examination. One hundred thirty-nine patients were eventually found to have a nasopharyngeal primary lesion, 23 an oropharyngeal primary lesion. The remainder were *assumed* to have their primary lesions in the nasopharynx.

Most authorities agree that metastases to cervical lymph nodes occur early while the primary lesion is still quite small. Teoh[29] found that, even at necropsy, the lesion in the nasopharynx might be very inconspicuous; in one of his cases, the tumor presented merely as a slightly raised and ill-defined granular patch on the nasopharyngeal mucosa.

In the face of a metastatic poorly differentiated epithelial neoplasm in a cervical lymph node, random biopsies or, better yet, a curettage of the nasopharynx are recommended, particularly on the side of the nodal metastasis. This measure should always be included in a search for a primary lesion in patients with metastatic squamous cell carcinoma and a so-called "unknown primary lesion." Given a neoplasm with the histological features of a lymphoepithelioma in the neck nodes, persistence in seeking a primary lesion in the nasopharynx and oropharynx is often rewarded. Struben[43] reports on the success of a "blind biopsy" of the nasopharynx yielding positive results in four of the five patients with cervical metastases and no visible primary tumor. Despite evident nasopharyngeal changes, the biopsy specimen may be negative. Therefore, it is important to make repeated biopsies. The extent of the cervical metastases bears no relationship to the size of the primary nasopharyngeal growth.

Much useful information can be gained by radiographic study of the base of the skull for neoplastic disease in the nasopharynx. Laing has outlined the value of different radiological studies.[37] Approximately one-third of patients with cancer of the nasopharynx will manifest some form of destruction of the base of the skull at the time of admission.[27] Involvement of the basisphenoid, petrous apex and the paranasal sinuses occurs in a little over one-fifth of these subjects.[27]

TREATMENT AND PROGNOSIS

Any attempt at a *surgical* control of cancer of the nasopharynx usually proves impossible. Complete surgical extirpation is hampered by the relative inaccessibility of the anatomical region, and its architecture does not lend itself to regional block resection of the malignancy.[44] Definite indications for surgical intervention do, however, exist. These are, however, restricted to the small percentage of cases presenting *limited* recurrent nasopharyngeal cancer following a full course of irradiation.[44] Radical neck dissection for the management of cervical lymph node metastases may also be used. Since the first relay of lymphatic spread is usually an inaccessible lymph node close to the skull's base, a too great expectation for neck dissection is not warranted.

At the present time the treatment of carcinomas of the nasopharynx is built around radiotherapy. In this respect, whatever the prognosis afforded a patient, it is largely due to radiotherapy. High-dose megavoltage irradiation and careful technique are necessary. If the lesions are small and no nodes are present, approximately half of these patients can be cured.[40]

Failures of therapy highlight the fact that the majority of patients with nasopharyngeal cancer present with far advanced disease when they are first seen. This establishes a difficult situation for local cancer control and enhances the opportunity for metastatic spread. Metastases occur in nearly 70% of cases, with the superior deep jugular and superior spinal accessory lymph nodes affected most frequently.[44] The stage of the disease (Table 8.2),[45] presence of metastases and the histological type of carcinoma obviously play significant roles in the ultimate salvage rate. It must be noted, however, that the fact that a patient with an advanced lesion (T3) may survive for a long period of time means that a relentless therapeutic approach can be rewarding.

The influence of stage of disease is seen by the observations that the prognosis is, of course, best in patients where the tumor is restricted to the nasopharynx when treatment is begun (Table 8.3).[46] More than half of the patients in this cate-

Table 8.2
Clinical Staging of Carcinoma of the Nasopharynx*

Tumor site

Tis Carcinoma in situ.

T1 Tumor confined to one site of nasopharynx, or no visible tumor (biopsy positive).

T2 Tumor involving two sites (both posterosuperior and lateral walls).

T3 Extension of tumor into oropharynx or nasal cavity.

T4 Invasion of skull or cranial nerves or both.

Lymph nodes

N0 No clinically positive node.

N1 Single clinically positive and homolateral lymph node; less than 3 cm.

N2 As above; 3 to 6 cm; or multiple clinically positive nodes; none more than 6 cm in diameter.

    2A. Single, 3 to 6 cm.

    2B. Multiple, all less than 6 cm.

N3 Massive homolateral node(s), bilateral nodes, or contralateral node(s)

    3A. Clinically positive homolateral node(s), one more than 6 cm.

    3B. Bilateral clinically positive nodes (stage both sides of neck separately).

    3C. Contralateral clinically positive node(s) only.

* Adapted from Beahrs.[45]

Table 8.3
5-Year Survival: Radiation Therapy of Carcinoma of Nasopharynx*

	Site (T)		Lymph Note Metastasis (N)		
	Over-all (%)	Without Disease (%)		Over-all (%)	Without Disease (%)
T1	54	44	N0	54	42
T2	27	24	N1	38	31
T3	26	17	N2	15	12
	—	—	N3	0	0
Total	39	31	Total	39	35

* Data from Wang and Meyer.[46]

gory survive 5 or more years. Cure rates are also found to be greater when the primary cancer originates on the posterior wall and in younger or middle age groups and in females. Metastasis to cervical lymph nodes lowers the survival figures to around one-quarter of the patients, and disease with cranial nerve palsies produced by infiltration by the neoplasm carries the worst prognosis.

Little et al.[47] report that 54% of patients reached a 5-year survival time when the neoplasm was located in the epipharynx; 40% when metastases were present in the cervical lymph nodes; and only 16% in cases when neurological symptoms were present. There were no survivors when distant metastases were found at the beginning of treatment. The significance of cell type in the neoplasms is clearly evident from Bloom's[37] study. He cites a 0% 5-year survival for mature (differentiated) squamous cell carcinomas. This dismal salvage is to be compared to a 16% survival rate for the more radiosensitive "immature" squamous cell carcinomas (partially differentiated) and a 32% 5-year survival rate for what he termed "embryonal cell" carcinomas (lymphoepitheliomas and "transitional cell" carcinomas). Similar impressions are gained from other studies.

The inclusion of *all* types of carcinomas of the nasopharynx to produce an *over-all* survival rate lowers the rate below that for the lymphoepithelioma and undifferentiated carcinoma groups alone. Of 467 patients treated in Hong King, Ho[48] reported a 25% 5-year survival. This compares well with the series of Godtfredsen[35] (266 cases) and Schnohr[36] (516 cases), who each reported a 22% 5-year survival. A survey of major reports from the world literature yields an overall 5-year survival of nearly 16%. Figure 8.4, modified from Shedd et al.,[49] compares the survival rates of patients with nasopharyngeal carcinoma and the survival rates of patients with hypo- and oropharyngeal carcinomas. Some improvement of survival statistics with radiation therapy have been recently recorded.[50, 51] Complications of such therapy, in-

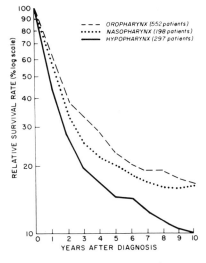

Figure 8.4. Relative survival rate of cancer of the nasopharynx compared with cancer of the hypopharynx and parts of the oropharynx (data modified from Shedd et al.[49]).

Table 8.4
Sites of Distant Metastases: Nasopharyngeal Carcinoma in 99 Patients*

Metastatic Site	No. of Patients	Frequency (%)
Bone	48	48.5
Lungs	30	30.3
Liver	29	29.3
Subclavicular lymph nodes	6	6.6
Soft tissues	5	5.5
Skin	3	3.3
Central nervous system	3	3.3

* From data presented by Khor et al.[53]

cluding immunosuppression are relatively frequent.[52]

Distant metastases occur in at least 20% of patients with carcinoma of the nasopharynx. There does not appear to be any difference in "risk" by age or sex. The predilection of nasopharyngeal carcinoma to develop *skeletal* metastases has been amply confirmed.[53] Pulmonary and hepatic involvement follow in frequency. Table 8.4 after data presented by Khor et al.[53] relates the distribution of metastases in 99 patients manifesting 124 metastatic sites. Both extent of primary tumor (T) and cervical lymph node status (N) exert a significant influence on the probability of metastases developing. In the large series of Khor et al.,[53] nearly two-thirds of the patients with distant spread had control of local disease. The discovery of metastases is nearly a death warrant with Khor et al.[53] reporting a median survival under 4 months and fatality rate of 91% within a year of first metastasis.

REFERENCES

1. Watson, C. R. R.: The anatomy of the post nasal space: its significance in local malignant disease. Aust. Radiol. 16: 118, 1972.
2. Yeh, S.: A histological classification of carcinomas of the nasopharynx with a critical review as to the existence of lymphoepitheliomas. Cancer 15:895, 1962.
3. Ali, M. Y.: Distribution and character of the squamous epithelium in the human nasopharynx. U.I.C.C. (Union Int. Cancer) Monogr. Ser. 1:138, 1967.
4. Martin, H., and Irean, S.: The racial incidence (Chinese) of nasopharyngeal cancer. Ann Otol. Rhinol. Laryngol. 60: 168, 1951.
5. Digby, K. H., Fook, W. L., and Che, Y. T.: Nasopharyngeal malignancy. Br. J. Surg. 28:517, 1941.
6. Bailar, J. C., III: Nasopharyngeal cancer in white populations—a world-wide survey. U.I.C.C. (Union Int. Cancer) Monogr. Ser. 1:18, 1967.
7. Martin, H., and Chakravorty, R. C.: Cancer of the nasopharynx. In Diseases of the Nose, Throat, and Ear, edited by C. Jackson and C. L. Jackson, p. 279. W. B. Saunders Co., Philadelphia, 1959.

8. Ormerod, F. C.: Malignant disease of the nasopharynx. J. Laryngol. 65:778, 1951.
9. Prasad, V.: Cancer of the nasopharynx: a clinical analysis with anatomicopathological orientation. J. Roy. Coll. Surg. Edinb. 17:108, 1972.
10. Buell, P.: Nasopharynx cancer in Chinese in California. Br. J. Cancer 19:459, 1965.
11. Klein, G.: The Epstein-Barr virus and neoplasia. New. Engl. J. Med. 293:1353, 1975.
12. Nadol, J. B., Jr.: Viral particles in nasopharyngeal carcinoma. Laryngoscope 87:1932, 1977.
13. Henle, W., and Henle, G.: Evidence for an etiologic relation of the Epstein-Barr virus to human malignancies. Laryngoscope 87:467, 1977.
14. Zeigler, J. L., Magrath, I. T., Gerber, P., and Levine, P. H.: Epstein-Barr virus and human malignancy. Ann. Int. Med. 86:323, 1977.
15. Uhlmann, C. H., Krueger, G. R. F., Sesterhenn, K., Rose, K.-G., Ablashi, D. V., and Wustrow, F.: Nasopharyngeal and adjacent neoplasms: a clinicopathologic and immunologic study. Arch. Otorhinolaryngol. 218:163, 1978.
16. Leading Article: Aetiology of nasopharyngeal carcinoma. Lancet 2:1393, 1976.
17. Henderson, B. E., Louie, E. W., Jing, J. S., and Alena, B.: Epstein-Barr virus and nasopharyngeal carcinoma: Is there an etiologic relationship? J. Natl. Cancer Inst. 59: 1393, 1977.
18. Scanlon, P. W., Rhodes, R. E., Jr., Woolner, L. N., Devine, K. D., and McBean, J. B.: Cancer of the nasopharynx, 142 patients treated in the 11 year period 1950–1960. Am. J. Roentgenol. Radium Ther. Nucl. Med. 99:313, 1967.
19. Perez, C. A., Ackerman, L. V., Mill, W. B., Ogura, J. H., and Powers, W. E.: Cancer of the nasopharynx: factors influencing prognosis. Cancer 24:1, 1969.
20. Svoboda, D. J., Kirchner, F. R., and Shanmugaratnam, K.: The fine structure of nasopharyngeal carcinomas. U.I.C.C. (Union Int. Cancer) Monogr. Ser. 1:163, 1967.
21. Michaels, L., and Hyams, V. J.: Undifferentiated carcinoma of the nasopharynx: a light and electron microscopical study. Clin. Otolaryngol. 2:105, 1977.
22. Shanmugaratnam, K., and Muir, C. S.: Nasopharyngeal carcinoma: origin and structure. U.I.C.C. (Union Int. Cancer) Monogr. Ser. 1:153, 1967.
23. Regaud, C., and Reverchon, L.: Sur un cas d'epithelioma epidermoide developpe dans le massif maxillaire superieur, et endu aux teguments de la face, aux cavities buccale, nasale et orbitaire, ainsi qa'aux ganglions du cou, gueri par la curietherapie. Rev. Laryngol. Otol. Rhinol. (Bord.) 42:369, 1921.
24. Schmincke, A.: Uber lympho-epitheliale geschwulste. Beitr. Pathol. Anat. Allg. Pathol. 68:161, 1921.
25. Quick, D., and Cutler, M.: Transitional cell epidermoid carcinoma; radiosensitive type of intra-oral tumor. Surg. Gynecol. Obstet. 45:320, 1927.
26. Ewing, J.: Lymphoepithelioma. Am. J. Pathol. 5:99, 1929.
27. Bloom, S. M.: Cancer of the nasopharynx: a study of ninety cases. J. Mt. Sinai Hosp. 36:277, 1969.
28. Loke, Y. M.: Lymphoepitheliomas of the cervical lymph nodes. Br. J. Cancer 19:482, 1965.
29. Teoh, T. B.: Epidermoid carcinoma of nasopharynx among Chinese; study of 31 necropsies. J. Pathol. Bacteriol. 78: 451, 1957.
30. Cappell, D. F.: Pathology of nasopharyngeal tumours. J. Laryngol. Otol. 53:558, 1938.
31. Larsen, R. R., Hill, G. J., II, and Ratzer, E. R.: Reticulum cell sarcoma in head and neck surgery. Am. J. Surg. 123: 338, 1972.
32. Giffler, R. F., Gillespie, J. J., Ayala, A. G., and Newland, J. R.: Lymphoepithelioma in cervical lymph nodes of children and young adults. Am. J. Surg. Pathol. 1:293, 1977.
33. Al-Saleem, T., Harwick, R., Robbins, R., and Blady, J.: Malignant lymphomas of the pharynx. Cancer 26:1383, 1970.
34. Yeh, S.: Histology of nasopharyngeal cancer. U.I.C.C. (Union Int. Cancer) Monogr. Ser. 147, 1967.

35. Godtfredsen, E.: Ophthalmologic and neurologic symptoms of malignant nasopharyngeal tumours: a clinical study comprising 454 cases, with special references to histopathology and the possibility of early recognition. Acta Psychiatr. Neurol. 34:1, 1944.

36. Schnohr, P.: Survival rates of nasopharyngeal cancer in California: a review of 516 cases from 1942 through 1965. Cancer 25:1099, 1970.

37. Laing, D.: Nasopharyngeal carcinoma. Otolaryngol. Clin. North Am. 2:703, 1969.

38. Lederman, M.: Cancer of the Nasopharynx: Its Natural History and Treatment. Charles C Thomas, Springfield, Ill., 1961.

39. Novick, W. H., Shimo, G., Ryder, D. R., Pirozynski, W. J., Hazel, J. J., and Bouchard, J.: Malignant neoplasms of the nasopharynx. Can. Med. Assoc. J. 93:303, 1965.

40. Wang, C. C., and Meyer, J. E.: Radiotherapeutic management of carcinoma of the nasopharynx: an analysis of 170 patients. Cancer 28:566, 1971.

41. Vilar, P.: Nasopharyngeal carcinoma: a report on 24 patients seen over 6 years. Scot. Med. J. 11:315, 1966.

42. Loke, Y. W.: Lymphoepitheliomas of the cervical lymph nodes. Br. J. Cancer 19:482, 1965.

43. Struben, W. H.: Lympho-epithelioma. Pract. Otorhinolaryngol. (Basel) 30:207, 1968.

44. Conley, J.: Concepts in Head and Neck Surgery, pp. 107–108. Georgthieme Verlag, Stuttgart, 1970.

45. Beahrs, O. H.: Clinical staging of cancer of the head and neck. Surg. Clin. N. Am. 57:831, 1977.

46. Wang, C. C., and Meyer, J. E.: Radiotherapeutic management of carcinoma of the nasopharynx. Cancer 28:566, 1971.

47. Little, J. B., Schultz, M. D., and Wang, C. C.: Radiation therapy for cancer of the nasopharynx. Arch. Otolaryngol. 77:621, 1963.

48. Ho, J. C.: Natural history and treatment of nasopharyngeal cancer. Presented at the International Cancer Congress, Houston, Texas, 1970.

49. Shedd, D. P., von Essen, C. F., Connelly, R. R., and Eisenberg, H.: Cancer of the pharynx in Connecticut, 1935–1959. Cancer 21:706, 1968.

50. Hoppe, R. T., Goffinet, D. R., and Bagshaw, M. A.: Carcinoma of the nasopharynx. Eighteen year's experience with megavoltage radiation therapy. Cancer 37:2605, 1976.

51. Urdaneta, A., Fischer, J. J., Vera, R., and Gutierrez, E.: Cancer of the nasopharynx. Review of 43 cases treated with supervoltage radiation therapy. Cancer 37:1707, 1976.

52. Wara, W. M., Phillips, T. C., Wara, D. W., Amman, A. J., and Smith, V.: Immunosuppression following radiation therapy for carcinoma of the nasopharynx. Radiology 123:482, 1975.

53. Khor, T. H., Tan, B. C., Chua, E. J., and Chia, K. B.: Distant metastases in nasopharyngeal carcinoma. Clin. Radiol. 29:27, 1978.

CHAPTER 9

Neoplasms of the Larynx

Studies of neoplastic disease of the larynx deal largely, if not exclusively, with carcinomas, particularly squamous cell carcinomas. The major part of this chapter conforms to this precedent, but additionally concerns itself with the primary supporting tissue neoplasms of the larynx that have not been presented elsewhere in this text.

According to World Health Organization statistics covering 35 countries, in the year 1961, an average of 1.2 persons out of every 100,000 inhabitants of these countries died of laryngeal cancer.[1] Kerr et al.[2] state that there is one new case of laryngeal carcinoma per 100,000 population per year. Table 9.1 presents the estimated cancer incidence (1972) for carcinoma of the larynx and relates it to similar statistics for cancer in the oral and upper respiratory regions.[3]

Epidemiological studies have incriminated a variety of underlying "causes" for carcinomas of the larynx. Two widely divergent factors are *smoking* and *irradiation* injury. Statistical studies have clearly demonstrated that cancer of the larynx only rarely develops among men who do not smoke.[4] Data also point to the fact that the risk of laryngeal cancer goes up as the amount of tobacco smoked increases. Cigar and pipe smoking are more closely associated with cancer of the larynx than with cancer of the lung.[5] Clinical "leukoplakia" and polypoid degeneration of the vocal cords are often associated with excessive smoking and often this "leukoplakia" may be noted to disappear after the cessation of the smoking.

A comparison of the microscopic sections from the larynges of nonsmokers with sections from the larynges of known excessive smokers reveals a thicker surface epithelium in smokers.[6] This thickness is due to: (1) excessive keratinization of the true cords; (2) an epithelial hyperplasia of the false and true cords and the subglottic area; (3) squamous metaplasia, edema and chronic submucosal inflammation in smokers' larynges.

Auerbach et al.[7] found significant laryngeal epithelial changes in smokers as compared with nonsmokers. Their findings were strikingly similar to previous findings in studies of the bronchial and esophageal epithelium. The most significant alterations were the occurrence of cells with atypical nuclei which are infrequent in nonsmokers, always found in cigarette smokers and increased in numbers with the amount of cigarette smoking. Other epithelial alterations included carcinoma in situ and invasive carcinomas. The deviations from normal were observed in the true vocal cord and, to a lesser degree, in the false vocal cord and the area of the larynx above the vocal cord.

The carcinogenic effect of irradiation on the larynx has been slowly established over a period of years.[8] In 1957, Goolden[9] reported on 25 cases of "radiation cancer" of the pharynx and larynx, with five of the cases occurring in the larynx and 20 in the hypopharynx. Many of his patients had received radiotherapy for thyrotoxicosis. The average time interval for the development of the upper airway carcinoma in his series was 25 to 30 years. Ten years was the shortest time span. In a study of 284 patients suffering from carcinomas of the larynx-hypopharynx, Van Dishoeck[10] found that no less than 8% had been treated by irradiation 10 to 20 years before the "benign lymphomata" of the neck. Other clinical investigations concerning irradiation and the larynx have been conducted by Majoros et al.,[11] and Rabbett[12] and Wlodyka.[13] Considering it unusual and unlikely to find *persistent* laryngeal carcinoma after 5 years of apparent freedom of the disease *after* irradiation therapy, Baker and Weissman[8] raise the specter that irradiation was the important carcinogenic factor.

The key to successful management of laryngeal carcinomas is early diagnosis and appropriate, curative treatment applied when the lesion is localized. The natural history of untreated carcinoma of the larynx indicates a median time to death from apparent onset of 12 months. Over 90% of untreated patients are dead within 36 months.[14]

As Daly[15] has pointed out, a number of variables and changing trends in the clinical approach to carcinoma of the larynx are constantly affecting our understanding of the disease. The surgical pathologist must be cognizant of these evolving concepts, or he will be relegated to a secondary role in the team management of patients. As a result, the pathologist *must* keep abreast of: (1) the evolving classifications of carcinoma of the larynx; and (2) the current trends in surgical, radiation and chemotherapeutic treatment for laryngeal cancer.

CLASSIFICATION OF LARYNGEAL CANCER

The anatomical limits of the larynx may be defined and divided into the following regions and/or sites:

1. *Anterior limit*: the posterior surface of the epiglottis, the anterior commissure, and the anterior wall of the subglottic region. It includes the anterior arch of the cricoid cartilage, the thyroid cartilage and the cricothyroid membrane.

2. *Superior lateral limit*: formed by the tip and the lateral margins of the epiglottis.

3. *Posterolateral limits*: include the aryepiglottic folds, arytenoid region, interarytenoid space or the posterior surface of the subglottic space (mucous membrane over the cricoid cartilage).

4. *Inferior limits*: defined by a plane passing through the inferior edge of the cricoid cartilage.

For consideration of appropriate treatment and prognosis, the endolarynx is further subdivided into the following anatomical areas:

1. The vestibular or *supraglottic compartment*. In this compartment are the lesions arising from the laryngeal surfaces of the arytenoid, laryngeal surface of the epiglottis (including the tip of the epiglottis), aryepiglottic fold, the ventricular bands (false cords) and the ventricle.

2. The *glottic compartment*. Neoplasms of the true vocal cords and the anterior commissure are considered as glottic in location.

3. The *subglottic compartment*. This region bears all of the lesions below the vocal cords to the level of the first tracheal cartilage.

The term *transglottic* was introduced by McGavran et al.[16] to describe tumors extending within the tissues above and below the ventricle.

The foregoing definitions of the "larynx" and the endolarynx allow clinical classifications of carcinomas arising from the mucosa of these sites and exclude those neoplasms arising from the lateral or posterior pharyngeal wall, posterior cricoid areas, vallecula or base of the tongue. The site of origin of a tumor in the three above-named anatomical compartments, including the T designations are presented in Table 9.2.

The need to develop and revise classifications for cancer of the larynx has arisen from the requirement for a common and universal means of communication. The TNM classification is a basic foundation and, by virtue of its basic format, is not suitable for every contingency that may be posed by carcinomas. The classification is clinically oriented and is formulated upon information such as location and extent of the primary lesion as determined by mirror and direct examination of the larynx, all diagnostic radiographic studies, examination of the neck, complete physical examination to establish the presence or absence of metastases and the results of the histopathological evaluation of the biopsy specimen.

The clinical judgment involved in determining the site of origin of extensive tumors of the pharynx and the larynx demands many arbitrary decisions. In addition, the presence or absence of cervical lymph node metastasis is notoriously unreliable by clinical palpation. Disagreement also is not uncommon in borderline lesions histologically designated as "dysplasia," carcinoma in situ, and microinvasive carcinoma (see Chapter 4). End result statistics undoubtedly will vary, depending on the subjective interpretation of these terms and on the significance attached to them.

These criticisms may apply to any form of classification, and Daly[15] states several problems connected with *all* forms of clinical classification of cancer. (1) Carcinomas are not respecters of ana-

Table 9.1
Estimated Cancer Incidence: 1972*

Site	Total No.	Males	Females
Lip	1,800	1,600	200
Tongue	2,800	2,000	800
Salivary glands			
Floor of mouth			
Other and not specified—oral	6,000	3,600	2,400
Pharynx	4,500	3,100	1,400
Larynx	6,800	6,000	800
Lung	76,000	62,000	14,000
Other and not specified—respiratory	2,500	1,400	1,100

* Reproduced from Silverberg and Holleb[3] by permission of the American Cancer Society.

Table 9.2
T Classification: Larynx*

Supraglottis

Tis	Carcinoma in situ.
T1	Tumor confined to site of origin; normal mobility
T2	Tumor into adjacent supraglottic site(s) or glottis, without fixation.
T3	Tumor limited to larynx with fixation and/or extension on postcricoid area, medical wall of pyriform sinus, or pre-epiglottic space.
T4	Massive tumor, beyond larynx, involving oropharynx or soft tissues of neck, or destruction of thyroid cartilage.

Glottis

Tis	
T2	Tumor confined to vocal cord(s); normal mobility (includes movement of anterior and posterior commissures).
T3	Tumor confined to larynx with fixation of cord.
T4	Massive tumor, beyond larynx and/or destruction of thyroid cartilage.

Subglottis

Tis	
T1	Confined to subglottic region.
T2	Extension to vocal cords, with normal or impaired cord mobility.
T3	Beyond larynx; cord fixation.
T4	Massive tumor with destruction of cartilage or extension beyond confines of larynx.

* From Beahrs.[17]

tomical boundaries, yet clinicopathological classifications are predicated on definitions of anatomical sites and regions. (2) Refinements of basic classifications are usually additive rather than subtractive, and, hence, there is a tendency to produce *clinically insignificant* subdivisions. (3) Anatomical boundaries are not universally accepted and are "shifted" to suit special purposes. (4) Application of the classification varies from user to user. (5) The principal weakness of all classifications is the lack of (a) measuring the biological malignancy of the tumor and (b) evaluating host-tumor relationships.

PATHOLOGICAL CONSIDERATIONS IN CARCINOMAS OF THE LARYNX

Over 90% of the epithelial malignancies of the larynx are squamous cell carcinomas, and the majority of these are usually at least moderately well differentiated. The varieties of squamous cell carcinomas, as well as other histological types of epithelial malignancy as presented in Table 9.3. This is the classification used by Ferlito[18] in his masterful study of 2,052 laryngeal and hypopharyngeal carcinomas.

The glottis far exceeds all other areas as a site of predilection. Subglottic primary carcinomas are unusual (vide infra). In this respect, the identification of the site of origin of the carcinoma and its spread are more significant than the histological grading of the squamous cell carcinoma.[19, 20]

Superficial and small lesions may be papillary or sessile (localized induration) and even verrucoid. The typical laryngeal carcinoma of moderate size (10 to 15 mm) consists of a central invasive mass with ulceration.[20] The lesion is surrounded by a nimbus of carcinoma in situ and an ill-defined border of atypism, metaplasia or both. The in situ carcinoma margin is usually of limited size, but it may be irregularly prolonged or relatively remote from the primary neoplasm. In carcinomas of the vocal cord, the in situ changes and epithelial dysplasias are commonly found in the proximal one-half of the laryngeal surface of the epiglottis and the adjacent anterior part of the false cords.[20] Toluidine blue has been used as a supravital stain during laryngoscopy as an aid in identifying the most likely site to obtain a positive biopsy. The dye stains areas of atypia, carcinoma in situ, and infiltrating carcinoma in a differential fashion.[21]

In Chapter 4, I discussed the considerable element of subjectivity that enters into the pathological diagnosis of *dysplasia, dyskeratosis* and *intraepithelial carcinoma*. A less subjective and more

Table 9.3
Classification and Frequency of Carcinomas of the Larynx and Pharynx as Studied by Ferlito[18]

	No. of Cases		Percentage of Primary Neoplasms
	Primary	Recurrent	
Carcinoma in situ	54	—	2.8
Squamous cell carcinoma	1605	110	84.0
Verrucous carcinoma	71	3	3.7
Pleomorphic (spindle cell)	12	3	0.6
Nonkeratinizing squamous cell (lymphoepithelioma)	1	—	0.05
Undifferentiated carcinoma	139	5	7.2
Oat cell carcinoma	1	—	0.05
Carcinoid	1	—	0.05
Adenocarcinoma	7	—	0.4
Giant cell carcinoma	1	—	0.05
Adenosquamous carcinoma	8	3	0.4
Mucoepidermoid carcinoma	10	1	0.5
Adenoid cystic carcinoma	1	—	0.05
Acinous cell carcinoma	1	1	0.05

Table 9.4
Squamous Cell Carcinoma of the Larynx*

	Nonkeratinizing	Keratinizing
Most common site	Supraglottic	Glottic and subglottic
Gross appearance	Central ulceration, may be papillary	Ulcerated or fungating with surrounding keratosis
Mucosal spread	Predominant mode	Infrequent
Surface margins of neoplasm	Often poor delimitation	Often sharp delimitation
Invasive pattern	Nearly half have pushing margins	Predominantly infiltrating margins
Carcinoma in situ	Common and extensive	Less common and usually in immediate periphery of tumor

* Modified from Bauer.[25]

exact differentiation must be established for these lesions, with criteria upon which all agree. This is especially important because of the present tendency toward conservation of function procedures that closely approach the clinical margins of tumors.

Squamous cell aberrations occurring in the larynx fall into the following categories: (1) benign hyperplasia; (2) benign keratosis (without atypia of the participating cells); (3) atypical hyperplasia; (4) keratosis with epithelial atypia (atypia or dysplasia of the cells of the deeper layers of the surface epithelium); (5) intraepithelial carcinoma; (6) microinvasive squamous cell carcinoma; (7) invasive squamous cell carcinoma.

The only cases which should be classified as in situ carcinomas are those which, in the absence of invasion, show as surface or glandular linings an epithelium in which, throughout its whole thickness, no differentiation or maturation takes place. The full-thickness involvement is required. but occasional cases may present a greater degree of differentiation. These cases are among the exceptions which no classification can include.

Most cases of carcinoma in situ of the larynx originate on the anterior end of the vocal cords. There is no clinical appearance, which strongly suggests the diagnosis. Miller and Fisher[22] consider the most suggestive lesion to be a thick, shaggy "leukoplakia" superimposed on an irregularly thickened and reddened mucosa; however, many lesions are indurated thickenings and swellings with or without a whitish plaque. The in situ lesion may remain as a discrete lesion; there may be extension across the anterior commissure to the other cord or the intraepithelial changes may be present in the supra or infraglottic regions. Carcinoma in situ is nearly always in continuity with areas of squamous metaplasia. There does appear to be a histogenic interdependence between the in situ cancer and atypical hyperplasia.[23]

Adequate and representative biopsies are essential for the evaluation of an intraepithelial carcinoma. "Nibbler" biopsies are to be condemned. In numerous instances, a biopsy specimen manifesting in situ change represents only the periphery of an invasive carcinoma. Altmann et al.[24] found that, in many cases, the more extensive the intraepithelial change, the more likely that there is an invasive carcinoma in adjacent areas. This is particularly true for supra and infraglottic lesions.

Bauer,[25] after a study of serial longitudinal step blocks of the laryngeal mucosa concluded: (a) biopsy findings of carcinoma in situ usually indicates the presence of an invasive carcinoma elsewhere in the mucosa; (b) carcinoma in situ is more commonly found and more widely spread from the edges of the invasive carcinoma in nonkeratinizing carcinoma of the larynx than in the keratinizing variety in which the extension is never far from the edge of the invasive carcinoma; and (c) carcinoma in situ is a common method of intramucosal spread of nonkeratinizing laryngeal carcinoma. Table 9.4, modified after Bauer[25] presents a synopsis of his findings.

Mention has been made above that tumor size and location play a more important role than histological grading in identifying the laryngeal carcinoma with high probability to have lymph node metastasis. That is not denigrate the value of histological grade and the pattern of infiltrative growth at the tumor's periphery. Rather successful tumor profiling has been obtained by Kashima[26] and Jakobsson.[27] While slightly different criteria for study were used by these workers, the characterization of the carcinoma falls into an evaluation of the tumor cell population and an assessment of the tumor-host relationship. Table 9.5 presents a suggested system of profiling based upon the recommendations of Kashima[26] and Jakobsson.[27] The level of differentiation of the carcinoma and the infiltrative pattern are the most important. Use of

Table 9.5
Histiological Evaluation of Squamous Cell Carcinoma of Larynx

Characteristics of the Tumor Cells

	I	*II*	*III*	*IV*
Structure	Verrucous Papillary	Exophytic-nodulo-infiltrative	Sessile-Ulceroinfil-trative	Marked cell disassocia-tion
Differentiation	Well (keratiniza-tion)	Moderate (some ker-atinization)	Poorly differen-tiated (includes pleomorphic or spindle cell)	
Mitotic index	Low (single)	Moderate	High (numerous)	

Characteristics of the Tumor-Host Relationship

Mode of invasion	Blunt borderline	Blunt borderline	Infiltrative	Diffuse
Stage of invasion	Early borderline	Microinvasion	Into connective tis-sue	Massive
Vascular and peri-neural invasion	Absent	Absent	Few	Many
Cellular response to neoplasm (plasma cell and lymphocytic)	Marked	Moderate	Slight	None

such a scheme in multivariate analysis may assist in prognostication.

In the evaluation of differentiation of the carcinoma, an over-all impression rather than cell count is considered more reliable. The assessment is based on the least differentiated parts of the tumor. Depending on the degree of prickle formation and keratinization together with an over-all resemblance of the carcinoma to normal squamous epithelium, the lesion is classified as (1) well, (2) moderately, or (3) poorly differentiated. Tumors of slow biological growth or growth restrained by anatomical barriers usually maintain or reconstitute the basement membrane at the foot of the differentiating cells and this yields a blunt or rounded lobular pattern of invasion. This usually parallels the level of differentiation. In contrast is the irregular infiltrative pattern. Therefore, biopsy specimens should be evaluated as either blunt or irregular in their invasion.

Complete evaluation of the patient will require histological evaluation of lymph nodes removed at the time of neck dissection. This too involves two factors: an assessment of the neoplastic metastasis and an assessment of the host response in the nodes. Neoplastic necrosis, level and change of differentiation, and extracapsular extension appear to be of some prognostic significance, especially extranodal growth. The host response has been presented elsewhere in this text and is based on the work of Berlinger et al.[28] and Van Nagell et al.[29]

The use of cytological material for the diagnosis of some dysplasias or carcinomas of the larynx continues to be debated.[30, 31] While suitable cytological material can be obtained by *direct* smears of the vocal cords and the larynx, the technique has not become popular with the practicing otolaryngologists, perhaps with justification. Heavily keratotic malignant or dysplastic lesions seldom yield *diagnostic* material, and these cases are a significant source of error.[30] Particular attention to technique is essential, as there is minimal secretion within the larynx and drying artefacts on the cytological preparations are a problem.[30]

Some of the varieties of epithelial laryngeal neoplasms that may present are discussed elsewhere in this text. Two special types merit mention here. These are the verrucous carcinoma and the carcinosarcoma.

Verrucous Carcinoma of the Larynx. Verrucous carcinoma of the larynx is a specific clinicopathological entity that should be recognized as such by both pathologists and laryngologists.[32-34] The lesion has an incidence of approximately 1 to 2% of laryngeal carcinomas.[35, 36]

Verrucous carcinoma of the larynx may present a difficult differential diagnosis because clinically it exhibits characteristics of an invasive carcinoma but, histologically, lacks the conventional features of neoplasia. Its often exhuberant growth may extend over a large area and may be mistaken for an extensive hyperkeratosis. The requirement of repeated biopsies to confirm the diagnosis underlines the necessity of close cooperation between the laryngologist and the surgical pathologist.

There is a heavy male predominance of this neoplasm, and approximately four-fifths of the patients are between the ages of 50 and 75 years of age. Cigarette smoking is a frequent historical finding. The initial symptom in nearly all patients is hoarseness. Duration of symptoms before diagnosis is variable; most patients tolerate the symptoms for over 1 year.

Grossly, verrucous carcinomas of the larynx are most likely to be pale, exophytic, warty tumors with multiple filiform-like projections. The majority are glottic in location with a lesser distribution in the supraglottic and transglottic regions. The warty, gray-white tumor seen grossly is composed of greatly thickened papillomatous folds of well-differentiated keratinizing squamous epithelium. Deceptively, the epithelial maturation sequence appears quite orderly. There is an active basilar layer and a thick parakeratotic superficial layer. Nucleoli are easily found in the large squamous cells, and individual dyskeratotic cells with atypical nuclei may be found. The expected, overt, cytological evidence of squamous cell malignancy is not found.

The neoplasm extends into soft tissues in a pushing or penetrating fashion by compressing the stroma with bulbous rete pegs (Fig. 9.1). A consid-erable inflammatory response in the form of lymphocytes and plasma cells surrounds the margins of the tumor. Often keratin debris provokes an acute inflammatory reaction and leads to the formation of micro- or even macroabscesses.[37] Pressure necrosis of cartilage follows extension of the neoplasm into the thyroid lamina. This invasion and the related chondritis may give rise to a painful soft tissue mass in the anterior neck.[37] There is some histochemical evidence that the grade of malignancy of the carcinoma is dependent upon the stromal reaction against the epithelial proliferation.[38]

With only a few dissenters,[39] it is accepted that verrucous carcinoma is not effectively managed by radiotherapy. In addition, anaplastic or sarcomatoid transformation after irradiation has been noted with sufficient regularity that it would appear to be contraindicated (Table 9.6). The failure of radiotherapy may be related to its lymphocytotoxic effects wherein lymphocytes and selectively T-lymphocytes decrease. As a result, there is an impaired cellular immunity which reflects on the host's response to tumor. Anaplasia following radiation therapy is less easily explained. In the examples recorded in the literature, the time interval between therapy and discovery of the anaplastic lesion has been between 2 to 7 months. Irradiation-produced perichondritis appears to enhance

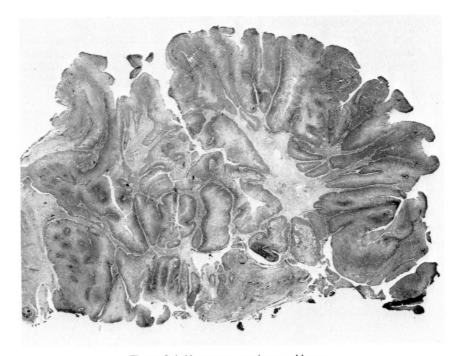

Figure 9.1. Verrucous carcinoma of larynx.

Table 9.6
Anaplastic Transformation of Verrucous Carcinoma

Author	No. of Patients Treated with Irradiation	No. with Anaplastic Transformation	Average time Interval from Treatment
Fonts et al.[40]	10	3	8 months
Kraus and Perez-Mesa[34]	17	4	1.5 months
Perez et al.[41]	8	3	7.5 months
Van Nostrand[42]	3	1	5 months
Biller and Bergman[43]	4	1	5 months
Ryan et al.[44]	3	0	—

Table 9.7
Verrucous Carcinoma of Larynx: Surgical Treatment

Author	No. of Patients	No. of Recurrences
Biller and Bergman[43]	25	2
Ryan et al.[44]	17	1
Kraus and Perez-Mesa[34]	12	0
Burns et al.[39]	8	0

local invasion of verrucous carcinomas of the larynx. The treatment is surgical with treatment directed toward total removal. Left untreated or inadequately excised, the verrucous carcinoma will continue its slow invasion and will ultimately kill the host. The surgical procedure employed is obviously determined by the extent of tumor involvement. Small vocal cord lesions have been cured by cord stripping, but partial laryngeal surgery and total laryngectomy are warranted for total removal. Curability is excellent, providing adequate resection is performed (Table 9.7). To date, laryngeal verrucous carcinomas have not metastasized. Although lymph node metastases from verrucous carcinoma of the larynx are unknown, the cervical nodes are often clinically enlarged, probably as a result of the inflammation associated with the tumor.[37]

Carcinosarcoma of the Larynx. Carcinosarcomas are rare neoplasms which occur in many organs. The diagnosis, properly applied, implies a mixed neoplasm containing both mesenchymal and epithelial elements, each of which displays the various histological and biological criteria of malignancy. As has been indicated elsewhere in this text, the diagnosis of an *apparently* mixed (mesenchymal and epithelial) neoplasm in the larynx is often controversial. The histologically malignant sarcomatous pattern in these tumors has usually been explained as either a unique, nonmalignant, connective tissue reaction to an epithelial cancer or simply as an anaplastic (spindle cell) carcinoma.[45]

My opinion is that most *apparently mixed* neoplasms of the larynx are in reality anaplastic carcinomas or carcinomas with a pseudosarcomatous reaction. Nevertheless, true carcinosarcomas do occur in the larynx. I have seen one example (a mixture of a rhabdomyosarcoma and a squamous cell carcinoma). An even more unique case of carcinosarcoma of the larynx has been reported by Minckler et al.,[46] who describe a lesion which metastasized as a carcinoma *and* a sarcoma and resulted in the death of the patient 15 months after detection.

CLINICOPATHOLOGICAL ASPECTS OF CARCINOMA OF THE LARYNX

The transmission of laryngeal cancer may be by direct mucosal and submucosal extension, by lymphatic or vascular permeation or by perineural spread. In view of the diverse ways the neoplasms may spread, there are distinctive peculiarities of laryngeal cancer behavior that have been utilized by surgeons and therapists to devise effective and yet conservative management.

Widespread mucosal spread, often unaccompanied by much submucosal infiltrative growth, is not an uncommon finding in carcinomas of the larynx. Kleinsasser[47] calls such lesions "carpet carcinomas." Different developmental derivations[48, 49] for portions of the larynx and submucosal compartmentalization[50] (Fig. 9.2) account for some of the observed patterns of the location and spread of cancer within the larynx (the rare tendency of glottic cancers to invade the supraglottic area and the tendency of supraglottic carcinomas to remain supraglottic).

Tucker and Smith[51, 52] have described the submucosal elastic tissue barriers and emphasized the importance of the paraglottic space as a feature of cancer invasion. The importance of the conus elasticus and the thyroid cartilage as barriers has also been well illustrated.[52, 53] Other anatomical predicators of laryngeal spread of cancer are the anterior commisure tendon[54] and the topography of the mucous glands in the anatomical region.[55] The former, a thickened band of fibrous tissue containing lymphatics and blood vessels, is an important link for the dissemination of cancer in the anterior commissure region.

Weak points in the laryngeal framework as barriers to the spread of cancer have been identified.[56-59] Glottic carcinomas with extralaryngeal spread do so at the anterior commissure through cartilage or penetration of the cricoarytenoid membrane. This facility may be related to the close relationship between mucosa and cartilage at the anterior commissure. Involvement of the commissure also allows subglottic spread, followed by penetration of the cricothyroid membrane. It has been well documented that once invasion of the laryngeal framework occurs, it is the ossified portions of cartilage that possess the least resistance. Frequent pre-epiglottic space invasion is a striking feature in carcinomas of the supraglottic group. Nearly *all* of these tumors involve the posterior surface of the epiglottis. The pre-epiglottic space is the laryngeal compartment bounded posteriorly by the epiglottic cartilage, anteriorly by the thyrohyoid membrane and hyoid bone, and superiorly by the hypoepiglottic ligament. The lateral parts are in direct continuity with the paraglottic space. The epiglottic cartilage with its fenestrations (dehiscences) facilitates extension into the pre-epiglottic space. Microfil angiography has further indicated the role the vasculature plays in tumor spread.[60] This form of spread is especially pertinent at the anterior commissure. In that region an extensive tubuloalveolar system of glands open into the subglottic surface of the anterior commissure.[61] These glands are within a condensation of the subepithelial elastic lamina, which here is intimately related to the cricovocal membrane and the cricothyroid ligament. Furthermore, the mucous glands, because of their secretory activity, are closely related to a rather rich vascular and lymphatic network, unlike the squamous epithelium of the vocal cord. Serial sectioning indicates the usual spread of glottic carcinoma reaching the anterior commissure is initially to the subglottis and later to the opposite vocal cord. This mode of invasion is due to a combination of the anterior commissure tendon, the microvasculature and mucous gland distribution. Spread of in situ carcinomas by glandular involvement has been emphasized by Bridger and Nassar.[62]

Lymph Node Metastases from Carcinomas of the Larynx. McGavran et al.[16] have shown that metastases to lymph nodes are more common when the primary neoplasm is greater than 2 cm in diameter, and are more frequent with poorly differentiated tumors than with well differentiated laryngeal carcinomas. These same workers also determined that the presence of cartilage invasion, penetration of the thyrocricoid membrane, pre-epiglottic space invasion, cervical soft tissue extension or vascular invasion is not associated with a significantly higher rate of cervical metastases than when these findings are absent. Staley and Herzon[63] have reaffirmed that nerve sheath invasion increases the probability of metastasis to lymph nodes and that carcinomas manifesting microscopically infiltrating margins produce lymph node metastases much more often than do carcinomas with so-called "pushing" margins.

In a series of 138 elective neck dissections for laryngeal cancer reported by several authors, pathologically positive lymph nodes were found in 16 to 26%. But, as McGavran et al.[16] point out, statements such as these are really of little value. To be of real value, a more specific localization of the site of the carcinoma is necessary. Such a topographical classification was introduced by McGavran et al.[16] They divided laryngeal carcinomas into four anatomical divisions: *glottic*, defined as cancers limited to the true cords; *infraglottic*, cancers involving the subglottis and glottis; *supraglottic*, cancers involving the false cords, fixed and free portions of the laryngeal surface of the epiglottis; and *transglottic*, cancers that cross the ventricle of Morgagni, thus involving two or three of the preceding sites. Their studies, as well as those of others, indicate that the latter three groups show a progressive increase in the incidence of lymph node metastases. In the report by McGavran et al.,[16] the progressive increase was 19, 33, and 52% respectively. Table 9.8 presents similar data.

The incidence of contralateral metastasis may

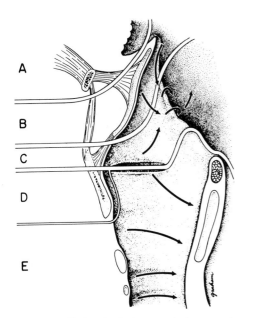

Figure 9.2. Embryological-anatomical compartmentalization of the larynx with lymphatic routes.

Table 9.8
Relation of Site of Laryngeal Carcinoma to Metastatic Frequency to Lymph Nodes

Author	Site	No. of Cases with Metastases	Percentage of Cases with Metastases
McGavran et al.[16]	Glottic	0/5	0
Ogura et al.[64]	Glottic (with fixed cord)	5/37	13
McGavran et al.[16]	Infraglottic	5/27	19
O'Keefe[65]	"Principally sub- glottic"	5/22	23
McGavran et al.[16]	Supraglottic	13/39	33
Ogura et al.[64]	Supraglottic	30/110	27
Bocca et al.[66]	Supraglottic	21/107	20
O'Keefe[65]	Supraglottic	9/28	32
Ogura et al.[64]	Transglottic	17/63	26
McGavran et al.[16]	Transglottic	13/25	52

be of such a magnitude that elective contralateral neck dissection may be indicated. Bocca[66] advocates bilateral neck dissection in *all* supraglottic cancers because of the high incidence of metastases, but he does not report specific data. McGavran et al.[16] reported that, in 15 patients with supraglottic or transglottic cancers having ipsilateral cervical node metastases, contralateral metastases developed in four (26%). Biller et al.[67] report a 2% incidence of contralateral metastases in 38 patients with fixed cord glottic carcinomas and a 5% incidence of contralateral metastases in 67 patients with transglottic carcinomas.

Glottic Carcinomas. Carcinomas arising in the glottic region of the larynx are the most numerous of all laryngeal carcinomas and are predominantly diseases of males. Over two-thirds of the patients are in their fifth to seventh decades. The initial complaint is usually an intermittent hoarseness, which becomes a constant hoarseness as the disease progresses. Continued growth of the neoplasm is accompanied by dyspnea resulting from fixation of the vocal cord and reduction of the glottic space. When the vocal cord is fixed, there is near certainty that invasion of muscle has occurred; therefore, the opportunity for lymphatic spread and metastases to lymph nodes is increased. Usually, however, the progress of a vocal cord carcinoma is slow and rather predictable. Spread from their origin on the free margin of the vocal cord is usually along the cord along the vocal ligament in the space of Reinke. Metastases are a late occurrence, and this is related to the limited lymphatic drainage of the cords. It may be said that metastases are possible only when the neoplasm has spread beyond the limits of the true cords.

We have mentioned above the relationship of fixation of the vocal cord and invasion of muscles. In nearly all such examples, the thyroarytenoid muscle is invaded. This may be alone or in association with the lateral cricoarytenoid muscle and interarytenoid muscle. Once there is invasion of the thyroarytenoid muscle, there is a decided tendency to intramuscular spread. A glottic lesion with a mobile cord is usually found to be superficial to the conus elasticus. A glottic carcinoma which transverses the anterior commissure and shows a normal or limited mobility of the cord is usually confined within the barrier formed by the anterior commissure tendons, the vocal ligament and the conus elasticus. Subglottic extension of more than 1 cm usually portends invasion of the cricothyroid membrane and overlapping soft tissue. Unless there is more than 1 cm subglottic extension, there is usually no invasion of the thyroid ala. Perineural and vascular invasion are found in approximately one-quarter of cases of glottic cancer. In most cases, the vessels inferior to the conus elasticus are involved. The recurrent laryngeal nerve fibers most often involved are medial to the lower border of the thyroid ala.

The majority of glottic squamous cell carcinomas are usually well differentiated. There is a predilection for the anterior half of the cord and the anterior commissure. Only rarely is the posterior commissure primarily involved. From these points of preference of origin, invasive carcinomas often extend in a radial fashion with submucosal extension toward the commissure. Once the commissure is reached, submucosal extension in several directions is facilitated. The larger the vertical direction of growth, the more often the opposite side of the glottis is involved.

MacComb et al.[20] have outlined the neoplastic ramifications from the commissure: (1) across the midline to involve the ventricular band, the vocal cord, or both; (2) into the inferior pre-epiglottic fat; (3) anteriorly, to the prelaryngeal connective tissue and often the thyroid cartilage at the notch; (4) superiorly, beneath the inferior wall of the ventricle toward the aryepiglottic fold. The homolateral false cord may be involved by retrograde extension from the commissure or by a part of a superior extension; (5) lateral extension to the perichondrium of the thyroid cartilage. Extensive neoplasms may penetrate the lateral expanse of the cricothyroid membrane; (6) inferior extension into the subglottis (rarely below the superior border of the arch of the cricoid); (7) posteriorly into the interarytenoid region. Posterior extension is not common in carcinomas arising in the anterior one-half of the vocal cords.

Early glottic carcinomas carry the best prognosis of all laryngeal carcinomas. High cure rates are obtained with either radiation therapy or by surgical resection in carcinoma of the vocal cords. Once the surrounding structures and laryngeal muscles are involved, 5-year survival figures drop from approximately 90 to 50% and about one-fourth of the tumors will metastasize to the cervical lymph nodes. The 5-year survival drops to 20% or less when there are positive lymph nodes at the time of admission.

Since the control of the neoplasm is equally satisfactory with either modality of treatment, the selection of the method of choice, for localized lesions, depends on the functional results desired, including the preservation of the larynx. A primary consideration is the confinement of the carcinoma.[68] Laryngographic studies are important preoperative tests in that they: (1) determine the degree of motility of the cords; (2) aid in the determination of involvement of the anterior commissure; and (3) assist in the evaluation of subglottic or transglottic extension.

There is no standardized treatment for carcinoma in situ of the vocal cord. The two main modalities are radiation and surgery. The latter has consisted of endoscopic stripping, thyrotomy and even biopsy excision. The ultraconservative management of superficially invasive carcinomas of the true cord by endoscopic biopsy requires the utmost cooperation by endoscopist and pathologist.[69]

The management of T1 and T2 glottic carcinomas is basically decided by the need for conservation of voice.[70-75] Vermund[70] has reviewed the results of both surgery and radiotherapy from more than 20 published reports and has summarized the therapeutic results achieved. For tumors involving the midportion of the margin of the cord, not extending to the anterior commissure and not impairing cord mobility, a partial laryngectomy *may* result in a good voice if normal motility of the arytenoid is maintained. However, the preservation of a near normal voice is more frequently achieved with radiation therapy.

Vermund's[70] conclusions, for glottic carcinomas, are as follows: (1) glottic carcinomas classified as T1N0 have a good prognosis and can be treated by laryngofissure and cordectomy or by radiotherapy with comparable cure rates. A high percentage of patients retain a practically normal voice after radiotherapy. (2) Lesions classified as T2N0 can also be cured by adequate radiotherapy with preservation of the voice. (3) The recurrence rate with radiotherapy is much higher with T3N0 lesions and laryngectomy must be done when tumor is suspected after irradiation. (4) The prognosis of T4N0 lesions with radiation treatment alone is poor. (5) Surgery is preferred in those cases with complete cord fixation. (6) Complete cord fixation hampers the radiotherapist more than it does the surgeon (29 versus 55% 5-year controls, respectively). (7) The prognosis of T4N0 lesions with radiation therapy alone is poor. (8) Surgical treatment is preferable in cases where there is complete cord fixation.

There is some debate over the treatment of glottic carcinomas involving and crossing the anterior commissure. Most surgeons observing patients with cancer of the vocal cords involving the anterior commissure believe that partial or total laryngectomy is the preferred method of treatment. In 1970, Kirchner[76] said: "Radiotherapy is not the treatment of choice for glottic cancer which crosses from one vocal cord to the other at the anterior commissure." In 1968, Som and Silver[77] came to the same conclusion. In 1971, Biller et al.[78] said: "Hemilaryngectomy is the modality of choice for true vocal cord cancers which extend beyond the confines of the membraneous vocal cord." Differences from these opinions have been presented by Olofsson et al.,[79] Jesse et al.[80] and Wang and Schulz.[81] It should be made clear that the favorable results obtained by the advocates in each camp are based on selection of patients and technical excellence in the use of the respective modality of treatment.

The Toronto experience with primary radiotherapy for glottic (T2) carcinomas involving or crossing the anterior commissure is as follows: a crude 5-year survival rate of 80% for all glottic tumors involving the anterior commissure, and 70% for true crossing tumors.

According to Biller et al.,[78] glottic T2 lesions with one or all of the following characteristics may be treated by hemilaryngectomy or by anterior commissure technique: (1) a true cord lesion which extends to involve the anterior commissure. Involvement of the anterior 30% of the opposite cord may be present; (2) a true cord lesion which involves the vocal process or the anterior and superior portions of the arytenoid; (3) a true cord lesion which extends to within 10 mm subglottic. Fixation of the cord should not be present. In the St. Louis series, tumor control was obtained in 45 of 58 patients (77%) at 3 years, and 23 of 33 (69%) at 5 years.[78]

According to Bardwil[68] a wide-field laryngectomy is advisable for the majority of patients with advanced cancer of the vocal cord as well as for those who have a recurrence after radiotherapy. If the carcinoma fulfills selective criteria, hemilaryngectomy may be applicable following radiation failure for carcinoma of the vocal cords.[82]

Supraglottic Carcinoma. Supraglottic cancer usually begins at the junction of the epiglottis and the false cords. Neoplasms of the supraglottic larynx do not invade the laryngeal framework unless the lower edge of the tumor extends below the anterior commissure.

Numerous studies have supported the concept of a rather tight barrier at the level of the anterior commissure and ventricle which prevents the downward extension of cancer of the epiglottis and false cords.[83–85] It has been observed that supraglottic carcinomas do not involve the larynx and that they are often bilateral or horseshoe in their distribution across the anterior larynx while remaining entirely above the ventricle. Others have confirmed the confinement of supraglottic cancers above the ventricle and that only ventricular growths spread to both the supraglottic and infraglottic larynx.[86, 87] One suggested reason for this restriction or confinement relates to the embryological development of the larynx. The supraglottic portion of the larynx develops from the buccopharyngeal anlage; the glottic and subglottic portions develop from the tracheobronchial anlage (Fig. 9.2).

Anatomical and experimental studies have added support to an embryological-anatomical demarcation.[88] The studies by Pressman et al.[50] demonstrated that the submucosal lymphatic network in the larynx is compartmentalized in accordance with the embryological development of the structure. Their studies showed that the ventricle is a compartment completely isolated from the false cord. Injections along the epiglottis spread to the false cord and were sharply terminated along its inferior border. The vocal cord with its sparse lymphatic system acts as a "barrier" to vertical lymphatic drainage. In addition, the left side of the larynx is independent from the right. Thus supraglottic lymphatics drain only through the thyrohyoid plexus to the cervical lymph nodes, and the infraglottic lymphatics drain only to the cricothyroid plexus and the cervical nodes.

Kirchner and Som,[83] after study of serial sections of laryngeal specimens, suggest that exophytic lesions of the supraglottic larynx are the kind that tend to remain above the ventricle and the anterior commissure and that they do not invade the thyroid ala. On the other hand, ulcerative lesions may extend downward across the anterior commissure or the anterior part of the ventricle. In this case, there is frequently invasion and destruction of the anterior portion of the laryngeal framework. Regardless of this invasion, microscopic involvement of the thyroid cartilage does not appear to occur unless the inferior edge of the neoplasm is visible below the level of the anterior commissure. When the thyroid cartilage is invaded, invasion is found to have been initiated in the tendon of the anterior commissure. These lesions are then classified as *transglottic* rather than T3 supraglottic.[83]

All of the foregoing studies have been instrumental in the advocacy of conservative laryngectomy for selected supraglottic carcinomas. For most supraglottic lesions of the larynx, sacrifice of the glottis by total laryngectomy does not increase the cure rate, and it additionally imposes an arduous rehabilitation on the patient. Supraglottic laryngectomy has conceptual and practical support for lesions of the false vocal cords, epiglottis and aryepiglottic folds. Pharyngeal lesions can also be resected with preservation of glottic function.[86] These include carcinomas of the pyriform fossa, vallecula and posterior one-third of the tongue.

Obviously, the extent of the laryngeal or hypopharyngeal cancer is of utmost importance when one evaluates patients for supraglottic resection. Kirchner and Som[83] have outlined several key criteria: (1) Supraglottic cancer *does not* invade the thyroid cartilage. (2) Involvement of perichondrium by cancer at the time of operation is an indication that the neoplasm is *transglottic* and, therefore, not suitable for conservative surgery. (3) Carcinomas of the epiglottis or false cord that extend downward below the anterior commissure are no longer supraglottic, but are transglottic and frequently invade the thyroid cartilage. (4) Extension below the anterior commissure requires total laryngectomy. (5) Gross examination of the inferior extent of the lesion after pharyngectomy is sufficient to define the limits of invasion. (6) Conservative surgery is not precluded by neoplastic extension along the medial surface of the aryepiglottic fold as far as the arytenoid.

Ogura[89] has divided the supraglottis further to facilitate indications for conservation surgery. He proposes that epiglottic, false cord and laryngeal ventricle lesions be named supraglottic, that pyriform sinus lesions be part of the hypopharynx, and that aryepiglottic fold lesions be called marginal. In a comparison of the marginal carcinomas with other supraglottic carcinomas, Ogura found that the aryepiglottic fold carcinomas had an overall survival rate of 53%, compared with an 82% survival of the other supraglottic lesions. Marginal lesions amendable by partial laryngopharyngectomy on a selection basis have a better prognosis, 65% no evidence of disease (NED) (with clinical nodes). With larger lesions, (T3 and T4) survival is reduced and dependent on tumor extent and presence of multiple nodes.[89]

Surgical techniques for supraglottic resection may be found in the reports of Ogura and Biller,[87] Kirchner,[53] and Calcaterra.[86] Because of neoplastic extension, excision of the pre-epiglottic space with the hyoid bone appears to be an essential part of the laryngectomy.[90]

Additional viewpoints concerning indications and limitations of conservative laryngectomy can be found in the published Workshop No. 6, of the Centennial Conference on Laryngeal Cancer.[91]

The value of preoperative irradiation for supraglottic carcinomas remains unsettled. Preliminary studies indicate that there is an enhancement of survival in hypopharyngeal carcinomas. No statistically significant series has emerged for supraglottic laryngeal carcinomas. Ogura et al.[92] indicate preoperative irradiation yields a better prognosis in patients with clinically positive nodes; 50% versus 64.5% survival. In Calcaterra's[87] opinion, the 5-year survival rates for patients treated by supraglottic laryngectomy compare favorably with those of patients treated by total laryngectomy and are better than those of patients treated by full-dose irradiation. When the carcinoma is confined to the epiglottis or the false cords, survival rates of better than 75% can be expected. While small, stage 1 lesions of the supraglottis can be controlled

equally well with radiotherapy or surgery. It is in the treatment of larger primary neoplasms that the superiority of surgery over radiotherapy becomes striking. In a survey of 544 supraglottic cancers classified as T2, T3 and T4 without clinical lymph node involvement, Vermund[70] reported a relative 5-year survival of 32% for primary radiation therapy and 64% for primary surgery.

Metastasis to the lymph nodes is the greatest single cause of failure of supraglottic laryngectomy. Baclesse[84] has described five subdivisions of the supraglottis, each differing from the others in prognosis and in regional lymph node metastases. In the more posterior sites of origin, the regional nodes are involved more than twice as often as in those arising anteriorly. There is no apparent relationship between the gross or histological appearance and the incidence of cervical metastases. In the series reported by Som,[93] 32% of 75 cases manifested lymph node metastases. Further, in 14 patients with positive palpable nodes of 2.0 cm or more, there was a 42% incidence of *contralateral* microscopically positive nodes.

Subglottic Carcinomas. The subglottic region is usually defined as the area between the inferior border of the vocal folds and the inferior margin of the cricoid cartilage, including the areas caudal to the anterior and posterior commissures. Alternatively, it may be considered to begin mucosally about 5 mm below the level of the free margin of the vocal cord. Arbitrary division can be further made into an upper mobile half and, where the mucosa and submucosa lie on the cricoid ring, a lower immobile half. Carcinomas occurring as primaries in the subglottis are relatively rare, constituting between 4 and 6% of all laryngeal carcinomas.[94, 95] The 5-year survival rate for primary subglottic cancer is low, whether the treatment is by radiotherapy or surgery. Vermund's[70] review of the literature disclosed a survival figure of approximately 40%. Harrison's experience is in keeping with that figure.[94]

Stridor and dyspnea are the most common presenting symptoms of a primary subglottic cancer. Hoarseness occurs only after invasion of the intrinsic musculature of the larynx or in cases where the carcinoma is transglottic (subglottic extension of a primary glottic carcinoma).[94] Early diagnosis of either primary or secondary subglottic carcinomas is hampered because the region beneath the cords may be difficult to visualize. Transconioscopy and microlaryngoscopy aid in the identification of the neoplasm and its extensions.

Martensson[96] stresses the value of transconioscopy in *all* patients with involvement of the vocal cords and cites the poor prognosis for patients with subglottic extension of glottic cancers. He reports a 5-year survival rate of 41% in a series of 29 patients.[97] Similar survival statistics have been reported by Shaw[97a] (37% and Martensson (36%)[96] and are similar to those for primary subglottic carcinomas.

Late discovery certainly accounts for this relatively poor survival. Subglottic carcinomas may invade deeply between the cricoid and thyroid cartilages without interfering with cord motility and may go unrecognized. The most common cause of failure in patients with subglottic carcinomas, however, is metastasis to lymph nodes.[94] This holds true whether they have been treated by irradiation and/or laryngectomy.

The subglottic lymphatics begin as a network in the mucous membrane on the inferior surface of the vocal cords. The *anterior union* of channels terminates in the lower deep cervical jugular chain or the prelaryngeal (Delphian) node. This is done after the lymphatic pedicle pierces the cricothyroid membrane. Drainage from the Delphian node is to the pretracheal and supraclavicular nodes.[94] The posterolateral (two) lymphatic pedicles pierce the cricotracheal membrane and end in the superior mediastinum.[94] The thyroarytenoid is commonly involved, as is the interarytenoid muscle with penetration of the cricotracheal space and posterior cricoarytenoid muscle.

Metastases to the paratracheal lymph nodes are clinically undetectable, although they are present in 50% of all larynges with primary subglottic carcinoma examined by serial section.[94] Harrison[98] has indicated that where the subglottis is involved, microscopically positive lymph nodes were found in 65% of cases.

Early diagnosis and removal of a lobe or the whole thyroid gland, in addition to a unilateral neck dissection with control of the paratracheal lymph nodes, are necessary to reverse the persistently low cure rates.[94]

General Therapeutic Considerations and Prognostic Factors. The preceding pages reiterate that at present there are three main ways of treating carcinoma of the larynx—radiotherapy, surgery, or both. Although there is still some debate about the exact place of each of these methods and about the systems of staging and classifying laryngeal neoplasms, highly effective routines of treatment have been established. In reaching this point, academically turbulent times have been transversed. "In the thirties, in the ebb and flow that took place as radiation sought to establish itself, the confusion that existed resembled a battle, so much so that it was common to refer to treatment of cancer of the larynx as Radiation vs. Surgery." Thus does Daly[15] summarize the events that led to present day principles for the selection of cases for radiation or surgery, or for combined therapy.

The method of treatment for a patient with carcinoma of the larynx, assuming he is a suitable candidate, depends largely on the exact site and extent of the carcinoma. Mucosal and submucosal extension and extralaryngeal spread dictate management more than does histological grading. The site of origin is particularly relevant at the upper and lower boundaries of the larynx, where the mucosa merges with that of the pharyngeal floor and trachea, respectively.

Cases of laryngeal carcinomas may be classified into three ill-defined therapeutic categories, which merge imperceptibly. In the first group are those patients with small and localized glottic carcinomas which do not fix the vocal cord. In most series there is a high successful cure rate with primary radiotherapy. Conservative surgery (partial laryngectomy) is most applicable to patients in the first group and therefore "competes" directly with radiotherapy. Laryngofissure, as a conservative surgical approach, has been criticized. It destroys the continuity of the thyroid cartilage, the natural barrier to the spread of disease, and may jeopardize the success of subsequent laryngectomy by allowing extralaryngeal spread at a relatively early stage. The choice of treatment of T2N0 glottic cancer may be difficult; the accent should be on conservatism. Laryngectomy will achieve an almost certain cure at the expense of the larynx. A subgroup of carcinoma deemed suitable for curative primary teleradiotherapy is that type occurring in women. These patients characteristically are "cured" by radiotherapy even when the lesion is not well localized.

The second category of patients includes those with carcinomas manifesting some destruction of laryngeal cartilages, extralaryngeal spread of neoplasm or involvement of lymph nodes. T3N0 glottic and the whole supraglottic group are also included in this category. At present, the tendency is to treat this second category by various combinations of radiotherapy and subsequent surgery. For those lesions destroying cartilage and with extralaryngeal spread, there is enthusiasm for preoperative irradiation followed by elective surgery. Laryngectomy, with or without block dissection of regional lymph nodes in the neck, is done no matter what the immediate outcome of the laryngectomy has been. Transglottic carcinomas are probably best treated by a definite program of radiotherapy followed by radical surgery. Radical neck dissection should be carried out at the same time as laryngectomy when there is a statistical likelihood of lymph node metastasis.[99]

The third group includes those patients with advanced carcinoma and gross spread of cancer into the neck, as well as distant metastases.[100] Palliative radiotherapy, tracheostomy, feeding gastrostomy, analgesics and cytotoxic agents may offer these patients with essentially terminal disease a small measure of comfort.

Patients with moderately advanced carcinomas of the larynx (T3N0M0) often pose problems over the most effective means of treatment. Vermund[70] lists the three alternatives: (1) planned preoperative radiation therapy followed by total laryngectomy and radical neck dissection; (2) initial radiotherapy followed by total laryngectomy and elective neck dissection in selective cases only; (3) initial total laryngectomy and elective radical neck dissection with or without preoperative radiation therapy. The combined treatment of plan 2 has the greatest number of protagonists.[101-105]

The influence of histological grade and clinical staging as generally reliable prognostic indicators has already been presented (Table 9.9). Other pathological factors affecting the survival of patients with carcinomas of the larynx follow. Futrell et al.[106] have observed that the patient's immune system response and host resistance changes in regional lymph nodes have little prognostic bearing on survival of patients with cancer of the larynx or hypopharynx. In an evaluation of sinus histiocytosis, McGavran and Bauer[107] came to similar conclusions. On the other hand, Berlinger et al.[108] and Ferlito[18] are of the opinion that useful prognostic indicators may be discovered by a careful examination of the type of lymph node reaction to squamous cell carcinomas of the larynx and other sites in the head and neck. Ferlito[18] regards

a lymph node pattern of "lymphocyte predominance," histologically expressed by a marked hyperplasia of T-lymphocytes located in the deep cortical regions, as an immune response of the cell-mediated type. This type is associated with a better prognosis than one in which a humoral immune response predominates. The latter is manifested by a "germinal center predominance" and may be appreciated by observing an expanded thymus-independent outer cortex area containing B-lymphocytes. The cortex and medulla of the lymph node are associated with humoral immunity, whereas the paracortex is responsible for cell-mediated immune response and, therefore, is considered a thymus-dependent area. According to Ferlito,[18] the presence of epithelioid cells is also an expression of a cell-mediated response. Berlinger et al.[108] emphasizing another modification of morphological grading of lymph nodes associated with carcinoma of the larynx, found that a definite relationship existed between such a marker of immunological activity and progression of the neoplasm and survival of the host. Investigations carried out in the Department of Pathology, University of Michigan by the author, however, point to the fallibility of such morphological assessments. Variations in the reaction patterns of lymph nodes at different levels from the primary carcinoma and even within single nodes makes categorization difficult. Additionally, preoperative irradiation to lymph nodes erases any significance to a morphological evaluation of the host response.

Table 9.9 from the experience of Bauer[36] expresses the influence of neoplastic differentiation on the tendency for metastasis. Significant prognostic correlation also exists with: (1) positive surgical wound washings; (2) the nearness of neoplastic involvement to the margins of surgical resection; (3) stomal recurrence after laryngectomy; and (4) the presence or absence of regional and distant metastases.

Experience with conservation surgery of the larynx (hemilaryngectomy) has allowed study of the meaning of surgical margins "involved" with carcinoma. This has been nicely done by Bauer et al.[109] in a retrospective review of 114 patients who underwent hemilaryngectomy for previously untreated infiltrating epidermoid carcinomas. Whatever the clinical impression of the adequacy of margins, a high incidence of involved margins was found in Bauer's study.[109] Thirty-five percent of all specimens were found to have either invasive cancer or intramucosal cancer at one margin. Two reasons for this are immediately apparent. The conservation surgeon cuts close to tumor and there

Table 9.9
Metastases and Level of Differentiation of Squamous Cell Carcinoma of the Larynx*†

Neoplasm	No. of Cases	Lymph Node Metastases	Dead of Cancer (10 years)
Well and moderately well differentiated carcinoma	62	12 (19%)	14 (23%)
Poorly differentiated carcinoma	38	20 (63%)	15 (40%)
	100	32	29

* Adapted from Bauer.[36]

† Carcinomas of the cord are not included.

is a limited amount of tissue that can be resected and still preserve function. This is particularly true of the anterior commissure and opposite cord. These are sites where most of the involved margins occurred in hemilaryngectomy specimens. The second factor, according to Bauer,[109] is the limitation inherent in the examination of any surgical specimens.

Follow-up of patients with positive margins yields rather surprising data. Patients with positive margins are three times more likely to have a local recurrence than patients with uninvolved margins. Practically, however, only 18% of Bauer's patients with positive margins developed a local recurrence if untreated.[109] Additionally, an uninvolved margin is no guarantee against a local recurrence. There is also a disappointing lack of correlation between recurrence rate and the type of involved margin (gross, close, and intraepithelial). Bauer's study further supports a conservative management of hemilaryngectomy patients with positive margins. No immediate therapy appears indicated. Careful follow-up, particularly directed to the anterior region as the most frequent site of recurrence *is* indicated. The recurrences can then be treated with either completion laryngectomy or full course irradiation. Use of this approach by Bauer et al.[109] has led to no deaths in a 5- to 12-year follow-up of patients with involved margins.

Stomal and peristomal recurrences of carcinoma and distant metastases from carcinoma of the larynx carry with them the onus of approaching death—often within 2 years after their discovery. The former, instrumental in the death; the latter usually coincidental with death. Both are heralds of therapeutic failure and yet despite therapeutic advances, each appears to be increasing in frequency, particularly the distant spread from carcinoma of the larynx.[110] The pathogenesis of the stomal recurrence (defined as neoplasm of stomal epithelium, i.e., mucocutaneous junction or, in tracheal mucosa, the peristomal soft tissues, or both) is unknown and the major postulates unproved. The increasing reports of distant spread (visceral and below the clavicles) must be related to the over-all enhanced survival of patients with laryngeal carcinoma brought about by surgical and radiotherapeutic advances.

In the following, we present a conspectus of these two postlaryngectomy failures.

Stomal and Peristomal Recurrence. Despite the adverse prognostic implications of persistence and/or recurrence of carcinoma in and about the tracheal stoma after laryngectomy, it has only been since 1962 that a concerted effort has been made to define the pathogenesis or treatment of this complication.

Judging from the published reports, the postlaryngectomy stomal recurrence is not a rare complication (Table 9.10). The divergence in statistics is not fully explainable; nor is there unanimity among authors on the predisposing clinicopathological factors.

Figure 9.3 depicts the several anatomical factors presumed to play a role in stomal and peristomal recurrence or persistence of cancer after laryngectomy. These are: (1) submucosal extension or undetected neoplasm at the margin of resection; (2) development of an additional primary neoplasm; (3) neoplastic cell implantation at the time of primary surgery; and (4) recurrence spawned by metastases to paratracheal and pretracheal lymph nodes.

For each of these factors there are proponents and detractors. The proximity of tumor to the surgical margins in permanent histological sections has a considerable predictive value for prognosis. Specimens with margins of 2 mm or less carry a 5-year survival equal to those with neoplasms at the resected end; i.e., 28 to 30%. Patients whose resected larynges have a margin of clearance greater than 2 mm do almost as well as patients with widely clear margins. The development of a second primary neoplasm deserves consideration because of the "field effect" phenomena. Of 20 stomal recurrences treated at the University of Michigan Medical Center, only one case fell into this category and this manner of generating stomal recurrences is not regarded as a prime factor by authors. The same cannot be said, however, for spread by implantation.[111, 114]

The inoculation of tumor cells in the tracheal wound and extension from involved paratracheal lymph nodes, although unproved, are the two most likely sources for stomal recurrences.

On the basis of statistics alone, implantation of residual cancer cells in the granulation tissue or

Table 9.10
Postlaryngectomy Stomal Recurrences

Authors	No. of Laryngectomies	No. of Recurrences	Percent
Bauer et al.[111]	86	6	7.0
Modlin and Ogura[112]	243	12	5.0
Keim et al.[113]	116	17	14.7
Stell and Van Den Broek[114]	130	7	5.0
Loewy and Laker[115]	138	4	3.0
de Jong[116]	114	2	1.7
Schneider et al.[117]	199	24	12.0

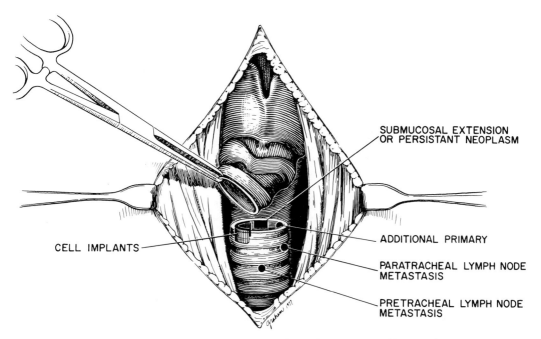

SUBMUCOSAL EXTENSION OR PERSISTANT NEOPLASM

CELL IMPLANTS

ADDITIONAL PRIMARY

PARATRACHEAL LYMPH NODE METASTASIS

PRETRACHEAL LYMPH NODE METASTASIS

Figure 9.3. Proposed causes for stomal and peristomal recurrences of laryngeal cancer.

exposed tissue around the tracheal stoma, either at the time of surgery or possibly at the time of preliminary tracheostomy, outweighs extension from adjacent lymph nodes.[111, 114] It is further our opinion that tracheostomy carried out before laryngectomy has a direct bearing on the probability of recurrent carcinoma around the tracheostoma. Endotracheal intubation does not appear to be pathogenetically important.[114]

Failure to identify lymphoid tissue does not exclude total replacement of such structures by metastatic carcinoma and in that event retrograde or extranodal extension is facilitated. Such a rationale may be applied to a genesis of stomal recurrence from metastases to adjacent lymphoid nodes. No proof, however, has been brought forth.

Size, laryngeal site, and level of differentiation of the primary carcinoma have not shown significant correlation to recurrence rates, again indirectly supporting the implantation hypothesis. Many authors, however, cite the danger of subglottic neoplasms.

The appearance of a stomal recurrence after laryngectomy varies from less than 6 months to over 6 years. Modlin and Ogura[112] found that approximately 50% occurred within 6 months.

Statistics relate that as a primary therapy, laryngectomy fails chiefly because of inapparent lymph node metastases, occasionally because of stomal recurrences, and very rarely because of distant metastases. They also demonstrate that salvage after laryngectomy failure is poor—approximately 20% of patients salvaged. Salvage after stomal recurrence is low and difficult to achieve. Most authors consider radiation therapy to be of little benefit, although there may be a temporary response.[122] Ogura and Biller[118] consider these lesions are not cured by radiotherapy and advise operative resection. This consists of resection of the manubrium and clavicular heads, formation of a new tracheostoma, and closure by regional flaps. Sisson[119] has had the greatest experience with operative treatment and reports a greater than 50% operative mortality. At best, surgical management yields only short survival and the mediastinal dead space created becomes a focus for infection, often with dire consequences. The best treatment is prevention.

Distant Metastases from Laryngeal Carcinoma. Reports of an increasing number of patients with cancer of the head and neck who manifest either clinical and/or necropsy evidence of distant metastases have dispelled an earlier impression that most of the neoplasms in this anatomical region tend to remain above the level of the clavicles. Crile[120] had underscored earlier observations by stating: "The collar of lymphatics about the neck forms an almost impassible barrier through which cancer rarely penetrates . . . ."

Every region studied has demonstrated an increased number of cases with distant metastases. Some indication of this may be seen in the report by Castigliano and Rominger.[121] In 1954 these authors reported 200 patients with fatal oral cavity cancer, who were treated from 1930 to 1954. Two percent of that group had distant metastases. In 120 patients with fatal oral cancer treated from 1943 to 1951, 10.7% had distant metastases.

Depending upon the site of the primary neoplasm and whether the statistics are based on clinical or necropsy findings, the percentage of patients with distant metastases varies from 15 to nearly 90%.

The incidence of distant metastases from laryngeal carcinoma also demonstrates this wide statistical variance. Harrer and Lewis[122] for example, report 16 of 18 patients with carcinoma of the larynx demonstrated diffuse metastases at necropsy. Abramson et al.[123] studied 650 patients with carcinoma of the larynx (75 with necropsy) and found that 34% had evidence of distant metastatic disease. At the time of necropsy, 80% of the patients with disseminated carcinomas also had local involvement in the neck. It is further evident that a pulmonary metastasis is a harbinger of more remote lesions. Abramson et al.[123] found only one patient in 26 with distant metastases, who did not also have pulmonary metastases. Eighteen of 29 patients (62%) with carcinoma of the larynx manifested distant metastases in the study by O'Brien et al.[124] In both of the above studies, it was noted that supraglottic carcinomas demonstrated the greatest potential for distant metastases. This propensity of the site has been further confirmed. In 107 cases of laryngeal and hypopharyngeal carcinomas with distant spread, Alonso[125] found a supraglottic primary in 63 (50%) and glottic primaries in 24%. If we assume that the latter account for 65% of all laryngeal carcinomas and supraglottic carcinomas for 30%, an extrapolation yields a rate of remote metastases from supraglottic carcinomas, 4 times that for glottic carcinomas. Others report this ratio as 2 to 8 times.[126, 127] Subglottic carcinomas are capable of wide dissemination, but their lower incidence renders information less available. They appear to occupy a position intermediate between the metastatic rates exhibited by supraglottic and glottic carcinoma.

No statistically clear relationship of tumor size and distant metastases is available. In a comparison of size of the primary lesion and metastases, Probert et al.[127] found no differences. Supraglottic lesions, however, tended to be larger.

Nearly three-fourths of patients manifesting distant metastases from their laryngeal carcinomas also have local involvement in the neck. This correlates with the observations by Braud and Martin[126] that patients with head and neck malignancies and cervical node involvement have a 2½ times greater chance of developing distant metastases than those patients without spread to cervical lymph nodes. Control of regional metastases, however, is no assurance that distant metastases will not occur.[123, 127, 128]

Closely related to regional lymph node involvement is persistence of the primary carcinoma. An uncontrolled primary with or without lymph node metastases has been found in 53 to 80% of patients with distant metastases.[123, 127, 128]

No correlation with distant spread has been found with the age, sex or general clinical condition of the host.

The histological differentiation of the primary squamous cell carcinoma has not been shown to have an influence on the ability to disseminate widely. In one study, over 90% of the distant metastases were histologically identical with the primary lesion.[123]

If the primary lesion in the larynx is controlled, the mode of initial treatment does not appear to be a correlative factor in the subsequent development of metastases. Even combined therapy does not seem to affect or alter the rate of distant spread.[125] It has not been shown that manipulation of the primary neoplasm contributes to widespread dissemination, although some support (similar to that for stomal recurrences) can be found for the possibility of seeding of the tracheobronchial tree by endoscopic maneuvers or tracheostomy.

In all series, whether they are based on clinical or necropsy data, the lungs are the most common site of infraclavicular spread of laryngeal carcinoma. These tend to be small and multiple. Most are less than 3 mm and difficult to detect by x-ray examination. In order of other visceral involvement, the mediastinal lymph nodes, skeletal system and liver follow. Osseous metastases are osteolytic and most frequently involve the lumbosacral spine and the ribs. The hepatic metastases, like those in the lung tend to be small and multiple. Metastases to the heart have been reported to occur in from 2 to 25% of necropsied cases.

Evidence of distant spread from carcinoma of the larynx is often delayed with nearly 40% of cases discovered after 5 years' primary treatment. Once found, however, the distant metastasis is an ominous prognostic sign. Ninety percent of these patients will die within 2 years of the detection of the remote disease. Certainly these metastases contribute to death, but the failure to eradicate local disease and regional metastases appears to be the principal determinant.[129]

PLEOMORPHIC CARCINOMA OF THE LARYNX

This unusual and rare lesion of the larynx has been called squamous cell carcinoma with sarcoma-like stoma, carcinosarcoma, spindle cell carcinoma and pseudosarcoma. Sites other than the larynx where the lesion may present are the upper and lower respiratory tracts, lips, oral cavity and esophagus.[130, 131] Discussion is presented here because of its potential confusion with primary supporting tissue neoplasms of the larynx. The spindle cell or pleomorphic carcinoma of the tongue has been ably reviewed by Someren et al.[131] (See also Chapter 6).

Pleomorphic pseudosarcomatous carcinoma of the larynx is both distinctive and yet enigmatic in regard to its structure and its biological behavior. With others,[131-134] I regard the neoplasm as most often a squamous cell carcinoma. This may be overshadowed or even completely overlooked by the unsuspecting physician because of the histologically dominating stroma which may suggest anything from a spindle cell carcinoma to a variety of sarcoma types or just a fibroblastic proliferation which is associated with a chronic inflammatory reaction. Pleomorphic carcinoma is differentiated from the highly unusual collision tumor or carcinosarcoma in that it is strictly an epithelial neoplasm with pleomorphism and not two neoplasms in juxtaposition or intermingled.

The term "pseudosarcoma," entirely appropriate as a qualifying but not diagnostic term, was introduced by Lane[135] to describe the anaplastic and sarcomatous-like stroma associated with a frequently inconspicuous intraluminal or invasive squamous cell carcinoma. He considered the stromal changes as part of reactive process and, as such, probably not neoplastic. Unlike Lane,[135] who doubted any transition between the carcinoma and the stroma, others have demonstrated the transition of the infiltrative carcinoma to the atypical spindled elements.[132, 136] A transmission electron microscopic study of spindle cell carcinomas of the skin and esophagus has suggested that the pseudosarcomatous component of the neoplasms originates from mesenchymal metaplasia of squamous cells and that collagen is produced by these metaplastic cells.[134]

After a review of the series from the University of Michigan, I consider the source of most of the anaplastic sarcoma-like cells to be the laryngeal epithelium. In some instances of laryngeal carcinoma, the neoplasm may possess such extreme powers of polymorphism that the cells tend to lose all traces of their epithelial origin and may become indistinguishable from connective tissue elements. This does not ignore or refute the participation in the mass by reactive and proliferating connective tissue, such as fibroblasts and angioblasts.[137] A diligent search and, quite often multiple sections are required to identify the squamous cell carcinoma. According to Hyams,[132] this element is usually reliably concentrated at the base or stalk of the tumor. All histological grades of squamous cell carcinomas may be encountered, and these may be quite variable even within the same tumor.

The epithelial lesion may vary from focal carcinoma in situ to an invasive moderately well differentiated squamous cell carcinoma. Metastases, when they occur, usually manifest only the definable epithelial component, but instances of only the spindle cell component in involved nodes have been recorded.[132] True carcinosarcomas or collision tumors, on the other hand, usually demonstrate both carcinomatous and sarcomatous components in the metastatic lesion.

In its gross presentation, pleomorphic carcinomas may present in two basic forms, polypoid or pedunculated and infiltrative. On occasion, a lesion may have both features. It is the gross configuration of the lesion which correlates with the clinical course and the biological behavior of the neoplasm. If the tumor is polypoid or pedunculated, regardless of the histological composition, the outcome is relatively more favorable. Any other configuration is associated with a prognosis not unlike infiltrative squamous cell carcinoma without pleomorphism. A polypoid configuration does not always imply a better prognosis and according to some investigators, the connotation is simply because clear margins can be more easily achieved at the base of a polypoid tumor than is an infiltrative type.[138]

Under the light microscope, all pleomorphic carcinomas of the larynx manifest a sarcoma-like growth pattern associated with small, often inconspicuous foci of obvious squamous cell carcinoma. In the report by Sherwin et al.,[136] this extraordinary growth pattern was thought to be caused by a polypoid structure resulting from mucosal ulceration and an overgrowth of granulation tissue, junctional change of the carcinoma overlying the mass, and a neoplastic and host-response spindle cell proliferation.

The inter-relationship of cells is usually one of an intermixture of invasive epithelial and sarcoma-like elements. This blending of patterns often consists of a loss of cellular cohesion with dropping of single cells or groups of squamous carcinoma cells into the underlying stroma. Comparison with the junctional change of nevi or melanomas is appropriate.

The distinctive epithelial cells are admixed with a proliferation of spindle cells, many of which are of epithelial origin but are difficult to separate from angioblasts or fibroblasts (Fig. 9.4). An associated deposition of collagen is, however, usually absent, and dense cytoplasmic keratinization may occasionally be seen in the spindle cell forms. While admixture of the two distinctive cell pat-

terns is the rule, an occasional lesion may appear to have little intermingling of the components. Osteoid, cartilage or bone formed by metaplasia may be present, and, in these instances, the tissues probably represent a response to previous radiotherapy and are not, then, an integral part of the neoplasm.

Virtually all examples have occurred in patients in the cancer age group for carcinoma of the larynx. The vast majority are in male patients. Metastases, particularly from the polypoid type are unusual (Table 9.11). The collected therapeutic experience with this neoplasm is too small to judge between surgical excision and irradiation. In half

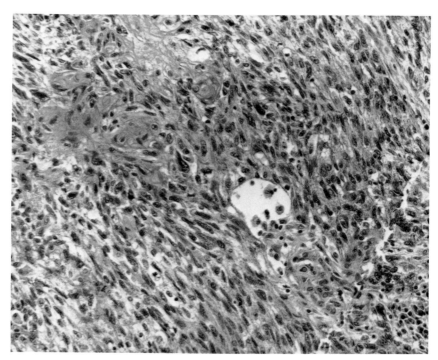

Figure 9.4. Pleomorphic carcinoma of larynx. So-called spindle cell or pseudosarcomatous squamous cell carcinoma.

Table 9.11
Pleomorphic Carcinoma of the Larynx: Clinicopathological Observations

Author	No. of Cases	Location in Larynx	Lymph node Metastases	Died of Tumor
Randall et al.[133]	9	3 glottic 6 supraglottic	3	2 (2 months –3 years)
Hyams[132]	39	23 glottic 8 supraglottic 2 subglottic	5	8 of 20 with follow-up (4 months–2 years)
Goellner et al.[137]	25	23 glottic 2 supraglottic	2	4 (6 months–2 years)
Appelman and Oberman[139]	11	6 glottic 5 supraglottic	2	8 (8 months–5.5 years)

of the cases treated by either forms of treatment, there have been local recurrences. It is further quite clear that pleomorphic carcinoma of the larynx is not a low-grade malignancy. Hyams[132] indicates a 2-year mortality of 40%.

SUPPORTING TISSUE TUMORS OF THE LARYNX

The total frequency of supporting tissue neoplasms among the primary neoplasms of the larynx probably does not exceed 2%.[45]

Fibrosarcomas. By 1969, 32 histologically recorded and acceptable examples of laryngeal fibrosarcoma had been reported. Approximately 70% of the patients were over the age of 50 years, and males dominated by a ratio of 4:1[45, 140] The majority arise from the anterior cords or commissure, or both; others are found at the level of the cricoid cartilage or ventricle. The majority present as a nodular or pedunculated mass. There is a marked correlation of histological grade and prognosis.[141]

Laryngeal fibrosarcomas rarely metastasize to cervical lymph nodes, and this tendency is shared by fibrosarcomas in other loci. Spread is vascular and most often by infiltration along the fascial planes or muscles in the environs of the larynx. There can be no generalizations over so-called appropriate treatment, but differentiated fibrosarcomas, if small and polypoid or pedunculated, may be adequately resected with a laryngofissure or partial laryngectomy or through the laryngoscope. Radical resection (wide-field laryngectomy) is reserved for either anaplastic or widely infiltrative fibrosarcomas.

Cartilaginous Tumors of the Larynx. These are unusual lesions. Between 1831 and 1968, only between 125 and 136 cartilaginous tumors of the larynx had been recorded in the world literature.[142, 143] Further indications of their rarity are statistics available from the Massachusetts Eye and Ear Infirmary[144] and the Armed Forces Institute of Pathology (AFIP)[145]. In the former institution, 10 cases among 5,000 primary laryngeal neoplasms (30 years) were reported. The AFIP series entails 31 cases between 1929 and 1969.

Anatomical sites of involvement in the larynx are presented in Table 9.12. This frequency distribution is in general agreement with other published reports. The greatest number develop from the cricoid cartilate with a predilection for the posterior lamina. The AFIP series also contains a relatively large number of tumors arising in the soft tissues of the vocal cord.[145] To my knowledge,

Table 9.12
Cartilaginous Tumors of the Larynx*

Site	Histological Classification	
	Chondroma	Chondrosarcoma
Cricoid cartilage	3	20
Thyroid cartilage	2	5
Arytenoid	0	4
Epiglottis	2	0
Vocal cord	9	0
	—	—
	16	29

* Based on the series of Hyams and Rabuzzi[145] and Huizenga and Balogh.[144]

no cartilage tumors have arisen from the corniculate, cuneiform or triticea cartilages.

Histogenetically, it is noteworthy that nearly all documented cases have arisen from hyaline cartilage and show no evidence of elastic tissue.

The tumors of the larynx are predominantly in patients in their fourth through sixth decades of life and manifest a distinct male predominance. This is in contrast to the cartilaginous neoplasms (particularly chondrosarcomas) of extralaryngeal origin which affect mainly young and middle aged adults. It is, however, in consort with the age incidence of cartilaginous neoplasms of the facial bones.

Clinical signs and symptoms are nonspecific and relate to a slow, yet progressive encroachment of the subglottic space, i.e., hoarseness, poor voice or dysphagia. Rarely mass growth is extralaryngeal. Cocke[143] records presentation in the neck from a chondromatous growth outward from the larynx in about 20% of these lesions. Because of their common location below the vocal cords, laterally or posteriorly, hoarseness may be minimized, and it is dyspnea which finally brings the patient to a physician.

Figure 9.5 presents the laryngeal distribution of 62 chondrosarcomas as reported by Hyams and Rabuzzi[145] and Huizenga and Balogh[144] and additional cases derived from the literature. The hyoid bone is not considered anatomically to be part of the larynx but it too may be the site of chondrosarcoma. Greer et al.[146] reported the fifth example (one with Gardner's syndrome). Of the five patients with chondrosarcoma of the hyoid bone, the three with any meaningful follow-up had recurrences and died as a result.

Primary chondrosarcoma of the trachea is even more rare. Daniels et al.[147] after a review of the literature, could find only one example.

At laryngoscopic examination, the tumors ap-

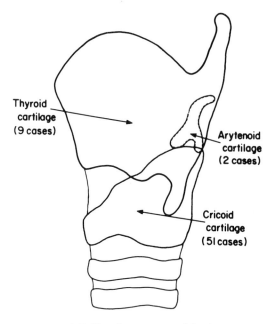

Thyroid cartilage (9 cases)

Arytenoid cartilage (2 cases)

Cricoid cartilage (51 cases)

Figure 9.5. Chondrosarcomas of the larynx.

pear as smooth and encapsulated masses located beneath the mucosa of the subglottis with the arytenoid or true cores pushed laterally. Roentogenograms of the soft tissue of the larynx, planograms and larynogograms are useful to delineate the lesion and its points of attachment. They demonstrate a smooth-surfaced, homogeneously dense, unilateral tumor which bulges into the airway. A mottled calcification in the region is seen in approximately 80% of the lesions. Tomograms may permit identification of tumor penetration through the cricoid lamina to the external perichondrium.

Biopsy of the tumors may be difficult or impossible, because of the hardness of the mass.

The histological definition of a chondroma given by Hyams and Rabuzzi[145] is that the tumor duplicates the histology of normal cartilage. While the chondroma may exhibit an increased cellularity, the individual cells retain a uniform morphology similar to those of normal cartilage.

The criteria for chondrosacromas are those of Lichtenstein and Jaffe[148] and Spjut et al.[149]: (1) pronounced irregularity in size of the cells and their nuclei; (2) presence of numerous cells and their nuclei; (3) pronounced hyperchromatism of the nuclei; and (4) any large or giant cartilage cells with single or multiple nulcei or with clumps of chromatin. To these I add a "cluster disarray" of cartilage cells. The presence of bone in the neoplasm does not alter the classification or prognosis.

All cartilage tumors of the larynx require wide local excision, encompassing a safe margin of normal tissue, including laryngectomy if necessary. Even the benign tumors in this area are potentially lethal. The cure rate of patients with no treatment is zero.

There is no other method of treatment except surgical removal. It is generally agreed that the surgeon should not be governed by the histological appearance of the neoplasm and that histologically benign chondromas and chondrosarcomas be treated in a similar manner. As conservative a procedure as the age of the patient and the size and location of the tumor permits is a wise guide to treatment. Cricoid involvement is the critical feature and the key to the extent of resection. At times, the neoplastic involvement of the cricoid is so extensive that laryngectomy is needed. However, preservation of this structure is important, since loss of this structure eliminates the upper fixation of the trachea and lower aspect of the larynx. If more than one-half of the cricoid lamina must be sacrificed, laryngectomy may be advised because of the potential of a resultant tracheal and laryngeal stenosis. Thyrotomy may allow adequate removal of the tumor in the majority of patients.

Chondrosacromas of the larynx are primarily local invaders, but metastases (to lungs) have been reported in five cases.[144, 145] Local recurrences occur in approximately one-quarter of the cases, but are not catastrophic and are locally treatable.

Hemangiomas of the Larynx. The most comprehensive survey of laryngeal hemangiomas was made by Ferguson.[151] He reviewed 125 instances and perpetuated the classification of adult and infantile types. Of the 125 examples 117 were of the adult type. The rarely occurring infantile form constituted less than 10% and was characterized as occurring below the level of the vocal cords, while the so-called adult form occurred on or above the vocal cords.

The adult form, if such a lesion can be truly separated from angiomatoid speaker's nodules or granulation tissue, presents with an entirely different set of signs and symptoms. These are not different from those associated with speakers nodules. The lesions occur on or above the true cords, are often pedunculated, well demarcated and reddish-blue in color.[152]

Infantile hemangiomas of the larynx may be either neoplasms or congenital malformations. Their exact incidence is difficult to determine since postmortem emptying of blood makes them difficult to recognize grossly. There is a female preponderance in the subglottic or infantile forms by a ratio of approximately 2:1. This contrasts sharply with the 90% incidence in men with the so-called adult form. Usually asymptomatic at birth, the infantile lesions produce signs and symptoms of respiratory distress before the patient reaches the age of 3 months.[153] Because of their subglottic location, laryngeal hemangiomas typically present with a history of dyspnea and inspiratory stridor, which may become biphasic. The cry and voice usually remain clear.

The fluctuating character of the respiratory distress, varying from day to day, or even more often, with an aggravation by excitement or infection is considered strongly diagnostic. Calcaterra[154] attributes this symptom pattern to be a response to varying venous pressures. Association with hemangiomatous lesions elsewhere, particularly dermal hemangiomas of the head and neck, should prompt suspicion of laryngeal involvement in a child with respiratory distress. Approximately 50% of affected children will manifest this relationship.

Infantile laryngeal hemangiomas usually appear as compressible, sessile masses between the true vocal cord and the lower limits of the cricoid cartilage. They usually present on only one side of the subglottic area but may circumscribe the entire lumen. They may be cavernous or simple or capillary in appearance. They only rarely extend to involve the true cords.

Treatment must be considered from two aspects. Relief of dyspnea often becomes an urgent necessity, and tracheostomy, performed as low as possible to avoid cutting the tumor, is the best procedure in acute instances. In less urgent situations, biopsy is generally condemned as not only dangerous but also unnecessary. The clinical history and endoscopic appearance are usually sufficient for diagnosis. After the report by Ferguson,[151] treatment has been almost exclusively low-dose irradiation, but doubts have been raised concerning the necessity and indeed the efficacy of this form of treatment.

A valid comparison has been made between cutaneous hemangiomas in infants and infantile laryngeal hemangiomas.[154] Noninvoluting cutaneous hemangiomas of infancy are exceptional and constitute only a small fraction. Growth usually ceases by 6 months of age and almost never persists beyond 1 year. In a similar manner, subglottic hemangiomas have been observed to increase in size and symptom severity until 6 months, after which spontaneous regression may be noted. Because of this biological course and the variable responsiveness to radiotherapy, combined with the inherent dangers of such treatment, tracheostomy

alone, if indicated, may be the primary treatment of choice. The philosophy of management and forms of treatment are reviewed by Charachon et al.[155] and Benjamin.[156] The authenticity of all cases reported to be hemangiosarcomas of the larynx is suspect.

Other Nonepithelial Tumors of the Larynx. Data in this chapter should underscore the fact that neoplastic disease originating from the mesenchyme of the larynx is an uncommon finding. In the following, I briefly review some of the unusual forms. Additional information on many of the entities can be found in chapters dealing with the generic tissue; i.e., skeletal muscle, paraganglia, etc.

Tumors of the Peripheral Nerves. Many reports of tumors of the peripheral nerves of the larynx have considered neurofibroma and neurilemoma as one entity and consequently it is difficult to obtain differences in biological behavior. The larynx, like the upper airway, is infrequently involved in patients with multiple neurofibromatosis. Chang-Lo[157] recorded the twentieth case in 1977. All were neurofibromas. The peripheral nerve tumors are usually solitary and lobulated. Unless there has been prior surgical intervention, the overlying mucosa is intact. The great majority of tumors take origin from the aryepiglottic fold or from the false cords. Adequate removal has not been followed by recurrence. I know of no neurogenous sarcomas of the larynx.

Tumors of Fibroadipose Tissue. In a 26-year review of 621 lipomas of various organs, it was found that 9% affected the respiratory tract and only 0.6% were localized in the larynx.[158] Liposarcomas, in keeping with their rarity in the head and neck, are extremely rare in the larynx.[159] Ferlito[160] reported the second case in the world literature in 1978.

Tumors of Skeletal Muscle. Rhabdomyoma and rhabdomyosarcoma of the larynx remain among the least common of that structure's supporting tissue neoplasms.[161] They are fully discussed in Chapter 14.

Tumors of Paraganglionic Tissue. While not unexpected because of the presence of paraganglionic tissue in the larynx (Chapter 19), paragangliomas are rarely found in that anatomical structure. Despite reports to the contrary, I have not accepted a malignant paraganglioma of the larynx.

Tumors of Lymphoreticular Tissue. Lymphoma involving the larynx is an unusual lesion and very likely accounts for less than 1% of laryngeal neoplasms. Primary, extranodal lymphomas in the larynx is even more unusual. DeSanto and Weiland[162] reported nine patients treated at the Mayo Clinic from 1952 to 1968 who had lymphoma involving the larynx. During the same period, 5,319 patients were seen for malignant lymphoma. Involvement of the larynx was less than 0.2%. Additional reviews have been provided by Dickson[163] and Anderson et al.[164] The majority of the lymphomas have presented as smooth *supraglottic* masses, usually of the epiglottis or aryepiglottic fold.

All of the reported examples of laryngeal involvement by lymphoma have been of the lymphocytic lymphoma type.

The presence of an apparent extranodal lymphoma in the larynx requires systemic evaluation of the patient since the majority of patients either have coexisting extralaryngeal disease or will develop it.

Radiation therapy is the best initial treatment for an isolated or apparently isolated lymphoma. Local tumor control, however, should not be interpreted as a cure.

The related lesion, plasmacytoma, is rare in the larynx. Pahor[165] has reviewed 32 cases. The epiglottis is the most commonly involved site, followed by the vocal cords, false cords and ventricles. Nearly one-half of the patients with plasmacytoma of the larynx have associated upper aerodigestive tract plasma cell lesions. As presented in Chapter 23, exclusion of multiple myeloma is required. Treatment of the localized plasmacytoma is essentially by radiotherapy.

Localized Amyloidosis. Localized (primary) amyloidosis of the laryngotracheobronchial tree is a relatively rare condition.[166, 167] Laryngeal amyloidosis is almost always a localized form. McAlpine and Fuller[168] were able to find only 10 of 118 cases in which systemic involvement was associated, and in none of these was the patient asymptomatic.

In the larynx, the lesion is associated with hoarseness as the most frequently encountered initial complaint. The true vocal cord is the most common site of involvement, followed by the subglottic region. A polypoid configuration is usual in the glottic and supraglottic forms while a diffuse submucosal lesion is the manner of presentation in the subglottis. The tumors are unencapsulated, firm, pale, wax-like, and homogenous beneath an intact mucosal surface.

In these tumors, as in the other forms of amyloidosis, diagnosis is based on biopsy and histological examination, using adequate methods for the identification of the amyloid. However, not all methods used are equally efficient and specific.

Amyloid appears homogenous and amorphous under the light microscope. It stains pink with hemotoxylin and eosin and metachromatically with methyl violet or crystal violet. Thioflavine T produces an intense yellow-green fluorescence with amyloid, but false positives occur. Congo red is widely used for staining, but it also stains collagen and elastic tissue as well as amyloid. However, Congo red does produce a green birefringence of amyloid when tissue is examined under polarizing microscope, and this is the most specific stain for the detection of amyloid.[169] Under the electron microscope, amyloid is seen to consist of rigid and nonbranching fibrils that are approximately 50 to 150 Å in width. The fibril length has been estimated to be in the order of 8,000 Å. Amyloid fibrils are arranged in an antiparallel conformation and beta-pleated sheet structure as revealed by low-angle x-ray diffraction. The fibrils are insoluble and generally resist proteolytic digestion.

Prognosis for patients with laryngeal amyloidosis appears favorable. Recurrences occur, especially in the diffuse submucosal form, but are localized to the larynx and may be treated conservatively.

REFERENCES

1. Laurema, S.: Treatment of laryngeal cancer: a study of 638 cases. Acta Otolaryngol. (suppl.) 225:1, 1967.
2. Kerr, R. C., Madigan, J. P., and Millar, H. S.: Carcinoma of the larynx in Melbourne, 1956–1965. Aust. N. Z. J. Surg. 40:19, 1970.
3. Silverberg, E., and Holleb, A. I.: Cancer statistics, 1972. CA 22:2, 1972.
4. Wynder, E. L., Bross, I. J., and Day, E.: A study of environmental factors in cancer of the larynx. Cancer 9:86, 1956.
5. Devine, K. D.: Pathologic effects of smoking on the larynx and oral cavity. Staff Meet. Mayo Clin. 35:349, 1960.
6. Ryan, R. F., McDonald, J. R., and Devine, K. D.: The pathologic effects of smoking on the larynx. Arch. Pathol. 60:472, 1955.
7. Auerbach, O., Hammond, E. C., and Garfinkel, L.: Histologic changes in the larynx in relation to smoking habits. Cancer 25:92, 1970.
8. Baker, D. C., and Weissman, B.: Postirradiation carcinoma of the larynx. Ann. Otol. Rhinol. Laryngol. 80:634, 1971.
9. Goolden, A. W.: Radiation cancer. Br. J. Radiol. 30:626, 1957.
10. Van Dishoeck, H. A. E.: Malignant tumours in the Leiden Ear-Nose-Throat Clinic. Pract. Otorhinolaryngol. (Basel) 30:248, 1968.
11. Majoros, M., Devine, K. D., and Parkhill, E. M.: Malignant transformation of benign laryngeal papillomas in children after radiation therapy. Surg. Clin. North Am. 43:1049, 1963.
12. Rabbett, W. F.: Juvenile laryngeal papillomatosis. Ann. Otol. Rhinol. Laryngol. 74:1149, 1965.
13. Wlodyka, J.: Carcinogenic effects of x-ray on the larynx. Arch. Otolaryngol. 76:372, 1962.
14. Shimkin, M. B.: Duration of life in untreated cancer. Cancer 4:1, 1951.

15. Daly, J. F.: Variations and trends in cancer of the larynx and supralarynx. In Cancer of the Head and Neck, edited by J. Conley, pp. 365–366. Butterworths, Washington, D. C., 1967.

16. McGavran, M. H., Bauer, W. C., and Ogura, J. H.: The incidence of cervical lymph node metastases from epidermoid carcinoma of the larynx and their relationship to certain characteristics of the primary tumor. Cancer 14:55, 1961.

17. Beahrs, O. H.: Clinical staging of cancer of the head and neck. Surg. Clin. N. Am. 57:831, 1977.

18. Ferlito, A.: Histological classification of larynx and hypopharynx cancers and their clinical implications. Pathologic aspects of 2052 malignant neoplasms diagnosed at the ORL Department of Padua University from 1966 to 1976. Acta Otolaryngol. Supp. 342, 1976.

19. Olofsson, J., and van Nostrand, A. W. P.: Anaplastic small cell carcinoma of the larynx. Ann. Otol. Rhinol. Laryngol. 81:284, 1972.

20. MacComb, W. S., Fletcher, G. H. Gallager, H. S., Healey, J. E., Jr., and Lehmann, Q. H.: Larynx. In Cancer of the Head and Neck, edited by W. S. MacComb and G. H. Fletcher, pp. 241–292. Williams & Wilkins Co., Baltimore, 1967.

21. Strong, M. S., Vaughan, C. W., and Incze, J.: Toluidine blue in diagnosis of cancer of the larynx. Arch. Otolaryngol. 91:515, 1970.

22. Miller, A. H., and Fisher, H. R.: Clues to the life history of carcinoma in situ of the larynx. Laryngoscope 81:1475, 1971.

23. Bridger, P., and Nassar, V. H.: Carcinoma in situ involving the laryngeal mucus glands. Arch. Otolaryngol. 94:389, 1971.

24. Altmann, F., Ginsberg, I., and Stout, A. P.: Intraepithelial carcinoma (cancer in situ) of the larynx. Arch. Otolaryngol. 56:121, 1952.

25. Bauer, W. C.: Concomitant carcinoma in situ and invasive carcinoma of the larynx. Canad. J. Otolaryngol. 3:533, 1974.

26. Kashima, H. K.: The characteristics of laryngeal cancer correlating with cervical lymph node metastasis. Canad. J. Otolaryngol. 4:893, 1975.

27. Jakobsson, P. A.: Histologic grading of malignancy and prognosis in glottic carcinoma of the larynx. Canad. J. Otolaryngol. 4:885, 1975.

28. Berlinger, N. T., Tsakraklides, V., and Pollack, K.: Immunologic assessment of regional lymph node histology in relation to survival in head and neck carcinoma. Cancer 37:697, 1976.

29. Van Nagell, J. R., Jr., Donaldson, E. S., and Parker, J. G.: The prognostic significance of pelvic lymph node morphology in carcinoma of the uterine cervix. Cancer 39:2624, 1977.

30. Frable, W. J., and Frable, M. A.: Cytologic diagnosis of carcinoma of the larynx by direct smear. Acta Cytol. 12:318, 1968.

31. Chandler, J. R.: The nonvalue of oral cytology. Arch. Otolaryngol. 84:527, 1966.

32. Ackerman, L. V.: Verrucous carcinomas of the oral cavity. Surgery 23:670, 1948.

33. Goethals, P. L., Harrison, E. G., Jr., and Devine, K. D.: Verrucous squamous carcinoma of the oral cavity. Am. J. Surg. 106:845, 1963.

34. Kraus, F. T., and Perez, C. A.: Verrucous carcinoma. Clinical and pathologic study of 105 cases involving the oral cavity, larynx and genitalia. Cancer 19:26, 1966.

35. Ferlito, A., Antonutto, G., and Silvestri, F.: Histological appearance and nuclear DNA content of verrucous carcinoma of the larynx. ORL 38:65, 1976.

36. Bauer, W. C.: Varieties of squamous carcinoma—biologic behavior. Radiat. Ther. Oncol. 9:164, 1974.

37. Biller, H. F., Ogura, J. H., and Bauer, W. C.: Verrucous cancer of the larynx. Ann. Otol. Rhinol. Laryngol. 80:1323, 1971.

38. Matsumura, T., and Kawakatsu, K.: Verrucous carcinoma of the oral mucosa: histochemical pattern and clinical behavior. Oral Surg. 30:349, 1972.

39. Burns, H. P., van Nostrand, A. W. P., and Bryce, D. P.: Verrucous carcinoma of the larynx. Management by radiotherapy and surgery. Ann. Otol. 85:538, 1976.

40. Fonts, E. A., Greenlaw, R. H., Rush, B. F., and Rovin, S.: Verrucous squamous cell carcinoma of the oral cavity. Cancer 23:152, 1969.

41. Perez, C. A., Kraus, F. T., Evans, J. C., and Powers, W. E.: Anaplastic transformation in verrucous carcinoma of the oral cavity after radiation therapy. Radiology 86:108, 1966.

42. van Nostrand, A. W. P., and Olofsson, J.: Verrucous carcinoma of the larynx. A clinical and pathologic study of ten cases. Cancer 30:691, 1972.

43. Biller, H. F., and Bergman, J. A.: Verrucous carcinoma of the larynx. Laryngoscope 85:1698, 1975.

44. Ryan, R. E., Jr., DeSanto, L. W., Devine, K. D., and Weiland, L. H.: Verrucous carcinoma of the larynx. Laryngoscope 87:1989, 1977.

45. Batsakis, J. G., and Fox, J. E.: Supporting tissue neoplasms of the larynx. Surg. Gynecol. Obstet. 131:989, 1970.

46. Minckler, D. S., Meligro, C. H., and Norris, H. T.: Carcinosarcoma of the larynx: case report with metastases of epidermoid and sarcomatous elements. Cancer 26:195, 1970.

47. Kleinsasser, O.: Microlaryngoscopy and Endolaryngeal Microsurgery. W. B. Saunders Co., Philadelphia, 1968.

48. Bocca, E., Oreste, P., and Oreste, M.: Supraglottic surgery of the larynx. Ann. Otol. Rhinol. Laryngol. 77:1005, 1968.

49. Hast, M. H.: Applied embryology of the larynx. Canad. J. Otolaryngol. 3:412, 1974.

50. Pressman, J., Simon, M. B., and Monell, C.: Anatomical studies related to the dissemination of cancer of the larynx. Trans. Am. Acad. Ophthal. Otolaryngol. 64:628, 1960.

51. Tucker, G. F., Jr., and Smith, R., Jr.: A histological demonstration of the development of laryngeal connective tissue compartments. Trans. Am. Acad. Ophthal. Otolaryngol. 66:308, 1962.

52. Tucker, G. F., Jr.: Some clinical inferences from the study of serial sections. Laryngoscope 73:728, 1963.

53. Kirchner, J. A.: One hundred laryngeal cancers studied by serial section. Ann. Otol. Rhinol. Laryngol. 78:689, 1969.

54. Broyles, E. N.: The anterior commissure tendon. Ann. Otol. Rhinol. Laryngol. 52:342, 1943.

55. Bridger, C. P., and Nassar, V. H.: Cancer spread in the larynx. Arch. Otolaryngol. 95:497, 1972.

56. Tucker, G. F., Jr.: The anatomy of laryngeal cancer. J. Otolaryngol. Soc. Austral. 3:617, 1974.

57. Micheau, C., Luboinski, B., Sancho, H., and Cachin, Y.: Modes of invasion of cancer of the larynx. A statistical, histological and radioclinical analysis of 120 cases. Cancer 38:346, 1976.

58. Olofsson, J., van Nostrand, A. W. P.: Growth and spread of laryngeal and hypopharyngeal carcinoma with reflection on the effect of preoperative irradiation: 139 cases studied by whole organ serial sectioning. Acta Otolaryngol. Suppl. 308, 1973.

59. Olofsson, J.: Growth and spread of laryngeal carcinoma. Canad. J. Otolaryngol. 3:446, 1974.

60. Freeland, A. P.: Microfil angiography: a demonstration of the microvasculature of the larynx with reference to tumor spread. Canad. J. Otolaryngol. 4:111, 1975.

61. Bridger, G. P.: Mucous gland involvement in cancer at the anterior commissure. Canad. J. Otolaryngol. 3:507, 1974.

62. Bridger, P., and Nassar, V. H.: Carcinoma in situ involving the laryngeal mucus glands. Arch. Otalaryngol. 94:389, 1971.

63. Staley, C. J., and Herzon, F. S.: Elective neck dissection in carcinoma of the larynx. Otolaryngol. Clin. North Am. 3:543, 1970.

64. Ogura, J. H., Biller, H. F., and Wette, R.: Elective neck dissection for pharyngeal and laryngeal cancers. Ann. Otol. Rhinol. Laryngol. 80:646, 1971.

65. O'Keefe, J. J.: Evaluation of laryngectomy with radical neck dissection. Laryngoscope 69:914, 1959.

66. Bocca, E., Pignataro, O., and Mosciaro, O.: Supraglottic surgery of the larynx. Ann. Otol. Rhinol. Laryngol. 77:1005, 1968.

67. Biller, H. F., Davis, W. H., and Ogura, J. H.: Delayed contralateral cervical metastases with laryngeal and laryngopharyngeal cancers. Laryngoscope 81:1499, 1971.

68. Bardwil, J. M.: Cancer of the vocal cord. Cancer 29:31, 1972.

69. Stutsman, A. C., and McGavran, M. H.: Ultraconservative management of superficially invasive epidermoid carcinoma of the true vocal cord. Ann. Otol. Rhinol. Laryngol.80:507, 1971.

70. Vermund, H.: Role of radiotherapy in cancer of the larynx as related to the TNM system of staging. A review. Cancer 25:485, 1970.

71. Lederman, M., and Dalley, V. M.: The treatment of glottic cancer. The importance of radiotherapy to the patient. J. Laryngol. Otol. 79:767, 1965.

72. Perez, C. A., Holtz, S., Ogura, J. H., Dedo, H. H., and Powers, W. E.: Radiation therapy of early carcinoma of the true vocal cords. Cancer 21:764, 1968.

73. Perez, C. A., Mill, W. B., Ogura, J. H., and Powers, W. E.: Irradiation of early carcinoma of the larynx: significance of tumor extent. Arch. Otolaryngol. 93:465, 1971.

74. Brand, W. N., and Moss, W. T.: Radiotherapy of the larynx. Otolaryngol. Clin. North Am. 3:581, 1970.

75. Sisson, G. A., Goldstein, J. C., and Becker, G. D.: Surgery of limited lesions of the larynx (past and present). Otolaryngol. Clin. North Am. 3:529, 1970.

76. Kirchner, J. A.: Cancer of the anterior commissure of the larynx. Arch. Otolaryngol. 91:524, 1970.

77. Som, M. L., and Silver, C. E.: The anterior commissure technique of partial laryngectomy. Arch. Otolaryngol. 87:138, 1968.

78. Biller, H. F., Ogura, J. H., and Pratt, L. L.: Hemilaryngectomy for T_2 glottic cancers. Arch. Otolaryngol. 93:238, 1971.

79. Olofsson, J., Williams, G. T., Rider, W. D., and Bryce, D. P.: Anterior commissure carcinoma: primary treatment with radiotherapy in 57 patients. Arch. Otolaryngol. 95:230, 1972.

80. Jesse, R. H., Lindberg, R. D., and Horiot, J.-C. Vocal cord cancer with anterior commissure extension: choice of treatment. Am. J. Surg. 122:437, 1971.

81. Wang, C. C., and Schulz, M. D.: Treatment of cancer of the larynx by irradiation. Ann. Otol. Rhinol. Laryngol. 72:637, 1963.

82. Biller, H. F., Barnhill, F. R., Jr., Ogura, J. H., and Perez, C. A.: Hemilaryngectomy following radiation failure for acrinoma of the vocal cords. Laryngoscope 80:249, 1970.

83. Kirchner, J. A., and Som, M. L.: Clinical and histological observations on supraglottic cancer. Ann. Otol. Rhinol. Laryngol. 80:638, 1971.

84. Baclesse, F.: Carcinoma of the larynx. Br. J. Radiol. (suppl.) 3:1, 1949.

85. Coates, H. L., DeSanto, L. W., Devine, K. D., and Elveback, L. R.: Carcinoma of the supraglottic larynx. A review of 221 cases. Arch. Otolaryngol. 102:686, 1976.

86. Calcaterra, T. C.: Supraglottic laryngectomy with preservation of laryngeal function. Am. Surg. 37:393, 1970.

87. Ogura, J. H., and Biller, H. F.: Conservative surgery in carcinomas of the head and neck. Otolaryngol. Clin. North Am. 1:641, 1969.

88. Hajek, M.: Anatomische Untersuchungen über das larynxödem. Arch. Klin. Chir. 42:46, 1891.

89. Ogura, J. H., Spector, G. J., and Sessions, D. G.: Conservation surgery for epidermoid carcinoma of the marginal area (aryepiglottic fold extension). Laryngoscope 85:1801, 1975.

90. Dayal, V. S., Bahri, H., and Stone, P. C.: Pre-epiglottic space: an anatomic study. Arch Otolaryngol. 95:130, 1972.

91. Workshop No. 6.: Roles with limitations of conservative surgical therapy for laryngeal carcinoma. Canad. J. Otolaryngol. 4:392, 1974.

92. Ogura, J. H., Sessions, D. G., and Spector, G. J.: Conservation surgery for epidermoid carcinoma of the supraglottic larynx. Laryngoscope 85:1808, 1975.

93. Som, M. L.: Conservative surgery for carcinoma of the supraglottis. J. Laryngol. Otol. 84:655, 1970.

94. Harrison, D. F. N.: The pathology and management of subglottic cancer. Ann. Otol. Rhinol. Laryngol. 80:6, 1971.

95. Lund, W. S.: Classification of subglottic tumors and discussion of their growth and spread. Canad. J. Otolaryngol. 3:469, 1974.

96. Martensson, B.: Transconioscopy in cancer of the larynx. Acta Otolaryngol. (suppl.) 224:476, 1967.

97. Martensson, B.: Aspects on treatment of cancer of the larynx. Ann. Otol. Rhinol. Laryngol. 76:313, 1967.

97a. Shaw, H. J.: Glottic cancer of the larynx. J. Laryngol. Otol. 79:1, 1965.

98. Harrison, D. F. N.: Cancer of the hypopharynx and cervical oesophagus. Br. J. Surg. 56:95, 1969.

99. Leading article: Treatment of carcinoma of the larynx. Br. Med. J. 2:417, 1971.

100. Lederman, M.: Radiotherapy of cancer of the larynx. J. Laryngol. Otol. 84:867, 1970.

101. Roswit, B., Spiro, R. H., Kolson, H., and Lin, P. Y.: Planned preoperative irradiation and surgery for advanced cancer of the oral cavity, pharynx and larynx. Ann. J. Roentgenol. Radium Ther. Nucl. Med. 114:59, 1972.

102. Lott, S., Anas, M. E.-M., and Hazra, T.: Supervoltage radiotherapy of carcinoma of the larynx. Johns Hopkins Hosp. Med. J. 130:244, 1972.

103. Bryce, D. P., and Rider, W. D.: Pre-operative irradiation in the treatment of advanced laryngeal carcinoma. Laryngoscope 81:1481, 1971.

104. Levitt, S. H., Beachley, M. C., Zimberg, Y., Pastore, P. N., DeGiorgi, L. S., and King, E. R.: Combination of preoperative irradiation and surgery in the treatment of cancer of the oropharynx, hypopharynx, and larynx. Cancer 27:759, 1971.

105. Goldman, J. L., and Friedman, W. H.: High dose preoperative irradiation in cancer of the larynx. Otolaryngol. Clin. North Am. 2:473, 1969.

106. Futrell, J. W., Bennett, S. H., Hoye, R. C., Roth, J. A., and Ketcham, A. S.: Predicting survival in cancer of the larynx or hypopharynx. Am. J. Surg. 122:451, 1971.

107. McGavran, M., and Bauer, W. C.: Sinus histiocytosis and cervical lymph nodal metastases from transglottic epidermoid carcinoma of the larynx. Canad. J. Otolaryngol. 4:903, 1975.

108. Berlinger, N. T., Tsakpraklides, V., Pollack, K., Adams, G. L., Yang, M., and Good, R. A.: Prognostic significance of lymph node histology in patients with squamous cell carcinoma of the larynx, pharynx, or oral cavity. Laryngoscope 86:792, 1976.

109. Bauer, W. C., Lesinski, S. G., and Ogura, J. H.: The significance of positive margins in hemilaryngectomy specimens. Laryngoscope 85:1, 1975.

110. Batsakis, J. G., Hybels, R., and Rice, D. H.: Laryngeal carcinoma: stomal recurrences and distant metastases. Canad. J. Otolaryngol. 4:906, 1975.

111. Bauer, W. C., Edwards, D. L., and McGavran, M. H.: A critical analysis of laryngectomy in the treatment of epidermoid carcinoma of the larynx. Cancer 15:263, 1962.

112. Modlin, B., and Ogura, J. H.: Postlaryngectomy tracheal stomal recurrences. Laryngoscope 79:239, 1969.

113. Keim, W. F., Shapiro, M. J., and Rosen, H. O.: Study of postlaryngectomy stomal recurrences. Arch. Otolaryngol. 81:183, 1965.

114. Stell, P. M., and Van Den Broek, P.: Stomal recurrence after laryngectomy: aetiology and management. J. Laryngol. 85:131, 1971.

115. Loewy, A., and Laker, H. I.: Tracheal stomal problems.

Arch. Otolaryngol. 87:477, 1968.

116. de Jong, P. C.: Intubation and tumor implantation in laryngeal carcinoma. Pract. Otolaryngol. 31:119, 1969.

117. Schneider, J. J., Lindberg, R. D., and Jesse, R. H.: Prevention of tracheal stoma recurrences after total laryngectomy by postoperative irradiation. J. Surg. Oncol. 7:187, 1975.

118. Ogura, J. H., and Biller, H.: Cysts and tumors of the larynx. In Otolaryngology, edited by M. Paparella and R. Shumrich, W. B. Saunders Co., Philadelphia, 1973.

119. Sisson, G. A.: Extended radical surgery for stomal recurrences. Otolaryngol. Clin. N. Am. 2:617, 1969.

120. Crile, G. W.: Cancer of jaws, tongue, cheeks, and lips. Surg. Gynec. Obstet. 36:159, 1923.

121. Castigliano, S. G., and Rominger, C. J.: Distant metastases from carcinomas of oral cavity. Am. J. Roentgenol. 71:997, 1954.

122. Harrer, W. V., and Lewis, P. L.: Carcinomas of the larynx with cardiac metastasis. Arch. Otolaryngol. 91:382, 1970.

123. Abramson, A. L., Parisier, S. C., and Zamansky, M. J.: Distant metastases from carcinoma of the larynx. Laryngoscope 81:1503, 1971.

124. O'Brien, P. H., Carlson, R., Steubner, E. A., and Staley, C. T.: Distant metastases in epidermoid cell carcinoma of the head and neck. Cancer 27:304, 1971.

125. Alonso, J. M.: Metastasis of laryngeal and hypopharyngeal carcinoma. Acta Otolaryngol. 64:353, 1967.

126. Braud, R. R., and Martin, H. E.: Distant metastasis in cancer of the upper respiratory and alimentary tracts. Surg. Gynecol. Obstet. 73:63, 1941.

127. Probert, J. C., Thompson, R. W., and Bagshaw, M. A.: Patterns of distant metastases in head and neck cancer. Cancer 33:127, 1974.

128. Mumma, C. S., and Chusid, L. A.: Distant metastases from primary malignancies of the endolarynx. Laryngoscope 71:524, 1961.

129. Ju, D. M. C.: A study of the behavior of cancer of the head and neck during its late and terminal phases. Am. J. Surg. 108:552, 1964.

130. Matsusaka, T., Watanabe, H., and Enjoji, M.: Pseudosarcoma and carcinosarcoma of the esophagus. Cancer 37:1546, 1976.

131. Someren, A., Karcioglu, Z., and Clairmont, A. A.: Polypoid spindle-cell carcinoma (pleomorphic carcinoma). Report of a case occurring on tongue and review of the literature. Oral Surg. 42:474, 1977.

132. Hyams, V. J.: Spindle cell carcinoma of the larynx. Canad. J. Otolaryngol. 4:307, 1975.

133. Randall, G., Alonso, W. A., and Ogura, J. H.: Spindle cell carcinoma (pseudosarcoma) of the larynx. Arch. Otolaryngol. 101:63, 1975.

134. Battifora, H.: Spindle cell carcinoma. Ultrastructural evidence of squamous origin and collagen production by the tumor cells. Cancer 37:2275, 1976.

135. Lane, N.: Pseudosarcoma (polypoid sarcoma-like masses) associated with squamous cell carcinoma of the mouth, fauces, and larynx. Cancer 19:19, 1957.

136. Sherwin, R. P., Strong, M. S., and Vaughn, C. W., Jr.: Polypoid and junctional squamous cell carcinoma of the tongue and larynx with spindle cell carcinoma ("pseudosarcoma"). Cancer 16:51, 1963.

137. Goellner, J. R., Devine, K. D., and Weiland, L. H.: Pseudosarcoma of the larynx. Am. J. Clin. Pathol. 59:312, 1973.

138. Friedel, W., Chambers, R. G., and Atkins, J. P.: Pseudosarcoma of the pharynx and larynx. Arch. Otolaryngol. 102:286, 1976.

139. Appelman, H. D., and Oberman, H. A.: Squamous cell carcinoma of the larynx with sarcoma-like stroma. Am. J. Clin. Pathol. 44:135, 1965.

140. Davies, D. G.: Fibrosarcoma and pseudosarcoma of the larynx. J. Laryngol. Otol. 83:423, 1969.

141. Flanagan, A., Cross, R. M., and Libcke, J. H.: Fibrosarcoma

of the larynx. J. Laryngol. Otol. 79:1049, 1965.

142. Barsocchini, L. M., and McCoy, G.: Cartilaginous tumors of the larynx: a review of the literature and report of four cases. Ann. Otol. Rhinol. Laryngol. 77:141, 1968.

143. Cocke, E. W.: Benign cartilagenous tumors of the larynx. Ann. Otol. Rhinol. Laryngol. 72:1678, 1962.

144. Huizenga, C., and Balogh, K.: Cartilaginous tumors of the larynx: a clinicopathologic study of 10 new cases and a review of the literature. Cancer 26:201, 1970.

145. Hyams, V. J., and Rabuzzi, D. D.: Cartilaginous tumors of the larynx. Laryngoscope 80:755, 1970.

146. Greer, J. A., Devine, K. D., and Dahlin, D. C.: Gardner's syndrome and chondrosarcoma of the hyoid bone. Arch. Otolaryngol. 103:425, 1977.

147. Daniels, A. C., Conner, G. H., and Straus, F. H.: Primary chondrosarcoma of the tracheobronchial tree: report of a unique case and brief review. Arch. Pathol. 84:615, 1967.

148. Lichtenstein, L., and Jaffe, H.: Chondrosarcoma of bone. Am. J. Pathol. 19:553, 1943.

149. Spjut, H. J., Dorfman, H. D., Fechner, R. E., and Ackerman, L. V.: Tumors of bone and cartilage. In Atlas of Tumor Pathology. Series 2, Fascicle 5. Armed Forces Institute of Pathology, Washington, D.C., 1970.

150. Goethals, P. L., Dahlin, D. C., and Devine, K. D.: Cartilaginous tumors of the larynx. Surg. Gynecol. Obstet. 117:77, 1963.

151. Ferguson, G. B.: Hemangioma of the adult and of the infant larynx. Arch. Otolaryngol. 40:189, 1944.

152. Bridger, G. P., Nassar, V. H., and Skinner, H. G.: Hemangioma in the adult larynx. Arch. Otolaryngol. 92:493, 1970.

153. Minnigerode, B.: Das subglottische Kehlokopfhamangiom des Neugeborenen. Zeit. F. Laryngol. 49:585, 1970.

154. Calcaterra, T. C.: An evaluation of the treatment of subglottic hemanangiomas. Laryngoscope 78:1956, 1968.

155. Charachon, R., Junien-Lavillauroy, C., Accoyer, B., Roux, O., and Frapport, P.: The place of cryosurgery in the treatment of subglottic angioma of the infant. Clin. Otolaryngol. 2:207, 1977.

156. Benjamin, B.: Treatment of infantile subglottic hemangioma with radioactive gold grain. Ann. Otol. 87:18, 1978.

157. Chang-Lo, M.: Laryngeal involvement in von Recklinghausen's disease: a case report and review of the literature. Laryngoscope 87:435, 1977.

158. Zakrzewski, A.: Subglottic lipoma of the larynx. J. Laryngol. Otol. 79:1039, 1965.

159. Hudson, C., Cove, P., and Adekeye, E. O.: Liposarcoma of the head and neck: report of case and review of the literature. J. Oral Surg. 36:380, 1978.

160. Ferlito, A.: Primary pleomorphic liposarcoma of the larynx. J. Otolaryngol. 7:161, 1978.

161. Frugoni, P., and Ferlito, A.: Pleomorphic rhabdomyosarcoma of the larynx. A case report and review of the literature. J. Laryngol. 90:687, 1976.

162. DeSanto, L. W., and Weiland, L. H.: Malignant lymphoma of the larynx. Laryngoscope 80:966, 1970.

163. Dickson, R.: Lymphoma of the larynx. Laryngoscope 81:578, 1971.

164. Anderson, H. A., Maisel, R. H., and Cantrell, R. W.: Isolated laryngeal lymphoma. Laryngoscope 86:1251, 1976.

165. Pahor, A. L.: Plasmacytoma of the larynx. J. Laryngol. 92:223, 1978.

166. Ryan, R. E., Jr., Pearson, B. W., and Weiland, L. H.: Laryngeal amyloidosis. Tr. Am. Acad. Ophth. Otol. 84:872, 1977.

167. Deodhare, S. G., and Dasgupta, G.: Primary amyloidosis of the trachea. J. Laryngol. 89:645, 1975.

168. McAlpine, J. C., and Fuller, A. P.: Localized laryngeal amyloidosis: a report of a case with a review of the literature. J. Laryngol. 78:296, 1964.

169. Kyle, R. A., and Bayrd, E. D.: Amyloidosis: review of 236 cases. Medicine 54:271, 1975.

CHAPTER 10

Teratomas of the Head and Neck

Teratomas are tumors or neoplasms composed of multiple tissues foreign to the part of the body in which they arise. Outside their principal sites of origin (genital organs, retroperitoneum and mediastinum), teratomas are generally regarded as pathological curiosities and, as such, elicit only isolated case reports without efforts made toward an over-all appraisal of their biological activity. This statement is particularly true for teratomas of the head and neck and is exemplified by the four scant lines given to their discussion in a monograph of neoplasms of the upper respiratory tract.[1]

An explanation of terminology is necessary. The term *teratoma* is used here in the generic sense to include teratoid tumors, epignathi and "dermoid" tumors. Teratoid has been used by some to indicate teratomatous neoplasms or acquired lesions that lack a trigerminal or complex histological appearance. In true teratomas, failure to demonstrate more than two germ-layer components may represent only a sectioning artefact and, hence, not justify a separate category. The term dermoid cyst is, unfortunately, frequently used as a synonym for benign cystic teratoma. That the same name is applied justifiably to unrelated sequestration cysts makes separation of the two types of lesions difficult. The dermoid cysts to be discussed here represent both types and, in fact, are numerically dominated by the nonteratomatous types.

The neck and nasopharynx are the most common sites for teratomas in the head and neck. Nearly 100 examples have been reported from each anatomical area.

True teratomas of this region, like those of the saccrococcygeal region and chest, very likely arise from embryonic tissue about the primitive streak and notochord after an escape from external governing influences.[2]

DERMOID CYSTS AND RELATED CYSTIC LESIONS

As implied above, the term "dermoid cyst" has been rather loosely applied to a number of presumably dysontogenetic cystic lesions wherever they occur in the body. New and Erich,[3] for example, included pilonidal cysts in their review of 1,495 patients with dermoid cysts. "Dermoid cyst" is also still preferred by clinicians to the more appropriate and correct "benign cystic teratoma of the ovary." In the head and neck, "dermoid cyst" may apply to three varieties of cysts: (1) epidermoid or epidermal cyst; (2) *dermoid* cyst; and (3) teratoid cyst.[4]

The epidermoid cyst is lined by a simple squamous epithelium with a fibrous wall and no adenexal structures. The dermoid cyst is an epithelial-lined cavity with variable numbers of skin appendages (hair, hair follicles, sebaceous glands, sudoriferous glands, etc.). The lining of the teratoid cyst ranges from simple stratified squamous epithelium to ciliated respiratory-type epithelium (Fig. 10.1). These different epithelia may coexist in the same cyst and are accompanied often by not only skin appendages, but derivations of the mesoderm and entoderm as well as the ectoderm. All three types may contain a cheesy keratinaceous material in their cavities. The epidermoid variety is most common; the dermoid is next in frequency and the teratoid cyst or teratoma is considered rare in the head and neck.

Pathogenesis of these lesions remains as obscure as it did half a century ago, and it serves no clinical purpose to relate the hypotheses. In general, two prevail. The dermoid cysts arise from epithelium that has been enclaved in the tissue either on closure of embryogenic processes or from traumatic implantation. A small, related group are the heterotopias or choristomatic cysts. We shall dispose of this class before discussing the larger group of "dermoid cysts."

Gorlin and Jirasek[5] analyzed 13 reported cases of oral cysts that contained gastric or intestinal mucosa in the tongue or in the floor of the mouth, which may communicate with the surface. Proximity of the undifferentiated primitive stomach to the anlage of the tongue in the embryogenic mid-neck region is related to the heterotopias.

Defined loosely, dermoid cysts of the head and neck account for nearly 7% of *all* dermoid cysts.[6] New and Erich[3] divided them into four categories according to their anatomical distribution and their presumed embryogenic derivation. Those of the midfacial region have been most intensively studied (Fig. 10.2).

Dermoid Cysts of the Nose

Less than 150 cases of median dermoid cysts of the nose have been reported. They constitute about 3% of all dermoids and approximately 7.6% of those occurring in the head and neck.[6] Clinical features are as follows.[6, 7]

Age. Often apparent shortly after birth, the age range is wide (3 months to 59 years), with an average age at time of diagnosis and treatment between 12 and 13 years.

Sex. There is an apparent predominance in the male in the ratio of 2:1.

Size. Because of their position, the cysts rarely exceed 4 cm in diameter.

Site. Several variations in a limited area have been described, but they are almost exclusively all in the midline: (1) dorsum or root of nose—most common site; (2) tip of nose; (3) columella.

There is a high incidence of primary surgical failure with one-fourth to one-half the total number of patients giving a history of one or more surgical attempts at correction of the lesion.[6]

The mode of presentation is dependent upon the location of the cyst. The first indication of a superficial dermoid of the nose may only be a small dimple on the bridge of the nose. Hairs may protrude from the dimple. The pit represents the opening of a sinus that may extend deeply between the nasal bones to the cribriform plate or into the nasal septum itself. These deeply placed cysts are constricted where they pass through the nasal bones, producing a "dumbbell" effect with a small

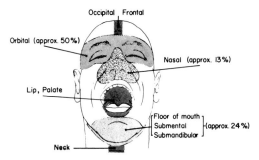

Figure 10.2. Dermoid cysts of the head and neck are predominantly found in the orbital, oral and nasal regions (over 80%). The remainder are found in the neck, occipital or frontal midline, or lip and palate. Note the sparing of the upper lip.

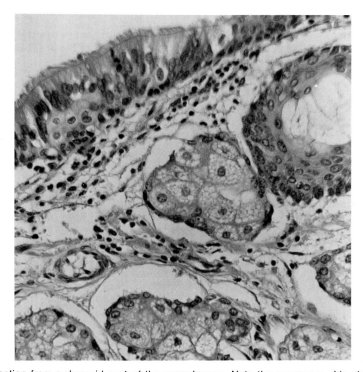

Figure 10.1. Section from a dermoid cyst of the nasopharynx. Note the accessory skin structures beneath respiratory epithelium.

subcutaneous mass over which the skin moves freely. Cysts involving the nasal bones produce a marked broadening of the nasal bridge. Cellulitis and purulent discharge following infection may also be presenting signs. Deeper cysts are liable to present with nasal obstruction, and, occasionally, there may be signs of an intracranial lesion.

The most important differential diagnosis is that of an encephalocele. When a nasal dermoid is suspected, radiographic examination of the skull and facial bones is essential.[6] This examination must include anteroposterior lateral and Water's projections. These may show a broadened or bifid nasal septum, and there may be evidence of bone destruction or separation of the nasal bones due to distortion by the cyst. If a sinus exists, accurate localization can be accomplished by contrast studies.

Because of progressive expansion, destruction of bone and the possibility of secondary infection, early surgical removal is recommended if feasible. Nearly half of the nasal dermoids extend deeply to the nasal bones, and this should be determined before surgical intervention. The relatively high recurrence rate is directly related to their inaccessibility during attempted removal. In recurring lesions, complete dissection of the epithelial lining may be difficult; such recurrences are less likely if the lining is destroyed by electrocoagulation.[8]

Dermoid Cysts of the Oral Cavity

When found in the oral cavity, dermoid cysts are usually in the anterior portion of the floor of the mouth. The incidence in this region is low, approximately 1.6% of all dermoids, but they form striking clinical entities.[9, 10] Nearly all examples in

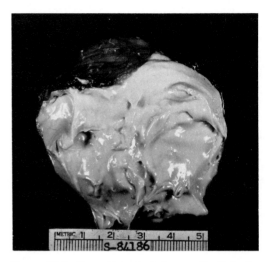

Figure 10.4. Dermoid cyst of the mouth. Note the apparent encapsulation and the thick cheesy (keratinaceous) material in the lumen.

the oral cavity are either acquired-implantation cysts or congenital enclaves of tissue.

In the simplest manner of classification, dermoid cysts of the floor of the mouth may present in either a sublingual or submental position (Fig. 10.3). They are invariably midline, and doubt exists to the authenticity of so-called true-lateral dermoids. Seward[9] describes in detail a complicated subclassification of these lesions. These cysts usually become manifest during the second or third decades of life but probably have been present since birth. There is no significant sex predominance.

Sublingual dermoids raise the tongue, simulate a ranula and may interfere with deglutition (Fig. 10.4). The sublingual dermoid may grow to sufficient size to present as a large pedunculated mass beneath the mandible. Submental dermoids usually present as external swellings just above the hyoid bone. Rare forms occur on the dorsum of tongue and hard and soft palate. Treatment is complete surgical removal.

Teratomas of the Nasopharynx

Most of these teratomas arise from the midline or lateral wall of the nasopharynx and are present at birth. Rarely is a patient seen for the first time after age 21. If so, the condition has probably been present, but undetected, for much longer than the clinical history indicates. Females are affected six times as often as males.[11] The dermoid or dermoid cyst is the most common nasopharyngeal teratoma.

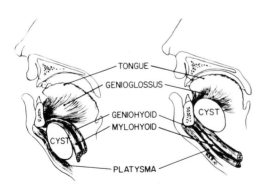

Figure 10.3. Two consistent localizations of dermoid cysts of the floor of the mouth. The cyst is either at the base of the tongue and above the muscle masses or lies between the platysma and the mylohyoid muscles. The latter presents in the neck as well as in the mouth.

The "hairy polyp," a dermoid often covered by hairy skin, appears at birth or later and is attached to the hard or soft palate, to the wall or vault of the pharynx or in or near the midline; it fills the nares or the oral cavity. Sometimes an intracranial portion is connected with the main mass through a perforation in the skull. The main mass consists largely of fibroadipose tissue with cartilage, bone and slips of skeletal muscle.

Complex teratoid tumors or teratomas differ from the more common dermoids not only in their histological appearance, but also in their frequent association with extensive deformities of the skull (e.g, anencephalies, hemicrania and palatal fissures). The least common variety, but the most striking, is epignathus, which consists of well formed organs and limbs of a parasitic fetus. The otolaryngologist rarely sees highly developed tumors, since the more highly developed the lesion (epignathus), the greater the chance of a stillborn fetus.

Signs and symptoms depend on the size and site of the tumor. Hairy polyps are usually pedunculated and, not infrequently, the pedicle is long enough to permit considerable mobility and, hence, intermittent symptomatology. Sessile tumors or those with short pedicles, which completely block the nasopharynx, not only obstruct the normal airway but may also impede mouth breathing as well. If the nasopharyngeal obstruction is only partial, symptoms will be milder and may impede correct diagnosis. Clinical diagnosis is not difficult with the larger tumors or when coughing brings a pedunculated tumor to view. Tumors appearing for the first time in later life may be mistaken for "fibromas" or papillomas.

The method of surgical removal depends on the type of gross presentation. Pedunculated tumors are removable with a snare. Sessile tumors in the nasopharynx have been grasped by forceps and avulsed.[12] As indicated earlier, the prognosis is related to the histological development of the tumor and to the association with cranial deformities. After review of 89 patients with dermoids of the nasopharynx, not one death could be attributed to the tumor itself.[11]

As stated above, teratomas of the nasopharynx and paranasal sinuses are almost always composed of well-differentiated tissues and present in infants and children. Neuroectodermal and neural tissues predominate. The presence of immature or differentiating neural cells in an otherwise benign teratoma is of little prognostic significance. If removable, these tumors rarely recur whether or not they contain immature foci.

In teratomas, there are anomalies of both the level of differentiation and also the type of differentiation. A low level of differentiation with a concentration of cells on a replicative rather than functional activity is seen in the malignant teratoma. In the nasopharynx and paranasal sinuses, *teratocarcinomas* arise high in the nasal cavity and in or around the ethmoid sinuses (Fig. 10.5). They also are diagnosed in an older group of patients—young and middle aged adults. Reported examples[13, 14] have contained representatives of all three so-called germ layers and a preponderance of neuroectodermal derivatives. Massive and rapid recurrence characterize these life-consuming lesions. Perhaps the rapidity of intracranial extension is accountable for the absence of lymphogenous and hematogenous spread of the teratocarcinomas of this region.

Teratoma of the Orbit

A subclassification of this rare teratoma has recently been offered.[15] My modication of this subclassification is as follows:

1. A complete fetus in the orbit, extremely rare (only two cases reported).

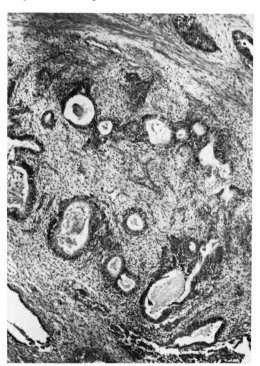

Figure 10.5. Malignant teratoma from the ethmoid sinus. In this instance, the glandular component is the malignant tissue. The teratomatous nature of the neoplasm was not evident until the resected specimen was examined.

2. A portion of a second fetus in the orbit (only one case reported).

3. A tumor containing derivatives of the germinal layer (two or three components) but without fetal configuration. This type is entirely analogous histologically to the gonadal teratomas of germinal origin.

4. Dermoid cysts containing only representatives of the ectodermal germ layer.

The dermoid cyst is the most common teratoid tumor in the orbit. The complex-mature teratoma is the next most frequently encountered type but, in reality, it is a rare tumor in the orbit. By 1965, only an estimated 21 trigerminal teratomas of the orbit had been reported.[16] The patient with a true teratoma of the orbit is born with exophthalmos caused by the mass behind the eye. Dermoid cysts, on the other hand, do not usually become obvious until later in life.[17] There is usually some degree of microphthalmos. The teratomas are almost invariably unilateral and almost always benign.

Intraorbital teratomas may extend through defects in the orbital bones into the nasal cavity, anterior and midline cranial fossae or temporal fossa. Such tumors have a cystic-dumbbell or hourglass shape. As with teratomas elsewhere, they show a great variety of tissues. Dermoid cysts have the usual histological appearance.

In the past, exenteration of the orbit of infants with teratomas was associated with a high mortality rate. In recent years, improvements in anesthetic and surgical techniques and in postoperative care have greatly improved the outlook. Nevertheless, the approach to and dissection of the orbital tumor require a high order of judgment. If there has been extension outside the orbit, a combined ophthalmological, neurosurgical and otolaryngological procedure is certainly indicated.

Teratomas of the Neck

Several investigators have presented clinical and pathological analyses of teratomas of the neck, each report dealing with more than 87 patients.[18, 19] Cervical teratomas are rare in patients over the age of 1 year, and are most commonly present at birth in full-term, premature or stillborn infants. Far fewer teratomas of the neck have been documented in adults.[20, 21] There is no significant sex difference.

The clinical presentation of a cervical teratoma is almost invariably that of a mass in the neck discovered at birth. Such infants usually have acute respiratory symptoms (e.g., stridor, apnea and cyanosis) due to compression or deviation of the trachea. Dysphagia may result from pressure on the esophagus. A few patients are asymptomatic at birth, only to develop symptoms in the first few weeks or months of life. There is no increased incidence of coexistent congenital abnormalities or anomalies. However, the association of maternal hydramnios is often a prominent feature; an incidence of 19.6% versus the usual 0.5% has been observed.[22]

Since the majority of soft tissue or lymphoreticular tumors which occur in the neck during childhood are not present at birth, the chief tumors to be distinguished from teratomas are cystic lymphangioma, congenital goiter, branchial cleft and thyroglossal cysts. Because of similarity in age and sex incidence, size, gross characteristics and localization, cystic lymphangioma presents the most difficult differential diagnosis. The hygroma, however, has a more limpid or cystic consistency and less well defined margins or borders, and it is readily transilluminated. Although lymphangiomas arise in the posterior triangle of the neck, such origin is usually obscured by the size of the tumor.

Proximity to and involvement of the thyroid gland has prompted a division of cervical teratomas into three categories[22]: "teratomas of the thyroid gland," which derive blood supply from thyroidal arteries; "teratomas in the region of the thyroid gland," which displace the thyroid gland but lack definite blood supply from thyroidal arteries; and "teratomas of the neck, probably in the region of the thyroid gland." This classification has been criticized as artificial, cumbersome and unnecessary except for teratological purposes.[23] Since only a small minority of these neoplasms are true teratomas of the thyroid gland, a preferable designation is teratoma of the neck or cervical teratoma. The thyroid gland is usually involved when there is a teratoma of the neck, but subdivision or classification, if necessary, must await examination of a larger number of tumors in which the known blood supply is available.

The majority of the neoplasms are large, measuring between 5 and 12 cm in longest axis. They are usually semicystic but may be solid or multiloculated. Overlying skin is usually freely movable. The bulk of the mass is usually unilateral, although the medial border often extends across the anterior midline in close relation to the thyroid gland and trachea. Encapsulation is the rule, facilitating dissection from surrounding tissue.

All varieties of tissue from the three germinal layers, sometimes as many as 15,[24] have been found in these tumors. Central nervous system tissue is often conspicuously abundant, but this is not unique to cervical teratomas. Overt histological malignant change in a gonadal teratoma is unusual in childhood, especially in those removed shortly after birth.[25] Similar clinical behavior has characterized cervical teratomas. Focal immaturity of tissue components may suggest malignant change, but such areas are usually in keeping with the immaturity of the host. Two infants with cervical teratoma had teratomatous tissue in cervical lymph nodes at the time of surgical excision.[18] The neoplasm in each contained areas of undifferentiated embryonic and nervous tissue, and, in each, "metastasis" to the lymph node contained embryonic nervous tissue. It should be emphasized, however, that the "metastasis" (if valid) in these two patients was exceptional.[26] There has been no instance of a benign teratoma of the neck in adults.[19]

Early surgical removal is mandatory in the management of these tumors in infants. Delay, when partial respiratory obstruction exists, usually results in retention of secretion, atelectasis and lobular pneumonia. Respiratory obstruction and its complications have been the most common cause of death in infants with cervical teratomas. Of 22 live newborns who were not treated by surgical excision of the tumor, all died. This disheartening death rate is compared to an estimated 9% mortality with surgical treatment.[23]

Although follow-up periods are short, documented malignant teratomas of the neck, are few in number and all have occurred in adults.[20, 21] Histological examination usually reveals a conspicious neural component accompanied by poorly differentiated carcinoma and/or sarcoma. Metastases (lymphatic and blood vascular) are common and prognosis is poor. Survival for malignant teratomas of the neck is expressed in terms of months rather than years.

Hamartomas

Hamartomas are simple and spontaneous growths composed exclusively of components derived from *local tissue*. The growths produce an excessive number of cells that reach maturity and then cease to reproduce, so that the growths are self-limiting. In many instances, the resulting lesions seem to represent a simple exaggeration of a normal physiological process. Hamartomas more often than not present many clinical features of a neoplasm although basically they are malformations.

In the sense of the above description, hemangiomas and angiomatosis may be considered as hamartomatous lesions, as well as congenital li-

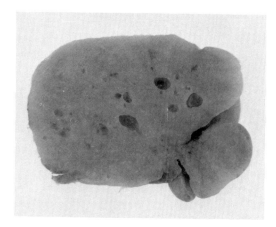

Figure 10.6. Nasopharyngeal hamartoma in a young child. Microscopically the lesion consisted of glands, ducts and supporting tissue elements indigenous to the area. Note the dilated ducts.

pomas, tuberous sclerosis and its congeners, multiple enchondrosis, multiple exostosis, neurofibromas and melanotic nevi.

Hamartomas in the upper respiratory tract are unusual, at least as judged by the literature.[27, 28] Cartilagenous hamartomas may arise in the larynx as well as trachea and lungs. They invariably contain other mesodermal components as well as epithelium. They are exceedingly rare in the paranasal sinuses. Glandular hamartomas are also unusual in the upper airway (Fig. 10.6).

REFERENCES

1. Ash, J. E., Beck, M. R., and Wilkes, J. D.: Tumors of the upper respiratory tract and ear. In Atlas of Tumor Pathology, Section IV, Fascicles 12 and 13. Armed Forces Institute of Pathology, Washington D.C., 1964.
2. Damjonov, I., and Solter, D.: Teratoma and teratocarcinoma. Animal model: Embryo-derived teratomas and teratocarcinomas in mice. Am. J. Path. 83:241, 1976.
3. New, G. B., and Erich, J. B.: Dermoid cysts of the head and neck. Surg. Gynecol. Obstet. 65:48, 1937.
4. Batsakis, J. G.: Non-odontogenic and fissural cysts. ORL. 33:19, 1971.
5. Gorlin, R. J., and Jirasek, J. E.: Oral cysts containing gastric or intestinal mucosa: unusual embryologic accident or heterotopia. J. Oral Surg. 28:9, 1970.
6. Taylor, B. W., and Erich, J. B.: Dermoid cysts of the nose. Mayo Clin. Proc. 42:488, 1967.
7. Khan, M. A., and Gib, A. G.: Median dermoid cysts of the nose: familial occurrence. J. Laryngol. Otol. 84:709, 1970.
8. Batsakis, J. G., and Farber, E. R.: Teratomas of the head and neck. Eye Ear Nose Throat Mon. 30:67, 1968.
9. Seward, G. R.: Dermoid cysts of the floor of the mouth. Br. J. Oral Surg. 3:36, 1965.
10. Meyer, I.: Dermoid cysts (dermoids) of the floor of the mouth. Oral Surg. 8:1149, 1955.
11. Foxwell, P. B., and Kelham, B. H.: Teratoid tumors of the nasopharynx. J. Laryngol. Otol. 72:647, 1958.
12. Sollee, A. N.: Nasopharyngeal teratoma. Arch. Otolaryngol. 82:49, 1965.
13. Patchefsky, A., Sundmaker, W., and Marden, P. A.: Malignant teratoma of the ethmoid sinus. Cancer 21:714, 1968.

14. Dicke, T. E., and Gates, G. A.: Malignant teratoma of the paranasal sinuses. Arch. Otolaryngol. 91:391, 1970.
15. Duke-Elder, W. S.: System of Ophthalmology, vol. 3, pp. 966–974. Henry Kimpton, London, 1964.
16. Ferry, A. P.: Teratoma of the orbit: report of two cases. Surv. Ophthalmol. 10:434, 1965.
17. Jones, S. T.: Dermoid and teratoid tumors of the eye and orbit. J. Arkansas Med. Soc. 60:66, 1963.
18. Batsakis, J. G., Littler, E. R., and Oberman, H. A.: Teratomas of the neck: a clinicopathological appraisal. Arch. Otolaryngol. 79:619, 1964.
19. Hajdu, S. I., and Hajdu, E. O.: Malignant teratoma of the neck. Arch. Pathol. 83:567, 1967.
20. Kemp, D. R.: Teratoma of the neck in the adult. Report of a case and review of the literature. Aust. N.Z.J. Surg. 36:320, 1967.
21. Rundle, F. W.: Cervical teratomata. J. Otolaryngol. 5:513, 1976.
22. Bale, G. F.: Teratoma of the neck in region of thyroid gland: review of literature and report of four cases. Am. J. Pathol. 26:565, 1950.
23. Keynes, W. M.: Teratoma of neck in relation to thyroid gland. Br. J. Surg. 46:466, 1959.
24. Potter, E. L.: Teratoma of thyroid gland. Arch. Pathol. 25:689, 1938.
25. Batsakis, J. G.: Tumors of testis in infancy and childhood. Arch. Pathol. 72:27, 1961.
26. Pupovac, D.: Ein Fall von Teratoma colli mit Veranderungen in dest regionaren Lymphdrusen. Arch. Klin. Chir. 53:59, 1896.
27. Majumder, N. K., Venkataramaniah, N. K., Gupta, K. R., and Goplakrishnan, S.: Hamartoma of nasopharynx. J. Laryngol. 91:723, 1977.
28. Baille, E. E., and Batsakis, J. G.: Glandular (seromucinous) hamartoma of the nasopharynx. Oral Surg. 38:760, 1974.

CHAPTER 11

Parenchymal Cysts of the Neck

Cervical cysts taking their origin from *parenchymal organs* other than the thyroid gland (thymic, parathyroid, thyroglossal and bronchogenic) constitute a small, but nevertheless important, category of lesions of the head and neck.

THYMIC CYSTS IN THE NECK

Small nodules of thymic tissues are not infrequently found in the neck at necropsy and, in view of the embryological path of descent of the thymus, it is surprising that "clinically significant" remnants of the thymus gland are not found more often than the literature would indicate.

The third pharyngeal pouch gives rise to the paired primordia of the thymus gland during the sixth week of fetal life. The paired anlagen migrate in the caudal and medial direction, and, since the two anlagen never completely fuse, the thymus remains, to some degree, a paired organ. Joining in the middle, the primordia attach to the pericardium and descend into the superior mediastinum. By the ninth week of development, the main thymic mass has descended below the level of the clavicles to its permanent position. During this descent, an attachment to the main mediastinal thymic mass may be left as an implant in the cervical path of descent.

If the superior end of the thymic anlage fails to regress (eighth embryonic week), sequestered solid or cystic nodules of tissue may be left along the migration course and have been found incidentally around the thyroid gland. Thymic tissue may, therefore, occur in the neck, either as separate nodules of mature and well-differentiated tissue or in association with ciliated or columnar epithelial remnants of the pharyngeal outpouching.

Lewis,[1] in a review of the literature in 1962, recorded 32 reports where thymic tissue was present in the neck. These presented as cysts, isolated masses, persistant cords, or some combination of these. As late as 1964, only 15 documented examples of cervical thymic *cysts* had been recorded, and most of these were reported in the preceding decade.[2] Since then additional cases have been reported.[3, 4] Ninety-five percent are said to be unilateral and 90% of the thymic ectopias in the neck are cystic.[4]

Thymic cysts in the neck may be located in any position along a line extending from the angle of the jaws medially to the midline of the neck. Since the thymus gland reaches its greatest relative size at 2 to 4 years of age and its greatest absolute size at puberty, it is to be expected that the majority of cervical thymic masses would be detected in the pediatric age group. Such is the case.

As it eventually comes to all congenital disorders, cervical prolongation of the thymus has been classified into seven types; type 0, *no* cervical prolongation; type 1, left or right prolongation, not reaching the thyroid gland; type 2, left or right prolongation reaching the thyroid gland; type 3, bilateral prolongation not reaching the thyroid gland; type 4, bilateral prolongations, one side reaching the thyroid gland; type 5, bilateral prolongations to the thyroid gland; type 6, unilateral prolongation beyond the thyroid gland; and type 7, discrete nodules of thymic tissue according to position with respect to the thyroid gland. According to Maisel et al.,[5] types 3 and 4 are the most common. Figure 11.1, modified from these authors, presents the variations.

The cysts may be uni- or multilocular and appear to occur almost exclusively unilaterally.[6] They are often asymptomatic, but the mass may be painful if it is infected or if there has been a period of rapid increase in size. Midline cysts are capable of producing dysphagia. Myasthenia gravis has not been found in these patients, in contrast to its occasional relationship to thymic cysts of the mediastinum. The preponderance of males with a cervical thymus is also at variance with the female dominance in myasthenia gravis.

Benign or malignant neoplasia of the ectopic

233

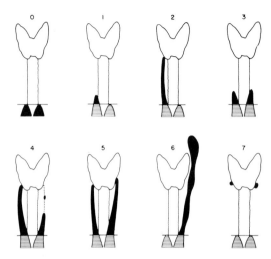

Figure 11.1. Types of cervical prolongation of the thymus.

thymic tissue has not been reported in cervical thymic *cysts.* Both forms of neoplastic changes have been reported in *solid* ectopic cervical thymuses.[7] A visible connection with a normal mediastinal thymus has been reported in about one-third of cases and suspected in the others. Extension in a medial direction between the internal and external carotid arteries does not occur in cervical thymic cysts as it does with branchial cleft cysts. The loculated cysts most often contain fluid varying from light amber to dark brown in color. The fluid may be clear or turbid due to cholesterol crystals in the cyst fluid. Size of the cysts has varied from 2.0 to 15 cm in major diameter.

On microscopic examination, squamous cells have been reported to line some thymic cysts, while other cysts have a cuboidal epithelial lining. Besides thymic tissue, cholesterol clefts and a foreign body reaction are frequent findings in the cyst wall (Fig. 11.2). The histological similarity between the cysts and the centers of Hassall's corpuscles and the variety of pathological features seen in the cervical masses that may be ascribed to degenerative changes in and/or rupture of Hassall's corpuscles is certainly more consistent with origin from ectopic tissue than from the epithelium of the pharyngeal out-pouchings.[8] The diagnosis of these most often asymptomatic cysts is almost never made preoperatively.[9]

Branchial cleft cysts may be found in identical positions, but they seldom extend to the clavicle. They characteristically lie along a line extending from the skin in the lower neck, through the carotid bifurcation to the upper tonsillar fossa. In addition, branchial cysts often present with signs

and symptoms of acute inflammation. The cystic hygroma is lateral, tends to be more diffuse, spongy in consistency, and seen in early in infancy. Cystic teratomas are exceedingly rare.[10] They may be lateral but are more often in the midline.

PARATHYROID CYSTS

Although microscopic cysts are frequent findings in the normal parathyroid glands, relatively few clinically significant cysts have been reported. By 1968, only 56 patients had been reported in whom surgical exploration of a palpable neck mass revealed a parathyroid cyst.[11] The clinically significant parathyroid cyst typically presents as a solitary mass in the region of the inferior lobe of either side of the thyroid gland. The cysts occur in both sexes, in a wide age range and *always* singly. No *case* has been reported in a child and most of the patients are between 30 and 50 years of age.[12]

Their presence may be asymptomatic, but usually symptoms relate to their physical mass and consist of tracheal deviation and some degree of respiratory obstruction or distress. The recurrent laryngeal nerve may be impaired by pressure, and hoarseness may ensue. In a number of patients the cyst may extend into the anterior mediastinum or be confined to that space. Physiologically, the cyst may be considered to be nonfunctional, despite the occasional report of clinical hyperparathyroidism in association with the lesion. In these instances, the cysts appear to have originated in a true parathyroid adenoma.[13]

At surgery, the cysts are usually found distinct from the lower pole of the thyroid gland, loosely adherent to the gland and pushing it forward. The

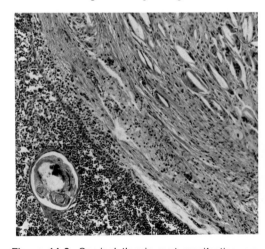

Figure 11.2. Cervical thymic cyst manifesting pronounced foreign body reaction to cholesterol and cholesterol esters. Note the degenerating Hassall's corpuscle.

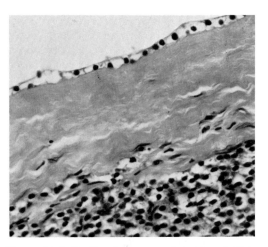

Figure 11.3. Section from a parathyroid cyst. Note parenchymal cells in the wall.

blood supply of the cyst is generally poor, and the cyst usually "shells out" from its relatively avascular covering. The cyst is unilocular, solitary and tense, averaging 4 cm in diameter (1 to 9 cm), and may resemble a hydrocele or a pericardial cyst.[12] The noncolloidal fluid is watery and opalescent or clear, and it is hormonally inactive.

Microscopically, the wall of the cyst is usually composed of a thin layer of fibrous connective tissue, covered by a single layer of flattened cuboidal or columnar epithelium, closely resembling cells of the normal parathyroid gland. Occasionally this epithelial lining is absent. The presence of nests of collections of typical parathyroid cells in the wall of the cysts is considered by most authors to be essential for the diagnosis (Fig. 11.3). Wasserhelle and chief cells are usually present, but one or the other may be dominant.

The origin of the cysts is obscure, but probably falls into two basic groups, congenital and acquired. Four possibilities then exist: (1) origin from vestigial structures in the neck, such as the thyroid or fourth gill pouches, ultimobranchial body or thymic remnants; (2) congenital enlargements of parathyroid vesicles or microscopic cysts due to retention; (3) coalescent degeneration; and (4) cystic degeneration in a parathyroid adenoma.

Of the benign noncystic parathyroid enlargements, only a very few present a palpable mass in the neck. On the other hand, the incidence of palpable neck masses in parathyroid carcinomas has been stated to be at least 45 to 50%.[14]

LESIONS OF THE THYROID PRIMORDIA

Reduced to its simplest considerations, the genesis of these lesions centers on the downward projection of the anlage of the thyroid gland from the region of the foramen cecum of the tongue in the 2.0- to 2.5-mm human embryo. In its descent, the primordium passes in front of the precursor of the hyoid bone and ventral to the thyroid and cricoid cartilages. At the hyoid bone the thyroglossal duct may pass closely in front of the developing bone, through it, or close behind it.

In normal development, the connection between the cervical thyroid gland and the point of origin at the foramen cecum is obliterated, usually during the sixth to eighth week. Only a small depression at the base of the tongue (foramen cecum) remains as evidence of this stage of development. Cell elements of the thyroidal primordium, may, however, remain at any site along this stem and give rise not only to cysts and fistulae, but also to accessory thyroid tissue and even neoplasms.

While there are many reports on the frequency with which thyroid epithelium is found in the midline thyroglossal remnants, the over-all incidence averages less than 5%. The presence of *histologically* identifiable thyroid epithelium may or may not have the same significance as the presence of *functioning* thyroid tissue.

The majority of lesions of the thyroglossal duct are midline in the neck and around the hyoid bone. Solid tumors of the thyroglossal duct vestiges, unlike the cysts, occur almost exclusively within the tongue and above the hyoid bone. (Fig. 11.4)

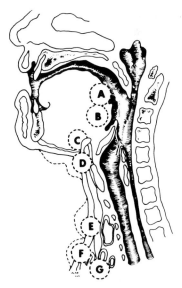

Figure 11.4. Potential sites of thyroglossal tract remnants. *A*, in front of the foramen cecum; *B*, at the foramen cecum; *C*, suprahyoid; *D*, infrahyoid; *E*, area of the thyroid gland; *F*, suprasternal; *G*, substernal. (Modified from Ward et al.[32])

Solid Thyroid Rests

Caution must be observed in the removal of this group of thyroglossal lesions. Located predominantly in the tongue and above the hyoid bone, these "ectopic" or lingual thyroids may or may not be associated with functioning thyroid tissue in the neck. Total removal may mean a lifelong replacement therapy of thyroid hormone to combat the surgically induced hypothyroidism and myxedema. It has been estimated that 70 to 80% of lingual thyroid patients have no other thyroid tissue.

Approximately 300 cases of lingual thyroid ectopia had been recorded prior to 1976.[15] Estimates from large thyroid clinics indicate this anomaly may account for one in every 4,000 cases of thyroid disease. This frequency represents those ectopia which are clinically significant. Ten percent of an auotpsy population studied by Sauk[16] manifested ectopic lingual thyroid tissue, ranging from a few acini to a 1.0 cm nodule. There is no doubt, therefore, that a significant number of lesions are never clinically diagnosed.[17]

Montgomery[18] has given us the most comprehensive review of lingual thyroids to date. He accepted 144 examples, of which 142 occurred in the dorsum of the tongue and two in the body of the tongue. The incidence is much higher in females, and the onset of symptoms relating to the mass may present at any time from birth to 60 years of age. Symptomatology is variable in severity and ranges from slight voice changes to severe dysphagia, interference with deglutition, orthopnea, severe dysphasia and even exsanguinating hemorrhage. Dysphagia is the most frequent complaint and may be so great in a few patients that inanition may result. Montgomery[18] considered four of the 144 cases he reviewed to manifest malignancy. Metastases occurred to the lungs and cervical lymph nodes in three of the four patients. All four examples were in men over 35 years of age.

Lingual thyroids are reddish, globular masses of varying size which occur in the median line of the base of the tongue between the foramen cecum and the epiglottis. The overlying mucous membrane is thin, and a network of large veins is common. The mass may be smooth or lobulated, intact or ulcerated, firm or soft.

The microscopic appearance of lingual thyroid nodules may be one of embryonic thyroid tissue, mature thyroid tissue, or a combination of the two.[19] The lingual thyroid tissue can further display any features characteristic of diseases in its normal locus. In at least one case, removal of parathyroid tissue in conjunction with the lingual thyroid resulted in postoperative tetany.

Biopsy of the lingual masses manifesting functional thyroid activity is not advised. Possible post-biopsy infection, slough and inflammation make subsequent excision unsatisfactory. Radioiodine studies to determine the functional activity of the mass and to determine the presence or absence of a normally placed gland in the neck are mandatory preoperative procedures. Similar precautions should be carried out for *all* anterior *midline* neck masses which suddenly appear during childhood.[20] These masses may arise from the enlargement of dysgenetic (ectopic) thyroid glands and may simulate thyroglossal duct cysts.

Approximately 40 cases of undescended thyroid gland in the anterior neck superficial to the hyoid bone had been documented by 1972.[19] Suprahyoid and infrahyoid anterior ectopias are not common and are often mistaken for thyroglossal duct cysts. As in the case of lingual thyroid, palpation may reveal easily felt tracheal rings where the normal thyroid gland should be. Haffly[15] states the literature is understandably reticent about ectopic thyroids in the midline of the neck removed in error since their removal usually results in myxedema. No more than one-third of thyroglossal duct cysts are detected in the first year of life. On the other hand, median ectopic thyroid representing the entire thyroid mass becomes palpable often within the first few months of life.

Ectopic thyroid masses in the intralaryngotracheal area are said to account for 7% of all primary intratracheal tumors. By 1975, approximately 115 reported cases, 90% of which were in persons living in middle European countries had been reported.[21] The ectopias may or may not be in continuity with the thyroid gland proper. The endotracheal ectopias affect females more often than males (3:1) and they present in third to fifth decades. The patients usually reside in endemic goiter areas. Symptoms develop in a gradual manner over a period of time and become accentuated at the time of menstruation or pregnancy.

The clinical course of these patients is similar to that of patients with "lingual goiter." Typically, the thyroid functions normally in early life, but increases in size during childhood or adolescence as functional inadequacy becomes apparent.

Therapy is dictated by the individual patient. Total excision in an athyroid patient requires continued supportive therapy. Subtotal removal generally does not prevent the development of myxedema, and regrowth, with a recurrence of symptoms, is possible. Ablation by I^{131} has only the advantage of being nonsurgical. It may cause incomplete regression of the tumor with persistence of symptoms, and continuing replacement therapy is necessary. Total removal with autografting or autotransplantation to the muscles of the neck or some more remote area has been suggested to restore thyroid function, while eliminating the hazards of a highly vascular and obstructive mass in the tongue.[22]

Thyroglossal Cysts, Sinuses and Fistulae

According to location, thyroglossal *cysts* may be classified as: (1) suprahyoid (20%); (2) at the level of the hyoid bone (15%); and (3) infrahyoid (65%). In a few patients, cysts may appear to be one side or the other of the midline; according to Judd,[23] most of these patients give a history of at least one previous operation which distorts the usual location.

The majority of thyroglossal duct cysts are subcutaneous, but fistulas from the duct do not normally occur. Fistulas are almost always the result of infection with either spontaneous or surgical drainage.[24] The incidence of spontaneous fistulization is not significant, and fistulas may occur without the presence of a cyst. When they occur, fistulae may be: (1) internal, with an opening into the pharynx; (2) external, with an opening into the skin; or (3) complete, with communications between the skin and the pharynx. Fistulae are, as a rule, simple and located in the midline, although more laterally situated branches may occur between the hyoid bone and the foramen cecum.

Several branching fistulae may rarely present at the base of the tongue, but these are considered to differ in their origin. In the third month of embryonic life, the lingual duct is formed from the foramen cecum. This duct is probably unrelated to the thyroglossal duct and derives from stratified squamous epithelium or the base of the tongue. If a communication is formed between a thyroglossal cyst and the lingual duct, it may result in a cyst with several ducts, all extending to the base of the tongue.

Murphy and Budd[25] have analyzed the age distribution of 1,044 patients with thyroglossal duct cysts (1890–1976). About half the patients have been under 10 years of age and only 14 patients (1.3%) have been over 60 years old. The male/female distribution is nearly equal and racial predominance is white.

Usually a midline lesion, the average thyroglossal duct cyst is 2 to 4 cm in diameter. The cyst may fluctuate in size, but, more commonly, the history is that of gradually increasing size. Microscopically, a squamous lining is the rule in the majority of the cysts and/or sinuses. Infrequently,

inflammatory changes obliterate the mucosa entirely, so the pathologist makes his diagnosis on presumptive and clinical evidence. As indicated above, thyroid tissue is not a common finding in the wall of the cyst.

Treatment is surgical and, in view of the embryological and anatomical conditions, the removal of all tissues along the duct as far as the foramen cecum is essential. Extirpation of a central portion of the hyoid bone and following of the tract behind the hyoid bone to the base of the tongue is considered of the utmost importance. If a remnant of a cyst or fistula is left behind, recurrence is inevitable. The applied anatomy dealing with removal of the whole thyroglossal duct tract has been presented by Ellis and van Nostrand.[26]

Thyroglossal Duct Carcinoma

Examples of carcinoma arising in a thyroglossal duct are not common, and Judd[23] regards the occasional reporting of a pipillary carcinoma of a thyroglossal duct cyst or sinus as erroneous: As of 1963, there was no proved example of a thyroglossal duct carcinoma in the Mayo Clinic files.[23] This is contrary to our experience and in 1977, there were 80 documented cases of carcinoma arising in thyroglossal duct remnants in the literature.[27–30] Carcinoma, however, occurs in less than 1% of thyroglossal duct abnormalities. Papillary thyroid carcinomas make up 75 to 80% of the carcinomas (Fig. 11.5). These arise from ectopic thyroid tissue in the remnants of the duct and not from the thyroglossal duct lining itself. The frequency of the ectopic remnants is much greater than cited in the literature. If sought for by sections, approximately 75% of thyroglossal ducts will show these rests. Approximately one-third of patients examined by radioactive iodine scan have shown evidence of functional thyroid tissue along the course of the tract.

The relative infrequency of malignancy in thyroglossal remnants is to be contrasted with the more frequent occurrence of carcinoma arising from aberrant lingual thyroid tissue.

Females are slightly in a majority of 1.5 to 1. The majority of patients are in the 40- to 60-year range, but examples have occurred in children and more elderly patients.

A benign appearing cystic mass is the initial symptom in nearly every case. The mass is nontender, painless and historically slow to enlarge.

Therapy consists of wide excision (Sistrunk procedure) in those cases localized to the duct remnant itself. Distant metastasis is extremely rare, having been reported in only three patients.[28]

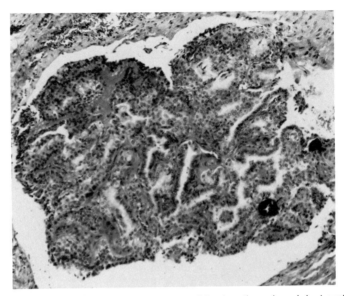

Figure 11.5. Papillary thyroid carcinoma arising in a thyroglossal duct cyst.

The possibility that a thyroglossal duct carcinoma is really a metastasis from a primary thyroid gland carcinoma must always be entertained and evaluated.

Primary squamous cell carcinoma and nonthyroidal adenocarcinomas have been rarely reported from thyroglossal duct remnants. In these instances, the carcinomas arise from the duct lining.

CUTANEOUS BRONCHOGENIC CYSTS

An unusual form of congenital cyst, the bronchogenic cyst in the skin and subcutaneous tissues usually makes its clinical presentation in the region of the suprasternal notch.[31] These cysts are noted at or soon after birth, appearing as asymptomatic nodules that slowly increase in size. In nearly one-third of the cases, there has been a recognizable sinus opening. In the series collected by Fraga et al.,[31] the lesions varied in diameter from 0.3 to 6.0 cm at the time of operation.

The cysts are located in the corium and/or subcutaneous tissue, and most contain a clear mucoid fluid unless there has been secondary infection. Microscopically, the lesions show the distinctive histological features of a bronchogenic cyst, lined by pseudostratified ciliated columnar epithelium containing mucous cells. Smooth muscle, collections of mucous and seromucous glands and, rarely, cartilage may also be found in the lesions.

A bronchogenic cyst is differentiated from the branchiogenic cyst by the presence of smooth muscle and seromucous glands and by an absence or paucity of lymphoid tissue. The anatomical region involved also rules out a diagnosis of branchogenic cyst. Thyroglossal duct cysts may be differentiated from bronchogenic cysts if thyroid follicles are identified. Furthermore, the thyroglossal duct cysts are not surrounded by smooth muscle and do not have cartilage in the wall even though hyoid bone may be present.[31]

It is postulated that the cutaneous bronchogenic cysts arise during embryological development as a result either of distant migration of sequestered cells from the respiratory tree or by displacement of a preformed cyst from its origin in the thorax.

REFERENCES

1. Lewis, M. R.: Persistance of the thymus in the cervical area. J. Pediat. 61:887, 1962.
2. Simons, J. N., Robinson, D. W., and Masters, F. W.: Cervical thymic cyst. Am. J. Surg. 108:578, 1964.
3. Mikal, S.: Cervical thymic cyst. Case report and review of the literature. Arch. Otolaryngol. 109:558, 1974.
4. Lewis, C. T.: Ectopic thymus of the neck—report of three examples in children. Postgrad. Med. J. 51:38, 1975.
5. Maisel, H., Yoshihara, H., and Waggoner, D.: The cervical thymus. Mich. Med. 74:259, 1975.
6. Fielding, J. F., Farmer, A. W., Lindsay, W. K., and Conen, P. E.: Cystic degeneration in persistent cervical thymus. Can. J. Surg. 6:178, 1963.
7. Laage-Hellman, J. E.: Accessory thymus tissue of the neck. Acta Otolaryngol. 42:375, 1952.
8. Speer, F. D.: Thymic cysts: report of a thymus presenting cysts of three types. N.Y. Med. Coll. Flower Hosp. Bull. 1:142, 1938.
9. Behring, Ch., and Bergman, F.: Thymic cyst of the neck. Acta Pathol. Microbiol. Scand. 59:45, 1963.
10. Batsakis, J. G., and Farber, E. R.: Teratomas of the head and neck. E.N.T. Digest 30:67, 1968.

11. Haid, S. P., Method, H. L., and Beal, J. M.: Parathyroid cysts: report of two cases and a review of the literature. Arch. Surg. 94:421, 1967.

12. McGinty, C. P., and Lischer, C. E.: The surgical significance of parathyroid cysts. Surg. Gynecol. Obstet. 117:703, 1963.

13. Weeks, P. M.: Clinically significant parathyroid cysts: case report and review of the literature. Am. Surg. 31:366, 1965.

14. Deeb, Z. E., Trible, W. M., Page, R., and Fernandez, M. G.: Parathyroid tumors as lateral pharyngeal masses: report of a case. Ann. Otol. 85:86, 1976.

15. Haffly, G. N.: The spectacular lingual thyroid and midline anterior cervical ectopic thyroid. Trans. Pacific Coast Oto-Ophth. Soc. 57:137, 1976.

16. Sauk, J. J., Jr.: Ectopic lingual thyroid. Pathology 102:239, 1970.

17. Monroe, J. B., and Fahey, D.: Lingual thyroid. Case report and review of the literature. Arch. Otolaryngol. 101:574, 1975.

18. Montgomery, M. L.: Lingual thyroid: comprehensive review. West. J. Surg. 43:661, 1935.

19. Baughman, R. A.: Lingual thyroid and lingual thyroglossal duct remnants. Oral Surg. 34:781, 1972.

20. Strickland, A. L., Macfie, J. A., WanWyk, J. J., and French, F. S.: Ectopic thyroid glands simulating thyroglossal duct cysts. J.A.M.A. 208:307, 1969.

21. Myers, E. N., and Pantangco, I. P., Jr.: Intratracheal thyroid. Laryngoscope 85:1833, 1975.

22. Myerson, M., and Smith, H. W.: Lingual thyroid—a review. Conn. Med. 30:341, 1966.

23. Judd, E. S.: Thyroglossal-duct cysts and sinuses. Surg. Clin. North Am. 43:1023, 1963.

24. Pollack, W. F., and Stevenson, E. O.: Cysts and sinuses of the thyroglossal duct. Am. J. Surg. 112:225, 1966.

25. Murphy, J. P., and Budd, D. C.: Thyroglossal duct cysts in the elderly. South. Med. J. 70:1247, 1977.

26. Ellis, P. D. M., and vanNostrand, A. W. P.: The applied anatomy of thyroglossal tract remnants. Laryngoscope 87: 765, 1977.

27. Joseph, T. J., and Komorowski, R. A.: Thyroglossal duct carcinoma. Hum. Pathol. 6:717, 1975.

28. Trail, M. L., Zeringue, G. P., and Chicola, J. P.: Carcinoma in thyroglossal duct remnants. Laryngoscope 87:1685, 1977.

29. LiVolsi, V. A., Perzin, K. H., and Savetsky, L.: Carcinoma arising in median ectopic thyroid (including thyroglossal duct tissue). Cancer 34:1303, 1974.

30. Widstrom, A., Magnusson, P., Hallberg, O., Hellquist, H., and Riiber, H.: Adenocarcinoma originating in the thyroglossal duct. Ann. Otol. 85:286, 1976.

31. Fraga, S., Helwig, E. B., and Rosen, S. H.: Bronchogenic cysts in the skin and subcutaneous tissue. Am. J. Clin. Pathol. 56:230, 1971.

32. Ward, G. E., Hendrick, J. W., and Chambers, R. G.: Thyroglossal tract abnormalities-cysts and fistulas. Surg. Gynecol. Obstet. 89:727, 1949.

CHAPTER 12

Metastatic Neoplasms to and from the Head and Neck

The diagnosis and management of metastatic disease from known head and neck primaries to cervical lymph nodes and the soft tissues of the region, while certainly not standardized, have had considerable documentation and fairly well-established guidelines. Unusual forms of metastatic patterns (i.e., to the bony structures of the face, the sinonasal tract, the skin of the head and neck and the metastasis from the occult primary) always pose not only therapeutic but often diagnostic problems of no mean order. In the following discussion, I have considered each of the above and present them in the form of a contemporary conspectus.

METASTATIC CARCINOMA OF THE JAWS

In contrast to a metastatic neoplasm within a cervical lymph node being most likely from a primary site in the confines of the head and neck, metastases to the bones of the jaws are almost always from regions below the clavicle. It is estimated that 1% of malignant neoplasms metastasize to the jaws and that 1% of all oral malignancies represent metastatic foci.

The number of cited examples of metastases to the jaw bones from distant primary sites, however, appears small. This is true, despite the fact that primary neoplasms of the breast, thyroid, prostate glands and ovaries commonly metastasize to bone. An anatomical factor bears on the relatively low incidence of secondary deposits in the jaw bones. For a metastatic lesion to become established in bone, there is at least a partial dependence upon the presence of red marrow. Here, thin-walled vascular channels provide a suitable site for the enlodgment and proliferation of neoplastic emboli.[1] In accordance with this, secondary lesions should most often be found in the molar region (vide infra).

The infrequency of mandibular involvement is further abetted by the physiological paucity of red marrow in the age group where carcinoma is most prevalent. Box,[2] after examining a series of mandibles, found that only 25% contained any red marrow, and this was distributed in small discrete patches.

For the present review of primary sites for a metastatic carcinoma to the jaws we have adhered to the criteria for inclusion established by Clauson and Poulsen.[3] All of the lesions are *true* metastases to bone as distinguished from direct or contiguous invasion by a primary carcinoma in proximity to the jaws. In each instance the metastasis has been verified microscopically, and in each the primary site of the neoplasm is known. From 1884 to 1965, 115 cases fulfill the aforementioned criteria. An additional 106 cases have been reviewed from 1966 to 1973.[4]

Metastases to the gingivae without osseous involvement is even more unusual than metastases to the jaws.[5] The sites of the primary lesions have been most often the kidney and lungs. Surprising in view of their infrequency, supraclavicular spread by germ cell neoplasms ranks third in frequency.

Table 12.1 presents the relative frequency of metastatic neoplasms. As might be expected from general prevalence and surgical pathological experience, neoplasms originating in the breasts, lungs and kidneys are leaders in this type of metastatic manifestation. The high number of breast carcinomas also accounts for the female predominance in the series. Between 20 and 30% of the group offered their jaw metastases as the first indication of harboring a malignant neoplasm. In the 103 cases where the age of the patient was given, the average age at the time of diagnosis was 56 years, with a range of 16 to 79 years. Forty-eight patients were over 60 years of age, 43 were between the ages of 50 and 60 years and 12 patients were younger than 40 years.

The mandible is by far the favorite metastatic site (92 cases), and, as Box[2] postulated, the highest concentration of metastatic sites was in the mandible, distal to the canines (75%). The maxilla was involved in 20 patients, and both jaws were involved in two patients. While mandibular and/or maxillary bone metastases may be the first evidence of an occult primary malignancy, jaw involvement is usually an accompaniment of generalized skeletal metastases.

Symptoms, when present, are those of pain and swelling of the affected area. Pain may precede radiological evidence of the lesion for as long as 15 months. When the mandible is involved, the earliest sign may be an anesthesia over the peripheral distribution of the inferior alveolar dental nerve on the affected side. Loosening of teeth without evidence of periodontitis and "pathological" fracture have also been stressed as early signs.[6] Radiological appearances are variable and may be simulated by a group of benign or malignant lesions. The majority of the metastases are osteolytic and appear in the molar area.

A patient manifesting carcinomatous metastases to the jaws has a grave prognosis. Treatment is chiefly palliative, with the intention of providing relief from pain and prolonging life. Resection of the mandible is too mutilating a procedure in these instances and does not significantly prolong the life of the patient. Radiation thereapy gives variable results and is dependent on the type and responsiveness of the neoplasm. Over two-thirds of patients manifesting metastatic carcinomas to the jaws are dead within 1 year. The 4-year survival is approximately 10%.[3]

METASTATIC CARCINOMA OF THE NOSE AND PARANASAL SINUSES

Metastases to the sinonasal tract are infrequent occurrences from primaries below the clavicle. The total number of reported cases to date is less than 100. There is, however, complete unanimity concerning the type of metastatic neoplasm most often encountered in these cases—renal cell carcinoma (Fig. 12.1).[6-11] In second position are metastases from the lung and the breasts. Considerably less frequent sites of origin are the gastrointestinal and distal urogenital tracts. The average age of patients with histological evidence of metastatic renal cell carcinoma to the nose and paranasal sinuses is at the end of the sixth decade, similar to those with carcinoma of the breast and a decade older than patients with metastases from bronchogenic and gastrointestinal neoplasms.

The clinical manifestations of metastases to the sinonasal tract are usually nonspecific, i.e., swelling, pain or nasal obstruction. Metastatic renal cell carcinoma however, has a significant propensity

Table 12.1
Metastatic Carcinomas to the Jaws
Tabulation of the site of origin of primary neoplasms (115 cases) that have manifested metastases to the bones of the jaws. The majority are mandibular metastases. This grouping does not include direct or contiguous invasion.

Primary Site of Neoplasm	No. of Cases	Percentage of Cases
Breast	35	30.4
Kidney	18	15.6
Lung	17	14.8
Colon and rectum	9	7.8
Prostate gland	8	7.0
Thyroid gland	7	6.1
Stomach	6	5.2
Melanoma	5	4.4
Testes	3	2.6
Bladder	1	0.87
Ovary	1	0.87
Cervix	1	0.87
Parotid gland	1	0.87
Submaxillary gland	1	0.87
Liver	1	0.87
Lip	1	0.87
	115	100%

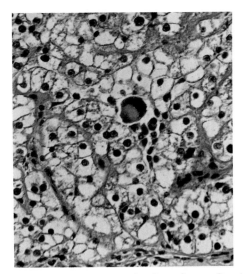

Figure 12.1. Metastatic renal cell carcinoma. Specimen was removed from the maxillary antrum.

for causing epistaxis. Bernstein et al.[7] found that epistaxis was the most common presenting complaint from patients with metastatic renal cell carcinoma to the nose or paranasal sinuses, and they attributed this to the richly vascular stroma associated with the neoplasm. Signs and symptoms referable to nasal or sinus disease very often precede discovery of the primary neoplasm. This is especially true with renal cell carcinoma (50 to 65%).[7, 9]

The prognosis for patients with metastatic carcinoma to the nose and paranasal sinuses is, in general, the same as for patients with generalized carcinomatosis. Possible exceptions are those instances where the upper respiratory tract lesion is the only metastatic focus. This is particularly true for renal cell carcinoma. Removal of the metastases *and* the primary may effect good results.[7] For those patients in whom the metastasis represents only one site of multiple areas of involvement, palliative therapy (irradiation, local arterial perfusion or chemotherapy) may be used.

Considerable variation exists in reports dealing with the frequency with which carcinoma of the prostate gland metastasizes to regions above the clavicle. In large series, it is surprisingly high in patients with extraglandular spread (41% in left supraclavicular fossa, 28% in right supraclavicular

fossa).[12] Butler et al.[12] consider that the diagnosis is suggested in the presence of metastatic carcinoma confined to the left supraclavicular area in a man over the age of 45 years, if the metastasis: (1) is an adeno- or poorly differentiated carcinoma; (2) does not have the appearance of carcinoma from some other primary site; (3) does not contain significant intracytoplasmic mucin as demonstrated by special stains (Fig. 12.2). As far as metastasis to the jaws is concerned, it has been estimated to occur in approximately 1% of patients with prostatic carcinoma.[13]

Like metastases from the prostate gland, the relative frequency of lung cancer as the occult primary tumor in patients *presenting* with cervical lymph node involvement varies with reporters (1.5 to 32%). This wide variation is probably attributable to the tendency to describe all adenopathy in the neck as involving a cervical lymph node without distinction as to the anatomical area. Given the skill of the surgical pathologist, considerably more information can be returned to the surgeon if the pathologist is provided with a reasonably accurate location of the lymph node. If supraclavicular metastases are excluded, a patient presenting with cervical metastases from an occult lung primary is unusual. Of 1,686 cases of bronchogenic carcinoma seen at the University of Louisville

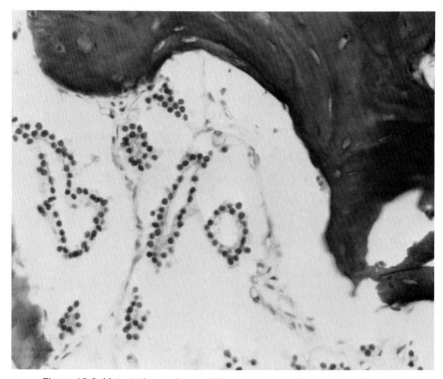

Figure 12.2. Metastatic carcinoma of the prostate gland to the mandible.

Hospitals only 26 (1.5%) patients presented with cervical node metastases.[14]

METASTATIC CARCINOMA OF THE TEMPORAL BONE

Schuknecht et al.[15] have reviewed the literature and discussed the clinicopathological manifestations of secondary neoplasms of the temporal bone. They indicate that metastatic involvement of this bony structure is much more common than their review would suggest, but the true incidence is overshadowed by other metastatic lesions.

The principal histological types of neoplasm are those involving the jaws, nose and paranasal sinuses, i.e., carcinoma of the breast, renal cell carcinoma and bronchogenic carcinoma.[16] Hearing loss is a common early sign of temporal bone involvement, but the bony otic capsule is quite resistant to invasion, and involvement of the inner ear is quite common. Clinically and radiographically, the metastasis may simulate chronic otitis media. The most frequent and usually most prominent symptom is pain. This may be intense and lancinating, many times disproportionate to clinical findings. The treatment of metastatic temporal bone lesions is palliative and all series report dismal survival figures.[17]

CUTANEOUS METASTASES TO THE HEAD AND NECK REGION

Cutaneous metastases from internal carcinomas are relatively rare. There is a tendency for the metastases to occur in the region of the primary growth, but the skin of the head and neck is a favorite site for metastatic deposits from remote primary neoplasms.[18] Here again, renal cell carcinoma is important not only from the standpoint of relative frequency, but also because of the diagnostic difficulties presented to the unsuspecting pathologist.

Cutaneous metastases from the kidney rank third or fourth behind those from the breasts, gastrointestinal tract and lung.[19] Connor et al.[18] found that the incidence of renal cell carcinoma, metastatic to skin, in surgical material was 6.8% as compared to a 3% incidence based on necropsy observations. In the Armed Forces series,[18] renal cell carcinoma manifested a striking predilection for the skin of the face and scalp. In 10 to 20% of patients, the cutaneous metastases were the first sign of carcinoma of the kidney.

The surgical pathologist must keep in mind the possibility of metastatic renal cell carcinoma, or misdiagnosis may be made. The metastases may simulate the appearance seen in sebaceous gland tumors and the eccrine porosyringoma. Connor et al.[18] consider that the presence of both glycogen and lipid in the metastatic lesion provides a reasonably firm histochemical basis for substantiating the diagnosis.

The statistical significance of metastatic renal cell carcinoma in the foregoing should serve to remind those dealing with head and neck lesions that the kidney is always worthy of investigation when one is presented with an apparent metastatic lesion to the head and neck for which no primary lesion can be found.[20] The University of Michigan Medical Center data serve to emphasize this point.[21] In a 6-year period (1958–1964), 105 patients with carcinoma of the kidney were seen at that institution (Table 12.2). Sixteen patients (15.2%) were found to have metastases to the head and neck region; in eight of the subjects (7.6%), the head and neck metastases accounted for the presenting complaint.

That renal cell carcinomas apparently bypass the fine pulmonary "filter bed" to metastasize to the head and neck is probably best explained by the rich venous plexuses and anastomoses of the vertebral and epidural systems. These are avalvular veins which should offer little resistance to the propagation of tumor emboli toward the head and neck with recumbency and with efforts which increase intra-abdominal and intrathoracic pressures.

METASTATIC CARCINOMA TO THE EYE AND ORBIT

Metastasis of carcinoma to the orbit occurs less often than metastasis to the eye. By 1976, 104 cases of metastasis to the orbit had been recorded.[22] As

Table 12.2
Distribution of Metastases in 105 Patients with Renal Cell Carcinoma*

Site of Metastasis	No. of Patients
Lung	43
Liver	18
Head and neck	16
Spine	15
Long bones	14
Pelvis	7
Ribs	7
Adrenal glands	4
Mediastinum	4
Skin	4
Heart	2
Miscellaneous	5

* The tabulated data are from the study by Boles and Cerny.[21]

of 1969, approximately 463 cases of intraocular metastasis had been collected, to which many smaller series and case reports have been added.[23] Breasts, lung and kidney primaries, in that order, are the most frequent seeders of the orbit. It should be emphasized that metastatic (not direct extension) squamous cell carcinoma in the orbit is exceptional.[22] The median survival of patients manifesting orbital metastases is approximately 15.5 months from the time of orbital surgery. This is much better than the median survival of patients with metastases to the eye and ocular adenexa (7.5 months).[22]

Secondary spread to the eye occurs in the following order of decreasing frequency from these primary sites: breast, lung, colon and prostate gland. At least 50% of intraocular metastases are from malignancies of the breast. Except for metastatic melanomas, the choroid is seeded more often than the retina. The majority of retinal metastases are melanomas. Useful findings to differentiate choroidal metastases from primary tumors include: (1) metastases are often bilateral; (2) metastases are commonly multifocal; and (3) metastatic tumors tend to be flat and infiltrative.

BRANCHIOGENIC CARCINOMA AND CERVICAL LYMPH NODE METASTASES FROM THE "OCCULT PRIMARY"

Discussion of these two perplexing lesions *must* be together since for the most part they are interrelated. Perhaps no other lesion in the head and neck has generated more controversy than branchiogenic carcinoma or branchial cleft carcinoma. The surfeit of publications concerning this highly controversial lesion since von Volkman's[24] description in 1882 certainly attests to its problematic nature. Too often, in my opinion, this diagnosis has been used as an "easy way out" for both pathologist and surgeon. Martin et al.[25] made the first serious attempt to reduce the confusion. These authors published *four* criteria whose fulfillment were required before the diagnosis of branchiogenic carcinoma was acceptable:

1. "The cervical tumor must occur on a line from anterior to the tragus to the anterior border of the sternocleidomastoid muscle.

2. The histological appearance must be consistent with an origin from tissue known to be present in branchial vestigia.

3. The patient must have survived and have been followed by periodic examination for 5 *years* without development of any other lesion which could possibly have been the primary lesion.

4. The best criterion would be the histological demonstration of cancer developing in the wall of an epithelial-lined cyst situated in the lateral aspect of the neck."

The fulfillment of these "postulates" may be regarded by some as akin to the labors of Heracles, and, in fact, Martin et al.[25] found great difficulty in applying the criteria to their own cases. From their review of previous reports, they accepted only *three* of 250 examples. They included in their report 15 cases of their own which they designated as "tentative branchiogenic carcinomas" since none of the lesions fulfilled their fourth criterion. Their doubt over the very existence of a primary branchiogenic carcinoma was expressed when they indicated that: (1) an occult primary may have been "cured" by location in the field of the tumoricidal dose of radiation given to the presenting cervical neoplasm; and (2) the possibility that spontaneous regression of a cryptogenic primary may have occurred.

A review of the literature since the report by Martin et al.[25] has yielded 15 *reputed* branchiogenic carcinomas.[26] While most recent authors have emphasized fulfillment of the fourth criteria, they have not complied to the third and, in my opinion, the most important prerequisite. Many of the recently compiled examples manifested a *second* neoplasm above the level of the clavicle during the course of follow-up studies. In *all* of these instances of hasty publication, the authors dismissed the second primary lesion as "unrelated to the presenting cervical mass" and evoked the "cancer field effect" to support their decision. Kolson and Akos[27] have reviewed this concept. These workers performed random biopsies of areas of the oral cavity, pharynx, larynx and esophagus in subjects with known primary epithelial neoplasms in the head and neck. Nine of 37 (24%) manifested second primary neoplasms. Five of these *nine* patients did not manifest grossly identifiable lesions in the sites of biopsy.

If we assume the criteria proposed by Martin et al.[25] are not too exclusively rigid, we must also propose that a *true* primary branchial cleft carcinoma rarely, if ever, occurs.[28, 29] The diagnosis certainly cannot be made with dogmatism in the presence of a second, histologically similar neoplasm. A *presumptive* or tentative diagnosis may be made with the complete understanding that a periodic surveillance of the patient must be made for a period of no less than 5 years after the original diagnosis.

With respect to the tentative examples of branchiogenic carcinoma, the following clinicopathological features are pertinent. The incidence is very low (0.3% of all malignant supraclavicular neoplasms). Sex distribution is almost equal, with the average age of subjects at the time of the tentative diagnosis being the late fifties. The average size of the cervical mass at time of initial examination is 4.0 cm in major dimension.

From a histological standpoint, the tentative examples have been predominantly squamous cell in type but may be adenocarcinoma or anaplastic carcinoma. Prima facie histological evidence for branchiogenic carcinoma is the demonstration of a carcinoma in situ evolving into invasive carcinoma within a branchial cleft cyst or sinus. This has never been documented with satisfaction. The mere histological presence of neoplasm "within the wall of the cyst" or a cystic carcinoma in a lymphoid stroma is not acceptable.

When, and if, a tentative diagnosis of branchiogenic carcinoma is made, the clinician must decide on a form of therapy, while *continuing* to search for an occult primary. Published series offer some form of therapeutic guidelines, but, certainly, treatment must be individualized.[25, 30] Squamous cell carcinoma is the dominant histological type of so-called branchiogenic carcinomas, and, from a statistical standpoint, irradiation alone, after biopsy or excisional biopsy, appears to offer the best prognosis. The patients reviewed by France and Lucas[30] had an average survival of 11.6 months after "surgery and irradiation" and 17.4 months after irradiation alone.

OCCULT PRIMARY AND CERVICAL METASTASES

It is highly probable that "branchiogenic carcinomas" actually represent cervical lymph node metastases of unknown origin at the time, and we have seen how important a significant follow-up period is to that diagnosis. There exists, however, a significant number of cases of metastatic carcinoma in cervical lymph nodes where, even after exhaustive clinical studies and follow-up periods, the primary lesion *never* declares itself (Table 12.3). The primary site remains elusive despite rather intensive clinical, biopsy and radiological evaluation of areas above and below the clavicles.

In a comparative study of several large series totalling 12,121 cases, the average incidence of cases of metastasis from an occult primary lesion was 4.7%.[31] That this phenomenon is not unique to cervical lymph nodes can be seen in a study of 254 patients with metastatic cancers at the Roswell Park Memorial Institute.[32] In these patients, the clinical *presentation* was commonly in the form of metastatic lesions in lungs, bone, liver or cervical lymph nodes. Diagnosis of the primary lesion could be established in only 77 patients (30%) and most often at necropsy. The most common origin of the primary lesion was the lung (40%); followed by pancreas, stomach, kidney, colon, ovary and other organs. The survival data (Table 12.4) from the Roswell Park study[32] is of particular interest to the head and neck surgeon in the different survival statistics according to level of cervical lymph node involvement.

The experience of the Head and Neck Service, Memorial Hospital, New York may be considered fairly representative.[33] Between 1950 and 1964, 123 patients manifesting no demonstrable primary cancer were treated for cervical node metastases. The primary neoplasm, despite considerable investigation, remained occult in 85 patients. The

Table 12.3
"Occult Primary" Neoplasms: Incidence of Subsequent Determinate Cases

Discovery of the primary neoplasm in the majority of instances occurred within a 5-year period after initial treatment of the metastases. Most of the discovered primary lesions were found in the upper respiratory tract.

Authors	Eventual Discovery of Primary
	% of cases
Comess et al.[35]	42
Marchetta et al.[34]	45
Jesse and Neff[42]	33
Smith et al.[37]	28
Barrie et al.[33]	30
Coker et al.[62]	30

Table 12.4
Life Table Analysis Survival Data—Rosewell Park Memorial Institute: According to Site and Histological Type of Metastases*

	No. of Patients	Median Survival (months)	5-Year (%)
Location of Metastases			
High and midneck lymph nodes	39	21	28.0
Low neck	53	7	8.3
All others	166	5–7	8.0
Histological classification			
Squamous cell carcinoma	37	13.7	13.5
Adenocarcinoma	103	6	5.0
Undifferentiated	85	7.7	9.4

Modified from Didolkar et al.[32]

source of the metastases in the remainder of the patients was discovered from 1 month to 5 years after the metastases were treated.

From a survey of several large series[33-39] dealing with metastatic carcinoma in cervical lymph nodes from cryptogenic carcinomas comes a number of clinicopathological consistencies that permit generalization:

1. A cervical lymph node should *not* be excised for diagnostic purposes until all other measures fail. Renewed activity in the neck of a patient with a previously excised lymph node invariably appears in the region from which the node has been excised for diagnostic purposes. This occurs whether the patient has been treated by radiotherapy or by operation. The same cannot be said for expert fine-needle biopsy of the lymph node. Whether an initial biopsy influences *survival* in patients who subsequently undergo curative resectional surgery is unclear. The data presented by Razack et al.[40] would indicate there is no adverse effect.

2. There is a significant predominance of males.

3. The peak age of patients at the time of initial diagnosis is between 50 and 69 years.

4. Various lymph nodes can be affected, but there is a predilection for the upper jugular chain.

5. Patients with a metachronous regional lymph node involvement appear to have a better prognosis than those with synchronous primary cancer and regional lymph node metastases.

6. Squamous cell carcinoma is the most common histological type encountered in the metastasis.

7. Apparently occult primary neoplasms of the naso-, oro- and laryngopharynx remain undetected longer than those in any other location. The possibility of subsequent discovery of a hidden primary tumor decreases with the passing of time.

8. Most of the primaries below the clavicles become apparent during the first year of observation.

9. The upper respiratory tract and oral cavity are the sites of origin for the majority of apparently occult metastases that are eventually classed as *determinate* secondaries (Table 12.5).

10. The majority of *detected* primary neoplasms *below* the clavicles are from the lungs or gastrointestinal tract.

11. The prognosis for the patient with a subsequently located primary neoplasm is apparently worse than in those patients in whom the primary remains indeterminate.

12. Patients with the involved lymph nodes limited to the upper one-half of the neck manifest a

Table 12.5
Site of Primary Neoplasm in Determinate Cases

Area of Primary Neoplasm	No. of Cases
Oral and nasal cavity and oronasopharynx	38
Larynx—hypo- and posterior pharynx	26
Lung	17
Gastrointestinal tract (including pancreas)	11
Thyroid gland	9
Miscellaneous neoplasm above clavicles	6
Miscellaneous neoplasms below clavicles	10
	117

better prognosis than those with lower node metastases.

13. The prognostic outlook is further enhanced for those patients manifesting a metastasis in a *single* node within the superior part of the neck.

14. Metastases to *supraclavicular* lymph nodes are an extremely poor prognostic indicator. A census of patients presenting with only supraclavicular nodes indicates that almost all have primary neoplasms below the clavicle.

15. Survival of patients with metastases in multiple or bilateral lymph nodes is generally brief regardless of treatment.

16. Metastatic adenocarcinoma (exclusive of thyroid carcinoma) to cervical lymph nodes carries a poor prognosis no matter where the lymph node is located in the neck.

17. There is no prognostic significance attached to histological type when the involved lymph node is in the lower one-half of the neck.

18. The site of the adenopathy may provide a clue to the location of the primary lesion. Speaking in general, lymph nodes high in the neck correspond to primary sites in the nasopharynx; the upper jugular region to sites in the oropharynx; the lower jugular region, to sites in the hypopharynx; and supraclavicular nodes, to subclavicular primary lesions.

A knowledge of the incidence and topographical distribution of lymph node metastases from mucosal squamous cell carcinoma in the head and neck can assist in determining possible primary sites for an occult lesion. This has been admirably evaluated by Lindberg[45] in his study 1,155 patients. His analysis by region follows:

1. *Oral Tongue.* Subdigastric nodes are most commonly involved. After the nodes in the submandibular triangle, the midjugular nodes are next. Submental, low jugular and posterior cervical lymph nodes are seldom involved.

2. *Floor of Mouth.* Because of the anterior location of most of the neoplasms the lymph nodes of the submandibular triangle are most commonly

involved. Unlike the subdigastric nodes, the submental lymph nodes are not often involved. Posterior cervical and low jugular lymph nodes are rarely the sites of metastases.

3. *Oropharynx.* The subdigastric lymph nodes are most commonly involved in all sites. Submandibular and submental lymph node involvement is unusual to rare. Lesions of the retromolar trigone, anterior faucial pillar and soft palate most often metastasize to the tonsillar node in the subdigastric group. The incidence of submandibular triangle and midjugular lymph node involvement is also high. Posterior cervical lymph nodes are rarely involved. Carcinomas of the soft palate manifest an involvement of the upper jugular nodes most often. There is also a high incidence of bilateral metastases. If the carcinoma is in the tonsillar fossa, the tonsillar node of the subdigastric group is almost always the first one to be invaded. The incidence of mid- and low jugular nodes is also significant. Metastasis to the posterior cervical nodes is common, both ipsi- and contralaterally. Bilateral metastases are quite common in base of tongue carcinomas. After the subgastric nodes, the midjugular nodes are involved (often bilateral). Only a few patients present with posterior cervical nodes. Low jugular and supraclavicular lymph nodes are rarely involved. Carcinomas of the oropharyngeal walls spread along the jugular chain bilaterally. The upper jugular lymph nodes are most commonly involved, followed by the midjugular nodes. The incidence of posterior cervical node involvement is high.

4. *Supraglottic Larynx.* Principal dissemination is along the jugular chain, with the upper jugular nodes most commonly affected, followed closely by the midjugular nodes. Bilateral metastasis may be frequent. Posterior cervical nodes are seldom, and submandibular and submental lymph nodes almost never involved.

5. *Hypopharynx.* the upper, mid-, and lower jugular chain node, in decreasing frequency, are the principal sites of metastases. Frequency of bilateral metastases is low. Ipsilateral posterior cervical lymph node involvement is occasionally seen. Submandibular triangle and submental involvement is rare.

6. *Nasopharynx.* Carcinomas from this site have the highest incidence of posterior cervical chain involvement and also bilateral metastases. The ipsi- and contralateral upper jugular nodes are most often involved. There is a significant incidence of supraclavicular metastases. Submental and submandibular lymph nodes are only rarely involved.

On a statistical basis, the primary site for a metastasis to a posterior cervical triangle lymph node, is most likely to be the nasopharynx. This site is followed by the oropharyngeal walls, hypopharynx and tonsillar fossa. On the other hand, this author has rarely seen a posterior cervical lymph node metastasis as a harbinger of an occult carcinoma. This observation is supported by Skolnick et al.[46] who found a 4% incidence of metastasis in the posterior triangle in 225 neck dissections. All of these, however, were associated with extensive clinical and microscopic involvement of the anterior triangle. By citing findings to indicate that laryngeal carcinomas relate primarily to the jugular, submandibular and paratracheal lymph nodes and carcinomas of the oral cavity and pyriform sinus rarely manifest posterior triangle metastases, Skolnik et al.[46] raise the question of preserving posterior triangle tissue in radical neck dissection.

The reader is also advised to consider that the posterior cervical lymph nodes may mimic metastases because of chronic scalp or nasopharyngeal infections. Further, rather than an occult carcinoma, a satellite lymphomatous node is a more likely reason for adenopathy in that triangle.

It follows that Lindberg's[45] excellent analysis would be tested by probability statistics. This has been quite admirably done by Molinari et al.[47] Figure 12.3 presents their lymph node divisions in the neck and one of their metastatic maps with probability percentages for site of the primary lesion.

As indicated in Table 12.5, the oropharynx (tonsils, soft palate, posterior third of tongue), the hypopharynx, and the nasopharynx account for two-thirds of the discovered primary cancers, followed in order by localizations in the larynx, oral cavity and paranasal sinuses.

The delay between initial evaluation and discovery of the primary can vary from a few months to several years. Generally, two-thirds of the upper aerodigestive lesions that will be discovered will declare themselves during the first 18 months.

The probability of metastasis from an oral or oropharyngeal squamous cell carcinoma as judged by anatomical site and level of neoplastic differentiation may also aid in discovery of the occult primary lesion (Table 12.6).

The mode and degree of aggressive treatment for patients with metastatic carcinoma to the head and neck with no detectable primary site has been controversial in the past. There can be no doubt, however, that some form of treatment is required, since the average survival of untreated patients is approximately 4 months. It is important to reemphasize that excision of the cervical node for

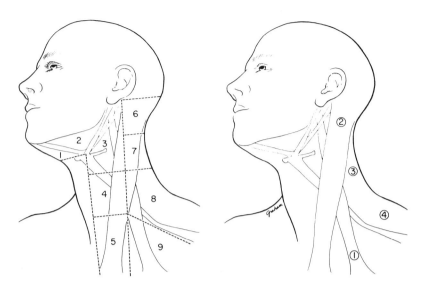

Figure 12.3. *Left,* divisions of the neck according to Molinari et al.: *1,* submental; *2,* submandibular; *3,* subdigastric; *4,* middle jugular; *5,* inner jugular region; *6,* upper spinal region; *7,* middle spinal region; *8,* inner spinal region; *9,* lateral supraclavicular region. *Right,* sites of primary lesion; frequency according to location of involved lymph nodes: *1,* Lung, 40%; thyroid gland, 23%; digestive tract, 12%; hypopharynx, 4%; larynx, 4%; base of tongue, 3.5%. *2,* Nasopharynx, 58%; tonsil, 10%; oropharynx, 8.5%; base of tongue, 8%; hypopharynx 8%, larynx, 4.6%. *3,* Nasopharynx, 55%; hypopharynx, 12%; base of tongue, 12%; oropharynx, 9%; tonsil, 9%; thyroid, 3%. *4,* Hypopharynx, 25%; nasopharynx, 24%; thyroid, 16%; tonsil, 10%, larynx, 8%; oropharynx, 5%; base of tongue, 4%; lung, 2.5%; floor of mouth, 1.5%; digestive tract, 1.5%.

Table 12.6
Oral Carcinoma—Influence of Site and Differentiation on Metastatic Rate (898 Cases)*

	Metastases to Lymph Nodes		No Metastases	
	No. of Cases	Per-cent	No. of Cases	Per-cent
I. Influence of site				
Oropharynx	195	78	56	22
Posterior tongue	97	83	20	17
Anterior tongue	107	59	74	41
Hard palate	9	53	8	47
Floor of mouth	77	52	66	48
Buccal mucosa	32	50	32	50
Gingiva	34	46	40	54
Lip	19	37	32	63
II. Influence of Differentiation				
Well	31	48	33	52
Moderate	324	57	243	43
Poor	215	81	52	19

diagnostic purposes follows a thorough clinical and radiographic study for primary sites.[41]

Most reports are surgical series, and the survival figures presented tend to support surgical treatment as being most effective. Radical neck dissection alone, for example, afforded a "cure" rate of almost 35% in Jesse and Neff's[42] series, and a nearly similar 3-year survival has been reported for treatment based almost solely on irradiation (Tables 12.7 and 12.8).

Radical surgical excision appears justified when the metastasis is a squamous cell carcinoma or melanoma, especially when the lymph node involved from the occult primary is high in the neck. In these instances radical neck dissection will produce an apparent control of the local disease. It is conjectural, however, whether neck dissection is at all effective in patients with metastases in the supraclavicular region, regardless of histological type, and in cases of metastatic adenocarcinoma from a presumed primary lesion below the clavicles.

A combined radical radiation-surgical attack may enhance survival in patients with multiple involved unilateral lymph nodes. Combined therapy in the form of preoperative irradiation and surgery may have the advantage of "treating" a hidden primary lesion in the naso-, oro- and hypopharynx, while at the same time decreasing the size of the involved lymph nodes prior to their surgical removal.[36, 43, 44] Certainly, combined therapy is indicated in those subjects with recurrence in the neck after radical dissection.

DISTANT METASTASES FROM CARCINOMAS OF THE HEAD AND NECK

The increasing incidence of distant metastases from head and neck cancer and a variety of clinical and necropsy studies have been important in dispelling the early belief that most head and neck cancers tend to remain above the level of the clavicles. In 1906, Crile[48] reported a study done by Hitchings on 4,500 patients who died of cancer of the head and neck, less than 1% of whom manifested visceral metastases. Later, he emphasized these findings by stating: "The collar of lymphatics about the neck forms an almost impossible barrier through which cancer rarely penetrates and every portion of this barrier is readily accessible to the surgeon."[49]

Improvements in diagnosis and treatment by 1941 changed the opinions of various workers in this field. Martin and Braund,[50] in 1941, considered that patients with malignancies of the head

and neck *and* cervical lymph node involvement had two and a half times greater chance of developing distant metastases than patients without spread to the regional lymph nodes.

Depending on the site of the primary in the head and neck and whether the studies are clinical or necropsy in type, the percentage of distant metastases found has ranged, in recent years, from 15% to nearly 90%. Ju's[51] study is important in that he excluded thyroid carcinomas from a portion of his analysis. With that exclusion, he concluded that 52% of 293 cases of cancer of the head and neck showed distant metastases at the time of necropsy.

Every region studied in the head and neck has manifested an increasing number of distant metastases. In 1954, Castigliano and Rominger[52] reported 200 patients with fatal oral cavity cancer, who were treated from 1930 to 1954. In this study, 2% had distant metastases, but, in 120 patients with fatal oral cavity cancer treated from 1943 to 1951, 10.7% had distant metastases.

These statistics for oral cancer, like those obtained for carcinomas of the larynx, are subject to considerable variance.[53, 54] Harrer and Lewis[55] for example, report that 16 of 18 patients with carcinoma of the larynx manifested *diffuse* metastases at necropsy. A more probable statistic is that obtained by Abramson et al.,[56] who studied 650 patients with laryngeal carcinomas (75 of whom had necropsies). These workers found that 34% had distant metastatic spread. Position of the neoplasm, i.e., glottic or supraglottic, did not appear to have a bearing on the probability of metastasis. At the time of necropsy, however, 80% of the patients with disseminated disease also had local neck involvement.

While the lungs, liver and skeletal system are the most common sites for secondary deposits from head and neck cancer, the visceral spread from the primary neoplasm is surprisingly wide.[57]

Table 12.7
Survival: Metastatic Cancer in Neck
Comparison of survival rates in six major series relating to the occult primary and cervical lymph node metastases. The patients of Marchetta et al.[34] represent a series treated almost solely by irradiation. The remainder of the authors report predominantly a surgically treated patient population.

Authors	No. of Patients	Time Period	Survival
			%
Comess et al.[35]	103	Unlimited	37
Marchetta et al.[34]	33	4 years	30
Robinson[36]	32	Unlimited	28
Jesse and Neff[42]	127	3 years	34
Smith et al.[37]	28	Unlimited	14
Barrie et al.[33]	123	3 years	30
		5 years	25.2
		10 years	15.0
		15 years	11.6

Table 12.8
Occult Primary: Mode of Treatment and Survival*

Treatment Center	Form of Treatment	No. of Patients	Survival (%)	
			3-Year	5-Year
M. D. Anderson	Radiation and surgery	259	38.5	—
Princess Margaret	Radiation	233	25.0	18.0
Instit Gustave-Roussy	Surgery and radiation	154	21.0	12.0
Memorial (New York)	Surgery	123	30.0	25.0
Royal Marsden	Radiation	96	26.0	16.0

* From data presented by Richard and Micheau.[31]

In the study of Abramson et al.,[56] the lungs were involved in 80% of the necropsy cases. These pulmonary metastases were usually multiple. Next in frequency were the mediastinal lymph nodes at 58% involvement. The skeletal system, most often the lumbosacral spine and the ribs, was involved in 35% of the cases. Twenty-five percent of the patients manifested hepatic metastases. Cardiac involvement (without contiguous spread) is, in my experience, uncommon.

Eighty of 215 patients with carcinoma of the hypopharynx studied by Stefani and Eells[58] manifested distant metastases. The anatomical distribution of the metastatic sites follows that of carcinoma of the larynx, with the lungs, mediastinal lymph nodes, skeletal system and liver being the predominant sites and in that order of frequency.

In a study of 779 patients with cancer of the oral cavity, oropharynx, nasopharynx, hypopharynx and larynx, Probert et al.[59] found 96 (12.3%) to have distant metastases. In that series, the nasopharyngeal and hypopharyngeal carcinomas manifested the highest rate of metastasis. The most advanced primary tumors (T_4) are most likely to have distant spread, but more than 50% of Probert's patients had primary lesions considered to be completely eradicated. Merino et al.[60] have presented similar findings in their evaluation of 5,019 patients with squamous cell carcinoma of the upper aerodigestive tracts. Five hundred forty-six subjects developed clinical evidence of distant metastases, an over-all incidence of 10.9%. This varied from 3.1% for vocal cord cancers to 28.1% for cancer of the nasopharynx. In both Probert's[59] and Merino's[60] series, the distant metastases occurred within 18 to 24 months after initial treatment. The 5-year actuarial survival of patients developing distant metastases is less than 5%.

Arlen et al.[61] have concentrated on *osseous* metastasis in relation to primary carcinoma of the head and neck, excluding salivary gland primary tumors and carcinomas of the skin. These authors investigated 93 carcinomas with metastases to bone. Tumors of the extrinsic larynx, followed by nasopharyngeal, pharyngeal and oral carcinomas were the neoplasms most often implicated.

The significance to prognosis of the distant metastases is difficult to glean from the reports in the literature. Ju's[51] study is pertinent in this respect, since it afforded the necropsy pathologist an opportunity to study the end stages of head and neck cancer. Failure of eradication of local disease and regional metastases appears to be the main contributor to death. Pneumonia was the "friend of the feeble" and the intractable, being the terminal event in approximately 60% of Ju's patients.[51]

In reference to the local pathological findings, 236 of 293 of Ju's patients had proved persistent local disease, and 168 patients were found to have direct extension of the neoplasm to surrounding organs and structures.[51]

REFERENCES

1. Stockdale, C. R.: Metastatic carcinomas of the jaws secondary to primary carcinoma of the breast. Oral Surg. 12: 1095, 1959.
2. Box, H.: Canadian Dental Research Foundation Bulletin, No. 20, 1935.
3. Clausen, F., and Poulsen, H.: Metastatic carcinoma to the jaws. Acta Pathol. Microbiol. Scand. 57:361, 1963.
4. McMillan, M. D., and Edwards, J. L.: Bilateral mandibular metastases. Oral Surg. 39:959, 1975.
5. Perlmutter, S., Buchner, A., and Smukler, H.: Metastasis to the gingiva. Report of a case of metastasis from the breast and review of the literature. Oral Surg. 38:749, 1974.
6. Meyer, I., and Shklar, G.: Malignant tumors metastatic to mouth and jaws. Oral Surg. 20:350, 1965.
7. Bernstein, J. M., Montgomery, W. W., and Balogh, K.: Metastatic tumors to the maxilla, nose and paranasal sinus. Laryngoscope 76:621, 1966.
8. Friedman, I., and Osborn, D. A.: Metastatic tumors in the ear, nose and throat region. J. Laryngol. Otol. 79:576, 1965.
9. Nahum, A. J., and Bailey, B. J.: Malignant tumors metastatic to the nose and paranasal sinuses: case report and review of the literature. Laryngoscope 73:942, 1963.
10. Miyamoto, R., and Helmus, C.: Hypernephroma metastatic to the head and neck. Laryngoscope 83:898, 1973.
11. Schantz, J. C., Miller, S. H., and Graham, W. A., III.: Metastatic hypernephroma to the head and neck. J. Surg. Oncol. 8:183, 1976.
12. Butler, J. J., Howe, C. D., and Johnson, D. E.: Enlargement of the supraclavicular lymph nodes as the initial sign of prostatic carcinoma. Cancer 27:1055, 1971.
13. Snyder, S. R., Merkow, L. P., and White, N. S.: Prostatic carcinoma metastatic to the mandible: report of case. J. Oral Surg. 29:205, 1971.
14. Davis, R. S., Flynn, M. B., and Moore, C.: An unusual presentation of carcinoma of the lungs: 26 patients with cervical node metastases. J. Surg. Oncol. 9:503, 1977.
15. Schuknecht, H. F., Allam, A. F., and Murakami, Y.: Pathology of secondary malignant tumors of the temporal bone. Ann. Otol. Rhinol. Laryngol. 77:5, 1968.
16. Hill, B. A., and Kohut, R. I.: Metastatic adenocarcinoma of the temporal bone. Arch. Otolaryngol. 102:568, 1976.
17. Stucker, F. J., and Holmes, W. F.: Metastatic disease of the temporal bone. Laryngoscope 86:1136, 1976.
18. Connor, D. H., Taylor, H. B., and Helwig, E. B.: Cutaneous metastases of renal cell carcinoma. Arch. Pathol. 76:339, 1963.
19. Brownstein, M. H., and Helwig, E. B.: Spread of tumors to the skin. Arch. Dermatol. 107:80, 1973.
20. Batsakis, J. G., and McBurney, T. A.: Metastatic neoplasm to the head and neck. Surg. Gynecol. Obstet. 133:673, 1971.
21. Boles, R., and Cerny, J.: Head and neck metastases from renal cell carcinomas. Mich. Med. 70:616, 1971.
22. Font, R. L., and Ferry, A. P.: Carcinoma metastatic to the eye and orbit. III. A clinicopathologic study of 28 cases metastatic to the orbit. Cancer 38:1326, 1976.
23. Fine, E., Tamura, H., Spraragen, S. C., Geltzer, A. I., Albert, D. M., and Bogaars, H. A.: Metastatic intraocular carcinoma: clinicopathologic study of a case. South. Med. J. 69:121, 1976.
24. von Volkmann, R.: Das tiefe Branchiogene Halskarcinom. Zentralbl. Chir. 9:49, 1882.
25. Martin, H., Morfit, H. M., and Ehrlich, H.: The case for branchiogenic cancer (malignant branchioma). Ann. Surg. 132:867, 1950.

26. Black, B., and Maran, A. G. D.: Branchiogenic carcinoma. Clin. Otolaryngol. 3:27, 1978.

27. Kolson, H., and Akos, R.: Multiple biopsies in head and neck cancer. Arch. Otolaryngol. 90:159, 1969.

28. Bernstein, A., Scardino, P. T., Tomaszewski, M.-M., and Cohen, M. H.: Carcinoma arising in a branchial cleft cyst. Cancer 87:2417, 1976.

29. Compagno, J., Hyams, V. J., and Safavian, M.: Does branchiogenic carcinoma really exist? Arch. Otolaryngol. 100: 311, 1976.

30. France, C. J., and Lucas, R.: The management and prognosis of metastatic neoplasms of the neck with an unknown primary. Am. J. Surg. 106:835, 1963.

31. Richard, J. M., and Micheau, C.: Malignant cervical adenopathies from carcinoma of unknown origin. Tumori 63: 249, 1977.

32. Didolkar, M. S., Fanous, N., Elias, E. G., and Moore, R. H.: Metastatic carcinomas from occult primary tumors. A study of 254 patients. Ann. Surg. 186:625, 1977.

33. Barrie, J. R., Knapper, W. H., and Strong, E. W.: Cervical nodal metastases of unknown origin. Am. J. Surg. 120: 466, 1970.

34. Marchetta, F., Murphy, W., and Kovaric, J.: Carcinoma of the neck. Am. J. Surg. 196:974, 1963.

35. Comess, M., Behars, O., and Dockerty, M.: Cervical metastasis from occult carcinoma. Surg. Gynecol. Obstet. 104: 607, 1957.

36. Robinson, D.: The management of metastases in lymph nodes when the primary cannot be found. Plast. Reconstr. Surg. 113:663, 1967.

37. Smith, P. E., Krementz, E. T., and Chapman, W.: Metastatic cancer with a detectable primary site. Am. J. Surg. 113: 663, 1967.

38. Lindberg, R.: Distribution of cervical lymph node metastases from squamous cell carcinoma of the upper respiratory and digestive tracts. Cancer 29:1446, 1972.

39. Sprio, R. H., Alfonso, A. E., Farr, H. W., and Strong, E. W.: Cervical node metastasis from epidermoid carcinoma of the oral cavity and oropharynx. A critical assessment of current staging. Am. J. Surg. 128:562, 1974.

40. Razack, M. S., Sako, K., and Marchetta, F. C.: Influences of initial neck node biopsy on the incidence of recurrence in the neck and survival in patients who subsequently undergo curative resectional surgery. J. Surg. Oncol. 9:347, 1977.

41. MacComb, W. S.: Diagnosis and treatment of metastatic cervical cancerous nodes from an unknown primary site. Am. J. Surg. 124:441, 1972.

42. Jesse, R. H., and Neff, L. E.: Metastatic carcinoma in cervical nodes with an unknown primary lesion. Am. J. Surg. 112: 547, 1966.

43. Jesse, R. H., Perez, C. A., and Fletcher, G. H.: Cervical lymph node metastasis: Unknown primary cancer. Cancer 31:854, 1973.

44. Frieo, M. P., Diehl, W. H., Jr., Brownson, R. J., Sessions, D. G., and Ogura, J. H.: Cervical metastasis from an unknown primary. Ann. Otol. 84:152, 1975.

45. Lindberg, R.: Distribution of cervical lymph node metastases from squamous cell carcinoma of the upper respiratory and digestive tracts. Cancer 29:1446, 1972.

46. Skolnik, E. M., Yee, K. F., Friedman, M., and Golden, T. A.: The posterior triangle in radical neck surgery. Arch. Otolaryngol. 102:1, 1976.

47. Molinari, R., Cantu, G., Chiesa, F., Podrecca, S., Milani, F., and Del Vecchio, M.: A statistical approach to detection of the primary cancer based on the site of neck lymph node metastases. Tumori 63:267, 1977.

48. Crile, G. W.: Excision of cancer of the head and neck. J.A.M.A. 47:1780, 1906.

49. Crile, G. W.: Cancer of jaws, tongue, cheek, and lips. Surg. Gynecol. Obstet. 36:159, 1923.

50. Martin, H. E., and Braund, R. R.: Distant metastases in cancer of the upper respiratory and alimentary tracts. Surg. Gynecol. Obstet. 73:63, 1941.

51. Ju, D. M. C.: A study of the behavior of cancer of the head and neck during its late and terminal phases. Am. J. Surg. 108:552, 1964.

52. Castigliano, S. G., and Rominger, C. J.: Distant metastases from carcinomas of the oral cavity. Am. J. Roentgenol. Radium Ther. Nucl. Med. 71:997, 1954.

53. Topazian, D. S.: Distant metastasis of oral carcinomas. Oral Surg. 14:705, 1961.

54. Alonson, J. M.: Metastasis of laryngeal and hypopharyngeal carcinoma. Acta Otolaryngol. 64:353, 1967.

55. Harrer, W. V., and Lewis, P. L.: Carcinoma of the larynx with cardiac metastasis. Arch. Otolaryngol. 91:382, 1970.

56. Abramson, A. L., Parisier, S. C., Zamansky, M. J., and Sulka, M.: Distant metastases from carcinoma of the larynx. Laryngoscope 81:1503, 1971.

57. O'Brien, P. H., Carlson, R., Steubner, E. A., Jr., and Staley, C. T.: Distant metastases in epidermoid cell carcinoma of the head and neck. Cancer 27:304, 1971.

58. Stefani, S., and Eells, R. W.: Carcinoma of the hypopharynx—a study of distant metastases, treatment failures, and multiple primary cancers in 215 male patients. Laryngoscope 81:1491, 1971.

59. Probert, J. C., Thompson, R. W., and Bagshaw, M. A.: Patterns of spread of distant metastases in head and neck cancer. Cancer 33:127, 1974.

60. Merino, O. R., Lindberg, R. D., and Fletcher, G. H.: An analysis of distant metastases from squamous cell carcinoma of the upper respiratory and digestive tracts. Cancer 40:145, 1977.

61. Arlen, M., Wanebo, H., Guerra, O., Higinbotham, N., Huvos, A., and Miller, T.: Osseous metastasis: Its relationship to primary carcinoma of the head and neck. Am. J. Surg. 128:568, 1974.

62. Coker, D. D., Casterline, P. F., Chambers, R. G., and Jaques, D. A.: Metastases to lymph nodes of the head and neck from an unknown primary site. Am. J. Surg. 134:517, 1977.

63. Shear, M., Hawkins, D. M., and Farr, H. W.: The prediction of lymph node metastases from oral squamous carcinomas. Cancer 37:1901, 1976.

CHAPTER 13

Fibrous Lesions of the Head and Neck: Benign, Malignant and Indeterminate

Mackenzie[1] lists three cardinal errors in the management of fibrous tumors: (2) the *surgeon* has accepted apparent encapsulation of the tumor as an indication of innocence; (2) the *pathologist* is lulled into a sense of false security by the cellular consistency of the tumor; and (3) neither surgeon *nor* pathologist understands the natural history of fibromatous tumors.

Much of what has been written about soft part lesions and about fibrous tumors in particular has been centered around morphological aspects, and therein lies a major source of confusion. Some fibrous tissue enters into the composition of almost all tumors or neoplasms as a supportive framework.[2] In addition, many cell types can act as facultative fibroblasts. A variety of cells—lipoblasts, rhabdomyoblasts, synovial cells, etc.—by exercising this ability, may be histologically mistaken for fibroblasts.

Morphological similarities between some of the supporting tissue tumors is another frequent source of error in diagnosis. Certain neurogenic sarcomas, for example, may be indistinguishable from leiomyosarcomas or even some aggressive fibromatoses.

Stout[2] cited another potent source of error and confusion derived from the fact that the term *fibrosarcoma* is often applied indiscriminately to both benign and malignant tumors, because of cellularity and histological features alone. The reliability of employing the usual histological criteria for determining the degree of malignancy of a fibrous tissue tumor has been questioned by Stout[2, 3] because, in some instances, they are similar. In these instances *clinical* evidence must be used to determine the degree of malignancy. Furthermore, the successful treatment of a fibrosar-

coma may depend more on size and location of the lesion than on the grade of malignancy as determined by histological evidence.

If the suffix, *sarcoma*, is limited to those fibrous neoplasms capable of generating metastases, it is a truism that the majority of fibrous neoplasms do *not* qualify. On the other hand, "fibroma," except for neoplasms occurring in the skin, is practically indefinable when it appears in the deeper soft tissues or oral and perioral regions. One is then left with a class of intermediate, also poorly defined tumors, including "fibromatoses, fasciitis, desmoid," etc. This form of classification, suggesting an obviously malignant, obviously benign and a larger "questionable behavior" group, is facile enough for statistical studies but more difficult to apply to everyday surgical practice.

Borderline cases, the number of which will vary with the experience of the microscopist, require a complete clinicopathological correlation (age, sex, duration, size, location, gross appearance and consultation with the surgeon) before diagnosis is rendered. The presence or absence of a detectable encapsulation is not reliable, for many clinically benign lesions appear to have no recognizable capsule and, in fact, may even appear locally invasive. Nuclear activity is also misleading, for in malignant lesions there may be only a small number of mitoses. Pleomorphism of cells, hyperchromatism of nuclei and apparent immaturity of cells are often features that may be misleading. By recalling the histological appearance of a lush reactive fibroblastic reaction, the pathologist can appreciate this.

Whatever may be said about Stout's[2-5] approach to fibrous tumors, it was one made by an intellectually honest pathologist who attempted to unravel some of the tangle of terms and classifications. He applied the term, "differentiated" fibrosarcoma to those fibroblastic proliferations whose cellularity was such that he could not completely exonerate them as benign. This leaves the designation "undifferentiated" fibrosarcoma for the malignant neoplasms that often metastasize. What the practitioner lacks, however, is a definition as to what degree of cellularity or other features are necessary or required to shift a lesion from an apparent *fibromatosis-fasciitis* group to the differentiated fibrosarcoma class of neoplasms.

As we have indicated above, fibrosarcomas and other malignant soft tissue neoplasms do not necessarily conform to the classical criteria used in the diagnosis of other forms of cancer. Mitotic activity, for example, is of limited value when dealing with soft part fibrous tumors in infancy. Other, and admittedly ancillary, histological features may play a decisive role. Immature blood vessels and areas of necrosis are more likely to occur in the malignant forms than in benign ones. Most of the neoplasms and "tumor-like" lesions of the soft parts show a conspicuous vascular participation. Desmoid tumors, juvenile fibromatoses, nodular and pseudosarcomatous fasciitis, proliferative myositis and myositis ossificans all manifest this feature. In the desmoid tumor and juvenile fibromatosis, the vascular pattern and arrangement are haphazard. In nodular fasciitis and myositis ossificans, the vessels align themselves in the direction of growth radially, like the spokes of a wheel, or show a branching configuration. The vessels are nearly all arterioles. The attendance to other cellular participants in the tumor, inflammatory cells included, in fibrous lesions is important for, in the final analysis, it may be these components and the lesion's resemblance to a reactive process, albeit florid at times, that may tip the diagnostic scale away from "malignant." Care must always be taken to separate *ab initio* reactive or necrotic changes from secondary effects due to trauma.

Classifications of this group of tumors (proliferations and neoplasms) have often been rambling monstrosities with terms such as fasciitis, nodular fasciitis, infiltrative fasciitis, pseudosarcomatous fibromatosis, aggressive fibromatosis, cellular keloid, differentiated or grade I fibrosarcoma and nonmetastasizing fibrosarcoma, either lumped together or sharply defined by ill-defined and often intangible criteria. The rather recent exploitation of an earlier recognized ability of the histiocyte to behave as a facultative fibroblast has opened up another Pandora's box of terms, which, without a qualifying commentary by the pathologist, serves only to confuse the harassed surgeon (Fig. 13.1).

If one pauses in his haste to apply a newly acquired and, for the moment, "fashionable" diagnosis to a fibrous lesion, he will recall that seldom, if ever, is the clinicopathological situation with fibromatous lesions "black and white." Most often, it is one in which there are various shades of gray. The surgeon confronted with an aggressively behaving and recurrent fibrous tumor in the supraclavicular fossa, for example, is not at all comforted or even aided by the apparent inconsistency and indecision shown by the pathologists,

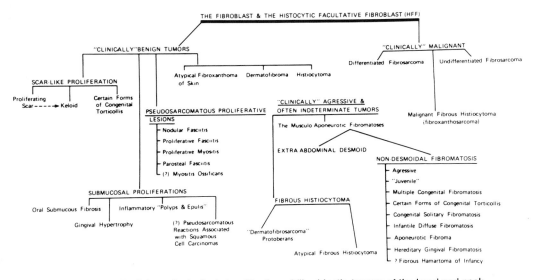

Figure 13.1. A clinicopathological classification of fibroblastic tumors of the head and neck.

when three different histological diagnoses—"fasciitis," "aggressive fibromatosis" and "well-differentiated fibrosarcoma"—are rendered by three consultants for the same lesion.

Even though our three (not so hypothetical) pathologists have used different diagnostic terms, the meaning they probably intended to convey was that the lesion in question, "is locally aggressive but very likely will not metastasize." One pathologist's extra-abdominal desmoid is another's grade I fibrosarcoma; another's well-differentiated fibrosarcoma is the same as his colleague's aggressive fibromatosis. In the end, it is the location and size of the lesion and its local biological activity that determine the form of treatment. An important modifier is the age of the patient.

THE FIBROMATOSES

The fibromatoses in aggregate include a wide histological range of lesions, from the often stubbornly recurrent, yet parvicellular, keloid (Fig. 13.2) to very cellular lesions which some authorities prefer to call differentiated sarcomas. Not only does their histological make-up vary, their locations in the body are also diverse. Wherever they occur, their diagnosis and management are always sources of concern.

The fibromatoses, in general, arise from the musculo-aponeuroses. A salient clinical feature is the regularity with which they appear to defeat

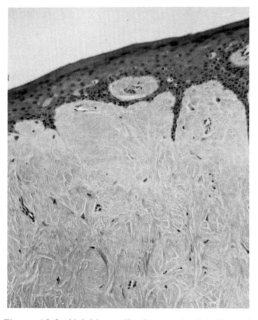

Figure 13.2. Keloid, manifesting parvicellularity and atrophy of overlying epithelium.

surgical efforts toward their removal. The most disconcerting aspect of the fibromatoses for the surgical pathologist (particularly so in the head and neck) is the impossibility of predicting how any of them will behave. Exceptions to this are the plantar and palmar fibromatoses and the fibrous reaction found in congenital torticollis (vide infra).

The fibromatoses form a spectrum of proliferative fibrous lesions whose kaleidoscopic histological appearances overlap or shade into one another to such an extent that the pathologist may be more influenced by the anatomical location of the neoplasm, sex of the patient and clinical behavior of the disease than by the morphology of the lesion in rendering his diagnosis. Table 13.1 presents a listing of the fibromatoses affecting the head and neck. It is to be noted, however, that for many of the lesions, the head and neck is not a common location.

In the head and neck, the keloid and "fibrosarcoma" lie at the two extremes of the histological scale. In between lie the diverse-appearing musculo-aponeurotic fibrous lesions (also called extra-abdominal desmoids). These fibromatoses range from lesions identical to the desmoid of the anterior abdominal wall to cellular fibrous proliferations, lacking any histological evidence of the "usual" desmoid tumor. Because the term *desmoid* does not convey the diversity of cellularity, I prefer to call the lesions fibromatoses. I usually qualify this diagnostic term by the adjectives *juvenile,* for those occurring in patients younger than 16 years of age, and *aggressive,* in deference to their local invasion and stubborness in response to treatment. For the most part, fibromatoses of the head and neck occur in children and in young adults.

The primary or initial surgical treatment should be as thorough as possible whenever a diagnosis of fibromatosis of the head and neck is made. Because these lesions may invade and recur so frequently, extensive resections do not obviate major and radical surgery. Although amputative or super-radical surgery will not be generally required, it is evident that the principle of en bloc resection of soft parts, including wide ablation of the surrounding grossly normal tissue and removal of entire muscle bundles, must be requisite if the results of surgical management are to be improved.

Musculo-aponeurotic Fibromatoses (Desmoid Tumor)

A *desmoid* tumor may be defined as a form of fibromatosis that presents as a circumscribed, locally infiltrative, usually well differentiated and firm overgrowth of fibrous tissue arising in the

Table 13.1
The Fibromatoses of the Head and Neck

Lesion	Age	Location
Fibrous hamartoma of infancy[6]	Birth, infancy	Usually in axillae and shoulder. Subcutaneous lower dermis and subcutaneous fat.
Fibromatosis colli[7]	Birth, infancy	Lower third of sternocleidomastoid muscle. May be bilateral. Associated with congenital anomalies.
Aggressive infantile and juvenile fibromatosis[8, 9]	First year of life through adolescence	Locally aggressive and tend to recur even after many years
Diffuse infantile fibromatosis[10]	First 3 years of life; occ. at birth	Arm-shoulder-neck area. Solitary and multicentric. Has inflammatory cell foci.
Congenital generalized fibromatosis[10, 11]	Multicentric mesenchymal dysplasia with onset in uterine life	Multiple lesions in subcutaneous tissues, muscle, bone, viscera.
Congenital solitary fibromatosis[10]	Infancy, childhood	Variant of generalized in soft tissues
Aponeurotic fibroma and cartilaginous analogue[12]	Infants, juveniles, adults	Rare in head and neck. Most often in palms, soles, limbs. Subcutaneous or deep fascia, tendons.
Extra-abdominal desmoid[13]	Young adult, adults	Shoulder girdle, extremities, neck.

musculo-aponeurotic structures of the body. The name is derived from the Greek desmos, signifying "band or tendon," and alludes to the tendon-like consistency of the tumor.

The tumors are most often found in the anterior abdominal wall, where they arise especially from the rectus sheath and usually in young or middle-aged parous women. Extra-abdominal desmoids are also recognized. In fact, the first microscopic description of a "desmoid tumor" was probably given from extra-abdominal forms by Bennett[14] in 1849. They have been described in the region of the shoulder girdle, which is the site of predilection, and in the muscular tissues of the legs, thighs, chest, head and neck. Those arising from the masseteric aponeurosis simulate parotid tumors. There is strong evidence that the anatomical location of the musculo-aponeurotic fibromatoses affects, to a significant degree, the clinical behavior and course of the lesion. The extra-abdominal desmoids, then, assume a greater clinicotherapeutic significance than do their abdominal wall counterparts.

In general, both abdominal and extra-abdominal desmoids present with identical histological appearances. The mature-appearing and relatively acellular form seen in Figures 13.3 and 13.4 is familiar to surgeons and pathologists. With an increasing cellularity, this classical desmoidal pattern is lost and the true fibromatous character of

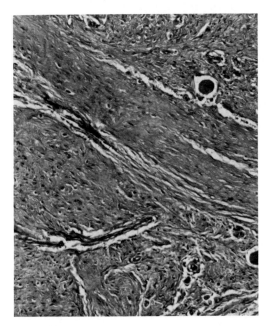

Figure 13.3. Desmoidal fibromatosis in the "classical" abdominal form.

the lesion is more apparent. There is often a striking discrepancy between their deceptively harmless microscopic appearance and their potential to attain a large size, to recur and to infiltrate structures in a manner like a fibrosarcoma.

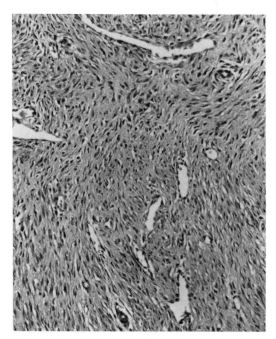

Figure 13.4. Fibromatosis in neck (extra-abdominal desmoid).

In my experience, and that of others, the extra-abdominal desmoid tumors have manifested a much more aggressive clinical behavior than those originating from the anterior abdominal wall.[7] As will be seen, this is particularly true for those occurring in the head and neck and in children or young adults. An appreciation of this aggressiveness may be found in the study by Enzinger and Shiraki.[15] Eight of their 30 patients with extra-abdominal desmoids of the shoulder girdle had their tumors located primarily in the supraclavicular fossa. In this location, the tumors involved, to varying degrees, the supraspinatus, the anterior scalene and the pectoralis minor muscles, usually together with the enveloping fascia. Complete removal in this location was often impossible without sacrificing a portion of the brachial plexus or the large vessels entrapped by the infiltrating tumor.

Because of this aggressive character, the desmoid tumor, in some institutions, is regarded as a fibrosarcoma, grade I (desmoid type).[16] Stout[2] suggested "differentiated fibrosarcoma" for the cellular desmoid and "desmoid fibromatosis" for the less cellular variety.

Fibromatoses in the Head and Neck

The frequency with which fibromatoses involve the head and neck is difficult to assess because of the pecularities of classification used by different authors. At the Mayo Clinic, head and neck desmoids constituted 12% of 284 desmoid tumors in all locations of the body.[17]

Masson and Soule[17] have presented the most comprehensive analysis of desmoid tumors in this region of the body. The fibromatoses, in the head and neck, present over a wide span of life, from early childhood to old age. Most tumors present before the patient is 50 years old. The generally recognized prevalence of desmoids in women also pertains to those arising in the head and neck. The neck, or, more precisely, the supraclavicular region, is the most common area of involvement (85% in the Mayo Clinic series).[17] The remainder occur on the scalp and face (Fig. 13.5). A primary involvement of the oral soft tissues, nasal cavity, paranasal sinuses and larynx is less common.[18] These structures are usually secondarily invaded by the aggressive behavior of a fibromatosis. In the nasal cavity and sinuses, the lesions tend to be located in the nasal turbinates and antrum where they infiltrate adjacent structures and tissues. In the sinus, they may completely fill the sinus cavity. The biological behavior follows that of those outside of the airway; recurrences are common and death may ensue due to a lack of control of the lesion. I know of no primary lesion lower in the airway.

Primary oral fibromatosis is also unusual and, like its counterparts elsewhere, requires an aggressive surgical treatment.[19]

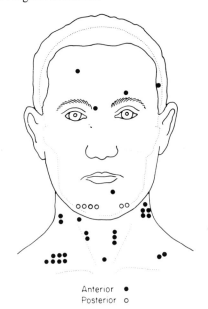

Anterior ●
Posterior ○

Figure 13.5. Location of head and neck fibromatoses (desmoid tumors) as studied by Masson and Soule.[17]

The mode of presentation and the initial clinical course of a desmoid tumor in the head and neck are not unlike those of desmoid tumors in other locations. A progressively enlarging, painless tumor, usually present for less than 1 year, causes the patient to seek medical attention. The slow growth sometimes manifested by desmoids in other anatomical regions is not necessarily valid for those presenting in the head and neck.

The gross appearance of a desmoid tumor, wherever it occurs, is that of an ill-defined, gray-white, firm mass with a propensity to infiltrate surrounding muscle and fibroadipose or connective tissue. The mass appears to encase neural and vascular elements. Erosion of bone or actual invasion of bone may occur. Recurrent lesions are similar in appearance and are often multiple. The degree of microscopic cellularity of a fibromatosis is variable, not only from tumor to tumor, but also from area to area. Some tumors present with a proliferation of mature fibroblasts and a dominating collagenous component (tendon-like) or lack the densely collagenized feature and manifest a conspicuously cellular fibroblastic component (Fig. 13.6). In both forms, cellularity is most evident at the peripheral advancing edges of the tumor.

Individual fibroblasts also vary in the appearance of their nuclei and cytoplasmic prominence.

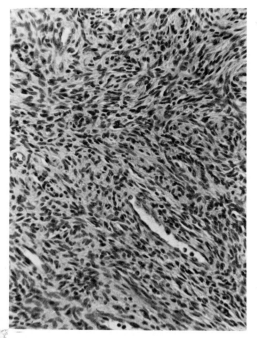

Figure 13.6. Cellular and "aggressive"-appearing extra-abdominal desmoid or fibromatosis from the lateral lower neck in a 7-year-old boy.

Mitoses, never atypical are found in the cellular regions. Primary lesions tend to be more cellular than the recurrent tumors. As indicated earlier, a random distribution of thin-walled vascular spaces is almost always present. The infiltrative edges of the fibromatoses replace skeletal muscle and induce atrophy and regenerative attempts in the muscle fibers. These changes account for the presence of multinucleated giant cells at the periphery of the lesions.

As far as the host is concerned, fibromatoses of the head and neck are serious lesions. The combination of an innate local aggressiveness, a high rate of recurrence and a relatively restricted and confined anatomical region not only compromises surgical excision but also brings the tumors dangerously close to vital vascular, neural and visceral structures. Seventy percent of the Mayo Clinic group of patients had one or more recurrences, as compared with a 50% incidence for patients with desmoid tumors from all locations.[17] Improper *primary* surgery certainly accounts for some of this morbidity. Das Gupta et al.[13] record only a 20% recurrence rate for extra-abdominal desmoids when the primary surgery was adequately carried out. With operations on patients who already had manifested recurrences, however, the percentage increased to one-third of the group.

En bloc resection of tumor and surrounding normal structures, if possible, should be carried out. Masson and Soule[17] believe that complete removal of the lesion in the neck is best accomplished by a radical neck dissection, regardless of the size of the tumor. A tumor considered inoperable in this region is capable of killing the host, witness the four deaths from the series of Masson and Soule[17] and Das Gupta et al.[13] There is some indication that irradiation may exercise a modicum of control over the tumor, and certainly it is advised when antomical restrictions preclude surgical control.

In my consideration, both abdominal and extra-abdominal desmoids are best designated as fibromatoses and, as such, are not true neoplasms. Acceptable examples of metastasis have not occurred, nor have I been impressed with an increasing anaplasia after repeated recurrences. In the young patient whose lesion has metastasized, the lesion *was* a fibrosarcoma at the onset and, because of the notorious difficulty in separating benign from malignant fibrous tumors in the child, was undercalled (misdiagnosed) at the initial examination.[20]

The lesion called "juvenile fibromatosis" by Stout[3] and "aggressive infantile fibromatosis" by

Enzinger,[9] I regard as a form of aggressive extra-abdominal desmoid, but I recognize that the lesion represents one of the most complex problems in the classification of fibrous tumors. Seen particularly in the infant and juvenile patient, this lesion and well-differentiated fibrosarcoma, if they can indeed be separated, have a tendency to occur in the head and neck and neck region, including the sinuses and oral cavity. Mitoses are not reliable indices for malignancy in this age group, but one of 13 cases classified in this category metastasizes.[20] Balsaver et al.,[21] recognizing this potential, consider the lesion when it occurs in the very young as "congenital fibrosarcoma." Recurrences after some time delay are common, and vital structures may be involved, thus precluding total removal. If complete removal can be accomplished, almost all cases will be cured.

The incidence of fibromatosis in neonates is second only to that of vascular tumors. Among these lesions may be included fibromatosis colli, recurrent digital fibromatosis, fibrous hamartoma of infancy, diffuse infantile fibromatosis, fibromatosis hyalinica multiplex juvenilis, juvenile aponeurotic fibroma, hereditary gingival fibromatosis and congenital solitary or generalized fibromatosis.[10]

Congenital generalized fibromatosis is a form of multicentric, focal mesenchymal dysplasia developing in the last few months of intrauterine life.[10] The multinodular lesions involve subcutaneous tissues and/or skeletal muscle and visera and/or skeleton and have often been fatal (Fig. 13.7). Some lesions on the other hand have shown spontaneous regression. The histological appearance of these lesions is that of a predominating and partly immature fibroblast-like cell population possessing pericytoma-like areas. Some solitary fibromatoses manifest an identical histological pattern and the solitary and generalized forms are likely related. Whether some of the so-called infantile fibrosarcomas are actually a localized congenital fibromatosis is not clear. The relationship to what we have termed aggressive extra-abdominal desmoid is also unclear.

Fibrous hamartoma of infancy is clearly distinguished from the fibromatoses by a characteristic organoid arrangement of traversing bundles of dense fibrocollagenous tissue, immature-appearing mucoid loose-textured cellular areas and mature fibroadipose tissue.[6] Moreover these lesions are situated in the lower dermis or subcutaneous fat. Infantile hemangiopericytoma (see p. 308) has some features in common with congenital generalized fibromatosis: a perivascular pattern, multinodular growth pattern, variable mitotic activity

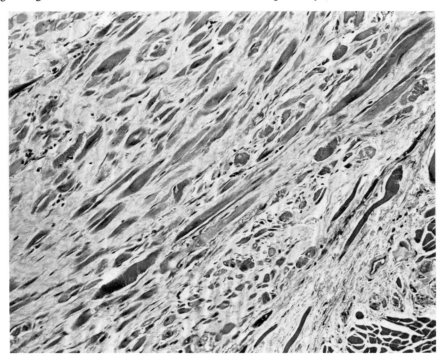

Figure 13.7. Congenital fibromatosis from a 2-month-old child. The lesion invaded the larynx, necessitating en bloc resection.

with occasional necrosis. However, in contrast the infantile hemangiopericytoma is exclusively a subcutaneous lesion, and is characterized by a prominent pericytoma and endothelial proliferation pattern throughout the lesion.

Goldman[22] has described the cartilage analogue of fibromatosis. This lesion's hallmark is a differentiation of peculiar chondroid conformations within the spindle cell stroma. These resemble fibrocartilage and are not unlike the fibrocartilaginous transformation in aponeuroses near their attachments to skeletal structures. The calcifying aponeurotic fibroma of Keasby is a modification of this lesion.[22] Primarily a lesion of the hands and feet, the cartilage analogue may present in the neck.

PSEUDOSARCOMATOUS PROLIFERATIVE LESIONS OF SOFT TISSUES WITH OR WITHOUT BONE FORMATION

The heading of this section indicates the close relationship that exists between nodular fasciitis, proliferative fasciitis and proliferative myositis. The descriptive term "pseudosarcomatous proliferative lesion of soft tissue" has been proposed for these lesions and mixed forms with or without bone formation.[23] In the discussion which follows, the terms, nodular fasciitis, proliferative myositis and proliferative fasciitis are retained as subtypes, with different gross structural patterns, light microscopic appearance and age distribution within the spectrum of pseudosarcomatous proliferative lesions of soft tissue. As will be seen also, some of the lesions are only infrequently found in the soft-tissues of the head and neck.

Proliferative myositis and fasciitis are considered distinguishable from nodular fasciitis, not only because of their gross features, but also because of their light microscopic appearance with large mono- and binucleated cells as predominating cell types. That this may not always apply has been considered by Dahl and Angervall.[23] In contrast to nodular fasciitis, which occurs in all ages, proliferative myositis and proliferative fasciitis do not affect children. This age difference may serve as a reason for separating the lesions or it merely may reflect different age-linked types of reaction to the same basic stimulus.

The presence of bone in this group of reactive processes is not common and when it occurs does not manifest the zoning-phenomenon of myositis ossificans.

Whether or not the lesions are pathogenetically related (and we believe they are), the most important consideration is to clearly separate them from sarcomas.

Nodular Fasciitis

Nodular fasciitis is singled out as a definite clinicopathological entity and *should not* be classified under the general heading of fibromatosis. There is a difference in its clinical behavior as well as its histological appearance. Nodular (pseudosarcomatous) fasciitis is most likely a reactive, non-neoplastic response to injury. The lesion is entirely benign but is deceptive in its rather rapid onset and in its histological appearance, which belies its innocent clinical behavior.

Nodular fasciitis may present over a wide range of life, from early childhood through the seventh decade of life. A peak incidence occurs between 30 and 40 years. Nearly half of the reported cases (293 between 1955 and 1969) have presented in the upper extremity, with the forearm being the area of predilection. Schreiber et al.[24] found the site breakdown to be as follows: upper extremity, 49%; trunk, 18%; lower extremity, 17%; *head and neck*, 13%; "elsewhere," 3%. A nearly identical incidence in the head and neck has been found by Allen[25] after a review of 829 cases of nodular fasciitis (Table 13.2). Nearly half of the number of head and neck tumors have occurred in children less than 15 years of age. Usually fast growing, the majority of lesions have been noted only for a short time before their excision. Sixty percent are removed within 4 months and 40% are excised less than 3 weeks after their onset. Only rarely does a patient wait for a year before seeking medical attention.

The tumor is usually a discrete soft tissue mass, somewhat tender and fixed to the subjacent structures but with a freely movable overlying skin. Size at the time of removal varies from 4 mm to 4

Table 13.2
Nodular Fasciitis: Locations in Head and Neck*

Site	No. of Cases
Neck	51
Face	49
Forehead	21
Scalp	13
Orbit	13
Conjunctiva	9
Eyelid	5
Buccal mucosa	2
	163
Percent of total	20%

* Adopted from Allen.[25]

cm in diameter. Depending on their histological make-up, they may clinically simulate anything from an abscess to a neurofibroma.

Nodular fasciitis may be loosely divided into three gross types according to its relation to the superficial fascia of the anatomical region. The most common (80%) grows from the fascia upward into the subcutaneous tissues, where it usually presents as a well-circumscribed round to oval nodule of less than 3 cm in diameter. The second type affects chiefly the fascia itself or its close environs. The third form grows downward from the fascia into the underlying muscle. All three types behave in a similar (benign) manner and do not show a tendency to recur. Characteristically, the lesions are unencapsulated yet fairly well circumscribed; herein may lie the reason for the low recurrence rate. The tumors formed by the fibromatoses, on the other hand, are larger, firmer, more deeply situated and more fixed to the deeper tissues. Even in the third gross type of nodular fasciitis, the nodule does not manifest the characteristic gross appearance of a fibromatosis, which is hard and rubbery and has a glistening, fibrous-appearing cut surface.

Histologically, the appearance of the lesion is characteristic and striking. If there is a single principal criterion for the diagnosis of nodular fasciitis, it may be the haphazard arrangement of irregular bundles or single fibroblasts in a mucoid matrix (Fig. 13.8). However, as indicated earlier and as will be shown, this feature alone does not

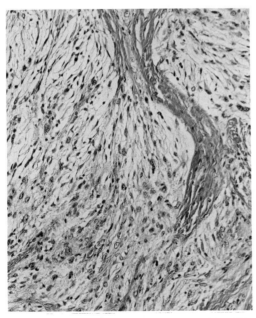

Figure 13.8. Nodular (pseudosarcomatous) fasciitis.

suffice for a consistently accurate diagnosis. An important and constant feature is the vasculature of the lesion, composed of a fine capillary network arranged in a radial pattern and apparently deriving its branching from the larger vessels of the adjacent tissue.

The predominant cells are large, often plump fibroblasts, not unlike those seen in tissue culture preparations or in a reactive granulation tissue. Mitoses are common but never plentiful. Variable quantities of fibroblastic products, i.e., collagen fibers and acid mucopolysaccharide, are the other components with which the fibroblasts are associated. Because of the rich acid mucopolysaccharide content of the intercellular matrix, it is readily stained by colloidal iron or alcian blue. Other cellular elements in the loosely textured, somewhat feathery-appearing lesion are scattered mononuclear inflammatory cells and, in those lesions of longer duration, absorptive-type giant cells and foamy histiocytes.

Price et al.[26] have divided nodular fasciitis into three histological subtypes. Type 1 nodules are moderately cellular with an abundant interstitial ground substance, giving the lesion a distinctly myxoid appearance. This ground substance is most abundant in the parvicellular center with increasing cellularity at the periphery of the lesion. Vascularity is prominent, and multinucleated giant cells are commonly seen. Type 2 nodules manifest less ground substance and a tendency toward greater cellularity with a less haphazard arrangement of the cells. Type 3 nodules are biologically more mature. There is increased collagen production with only a small amount of interstitial ground substance. The vascularity of the lesion is still maintained but is of a more mature type. The young patient may have a tendency to harbor lesions of the type 2 variety.

Ultrastructural study confirms and extends the morphological description based on light microscopy. Also the findings reveal that myofibroblasts participate in the lesion.[27] These cells, found in hypertrophic scars, granulation tissue and other inflammatory and trauma-related conditions have the basic appearance of a fibroblast but also contain peripherally located bundles of filaments, like those of smooth muscle.

As we have seen, the histological features of nodular fasciitis may vary considerably, but four features are common to nearly all cases. These are: (1) spindle-shaped fibroblasts that tend to be arranged in long fascicles which are slightly curved, whorled or S-shaped; (2) small clefts or slit-like spaces that often separate the fibroblasts; (3) a few extravasated erythrocytes; and (4) mucoid interstitial ground substance. These are elaborated in greater detail by Allen.[25]

Accurate histopathological identification of this entity is necessary to prevent mutilation and morbidity resulting from a false diagnosis of fibrosarcoma or other malignancy. In addition, the surgeon must be aware of the benign nature of this entity. Soule[28] and Price et al.[26] have emphasized the frequency with which these lesions are erroneously interpreted as malignant. One-fourth of Soule's[28] cases had undergone wide excision or radiation therapy. Twenty of Price's[26] 65 cases were originally diagnosed as either fibrosarcoma or angiosarcoma. Phelan and Jurado[29] cautioned against an erroneous diagnosis of liposarcoma or fibrosarcoma.

If the diagnosis is a correct one, the surgeon and patient can be reassured that prognosis is excellent. The studies of Hutter et al.[30] and Stout[31] have conclusively shown the benign nature of this condition and its relatives in the periosteum and in skeletal muscle (vide infra). Simple local excision is the recommended treatment for the more superficial lesions. As the deeper nodules tend to be somewhat larger and less well demarcated, a wider local excision is advisable.

As to prognosis, none of the patients followed by Hutter et al.[30] including 26 cases followed for 5 to 20 years, developed a recurrence or metastasis after local excision. In those patients in whom *no excision* was carried out, the nodules regressed and disappeared, supporting the concept of a benign and self-limiting inflammatory reaction of fascia. Allen's[25] review of the literature indicates a reported recurrence rate of approximately 6%, but in his personal series of 895 cases, he records only a 1% recurrence.

Proliferative Myositis

A pseudosarcomatous lesion, proliferative myositis may occasionally present in the head and neck (particularly in the sternocleidomastoid muscle) but has a predilection for the flat muscles of the shoulder girdle. Children do not appear to be affected, and the highest incidence is in patients between 45 and 65 years of age. There appears to be a slight female predominance.

The lesion was first described by Kern[32] in 1960. He named the lesion in analogy to myositis ossificans, to which there is a possible relationship. Bullock,[33] in fact, has interpreted these lesions as a "green stage" in the development of myositis ossificans. Others, however, are not convinced of this relationship and prefer, for the present, to consider the disorder a clinicopathological entity. Trauma or other forms of injury to the fascia, muscle or blood supply to muscle probably are the underlying causes.

Clinical onset, many aspects of the microscopic appearance, and the benign course of proliferative myositis make it more aligned with nodular fasciitis than any of the other fibroproliferative disorders. The importance of accurate diagnosis is the same as that for nodular fasciitis—to avoid misinterpreting the pseudosarcomatous reaction as a sarcoma. In this respect, a diagnosis of malignancy was initially made in 14 of 33 cases reviewed by Enzinger and Dulcey[34]; in eight of the 14, the primary diagnosis was rhabdomyosarcoma!

Like other pseudosarcomatous processes, proliferative myositis is a rapidly growing lesion. There is only a short interval between onset and treatment, not unlike nodular fasciitis or myositis ossificans. Unlike nodular faciitis or myositis ossificans, however, the lesion involves muscle in a diffuse manner and primarily affects interfascicular connective tissue. The lesion also differs from these two pseudosarcomatous lesions by its infiltrative diffuse growth pattern, the presence of bizarre giant cells and the high incidence in patients older than 45 years.

On gross inspection the lesion is almost scarlike, and often is poorly circumscribed and gray-white. The involved areas measure from 1.5 to 5.0 cm in greatest dimensions. Microscopically, the fibrosis involves chiefly the perimysium, epimysium and the fascia. Residual muscle is relatively unaffected. A significant degree of inflammation is never a conspicuous feature. The perimysial and endomysial cellular proliferation, alternating with remnants of skeletal muscle, imparts a "checkerboard effect" under low-power microscopic examination.[34] Giant cells with prominent nucleoli and deeply staining basophilic cytoplasm are the hallmark of proliferative myositis (Fig. 13.9). The resemblance of these cells to ganglion cells and/or rhabdomyoblasts is particularly noteworthy for the microscopist. There is no convincing evidence that these giant cells are osteoblasts, and, although a rhabdomyoblastic origin for these cells has been suggested, they are more likely modified fibroblasts.[35]

Complete spontaneous regression (on occasion), the clinical benignancy of the lesion (nonrecurrence) and the apparent self-limited course certainly indicate that surgical treatment should be conservative. Enzinger and Dulcey[34] state "no further surgery is necessary after the diagnosis has been established on material gained by simple

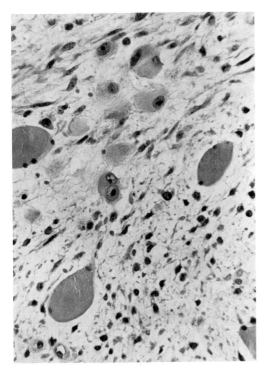

Figure 13.9. Proliferative myositis, a pseudosarcomatous lesion, is characterized by the ganglion cell-like appearance of fibroblasts.

excision or biopsy." Kern's[32] suggestion that some of these lesions might terminate as extra-abdominal desmoids has not been endorsed by follow-up studies for as long as 16 years.

Proliferative Fasciitis

Closely related to proliferative myositis, this lesion, despite its rapid growth and often bizarre microscopic appearance pursues a benign clinical course. To date, its recognition in the head and neck is limited. Preferential sites are the extremities and the trunk. These lesions involve the fascia and interlobular fibrous septa of the *subcutaneous* fibroadipose tissue and occur exclusively in adults.[36] The lesion is usually present from 2 to 6 weeks in the great majority of cases. A history of trauma to the area can be elicited in only a quarter of the cases. The lesions are usually poorly demarcated and situated primarily between the subcutis and underlying muscle in the region of the superficial fascia. They are rarely attached to or superficially infiltrate the underlying skeletal muscle. The average size of the lesion in the series studied by Chung and Enzinger[36] was 2.6 cm. Microscopically, the features characteristic of proliferative myositis are a mixture of large basophilic

"giant" cells and fibroblast-like spindle cells in a more or less prominent myxoid matrix. The cellular proliferation is largely confined to the fascial plane. The histological features are nearly those of proliferative myositis and some have considered the lesion to be no more than a subcutaneous variant of proliferative myositis. The ganglion-like cells in both lesions represent modified fibroblasts of unusual size and shape. These giant cells are not those of the reactive multinucleated giant cells, the latter, a relatively common finding in nodular fasciitis, are exceedingly rare in the proliferative variants.

Parosteal Fasciitis

The pathological features of *parosteal* fasciitis are the same as those of fasciitis occurring in any other location except for an adjacent reactive cortical bone formation.[37] Like nodular fasciitis and proliferative myositis, the histopathology is unique and distinctive. The essential features are a fibroblastic proliferation in a myxoid or collagenous matrix which contains a rich capillary network and a sparse round cell infiltrate (Fig. 13.10). The fibroblasts may take various forms—large, triangular or roughly stellate with tapering cytoplasmic ends. When closely packed, they are spindled. The

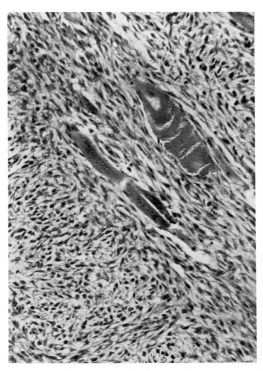

Figure 13.10. Parosteal fasciitis; in this area the lesion has extended into adjacent skeletal muscle.

nuclei in all forms of fasciitis are vesicular with one or two prominent nucleoli. Mitoses may be frequent, yet not atypical. Reactive bone formation in the adjacent cortex is a feature of parosteal fasciitis. This is not to be confused with the occasional foci of osteoid, bone and cartilage found in fasciitis of the soft tissues where there is no adjacent bone.

Parosteal fasciitis resembles neither the so-called periosteal desmoid or periosteal fibrosarcoma. Both of these lesions may be histologically quite benign yet clinically quite aggressive, and numerous re-excisions are the rule. Fasciitis, antithetically, is histologically aggressive yet clinically innocuous.

Myositis ossificans may be a more difficult differential diagnosis. Myositis ossificans has a periphery of well-formed bone that traces to a less mature central position. It is predominantly a bone-forming lesion. Fasciitis is basically a spindle cell lesion in which *small* foci of metaplastic bone and/or cartilage may be present. Growth rate, age range and clinical findings of parosteal fasciitis are similar to other types of fasciitis. Simple surgical excision after diagnosis is adequate therapy for this form of fasciitis, as it is for all other forms of fasciitis.

MYOSITIS OSSIFICANS

This disorder occurs in at least two clinical forms: a systemic, progressive disorder and a localized, presumably traumatic variety.

The former, *myositis ossificans progressiva,* affects young growing children as well as young adults. It involves not only skeletal muscle, but also tendons, fascia, aponeuroses and ligaments as well. The condition is frequently associated with various assorted congenital anomalies, commonly congenital anomalies of the toes and thumbs with ankylosis of the digits.[38] There is often a past history of pain and swollen joints. A clear-cut traumatic incidence is seldom found. The disease is nearly always manifest before the age of 10 years.

Ossifications frequently are recognized first in the tongue, face or neck, and the shoulder girdle muscles. The disease progresses rapidly to involve noncontiguous areas, until the entire voluntary muscular system may eventually be affected. Death is ushered in through involvement of the thoracic musculature and/or the masseter and temporalis muscles.

Examination of the literature from 1700 to the present date by Trestor et al.[39] indicates that there are almost 260 cases with sufficient documentation for the diagnosis of myositis ossificans progressiva.

Traumatic myositis ossificans is characterized by ossifications in a muscle which appear after either a single, acute trauma or after a chronic and repetitive series of minor traumatic injuries to a muscle. The musculature of the head and neck is an uncommon area for the development of localized myositis ossificans, but when the lesion occurs, it is usually in the masseter and sternomastoid muscles.[40] An exact incidence of the occurrence is not possible to relate since many are asymptomatic and are discovered only incidentally. We doubt that the few (seven) cases of traumatic myositis ossificans of the masseter muscles are representative of the true incidence.[41]

Masseteric lesions have been associated with a *single* severe trauma. This is followed by a painful mass in the injured area within 1 to 4 weeks. Organization of a hematoma is considered the most likely genesis, but implantation of periosteum in muscle and escape of osteogenic cells into muscle have also been suggested.

Two radiographic features may be presented. Feathery opacities, caused by ossifications along muscle fibers or irregular, more solid radiodensities, appear approximately 2 weeks after the muscle injury. It should be noted that the lesions lie adjacent to the facial bones but are not firmly attached to them.

Ackerman[42] has beautifully described the key differential diagnostic features of the localized form of myositis ossificans. In brief, a "zoning phenomenon" is of great histological importance. There is a central, undifferentiated zone that may be impossible to distinguish from a sarcoma. This atypical zone merges into oriented osteoid formation and finally into well-formed bone in the periphery of the lesion. If these zones are present, they are of paramount importance in the making of a diagnosis of a *benign* process and may save the patient from multilating and needless surgery. Both forms of the ossification tend to recur locally.

FIBROMA

Pure benign neoplasms of the fibrocyte are rare in any part of the body, and, as we have indicated in our discussion of localized fibrous overgrowths of the oral cavity, there is even doubt as to whether such an entity even exists. The term "fibroma" has occasionally been applied to a group of subcutaneous lesions of disputed etiology and varied nomenclature. These include fibroma durum, dermatofibroma, histiocytoma cutis and sclerosing hemangioma. These lesions are probably all variants of a single pathological process in which the microscopic appearance is dependent on the age of the lesion (vide infra).

"Fibroma" has also been incorrectly applied, but without danger, to certain pedunculated lesions of the skin which are either malformations or more likely hyperplastic proliferations secondary to injury or inflammation. The same absence of hazard cannot be said for the use of the term for deeper soft tissue tumors, where a histological diagnosis of "fibroma" is always suspect. In this location, such fibrous lesions represent reactive processes, fibromatoses, fibrosarcomas or other types of soft tissue neoplasms, benign or malignant.

Suspicion should also be attached to a diagnosis of "fibroma" given to a supporting tissue lesion of the upper respiratory tract and hypopharynx. The dramatic mode of presentation of some of the pedunculated fibromatous lesions of the hypopharynx have beclouded the fact that they are, in reality, extremely rare. Sohn and Feuerstein[43] have reviewed these so-called "fibromatous polyps" of the hypopharynx, and Hara[44] has reviewed similar tumors of the tonsil.

In the hypopharynx, fibromatous "polyps" are mostly the result of local injury or inflammatory reaction causing damage to the elastic fibers within the submucosal layers of the pharyngeal wall, leading to herniation of fibrous or adipose tissue (hence "lipomatous" polyp). The polypoid lesions vary greatly in size and often arise from the posterior wall of the pharynx. They may be sessile or, more often, polypoid. In consistency, they vary from soft and fibrillar to dense, firm masses. Mechanical obstruction is rare, but larger tumors may act as a ball-valve.

The lesions are quite unlike angiofibromas in their appearance and clinical behavior. If completely excised, the prognosis is excellent, with little chance of recurrence. They do not exhibit any of the local invasiveness seen in angiofibroma of the nasopharynx.

HISTIOCYTIC TUMORS (BENIGN AND MALIGNANT)

The acceptance of the histiocyte as a potential facultative fibroblast and convincing in vitro tissue culture studies have called forth a significant revision of the nomenclature formerly attached to a variety of superficial and deep supporting tissue tumors. The histiocytic character and unity (modified primarily by the biological age) of the lesion

known as sclerosing hemangioma, dermatofibroma and recurrent dermatofibroma have previously been postulated on the basis of histological observations and have been accepted by nearly all pathologists.

The unitarian concept has now been extended to include tumors such as dermatofibrosarcoma protuberans, giant cell tumors of tendon and fascia and villonodular synovitis. Replacement terms now are: histiocytic tumors, fibrous xanthoma, histiocytoma, atypical fibroxanthoma and *malignant* histiocytoma or fibrous xanthosarcoma. The justification for this re-orientation is the assumption that the histiocyte can form connective tissue fibers as well as act as a phagocyte. In the pure histiocytoma, no fibers are formed by the cell. In the fibrous xanthoma, the histiocyte performs both functions. These lesions, particularly the fibrous xanthoma, are to be distinguished from "pure" xanthomas and xanthelasmas, which are probably not neoplastic.

It is beyond the purpose and scope of this chapter to delve further into the experimental and hypothetical reasoning for the histiocytic origin of several "fibromatous lesions." The reader can satisfy his needs in several excellent reports.[45-48] Several points are, however, important to review before we consider the tumors of this type of importance to the head and neck surgeon.

1. The generic term of fibrous histiocytoma is used to include a heterogenous group of tumors proposed to have a common origin from the tissue histiocyte. Table 13.3 presents this group of lesions.

2. The fibrous histiocytoma is a tumor that can

Table 13.3
Classification of the Fibrous Histiocytomas

Benign
    Nodular tenosynovitis (giant cell tumor of tendon sheath)
    Dermatofibroma, sclerosing hemangioma, subepidermal nodular fibrosis
    Atypical fibroxanthoma of skin
    Pigmented villonodular synovitis
    Juvenile xanthogranuloma
    Xanthoma
    Xanthofibroma

Locally Aggressive or Malignant
    Storiform fibroxanthoma (dermatofibrosarcoma protuberous)
    Histiocytoma
    Atypical fibrous histiocytoma
    Malignant histiocytoma of bone and soft tissue (fibroxanthosarcoma)

assume many forms. This diversity accounts for the several names it is often given.

3. In many examples, the "fibroblast" of the tumors (accompanied by reticulin fibers), instead of being sinuously intertwined as in the fibromatoses, tend to be arranged in a spiral nebula or flower pattern, perhaps best described by the term "storiform," meaning matted. A Laidlaw stain will enhance this histological feature (Fig. 13.11).

4. In other lesions of the family, the fibrous elements lack a storiform arrangement and display, instead, varying numbers of multinucleated histiocytic phagocytes in company with the fibroblastic cells (Fig. 13.12).

5. Histological combinations of points 2 and 3 above are found, and the tumors are then called "mixed fibrous histiocytoma."

6. Atypical fibroxanthoma (pseudosarcoma) of the skin is a lesion of considerable microscopic pleomorphism, numerous mitoses and a high degree of cellularity. This tumor has been and will probably continue to be misdiagnosed as malignant by the unwary or unknowing.

7. Like the atypical fibroxanthoma of skin, the vast majority of the histiocytic-fibrous xanthomas are benign. Only approximately 1% of fibrous histiocytomas are malignant.[46]

8. There are no reliable criteria which will per-

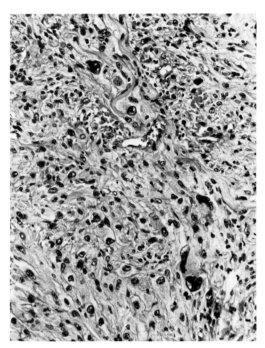

Figure 13.12. Fibrous histiocytoma containing a mixture of fibroblast-like cells and histiocytes with large nuclei.

mit the pathologist to recognize malignancy in this group of tumors from their light microscopic features alone.[46]

Dermatofibrosarcoma Protuberans and Malignant Fibrous Histiocytoma (Fibroxanthosarcomas)

The uncommon tumor of the superficial soft tissue parts, dermatofibrosarcoma protuberans, is considered by some authorities to be a form of fibrous histiocytoma of indeterminate malignant potential.[47] The tumor has been considered to have a fibrous, neural and histiocytic origin.[49] Of the ultrastructural studies of this lesion, the ones by Hashimoto et al.[50] and Alguacil-Garcia et al.[51] have been the most scholarly. These authors suggest the cell of origin is a modified fibroblast with perineural and endoneural cell features. Furthermore, there are ultrastructural suggestions that dermatofibrosarcoma protuberans should not be included in the fibrous histiocytic category. For our purposes, however, and until further proof is evolved, the lesion is included here.

The majority of these tumors present as nodular or multinodular masses on the trunk or scalp and only rarely occur below the knees. A significantly large number occur in the region of the head and

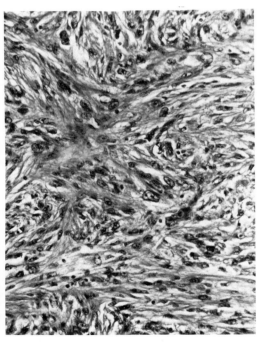

Figure 13.11. Fibrous histiocytoma with fibroblasts and histiocytes arranged in a storiform or matted arrangement.

neck, in the infra- and/or supraclavicular areas.[52] Reported series vary in their sex dominance, but men (40 to 50 years) are most often afflicted. Pain is a variable symptom and, for the most part, the tumors are painless, slowly growing masses. Possessing an indolent disposition, a dermatofibrosarcoma protuberans usually grows slowly over many years, but the duration of the tumor may vary from only a few months to many decades.

For succinctness, Borrie's[53] gross description is a minor classic: "The fundamental lesion is a firm, flat, skin-covered nodule, 5 mm in diameter, which by coalescence with other similar nodules forms a continuous plaque usually level with the skin surface to which it is fixed, though freely movable over the deeper structures. The plaque may remain in this state for anywhere from 5 to 50 years, but in time, firm, sessile or pedunculated tumors grow in the surface, varying in size from a pea to a fist. Ulceration may take place or the tumor may become soft, necrotic or hemorrhagic."

The large tumors, most often of a multiple and conglomerate character, may be greater than 20 cm in diameter. Most are firm and gray-white. On occasion, myxoid areas may simulate a liposarcoma, both grossly and microscopically. Infiltration of the adjacent tissues is a constant finding. In practically every case, microscopic evidence of the neoplasm will be found to have extended well beyond the clinically definable borders.

Microscopically, the lesion consists basically of a proliferation of fibroblastic-like cells. An alignment around a central acellular zone, or rarely around a blood vessel, produces a cartwheel effect, or "storiform" matted pattern (Fig. 13.13). This radial arrangement of the cells is a highly characteristic pattern and has been considered "diagnostic" by some authorities.[49] In other areas of the tumor, the fibroblastic cells manifest an interlacing fasicular pattern. The amount of collagen and reticulin fibers present in a tumor appears universally to be proportioned to the cellularity of the lesion. Recurrent tumors are less cellular than primary tumors. Nuclear variation is common with the majority assuming a spindle shape. Mitotic figures are never numerous but may be found without difficulty in the more cellular lesions. Giant cells are rare.

Like its presumed relative, the dermatofibroma, all dermatofibrosarcomas are quite vascular. Myxoid foci, particularly in recurrent lesions, may pose a problem in differentiation from liposarcomas. Large, long-standing tumors manifest necrotic areas. The presumed parent cells (histiocytes) and other chronic inflammatory cells may

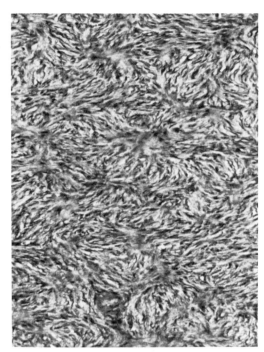

Figure 13.13. Dermatofibrosarcoma protuberans. Note the prominent cartwheel or storiform effect.

be found at the periphery of the lesions, particularly in recurrences. An apparent encapsulation may be present, but this is deceiving and most likely represents compression of adjacent tissues. A transition with the adjacent dermis is found in all cases.

Recurrences are frequent (as high as 60%) and are often repeated. Persistence, rather than recurrence, is more appropriate, and this is attributable to the microscopic spread of the lesion from the main body of the tumor. This local invasiveness accounts for the aggressive behavior of this slow-growing tumor, and any surgical procedure which does not take into account this feature is *inadequate* and doomed to "recurrences."

In the head and neck, because of the proximity of the tumors to the great vessels and nerves, each patient's therapy must be individualized, but, hopefully, it will encompass the clinically not detectable extensions of the tumor. An added incentive to complete surgical removal is the fact that a small number of dermatofibrosarcoma protuberans unpredictably metastasize in the fashion of a fibrosarcoma.

Histiocytic tumors in children have a more decided predilection for the head and neck. Twelve of 39 histiocytic tumors (benign fibrous xanthomas, benign histiocytomas and malignant or questionably malignant variants) presented by Kauffman and Stout[48] occurred in the head and neck. In children, the great majority are benign and do not exhibit any evidence of biological malignancy. A latent biological malignant potential presumably exists, but it is rare. There are no assignable criteria that definitely separates these tumors into benign and potentially malignant groups, even in a retrospective study such as that by Kauffman and Stout.[48]

Atypical Fibroxanthoma of Skin. The term *atypical fibroxanthoma* was coined by Helwig[54] for a group of skin tumors, which have cytological features suggesting malignancy, but which behave in a benign fashion. Independently, Bourne[55] described similar tumors under the name *paradoxical fibrosarcoma* of skin (pseudosarcoma). By 1976, some 300 cases of atypical fibroxanthoma of the skin had been recorded in the literature (Table 13.4).[56] Atypical fibroxanthoma may occur on any part of the body's surface. It is most commonly seen in the sun-damaged skin of the head and neck in elderly patients. In the younger patient it occurs more frequently on the trunk and the limbs.[57] The lesion is extremely rare in children. It appears as a solitary firm nodule, sometimes ulcerated and usually about 1 cm in diameter, although the range is from 0.2 cm to 12 cm. Apart from the ulceration they are mostly asymptomatic.

The lesion has been considered to be an inflammatory reactive process associated with actinically damaged skin and/or previous trauma, or irradiation of the area. However, as Dahl[56] points out, these have been found pertinent in only 20% of the reported cases.

In patients with atypical fibroxanthoma of the skin the clinical course is almost always benign and recurrence is infrequent (9.5%) as recorded in the literature. Malignant fibroxanthosarcoma of the *skin* seems to be extremely rare. Dahl[56] accepts four cases.

Table 13.4
Atypical Fibroxanthoma of Skin: Demographics of 287 Cases*

	No. of Cases
Sex	
Male	183
Female	104
Head and neck location	241
History of trauma	17
History of radiation	38
Recurrence	28
Metastases	4

* Modified from Dahl.[56]

Microscopically the lesions are located entirely, or almost entirely, in the corium. They are not encapsulated. The tumors contain cells which are principally of two types; one, fibroblast- and the other, histiocyte-like. Nuclear changes may be bizarre and nucleolar prominence is always a feature. Multinucleated, large, pleomorphic cells with homogeneous or foamy cytoplasm and mitoses may be numerous (Fig. 13.14). A variable degree of lipidosis of histiocytes is present. Hemosiderin and chronic inflammatory cells may be intermingled with the tumor cells. The ultrastructure of these unique dermal lesions has been presented by Alguacil-Garcia[58] among others. A differential diagnosis of the histiocytic infiltrates of the skin has been prepared by Mihm et al.[59]

Fibrous Histiocytomas of the Deep Tissues. Despite the often bizarre histological appearance of the atypical fibroxanthomas of skin, both pathologist and surgeon can take comfort in their usually benign course. The same cannot be said of the fibrous histiocytomas of the deep structures and bone. The experience of most workers in the field is that these lesions are more aggressive than are the dermal lesions regardless of their histological appearance.[60–63]

Blitzer et al.[62] recorded the 32nd case of fibrous histiocytoma of the deep structures of the head

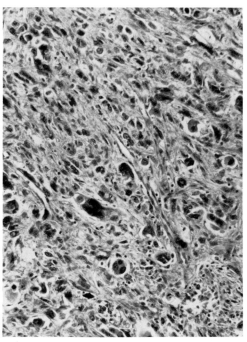

Figure 13.14. Atypical fibroxanthoma of skin. The polymorphic tumor cell population aids in differentiating this tumor from a malignant neoplasm.

and neck in 1977. Eight were intraosseous (three in mandible, one in maxilla, one in skull bone and one in the temporal bone). A discussion of fibrous histiocytoma of bone is given below. Seven were in the paranasal sinuses, four in the major salivary glands, three in the airway, five in the oral cavity, four in the neck, and three in the temporomandibular joint (Fig. 13.15).

Histologically, a wide spectrum of lesions is presented by the deep-seated fibrous histiocytomas. The malignant potential of these lesions cannot be predicted solely from their histopathology although anaplastic giant cells and numerous mitoses correlate with malignancy. Soule and Enriques[60] consider tumors with anaplastic stromal cells as malignant but admit the uncertainty of criteria. A myxoid change in a fibrous histiocytoma imparts a better prognosis with a lower metastatic rate.[64] On the other hand, a diffuse and at times intense neutrophilic infiltrate unassociated with necrosis decreases survival.[65] Merkow et al.[66] and Fu et al.[67] have characterized the ultrastructural features of the malignant fibrous histiocytoma.

The majority of fibrous histiocytomas are benign (incapable of metastasis) yet recurrences are frequent. The initial approach to these tumors should be an aggressive and wide local excision. Radiotherapy seems to have limited effect on these tumors. The statistics for recurrences after surgical excision alone are the same as that after combined therapy.

In the deep structures of the head and neck, irrespective of the histological appearance, these tumors manifest a definite tendency to local invasion. In the 32 cases reviewed by Blitzer et al.,[62] long term follow-up was absent. Even with that deficit, they recorded a 22% incidence of metastasis (lymph nodes, bone, lungs). The fallibility of microscopic evaluation of malignancy was clearly evident in their series since only four of the seven cases manifesting metastases were originally classified as malignant. The tumors in the soft tissues seem to have a smaller percentage of metastases than tumors originating in bone.[68]

Fibrous histiocytoma arising in bone is rare, while its malignant counterpart is more common.[69, 70] The distinction is important since in several series, malignant fibrous histiocytoma of bone is a highly lethal neoplasm. According to Dahlin et al.,[69] malignant (fibrous) histiocytoma is a valid diagnosis for a bone tumor if thorough sampling proves that another definable bone malignancy is not present (fibrosarcoma, osteosarcoma, dedifferentiated chondrosarcoma and even metastatic carcinoma). These authors emphasize the capability of some of the tumor cells to resemble epithelial cells and even to grow in an alveolar pattern. As it is with its soft tissue counterpart, malignant fibrous histiocytoma of bone presents many and varied histological faces. Multinucleated tumor cells or malignant giant cells are a constant finding. Fibrosis varies from prominent throughout many fields to scant, but is present in all lesions. A storiform pattern of the fibrogenic cells is frequently noted. Foamy (lipid containing) cells may or may not be present. If found, they appear to be histiocytes or modified fibrocytes.

Some differences of opinion exist as to the degree of malignancy of malignant fibrous histiocytoma of bone. In 32 detailed cases, 14 patients died in 2 to 24 months (average 12 months) after primary treatment.[70] In the same series only eight patients were alive without metastases 2 to 20 years later. The patients surveyed by Dahlin et al.[69] had a somewhat more favorable prognosis.

The malignant fibrous histiocytoma of bone is principally a tumor of long-tubular bones; six of 35 cases in the Mayo Clinic series were in the skull and facial bones.[69]

A neoplasm appearing to be closely related to

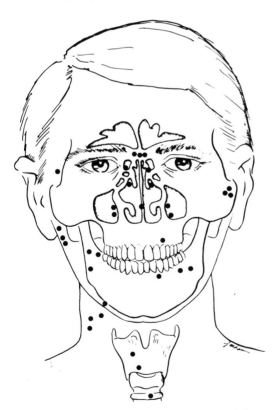

Figure 13.15. Location of reported fibrous histiocytomas in the head and neck according to the survey by Blitzer et al.[62]

the malignant fibrous histiocytoma is the malignant giant cell tumor of soft parts. It is rare anywhere in the body and especially so in the head and neck region. The abundance of multinucleated giant cells and small amounts of neoplastic osteoid or bone are the principal histological differences between this tumor and the malignant fibrous histiocytoma. A paucity of xanthomatous cells and a storiform growth pattern further serve to distinguish the malignant giant cell tumor of soft parts. These tumors may be divided into superficial and deep groups with a far greater lethality attached to the deep tumors.

Considerable light and microscopic evidence supports a histiocytic origin for these tumors and they are probably a variant of mesenchymal fibrohistiocytic sarcoma.[71, 72]

FIBROSARCOMA

Fibrosarcoma as a category of fibroblastic lesions is presented late in this presentation, not only because fibrosarcomas are relatively uncommon in the head and neck, but also so that the reader will have gained an appreciation of the pathologist's difficulty in so designating a fibrous tumor presented for his evaluation. Neoplasms labeled fibrosarcomas used to dominate the statistics in many early studies dealing with soft tissue sarcomas. Probably erroneous diagnosis accounted for this preponderance, since the tumors were confused with other soft tissue malignancies. Improvement of diagnostic acumen has markedly reduced the apparent incidence of fibrosarcoma. These neoplasms now constitute only about 0.5% of all malignancies and 5.5% of the malignant soft part sarcomas.[73]

The histological features of fibrosarcomas are conveniently, yet arbitrarily, described as of a *differentiated* or *undifferentiated* character.[2, 4] This rather loose characterization encompasses tissue forms indistinguishable from fibromatosis to those of very undifferentiated (pleomorphic sarcoma of fascia) appearance and a highly malignant disposition.

A differentiated fibrosarcoma infiltrates and recurs after removal, but only rarely spreads by metastases. The undifferentiated type, in addition to a locally aggressive behavior, also manifests a propensity to metastasize. It cannot, however, be emphasized enough that only in the most general terms can it be said that the metastasizing proclivity of a fibrosarcoma is directly proportional to its most undifferentiated portions.

Differentiated fibrosarcomas manifest an interwoven texture of differentiated cells and fibers. The fibroblasts appear relatively uniform in size and shape, do not display much hyperchromatism and lie surrounded by well-developed collagen. They are arranged in bands and bundles. Mitoses are seldom seen.

Moderately differentiated fibrosarcomas are more cellular and present a "herringbone" arrangement of their spindle cells. Mitoses are still sparse. Some correlation between the mitotic index and the rate of proliferation appears to exist. Usually behaving like its well differentiated cousin, this form of fibrosarcoma can metastasize and cause death through its dissemination.

Approximately 20% of soft part fibrosarcomas are undifferentiated and are richly cellular. Intercellular matrix and fibroblastic products are relatively sparse in the poorly differentiated fibrosarcomas. There is an inverse relationship between the degree of cellularity and the intercellular ground substance. Mitoses are frequent (Fig. 13.16). The pleomorphic giant cell sarcoma represents the epitome of poorly differentiated fibrosarcomas.

Despite their ugly and anaplastic appearances, often bearing no evidence of a fibroblastic origin, only about 25% of undifferentiated fibrosarcomas metastasize, principally by hematogenous routes.

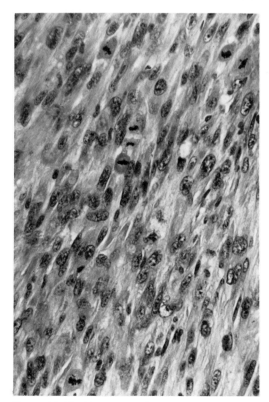

Figure 13.16. Numerous mitoses and sparse intercellular matrix in a poorly differentiated fibrosarcoma.

Other authors have expanded this simple but effective classification into grades one through four, based on the degree of cellular differentiation.[1, 74]

Superficial fibrosarcomas in the skin and the subcutaneous tissues are generally of a well-differentiated appearance and, although they are locally aggressive, rarely metastasize. A well-differentiated appearance also holds true for most of the more deeply situated fibrosarcomas. These fibrosarcomas occur most frequently in the extremities and less often in the head and neck region, back and abdominal wall. The tissues of origin for these deeper fibrosarcomas are the fascia, fibrous septae of skeletal muscle and the deep connective tissue, sites not unlike those for the fibromatoses.

Fibrosarcomas tend to occur more frequently in males, although some authors have reported a predominance of females. While any age group may be affected, the greatest incidence occurs in the fourth through the sixth decades.

Local recurrence is the main problem encountered in the management of fibrosarcomas; it has ranged from nearly 30 to nearly 60%.[73] It has been stated that fibrosarcomas have the highest rate of persistence of tumors of all soft tissue sarcomas. The presence of local recurrence more than doubles the probability that the patient will die of his sarcoma.[75]

Many attempts have been made to correlate a variety of factors with the prognosis of fibrosarcoma.[1, 4, 76–78] These have included the patient's age, duration of signs and symptoms before treatment, microscopic appearance and size of the neoplasm, aggressiveness of surgical treatment, etc. Some of these modifying factors are presented in Tables 13.5, 13.6 and 13.7. As Thompson et al.[73] point out, however, such correlations are often less than convincing, for it remains difficult to explain

why one patient treated vigorously with super-radical surgery will die early with metastases while another will survive for many years with numerous local recurrences.

The recommended treatment of fibrosarcoma, regardless of site, is local excision, radical en bloc excision or amputation. The infiltrative behavior of its growth makes it mandatory that all of the tumor be removed at the first surgical intervention.[79] Most authors believe that radiotherapy is of little benefit in curing these tumors.

Fibrosarcoma of the Head and Neck

The study of fibrosarcomas most germaine to the head and neck surgeon is the one by Conley,

Table 13.6
Influence of Histological Differentiation in Fibrosarcoma and Survivorship

Author(s)	Classification	No. of Cases	5-Year Survival
			%
Meyerding et al. (1936)[74]	Broders'		
	Grade I	22	45.4
	Grade II	30	36.6
	Grade III	18	16.6
	Grade IV	5	0.0
Ivins et al. (1950)[77]	Broders'		
	Grade I	14	57.0
	Grade II	13	38.0
	Grade III	26	31.0
	Grade IV	10	20.0
MacKenzie (1964)[1]	Grade I	29	82.8
	Grade II	60	55.0
	Grade III	16	35.5
Stout (1948)[4]	Poor differentiation	41	26.8
	Good differentiation	104	52.8

Table 13.5
Influence of Type of Excision on Recurrences and Survival in Fibrosarcoma*

Radical excision was defined as resection of neoplasm with a 4- to 6-cm margin of normal tissue in three planes, and it included en bloc regional node dissection if the position of the primary tumor was close to its regional lymph node basin. In several cases, this necessitated amputation or quarterectomy because of the size and position of the fibrosarcoma.

Treatment	No. of Patients	Recurrences	5-Year Survival
No treatment	14		
Local excision	23	17 (74%)	7 (30%)
Radical excision	27	8 (30%)	21 (78%)
Total	64		28 (44%)

* Statistics from Bizer.[76]

Table 13.7
Influence of Site of Origin on Survival of Patients with Fibrosarcoma*

Site of Origin	Percent Survivors (N = 139)			
	5-year	10-year	15-year	Median
				years
Head and neck	36	15	15	2.9
Upper limb	69	57	49	13.9
Lower limb	59	37	30	6.3
Trunk	51	34	34	5.5
Retroperitoneum	24	0	0	0.8
Breast	92	92	92	≧15.0

* Reproduced from van der Werf-Messing and van Unnik[78] by permission of the J. B. Lippincott Co.

Stout and Healey.[79] Stout, the pathologist of the group, *reclassified* 84 cases bearing an original surgical-pathological diagnosis of "fibrosarcomas of the head and neck." There was an 85% accuracy of the original diagnosis. Thirteen of the tumors represented other histological types of tumors. Stout further reclassified the other fibroblastic lesions of the head and neck in their study as: infiltrative fibromatoses (low-grade fibrosarcoma), 42 cases; and undifferentiated fibrosarcoma, 12 cases. Thus, nearly three-quarters of the final group might fall into the group I have described as aggressive fibromatosis (vide supra) rather than fibrosarcoma.

The 54 patients forming the basis of their study were also subdivided into four chronological subgroups. In the prepubertal groups (birth to 14 years), the diagnosis of fibromatosis was made six times. Two of these children died as a result of local extension of the process, and one died as an outcome of distant metastases. This varying biological behavior certainly emphasizes the difficulty in equating clinical behavior with histological appearances, particularly in this age group.

The largest number of patients were adults (22 to 49 years). Of 24 adults with lesions called fibromatosis, 19 manifested no recurrences, but five died from the results of local invasion. Eight adults were the hosts of undifferentiated fibrosarcomas; five of these patients died of local and/or widespread metastasis. Sixty-nine percent of the 54 patients were apparently cured, and 31% were either dead from, or living with, incurable disease.

Nearly 80% of the patients with fibromatoses were considered as being apparently cured, and 21% were either dead or dying as a result of local disease. One patient, in addition, manifested distant metastases. Undifferentiated fibrosarcomas presented an aggressive and relentless course and behaved clinically as a high-grade malignancy, with 67% of the patient group dead as an outcome of persistent, local invasion or widespread metastases. Only 33% of the patients with undifferentiated fibrosarcomas were apparently cured of their disease. The level of differentiation of the fibrosarcoma and its impact on prognosis is also stressed by others.[18, 80]

The sites of origin of fibrosarcoma of the head and neck, in order of frequency, are: soft tissues of the face and neck; maxillary antrum; other paranasal sinuses; and nasopharynx.

In comparison to several other malignant soft tissue tumors which may involve this area, fibrosarcomas appear to grow more slowly, infiltrate less extensively, metastasize less frequently and

are associated with a better prognosis. These features, however, do little for the individual patient.

Patients with fibrosarcoma of this anatomical area do best when their initial treatment has been large en bloc (widefield) surgical excision. Local recurrence is associated with inadequate resection and these recurrences may be so bulky as to negate curative resection. Death is due to uncontrolled local growth and metastases are relatively infrequent. Experiences with various modalities of therapy and their indictions are discussed by Swain et al.[80]

Fibrosarcomas of the Oral Regions

Because of the small number of authenticated cases and few extant analyses of series of cases, it is not possible to characterize accurately fibrosarcomas of the oral regions. The rarity of documented cases of oral soft tissue fibrosarcoma is underlined by the study of O'Day et al.[81] These workers were able to find only 15 examples in the literature and they added six additional cases. In their experience, fibrosarcomas made up approximately 2% of the malignant mesenchymal neoplasms of the oral cavity. This is compared to an over-all incidence (in the head and neck) of 5 to 10 or 15%[82] (Table 13.8).

I recognize the periosteal soft tissues, the periodontal membranes and the endosteum as legitimate potential sources of fibrosarcoma of the jaws. Not all pathologists (oral and general) concur. Some have divided fibrosarcomas of the jaws into odontogenic and osteogenic types. Other authorities deny the existence of an endosteal or so-called medullary fibrosarcoma and consider the purported examples as undifferentiated chondro- or osteogenic sarcomas.

All authors agree on the category of periosteal fibrosarcoma, arising either from the periosteum itself or from the periosteal tissues. The latter are said to be more malignant and exhibit a greater

Table 13.8
Anatomical Distribution of Fibrosarcomas*

Site	No.	Percentage
Head and neck	52	15
Upper limb	47	14
Lower limb	136	39
Trunk	87	23
Retroperitoneum	8	2
Breast (from cystosarcoma phyllodes)	14	4
	—	—
Total	344	100

* From figures supplied by van der Werf-Messing and van Unnik[78] and Mackenzie.[1]

tendency to invade bone.[83] There is further agreement that, even though their number is small, the majority of *oral* fibrosarcomas are *not* of soft tissue origin, but, rather, are periosteal fibrosarcomas. The less common fibrosarcomas of the perioral soft tissues occur in the subcutaneous tissues, especially in the region of the chin and the angle of the mandible. These fibrosarcomas occur particularly in children or young adults and tend to more malignant than the periosteal fibrosarcomas.

Histological grading and the mitotic index are of some aid in predicting the general degree of clinical malignancy, but as previously noted, the successful management of oral fibrosarcoma depends to a greater extent on the size and location of the tumor.

Fibrosarcoma of the tonsil and hypopharynx are exceedingly rare. This rarity is in sharp contrast to the incidence in the larynx, where fibrosarcoma is the most commonly reported malignant mesenchymal tumor.[84]

As indicated above, fibrosarcomas arising in bone (of endosteal origin-medullary fibrosarcomas) are debatable lesions. Along with others, I consider the neoplasm as a distinct pathological entity worthy of separate consideration.[85, 86] Medullary fibrosarcomas have a reported incidence relative to all bone sarcomas of 2 to 10%. The neoplasm favors long bones in its distribution and is reported to occur about the knee joint in as high as 77% of cases.[85]

In its age distribution, medullary fibrosarcoma resembles the soft tissue fibrosarcoma more than osteogenic sarcoma. The average age has been given as near 40 years. The median age for osteogenic sarcoma is younger than 20 years, while that for soft part fibrosarcomas ranges from 39 to 44 years. Huvos and Higinbotham[86] record 19 instances in which the bones of the head and neck area were the primary site. Mandible and maxilla were nearly equally represented and endosteal and periosteal sites were also nearly equal. The tumors may arise de novo or may be associated with fibrous dysplasia, Paget's disease, osteomyelitis or giant cell tumor. They may be induced by previous irradiation.

The best study to date issues from the Mayo Clinic.[85] Workers there studied 13 cases, reviewed the literature and reaffirmed that fibrosarcoma of the mandible is a distinct entity. Two additional patients had fibrosarcomas that apparently arose in the maxilla, but positive proof of intraosseous origin was lacking.

There are no distinguishing roentgenological features of this osteolytic neoplasm. Every patient in the Mayo Clinic series had a radiolucent defect of variable size, without evidence of nodular or diffuse calcification. In gross appearance, the tumors are generally densely firm, gray-white masses. If highly cellular or myxomatous foci are present, the tumor may manifest zones of softening and fluctuance. Perforations of the medial and lateral cortical plates produce contiguous soft tissue masses that require wide surgical excision.[85] The neoplasm most often involves the body and the angle regions of the mandible.

The rare clinicopathological entity, multiple diffuse fibrosarcoma of bone may involve skull and facial bones.[87]

From a histopathological aspect, fibrosarcoma of bone has features like those of its soft tissue counterparts. Collagen is produced in variable amounts, and the cells have spindle-shaped nuclei. The tumors manifest a wide variation in cellular differentiation as well as in the amount of collagen formed. The site of origin within the jaws is obscure. Van Blarcom et al.[85] review the prevailing theories.

Perhaps the most important differences between osseous and soft part fibrosarcomas are in their clinical behavior. While lymph node metastases are uncommon in either group, the soft part fibrosarcoma is predominantly a problem in local control. In bones and in the mandible the neoplasm is highly lethal because of its tendency to recur locally and to metastasize. Prognosis is enhanced by a periosteal location. Such lesions, in contrast to the endosteal fibrosarcoma have nearly twice the number of 5-year survivors.

Fibrosarcoma of the Head and Neck in Children

The head and neck region is an area of relative predilection for fibrosarcomas presenting in the first 15 years of life. Nearly 20% of 110 cases of fibrosarcoma in infants and children reviewed by Soule and Pritchard[88] were primary in that anatomical region. Thirteen percent of 53 cases in an Armed Forces Institute of Pathology (AFIP) series of infantile fibrosarcomas presented in the head and neck.[89]

Nearly all workers in this field agree that there is little histological difference between the childhood and adult forms of fibrosarcoma. Chung and Enzinger[89] believe the tumor cells tend to be less mature. A primitive mesenchymal sarcoma appearance is sometimes displayed. Nuclear pleomorphism is not a feature. Mitoses are common, but their number varies from tumor to tumor and within different areas of a given tumor. Similarly, the degree of fibroblastic differentiation and production of collagen varies. Chronic inflammatory cell foci are said to be prominent in these fibrosarcomas. There have been attempts also to grade the fibrosarcomas of the young according to their growth and cellular patterns: desmoplastic and medullary forms. No histological feature or group of features has been successfully related to clinical behavior and prediction of biological course.

There is fairly general agreement that children who are less than 5 years of age manifest a more favorable prognosis. In the Mayo Clinic series, these children were said to have a 7.3% chance of dying of their tumor, even though there is a significant recurrence rate of 43%.[88] Chung and Enzinger[89] record a 5-year survival rate of 84% in their patients with fibrosarcoma. Children older than 5 years of age may be expected to have clinical courses and prognoses of adult patients.

Wide local excision appears to be the treatment of choice for primary and recurrent tumors. To date, little support for radiation therapy has been given.

Myxofibrosarcoma

Discussed elsewhere in this book are the myxoma and a lesion we have designated as myxofibroma (see pp. 359 and 410). If the myxofibroma is accepted, the probability of a malignant counterpart is high. Such a lesion has been described by Angervall et al.[90]—*myxofibrosarcoma*. Myxofibrosarcoma is sometimes used in the literature and in daily surgical pathology practice as a *descriptive* term for lesions which have or have not been defined as specific and otherwise recognizable entities. The diagnostic use of the term should be reserved for fibroblastic and histiocytic malignant soft tissue tumors characterized by their mucoid and nodular appearance and manifesting no evidence of lipoblastic, myoblastic or chondroblastic differentation. Thus defined, the tumor is one of elderly patients (in contrast to the fibromyxoma) and most often found in the subcutaneous tissues of the extremities. On occasion they may be deep seated in muscle. Recurrences, often multiple, and a significant frequency of metastases characterize their clinical behavior.

Histologically the tumors present fibroblast and/or histiocytic-fibroblast-like cells in a myxoid nodular pattern. The vascular pattern is plexiform and capillary. Angervall et al.[90] graded the malignancy according to cellularity, cellular atypia and mitoses. Grade IV lesions manifest pronounced atypia, often presenting bi- and multinucleated giant tumor cells and occasionally Touton type giant cells. This suggests a relationship to malig-

nant fibroxanthoma. The differential diagnosis is broad and includes rhabdomyosarcoma, liposarcoma, spindle cell lipoma, extraskeletal chondrosarcoma and even chordoma. Two lesions especially may be difficult, the myxoid form of nodular fasciitis and myxoma. A radiating vascular pattern, instead of the plexiform capillary pattern and the presence of inflammatory cells, may serve to distinguish nodular fasciitis from myxofibrosarcoma. Myxomas are either in the skin or are deep-seated, but are rarely located subcutaneously. The myxoma is less cellular, lacks fibroblastic differentiation and does not have the prominent plexiform vascular pattern of myxofibrosarcoma.

MISCELLANEOUS FIBROUS LESIONS

Localized Fibrous Overgrowth of the Oral Mucosa

Localized fibrous lesions of the oral regions are probably the most common soft tissue lesions with which the oral and head and neck surgeon has to deal. There is considerable diversity of opinion as to their exact nature, and this is manifested in the variety of names applied to them: fibrous epulides, fibromas, fibrous hyperplasias, fibroepithelial polyps or similar titles. Controversy exists as to whether the majority are neoplasms or hyperplasias; or, if both exist, what is the distinction between them? A considerable number of authors consider true oral fibromas to be rare. Others claim fibromas are common. Still others ride the diagnostic fence and consider that both neoplastic and hyperplastic fibrous lesions exist, but they doubt whether a distinction can be made histologically. In this, I agree.

Barker and Lucas[91] attempted to resolve the problem through examination of 171 fibrous lesions—62 from the cheek, 39 from the lip, 45 from the palate and 25 from the tongue. Only two qualified, in their opinion, for the histological diagnosis of a neoplasm, i.e., fibroma. The remainder were considered fibrous hyperplasias, such as gingival reparative lesions associated with irritation from dentures. Fibromas, in the opinion of Barker and Lucas,[91] manifest a distinct separation from the surrounding tissue and a different internal structure. The latter may be characterized by a circular arrangement of individual fibers with a suggestion of whorling.

In my opinion, benign *neoplastic* fibrous lesions of the oral cavity are very unusual. Unlike lesions of the peripheral soft tissues, the diagnosis of "fibroma" of the oral soft tissues, if not accurate, is at least not dangerous.[1] Their clinical and histological course is entirely benign. Thus it would seem that there is an appreciable divergence of behavior between lesions diagnosed as fibromas when they occur in the oral tissues and when they occur elsewhere.[91] This speaks further for the reactive basis for the vast majority of the localized fibrous lesions. Depending on the initiating irritation, the lesions may be pendunculated, sessile, keratinizing, hard, soft or with a granulation tissue surface. Recurrence is not a feature following the removal of stimulus.

The reactive fibroblastic lesions may occur at any site in the oral tissues but are most common in the gums. In the gingiva, an interdental papilla is the usual site for these lesions, but they may originate more deeply (from the periodontal membrane or the periosteum). Removal of the related tooth, in the latter instance, may be required to ensure total removal of the lesion. In the lips, tongue, palate and buccal mucosa, the tumors are usually circumscribed and may often be polypoid. Irritative and post-traumatic fibrosis of the region of the upper molars and the tuberosities, if bilateral, may simulate hereditary gingival fibromatosis.

Dentures are often the offenders leading to the formation of localized fibroblastic lesions. The most common denture-lesion occurs in the buccal sulcus where it has been known as "denture fibrosis," "fibroma" or "denture hyperplasia."

Microscopically, the lesions most often consist of collagen bundles coursing haphazardly in all directions and continuous with the surrounding normal connective tissue. Those in the cheek, deep lips or tongue may have an outer mantle of concentric layers of collagen. Calcification and, less frequently, ossification may be present in the lesions of the palate and the gingiva. Acute and chronic inflammatory cells are variably seen and variable in their members. Those subject to trauma may manifest superficial ulceration.

Gingival Fibromatosis

The gingival fibromatoses are a peculiar family of gum tumors which, as a group, are characterized by an abnormal increase in the connective tissue elements of the gingival corium. The entire group may be conveniently subdivided, on the basis of etiology, into: irritative, chemical, anatomical, and idiopathic or hereditary fibromatoses.[92] Clinically, they are nonpainful protrusive gingival masses which are firm, hard and cover varying portions of the erupted crowns of teeth included within the lesions. The patient's complaint is usually that of concern with the cosmetic appearance of the lesions or with interference with mouth functions.

The irritative form results from the effects of a chronic local irritation on the tissues of the gingiva. The fibromatous lesion is almost invariably preceded by an intensive and abundant inflammatory reaction in the gingiva. Irritative fibrous reactions of the gingiva are localized phenomena. The other forms may be either generalized or localized.

Classification of Gingival Fibromatosis:
  I. Generalized gingival fibromatosis
     A. Hereditary types
     B. Drug influenced
     C. Idiopathic
  II. Localized gingival fibromatosis
     A. Hereditary
     B. Idiopathic
     C. Irritative or traumatic

Generalized gingival fibromatosis has also been called elephantiasis gingivae, gigantism of the gingiva, multiple epulides and chronic hypertrophic gingivitis.

Although complete knowledge concerning the etiology is lacking, several "types" of generalized gingival fibromatosis have been noted. Hereditary, generalized (both maxillary and mandibular) gingival fibromatosis is transmitted as an autosomal dominant trait with variable, although moderate, penetrance. As both sexes are equally affected, the genes are not sex-limited. The age of the patient when the disease begins varies considerably. In most instances, however, the disease is not noticed until the eruption of permanent teeth.

A number of abnormalities have been reported in association with the idiopathic variety, chiefly hypertrichosis. It is an accompaniment of several syndromes, including occasional cases of cherubism. Like the other forms of gingival fibromatosis, the predominant histological feature is collagenous fibrous connective tissue and is nearly identical to fibrous reactive hyperplasia and/or a "fibroma." Although the role of hereditory in the etiology of this disease has been well documented, sporadic or *idiopathic* cases also occur.

Treatment in early cases should be conservative. In severe cases removal of the teeth may be all that is required, with the gingiva returning to normal after this procedure.[92]

Diphenylhydantoin Gingival Hyperplasia and Hypertrophy. Drug-influenced fibromatosis has come to be synonymous with Dilantin "gingivitis." Sodium diphenylhydantoinate (Dilantin) is probably the only chemical capable of stimulating a gingival fibromatosis.

The mechanism or mechanisms involved in the causation of the lesion have by no means been clearly defined or established. There is no evidence that diphenylhydantoin causes similar tissue alterations in any other parts of the body.[93] The reported incidence of diphenylhydantoin gingival hyperplasia ranges from 3 to 78% of users of the drug. A more realistic figure is 40%.[94] The lesion occurs with much greater frequency in the young than in the adult. There is neither sex nor racial predilection.

Gingival enlargement, in most patients, appears 2 to 3 months after the initial administration of the drug and reaches its maximal severity in 9 to 12 months. The occurrence and severity are generally not related to the drug dosage or blood levels. This is in contrast to the signs and symptoms of intoxication by the drug, and suggests that the drug-related gingival fibrosis is perhaps due to a specific hypersensitivity to the drug per se, or to one of its metabolites. It is of interest to note, however, that almost identical alterations may occur in some epileptics who do not take the drug. Another important predisposing factor is poor dental hygiene. In this respect, diphenylhydantoin hyperplasia does not occur in edentulous areas.

Clinically, the lesion generally occurs in a semilunar distribution circumscribing the necks of the individual teeth.[94] It begins as a painless, discrete projection of the gingival mucosa (often mulberry-shaped) and is firm, pale and resilient. There is no special tendency for the lesion to bleed. Microscopically, there is a delicate strand-like acanthosis overlying interlacing and prominent collagen bundles, separated only infrequently by small vascular channels. Local irritants modify the clinical and microscopic appearance, as they may for all forms of gingival fibromatosis.

The best and most satisfactory treatment is withdrawal of the drug. This is followed by spontaneous recovery, usually within 3 to 5 months. If drug therapy continues, there will be recurrent enlargement and progression to the previous magnitude, usually within 6 months. Forms of management are outlined by Livingston and Livingston.[94]

Localized Gingival Fibromatosis. This is a clinically independent lesion and is often called "fibroma." It is a localized, unilateral or, more often, bilateral collagen tissue mass of the maxillary or mandibular tuberosity mucosa. Zegarelli et al.[95] refer to these lesions as "anatomic fibromatosis." They may be hereditary or idiopathic. The bilaterality assists in separating these lesions from reactive processes. Microscopic distinction, however, may be impossible.

Oral Submucous Fibrosis

First described in the Indian medical literature just under 20 years ago, submucous fibrosis is an insidious and chronic disease with many intriguing facets, not the least of which is its role as a probable precancerous condition. All recorded cases have been in Indians, apart from a few Asians and Europeans living in India, occasional reports from East Africa and Caucasian women married to Indians.[96] There is no doubt that submucous fibrosis is largely indigenous to India, where the prevalence rate is 0.5% or an estimated 2,000,000 cases. There is, however, an indication that the subcontinent is not peculiarly affected.[96]

Females are more susceptible, and the age range is relatively wide, 10 to 70 years, with maximum frequency in the 20- to 40-year-old groups. A considerable number of patients have an associated marked microcytic anemia. Early signs and symptoms are a burning sensation in the mouth, ulceration and recurrent stomatitis and inability to tolerate spicy foods within the mouth. Later problems are stiffness of oral musculature, trismus, reduced mobility of the tongue and soft palate and, rarely, deafness due to occlusion of the eustachian tubes.

It was previously thought that the palate and the faucial pillars were the primary affected areas, but the buccal mucosa and lips (especially the lower) are also frequently involved. Actually, any part of the oral cavity is susceptible, with occasional extension down to involve the pharynx and pyriform fossae.

Clinical onset is very often heralded by painful subepithelial vesicles in areas of redness. Rupture of the vesicles promotes superficial ulceration, which is succeeded by a blanching of the mucosa and the appearance of white fibrous bands. The involvement is most often symmetrical.[96]

The fibrous bands in the buccal mucosa course in a vertical direction, and the ensuing fibrosis may become so marked as to immobilize the cheek. In the soft palate, the fibrous bands have a scar-like appearance. The uvula is almost always involved and, in the later stages, may be reduced to a small fibrous "bud." As the fibrosis progresses and infiltrates into underlying muscles, a gradual and unrelenting trismus ensues. The entire isthmus faucium is reduced, which may give rise to speech, mastication and swallowing difficulties.[97] Pindborg and Sirsat[96] have described four histological stages in the disease from very early to advanced. The similarity to scleroderma and its developmental stages is noteworthy.

While there is unanimity concerning the collagenization, there is divergence concerning the epithelial changes associated with submucous fibrosis. Wahi et al.[98] describe a hyperplasia, while Pindborg and Sirsat[96] found a markedly atrophic mucosa with loss of rete pegs in more than 90% of cases. These different opinions may be related to the time biopsy specimens were taken.

The relationship of submucous fibrosis to oral epithelial dysplasia in India is highly significant, 27% with submucosal fibrosis as compared to 3% without.[96] The incidence of a slowly growing squamous cell carcinoma superimposed on the affected areas is from 33%[99] to 25% of cases.[96]

Once diagnosis is made, it is difficult to effect any satisfactory treatment. Surgery is usually impossible due to the mass of fibrous bands in the cheeks, circumorally and in the pterygomandibular raphe. Furthermore, the trauma of surgery leads to additional fibrosis. A combination of systemic and local corticosteroids may, on occasion, be effective in controlling progression of the disease.

Congenital Muscular Torticollis (Fibromatosis Colli, Wry Neck)

Congenital muscular torticollis is a condition characterized by the formation of a fibrous tumor in the sternocleidomastoid muscle at or soon after birth. The genesis is unknown, and there is no good evidence that birth injuries are at fault. The disorder has no relationship to spasmodic torticollis in older patients or with other congenital disorders involving the neck.

The incidence of the disorder is low, less than 1% of live births.[100] There does not appear to be a sex predisposition, and both sides of the neck are almost equally involved. The lesion is rarely bilateral. The median age of discovery is about 2.5 months, with nearly half discovered at birth. There is a high incidence of complicated deliveries and a prevalence of breech presentations. Japanese workers have recorded an association of the disorder with various other congenital anomalies, principally an ipsilateral dislocation of the hip.[101] Some facial asymmetry is always present.

Located principally in the lower third of the involved sternocleidomastoid muscle, most examples differ from the usual desmoidal type of fibromatosis not only in microscopic appearance, but also in their often unique involution and lack of aggressive infiltration beyond the muscle.

The tumor is not a neoplasm but a diffuse fibrous replacement of muscle. The relatively large numbers of interspersed residual muscle fibers and the relationship of age of lesion to the relative amount of collagen constitutes the major histological difference from the desmoid tumor (Fig. 13.17).

Most patients recover spontaneously. The tumor

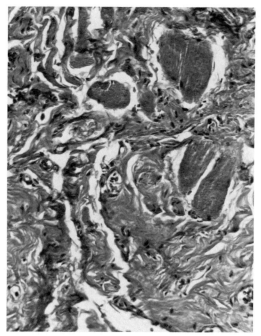

Figure 13.17. Torticollis of the usual type. This should not be considered a form of fibromatosis.

gradually disappears, and by 1 year of age no residual mass or torticollis remains. For unknown reasons, a few patients do not fully recover but have a permanent wry neck deformity. The fixed torticollis is the result of continued fibrosis and contraction of the involved muscle. Because of the involution of the disorder in so many subjects, any surgical correction should be postponed until after 1 year of age.[100] Surgical correction of the residual deformity is indicated in the occasional subject who manifests a persistence of the torticollis deformity after this time.

Care must be made clinically to distinguish the above type of torticollis from a desmoid-like or differentiated fibrosarcoma-like lesion appearing in the same region shortly after birth and up to 1 year of age. Two of these tumors in Stout's[3] series penetrated deeply into the neck as far as the larynx and one caused death of the host by extensive local infiltration.

Sclerosing Cervicitis

This histologically benign, yet potentially lethal lesion is considered to be the cervical (neck) homologue of sclerosing retroperitonitis and mediastinitis.[102] In the region of the head and neck, only two other areas have been sites of similar lesions; the thyroid gland and the orbit. Whatever the inciting agent or agents may be, it is histologically a clear response to injury, not unlike the formation of keloids. The local behavior of these lesions is more like the fibromatoses than the pseudosarcomatous proliferative disorders. The relative acellularity and inflammatory features of sclerosing cervicitis, retroperitonitis, and mediastinitis are, however, foreign to the fibromatoses.

Myofibroblast

The myofibroblast, which combines ultrastructural features of both fibroblasts and smooth muscle cells is being increasingly recognized in a variety of supporting tissue lesions. The salient features of this cell are: (1) nuclear indentations and folds that are indirect evidence of a contractile cell; (2) bundles of microfilaments arranged parallel to the long axis of the cells and showing multiple dense bodies similar to those seen in smooth muscle cells; (3) intercellular connections through desmosomes and the formation of basal lamina-like material surrounding the cells; and (4) abundant cisternae of rough endoplasmic reticulum and a prominent Golgi apparatus; features typical of a fibroblast.[103]

Most of the lesions in which the myofibroblast has been described are non-neoplastic and have consisted of granulation tissue, atheromatous plaques, ganglia of soft tissues, tenosynovitis and the stroma of tubular carcinoma of the breast. Additional soft tissue lesions in which the myofibroblast is said to participate are: various forms of fibromatosis and nodular fasciitis. Only a few reported examples of neoplasms (benign and malignant) have had myofibroblasts described.[103] All of the documented malignant tumors containing myofibroblasts have been classified as fibrosarcomas.

Any biological or clinical significance of the presence of myofibroblasts in fibrous lesions is doubtful. It is very likely the cell is an expression of a limited potential in fibroblasts for determination along myoid lines.

REFERENCES

1. Mackenzie, D. H.: Fibroma: a dangerous diagnosis: a review of 205 cases of fibrosarcoma of soft tissues. Br. J. Surg. 51:607, 1964.
2. Stout, A. P.: Fibrous tumors of the soft tissues. Minn. Med. 43:455, 1960.
3. Stout, A. P.: Juvenile fibromatosis. Cancer 7:953, 1954.
4. Stout, A. P.: Fibrosarcoma. The malignant tumor of fibroblasts. Cancer 1:30, 1948.
5. Stout, A. P.: Tumors of the soft tissues. In Atlas of Tumor Pathology, Section II, Fasicle 5. Armed Forces Institute of Pathology, Washington, D.C., 1953.
6. Enzinger, F. M.: Fibrous hamartoma of infancy. Cancer 18: 241, 1965.
7. Coventry, M. B., Harris, L. E., Bianco, A. J., and Bulbullan, A. H.: Congenital muscular torticollis (wryneck). Postgrad. Med. 28:383, 1960.
8. Stout, A. P.: Juvenile fibromatosis. Cancer 7:953, 1954.
9. Enzinger, F. M.: Fibrous tumors of infancy. In Tumors of Bone and Soft Tissue, pp. 375-396. Year Book Medical Publishers, Chicago, 1965.
10. Kindblom, L.-G., Termen, G., Save-Sodenbergh, J., and Angervall, L.: Congenital generalized fibromatosis. Acta Pathol. Microbiol. Scand. (A) 85:640, 1977.
11. Dehner, L. P., and Askin, F. B.: Tumors of fibrous tissue origin in childhood. A clinicopathologic study of cutaneous and soft tissue neoplasms in 66 children. Cancer 38:888, 1976.
12. Specht, E. E.: Juvenile aponeurotic fibroma. The cartilage analogue of fibromatosis. J. A. M. A. 234:626, 1975.
13. Das Gupta, T. K., Brasfield, M. D., and O'Hara, J.: Extra-abdominal desmoids: A clinicopathological study. Ann. Surg. 170:109, 1969.
14. Bennett, J. H.: On Cancerous and Cancroid Growths, p. 176. Sutherland and Knox, Edinburgh, 1849.
15. Enzinger, F. M., and Shiraki, M.: Musculo-aponeurotic fibromatosis of the shoulder girdle (extra-abdominal desmoid). Cancer 20:1131, 1967.
16. Butler, J. J.: Fibrous tissue tumors: nodular fasciitis, dermatofibrosarcoma protuberans, and fibrosarcoma, grade I, desmoid type. In Tumors of Bone and Soft Tissues, p. 397. Year Book Medical Publishers, Chicago, 1965.
17. Masson, J. K., and Soule, E. H.: Desmoid tumors of the head and neck. Am. J. Surg. 112:615, 1966.
18. Fu, Y.-S., and Perzin, K. H.: Nonepithelial tumors of the nasal cavity, paranasal sinuses, and nasopharynx. A clinicopathologic study. VI. Fibrous tissue tumors (fibroma, fibromatosis, fibrosarcoma). Cancer 37:2912, 1976.
19. Wilkins, S. A., Jr., Waldron, C. A., Mathews, W. H., and Droulias, C. A.: Aggressive fibromatosis of the head and neck. Am. J. Surg. 130:412, 1975.
20. Stout, A. P.: Fibrosarcoma in infants and children. Cancer 18:1028, 1968.
21. Balsaver, A. M., Butler, J. J., and Martin, R. G.: Congenital fibrosarcoma. Cancer 20:1607, 1967.
22. Goldman, R. L.: The cartilage analogue of fibromatosis (aponeurotic fibroma). Further observations based on seven new cases. Cancer 26:1325, 1970.
23. Dahl, I., and Angervall, L.: Pseudosarcomatous proliferative lesions of soft tissues with or without bone formation. Acta Pathol. Microbiol. Scand. (A) 85:577, 1977.
24. Schreiber, M. M., Shapiro, S. I., and Sampsel, J.: Pseudosarcomatous fibromatosis (fasciitis). Arch. Dermatol. 92: 661, 1965.
25. Allen, P. W.: Nodular fasciitis. Pathology 4:9, 1972.
26. Price, E. B., Jr., Silliphant, W. M., and Shuman, R.: Nodular fasciitis: a clinicopathologic analysis of 65 cases. Am. J. Clin. Pathol. 35:122, 1961.
27. Wirman, J. A.: Nodular fasciitis, a lesion of myofibroblasts. An ultrastructural study. Cancer 38:2378, 1976.
28. Soule, E. H.: Proliferative (nodular fasciitis). Arch. Pathol. 73:437, 1962.
29. Phelan, J. T., and Jurado, J.: Pseudosarcomatous fasciitis. N. Engl. J. Med. 266:645, 1962.
30. Hutter, R. V. P., Stewart, F. W., and Foote, F. W., Jr.: Fasciitis: a report of 70 cases with follow-up proving the benignity of the lesion. Cancer 15:992, 1962.
31. Stout, A. P.: Pseudosarcomatous fasciitis in children. Cancer 14:1216, 1961.
32. Kern, W. H.: Proliferative myositis: a pseudosarcomatous reaction to injury. Arch. Pathol. 69:209, 1960.
33. Bullock, W. K.: Personal communication, cited in Kern, W. H. Proliferative myositis; a pseudosarcomatous reaction to injury. Arch. Pathol. 69:209, 1960.
34. Enzinger, F. M., and Dulcey, F.: Proliferative myositis; report of thirty-three cases. Cancer 20:2213, 1967.
35. Gokel, J. M., Meister, P., and Hubner, G.: Proliferative myositis. A case report with fine structural analysis.

Virchows Arch. (Pathol. Anat.) 367:345, 1975.

36. Chung, E. B., and Enzinger, F. M.: Proliferative fasciitis. Cancer 36:1450, 1975.

37. Hutter, R. V. P., Foote, F. W., Jr., Francis, K. C., and Higinbotham, N. L.: Parosteal fasciitis: a self-limited benign process that simulates a malignant neoplasm. Am. J. Surg. 104:800, 1962.

38. Grewal, K. S., and Das, N.: Myositis ossificans progressiva. J. Bone Joint Surg. 35-B:244, 1953.

39. Trestor, P. H., Markovitch, E., Zambito, R. F., and Stratigos, G. T.: Myositis ossificans, circumscripta and progressiva, with surgical correction of the masseter muscle: report of two cases. J. Oral Surg. 27:201, 1969.

40. Goodsell, J. O.: Traumatic myositis ossificans of the masseter muscle: review of the literature and report of a case. J. Oral Surg. 20:116, 1962.

41. Parnes, E. I., and Hinds, E. C.: Traumatic myositis ossificans of the masseter muscle. Report of case. J. Oral Surg. 23: 245, 1965.

42. Ackerman, L. V.: Extra-osseous localized non-neoplastic bone and cartilage formation (so-called myositis ossificans). J. Bone Joint Surg. 40-A:279, 1965.

43. Sohn, D., and Feuerstein, S. S.: Fibromatous polyp of hypopharynx presenting from the mouth. Arch. Otolaryngal. 86:61, 1967.

44. Hara, H. J.: Benign tumor of the tonsil with special reference to fibroma. Arch. Otolaryngal. 18:62, 1933.

45. Ozello, L., Stout, A. P., and Murray, M. R.: Cultural characteristics of malignant histiocytomas and fibrous xanthomas. Cancer 16:331, 1963.

46. O'Brien, J. E., and Stout, A. P.: Malignant fibrous xanthomas. Cancer 17:1445, 1964.

47. Stout, A. P., and Lattes, R.: Tumors of the soft tissues. In Atlas of Tumor Pathology, 2nd series, Fascicle I. Armed Forces Institute of Pathology, Washington, D.C., 1967.

48. Kauffman, S. L., and Stout, A. P.: Histiocytic tumors (fibrous xanthoma and histiocytoma) in children. Cancer 14:469, 1961.

49. Taylor, H. B., and Helwig, E. B.: Dermatofibrosarcoma protuberans: a study of 115 cases. Cancer 15:717, 1962.

50. Hashimoto, K., Brownstein, M. H., and Jakobiec, F. A.: Dermatofibrosarcoma protuberans: A tumor with perineurial and endoneural cell features. Arch. Dermatol. 110:874, 1974.

51. Alguacil-Garcia, A., Unni, K. K., and Goellner, J. R.: Histogenesis of dermatofibrosarcoma protuberans. An ultrastructural study. Am. J. Clin. Pathol. 69:427, 1978.

52. Phelan, J. J., and Juardo, J.: Dermatofibrosarcoma protuberans. Am. J. Surg. 106:943, 1963.

53. Borrie, P.: Dermatofibrosarcoma protuberans. Br. J. Surg. 39:452, 1952.

54. Helwig, E. B.: Atypical fibroxanthoma. In Tumor Seminar, Proc. 18th Tumor Seminar, San Antonio Soc. Path., 1961, Texas J. Med. 59:664, 1963.

55. Bourne, R. G.: Paradoxical fibrosarcoma of skin (pseudosarcoma): A review of 13 cases. Med. J. Aust. 1:504, 1963.

56. Dahl, I.: Atypical fibroxanthoma of the skin. Acta Pathol. Microbiol. Scand. (A) 84:183, 1976.

57. Milberg, P., Nichols, G., and Weiner, L. J.: Cutaneous atypical fibroxanthoma. Br. J. Plast. Surg. 30:146, 1977.

58. Alguacil-Garcia, A., Unni, K. K., Goellner, J. R., and Winkelmann, R. K.: Atypical fibroxanthoma of the skin. An ultrastructural study of two cases. Cancer 40:1471, 1977.

59. Mihm, M. C., Jr., Clark, W. H., and Reed, R. J.: The histiocytic infiltrates of the skin. Hum. Pathol. 5:45, 1974.

60. Soule, E. H., and Enriques, P.: Atypical fibrous histiocytoma, malignant fibrous histiocytoma, malignant histiocytoma, and epitheliod sarcoma. A comparative study of 65 tumors. Cancer 30:128, 1972.

61. Kempson, R. L., and Kyriakos, M.: Fibroxanthosarcoma of soft tissues. A type of malignant fibrous histiocytoma. Cancer 29:961, 1972.

62. Blitzer, A., Lawson, W., and Biller, H. F.: Malignant fibrous histiocytoma of the head and neck. Laryngoscope 87: 1479, 1977.

63. Rice, D. H., Batsakis, J. G., Headington, J. T., and Boles, R.: Fibrous histiocytomas of the nose and paranasal sinuses. Arch. Otolaryngol. 100:398, 1974.

64. Weiss, S. W., and Enzinger, F. M.: Myxoid variant of malignant fibrous histiocytoma. Cancer 39:1672, 1977.

65. Kyriakos, M., and Kempson, R. L.: Inflammatory fibrous histiocytoma. An aggressive and lethal lesion. Cancer 37: 1584, 1976.

66. Merkow, L. P., Frich, J. C., Jr., Slifkin, M., Kyreages, C. G., and Pardo, M.: Ultrastructure of a fibroxanthosarcoma (malignant fibroxanthoma). Cancer 28:372, 1971.

67. Fu, Y.-S., Gabbiani, G., Kaye, G. I., and Lattes, R.: Malignant soft tissue tumors of probable histiocytic origin (malignant fibrous histiocytomas): General considerations and electron microscopic and tissue culture studies. Cancer 35:176, 1975.

68. Slootweg, P. J., and Müller, H.: Malignant fibrous histiocytoma of the maxilla. Report of a case. Oral Surg. 44: 560, 1977.

69. Dahlin, D. C., Unni, K. K., and Matsuno, T.: Malignant (fibrous) histiocytoma of bone—fact or fancy? Cancer 39:1508, 1977.

70. Spanier, S. S., Enneking, W. F., and Enriquez, P.: Primary malignant fibrous histiocytoma of bone. Cancer 36:2014, 1975.

71. Guccion, J. G., and Enzinger, F. M.: Malignant giant cell tumor of soft parts. An analysis of 32 cases. Cancer 29: 1518, 1972.

72. van Haelst, U. J. G. M. and de Haas van Dorsser, A. H.: Giant cell tumor of soft parts. An ultrastructural study. Virchows Arch. (Pathol. Anat.) 371:199, 1976.

73. Thompson, D. E., Frost, H. M., Henrick, J. W., and Horn, R. C., Jr.: Soft tissue sarcomas involving the extremities and the limb girdles. South. Med. J. 64:33, 1971.

74. Meyerding, H. W., Broders, A. C., and Hargrave, R. L.: Clinical aspects of fibrosarcoma of the soft tissue of the extremities. Surg. Gynecol. Obstet. 62:1010, 1936.

75. Cantin, J., McNeer, G. P., Chu, F. C., and Booher, R. J.: The problem of local recurrence after treatment of soft tissue sarcoma. Ann. Surg. 168:47, 1968.

76. Bizer, L. S.: Fibrosarcoma: report of 64 cases. Am. J. Surg. 121:586, 1971.

77. Ivins, J. C., Dockerty, M. B., and Ghormley, R. K.: Fibrosarcomas of the soft tissues of the extremities: a review of 78 cases. Surgery 28:495, 1950.

78. van der Werf-Messing, B., and van Unnik, J. A. M.: Fibrosarcoma of the soft tissues: a clinicopathologic study. Cancer 18:1113, 1965.

79. Conley, J., Stout, A. P., and Healey, W. V.: Clinicopathological analysis of 84 patients with an original diagnosis of fibrosarcoma of the head and neck. Am. J. Surg. 114: 564, 1967.

80. Swain, R. E., Sessions, D. G., and Ogura, J. H.: Fibrosarcoma of the head and neck: a clinical analysis of forty cases. Ann. Otol. 83:439, 1974.

81. O'Day, R. A., Soule, E. H., and Gores, R. J.: Soft tissue sarcomas of the oral cavity. Mayo Clin. Proc. 39:169, 1964.

82. Vickers, R. A.: Mesenchymal (soft tissue) tumors of the oral region. In Thoma's Oral Pathology, 6th Ed., edited by R. J. Gorlin and H. M. Goldman, p. 868. C. V. Mosby Co., St. Louis, 1970.

83. Reade, P. C., and Radden, B. G.: Oral fibrosarcoma. Oral Surg. 22:217, 1966.

84. Batsakis, J. G., and Fox, J. E.: Supporting tissue neoplasms of the larynx. Surg. Gynecol. Obstet. 131:989, 1970.

85. Van Blarcom, C. W., Masson, J. K., and Dahlin, D. C.: Fibrosarcoma of the mandible. Oral Surg. 32:428, 1971.

86. Huvos, A. G., and Higinbotham, N. L.: Primary fibrosarcoma of bone. A clinicopathologic study of 130 patients. Cancer 33:837, 1975.

87. Hernandez, F. J., and Fernandez, B. B.: Multiple diffuse fibrosarcoma of bone. Cancer 37:939, 1976.

88. Soule, E. H., and Pritchard, D. J.: Fibrosarcoma in infants and children. A review of 110 cases. Cancer 40:1711, 1977.

89. Chung, E. B., and Enzinger, F. M.: Infantile fibrosarcoma. Cancer 38:729, 1976.

90. Angervall, L., Kindblom, L.-G., and Merck, C.: Myxofibrosarcoma. A study of 30 cases. Acta Pathol. Microbiol. Scand. (A) 85:127, 1977.

91. Barker, D. S., and Lucas, R. B.: Localized fibrous overgrowths of the oral mucosa. Br. J. Oral. Surg. 5:86, 1967.

92. Zackin, S. J., and Weisberger, D.: Hereditary gingival fibromatosis. Oral Surg. 14:828, 1961.

93. Simpson, G. M., Kuntz, E., and Slafta, J.: Use of sodium diphenylhydantoin in the treatment of leg ulcers. N.Y. J. Med. 65:886, 1965.

94. Livingston, S., and Livingston, H. L.: Diphenylhydantoin gingival hyperplasia. Am. J. Dis. Child. 117:265, 1969.

95. Zegarelli, E. V., Kutscher, A. H., and Lichtenthal, R.: Idiopathic gingival fibromatosis: report of 20 cases. Am. J. Dig. Dis. 8:782, 1963.

96. Pindborg, J. J., and Sirsat, S. M.: Oral submucous fibrosis. Oral Surg. 22:764, 1966.

97. Simpson, W.: Submucous fibrosis. Br. J. Oral Surg. 6:196, 1969.

98. Waki, P. N., Luthra, V. K., and Kapur, V. L.: Submucous fibrosis of the oral cavity: histopathological studies. Br. J. Cancer 20:676, 1966.

99. Paymaster, J. C.: Cancer of the buccal mucosa: a clinical study of 650 cases in Indian patients. Cancer 9:431, 1956.

100. Coventry, M. B., Harris, L. E., Bianco, A. J., and Bulbulian, A. H.: Congenital muscular torticollis (wryneck). Postgrad. Med. 28:383, 1960.

101. Iwahara, T., and Ikeda, A.: On the ipsilateral involvement of congenital muscular torticollis and congenital dislocation of the hip. J. Jap. Orthop. Assoc. 35:1221, 1962.

102. Rice, D. H., Batsakis, J. G., and Coulthard, S. W.: Sclerosing cervicitis. Homologue of sclerosing retroperitonitis and mediastinitis. Arch. Surg. 110:120, 1975.

103. Vasundev, K. S., and Harris, M.: A sarcoma of myxofibroblasts. An ultrastructural study. Arch. Pathol. Lab. Med. 102:185, 1978.

CHAPTER 14

Neoplastic and Non-neoplastic Tumors of Skeletal Muscle

Tumors of skeletal muscle, particularly rhabdomyosarcomas, have always been a source of fascination and frustration for pathologists. Their diverse patterns, ranging from the seemingly innocuous to the bizarre and pleomorphic types, have "trapped" the unwary into either positive or negative errors of diagnosis. Some surgical pathologists have an extremely low diagnostic threshold; others have a high one and do not deign to make the diagnosis unless cross-striations can be demonstrated in the neoplastic cells.

Frequently masquerading as an inflammatory polyp, oral, aural or nasal, the neoplasms, if unchecked, manifest a high lethality and until recently were resistant to even the most aggressive surgical management. In addition, their heavy preponderance in the young child and potential life-consuming behavior accentuated the frustrations of therapists. In recent years, however, the dismal prognosis for patients with rhabdomyosarcoma (all sites) has been remarkably changed. This has been accomplished as the result of many factors that include a better understanding of the natural history of the disease, careful clinical staging, an awareness of histological features, new techniques for accurately defining disease extent, effective chemotherapy co-ordinated with improved radiation therapy and surgery to derive the most benefit of each, and finally vigorous supportive therapy.[1]

The other two lesions considered in this section are benign lesions of skeletal muscle: rhabdomyoma and hypertrophy of the masseter muscles.

RHABDOMYOSARCOMA

From histomorphological considerations, rhabdomyosarcoma is the neoplastic analogue of the embryogenesis of skeletal muscle. The normal development of skeletal muscle progresses by a series of stages from a primitive, small round cell through a spindle cell form to a multinucleate muscle fiber with characteristic transverse and longitudinal striations.[2, 3] The myocyte of the 7- to 9-week fetus is a small cell with little cytoplasm and a deeply stained, homogeneous ovoid or spherical nucleus. During the early stage, a few cells also manifest bipolar cytoplasmic extensions. By the 10th week of fetal life, the myocytes have acquired more cytoplasm, and myofibrils and cross-striations make their appearance a short time later. Cross-striations are never prominent until the 14th week of development. Following this stage, the central cytoplasmic zone remains relatively clear, imparting to the developing cell the appearance of a hollow tube. Myofibrils gradually increase in number, fill the cytoplasm of the cells and eventually push the nucleus to its adult peripheral position.

Rhabdomyosarcomas, in a sense, recapitulate this embryonic process, but in a disorganized manner. The malignant myoblast may assume, in accordance to its resemblence to developing muscle, several forms: small round (primitive mesenchymal) cells, a mesenchymal syncytium-like cell, a tubular form, raquet-shaped cell, strap-shaped cells and spider-shaped cells (Fig. 14.1 to 14.3). With the preceding in mind, it may be seen that cross-striations, while helpful for diagnosis, are not essential. Certainly the failure to demonstrate them in a suspect lesion does not exclude the diagnosis.

The first detailed description of rhabdomyosarcoma was given by Stout[4] in his report of 121 cases in 1946. The neoplasm described in his paper is one of several variants of rhabdomyosarcoma—the pleomorphic or adult type. The other subtypes are: embryonal, alveolar and botyroid.

The *pleomorphic rhabdomyosarcoma* is the most "differentiated" of the group and also the most readily recognized because of the numerous cells

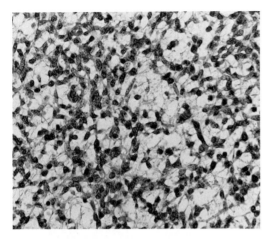

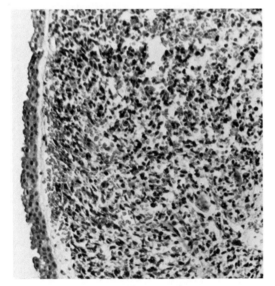

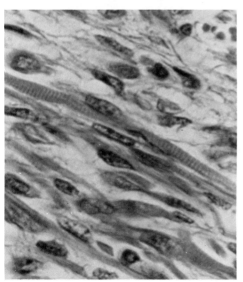

containing cross-striations (Fig. 14.4). Pleomorphic rhabdomyosarcomas do not correspond to a stage of development of normal muscle, but resemble dedifferentiated, adult striated muscle. Even in this form, striations may be absent in a considerable number of cases.

Embryonal rhabdomyosarcoma was first described in 1950.[5] Prior to that time, this variant was rarely recognized as a rhabdomyosarcoma. Embryonal rhabdomyosarcoma closely resembles developing muscle in the 7- to 10-week fetus. It is characterized by round and spindle cells of small to moderate size. The scant cytoplasm of the round cells may lead the unwary observer to consider them as lymphoid cells (Fig. 14.5). Other mistaken diagnoses liable to be rendered are: neuroblastoma, retinoblastoma, "hemangioendothelioma," melanoma, "myxosarcoma" or fibrosarcoma.

A careful search of an embryonal rhabdomyosarcoma will usually reveal areas of diagnostic assistance, i.e., an alveolar arrangement of the rhabdomyoblasts or areas in the neoplasm where the cells assume a spindle shape. The cells here have a central ovoid or elongated nucleus and bipolar cytoplasmic processes in which fibrils and, occasionally, even cross-striation can be seen. The

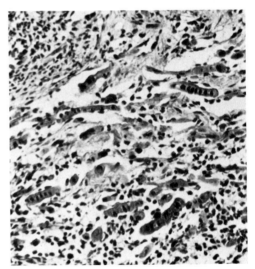

Figure 14.4. Rhabdomyosarcoma of the pleomorphic adult type. Cross-striations are readily visible.

Figures 14.1 to 14.3. Sections from several rhabdomyosarcomas of the head and neck region. The wide diversity in appearance, from primitive mesenchymal foci, through stages that abortively recapitulate myogenesis, to striated, pleomorphic cells is clearly evident.

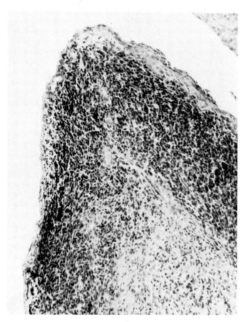

Figure 14.5. Embryonal rhabdomyosarcoma present beneath the attenuated squamous epithelial surface of the external auditory canal.

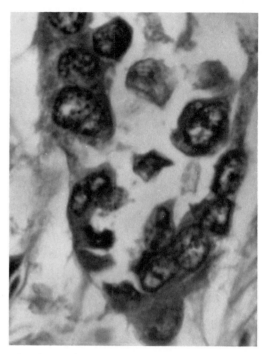

Figure 14.6. Alveolar rhabdomyosarcoma cells aligning themselves in a pseudoglandular pattern.

general pattern of the neoplasm may be loose and myxoid or compact. The embryonal rhabdomyosarcomas are most commonly seen in children.

Alveolar rhabdomyosarcoma was designated as a variant in 1956[6] and derives its name from the alveolar arrangement of its cells, imparting to the neoplasm a very superficial resemblance to an adenocarcinoma. The alveolar spaces are either round or elongated and often show "outpouching." The cells lining the spaces do not form a regular or continuous surface but are often few in number with considerable space between the cells (Fig. 14.6). Their cytoplasm is usually continuous with the core of the alveolar wall. According to Patton and Horn,[3] the latter is, in reality, a giant muscle cell with its nuclei placed laterally along the surface. Alveolar rhabdomyosarcomas are the least common of the subtypes and may not merit identification as a subclass since some consider them to be variants of embryonal rhabdomyosarcoma.

Subclass status of the fourth form, the so-called *botyroid rhabdomyosarcoma* is also probably not justified.[7] Whenever *any* embryonic sarcoma involves the mucosal surface of a hollow structure, it will usually assume a botyroid configuration. Intended originally to do no more than characterize a gross form, the term has evolved into a histogenetic and histological noncommital term

for a heterogenous group of tumors, regardless of their level of differentiation or variation in the constituent elements. "Sarcoma botyroides" is an inappropriate diagnostic term unless it is used parenthetically to denote only gross appearance. In the instance of rhabdomyosarcoma, virtually all botyroid forms are embryonal rhabdomyosarcomas.

Another distinctive, but by no means constant, histological feature of botyroid embryonal rhabdomyosarcoma is the presence of a more or less compact layer of parallel rows of cells immediately beneath the mucous membrane (Fig. 14.5), below which the neoplasm assumes a loose and more sparse cellular arrangement with the cells presenting in a more haphazard manner.

The ultrastructure of normal skeletal muscle and rhabdomyosarcoma have been well documented.[8, 9] Also evaluated is the diagnostic usefulness of electron microscopy in the diagnosis of rhabdomyosarcoma.[10].

In the head and neck, the botyroid presentation of a rhabdomyosarcoma from the ear, nasopharynx or oral cavity must not be confused with an inflammatory mass, viz., aural polyp in the external auditory canal or other orifice. The combination of superimposed inflammation, small, unrecognized rhabdomyoblasts and a loose stromal arrangement of deeper lying cells has led to the underdiagnosis of the neoplasm as granulation tissue. Conversely, overzealous interpretation of innocent inflammation as rhabdomyosarcoma must also be guarded against.

In surgical-pathological practice, individual rhabdomyosarcomas often contain more than one of the aforementioned patterns. In all cases, however, a predominant pattern is present.

The majority of rhabdomyosarcomas take their origin in the peripheral soft tissues. In children, however, there is a marked predilection for rhabdomyosarcoma to present in the head and neck.[11] This neoplasm is the *most common* malignant soft tissue neoplasm of that anatomical region in children.

Most rhabdomyosarcomas arise from unsegmented and undifferentiated mesoderm, and only a relatively small number arise from myotome-derived skeletal muscle. This genesis is particularly true for those rhabdomyosarcomas occurring in the head and neck, retroperitoneum and the urogential tract, where the embryonal type of rhabdomyosarcoma is predominant. Less than 5% of all embryonal rhabdomyosarcomas are encountered in the extremities.[12]

Stobbe and Dargeon[5] were the first to consider rhabdomyosarcoma of the head and neck as a clinical or pathological group. Earlier, Pack and Eberhart[13] had proposed that visceral and lingual rhabdomyosarcoma be placed in a separate category. Dito and Batsakis[11] were the first to consider the biological activity of the rhabdomyosarcoma of the head and neck as distinctive apart from other rhabdomyosarcomas.

Rhabdomyosarcoma of the Head and Neck

Rhabdomyosarcoma, primary in the orbit, is the most commonly encountered myogenic neoplasm in the head and neck, comprising almost one-third of the total number of reported cases. Reese[14] has shown that this neoplasm is the most common malignant mesenchymal neoplasm of the orbit. The second most frequent site of origin in the head and neck is the soft tissues of the neck itself. Neoplasms arising in the nasopharynx, soft tissues of the face, ear and mastoid, tongue and palate are next in order of decreasing frequency, although they each make up between 7 and 10% of the total.

Rhabdomyosarcoma of the head and neck is primarily a disease of the first decade of life. This is in contrast to the malignant rhabdomyomatous neoplasms of the peripheral musculature where they are seen predominantly in the fifth and sixth decades. The age distribution of 166 patients studied by Dito and Batsakis[11] is depicted in Fig. 14.7. Of this series of patients, 77% were 12 years old or younger at the time of diagnosis. Almost one-half of this number were younger than 6 years of age.

Visceral rhabdomyosarcomas in sites such as the bladder, prostate gland, cervix and vagina also manifest an age distribution closely akin to that for rhabdomyosarcomas of the head and neck.[7] The age spread for all areas of the head and neck is, however, quite wide, from birth to 80 years. Five of the 170 patients presented by Dito and Batsakis[7] had lesions which were presumed to be present at birth. The sites or origin of these "congenital" neoplasms included the floor of the mouth, the tongue and the temple.

The racial extraction of patients with rhabdomyosarcoma of the head and neck is infrequently recorded. Where race has been noted, it is pertinent to note that few Negroes have been listed. All of Pinkel and Pickren's[15] head and neck tumors were in Caucasians, as were those of Stobbe and Dargeon[5] and Horn and Enterline.[16]

The almost universal mode of presentation is that of a mass or symptoms leading to the detection of a mass by the examining physician. Neoplasms of the external auditory canal, middle ear or mastoid usually manifest symptoms referable to as "otitis media" or with a frequently bloody aural discharge. Cranial nerve palsies are very common in this group (vide infra). Tumors of the eyelids present as nontender masses, but intraorbital rhabdomyosarcomas most commonly produce a unilateral proptosis with little change in visual acuity. Almost all rhabdomyosarcomas of the head and neck possess a sufficiently rapid rate of growth

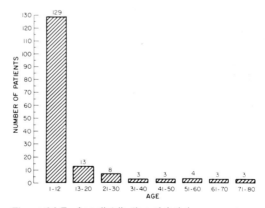

Figure 14.7. Age distribution of rhabdomyosarcomas of the head and neck. Of the 166 patients investigated, 129 were younger than 12 years of age at the time of pathological diagnosis. Rhabdomyosarcoma is the predominant malignant supporting tissue neoplasm in the head and neck of children.

that medical attention is sought within a 6-month period and, most often, before 2 months have elapsed. Slower growing neoplasms have a significantly longer survival after diagnosis.

Histologically, the most common variety of rhabdomyosarcoma of the head and neck is the embryonal or botyroid embryonal form, depending on whether or not the neoplasm is associated with the mucous membrane surface of a cavity. Next in frequency is the adult pleomorphic type. In the oral regions, the latter is quite frequent, and rhabdomyosarcomas of the tongue have been almost exclusively of this histological type. Neoplasms composed predominantly of an alveolar pattern are unusual in our experience.

In the past, authors have given the impression that each microscopic variant had a different prognosis. While there may be an element of difference in adults and in rhabdomyosarcomas in areas other than the head and neck, there is little prognostic value in differentiating histological types in the tumors of childhood or in the head and neck.[17-19]

For the sake of clinical comparison, rhabdomyosarcomas of the head and neck may be divided into five major groups on the basis of their anatomical site of origin. Certain common biological and anatomical characteristics serve to group these lesions. Orbital neoplasms are considered as a clinicopathological entity, not only because of their unique anatomical location, but also because of their numbers and other clinical features. They constitute group I. Group II consists of tumors arising in the soft tissues of the temple, face and neck. Intraoral, intranasal and pharyngeal rhabdomyosarcomas make up group III. Group IV is comprised of those rhabdomyosarcomas taking their origin from, or intimately associated with, the air-containing spaces of the skull. The remaining rhabdomyosarcomas of the head and neck, because of their small numbers and their miscellaneous sites, are arbitrarily placed in group V. One hundred seventy cases reviewed by the author are grouped in this fashion (Table 14.1).

Survival of patients with rhabdomyosarcoma of the head and neck *has* been depressingly and uniformly poor. Until the early 1970's there was a surprising constancy in survival figures in reports from many centers treating this neoplasm. Survival according to our group classification was expressed in months rather than years. If we relate to the precombination therapy experience as presented by Dito and Batsakis,[11] the following survival data evolve. In all, 27 of 170 patients were recorded as living 3 or more years after diagnosis,

Table 14.1
Rhabdomyosarcomas of the Head and Neck: Distribution of 170 Cases by Location

Group	Location of Tumor	No. of Cases
I	Orbit and eyelid	54 (31.6%)
II	Neck	18
	Face	15
	Temple	7
		40 (23.6%)
III	Nasopharynx	16
	Tongue	12
	Palate and uvula	12
	Hypopharynx	3
	Tonsil	3
	Floor of mouth	2
	Gingiva	1
		49 (28.8%)
IV	Ear, mastoid	12
	Maxillary sinus	3
		15 (8.8%)
V	Mandibular region	6
	Salivary gland region	5
	Occiput	1
		12 (7.2%)

an incidence of only 15.8%. Fourteen, or 8.2% of these patients were alive after 5 years. Only 10 patients of this group, however, were *free* of malignancy after 5 years, representing only 5.9% of the entire study group. It is significant that seven of these 5-year survivors had their primary neoplasms in the orbit. No patient in Dito and Batsakis'[11] group II and IV lived for 5 years. Over the same period of study, Pack and Eberhart[13] quoted a 5-year survival of 33.8% for peripheral rhabdomyosarcomas, a considerable difference when compared to the rather dismal survival in head and neck cases.

The comparative prominence of 5-year "cures" in the orbital groups of rhabdomyosarcoma has continued into the combination therapy era. Although capable of local recurrence and local invasion, orbital rhabdomyosarcomas are less likely to metastasize. In this respect, confirmed metastases to lymph nodes from an orbital rhabdomyosarcoma are unusual. The dissemination of rhabdomyosarcomas is primarily by hematogenous routes to lungs, bone, brain and other viscera. Rhabdomyosarcomas of certain peripheral locations manifest, in addition, a goodly frequency of regional lymph node metastasis. In my experience, the rhabdomyosarcoma, more than any other sarcoma, exhibits this morbidity. In the head and neck, however, the incidence of nodal metastasis is considerably less than that of tumors of the extremities.

In the precombination therapy era, total excision (radical removal) was the aim of surgical management for rhabdomyosarcomas. Now, the co-ordination of surgery, irradiation, and chemotherapy has reduced the need for ultraradical extirpative procedures.[20].

Maurer[1] has outlined the concepts of therapy that have contributed to the over-all improvement in prognosis in rhabdomyosarcoma. These are: (1) Combined modality therapy is superior to therapy with any single modality by itself; (2) adjuvant chemotherapy, radiation therapy and immunotherapy are of maximum benefit when the body burden of tumor cells is least. Thus, surgical "debulking," if feasible, is an important component of management; (3) chemotherapy for micrometastases (prophylactic chemotherapy) prolongs remission and increases survival; (4) combination chemotherapy is superior to single agent chemotherapy; (5) maintenance chemotherapy during high risk recurrence periods prolongs remissions and survival; (6) intermittent chemotherapy schedules are superior to continuous programs; (7) drug and treatment schedule selections should be predicated on the proliferative behavior of the malignant cell and the cell cycle specificity of the drug whenever possible.

The tailoring of combination therapy to anatomical regions must take into consideration the stage of disease. The anatomical site, while appearing to influence prognosis is secondary to clinical stage. For staging, a complete work-up of the patient, stylized according to the site of the primary lesion, is necessary. Several staging schemes have been proposed. The M. D. Anderson method (Table 14.2) is offered as a model.[19] To the T–N stage can be added distant metastasis with or without local control. Because of the infiltrative character of the rhabdomyosarcomas, a complete evaluation is necessary. This is reflected in Donaldson's[19] experience that while some patients appeared to have localized disease, a considerable number fall into a T3 stage after extensive evaluation because of soft tissue or bone invasion.

A comparison of survival statistics gives an indication of the impact on prognosis by combination therapy of rhabdomyosarcoma (Fig. 14.8). In an actuarial presentation of data from Memorial Hospital, New York, Ghavimi et al.[20] demonstrated a significant prolongation of survival in a group of patients treated by a multidisciplinary protocol between 1970 and 1974 over the survival of patients treated by a variety of modalities between 1960 and 1970. Excluding stage and site, the earlier treatment group had 2- and 3-year survivals of 37% and 28% respectively. The later group manifested a 2-year survival rate of 81% and all survived to 3 years. Excluding again stage of disease, patients with rhabdomyosarcomas of the head and neck demonstrated between 1960 and 1970 2- and 3-year survivals of 37% and 28%. In the 1970 to 1974 treatment group the 2- and 3-year survivals were 67%. Similar improvement in survivals with the use of combined therapy is reported by others.[22–24]

The combined modality treatment and intensified multidrug regimens appear to have succeeded where radical surgery had failed in respect to a disease-free survival. The chances for ultimate survival, however, are still poor in children who fail on primary therapy and develop metastases or local recurrences. In a study by Okamura et al.[25]

Table 14.2
Clinical Staging: Rhabdomyosarcoma of Head and Neck*

Stage	
T1	Neoplasm localized to one region or site.
T2	Neoplastic extension to adjacent structures or two or more sites.
T3	Radiographic evidence of bone destruction, or involvement of cranial nerves.
N0	No clinical evidence of nodal metastasis.
N1	Single, clinically positive lymph node less than 3 cm in diameter.
N2	Single lymph node over 3 cm in diameter, or multiple ipsilateral palpable nodes.
N3	Fixed lymph nodes or bilateral palpable nodes.

* From Donaldson et al.[19]

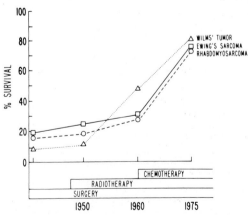

Figure 14.8. Influence of combination therapy on 2-year survival of rhabdomyosarcoma (all sites) compared with survival in patients with Wilm's tumor and Ewing's sarcoma.

the median duration of life after distant metastases were recognized was less than 12 months. Nineteen percent of their patients with rhabdomyosarcomas of all sites had distant metastases at the time of diagnosis. In their patients who later developed distant metastases, the frequency of this morbidity varied according to site of the neoplasm: extremity, 82%, trunk, 50%; head and neck (exclusive of orbit), 47%.

Encouraging statistics are provided by Okamura and associates[25] in their ability to markedly increase the disease-free and nonmetastatic interval in head and neck rhabdomyosarcomas by VAC-type chemotherapy.

Orbital Rhabdomyosarcomas. Porterfield and Zimmerman[26] have published the largest series to date of this group of rhabdomyosarcomas. It is their conclusion that the neoplasm is the most common malignant orbital tumor occurring in childhood. Ninety-one percent of their patients (55 cases) were under 15 years of age, and the oldest patient was only 25 years old. Forty of the neoplasms were of the embryonal type, six of the differentiated (adult pleomorphic variety) and nine were classified as alveolar rhabdomyosarcomas. The most common presenting sign was a rapidly developing proptosis. Usually the displacement of the eye is in a downward and temporal direction; this corresponds to the most frequently stated location of these tumors—the upper inner quadrant of the orbit.

Elusiveness of the correct diagnosis of rhabdomyosarcoma is exemplified by the original histological diagnosis rendered on this group of orbital neoplasms. The diagnosis of rhabdomyosarcoma was seldom made by the original contributor or consultant. Their most frequent diagnoses included angiosarcoma, reticulum cell sarcoma, undifferentiated carcinoma, neuroblastoma, retinoblastoma and paraganglioma.

The orbital rhabdomyosarcoma possesses the most favorable prognosis, possibly because of a paucity of lymphatics in the orbit, allowing diagnosis while the tumor is still localized.[18] In accordance with Ashton and Morgan,[27] I do not believe that histological subdivision of the rhabdomyosarcoma materially influences response to treatment or ultimate outcome. Local control of the neoplasm appears to be quite good by irradiation, either alone, or in combination therapy.

Intraoral, Pharyngeal and Nasopharyngeal Rhabdomyosarcomas. Approximately 29% of head and neck rhabdomyosarcomas have their origins in intraoral or pharyngeal structures.[28] The greatest number involve the nasopharynx and comprise

approximately one-third of the cases described from these regions. The tongue, palate and uvula are next in order of frequency (Table 14.3).

Within these antomical confines, the embryonal rhabdomyosarcoma is most frequently encountered. The botyroid variant has origin usually from the nasopharynx. Tumors with a primary site in the tongue are almost exclusively pleomorphic in type. In view of the more "adult" morphology of lingual rhabdomyosarcomas, these neoplasms may arise from a more differentiated tissue, as compared to the embryonal rhabdomyosarcoma, with origin from other oral, pharyngeal and nasopharyngeal structures. The mean age of 49 subjects studied by Dito and Batsakis[28] was 6 years. Of 49 patients, 36 (78.9%) were less than 12 years old.

There is an inverse relationship between the duration of symptoms prior to treatment and survival. Local recurrences and distant metastases are pronounced findings with rhabdomyosarcomas of this region. Recurrences occur in approximately one-half of the reported cases, and distant metastases are manifested in about one-third of the patients. These metastases may be either by hematogenous or lymphogenous dissemination. Lymph node involvement occurs in a high percentage (50%), but these have not necessarily been regional nodes. The lungs and bones are the secondary sites of favor.

Survival after diagnosis, regardless of the mode of treatment, is poor. Dito and Batsakis[28] quote a 12.5% 5-year survival. Early wide resection of the primary tumor *with* regional lymph node dissection, in conjunction with radiation therapy, offers the "best" prospect for "cure." Fu and Perzin[30] agree indicating this mode of therapy for lesions growing in the nasal vestibule, ala nasi or turbinate. These tumors tend to be relatively small when diagnosed and are thus more amenable to resection. They also point out that eight of their 16 rhabdomyosarcomas of the nasal cavity, para-

Table 14.3
Anatomical Distribution of Rhabdomyosarcomas of the Intraoral, Nasopharyngeal and Pharyngeal Soft Tissue*

Site	No.
Nasopharynx	31
Palate and uvula	15
Tongue	15
Hypopharynx (including tonsils and tonsillar fossae)	5
Floor of mouth	2
Gingiva	1

* Data are from Dito and Batsakis[28] and Masson and Soule.[29]

nasal sinuses and nasopharynx had metastases to cervical lymph nodes. Radiotherapy, chemotherapy, or both, probably should be used postoperatively in all these patients.

Rhabdomyosarcoma of the Larynx. About 60% of the cases of rhabdomyosarcoma in the head region will involve the orbit, nasopharynx or nose. In the larynx, rhabdomyosarcoma must certainly be close to, if not, the least common of laryngeal sarcomas.[31] Batsakis and Fox,[32] adding one case, were able to accept only five documented cases of rhabdomyosarcoma of the larynx from the literature (1949 to 1968). Canalis et al.[33] extended the review and by 1976 identified 24 examples in the world's literature.

Although the acceptable cases are admittedly few in number, several clinicopathological features are definable. All rhabdomyosarcomas of the larynx have been of the embryonal type or pleomorphic types. They tend to be bulky, sessile or pedunculated tumors and usually covered by epithelium unless secondarily ulcerated. They may arise from any area of the larynx or hypopharynx, but appear to be more prevalent in the glottic region (Fig. 14.9). The neoplasm has occurred twice as frequently in males as in females. One-third have occurred in children. Follow-up studies have not been lengthy, but there is a suggestion that the biological course for *laryngeal* rhabdomyosarcomas is less aggressive than that exhibited by other rhabdomyosarcoma in the head and neck. Early diagnosis and total laryngectomy may be responsible.

Rhabdomyosarcoma of the Middle Ear and Mastoid. Jaffe et al.[34] and Prat and Gray[35] and Pahor[36] have been among the more recent investigators of this lethal neoplasm. Their cases have brought to over 70 the number of cases reported in the literature.

Frustrating the surgeon in his efforts to control this disease is the fact that early diagnosis is nearly impossible. Surgical management must take into account destructive extension into the temporal bone, inferior extension into the neck, infratemporal fossa and parapharyngeal space. Extramural invasion into the posterior cranial fossa must also be considered. With the above considered, surgical excision, if ever contemplated for "cure," should be no less than a combined total temporal bone resection, exploration of the posterior cranial fossa, radical neck dissection and dissection of the parapharyngeal space and the infratemporal fossa.

One gross and microscopic feature of rhabdomyosarcoma in the region of the middle ear and also of the sinonasal tract merits re-emphasis. The presentation of a rhadomyosarcoma may simulate an inflammatory disease process both to clinicians and pathologists because of the accompanying discharge and polypoid configuration of the tumor at an orifice, or because secondary necrosis and inflammation may obscure the malignancy, especially if biopsy specimens are superficial. At least one-sixth of the reported examples of rhabdomyosarcoma of the middle ear were intially diagnosed as "granulation tissue," "granuloma" or "chronic inflammation."

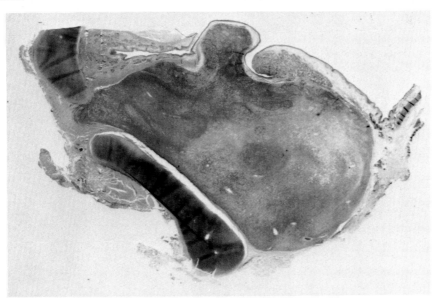

Figure 14.9. Rhabdomyosarcoma of larynx in a young child.

Although the average survival time has increased over the last four decades, it is still low and the lesion is uniformly fatal. Prat and Gray[35] indicate a patient in the 1930's survived 4 months; in the 1940's, 4.2 months; the 1950's, 8.8 months; and in the current decade, 27.6 months.

Rhabdomyoma

Extracardiac rhabdomyomas are benign tumors of skeletal muscle that have a predilection for the head and neck. Unlike the cardiac rhabdomyomas, the extracardiac tumors are not associated with any of the phakomatoses.[37] It is now generally accepted that rhabdomyomas of the heart are developmental malformations and/or examples of localized glycogen storage diseases. While more than half of the cardiac rhabdomyomas have been associated with tubersclerosis, this association has *not* been reported in any of the extracardiac rhabdomyomas.

Whether or not the extracardiac rhabdomyoma is a neoplasm is debatable. Nevertheless, it is a benign tumor and should not be confused with the granular cell myoblastoma, rhabdomyosarcoma, or harmartoma of skeletal muscle.

As of early 1978, 29 acceptable cases of extracardiac, *adult* rhabdomyoma had been reported.[38] Of this number, 26 presented in the head and neck, amply confirming this region as an area of predilection. Six of the head and neck rhabdomyomas have been laryngeal in origin. The larynx is followed by the submandibular region and pharyngeal regions as sites of preference. Fu and Perzin[30] have reported three examples from the nasopharynx.

Signs and symptoms, which are nonspecific are exclusively dependent upon the location and size of the tumor. Reported sizes have ranged from 7 mm to 13 cm in major dimension. All have been described as well-delimited. There is a slight male predominance, but there does not appear to be a predilection for any age group. The duration of signs and symptoms before removal of the tumor has varied considerably, from 11 months to 30 or 55 years.

Extracardiac tumors and those occurring in the myocardium possess more than just a superficial similarity. Cross-striations are more numerous in the cardiac type, but both contain glycogen and both demonstrate a vacuolization. The vacuolization is more uniform in the former, and cardiac rhabdomyomas also have larger cells.

The typical extracardiac rhabdomyoma is composed of large, round to oval cells with pale, pink-staining and faintly granular cytoplasm. Many cells are vacuolated (Fig. 14.10). In a few cells, definite cross-striations may be found and, in isolated cells, a haphazard arrangement of crystal-like particles is observed. The nuclei are uniform, round or oval and vesicular with fairly prominent nucleoli, usually centrally located. Slender, vascularized connective tissue septae traverse the lesion. Ultrastructurally, the "crystals" seen by light microscopy represent abnormal, hypertrophied Z-bands similar in size and type to those seen in nemaline myopathy.[39, 40]

What, at first glance, appears to be a superficial resemblance of rhabdomyoma to granular cell tumor is not indicative of any relationship. Cross-striations have never been found in granular cell myoblastomas, and histochemical and histogenetic evidence points to a marked difference between these two lesions. Despite this, the two continue to be confused. Climie et al.[41] rightly consider that most of the older reports of rhabdomyomas of the tongue were, in fact, examples of granular cell tumors.

The tumors are benign, both histologically and biologically, but recurrences may be expected if the initial excision is incomplete.

Fetal Rhabdomyoma. This uncommon and distinctive lesion of soft tissue is very likely an immature or fetal counterpart of the benign rhabdomyoma. The precise nature and origin of the tumor is unknown. The lesion may be a hamar-

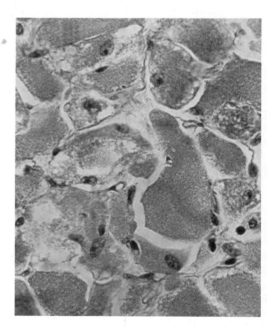

Figure 14.10. Rhabdomyoma of the larynx, a benign tumor of skeletal muscle.

toma and not a true neoplasm, as suggested by the presence in the tumor of myoblasts in early stages of differentiation analogous to striated muscle at the 6- to 10-week stage of development. There is no evidence that these lesions are a part of the tuberous sclerosis complex. The fetal rhabdomyoma usually presents shortly before birth and although cases have been recorded in adults, patient's are usually less than 3 years of age. There is a prominent male dominance with the Armed Forces Institute of Pathology (AFIP) series[42] indicating an 8:1 ratio over females. The lesion is benign.

The fetal rhabdomyoma has a rather striking predilection for the head and neck, expecially for the postauricular area. The tumor has been located always in the subcutaneous tissues and is well circumscribed, nontender, fluctuant to rubbery, and freely movable on examination.[43] They are nearly always solitary.

Fetal rhabdomyomas are moderately well circumscribed and may have a pseudocapsule. Their size has ranged from 1.2 to 8 cm in greatest diameter (median 5 cm). The outer surface is lobulated and pale gray to pink. Cut surfaces are glistening and mucoid in character.

The tumors are composed of *two* basic elements: immature skeletal muscle in varying stage of development, and small oval to spindle-shaped undifferentiated mesenchymal cells. One or the other of these elements may predominate.

These immature muscle cells and scattered mesenchymal cells lie in a vacuolated and edematous stroma. Ultrastructure of the cells shows well organized myofibrils with Z-bands, not unlike those of normal striated muscle.[42, 43] By contrast the "adult" rhabdomyoma manifests a haphazard distribution of myofibrils which are spread throughout the cytoplasm and mingled with other organelles.[44] Many of the myofilaments are found to be attached to a single hypertrophied Z-band forming crystalline bodies.

Benign Masseter Muscle Hypertrophy

Masseteric hypertrophy is a relatively uncommon condition which can occur unilaterally or bilaterally. The etiology is unclear in the majority of the patients. Associated with the enlargement of the masseter muscle, there is usually a bony overgrowth at the angle of the mandible. The combination of the bone and muscle overgrowth, if bilateral, produces a characteristic quadrangular appearance to the face.

Although rare and harmless, the lesion is apparently worldwide in distribution and is of importance in the differential diagnosis of head and

neck tumors. Breustedt[45] noted that most cases are found in the age group from 15 to 25 years. It rarely occurs in small children or in patients past the age of 30 years.

Waldhart and Lynch[46] have reviewed the several theories concerning the etiology. There are probably two fundamental forms of the disorder: (1) a congenital or familial type in which the muscles are prominent because of a thin bony face and where asymmetry of the bite, abnormal chewing habits and roentgenographic changes are not usually found; and (2) an acquired hypertrophy. The latter takes many etiological forms, particularly in unilateral hypertrophy.[47]

The usual history is that of a slow onset of either a unilateral or bilateral swelling over the ramus of the mandible. The mass is rarely painful and is not tender to palpation. Findings on radiographic examination include a flaring of the angles of the mandible and the presence of a bony spur at the lower border of the angle on the affected side.[48]

Once the disorder has been established as representing masseteric hypertrophy, the patient should be reassured, and this may be all that is required. If, however, there is asymmetry or the patient desires surgical correction for cosmetic reasons, the resection should include the enlarged bony portion of the angle of the mandible in addition to a portion of the lower inner part of the masseter muscle. Microscopic examination of the resected muscle may demonstrate normal-appearing muscle or muscle manifesting true work hypertrophy.

REFERENCES

1. Maurer, H. M.: Rhabdomyosarcoma in childhood and adolescence. Curr. Probl. Cancer 2:3, 1978.
2. Cappell, D. F., and Montgomery, G. L.: On rhabdomyoma and myoblastoma. J. Pathol. Bacteriol. 44:517, 1937.
3. Patton, R. B., and Horn, R. C., Jr.: Rhabdomyosarcoma: clinical and pathological features and comparison with human fetal and embryonal skeletal muscle. Surgery 52: 572, 1962.
4. Stout, A. P.: Rhabdomyosarcoma of skeletal muscles. Ann. Surg. 123:447, 1946.
5. Stobbe, G. D., and Dargeon, H. W.: Embryonal rhabdomyosarcoma of the head and neck in children and adolescents. Cancer 3:826, 1950.
6. Riopelle, J. L., and Theriault, J. P.: Sur une forme meconnue de sarcome des parties molles: le rhabdomyosarcome alveolaire. Ann. Anat. Pathol. 1:88, 1956.
7. Batsakis, J. G.: Urogenital rhabdomyosarcoma: histogenesis and classification. J. Urol. 90:180, 1963.
8. Vye, M. V.: The ultrastructure of striated muscle. Ann. Clin. Lab. Sci. 6:142, 1976.
9. Morales, A. R., Fine, G., and Horn, R. C.: Rhabdomyosarcoma: an ultrastructural appraisal. Pathol. Ann. 8:81, 1973.
10. Cori, G., Faraggiana, T., Granili, C., and Nardi, F.: The diagnostic usefulness of electron microscopy investigation of orbital rhabdomyosarcoma. Tumori 63:205, 1977.
11. Dito, W. R., and Batsakis, J. G.: Rhabdomyosarcoma of the head and neck: an appraisal of the biologic behavior in

170 cases. Arch. Surg. 84:582, 1962.

12. Enzinger, F.: Recent trends in soft tissue pathology. In Tumors of Bone and Soft Tissue, p. 315. Year Book Medical Publishers, Inc., Chicago, 1965.

13. Pack, G. T., and Eberhart, W. F.: Rhabdomyosarcoma of the skeletal muscle: report of 100 cases. Surgery 32:1023, 1952.

14. Reese, A. B.: Tumors of the eye and adenexa. In Atlas of Tumor Pathology. Armed Forces Institute of Pathology, Washington, D. C., 1956.

15. Pinkel, D., and Pickren, J.: Rhabdomyosarcoma in children. J. A. M. A. 175:293, 1961.

16. Horn, R. C., Jr., and Enterline, H. T.: Rhabdomyosarcoma: a clinicopathological study and classification of 39 cases. Cancer 11:181, 1958.

17. Bale, P. M. and Reye, R. D. K.: Rhabdomyosarcoma in childhood. Pathology 7:101, 1975.

18. Liebner, E. J.: Embryonal rhabdomyosarcoma of head and neck in children. Correlation of stage, radiation close, local control, and survival. Cancer 37:2777, 1976.

19. Donaldson, S. S., Castro, J. R., Wilbur, J. R., and Jesse, R. H., Jr.: Rhabdomyosarcoma of head and neck in children. Combination treatment of surgery, irradiation, chemotherapy. Cancer 31:26, 1973.

20. Johnson, D. G.: Trends in surgery for childhood rhabdomyosarcoma. Cancer 35:916, 1975.

21. Ghavimi, F., Exelby, P. R., D'Angio, G. J., Cham, W., Lieberman, P. H., Tan, C., Mike, V., and Murphy, M. L.: Multidisciplinary treatment of embryonal rhabdomyosarcoma in children. Cancer 35:677, 1975.

22. Razek, A. A., Perez, C. A., Lee, F. A., Ragab, A. H., Askin, F., and Vietti, T.: Combined treatment modalities of rhabdomyosarcoma in children. Cancer 39:2415, 1977.

23. Freeman, J. E.: Changing concepts in the management of Wilm's tumour and rhabdomyosarcoma. Proc. Roy. Soc. Med. 68:14, 1975.

24. Maurer, H. M., Moon, T., and Donaldson, M.: The intergroup rhabdomyosarcoma study. A preliminary study. Cancer 40:2015, 1977.

25. Okamura, J., Sutow, W. W., and Moon, T. E.: Prognosis in children with metastatic rhabdomyosarcoma. Med. Ped. Oncol. 3:243, 1977.

26. Porterfield, J. F., and Zimmerman, L. E.: Rhabdomyosarcoma of the orbit: a clinicopathological study of 55 cases. Virchows. Arch. (Pathol. Anat.) 335:329, 1962.

27. Ashton, N., and Morgan, C.: Embryonal sarcoma and embryonal rhabdomyosarcoma of the orbit. J. Clin. Pathol. 18:699, 1965.

28. Dito, W. R., and Batsakis, J. G.: Intra-oral, pharyngeal, and nasopharyngeal rhabdomyosarcoma. Arch. Otolaryngol. 77:123, 1963.

29. Masson, J. K., and Soule, E. H.: Embryonal rhabdomyosarcoma of the head and neck. Report of eighty-eight cases. Am. J. Surg. 110:585, 1965.

30. Fu, Y. -S., and Perzin, K. H.: Nonepithelial tumors of the nasal cavity, paranasal sinuses, and nasopharynx. A clinicopathologic study. V. Skeletal muscle tumors (rhabdomyoma and rhabdomyosarcoma). Cancer 37:364, 1976.

31. Batsakis, J. G., and Fox, J. E.: Supporting tissue neoplasms of the larynx. Surg. Gynecol. Obstet. 131:989, 1970.

32. Batsakis, J. G., and Fox, J. E.: Rhabdomyosarcoma of the larynx. Arch. Otolaryngol. 91:136, 1970.

33. Canalis, R. F., Platz, C. E., and Cohn, A. M.: Laryngeal rhabdomyosarcoma. Arch. Otolaryngol. 102:104, 1976.

34. Jaffe, B. F., Fox, J. E., and Batsakis, J. G.: Rhabdomyosarcoma of the middle ear and mastoid. Cancer 27:29, 1971.

35. Prat, J., and Gray, G. F.: Massive neuraxial spread of aural rhabdomyosarcoma. Arch. Otolaryngol. 103:301, 1977.

36. Pahor, A. L.: Rhabdomyosarcoma of the middle ear and mastoid. J. Laryngol. 90:585, 1976.

37. Wyatt, R. B., Schochet, S. S., and McCormick, W. F.: Rhabdomyoma: light and electron microscopic study of a case with intranuclear inclusions. Arch. Otolaryngol. 92: 32, 1970.

38. Ferracini, R., Cavina, C., and Morrone, B.: Rhabdomyoma (adult type) of the sublingual region. Tumori 63:43, 1977.

39. Czernobilsky, B., Cornog, J. L., and Enterline, H. T.: Rhabdomyoma: report of case with ultrastructural and histochemical studies. Am. J. Clin. Pathol. 49:782, 1968.

40. Albrechtsen, R., Ebbesen, F., and Vang Pedersen, S.: Extracardiac rhabdomyoma. Light and electron microscopic studies of two cases in the mandibular area with a review of previous reports. Acta Otolaryngol. 78:458, 1974.

41. Climie, A. R. W., Moscovic, E. A., and Kommel, R. M.: Rhabdomyoma of the larynx. Arch. Otolaryngol. 77:409, 1963.

42. Dehner, L. P., Enzinger, F. M., and Font, R. L.: Fetal rhabdomyoma. An analysis of nine cases. Cancer 30:160, 1972.

43. Dahl, I., Angervall, L., and Save-Soderbergh, J.: Foetal rhabdomyoma. Case report of a patient with two tumours. Acta Pathol. Microbiol. Scand. (A) 84:107, 1976.

44. Walter, P., and Guerbaoui, M.: Rhabdomyome foetal. Etude histologique et ultrastructurale d'une nouvelle observation. Virchows Arch. (Pathol. Anat.) 371:59, 1976.

45. Breustedt, A.: Ein Beitrag zur Clinik und Pathogenese der Masseter-Lypertsophie. Dtsch. Stomatol. 12:404, 1962.

46. Waldhart, E., and Lynch, J. B.: Benign hypertrophy of the masseter muscles and mandibular angles. Arch. Surg. 102: 115, 1971.

47. Wade, W. M., Jr., and Roy, E. W.: Idiopathic masseter muscle hypertrophy. J. Oral Surg. 29:196, 1971.

48. Bloem, J. J., and van Hoof, R. F.: Hypertrophy of the masseter muscles. Plast. Reconstr. Surg. 47:138, 1971.

CHAPTER 15

Vasoformative Tumors

Vasoformative tumors of the soft tissues and mucous membranes of the head and neck constitute a distinctive, yet clinically and often pathologically frustrating, class of lesions (Table 15.1). The exact nature of many, if not all the benign variants, whether true neoplasm, tumor-like malformations or responses to injury, remains controversial. Often, particularly in the oral cavity, distinction between granulation tissue with a rich, well-formed vascular component and "neoplasm" or malformation may be impossible.

The malignant vasoformative tumors are true neoplasms, but they arise de novo without going through a biological period as a benign lesion. Even here, however, histopathological diagnosis is difficult, and indications are that the interpretation of malignancy, in the sense of being able to disseminate, is overdone. Atypical and exuberant vascularity often accompanies epithelial and soft tissue malignancies, and, if the former are poorly differentiated, an inappropriate diagnosis of vasoformative malignancy may be made. This is particularly true if the histopathological preparations are substandard or if the observer has too low a threshold for these types of lesions.

Clinical frustration occurs in selecting the appropriate management for the diverse benign lesions. Most often location, accessibility, age of host and the ultimate cosmetic result dictate therapy. Once treatment has been instituted, an unpredictable biological course may ensue, with stubborn recurrences and locally aggressive activity thwarting a happy outcome for the patient.

In another section, I have presented clinicopathological information concerning vascular tumors of the bony structures of the face. While it is always advisable to check preoperative x-rays of the mandible and maxilla in any vascular lesion of the skin or soft tissues of the head and neck, it is not too artificial a separation to consider the latter group apart from the osseous lesions.

Before proceeding to detailed descriptions of vasoformative tumors in the head and neck, a clarification of nomenclature and some generalizations are indicated. Hemangiomas, whether malformations or neoplasms, are invariably classified according to their histological appearance, primarily architecture, into the following categories: capillary, cavernous, mixed and hypertrophic or "juvenile." In part, this is artifical and somewhat academic. There is considerable overlap with features of each, particularly, capillary and cavernous in any given lesion. Zones of transition lend some support to the supposition that the hypertrophic form of hemangioma is an immature form of capillary hemangioma and that the cavernous lesions result from "maturation" of the capillary variety. It has been suggested that pulsatile flow in end arteries over a long period may lead to cavernous enlargement of formerly capillary-sized vessels. Although hypertrophic forms may display a more aggressive behavior, no significant prognostication can be made on histological appearance alone.

Recurrences, failure to involute spontaneously and local infiltrative characteristics are more a reflection of: (1) anatomical site; (2) size and extent of the lesion, particularly with respect to depth; and (3) selection of the primary treatment when the patient is first seen.

We decry the use of the term *hemangioendothelioma*, except for the peculiar and rare hepatic vascular lesions. The term has been used to describe the hypertrophic form of capillary hemangioma. Other adjectives are "juvenile," cellular or aggressive (Fig. 15.1). While it is common for this type of hemangioma to be less circumscribed and more locally infiltrative, this is not invariably the case. Some users of the term hemangioendothelioma consider it the benign analogue of angiosarcoma (also called "malignant hemangioendothelioma"), but misuse and misunderstanding have

Table 15.1
Classification of Vasoformative Tumors—Head and Neck

I. Benign tumors (hamartomas, neoplasms or malformations?)
   A. Localized
      1. Hemangioma
         a. Capillary
         b. Cavernous
         c. Mixed
         d. Proliferative ("juvenile")
      2. Lymphangioma
         a. Capillary (simplex)
         b. Cavernous
         c. Mixed
      3. Angiofibroma
   B. Generalized or extensive
      1. Angiomatosis
         a. Macrochelia
         b. Macroglossia
         c. Diffuse
      2. Cystic hygroma
   C. Inflammatory or responsive versus neoplastic
      1. Granuloma pyogenicum
      2. Granuloma graviderum (angiogranuloma of pregnancy)
      3. "Hemangioma" of nasal septum
   D. Arteriovenous fistulae; aneurysm
   E. Phlebectasia and telangiectasia
II. Syndromes with vascular head and neck lesions (oral)
   A. Osler-Rendu-Weber (telangiectasia)
   B. Sturge-Weber
   C. Mafucci
   D. Von Hippel-Lindau
III. Malignant neoplasms
   A. Angiosarcoma
      1. Kaposi's sarcoma
   B. Hemangiopericytoma
   C. Malignant lymphogenous neoplasm (if recognizable)

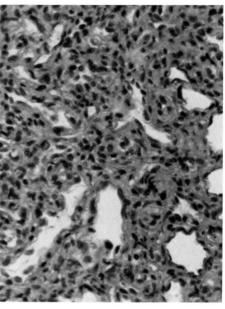

Figure 15.1. Cellular or "juvenile" hemangioma.

given similarly called benign lesions an unwarranted malignant connotation that has been a source of confusion.

The majority of angiomatous tumors are most often noticed at or shortly after birth or during early infancy. Discovery in adults is less frequent. In the latter they may often appear in ostensibly normal tissues.

Very like the growth of some capillary and cavernous hemangiomas, the growth of lymphogenous tumors may be self-limited. I have, however, observed a tendency for definable lymphogenous tumors to be less prone to this phenomenon and also somewhat more resistant to management.

Benign vasoformative lesions may be solitary, multiple, diffuse or small to extensive. They may also be only a part of a hemangiomatous syndrome.

Some of the clinical vascular lesions are not always tumor-like anomalies. Spider nevi associated with pregnancy or cirrhosis of the liver are merely localized dilations of capillaries, showing no evidence of cellular proliferation and usually without clinical import to the head and neck surgeon. Similarly, phlebectasias of the oral mucosa and tongue ("caviar spot") are manifestations of a decreased connective tissue tone in older patients and should not present diagnostic problems.[1] Other forms of multiple telangiectasis, however, may have considerable significance for the surgeon. A prototype is hereditary hemorrhagic telangiectasia.

HEREDITARY HEMORRHAGIC TELANGIECTASIA (OSLER-WEBER-RENDU DISEASE)

This telangiectatic bleeding disorder is characterized by familial occurrence and is transmitted as an autosomal dominant affecting both sexes equally. Diagnosis is usually based upon a clinical triad of characteristic telangiectatic lesions, the hereditary incidence and a hemorrhagic diathesis. The latter is usually accompanied by normal levels of measured hemostatic factors.[2]

The head and neck surgeon is often the initial physician contact made by the patient because of the presenting symptoms. Hemorrhage from the oral mucosa is a significant component of the disease and is second only to epistaxis, often beginning in early youth, with cutaneous and oral mucous membrane lesions appearing in the second and third decades of life. In respect to the former, telangiectases are frequently observed on the facial skin, especially at the nasal orifices and over the cheeks; less commonly, the scalp, ears, fingers, toes and nail beds are involved. The skin of the trunk and extremities is only rarely involved. The mucocutaneous junction of the lips and tongue (particularly the tip and anterior dorsum) are the dominant sites in the oral region.

The angiomatous skin or mucous membrane lesions pathognomonic of this malady may present in one of three forms: spider-like, punctiform or nodular. All have a tendency to bleed either spontaneously or when traumatized. The nodular type of telangiectasis is tumor-like and may reach 2 to 3 cm in diameter. Usually however, the lesions are macular in conformation and, when present in the mouth, appear as bright red, violaceous or purple spots that increase in size with increasing age. Pressure on the lesions produces blanching.

Histopathologically, the telangiectases are found just beneath the dermis or mucous membrane and consist merely of dilated vessels, lined by a single layer of endothelium and without elastic tissue. Electron microscopic evaluation has identified the affected vessels as venules.[3]

Management of expistaxis in this disorder may be found in the reports of McCaffrey et al.[4] and Stell.[5]

HEMANGIOMAS

Definable hemangiomas comprise the most common single tumor in the region of the head and neck in childhood. Together with lymphangiomas, they make up approximately 30% of all *oral* tumors in children.[6] The incidence in adults is considerably lower.

Cutaneous. In the skin of the head and neck, the scalp, neck and face are primary sites arranged in descending order of frequency of involvement. Females are affected more than males, and the lesions most often are solitary (Fig. 15.2).

The cutaneous birthmark (nevus flammus) is a capillary hemangioma characteristically in the dermis. The so-called strawberry nevus usually presents in the subcutis. It occurs primarily in infants and children and histologically conforms to the hypertrophic type of capillary hemangioma. The lesion is rare in adults. After an early period of evolution, the lesion may develop suddenly and assume considerable size. If involution occurs, the

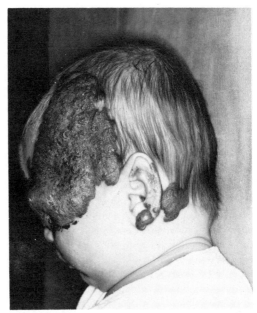

Figure 15.2. Extensive and deforming hemangioma in a child.

locally expansive stage is followed by involuting changes which ultimately produce regression of the angioma.

Cavernous hemangiomas of the skin or deeper structures are more permanent in their existence than the usual capillary hemangiomas. Spontaneous regression may be anticipated in a significant percentage of those present at birth, whereas it is less likely to occur when the lesion is not present at birth. Phleboliths are commonly seen in soft tissue *cavernous* hemangiomas.

A rather distinctive vasoformative lesion, the *arteriovenous hemangioma*, has a predilection for the lips and perioral skin and occurs almost exclusively in adults.[7] Regarded as hamartomas with numerous arteriovenous shunts, these lesions are throught to arise from the subpapillary vascular plexus of the skin. The essential histopathological features are multiple dilated vascular channels located in the corium or submucosa and without significant epidermal participation. Anastomosing vascular spaces are lined by endothelial cells and their thin-walled veins contrast sharply with arteries showing thick fibromuscular walls. There is a striking decrease to absence of elastic fibers and from their pattern, the vessels appear to be of multicentric origin.

Mucosal. Hemangiomatous lesions may develop anywhere in the mucosa of the oropharyngeal and upper respiratory tracts. The oral and nasal cavities are the most frequent sites.

Granulation tissue and other forms of inflammatory "pseudotumors" may not always be capable of being differentiated. These are most common on the lower portions of the nasal septum, a site readily subjected to trauma. Larger, inflammatory vascular masses may occur in the nasal cavity and sinuses, particularly the maxillary sinus.

Several inflammatory lesions with a dominant vascular component are important to the head and neck surgeon. "Hemangioma" of the nasal septum, or so-called "bleeding polyp," develops predominantly as a polypoid or sessile lesion in the mucosa of the cartilaginous system within Little's triangle.[8] Less frequently, it arises posterior to the triangle or in accessory sinuses. The lesion is rare before puberty (most common between 16 and 17 years) and is almost always heralded by epistaxis. Microscopically the lesion is composed of dilated thin-walled vessels in relatively little stroma. Large vessels are invariably present at the base. Persistence is possible, if the lesion is not completely destroyed down to and including the epichondrium.

Like the foregoing, *granuloma pyogenicum* is the result of an exaggerated response to relatively minor trauma.[9] Found in a universal distribution of the body, it is very common in the oral mucosa (Fig. 15.3). Following intubation, pyogenic granulomas may occur on tonsils or the laryngeal mucosa. Granuloma graviderum, predominantly

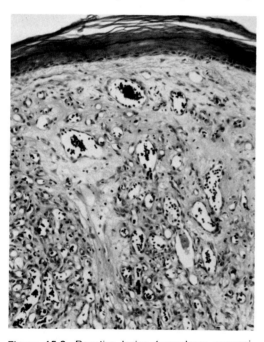

Figure 15.3. Reactive lesion (granuloma pyogenicum) virtually indistinguishable from hemangioma.

a lesion of the gingiva, is *identical* in appearance to the pyogenic granuloma.[9] The palate and nasal septum are occasional sites of involvement. Appearing in the early months of pregnancy, it usually disappears at the termination of gestation.

Noninflammatory hemangiomas can occur anywhere in the oral cavity, at any age and without sexual or racial predisposition. While certainly more common in children, many are identified in patients past the age of 40 years. In children, the lips, cheek and tongue are the most common areas of involvement.

Oral hemangiomas may exist as small superficial lesions, as larger superficial lesions with some depth extension or as extensive tumors involving large areas of mucosa or connective tissue resulting in gross deformity of the oral region. They may be multicentric with clustering in a given area.

Superficial hemangiomas of the oral mucous membranes tend to be blue or reddish-blue, compressible, partially submerged lesions which are easily diagnosed. The more deeply situated lesions tend to be firm, more diffuse and less circumscribed. Patients manifesting the deep type of hemangioma are usually under 5 years of age.[10] True cavernous hemangiomas of the oral and hypopharynx are very rare. Only 10 cases has been reported from 1887 to 1961.[11] Management of oral hemangiomas is discussed by Woods and Tulumello.[12] Hemangiomas of the salivary glands and the larynx are presented elsewhere in this text (Chapters 1 and 9).

So-called "Invasive" Hemangiomas

Circumscription is not an outstanding architectural characteristic of many hemangiomas; hence, in a sense, many appear invasive. Fortunately, the majority of cutaneous and mucosal hemangiomas, by virtue of their papular, nodular and polypoid features, do not manifest excessive infiltrative qualities. More deeply situated lesions, however, regardless of their subtype, exhibit a histological and clinical invasiveness that may be difficult to control. These occur in the deep subcutaneous tissues, deep fascial layers and muscles (Fig. 15.4). While cutaneous involvement may be present, it is the deep mass that brings the patient to the physician and serves as a problem to the therapist.

The experience of the Mayo Clinic is fairly representative of this group of lesions.[13] Between 1917 and 1969, 52 cases of deep lying hemangiomas were treated at that institution. In all cases, the mass was the presenting complaint, and almost all patients were specifically alarmed by a recent rapid enlargement. Twelve of the 52 had coexistent

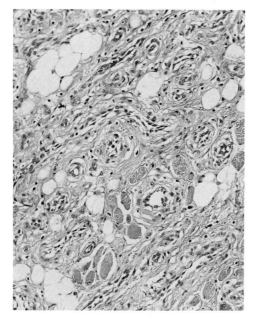

Figure 15.4. Deep lying hemangioma infiltrating between skeletal muscle fibers.

skin involvement. Children exceeded adults by a ratio of 2.5:1. Our personal experience with respect to age is approximately 10:1 in favor of children. All histological types were present and fairly well divided among each type. Again, my own experience differs, in that the invasive lesions have been predominatly capillary or hypertrophic in type. Persistence of lesion despite various modalities of treatment is "impressive." In only 16 of the 52 cases (Mayo series) was the initial care effective 5 years or longer, and in only seven cases was it adequate for 10 years or more. There was never any evidence of true malignant change, nor was any distant metastasis discovered in the follow-up periods.

The hemangioma of skeletal muscle (intramuscular hemangioma) has been singled out by rather intensive study.[14-16] It is a distinctive lesion originating for the most part in normal skeletal muscle and represents less than 1% of all hemangiomas. Very likely some of the invasive hemangiomas of the head and neck described by Hoehn et al.[13] were examples of this lesion since the biological behavior is the same.

The great majority of these lesions occur in muscles of the upper and lower extremity. Only approximately 14% of the lesions have presented in the head and neck where the masseter and trapezius muscles are most often the sites of involvement.

The intramusuclar hemangioma may be found at any age but has its highest incidence in young adults, particularly those in their third decade of life.

The most common presenting sign is a localized, rubbery swelling with distinct margins and a smooth surface. A palpable mass occurs in 98% of cases. Most often the mass is mobile but is rarely compressible. Pulsations, thrills and bruits are infrequent. A coincidental cutaneous involvement may be present, but is uncommon. Pain is present in more than half of the cases; it is thought to be due to compression. Loss of function of the involved muscle may occur.

Allen and Enzinger[15] formulated a classification based on vessel size in the lesions which correlated well with locations and prognosis for recurrence. Capillary or "small vessel" intramuscular hemangiomas are noted most commonly in the trunk and head and neck regions. They have a recurrence rate of 20%. "Large vessel" (cavernous) hemangiomas are most common in the lower limbs, followed by the head and neck. A 9% recurrence rate is given for these lesions. Over one-fourth of mixed type hemangiomas will recur. They are not common in the head and neck.

Optimal treatment should be complete excision with ligation of feeding vessels. Incomplete removal is followed by recurrence and deeper invasion.

Treatment

Two general patterns of management have evolved for benign hemangiomas of the head and neck region.[13,17] The simpler is predicated on the observations that the majority of congenital hemangiomas involute spontaneously. Here parental pressure to treat the affected child is combated by reassurance that the tumor will undergo spontaneous regression if given sufficient time. Hoehn et al.[13] relate the sequence in the second form of management, usually followed in cases of a tumor exhibiting an initial rapid growth. Initially there is some form of radiation therapy, injection of sclerosing agents, conservative excision and, ultimately, a radical surgical attack on a by now extensive tumor. The reports of Margileth and Museles,[18] Lampe and Latourette,[19] Martin[20] and Hoehn et al.[13] offer guidelines for appropriate management. Obviously the key to successful therapy is complete individualization. The choice of the mode of therapy is dependent upon several factors, including age of the patient, size of the lesion, site of involvement, depth of extension and general clinical characteristics. For the oral hemangiomas, small solitary tumors may be successfully surgically excised. Some prefer electrosurgery to the scalpel for the smaller hemangiomas. Active treatment can be deferred for the small oral lesions. Resolution following trauma, hemorrhage and organization often produces a very satisfactory cosmetic result. Shklar and Meyer[10] deplore the use of any form of radiation for the treatment of oral and perioral hemangiomas. These authors also recommend deferring surgical intervention for large, deep hemangiomas until the patient is at least 8 to 10 years old.

For deep-seated hemangiomas of the head and neck, wide-field surgical excision appears the treatment of choice. Elective sacrifice of normal structures, however, is never justified. Excessively radical surgery may, at times, be necessary. I recall an invasive hemangioma occurring in a 4-year-old girl in the posterior cervical triangle. The patient experienced four recurrences in 1.5 years, until the tumor was out of control of conservative surgery. Extension into the brachial plexus and around major vessels required a forequarter amputation. Admittedly such radical steps are uncommon, but they do illustrate the difficulties encountered in the management of these lesions.

According to Hoehn et al.,[13] radiation is a secondary form of treatment. In combination with surgical excision, it may suppress tumor growth, but probably will not effect a cure if used alone.

ARTERIOVENOUS FISTULAS AND CERVICAL PSEUDOANEURYSMS

Arteriovenous fistulas are usually the result of trauma; in rare instances the abnormality is apparently congenital and due to persistence of embryonic channels. Some authorities claim that the head and neck area is the most common location for congenital arteriovenous fistulas. Certain differences exist between congenital and acquired fistulas. In the congenital type, there may be multiple communications between the arteries and veins, as compared to a single union in the traumatic fistulas (cardiac hypertrophy and decompensation are unusual in congenital fistulas[21]).

The prognosis of untreated fistulas is uncertain, although it is claimed that those of the head and neck are better tolerated than those occurring in the extremities. The potential complications of rupture with hemorrhage, sudden enlargement, disfigurement and endarteritis with septicemia dictate an active approach to management.

Devine et al.[22] were struck by the frequency of only partial success in the treatment of the congenital fistula. Because of frequent multiple communications, simple ligation of the large arteries proximal to the fistula rarely, if ever, suffices to cure the lesion. A *direct attack* on the fistula, often preceded by a ligation of proximal arteries, offers the best potential for cure.

True aneurysms of arteries in the cervical region, not secondary to trauma or lues, are rare.[23] Redundant, buckled and tortuous carotid and innominate arteries often appear as pulsatile masses in the base of the neck. Bergen and Hoehn [24] call them "evanescent cervical pseudoaneurysms." Treatment is directed to reducing the obesity and hypertension that underlie the changes in the arteries.

Primary venous aneurysms are rare lesions. Between 1928 and 1977, 11 cases of primary venous aneurysms of the jugular and great mediastinal veins have been reported.[25] Clinically *significant* jugular vein dilation is also very uncommon.[26]

INTRAVASCULAR ANGIOMATOSIS

The lesion, intravascular angiomatosis, is a benign intravascular process which may be misdiagnosed as angiosarcoma by the unsuspecting pathologist. The lesion has its greatest incidence in the extremities and the head and neck where there is predilection for the subcutaneum of the perioral region.

Described over a half-century ago, these lesions have spawned a considerable literary effort, particularly to alert the microscopist against the diagnosis of angiosarcoma.[27–29] The lesion has acquired several names in the telling: vegetante intravascular hemangioendothelioma, endovasculaite proliferante thrombopoietique, intravascular angiomatosis, intravenous atypical vascular proliferation and Masson's pseudoangiosarcoma. By any name, it is nothing more than an unusual form of an organizing thrombus. While I consider that an unfamiliarity with the lesion more than histological atypism is cause for misdiagnosis of angiosarcoma, diagnostic assistance can be had by a comparison of intravascular angiomatosis and angiosarcoma (Table 15.2). Intravascular localization, absent to rare mitoses and necrosis and rare solid areas without vascular differentiation serve best to exclude angiosarcoma (Fig. 15.5).

ANGIOFIBROMA

The angiofibroma is an uncommon, highly vascular, locally invasive, nonencapsulated tumor with a sharp, if not almost exclusive, predilection for origin in the posterior nares or nasopharynx of adolescent males. The lesion produces its principal clinical effects during the adolescent years. Because of these clinicoanatomical characteristics, the adjective "juvenile" has been prefixed to the diagnostic designation of nasopharyngeal angiofibromas in most reports concerning the tumor. The use of the qualifying prefix, should not, however, imply that the lesion is restricted to adolescence.

Table 15.2
Microscopic Features of Intravascular Angiomatosis versus Angiosarcoma*

Histopathological findings	Intravascular Angiomatosis	Angiosarcoma
Intravascular location	Always	Rare
Central zone of thrombus	Common	Uncommon
Solid cellular areas	Uncommon	Common
Necrosis	Rare	Common
Layering of endothelium	Uncommon, usually focal	Common
Cellular pleomorphism	Not pronounced and more often only focal	Often pronounced
Mitoses	Rare	Common

* Modified after Clearkin and Enzinger.[27]

The incidence of this tumor has been estimated at 1:5,000 or 1:6,000 otolaryngological admissions to hospital clinics.[30] The entire clinical experience of the Head and Neck Service of the Sloan-Kettering Memorial Cancer Center over a 31-year period (1932 to 1963) was reported as 40 cases.[31] It has been estimated that the tumor accounts for 0.5% of all neoplasms of the head and neck.

The onset of signs and symptoms usually varies from 7 to 21 years of age, with an average of 14 or 18 years, depending on the series reported. Symptoms include nasal obstruction, recurrent severe epistaxis, purulent rhinorrhea, facial deformity and nasal speech. Schiff[32] considers the clinical manifestations to have a "general march of progression" with an order of occurrence as follows: nasal obstruction, recurrent epistaxis, progressive deformity of the palate, face and throat, rhinolalie and anosmia. Not infrequently, however, severe epistaxis is the first complaint. Rarely, signs and symptoms produced by extranasopharyngeal extension of the tumor are the initiating complaints.

With respect to the overwhelming male predominance, the view of many otolaryngologists is expressed in the categorical assessment by Capps et al.[33]: "It has been established that nasopharyngeal angiofibroma does not occur in females. The few

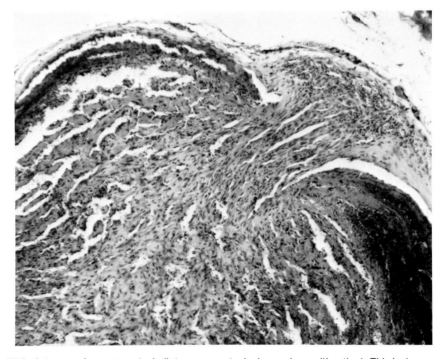

Figure 15.5. Intravascular angiomatosis (intravenous atypical vascular proliferation). This lesion was removed from the lateral neck of a 71-year-old woman. This section clearly identifies the lesion as an organization of thrombus.

cases reported in females have invariably turned out to be a pedunculated fibroma or polyp on histological examination." While the latter assessment is instructive in differential diagnosis of polypoid vascular lesions in the nasopharynx, the former is incorrect. I have personally seen two examples in young females and a few other cases have been well documented.[34–36] One angiofibroma in a female has been studied with the electron microscope and found to be similar ultrastructurally to those in males.[35] Assuredly, however, these examples are very rare. Apostol and Frazell[31] highlight this by stating that sex chromosome studies are indicated if the diagnosis is confirmed in a female. Angiofibromas manifest a pattern of geographical distribution with a higher incidence in Egypt, India, Southeast Asia and Kenya than in the United States and Europe.

The tissue of origin remains elusive and many theories remain now as only historical.[37, 38] Most likely the tumor arises from the distinctive fibrovascular stroma normally present in the nasal cavity and nasopharynx. Frequently, the angiofibroma duplicates this tissue.[39]

The site of origin is usually broadly based and situated on the posterolateral wall of the nasal cavity where the sphenoidal process of the palatine bone meets the horizontal ala of the vomer and the pterygoid process. This forms the superior margin of the splenopalatine formamen and the posterior end of the middle turbinate, thus explaining the ease with which spread occurs to sphenoid, nasopharynx and pterygomaxillary tissue and fosa (vide infra). Because of secondary attachments and additional blood supply, and spreading capabilities it is erroneous to restrict the site or origin to the nasopharynx.[40]

Hubbard,[41] in a classic paper, considers the nasopharyngeal angiofibroma to be a distinctive type of hemangioma. The diagnosis of nasopharyngeal angiofibroma can usually be readily made on the basis of the history, physical examination and appropriate radiographic examination. Biopsy of the mass is seldom necessary and is contraindicated as an office procedure because of the hazard of extensive hemorrhage.

The plainfilm and angiographic appearance of these tumors are consistent. On the plainfilms, "bowing" of the posterior wall of the maxillary sinus is the most consistent and reliable finding. The carotid arteriographic appearance is consistently typical and can be relied upon for diagnosis.[42, 43] It is to be noted that the lesion may be seen most clearly on lateral and verticosubmental views. Angiographic studies not only yield a char-

acteristic picture, they are invaluable for definition of the exact extent of the tumor and to diagnose the feeding vessels in order to determine if there is a one-sided or bilateral vascularization. The pattern of vessels is rather characteristic in the arterial phase where filling of an excessive number of dilated and tortuous vessels occurs. In the capillary phase, the configuration changes to a homogeneous vascular staining, enabling one to determine the extent of the tumor. The angiographic pattern closely resembles that of a meningioma.

Studies with angiography and subtraction technique demonstrate that the main blood supply of most angiofibromas comes from an enlarged internal maxillary artery but may come from both sides, particularly when the external carotid artery has been ligated.[44] Arterial supply has been identified from dural, sphenoidal, and ophthalmic branches of the internal carotid and the vertebral artery and thyrocervical trunk.[44]

Grossly the tumor is located on one side or the other of the posterior nares and nasopharynx, or it may completely fill the nasopharynx. A considerable number already have extensions into paranasal regions at the time of diagnosis. These include the sphenoid, ethmoid and maxillary sinuses, the retroantral space, orbit and intracranial space. The tumor is usually described as pink-gray to purple-red, lobulated and rubbery. Ulceration of the overlying mucosa in uncommon. More often sessile than polypoid, it is unencapsulated and infiltrates surrounding tissues. Because of their wide base of origin and secondary attachments, resection in continuity may be impossible. Occasionally, there may be only a narrow attachment stalk.

A description of the natural course of an angiofibroma has been provided by Neel et al.[44] The tumor first grows beneath the mucosa just inside the posterior choanal margins on the roof laterally. With increasing size, there is submucosal extension along the roof to the posterior border of the septum and thence downward where it forms a mass in the roof of the posterior nasal cavity. The nasal cavity is then filled, crowding the septum into the opposite nasal cavity and compressing the turbinates. Neel et al.[44] point out that the tumor does not enter the maxillary sinus through the lateral wall of the nose, but comes out of the posterior choana, where it may fill the nasopharynx, displaces the soft palate and be visible below the free edge. Destruction of the medial wall of the antrum may also occasionally occur. Lateral growth is through the sphenopalatine foramen with expansion of the posterior end of the middle turbinate.

Once into the pterygomaxillary fossa, the tumor presses on the surrounding bony walls and destroys the root of the pterygoid process of the sphenoid bone. The bulging of the cheek that is often an accompaniment of the angiofibroma is produced by extension into the infratemporal fossa and expansion of the pterygomaxillary fissure.

If the tumor is sufficiently large, it may bulge into a lower part of the temporal fossa and produce a swelling above the zygoma. Following this, the tumor usually moves into the inferior orbital fissure, which opens into the upper anterior third of the pterygomaxillary fossa, and enters the lower end of the superior orbital tissue, which meets the inferior orbital fissure in the posterosuperior wall of the pterygomaxillary fossa. At this site, the angiofibroma destroys the great wing of the sphenoid bone. This produces the characteristic widening along the lower lateral margin of the superior orbital fissure and proptosis. The lesion enlarges in the pterygomaxillary and temporal fossae destroying the base of the pterygoid process. Destruction of this bone brings the angiofibroma against the dura of the middle cranial fossa, anterior to the foramen lacerum and lateral to the cavernous sinus.

The above extensions are possibly concomitant with growth of the tumor from its point of origin through the floor of the sphenoid sinus. Continued expansion from this point fills the sinus and eventually into the sella turcica. Thus the angiofibroma may enter the cranial cavity in the middle fossa either anterior to the foramen lacerum and lateral to the cavernous sinus and carotid artery or through the sella medial to the carotid artery and lateral to the pituitary or by both paths. For a lesion as yet not defined as neoplastic, it clearly manifests biological aggressiveness.

The tumor is histologically benign and is composed of spindle or stellate fibrocytes in a varying amount of connective tissue stroma. An obligatory feature is the presence of a fairly wide and thin-walled vessels (Fig. 15.6). These are lymphatic-like endothelial spaces or channels. The picture varies from one of erectile-like tissue or a cavernous hemangioma with fibrous stroma to that of a cellular or, occasionally, partially myxomatous fibromatosis.

The cellularity and quality of the fibrous matrix are variable even within the same lesion. Hubbard[41] claims that there is an increase in fibrous elements in older patients, whereas there is a predominance of increased vascularity in the lesions of younger patients. McGavran[45] does not agree that this form of maturation occurs with increasing

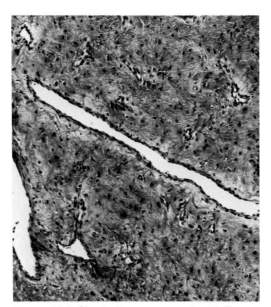

Figure 15.6 Classical appearance of angiofibroma. Mature connective tissue surrounds cleft-like endothelial-lined spaces.

age. My personal experience coincides with Hubbard's. Serial sections indicate that the classical appearance is to be found in the interior parts of the tumor. Surface areas, because of the common ulceration, manifest increased vascularity and less stroma. The vessels in this zone, however, do not have the appearance of passive participation, but, as expected, appear like the vessels accompanying granulation tissue. Sometimes vessels throughout the lesion show evidence of a vasculitis or thrombosis. In these areas, the connective tissue stroma is distinctly hyalinized. Depending on the area and superimposed reactivity, the proportion of vascular and stromal components varies. Electron microscopic evaluation has yielded minor controversies, but McGavran[45] claims evidence that the predominant stromal cell is the fibroblast.

Recent electron microscopic evaluations have raised new possibilities concerning the stromal cells in the angiofibroma.[46–48] Numerous, round, electron dense inclusions of uncertain compositions have been demonstrated in the nuclei of the stromal cells. The ultrastructural identity of the stromal cell to the fibroblast on the basis of collagen production, a well-developed rough endoplasmic reticulum (RER) and intracytoplasmic filaments has been challenged by Taxy[47] who raises the possibility that the cells may be myofibroblasts. Support for this idea has been given by Stiller et al.[46] These workers subdivided the fibroblasts on the basis of their organelle content: (1) activated "classical" fibroblasts; (2) activated fibroblasts with resemblance to histiocyte-like cells due to subplasmalemmal vesicles and lysosomal bodies; and (3) fibroblasts with a myoid differentiation. The latter range in appearance from typical myofibroblasts to cells indistinguishable from smooth muscle cells. The same investigators consider that cells of the capillary vessel may change into stromal cells.

By light microscopy, the effects of exogenous estrogen administration on the tumor may be summarized as follows: (1) increased collagenization of the stroma; (2) a decrease in blood vessels; and (3) an increase in the thickness of blood vessels with attenuation of the endothelia. Ultrastructural alterations described by Walike and MacKay[48] may suffer from sampling error according to Taxy[47] who could not confirm their findings.

The existence of a sarcomatous form of angiofibroma is denied by most authors. The patients reported by Batsakis et al.[49] and Hormia and Koskinen[50] appear to be legitimate. In the former, radiation was considered the provoking stimulus. In the latter patient, an 8-year-old boy, metastases occurred to regional lymph nodes and bone. This complication of angiofibroma must be considered as nearly negligible.

The management of angiofibroma has been as varied as the hypotheses concerning the lesion's histogenesis and biological behavior. Hemorrhage, local extension and recurrences further complicate decisions relative to the "appropriate" therapy.

Although considerable ink has been expended in relating the "natural regression" of the tumor, very few authorities have actually observed this phenomenon. Pressman[51] was unable to find a single case of angiofibroma, which had produced serious hemorrhage and was left unremoved, that disappeared upon the advent of adulthood. Neither did symptoms diminish so that treatment was unnecessary. Watchful expectancy, therefore, must be vigorously and categorically condemned as a form of primary management for an angiofibroma.

Advocacy of hormonal therapy waxes and wanes. Testosterone has not been very successful and cannot be recommended even as an adjunct to other forms of treatment. Schiff[32] and others have had success with stilbestrol. The secondary effects, however, negate its use on a long-term basis. Recommended uses of stilbestrol appear to be limited to preoperative administration to facilitate surgical removal by decreasing the tumor's size and vascularity.

Radiation-type therapy is no longer used as a primary form of treatment. Although irradiation can routinely be expected to produce a regression in an angiofibroma, the temporary nature of this regression and the functional morbidity, as well as the long-term hazard of induction of sarcoma (vide supra), place this form of treatment in an adjunctive role, if indicated. Martin et al.[52] have emphasized the complications attendant to radiation therapy.

The preferred treatment is surgical. Neglect of this, or any form of treatment, permits the persistence of epistaxis, which may be life-threatening, bone destruction with bulging of the cheek, exopthalmus and erosion of the base of the skull by local growth of the angiofibroma. Surgical approaches have ranged from conservative to radical and from avulsion to cryosurgical removal. Whichever technique is proposed, in any given patient the surgical approach to the tumor must be tailored to provide adequate exposure and to allow a controlled removal of the tumor. The contemporary management and evolution of treatment have been considered by Harrison[40] and Boles and Dedo.[53]

The prognosis for patients with angiofibroma is good, despite the fact that the tumor may be locally invasive and recurrences or, more aptly, persistence occur in approximately one-half of series of cases. The life-consuming character of angiofibroma relates largely to the bleeding from the lesion and less from a local aggressiveness. There is an estimated over-all mortality of 3%,[30] which I consider on the high side.

On many occasions after treatment, small asymptomatic areas of tumor persist but do not require further treatment. Symptomatic recurrences are manifested in the first 12 months after primary treatment and are unusual after 2 years. Smith et al.[54] report a recurrence rate of 2.5 in 19 of 40 patients. One of these patients had as many as 12 recurrences.

The relatively high recurrence rate is testimony to failure of the initial operator to fully encompass the lesion in his excision. This may be due to a conservatism on the part of the surgeon, but it is more likely related to (1) the multilobular nature of the tumor and its ability to invade adjacent sinuses and insinuate into potential fascial spaces and (2) anatomical irregularities of the nasopharynx.

There is no obvious relation between the age of onset and the clinical disease course. Cases reported in middle-aged males are not dissimilar to those in the adolescent male.

TUMORS OF LYMPHATIC ORIGIN

Lymphangiectasia, "lymphangiomas" and lymphangiosarcomas are the three principal tumorous disorders of the lymphatic system. The latter is a rare malignant neoplasm arising from the endothelium of lymphatic spaces. Although it has been described as arising de novo, as well as in association with irradiated lymphangiomas, it is most commonly associated with chronic lymphedema of an extremity. I know of no documented case occuring in the head and neck. Whether or not "lymphangiomas" are malformations, angiectases, hamartomas or benign neoplasms cannot be stated with certainty, and often their characterization is determined by their proliferation and growth rate.

The overwhelming majority of large cystic types of "lymphangioma" occur in the cervical region where they have been placed in a special category: hygroma colli. These cystic hygromas of the neck and upper parts of the body are generally considered as malformations rather than true neoplasms. Lymphangiomas and cystic hygromas have been classified into three groups[55]: (1) lymphangioma simplex, composed of thin-walled, capillary-sized lymphatic channels; (2) cavernous lymphangioma, composed of dilated lymphatic spaces, often with a fibrous adventitia; and (3) cystic lymphangioma or cystic hygroma, composed of cysts varing in size from a few millimeters to several centimeters in diameter.

Instead of considering these three categories as separate and distinct, a unified concept seems more appropriate.[56] The morphological differences between lymphangioma and cystic hygroma, may, in part, be due to differences in anatomical locations. The smaller, "angiomatous" and noncystic lesions occur in the lips, cheek and tongue and, to a lesser degree, in the floor of the mouth. Cystic hygromas occur where there are clearly definable tissue planes and loose areolar tissue, permitting space for expansion of the endothelial-lined spaces and insinuation of the tumor among vessels and nerve trunks. There is some evidence that cystic hygromas might first have been cavernous lymphangiomas.

In addition to the above, combinations of patterns are frequently seen; cystic areas and lymphangiomatous zones occupy separate, but nevertheless neighboring, parts of a tumor. In this respect, lymphangiomatous malformations of the tongue are often seen in association with cystic hygromas of the neck.

While a number of "lymphangiomas" and cystic hygromas have been reported in adults, between 50 and 60% are present at birth and 80 to 90% are detected by the end of the second year of life, during the period of greatest lymphatic growth.

The *lymphangiomyoma* has escaped only recently from being considered a lymphangiopericytoma. It is a lesion composed of smooth muscle and lymphatic channels. It occurs exclusively in females, is not infrequently associated with endocrine disorders, has some features analogous to tuberous sclerosis and may represent an incomplete expression or forme fruste of Bourneville's disease. The name has been extended to "lymphangiomyomatosis syndrome" by some authors in deference to presentation with multiple nodules or involvement of the lungs, in addition to masses in the mediastinum and/or retroperitoneum.[57] The aforementioned anatomical sites are the most frequent locations. The tumor has only rarely been found in the head and neck. Clinically lymphangiomyoma(s) is associated with chylothorax or chylous ascites.

CYSTIC HYGROMA

Cystic hygromas arise from the same primordia as do normal lymph vessels. They are found predominantly in the neck and are noticed at birth or shortly thereafter. They are more common in the posterior triangle of the neck, but larger masses extend beyond the sternocleidomastoid muscle, into the anterior compartment and often cross the midline. Hygromas in the posterior neck tend to reach up into the cheek and parotid gland region or down toward the mediastinum or axilla. Anterior masses tend to involve the floor of the mouth and base of the tongue. There is no sex predominance, and there is an even distribution as to the side of involvement.

Lynn[58] states that it is usually parental anxiety that first brings the patient to the attention of the physician. Some infants, however, do manifest difficulty in nursing, with choking and regurgitation. Other signs and symptoms may include: (1) distortion of the face or neck; (2) respiratory stridor with cyanosis by compression or mediastinal extension; (3) sudden increase in size by spontaneous hemorrhage which may be fatal; and (4) brachial plexus compression with pain or hyperesthesia.

The natural history of cervical lymphangiomas varies according to their histological configuration and may be progressive, static or intermittent in growth to regressive or spontaneous disappearance. Although rapid increase in size may occur, in the majority of cases the tumor seems to grow with the infant and, thereby, only gradually becomes more prominent.

Small lesions are unilocular and manifest a fairly firm consistency. The extensive, large tumors are obviously loculated and fill the side of the neck and cheek. The cavernous lymphangioma and cystic hygroma are usually compressible and capable of being shifted. The overlying skin is usually normal. The hygroma commonly transilluminates. Usually located beneath the platysma, the tumor may penetrate deeply into the neck and perhaps extend into the mediastinum and axilla.

Hygromas compress or stretch surrounding tissues. The cyst walls are usually tense except when collapsed. The majority of the large loculi intercommunicate, and the rupture of one locule can cause a partial collapse of the entire mass at the time of surgery. The fluid content of the hygroma is watery, serous, clear or straw-colored. Occasionally chylous, the fluid does not coagulate and contains cholesterol, leukocytes and phagocytic cells. If hemorrhage occurs or if there is secondary infection, the cyst fluid becomes discolored.

Cystic hygromas manifest tiny sprouts or buds of lymphangiomatous tissue that extend into adjacent tissues, but these are considerably less numerous than with the more solid type of cavernous lymphangioma.[59] The latter has definite invasive tendencies and frequently penetrates underlying muscle and other contiguous structures.

The classic cystic hygroma presents as a honeycomb of multiple dilated lymphatic channels lined by a single layer of flattened endothelium. In the noninfected tumors, there are only small amounts of connective tissue and muscle along with foci of lymphocytes (Fig. 15.7). Mixed hemangiomas and lymphangiomas may occur and are particularly common in the region of the upper neck, pharynx and parotid gland. All three types of lymphangioma are not infrequently found together in the same lesion.

While there is an apparent clinical difference between the cystic hygroma and the cavernous lymphangioma, I have found it difficult to separate the two on microscopic appearance alone. Features of assistance are large, thin-walled cysts in the former and more solid, small to microscopic cysts in the cavernous lymphangioma.

The treatment of cervical hygromas is moderately controversial and somewhat confused by the differences in behavior of the cystic hygroma and its more aggressive counterpart, the cavernous lymphangioma. The definite tendency of the latter

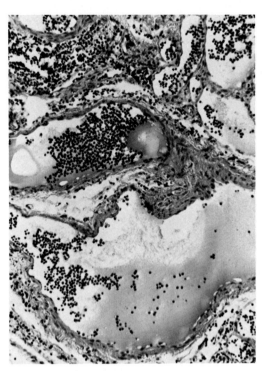

Figure 15.7. Cavernous lymphangioma. Spaces contain lymph and lymphocytes.

to recur following local excision constitutes the most difficult problem in its management.[59] Pott's[60] admonition must always be kept in mind: "The objectives in surgery of cystic hygromas are relief of obstruction upon vital structures and a good cosmetic result. Good judgment must control the extent of the operation. Inadequate operation is just as inexcusable as a daring operation, and nowhere does this maxim apply more forcefully than in the surgical treatment of large cystic hygroma of the neck."

Surgical excision is the mainstay of treatment, but the progress of any one lesion is difficult to forecast.[61, 62] In the early days and weeks of illness, treatment should be directed at relief of respiratory and alimentary obstruction, hemorrhage and infection. Aspiration may be indicated if tension within the hygroma is excessive. High mortality rates are associated with extensive lesions, expecially when emergency treatment is necessary during the early days or weeks of life. The optimum age for surgery is 18 months to 2 years. Watchful waiting until adolescence, aspirations, injection of sclerosing substances and radiotherapy have all been used as definitive treatment, but all except the first should *not* be considered as alternatives to careful and adequate surgical removal, even if a staged excision is required to remove all of the invasive ramifications of the lymphangioma/cystic hygroma.

In most cases, the hygroma does not follow the natural planes of cleavage but insinuates into and around adjacent structures. Dissection should be done with care to avoid leaving islands of tissue to act as foci for recurrence. There is little inclination for cystic hygroma or cavernous lymphangioma to be "shelled out."

Recurrences are possible following incomplete excision and, in general, tumors which extend over several adjacent anatomical regions are more prone to recurrence or persistence than are localized lesions (Figs. 15.8 and 15.9). Lesions with a considerable "lymphangiomatous" component are twice as difficult to eradicate as one consisting primarily of cystic elements.[59] Harkins and Sabiston[59] relate the high incidence of cure and low recurrence rate for cystic hygroma as compared to the cavernous type of lymphangioma. Lymphangiomas of the lips, cheek and tongue, even though small and localized, often require multiple operative procedures. This aggressive quality is most likely due to the insinuation of lymphangiomatous buds into skeletal muscle bundles. If the surgeon is forced to leave lymphangioma in tissue because complete removal would yield considerable cosmetic deformity, viz., lymphangiomas of the cheeks, the patient and his physician must be prepared for recurrent cellulitis and infection due to the poor lymphatic drainage.

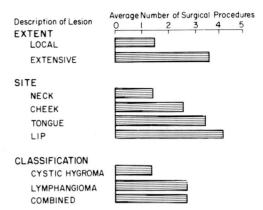

Figure 15.9. Relative recurrence rate of lymphangioma of the head and neck. Modified from Bill and Sumner.[56] Recurrences are dependent upon size, site of involvement and histological classification.

Although there are reports of lymphangiomas of the gastrointestinal tract occurring from the esophagus to rectum, *primary* lymphangiomas of the hypopharynx and upper airway are nearly nonexistent as judged by the literature. This contrasts to the relatively frequent occurrence in the lungs. A form of vallecular or pre-epiglottic cyst is attributed to angiomatous malformation (blood or lymph vessels).

ORAL AND PARORAL LYMPHANGIOMAS

Lymphangiomas of the oral regions are reasonably common lesions and are considered to be hamartomatous or malformations rather than true neoplasms. They are usually found at birth or shortly after. The tongue, cheek, floor of mouth and lips are the principal sites of involvement. Small, single lymphangiomas may occur as pale white or pink, soft fluctuant lesions in any area of the oral mucosa, or they may exist as lesions of the deeper submucosal tissue and present in the mouth as slightly elevated, but generally submerged, rubbery masses. The cavernous type of lymphangioma is by far the most common, and over two-thirds of the lymphangiomas of the tongue are of this type.

Extensive involvement of the tongue may result in notable enlargement of this structure (macroglossia). Giunta et al.[63] prefer to call this lesion "diffuse angiomatosis" of the tongue, not only because of the extent of the lesion, but also because individual lesions may be composed of both lymphatic vessels and blood vessels or each separately. Litzow and Lash[64] have reported a large series of similar cases. A 7% association with cystic hygroma was noted in their patients.

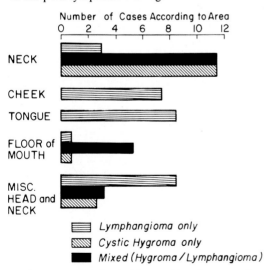

Figure 15.8. Relative incidence of lymphogenous tumors of the head and neck. Modified from Bill and Sumner.[56] Where the tumors are definable as cystic hygroma, lymphangioma and mixed forms, there is a tendency to geographic predilection.

Macrochilia may result from extensive angiomatosis of the lip, and it invariably involves the upper lip. Enlargement of the lower lip is usually the result of inflammatory obstruction of labial mucous ducts. The clinical appearance of the tongue is characterized by multiple small, transparent, clear fluid-filled vesicles. Lingual papillae are markedly increased in size. Most of the lingual tumefaction seems to be localized to the anterior two-thirds of the tongue. If the lingual tumor has been of long duration, a true open-bite malocclusion may occur and cephalometric analysis may show anterior incisal displacement. Lymphangiomas of the tongue run a slow, chronic course. Although there is no spontaneous regression, growth usually ceases at puberty unless infection intervenes. Therapy of the lingual lymphangioma is discussed by Dinerman and Myers.[65]

MALIGNANT VASCULAR TUMORS

Two general classes of malignant vasoformative neoplasms exist: angiosarcoma and hemangiopericytoma. The former, difficult to diagnose, is, nevertheless, easy to define. It is a malignant tumor of the vascular endothelial cell and includes hemangiosarcoma and lymphangiosarcoma. Since the level of differentiation is so poor, division into the two subclasses is not appropriate and, at the most, cumbersome and confusing. Kaposi's sarcoma, a variant of angiosarcoma, because of its multicentricity and unique features is discussed separately (vide infra).

Angiosarcoma. This lesion is extremely rare in the head and neck, especially when contrasted to its benign counterparts. Few institutions have sufficient experience with angiosarcomas of the head and neck to allow significant generalizations. The M. D. Anderson Hospital (Houston) recorded seven cases of angiosarcoma in the head and neck in the time span between 1945 and 1963.[66] In a 39-year period, the Memorial Hospital (New York City) treated 27 malignant vascular tumors of the head and neck.[67] Twenty-one of these were the subject of a recent report. Ten were classified as angiosarcomas and 11 as hemangiopericytomas. From these reports and isolated case reports, the following clinicopathological correlations can be made. The scalp is the predominant site of origin, with 3 of 10 from the Memorial series and 6 of 7 from the M. D. Anderson series arising from this area. The neck, mouth and antrum follow in distant order. The reported examples of malignant vascular tumors of the oral regions (Fig. 15.10) exceeds reported examples in the upper airway by nearly four times.[68] The majority of cases occur during the middle part of life, but patients have been as young as 9 and as old as 74 at the time of diagnosis. Angiosarcomas of the face and scalp

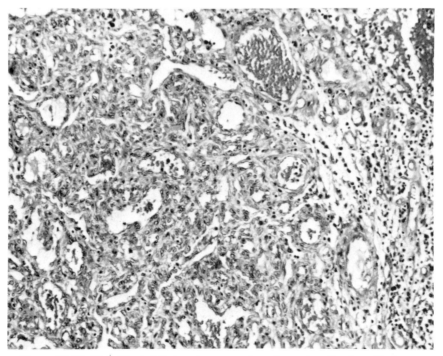

Figure 15.10. Well-differentiated angiosarcoma from the oral cavity of an elderly man.

show a rather marked predilection for elderly patients, a mean age of 60 to 70 years.[69]

In general, angiosarcomas are rapidly growing neoplasms with an insidious onset and minimal symptoms. Only the angiosarcomas of the scalp have had sufficient gross documentation. Here they are painless, soft and usually compressible masses with indistinct margins. They are mottled purple or violet and have ranged in size from 0.5 to 5.0 cm before treatment (Fig. 15.11). At the time of surgical treatment, there is no visible capsule or apparent clear demarcation of tumor from normal tissue. One of the characteristics of angiosarcomas, especially of the scalp, is a deceptive horizontal extension into the dermis. This is often definable only by microscopic examination. Regional cervical lymph node involvement occurs during the course of the disease in 30 to 50% of cases.

The clinical course is a relatively rapid one. The patient is either cured by primary surgical excision (approximately 50%) or he succumbs to the disease within 3 years.[67] Death is associated with regional lymph node and distant metastases or painful and ulcerohemorrhagic local recurrences into fascial planes, bone or cartilage. The survival rate for angiosarcoma of the head and neck is somewhat better than that for angiosarcomas not specifically limited to a specific region of the body.

When feasible, the treatment of choice for angiosarcoma is complete excision controlled by frozen sections for adequacy of margins. Radical neck dissection should be considered only for patients with metastases to cervical lymph nodes or whose primary lesion is under control or is resectable. As with any form of cancer, and especially those in the head and neck, the first therapeutic effort should attempt to be curative. Cure rates decline with secondary or tertiary attempts. Radiotherapy appears quite effective as palliation, but long-term results have not been encouraging. Chemotherapy has been quite ineffective.

Kaposi's Sarcoma. This uncommon disorder, also known as idiopathic multiple hemorrhagic sarcoma, is now considered an unusual, multifocal, neoplastic disease of the vascular system, with a rare tendency for metastasis. There appears to be more than a chance relationship between Kaposi's sarcoma and malignant lymphoma, with both neoplasms occurring in a large number of patients.

Exclusive of the heavy concentration of cases in equatorial Africa, Kaposi's sarcoma is primarily a disease of patients of Mediterranean extraction (Italian, Greek and Jewish). Contrasting with its rarity in temperate zones, Kaposi's sarcoma is a common disease in Africa south of the Sahara. The greatest incidence appears to be in the Congo, where the disease accounts for 9% of all cancers. In South Africa, the incidence of the disease among the Bantus is 10 times greater than among the white population of the same region.

Regardless of geographical differences, Kaposi's sarcoma is predominantly a disease of males (90%), who are usually in their fifth to seventh decades of life (60%). Children presenting with the disease are distinctly uncommon. In 1960 Dutz and Stout[70] culled only 40 childhood cases from the world literature. African dominance is present even in this age group, with 18 of Dutz and Stout's[70] cases being African children.

Olweny et al.[71] have reviewed the clinical features and therapy of childhood Kaposi's sarcoma.

The clinicoanatomical onset of the disease is overwhelmingly cutaneous. Rarely, the initial lesions may present in the oral cavity; usually, however, oral involvement is a part of generalized disease.[72] Visceral lesions, principally within the gastrointestinal tract, occur in over one-half of subjects manifesting Kaposi's sarcoma.[73] Lymphadenopathy and lymphedema are common accompaniments, with the latter occasionally preceding the appearance of cutaneous lesions.

The lesions of the skin classically appear as bluish-red maculae on the lower extremities. Very few patients herald the disease by an initial presentation in the skin of the head and neck. The skin lesions vary in size, up to 9 cm in diameter, and are often elevated, but not especially well

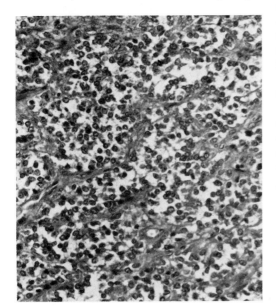

Figure 15.11. Poorly differentiated angiosarcoma of scalp.

defined. Pain and tenderness are not prominent features of the cutaneous forms. On the other hand, the oral lesions are often ulcerated, painful and tender. In both sites, either pyogenic granuloma or malignant melanoma may be simulated.

Lymph node enlargement may be due either to inflammatory reactivity or tumor deposition.[74] In the African child with Kaposi's sarcoma, gross enlargement of lymph nodes may be a striking feature and may antedate the skin manifestations of the disease. These features are distinctly unusual for non-African children and adults. On the other hand Kaposi's sarcoma in non-Africans is associated with an unusually high incidence of lymphoma.[75, 76] Such an impressive association is not found in African cases and may be due to the involvement of a younger age group and a greater number of fatal cases. Kaposi's sarcoma has also been observed in association with various paraproteinemias and immunosuppression in homograft recipients. Because of these relationships, it has been suggested Kaposi's sarcoma is the result of a chronic immunological reaction between antigenically altered or transformed lymphoid cells and normal lymphocytes.

From a histopathological viewpoint, four stages of evolution have been recognized: inflammatory, angiomatous, granulomatous and sarcomatous.[73]

The early lesions may be mistaken for nonspecific inflammation or a granulomatous lesion. Eventually, the histopathological pattern becomes more diagnostic, but, by that time, other lesions have *clinically* indicated the diagnosis. O'Connell[77, 78] has presented masterful histopathological studies of the disease.

Classically, hemorrhage and endothelial proliferation dominate the appearance of the lesion. There is an overgrowth of spindle cells set in characteristic intervening bundles, with poorly formed dilated or cleft-like vascular spaces. Many of these contain erythrocytes and there is considerable hemorrhage into the surrounding stroma (Fig. 15.12).

Mitoses, while present, are not in great numbers. Larger, thin-walled vessels and endothelial-lined spaces are found mainly at the margins of the tumor. There is usually a well-marked inflammatory and plasma cell infiltrate at the periphery of the lesion. There is no histological difference between those lesions associated with an indolent course and those associated with fulminant progression of the disease. Electron microscopy reveals a proliferation of capillaries with or without lumina. Two principal cells are found: poorly differentiated endothelial cells and fibroblast-like cells, possibly derived from pericytes.[79]

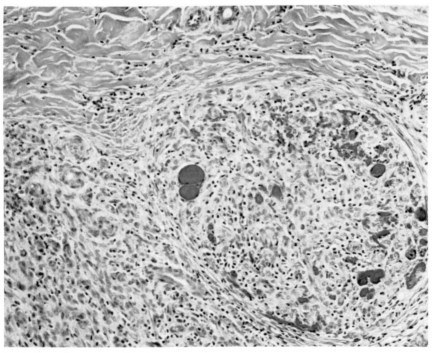

Figure 15.12. Kaposi's sarcoma. Specimen was excised from the tonsillar region in a patient with visceral and cutaneous disease.

Table 15.3, after Abramson and Simons,[80] presents data of *head and neck involvement* by Kaposi's sarcoma. This involvement was associated with simultaneous skin involvement of other regions in 84% of the reported cases. The malignant potential of this vascular neoplasm is considerably less than that of angiosarcoma. Twenty percent of patients manifest neoplastic involvement of lymph nodes, but most of the new lesions are considered as multicentric rather than as metastatic spread from a single, primary site.

Death is usually due to a generalized debilitation, secondary infection, or gastrointestinal hemorrhage from alimentary tract lesions. In patients dying *from* their disease, i.e., hemorrhage, the average duration of life after diagnosis is approximately 30 months. Treatment, because of the multiple and widespread involvement, is primarily by radiotherapy. The early, solitary lesions, without coexistent edema, may be widely excised.

Hemangiopericytoma. In 1942, Stout and Murray[81] separated the neoplasm, hemangiopericytoma, from other types of vascular tumors. They characterized the neoplasm as being composed of capillaries surrounded by an accumulation of spindled or round to oval cells. They further demonstrated, in tissue culture, that the perithelial spindle and round cells came from Zimmermann's pericyte and that the histogenesis of the neoplasms was similar and closely related to that of the glomus tumor.[82]

Since the original description and classification, hemangiopericytoma has had a troubled history. The neoplasm is histologically complex and demonstrates great variability. The anatomical distribution seems as wide as the distribution of capillaries in the body. Even Stout, in later years, confided "the hemangiopericytoma is an exasperating tumor."[83] If there is one common denominator for hemangiopericytomas, it is the lack of uniformity in appearance, growth and biological behavior. Despite these difficulties, some pathologists, either from frustration or a penchant for the unusual, seem to make the diagnosis with surprising facility. In many such instances, the diagnosis is in error.

Hemangiopericytomas may arise wherever capillaries are found. The musculoskeletal system and skin are regions of predilection, with approximately half of the reported cases occurring in these regions. The region of the head and neck accounts for approximately one-quarter of the total number, in both adults and children. In 98 cases involving external tissues, Stout[84] reported that 24 occurred in the head and neck (scalp, face, auricle of ear and neck). Eleven of 31 hemangiopericytomas in childhood were from this anatomical region, and, in fact, the soft tissues of the head and neck are a favorite site of origin in this age group. The orbit and oronasopharyngeal region and sinuses account for approximately 5% of the total number of reported hemangiopericytomas.[85] I am aware of only one authentic case from the larynx.

The age distribution for the neoplasm parallels the wide scope of anatomical distribution, from birth to 92 years.[86] There is a modest peaking of incidence in the middle ages of life. There is no unusual sex distribution. Hemangiopericytomas are seldom painful, and they are usually noticed because of rapid growth of a mass or appearance at a site of previous trauma. The glomus tumor, in contrast, is a painful, *cutaneous* nodule. This close relative of the hemangiopericytoma is *very rare* in the head and neck and face regions.

In the air passages, symptoms produced by a hemangiopericytoma are dependent on the site and size of the tumor and consist primarily of nasal obstruction of epistaxis or both. The period of growth of hemangiopericytomas of the head and neck is usually short before removal.

Partial or complete encapsulation and demarcation characterizes the configuration of the neoplasm when it occurs in the external soft tissues. Usually soft to rubbery, gray-white or translucent, the appearance of the hemangiopericytomas often belies its vascular nature. The lack of discoloration is explained by the compression of capillary lumina by proliferating pericytes. The more aggressive tumors may manifest gross evidence of infiltration and may have a friable, hemorrhagic char-

Table 15.3
Kaposi's Sarcoma of the Head and Neck*

As indicated from the tabulation of cases, mucosal or visceral involvement in the head and neck is almost always associated with coexistent skin lesions that have usually preceded the head and neck presentations.

Site	No. of Cases	Coexistent Cutaneous Lesions on Extremities
Oropharynx	14	14
Larynx	13	13
Skin of head and neck	13	13
Ear	12	8
Nose	8	7
Generalized lymphadenopathy	6	3
Cervical lymph nodes	4	2
Tongue	4	2
Tonsils	2	1

* Modified from Abramson and Simons.[80]

acter. Size at the time of surgical removal ranges from a few millimeters to 10.0 cm. In the upper airway, the neoplasm may present as a moderate-sized polyp, that partially occludes the affected side, or as a large, infiltrative lesion producing complete nasal obstruction.[87] Hypoglycemia and hypertension associated with hemangiopericytoma have been recorded for those neoplasms occurring in the retroperitoneum and pelvis, but not for those in the head and neck.

It may be said, at this juncture, that a prehistological diagnosis of hemangiopericytoma has never been made. The histopathological diagnosis is, at best, difficult and is made either with abandon by the unsuspecting or with extreme reluctance. Since Stout was the most active in the definition of this neoplasm, it is wise to relate to his microscopic descriptions of the lesion. The basic pattern is that of many capillaries, lined by flattened epithelium, lined by an intact reticulin sheath. The pericytes are around the vessels and in the spaces between the capillaries. They are oriented outside the reticulin sheaths but are characteristically enclosed by reticulin. The majority of the tumor cells possess a well-defined nucleus that stands out against a poorly defined cytoplasm (Fig. 15.13 A and B).

This general description, however, does little justice to the great variation and complexity of the hemangiopericytoma. At times, even the basic vascularity of the neoplasm may be hidden, requiring a reticulin stain in order to define the cell-vessel relationships. Some neoplasms may even lack this histological feature, and there is a suggestion that poorly defined or absent reticulin portends malignancy. Stout and Murray[81] have explained the variability of the number and thickness of the connective tissue fiber component in hemangiopericytomas on the basis of fibroblastic activity of the parent mesenchyme.

More contemporary studies have not improved greatly on the microscopic descriptions of the hemangiopericytoma. Notable among these, however, is the study by Enzinger and Smith.[88] These authors emphasized the following: (1) circumscription and pseudoencapsulation of the tumor; (2) a continuously ramifying vascular pattern with large channels extending from the pericapsular tissue into the tumor in a radical fashion and branching into dilated sinusoidal-like spaces or vessels of precapillary and capillary size (the vessels, regardless of size are thin-walled and thick muscular coats are unusual); (3) the reticulum preparations (Wilder or Snook) impart a pattern that is not only variable from tumor to tumor, but within different parts of a given tumor; (4) fibrosis is nearly always present and may be diffuse, localized, or primarily perivascular; (5) osseous and cartilaginous metaplasia may be occasionally noted; (6) necrosis, hemorrhage and thrombosis are seen chiefly in cellular and rapidly growing neoplasms; and (7) peripheral satellitosis and vascular invasion may be seen.

The infantile or congenital hemangiopericytoma is now regarded as a clearly separate variant.[88, 89] In contrast to the adult form of hemangiopericytoma, these tumors are biologically benign, occur in newborns or infants, occur mostly in the subcutis, and are multilobulated. The histology of this lesion is characterized by a collagen matrix, a rather irregular distribution of the vascular pattern, and most significantly, features suggesting a transition between hemangiopericytoma and cellular hemangioma. Despite the presence of an increased mitotic activity and focal necrosis in the tumor the tumor is benign. Paradoxically, in that respect there is often evidence of intra- or perivascular growth outside the main mass of the tumor. In this author's experience, the infantile hemangiopericytoma has a predilection for the neck.

The clinical course which a hemangiopericytoma will follow cannot be foretold from its histological appearance. Barkwinkel and Diddams[86] consider attempts to classify hemangiopericytomas into benign and malignant forms to be futile, with histological criteria of unreliable prognostic value. Mitoses and anaplasia may be only suggestive of malignancy in primary lesions and are usually absent in metastatic hemangiopericytomas.

Here again, Enzinger and Smith[88] have provided some not infallible criteria. Prominent mitoses, necrosis, hemorrhage and increased cellularity often associated with thrombosis may be ominous features usually observed in tumors that later recur or metastasize. Survival is also said to be less favorable for those tumors without a lymphocytic infiltrate, few vascular spaces and little desmoplasia. Malignancy is, however, also associated with tumors manifesting only a few mitotic figures and moderate cellular anaplasia, or moderate numbers of mitoses and slight cellular anaplasia. An improved prognosis is associated with tumors measuring less than 6.5 cm in major dimensions. Recurrence is clearly ominous, not only for metastases, but also for survival.

Electron microscopic studies of tumors arising from pericytes, glomus tumor and hemangiopericytoma, indicate that the parent cell, the pericyte, is a vascular satellite related to vascular smooth

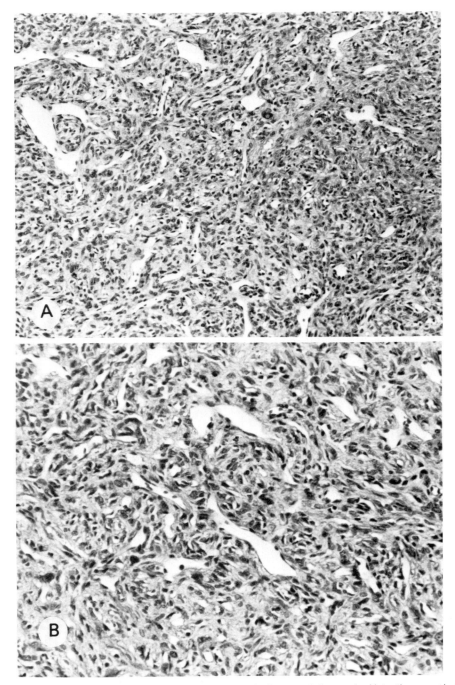

Figures 15.13. *A* and *B*, hemangiopericytoma of the soft tissues of the neck. Note the vascularity and arrangement of cells in a perithelial location.

muscle.[90, 91] The pericyte of the glomus tumor is better differentiated, whereas the large irregular nuclei and little, poorly developed cytoplasm present in the hemangiopericytoma indicate a poor differentiation of these cells. This finding may be used to explain the inherent malignant behavior of the hemangiopericytoma.

A lack of sufficiently long follow-up periods prohibits definite correlation of the clinicopathological features with biological activity of the neoplasm. All in all, hemangiopericytomas must be regarded as unpredictable neoplasms and as malignant, not in the usual 5-year survival sense, but over the lifetime of the host. They are locally aggressive and infiltrative and manifest a high recurrence rate, frequently persisting for years. Barkwinkel and Diddams[86] found a total recurrence rate, local and distant, of 52.2% in 224 cases. Blood-borne metastases have occurred in 20 to 45% of recorded series. Regional lymph node involvement is unusual.

Location of the neoplasm, more than histological features, is important in establishing guidelines to treatment and prognostication. Considering "malignancy" only in terms of metastases, the deep thigh and leg muscles and the retroperitoneum are among the favored sites of "malignant" tumors in adults; the same is probably true for children.[83] A lower grade of this type of "malignancy" appears to be associated with hemangiopericytomas in the upper air passages. Similarly, a small, superficial tumor, particularly in a child or infant, has very little potential for "malignant" behavior. In this respect, there is an increasing malignancy in the preadolescent and adolescent groups to adulthood. A comparison of recurrence rates by organ system, however, indicates that there is little to choose from with respect to this criterion of "malignancy" (Table 15.4).

At the present time, there is confusion concerning the biological activity of *intranasal* hemangiopericytomas. This state is due largely to an AFIP report of 23 cases, designated by the authors as "hemangiopericytoma-like tumors."[92] In that report, it was noted that these tumors most often originate in the paranasal sinuses and secondarily extend into the nasal cavity; appearing clinically as nasal polyps. The patients were primarily in their sixth or seventh decades. No form of aggressive behavior or metastases were observed in any of the 23 patients and 19 of the patients did not even manifest a recurrence regardless of the form of treatment! Such an effete behavior has not been the experience of others dealing with nasal, paranasal and nasopharyngeal hemangiopericytomas.[39, 93] Taken in aggregate, hemangiopericytomas in the head and neck appear to carry as much morbidity for recurrence but less mortality from metastases, when compared to their counterparts elsewhere. In a tabulation of 45 cases of head and neck tumors, 40% recurred locally and 10% metastasized to distant sites.[93]

The treatment of choice is wide surgical excision. While this dictum is appropriate for those neoplasms in the soft somatic tissues, the inherent problems related to the anatomy of the nasal and paranasal cavities often preclude effective removal. The results of high-voltage radiotherapy range from moderate to prolonged palliation and cure to no response at all. Adjunctive radiotherapy, with the limited data at hand, has not appeared to improve the results of surgery, but, at present, this is not a fair assessment.[94]

In an assessment of 224 cases of hemangiopericytomas from diverse sites,[86] a 5-year cure rate of 53.1% was achieved by surgical removal alone, as compared to a 13.3% cure rate for radiation and a 0% rate if cautery was the only method of treatment. These statistics are misleading, however, because recurrences are not considered.

The over-all mortality of hemangiopericytoma is high (50%), but mortality by regional sites shows considerable variation. The importance of more than a 5-year follow-up is highlighted by the fact that despite the high mortality, few deaths occur *during* the first 5 years after treatment. Four of O'Brien and Brasfield's[95] seven patients died from their disease, but the 5-year survival for this group was 100%.

Table 15.4
Recurrence Rates of Hemangiopericytoma*

Location of Neoplasm	No. of Cases	Total No. Recurrent†	Percentage
Musculoskeletal and skin	103	50	50.5
Intra-abdominal and retroperitoneum	39	16	41.0
Lung-mediastinum	22	10	45.3
Orbit, mouth and nasosinus tract	21	12	57.1
Central nervous system	15	12	80.0

* Modified from Barkwinkel and Diddams.[86]

† The percentage of recurrence represents observations over a 5-year period. In many instances, recurrences increased in number as follow-up time increased. For the hemangiopericytoma of the head and neck (orbit, mouth and nasosinus tract) there was a 4.7% recurrence in the first year, a 19% recurrence in 1 to 5 years and a 33% rate at 5 years.

REFERENCES

1. Rappaport, I., and Shiffman, M. A.: The significance of oral angiomas. Oral Surg. 17:263, 1964.
2. Killey, H. C. and Kay, L. W.: Hereditary haemorrhagic telangiectasia. Br. J. Oral Surg. 7:161, 1970.
3. Menefee, M. G., Flessa, H. C., Glueck, H. I. and Hogg, S. P.: Hereditary hemorrhagic telangiectasia (Osler-Weber-Render disease). Arch. Otolaryngol. 101:246, 1975.
4. McCaffrey, T. V., Kern, E. B., and Lake, C. F.: Management of epistaxis in hereditary hemorrhagic telangiectasia. Review of 80 cases. Arch. Otolaryngol. 103:627, 1977.
5. Stell, P. M.: Epistaxis. Clin. Otolaryngol. 2:263, 1977.
6. Bhaskar, S. N.: Oral tumors of infancy and childhood: a survey of 293 cases. J. Pediatr. 63:195, 1963.

7. Girard, C., Graham, J. H., and Johnson, W. C.: Arterio-venous hemangioma (arteriovenous shunt). A clinicopathological and histochemical study. J. Cutaneous Pathol. 1: 73, 1974.

8. Ash, J. E., and Old, J. W.: Hemangiomas of the nasal septum. Trans. Am. Acad. Ophthalmol. Otolaryngol. 54:350, 1950.

9. Kerr, D. A.: Granuloma pyogenicum. Oral Surg. 4:158, 1951.

10. Shklar, G., and Meyer, I.: Vascular tumors of the mouth and jaws. Oral Surg. 19:335, 1965.

11. Cocke, E. W., Jr.: Cavernous hemangioma of the oral and hypopharynges. Am. J. Surg. 102:798, 1961.

12. Woods, W. R., and Tulumello, T. N.: Management of oral hemangioma. Review of the literature and report of a case. Oral Surg. 44:39, 1977.

13. Hoehn, J. G., Farrow, G. M., Devine, K. D., and Masson, J. K.: Invasive hemangioma of the head and neck. Am. J. Surg. 120:495, 1970.

14. Conley, J. J., and Clairmont, A. A.: Intramuscular hemangioma of the masseter muscle. Plast. Reconstr. Surg. 60: 121, 1977.

15. Allen, P. W., and Enzinger, F. M.: Hemangioma of skeletal muscle. Cancer 29: 8, 1972.

16. Clemis, J. D., Briggs, D. R., and Changus, G. W.: Intramuscular hemangioma in the head and neck. Canad. J. Otolaryngol. 4:339, 1975.

17. Green, B. E., Jr.: Treatment of hemangioma. South. Med. J. 68:383, 1975.

18. Margileth, A. M., and Museles, M.: Cutaneous hemangiomas in children. J. A. M. A. 194:523, 1965.

19. Lampe, I., and Latourette, H. B.: Management of cavernous hemangiomas in infants. Pediatr. Clin. North Am. 6:511, 1959.

20. Martin, L. W.: Angiomas in infants and children. Am. J. Surg. 107:511, 1964.

21. Rappaport, I., and Rappaport, J.: Congenital arteriovenous fistula of the maxillofacial region. Am. J. Surg. 134:39, 1977.

22. Devine, K. D., Beahrs, O. H., Lovestedt, S. A., and Erich, J. B.: Congenital arteriovenous fistulas of the face and neck. Plast. Reconstr. Surg. 23:273, 1959.

23. Rhodes, E. L., Stanley, J. C. and Hoffman, G. L.: Aneurysms of extracranial carotid arteries. Arch Surg. 111:339, 1976.

24. Bergan, J. J., and Hoehn, J. G.: Evanescent cervical pseudoaneurysms. Ann. Surg. 162:213, 1965.

25. Harolds, J. A., and Friedman, M. H.: Venous aneurysms. South. Med. J. 70:220, 1977.

26. LaMonte, S. J., Walker, E. A., and Moran, W. B.: Internal jugular phlebectasia. A clinicoroentgenographic diagnosis. Arch. Otolaryngol. 102:706, 1976.

27. Clearkin, K. P., and Enzinger, F. M.: Intravascular papillary endothelial hyperplasia. Arch. Pathol. Lab. Med. 100:441, 1976.

28. Kuo, T., Sayers, C. P., and Rosai, J.: Masson's "Vegentant intravascular hemangioendothelioma." A lesion often mistaken for angiosarcoma. Cancer 38:1227, 1976.

29. Salyer, W. R., and Salyer, D. C.: Intravascular angiomatosis: development and distinction from angiosarcoma. Cancer 36:995, 1975.

30. Hora, J. F., and Brown, A. K.: Paranasal juvenile angiofibroma. Arch. Otolaryngol. 76:457, 1962.

31. Apostol, J. V., and Frazell, E. L.: Juvenile nasopharyngeal angiofibroma. Cancer 18:869, 1965.

32. Schiff, M.: Juvenile nasopharyngeal angiofibroma. A theory of pathogenesis. Laryngoscope 69:981, 1959.

33. Capps, F. C. W., Irvine, G., and Timmis, P.: Four recent cases of juvenile fibroangioma of the post nasal space. J. Laryngol. Otol. 75:924, 1961.

34. Osborn, D. A., and Sokolovski, A.: Juvenile nasopharyngeal angiofibroma in a female. Arch. Otolaryngol. 82:629, 1965.

35. Svoboda, D. J., and Kirschner, F.: Ultrastructure of nasopharyngeal angiofibroma. Cancer 19:1949, 1966.

36. Fitzpatrick, P. J.: Nasopharyngeal angiofibroma. Canad. J. Surg. 13:228, 1970.

37. Patterson, C. N.: Juvenile nasopharyngeal angiofibroma. Otolaryngol. Clin. N. Am. 6:839, 1973.

38. Girgis, I. H., and Fahmy, S. A.: Nasopharyngeal fibroma: its histopathological nature. J. Laryngol. 87:1107, 1973.

39. Fu, Y.-S., and Perzin, K. H.: Non-epithelial tumors of the nasal cavity, paranasal sinuses, and nasopharynx: a clinicopathologic study. I. General features and vascular tumors. Cancer 33:1275, 1974.

40. Harrison, D. F. N.: Juvenile postnasal angiofibroma—an evaluation. Clin. Otolaryngol. 1:187, 1976.

41. Hubbard, E. M.: Nasopharyngeal angiofibroma. Arch. Pathol. 65:192, 1958.

42. Sessions, R. B., Wills, P. I., Alford, B. R., Harrell, J. E., and Evans, R. A.: Juvenile nasopharyngeal angiofibroma: radiographic aspects. Laryngoscope 86:2, 1976.

43. Den Herder, B. A.: The vascular tree in the juvenile nasopharyngeal angiofibroma. Radiol. Clin. 45:27, 1976.

44. Neel, H. B., Whicker, J. H., Devine, K. D, and Weiland, L. H.: Juvenile angiofibroma—review of 120 cases. Am. J. Surg. 126:547, 1973.

45. McGavran, M. H., Sessions, D. G., Dorfman, R. F., David, D. O., and Ogura, J. H.: Nasopharyngeal angiofibroma. Arch. Otolaryngol. 90:94, 1969.

46. Stiller, D., Ketenkamp, D., and Kuttner, K.: Cellular differentiation and structural characteristics in nasopharyngeal angiofibromas; an electron-microscopic study. Virchows Arch. (Pathol. Anat.) 371:273, 1976.

47. Taxy, J. B.: Juvenile nasopharyngeal angiofibroma: an ultrastructural study. Cancer 39:1044, 1977.

48. Walike, J. W., and MacKay, B.: Nasopharyngeal angiofibroma: light and electron microscopic changes after stilbesterol therapy. Laryngoscope 80:1109, 1970.

49. Batsakis, J. G., Klopp, C. T., and Newman, W.: Fibrosarcoma arising in a "juvenile" nasopharyngeal angiofibroma following extensive radiation therapy. Am. Surg. 21:786, 1955.

50. Hormia, M., and Koskinen, O.: Metastasizing nasopharyngeal angiofibroma: case report. Arch. Otolaryngol. 89:523, 1969.

51. Pressman, J. J.: Nasopharyngeal angiofibroma. Arch. Otolaryngol. 76:167, 1962.

52. Martin, H., Ehrlich, H. E., and Abels, J. C.: Juvenile nasopharyngeal angiofibroma. Ann. Surg. 127:513, 1948.

53. Boles, R., and Dedo, H.: Nasopharyngeal angiofibroma. Laryngoscope 86:364, 1976.

54. Smith, M. F. W., Boles, R., and Work, W. P.: Cryosurgical techniques in removal of angiofibromas. Laryngoscope 74:1071, 1964.

55. Landing, B. H., and Farber, S.: Tumors of the cardiovascular system. In Atlas of Tumor Pathology. Armed Forces Institute of Pathology, Washington, D.C., 1956.

56. Bill, A. H., Jr., and Sumner, D. S.: A unified concept of lymphangioma and cystic hygroma. Surg. Gynecol. Obstet. 120:79, 1965.

57. Wolff, M.: Lymphangiomyoma: clinicopathologic study and ultrastructural confirmation of its histogenesis. Cancer 31:988, 1973.

58. Lynn, H. B.: Cystic hygroma. Surg. Clin. North Am. 43:1157, 1963.

59. Harkins, G. A., and Sabiston, D. C., Jr.: Lymphangioma in infancy and childhood. Surgery 47:811, 1960.

60. Potts, W. J.: The Surgeon and the Child, p. 245. W. B. Saunders Co., Philadelphia, 1959.

61. Stromberg, B. V., Weeks, P. M., and Wray, R. C.: Treatment of cystic hygroma. South. Med. J. 69:1333, 1976.

62. Saijo, M., Munro, I. R., and Mancer, K.: Lymphangioma. A long-term follow-up study. Plast. Reconstr. Surg. 56:642, 1975.

63. Giunta, J., Shklar, G., and McCarthy, P. L.: Diffuse angiomatosis of the tongue. Arch. Otolaryngol. 93:83, 1971.

64. Litzow, T. J., and Lash, H.: Lymphangiomas of the tongue. Mayo Clin. Proc. 36:229, 1961.

65. Dinerman, W. S., and Myers, E. N.: Lymphangiomatous macroglossia. Laryngoscope 86:291, 1976.

66. Bardwil, J. M., Mocega, E. E., Butler, J. J., and Russin, D. J.: Angiosarcoma of the head and neck region. Am. J. Surg. 116:548, 1968.

67. Farr, H. W., Carandang, C. M., and Huvos, A. G.: Malignant vascular tumors of the head and neck. Am. J. Surg. 120: 501, 1970.

68. McClatchey, K. D., Batsakis, J. G., and Rice, D. H.: Angiosarcoma of the maxillary sinus: report of a case. J. Oral Surg. 34:1019, 1976.

69. Rosai, J., Sumner, H. W., and Kostianovsky, M.: Angiosarcoma of the skin. A clinicopathologic and fine structural study. Hum. Pathol. 7:83, 1976.

70. Dutz, W., and Stout, A. P.: Kaposi's sarcoma in infants and children. Cancer 13:684, 1960.

71. Olweny, C. L. M., Kaddumukasa, A., Atine, I., Owor, R., Magrath, I., and Ziegler, J. L.: Childhood Kaposi's sarcoma: clinical features and therapy. Br. J. Cancer 33:555, 1976.

72. Howland, W. J., Armbrecht, E. C., and Miller, J. A.: Oral manifestations of multiple idiopathic hemorrhagic sarcoma of Kaposi: report of two cases. J. Oral Surg. 24:445, 1966.

73. Cox, F. H., and Helwig, E. B.: Kaposi's sarcoma. Cancer 12: 289, 1959.

74. Ramos, C. V., Taylor, H. B., Hernandez, B. A., and Tucker, E. F.: Primary Kaposi's sarcoma of lymph nodes. Am. J. Clin. Pathol. 66:998, 1976.

75. Warner, T. F. C. S., and O'Loughlin, S.: Kaposi's sarcoma: a byproduct of tumour rejection. Lancet 2:687, 1975.

76. Law, I. P.: Kaposi's sarcoma and plasma cell dysplasia. J. A. M. A. 229:1329, 1974.

77. O'Connell, K. M.: Kaposi's sarcoma: histopathological study of 159 cases from Malawi. J. Clin. Pathol. 30:687, 1977.

78. O'Connell, K. M.: Kaposi's sarcoma in lymph nodes: histological study of lesions from 16 cases in Malawi. J. Clin. Pathol. 30:696, 1977.

79. Braun-Falco, O., Schmoeckel, C., and Hubner, G.: Zur Histogenese des Sarcoma isiopathicum multiplex haemorrhagicum (Morbus Kaposi). Virchows Arch. (Pathol. Anat.) 369:215, 1976.

80. Abramson, A. L., and Simmons, R. L.: Kaposi's sarcoma of the head and neck. Arch. Otolaryngol. 92:505, 1970.

81. Stout, A. P., and Murray, M. R.: Hemangiopericytoma: vascular tumor featuring Zimmermann's pericytes. Ann. Surg. 116:26, 1942.

82. Murray, M. R., and Stout, A. P.: The glomus tumor—investigation of its distribution and behavior, and the identify of its "epitheloid" cell. Am. J. Pathol. 18:183, 1942.

83. Kauffman, S. L., and Stout, A. P.: Hemangiopericytoma in children. Cancer 13:695, 1960.

84. Stout, A. P.: Tumors featuring pericytes: glomus tumors and hemangiopericytomas. Lab. Invest. 5:217, 1956.

85. Stenhouse, D., and Mason, D. K.: Oral hemangiopericytoma—a case report. Br. J. Oral Surg. 6:114, 1968.

86. Barkwinkel. K. D., and Diddams, J. A.: Hemangiopericytoma report of a case and comprehensive review of the literature. Cancer 25:896, 1970.

87. Rhodes, R. E., Jr., Brown, H. A., and Harrison, E. G., Jr.: Hemangiopericytoma of nasal cavity: review of literature and report of three cases. Arch. Otolaryngol. 79:505, 1964.

88. Enzinger, F. M., and Smith, B. H.: Hemangiopericytoma. An analysis of 106 cases. Hum. Pathol. 7:61, 1976.

89. Eimoto, T.: Ultrastructure of an infantile hemangiopericytoma. Cancer 40:2161, 1977.

90. Murad, T. M., von Haam, E., and Murthy, M. S. N.: Ultrastructure of a hemangiopericytoma and a glomus tumor. Cancer 22:1239, 1968.

91. Battifora, H.: Hemangiopericytoma: ultrastructural study of five cases. Cancer 31:1418, 1973.

92. Compagno, J., and Hyams, V. J.: Hemangiopericytoma-like intranasal tumors. A clinicopathologic study of 23 cases. Am. J. Clin. Pathol. 66: 672, 1976.

93. Walike, J. W., and Bailey, B. J.: Head and neck hemangiopericytomas. Arch. Otolaryngol. 93:345, 1971.

94. Mira, J. G., Chu, F. C. H., and Fortner, J. G.: The role of radiotherapy in the management of malignant hemangiopericytoma. Report of eleven new cases and review of the literature. Cancer 39:1254, 1977.

95. O'Brien, P., and Brasfield, R. D.: Hemangiopericytoma. Cancer 18:249, 1965.

CHAPTER 16

Tumors of the Peripheral Nervous System

Peripheral nerve tumors may be categorized into those of the sympathetic nervous system and those of nerve sheath origin.[1] The nerve sheath tumors include schwannoma, neurofibroma and neurogenous sarcoma. Discussion of the clinicopathological features of these three lesions forms the major part of this section. A complete classification is presented in Table 16.1.

NOMENCLATURE AND HISTOGENESIS

Prior to Virchow's classical study on tumors (1863 to 1867), the term *neuroma* was applied to all new growths from any nerve. In the course of time, a number of terms have been proposed and used as synonyms or replacements for this non-commital term. These include: perineural fibroma, fibroblastoma, neurofibroma, peripheral glioma, fibroglioma, neurofibroglioma, neurinoma, neurilemmoma, neurolemmoma and schwannoma. Several of these terms are definitely inaccurate, since it has now been established that these neurogenous tumors arise from *sheath* cells, not from nerve cells. But, other problems in terminology persist.[2]

The normal nerve fiber is ensheathed by Schwann cells, but it is also surrounded by the more loosely distributed endoneurial fibroblasts. Masson[3] was among the first to indicate that nerve sheath tumors were likely derived from Schwann cells. Accordingly, he called such tumors schwannomas. Schwannian origin has also been supported by Stout,[4] Murray and Stout,[5] Rio-Hortega[6] and Fisher and Vuzenski.[7]

The chief objection to the Schwann cell theory has been based on the presence of collagen in these tumors. Since collagen was assumed to be produced only by fibroblasts, the presence of collagen in the tumors was considered to prove the presence of fibroblasts, and the tumors were for that reason assumed to arise from fibroblasts. This objection has been successfully countered by experimental (tissue cultures) and electron microscopic studies which show that the Schwann cell can also produce collagen. Similar types of studies have shown that the Schwann cell is the parent cell of both of the clinically recognized tumors—*schwannoma* and *neurofibroma*.[7]

Other studies implicate the perineurial fibroblast. Since the protagonists are the Schwann cell and the perineurial fibroblast, a brief characterization of these cells is indicated.

The Schwann cells are regarded by many neuropathologists as homologous with the oligodendroglia of the central nervous system. In addition, the Schwann cell is generally accepted as being derived from the neural crest and, therefore, of neuroectodermal origin. The perineurial cell forms the inner layer of the perineurial sheath. Like Schwann cells, these cells possess a prominent basement membrane. Micropinocytotic vesicles, found in large numbers in the perineurial cell, are absent in the Schwann cell. The cells are surrounded by fibroblasts of the epineurian and endoneurian, but it is unclear whether they themselves can produce collagen.

Ultrastructural identification of individual cell types in nerve sheath tumors can be difficult. The main characteristic of Schwann cells—their relationship to axons—is mostly lost in peripheral nerve tumors and can usually only be found in the vicinity of nerve bundles entering the tumor. In neurofibromas a variable content of other cells besides Schwann cells are identified.[8] This observation adds credence to the hypothesis that all elements of normal peripheral nerves are involved in the formation of neurofibromas.

Clinical experience combined with repeated histochemical and ultrastructural studies have raised the question of whether the distinction between neurofibroma and schwannoma is a valid one. The proved point of cytogenesis aside, I feel that the two lesions should retain their *clinical* identity. Further, I am of the conviction the lesions are different and not simply different morphological expression of a Schwann cell proliferation, be that hamartomatous or neoplastic.

Table 16.1
Tumors of the Peripheral Nerves

Benign
    A. Neurofibroma
        1. Solitary (neurofibroma)
        2. Multiple (neurofibromatosis, von Recklinghausen's syndrome)
            a. Plexiform neurofibroma
            b. Elephantiasis neuromatosa
            c. Molluscum fibrosum
        3. Storiform neurofibroma
        4. Pacinian neurofibroma
    B. Schwannoma (neurinoma, neurilemmoma, perineural fibroblastoma)
    C. Granular cell "myoblastoma"
    D. Neurogenous nevi
    E. Neuroma (amputation neuroma, traumatic neuroma)

Malignant
    A. Neurogenous sarcoma
    B. Neuroepithelioma
    C. Malignant melanoma
    D. ? Malignant granular cell tumor

Gratifying in that respect is the acceptance of this concept by neuropathologists. Because of the controversy and attendant confusion, they advise a classification based on the histological appearance of the tumors. Table 16.2, modified from Lassmann et al.,[8] presents a review of the nomenclatures applied to benign tumors of the peripheral nerve sheath.

Before going on to the *clinical* differences between neurofibroma and schwannoma, a brief explanation justifying the use of the term *schwannoma* is necessary. Neurinoma, neurilemmoma, neurolemmoma and schwannoma have all been used to describe this nerve sheath tumor. Which is correct? The term neurinoma is improper since it implies origin from nerve fibers rather than from the schwann cells. Before Schwann, the term neurilemma defined a connective tissue sheath which covered the nerve. However, Schwann demonstrated that the covering of the nerve consisted of both the Schwann (sheath) cells and an outer, thin covering membrane. This *outer* membrane had no specific name and was subsequently called the neurilemma. The *inner* sheath was called the sheath of Schwann (or neurolemma). Stout[4] agreed with this interpretation but introduced the term neurilemmoma. This designation implies that the tumor is derived from the entire neurilemma sheath (including the thin membrane) instead of from the sheath of Schwann (or neurolemma) alone, which does not include the thin membrane.

Table 16.2
Evolution of nomenclature of Benign Nerve Sheath Tumors*

Zulch 1962[93]	Haferkamp 1960[94]	Harkin and Reed 1965[95]	Krucke 1974[96]	Russell and Rubenstein 1977[97]	Batsakis 1978
Neurinoma	Neurinoma	Schwannoma	Neurinoma	Schwannoma	Schwannoma (neurilemoma)
	Encapsulated neurofibroma			Neurofibroma	
	Diffuse neurofibroma	Diffuse neurofibroma	Type I (plexiform neurofibroma)		Diffuse neurofibroma
	Plexiform neurofibroma	Plexiform neurofibroma	Type II (diffuse neurofibroma)		Plexiform neurofibroma
			Type III (neurofibroma with tactile corpuscles)		Storiform neurofibroma
					Pacinian neurofibroma
	Argyrophilic neurinoma				
		Myxoma	Myxoma		

* Compiled from the classifications of Zulch,[93] Haferkamp,[94] Harkin and Reed,[95] Krucke[96] and Russell and Rubenstein.[97]

The term neurolemmoma reflects the cell of origin accurately and is an acceptable diagnostic term. However, it is too likely to be confused with neurilemmoma and is best discarded in favor of the term schwannoma.

GENERAL CLINICAL AND PATHOLOGICAL DIFFERENCES BETWEEN SCHWANNOMAS AND NEUROFIBROMAS

The schwannoma is a solitary and encapsulated tumor usually attached to, or surrounded by, a nerve and is almost never associated with von Recklinghausen's disease or malignant change. Neurites do not transverse the tumor, and degenerative changes such as cystic alterations or hemorrhagic necrosis are usually present (Figs. 16.1 and 16.2).

In contrast, neurofibromas are nonencapsulated and usually multiple. They are the prototype tumor of von Recklinghausen's disease, and, in approximately 8% of patients, one of these tumors is said to undergo malignant change.[9] Neurites pass through this tumor, and retrogressive changes are less common.

The schwannoma appears to push axons aside, while the neurofibroma incorporates them, suggesting neurofibromas are a diffuse reactive or hamartomatous process arising in the endoneurium.

Several other clinical and light microscopic features have also been used to separate (in the nosological sense) neurofibromas and schwannomas. Clinically, they usually demonstrate differences in distribution, prognosis and symptomatology. Schwannomas are predominantly centrifugally distributed, whereas neurofibromas are primarily centripetally located. The malignant potential of the schwannoma is considered slight and indeed questionable, whereas a variable percentage of neurofibromas undergo malignant change. Neurofibromas are characteristically asymptomatic, whereas schwannomas are often painful and tender.

The pain associated with schwannomas is characteristic and may be used to help distinguish it from other painful tumors of the skin. In the majority of instances, the pain remains localized to the tumor, but, on occasion, a characteristic sharp radicular pain and/or paresthesia occurs distal to the tumor. The pain may often be provoked by pressure.

With light microscopy, the differentiation of schwannoma and neurofibroma usually presents no difficulty. The schwannoma is an encapsulated

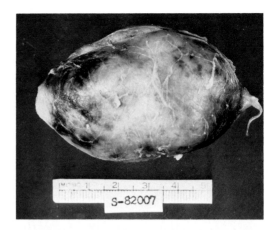

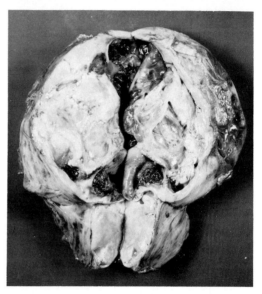

Figures 16.1 and 16.2. Schwannomas from the lateral neck. Note the apparent encapsulation and portion of nerve at one pole of the tumor. The sectioned schwannoma manifests advanced cystic degeneration.

tumor with a distinctive pattern formed by well developed cylindrical structures (Antoni type A tissue) which on cross-section produce a palisading pattern of nuclei about a central mass of cytoplasm (Verocay body) (Fig. 16.3). These structures are embedded in a loose-textured stroma in which the fibers and cells from no distinctive pattern (Antoni type B tissue). Retrogressive changes, including necrosis, cystic degeneration, lipidization and angiomatous clusters of blood vessels with focal thrombosis, are prominent and do not bear relation to the size or location of the tumor. The Antoni B pattern is commonly intermixed with the Antoni A, but an entire tumor may have this arrangement. In this histological variant of

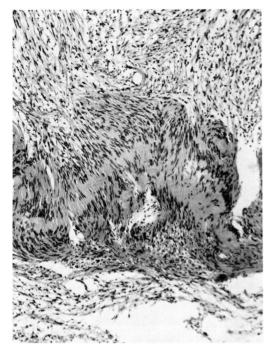

Figure 16.3. Schwannoma. Antoni A and B tissue in juxtaposition.

schwannoma, the important diagnostic features are the congeries of dilated blood vessels with thickened hyaline walls, perivascular hyaline deposits and fibrinous mural thrombi. Areas of recent and old hemorrhage are also common.

Most cells are usually present in relatively high concentration in neurofibromas.[10] They are found in smaller numbers in schwannomas and then only in Antoni B tissue.

Occasionally nonencapsulated schwannomas occur in both visceral and peripheral locations. Also, well developed Verocay bodies, typical of schwannomas, may be encountered in lesions otherwise consistent with neurofibromas. This occurrence and the presence of schwannomas in patients with classic neurofibromatosis should not be disconcerting, since the progenitor cell is the Schwann cell for both lesions.

Abell et al.[1] point out that the variety of secondary changes, so commonly seen in schwannomas, is responsible for certain descriptive adjectives accompanying the diagnosis of schwannoma. *Cystic* schwannomas manifest spaces filled with serous fluid or with a proteinaceous material rich in histiocytes. The so-called *ancient* schwannoma is one in which there has been extensive hyalinization with or without lime-salt impregnation.[11] *Pleomorphic* schwannomas are characterized by foci of large hyperchromatic mono- and multinu-

cleated Schwann cells. It is important to recognize that these cellular changes are the result of retrogressive changes and not to be misled into a diagnosis of neurogenous sarcoma arising from a schwannoma. The retrogressive changes are the result of the peculiar vascularity of the schwannoma and its tendency for intravascular thrombosis.

Neurofibromas may occur as part of the syndrome of neurofibromatosis, as solitary neurofibromas or, very rarely, as multiple neurofibromas without von Recklinghausen's disease. The first association is by far the most common. Histologically they are not encapsulated and manifest a spindle cell pattern of growth. They lack the many retrogressive foci seen in the schwannoma, and the cells commonly manifest a serpentine nucleus. Vascular proliferation and associated vascular changes are also not commonly seen.

The streams and twists of the elongated and spindled Schwann cells with variable numbers of axons and fibroblasts that make up the tumors are generally more compactly arranged in the solitary neurofibroma as compared to those associated with neurofibromatosis (Fig. 16.4). Depending on the size, depth and numbers of the neurofibromas, clinical presentation may occur in a variety of ways:

1. Cutaneous and Subcutaneous Neurofibromas. These neurofibromas are unencapsulated but often circumscribed tumors that arise at or near

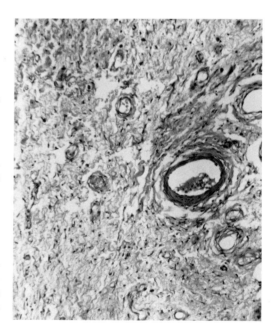

Figure 16.4. Neurofibroma removed from subcutaneous tissue in a patient with multiple tumors.

the terminations of small cutaneous nerves. They are soft, raised, nodular or pedunculated lesions with an increase in melanin in the overlying epidermis. Microscopically, these lesions are composed of proliferating Schwann cells, nerve fibers and fibroblasts.

2. Plexiform Neurofibromas. These lesions are usually deeply seated and involve major nerve trunks. They consist of nerve sheath cells and nerve fibers, initially within the epineurium of large nerves resulting in fusiform swellings, tortuosities, and irregular nodular enlargements which extend peripherally and proximally along the nerves. Their configurations account for the descriptive phrases, "beads of pearl," "worm-like" and "peas in a pod" (Fig. 16.5).

3. Elephantiasis Neuromatosa. The region affected by this diffuse proliferation of Schwann cells and accompanying axons shows a thickened, loose, redundant and often hyperpigmented skin overlying the neuromatous lesions. When an extremity is involved, there may be an associated hypertrophy of bones and an increased local vascularity resulting in gigantism.

4. Molluscum Fibrosum. This lesion is a dermal proliferation of small nerve fibers and sheath cells that characteristically surround yet do not displace the skin appendages. Grossly the tumors present as soft plaques and nodules of varying size.

Although these various lesions are all considered to be characteristic of neurofibromatosis, a number of other neurogenous tumors, including ganglioneuroma, schwannoma, gliomas, meningiomas, paragangliomas and neuronevi, occur much more frequently in patients with neurofibromatosis than in the normal population. In addition, the occasional finding of ganglion cells or ganglioneuromatous elements in neurofibromatous material from patients with neurofibromatosis has led some authors to theorize that the lesions of neurofibromatosis, in some instances, are derived from a disseminated neuroblastoma or aberrantly migrating neural crest cells, particularly so in the syndrome of congenital neuroblastomas with multiple regressing skin and visceral metastases.[12]

5. Multiple Neurofibromatosis. This hamartomatous disorder is also known as von Recklinghausen's disease. An autosomal dominant trait with variable penetrance and a very high rate of mutation, neurofibromatosis has a frequency of one case per 2,500 or 3,300 births.[13] Spontaneous mutation is said to explain why positive family histories are obtained in only 50% of cases. Some affected relatives may show only cutaneous pigmentation.

Nearly 50% of patients manifest physical signs of the disease at birth, and nearly two-thirds do so by 1 year of age.[13] Cafe-au-lait spots or tumors are the most common initial findings. In childhood they occur separately much more often than together. Pedunculated skin tumors and acoustic "neuromas," which are relatively common in adults, are not seen with any frequency in childhood. In the child, subcutaneous sessile or deeper plexiform masses predominate.

Pigmentation of the skin in the form of cafe-au-lait spots or patches may be evident at birth or develop during the first and second decades. It presents most often on the trunk and may vary from a faint light brown to quite dark pigmentation. However, it is not always present in von Recklinghausen's disease, and its incidence is quoted in figures as widely separated as 25 to 90%.[14] Vitiligo is a further anomaly of pigmentation which is not infrequently encountered in addition to cafe-au-lait spots.

The disease is often associated with other neurological abnormalities or developmental defects such as gliomas, meningiomas, acoustic "neuromas" and spina bifida. Syndactyly and hemangiomas also occur, and retinal or visceral manifestations of the disease are sometimes present. The neuropolyendocrine syndrome of mucosal neuromas, pheochromocytoma and medullary thyroid carcinoma is an interesting association recently discovered.[15] The extent to which various organ systems are involved determines other modes of clinical presentation.

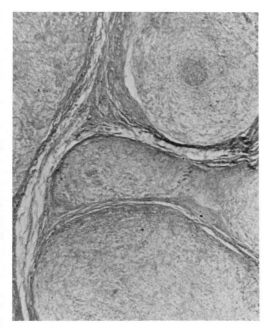

Figure 16.5. Plexiform neurofibroma.

The osseous manifestations of neurofibromatosis are well recognized. Heard[16, 17] considers that bony changes should be included as a feature upon which a diagnosis of the disease is dependent, as probably one-third of patients with neurofibromatosis have abnormalities of bone. The lesions of bone have been tabulated by Hunt and Pugh[18] and include spinal deformities, bowing of the lower limbs, erosive defects of bone due to contiguous tumors and various disorders of bone growth.

In the majority of patients, multiple neurofibromatosis runs a benign course, the tumors often increasing slowly in size and number, especially at puberty. There is, however, a definite mortality associated with the disease, which may occur as a result of the associated abnormalities or of the supervention of malignancy. Sarcomatous changes in neurofibromas or concomitant neurogenic sarcoma has been said to occur from 5.5[19] to 16%[20] of patients. It is in the deep lesions that sarcomas are most liable to occur, and the peak age incidence in Heard's series was between 20 and 30 years.[16] The prognosis is poor; of Heard's 14 patients there were only five alive after 5 years and only 2 of these were free from recurrence.

NEUROGENOUS SARCOMAS

The majority of malignant neoplasms of the peripheral nerves are probably of Schwann cell origin. The possibility that some may arise from perineural fibroblasts cannot be excluded.[1] Neuroepitheliomas are very rare and are presumed to take origin from neuroepithelium since they often reproduce growth patterns suggestive of the developing neural crest. For the peripheral nerve malignancies, I prefer the designation neurogenous sarcoma for use in surgical diagnosis. Synonyms are malignant neurilemmoma, malignant schwannoma or neurofibrosarcoma.

There has been a rather uniform failure by authors to establish criteria by which the diagnosis of primary neurogenous sarcoma can be established without gross evidence of origin in a nerve and microscopic evidence of epineural invasion. It is important to emphasize that the *only* feature distinguishing a neurogenous sarcoma from a fibrosarcoma is its origin from a nerve trunk (Fig. 16.6).

A strict dependence on the nature and the degree of involvement of nerve is very necessary, since extraneural, soft tissue sarcomas may completely surround a nerve, may infiltrate the epineurium and, on rare occasions, may actually invade the nerve longitudinally for some short dis-

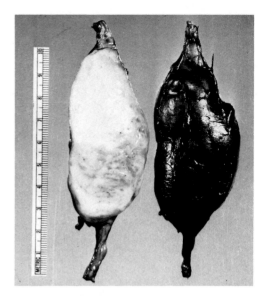

Figure 16.6. Neurogenous sarcoma in an intimate association with a nerve from the neck. Note the white sarcomatous area in the mass.

tances.[21] Stout[22] has written that it is unwise to classify a tumor as neurogenous sarcoma solely by its histological pattern; he preferred reasonable gross evidence of an origin from a nerve to substantiate such a diagnosis. Only when a circumscribed swelling has nerve fibers spread out over its surface or intertwined with its mass and is apparently developing as an expansile mass within a nerve can one be reasonably sure of its neural origin.[7]

The majority of authors have been unable to demonstrate any relationship between the benign and encapsulated schwannoma and neurogenous sarcoma. None of the 24 tumors studied by D'Agostino et al.[21] revealed any trace of a pattern reminiscent of a benign schwannoma. Encapsulated tumors arising in nerves and exhibiting a recognizable pattern of Antoni types A and B tissues behave in a benign clinical fashion, despite the occasional mitotic figure and borderline pleomorphism of cells related to obvious areas of degeneration. Atypical foci, where the cells of a schwannoma possess large, deeply staining nuclei, should not be used as evidence of "malignification" of a schwannoma.

On the other hand, the long observed association of multiple neurofibromatosis and sarcoma has resulted in the acceptance of a causal relationship between these two entities. The incidence of sarcoma of nerve and of the somatic tissue arising in association with multiple neurofibromatosis has never been firmly established. Stout[22] offered an "enlightened guess" of 5%, while Preston et al.[20] reported an incidence of 16.4% (10 examples of concomitant sarcomas in 61 male patients with neurofibromatosis).

A thorough microscopic examination of a neurofibroma is mandatory, as focal malignancy may be overlooked. Recurrences, rapid growth, necrosis, focal hypercellularity or mitotic activity in a neurofibroma should always alert the pathologist to an early malignant change and should occasion a wide excision of the tumor (Fig. 16.7). Sarcomatous transformation is more likely to occur in deeply situated neurofibromas and is more often observed in male patients. Malignancy is suggested by a sudden increase in growth of a neurofibroma or by a more luxuriant cellular composition of a recurrent lesion. Although in some instances neurofibromatous lesions appear malignant *ab initio*, it is more usual for many recurrences to take place before metastases occur. There is little evidence to support the thesis that surgical intervention in cases of neurofibromatosis predisposes the patient to sarcoma.

The sarcomas cause few symptoms other than those attributed to an expanding mass. Pain and paresthesias may occur when a large nerve is involved. The majority of neurogenous sarcomas are firm and lobulated and roughly circumscribed. Others manifest a softness brought about by necrosis, hemorrhage and cystic degeneration. Neurogenous sarcomas exhibit various patterns of small or plump spindled cells with varying degrees of pleomorphism. A cellular arrangement in streams or cords with tandem nuclei is a common finding. A suggestion of palisading or organoid foci may be present in some lesions. Neurofibromatous nerve bundles and neuraxons are sometimes identifiable in the smaller malignant tumors but are seldom seem in the larger variants. The degree of collagenization is variable, but most of the malignant tumors of the peripheral nerves are richly cellular, at least in some areas, and mitoses are usually conspicuous (Fig. 16.8).

The neoplastic spindle cells may manifest a rather remarkable uniformity, but more often there are pleomorphic foci and even giant cell forms. The cellular pleomorphism may at times become extreme. The use of stains to demonstrate so-called "straight wire" reticulin fibers parallel to the axes of the cells has been proposed to aid in distinguishing a fibrosarcoma from neurogenous sarcoma.[22] I have not found this a reliable index. The feature of palisading is also not very helpful

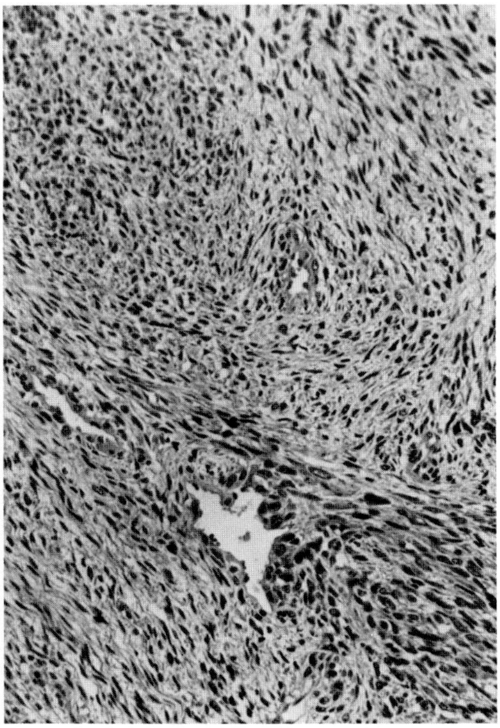

Figure 16.7. Neurogenous sarcoma arising in a neurofibroma from a patient with neurofibromatosis.

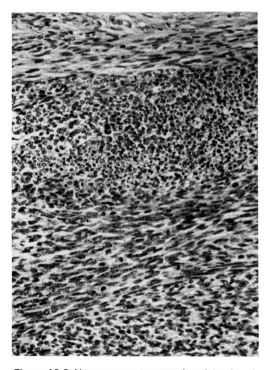

Figure 16.8. Neurogenous sarcoma from lateral neck.

in determining a neurogenous origin for a supporting tissue neoplasm, unrelated to nerves. The confusion between benign and malignant smooth muscle neoplasms and tumors originating from nerves in the intestinal tract attests to this fact.

The recurrence rates for neurogenous sarcomas are high (12 of 19 cases in the Mayo Clinic Series)[21] after enucleation, simple excision of nerve and tumor or even radical excision. The neoplasms are difficult to control and are prone to grow along the involved nerve, making complete surgical removal difficult to accomplish. Radical local excision should be reserved for those lesions not amenable to amputation. The admonition of the Mayo group is appropriate: "The occasional experience of curing a patient by lesser procedures than amputation or radical local excision, while very gratifying, should not lull one into a false sense of security and becloud good surgical judgement."[21] Metastases occur through blood vessels, and survival rates are poor.[21, 23, 24]

In addition to the neurogenous sarcomas that complicate multiple neurofibromatosis, there are a host of other malignant neoplasms. These include gliomas of the optic nerves, astrocytomas of the brain, gliomas of the spinal cord, pheochromocytomas and other endocrine tumors and a variety of soft tissue sarcomas (rhabdomyosarcomas, liposarcomas, etc.). The finding of the latter neoplasms does not exclude the outside possibility of Schwann cell origin, since a wide spectrum of metaplasia (fat, bone, cartilage, striated muscle) has been attributed to the Schwann cell. The pluripotential differentiation by the schwannian elements in peripheral nerve tumors is usually seen in the lesions from patients with von Recklinghausen's disease and is ominous for the host. Rhabdomyosarcomatous, glandular and malignant spindle cell and epithelioid differentiation in these tumors indicate them to be highly malignant.[25-28]

PERIPHERAL NERVE TUMORS OF THE HEAD AND NECK

The majority of tumors of neurogenous origin occurring in the head and neck are benign. Although a multiplicity of major and minor nerves pass through or are distributed within the deep tissues above the region of the level of the clavicles and below the cranial cavity and could provide ample sources of neurogenous neoplasms, the actual number of reported cases is not high.[29] They are of sufficient number, however, that at least one neurogenous tumor in the neck has been reported annually since the Ear, Nose and Throat edition

of *Excerpta Medica* was first published in 1948 From the point of view of number of times volved, the lateral neck is the site of preferen

About 25% of all reported schwannomas found in the head and neck region.[29] They occ in the face and scalp, intracranial cavity, orb nasal and oral cavities, parapharyngeal spa middle ear and mastoid, larynx and medial a lateral regions of the neck.

Neck. Schwannomas arising in the neck may divided into medial and lateral groups.[31, 32] T medial group arises from the last four cran nerves and the cervical sympathetic chain; t lateral group arises from the cervical neck tru cervical plexus and the brachial plexus. A schwa noma arising from or involving the cranial ner trunks may extend through the spinal foram into the spinal canal, where it forms a dumbb type of tumor. The intraspinal portion may diagnosed by pressure signs on the cord and enlargement of the spinal foramen. A similar gr configuration of the tumor has also been report for the tumors of the trigeminal nerve. Neuro nous tumors of the medial cervical group are interest because of their locations in the upp deep spaces of the neck. Here they may arise fr the vagus, hypoglossal, accessory, glossoph ryngeal or the cervical sympathetic nerves. The tumors have been reported as parapharyng "neurilemmomas."

The frequency with which the tumors associat with neurofibromatosis (von Recklinghausen syndrome) involve the head and neck cannot ascertained with certainty, since reported ser describing these cases are biased because the i volvement of the skin and subcutaneous tissues the face and neck is the most conspicuous defor ity presenting in these patients. The Mayo Cli experience is illustrative.[33] Between 1945 and 19 inclusively, 328 patients with diffuse neurofib matosis were examined at that institution. For seven patients had neurofibromatous tumors moved from their head and neck areas. Most of the lesions were small and sessile or pedunculat (fibroma molluscum) and were removed for eit cosmetic reasons or because they were painful.

One-fourth of the patient series reported Oberman and Sullenger[34] manifested stigmata von Recklinghausen's syndrome. This relativ low incidence certainly does not accurately refl the state of clinical practice, and it must be reme bered that *solitary* neurofibromas in the head a neck, or elsewhere, are less common. A solita benign, peripheral nerve tumor (especially neu fibroma) is relatively unusual. Before being sat fied with this diagnosis or with the diagnosis of malignancy in a solitary neurogenous neoplasm, the patient should be thoroughly investigated for stigmata of von Recklinghausen's syndrome, meager though they may be.

Das Gupta et al.[35] have reported a study of 303 patients with solitary, benign neurofibromas-schwannomas at various sites of the body. The anatomical distribution of the lesions in their study is presented in Table 16.3. Of great interest to the head and neck surgeon is the fact that 44.8% (136 cases) of these tumors were located in the region of the head and neck.

In the head and neck, the benign solitary neurogenous tumors are most often found in the lateral part of the neck, where they always pose a clinical diagnostic problem. They present initially as a visible and palpable mass. The association of pain along a peripheral nerve with the presence of a slowly growing submucous or subcutaneous tumor is suggestive of a schwannoma.

The size of the solitary tumor is quite variable and may range from a few millimeters to over 20 cm in diameter. Small tumors are usually white, fusiform, firm and circumscribed. The larger tumors are irregularly lobulated and grayish or yellowish-white, and they manifest retrogressive changes.

There may be considerable difficulty in distinguishing these tumors from the variety of tumors arising in the lateral part of the neck. This is especially true, since, in the majority of patients, the nerve of origin is often not demonstrable. The plexiform neurofibroma, with its characteristic "bag of worms" sensation to palpation usually presents no problem in diagnosis.[36] During exploration of the mass, a nerve trunk or branch may enter or its sheath may envelop the mass.

Neurogenous tumors in the lateral neck do not characteristically produce neurological signs or symptoms. When the site of origin is a sensory nerve, usually from the branches of the cervical plexus, excision results in little or no deficit. Brach-

ial plexus, cervical sympathetic or cranial nerve involvement is more serious.

Kragh et al.,[37] in discussing 77 cases of neurogenous tumors arising in the lateral cervical region, could identify the nerve of origin in 22 instances. Five tumors were from the vagus nerve, and seven arose from the sympathetic chain. Neurogenous tumors of the vagus nerve in the neck are unusual. Primary neurogenous tumors of the facial nerve are also rare and, in both instances, are primarily schwannomas. Schwannomas developing on cranial nerves containing only motor nerve fibers are extremely rare.

The clinical presentation is a mass and/or associated complications because of the tumor. In the nose or nasal cavity, the tumor produces difficult breathing, in the pharynx, difficulty in swallowing and in the larynx, hoarseness.

The majority of neurogenous tumors in the head and neck can safely and adequately be removed.[38, 39] On occasion, the lesions may be large enough to require sequential excision. A pharyngotomy or laryngofissure may be necessary for those in the pharynx or larynx. After excision of a solitary neurofibroma or schwannoma, the prognosis is excellent. In some incomplete excisions, the lesions may "recur," but the growth rate is usually very slow and most of the tumors can be excised. Cutler and Gross[40] and Das Gupta et al.[35] are in complete agreement that the benign forms of peripheral nerve tumors can easily be separated from their nerve trunks which can and must be left intact. A nerve graft should be employed when an important nerve is involved with a benign tumor which cannot be enucleated.

An additional finding by Das Gupta et al.[35] has not had sufficient exposure. In their previously mentioned study of 303 patients with solitary, extracranial schwannomas, they reported 49, or 16% also had an unrelated malignant tumor. This association should make the thorough examination of all patients with solitary schwannoma a requirement.[41]

Malignant nerve sheath tumors in the head and neck are rare. Anatomically, in order of descending frequency, the sites of preference for neurogenous sarcomas are: the lower extremity, upper extremity, chest wall, abdominal wall, head and neck, buttocks, axilla, groin and scalp. The nerves most frequently involved are the femoral, sciatic, ulnar, median, radial, brachial plexus, anterior cervical, popliteal, lumbosacral plexus, cervical sympathetic, fifth cranial nerve and the scapular region nerves.

The relation of benign neurofibromas and

Table 16.3
Location of Solitary (Benign) Perineural Nerve Tumors (Neurofibroma / Schwannoma)*

Site	No. of Cases
Head and neck	136
Upper extremity	58
Trunk	26
Lower extremity	41
Miscellaneous	42

* From data presented by Das Gupta et al.[35]

schwannomas to neurogenous sarcomas has already been presented. In Das Gupta's[35] series of *solitary* lesions, only one patient developed a sarcoma at the site of a previously excised benign neurofibroma. He also records a single possible case arising in a schwannoma.[35]

Facial Nerve. Tumors may affect the facial nerve in its intracranial, intratemporal or extratemporal course. In its intracranial part, the nerve is usually affected by tumors of the surrounding structures, i.e., acoustic neuromas or cholesteatomas of the temporal bone. In the intratemporal part, tumors may originate from the facial nerve proper, or the nerve may be involved by neoplasms in the surrounding structures, i.e., carcinomas or glomus jugulare tumors. Primary neurogenous tumors of the nerve may also present in the extratemporal course of the nerve, but most of the neoplastic involvements of the facial nerve occur after the nerve exits from the stylomastoid foramen. In this location, it is susceptible to secondary involvement from the surrounding structures, mainly lymph nodes at the angle of the jaw and tumors of the parotid gland.

In comparison to secondary involvement of the facial nerve by neoplastic processes, the frequency of primary neurogenic neoplasms is very low. The majority are schwannomas. The clinical presentation and symptoms of a schwannoma of the facial nerve differ according to its location. The main symptom is the occurrence of a progressive, peripheral facial palsy over a period of months. Associated findings and symptoms assist in localizing the site of the tumor.[42] A sensory neural hearing loss secondary to auditory nerve pressure occurs if the origin of the tumor is in the internal auditory canal. This *follows* the onset of the facial palsy. If the point of origin is located in the middle ear, at the height of the horizontal part of the facial canal, auditory symptoms (conductive hearing loss) secondary to involvement of the ossicles *precede* a progressive peripheral facial palsy. The mass may be visualized through the ear drum. Origin from the mastoid portion of the nerve leads to a facial palsy, followed by the formation of an aural polyp located in the posterior wall of the external auditory meatus; otorrhea may be present.[43, 44] The ear drum and the middle ear are usually unimpaired. A loss of taste in the anterior two-thirds of the tongue and a decreased salivary flow from the submaxillary gland on the same side of the tumor occur following involvement of the chorda tympani. Intracranial extension of the neoplasms may also produce signs and symptoms of an intracranial lesion and be clinically confusing.

The symptom-complex by which these tumors may be suspected while still confined to the middle ear or the mastoid should permit fairly accurate clinical diagnoses. Diagnosis should be made in the early stages, not only to prevent complications, but also to offer a better chance to restore function of the facial nerve (Fig. 16.9). The only treatment is surgical removal; when possible, a nerve graft should be done. Prognosis for survival with this benign tumor is good, but it is poor regarding the alleviation of the facial palsy.[45, 46]

Schwannoma of the Brachial Plexus. Fortunately, neurogenous tumors of the brachial plexus occur infrequently. A review of the literature (1960 to 1970) has failed to uncover a single reported case.[47]

Oral Cavity. Benign nerve sheath tumors are frequently encountered in oral and perioral locations. This is in accordance with the observation that the head and neck region is the most common site for benign nerve sheath neoplasms. A partial listing of sites favored by benign nerve sheath tumors in and around the oral cavity shows that the tongue, submandibular region and the mandible are regions of predilection. Malignant nerve sheath tumors (neurogenous sarcomas), on the other hand, are much less frequent. An exhaustive review by DeVore and Waldron[48] uncovered two cases of malignant neurogenous tumors involving the maxilla and seven involving the mandible and/or the inferior alveolar nerve.

The oral manifestations of multiple neurofibromatosis may consist of solitary or multiple nodules arising anywhere in the mouth, a diffuse soft tissue involvement or bone lesions. Pigmentation of the oral mucous membranes seems to be rare, and it is doubtful whether the teeth are affected as part of the disease. It is, however, noteworthy that several apparently solitary intraosseous neurofibromas have appeared near or in the vicinity of congenitally missing permanent teeth.

The incidence of oral involvement is given as 6.5%. Baden et al.,[49] in 1955, presented a complete review and were able to analyze the 42 cases with oral involvement that had been reported at that time. Involvement of the oral mucous membranes can occur at any site; it usually consists of one or two nodules but, occasionally, multiple lesions occur. The tongue is most frequently affected, and a unilateral macroglossia is the characteristic finding (Figs. 16.10 and 16.11). Macroglossia fibromatosa may be associated with infiltration by the tumor into the deep structures of the neck, thereby presenting considerable operative difficulties.[50] A diffuse involvement of the gingiva also occurs and

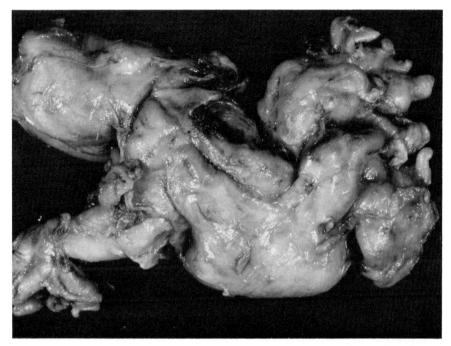

Figure 16.9. Plexiform neurofibroma of the facial nerve in a 60-year-old patient who had sustained six "recurrences" over 8 years.

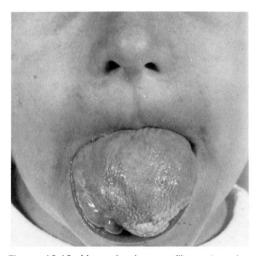

Figure 16.10. Macroglossia neurofibromatosa in a child.

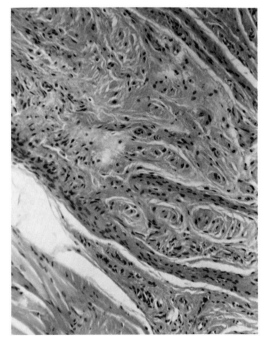

Figure 16.11. Neurofibroma of the tongue manifesting a plexiform and hamartomatous pattern.

may affect greater or smaller areas. After the tongue and the gingiva, the buccal muscosa and floor of the mouth follow next in frequency of soft tissue involvement. The mucosal surface of the lips is only rarely involved. Plexiform neurofibromas are occasionally found infiltrating the floor of the mouth and the buccal mucosa, but they are usually contiguous with an extraoral tumor.

The intraoral nodules of neurofibromatosis do not usually give rise to symptoms. They are, however, subject to chronic irritation and trauma. They may also interfere with mastication, speech, swallowing, etc. Normal oral hygiene is also hampered, and, in the edentulous patient, prosthetic difficulties are encountered. Because diffuse gingival enlargements predispose to periodontal disease, surgical intervention is indicated. Complete removal, if surgically accessible, is indicated in all cases. The neurofibroma is radioresistant; therefore, surgical removal is the only available method of treatment.

The schwannoma is the most frequently encountered peripheral nerve sheath tumor in the oral cavity, but its over-all incidence is, nevertheless, low. One hundred fifty-two cases had been reported by 1977[51]. The lesions may be present at any age, but most have been diagnosed in patients who are in their second or third decades of life.

The tongue is the most common site of involvement, and the mobile portion of the tongue is an area of predilection. The palate, floor of the mouth and buccal mucosa follow in order of involvement. In the majority of patients, the tumors are asymptomatic and solitary. It is not unusual for the tumor to be detected only because of its physical presence. Slow growing, the tumors have ranged from a few millimeters in size to several centimeters at the time of surgical removal.

The oral schwannoma, like its peripheral counterparts, is not a particularly serious tumor. Local excision is usually curative. Uncontestable neurogenous sarcomas arising in the oral soft tissues are very rare. Most of the acceptable examples in the oral regions have been within the jaw bones (intraosseous).

Nasal Cavity and Paranasal Sinuses. Primary nerve sheath tumors arising in the nasal cavity and paranasal sinuses are unusual entities, at least as judged by the reports in the literature.[52-54] That the slightly more than 60 cases recorded in the world literature at this writing do not accurately reflect the true incidence is my personal experience with five neurilemmomas of this region in the past 5 years. The great majority of the reported cases have been those dealing with neurilemmomas. Isolated neurofibromas without an association with von Recklinghausen's disease are rare and neurogenous sarcomas even more unusual. Intranasal nerves, the ophthalmic and maxillary branches of the trigeminal nerve, and branches of the autonomic nervous system give rise to the tumors. The olfactory nerve can be excluded as a possible origin for these tumors, since the olfactory nerve contains no Schwann cells.

Combined nasal-ethmoid involvement is most frequent. This is followed, in order, by maxillary sinus, intranasal, and sphenoid sinus. Nearly all examples have been solitary tumors. It appears that involvement of the ethmoid sinus has never been associated with von Recklinghausen's disease.

These peripheral nerve tumors usually occur in subjects who are between 25 and 55 years of life. Signs and symptoms are dependent on the involved site. Epistaxis is seen with involvement of the nasal fossa and ethmoid sinuses; pain is associated with maxillary sinus tumors. If situated in the nasal fossa, the tumor may clinically mimic an angiofibroma or fibrotic nasal polyp. The similarity to angiofibroma is strengthened by the complication of severe bleeding on biopsy. This is due to the rich vascularization of neurilemmomas. The vascularity, hemorrhagic necrosis and thrombi in the neurilemmoma are also responsible for misleading the pathologist to an erroneous diagnosis of a vascular rather than a neurogenous tumor.

Early diagnosis and complete surgical excision are key to cure. Adequate surgical removal is rarely followed by recurrence in the case of the neurilemmoma.

PHARYNX AND THE PARAPHARYNGEAL SPACE

The parapharyngeal space is an anatomical recess encased by the ascending ramus of the mandible, the parotid gland, the mastoid bone, the vertebral column and the pharyngeal wall. The importance of this region has been well outlined by McIlrath et al.[55]

Tumors of the parapharyngeal space are similar in their clinical manifestations, but range widely in their pathological features. Clinical similarity is due to their occurrence in a confined space, which is surrounded by bone on all sides with the exception of the medial wall, a wall formed by the superior constrictor muscle of the pharynx, and the inferior border beneath the ramus of the mandible. "Escape" from the space is through one or both of these boundaries. As a result, the predominant finding on oral examination is a mass displacing the lateral or posterior wall of the oropharynx. There may be a contiguous mass beneath the angle of the mandible.

The variety of structures within the parapharyngeal space accounts for the different lesions that may involve the area. These include sympathetic and cranial nerves, chemoreceptor tissue, "ectopic" salivary gland tissue, so-called embryonic remnants and lymphoid tissue. Primary neurogenous neoplasms of the parapharyngeal space may arise from any of the last four cranial nerves or m the sympathetic and parasympathetic nerves the area.[56] The primary neural source of the mors has been said to be the vagus nerve or the rvical sympathetic nerves.[57] The cranial nerves, her than the vagus, are rarely affected in the ck.[58]

In the parapharyngeal space, a schwannoma oduces its symptoms by involvement of the surunding structures. A Horner's syndrome freently follows trauma at the time of removal of e tumor, but it may also be produced by pressure the tumor on the postganglionic fibers of the perior cervical ganglia. In common with other hwannomas, the lesions here are slow growers d usually remain small in size, seldom exceeding any centimeters in diameter. In the largest tuors, encroachment on the fauces, choana, esophus and larynx, with displacement of vascular uctures, may be seen.

As a general rule, neurogenous tumors in the rapharyngeal space are solitary and are schwanmas. Multiple forms are infrequent, and invement of the space is not especially associated h neurofibromatosis. Conservative surgical reval is the method of choice. The trend in recent ars is to avoid transoral removal and secure od exposure and identification of structures via external neck excision.[56] Horwich and Hawe[58] licate that the chances of ipsilateral vocal cord ralysis after enucleation is high.

LARYNX

Neurogenic tumors (neurofibroma and schwanma) of the larynx are rare. El-Serafy[59] records at there have been 89 cases reported in the erature. Cummings et al.,[60] after reviewing the cords of the Massachusetts Eye and Ear Infirry (1940 to 1969), found only nine histologically oved cases of neurogenic tumors of the larynx. the 89 cases available in the literature,[59] 14 re associated with von Recklinghausen's dise. The majority of the neurogenous tumors of e larynx are solitary schwannomas.[61]

No age group has been spared, and the sympns are those of any slowly growing lesions. The eat majority of the tumors involving the larynx ginate from either the aryepiglottic fold or from false vocal cords, where they bulge into the praglottic space. Vocal cord paralysis is usually t a feature, but the size of the lesion may intere with movement of the vocal cords. The neugenous tumors are always submucosal and are ually smooth in their configuration. An excepn to the latter characteristic may be the neuro-

fibroma, which is more apt to be multinodular and diffuse.

Biopsy of these lesions is almost always difficult because of their resistance to the biopsy forceps. Nevertheless, biopsy by the endolaryngeal route should be attempted and, if unsuccessful, the lesion should be approached externally (lateral thyrotomy) with complete removal. I know of no example of a neurogenous sarcoma of the larynx.

SALIVARY GLANDS

There have been occasional reports of tumors of Schwann cell origin occurring in the major salivary glands. Undoubtedly some of the case reports of "neurilemmoma" actually represent "basket cell" or myoepithelial cell variants of benign mixed tumors. However, definite instances of plexiform neurofibromas associated with neurofibromatosis have been found in the parotid gland.

INTRAOSSEOUS NERVE SHEATH TUMORS

Traumatic neuromas, neurofibromas and schwannomas may present as central benign tumors of the jaws. Of the three, the schwannoma is the most commonly encountered. With infrequent exceptions, the majority of the intraosseous tumors appear in the mandible, particularly in the body and the ramus.[62-64] All present as radiolucent areas with the solitary neurofibromas and the schwannomas all destroying bone with varying degrees of severity. Schwannomas and neurofibromas expand the cortical plate and many perforate the cortex to produce a soft tissue swelling. Since their growth rate is slow, the tumors may obtain a considerable size, thus producing facial deformities.

The x-ray characteristics of these central osseous tumors are not distinctive. Bone destruction usually occurs distal to the mental foramen. Care must be taken, however, not to misinterpret the normal anatomical enlargement of some portion of the canal as evidence of a pathological condition. Deformities of the mandible and maxilla may also follow pressure from an overlying or adjacent nerve sheath tumor.

A review of the literature to 1970 has revealed only four cases of traumatic neuroma located centrally in the jaws. In the same review, it was found that there had been 18 central schwannomas of the jaws and 11 cases of solitary central neurofibromas.[62] Additional cases and an up-dating of the literature review have been provided by Ellis et al.[65] Neurofibromas that occur centrally, and which are also associated with multiple neurofibromatosis, are infrequent.[66] Bone involvement, when encountered in von Recklinghausen's disease, is usually the result of a subperiosteal neurofibroma that has caused cortical erosion.

No large reported series is available for central, intraosseous neurogenic sarcoma. Eversole et al.[67] reviewed 19 cases of primary neurogenic sarcoma of the oral regions. Seven were peripheral, six both central and peripheral and six arose centrally within the jawbones. The central/peripheral lesions were more common in the mandible, involving the inferior alveolar nerve and mental nerve. Pain and/or anesthesia or paresthesia of the upper lip and jaw is a consistent clinical finding in these cases. Eversole et al.[67] re-emphasize the propensity for neurogenic sarcomas involving the inferior alveolar nerve and mental nerve to proliferate longitudinally. This feature is held responsible for a high rate of recurrence. Occult foci may be present in areas of a nerve far removed from apparent clinical involvement. Therefore, it is recommended that resection of gnathic neurogenic sarcomas be accompanied by neurectomy of what may appear to be grossly normal nerve proximal to the excised tumorous tissue. Middle-aged persons are most often affected, but the neurogenic sarcoma has no age limitations.

The dominance of mandibular involvement in nerve sheath tumors is attributed to the unique anatomy of the mandible. No other bone in the body contains a canal that transmits a neurovascular bundle of such length and size as does the mandible, and this uniqueness accounts for the prevalence of central nerve sheath tumors at this site.

Treatment for the benign tumors is conservative excision. Radical surgical removal is the treatment for the neurogenous sarcomas.

TRAUMATIC NEUROMAS

These lesions represent exaggerated responses to nerve injury and are reactive hyperplasias resulting from abortive attempts at regeneration. Traumatic neuromas are prone to occur in areas of previous surgery and are not confined to either the superficial or deep tissues. Probably the most accurate description of what is normally considered to be a traumatic neuroma has been offered by Huber and Lewis.[68] They give the following description: "A neuroma (traumatic) indicates an attempt, which is thwarted or blocked by scar tissue, on the part of the neuraxes of a divided nerve to seek the distal segment and thus complete

nerve repair. When blocked, the regenerating neuraxes form spirals and end disks and become irregularly dispersed throughout the connective tissue of the bulb. The regenerating neuraxes react on the connective (tissue) elements of the bulb, which, as a consequence, increase in number and maintain their embryonal characteristics longer than is normally the case."[68]

Grossly, traumatic neuromas are generally oval or oblong in shape and are generally gray, white firm or rubbery and circumscribed but not encapsulated. They rarely exceed 2.0 cm in major dimension. On section, there is dense fibrous appearance, little vascularity and a nonuniform disposition of nerve fibers. In some instances, a nerve terminates at the upper pole of the mass; in others, the nerve fibers spread and become incorporated with the fibrous elements of the neuroma. The mass may even be situated several centimeters above the site of injury. The proximal portion of the nerve is usually relaxed. This is due to the elasticity of the nerve and its retraction upon being divided.

Histologically, amputation neuromas consist mainly of tangled and interwoven proliferations of endoneural and perineural connective tissue, neurilemmal cells and regenerating neuraxes (Fig. 16.12). Neurons follow a more or less straight course as they enter the proximal part of the neuroma, but the fibers then interlace and turn back on themselves. A few fibers may penetrate the "connective tissue cap," which forms at the

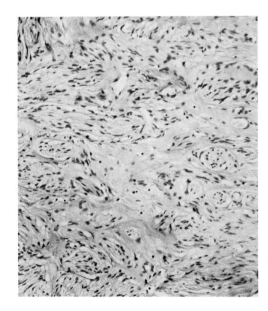

Figure 16.12. Traumatic neuroma.

end of the nerve, and escape into the surrounding tissue. Many end disks and bulbs (growth cones) are seen; these frequently become very large and manifest many branching fibrils. The end disks and fibrils show the regenerative power of the neuraxes. Upon encountering resistance, the fibrils turn back on themselves, forming spirals within the neurilemmal sheath, and curl around the neuraxes from which they have arisen. The amount and density of the resistance determine, to a large extent, the size and shape of the neuroma.[69] With age of the lesion, there is scarring and contraction of the neuroma.

When traumatic neuromas occur in certain locations, they give rise to a variety of symptoms. In oral surgery, the symptoms may arise following injury to the inferior dental nerve, the auriculotemporal nerve, the peripheral branches of the maxillary division of the trigeminal nerve, nerve fibers pressed against bone, inclusion of nerves in the ligation of an artery, and the involvement of nerves in scar tissue. Neuromas have also been known to occur as the result of the removal of teeth. Occasionally, this condition is observed after a Caldwell-Luc operation, in the course of which the infraorbital nerve may be traumatized by retraction of the lip or by an excessive separation of the periosteum in the area surrounding the infraorbital foramen. Severe blows to the head, especially those associated with basilar skull fractures, may injure the Gasserian ganglion and produce a chronic pain syndrome. As a rule, persistent, unpleasant paresthesia in the area surrounding the mental foramen is a "diagnostic" sign of the presence of a traumatic neuroma.[69] Swanson[69] has presented a superb review of the genesis and management of head and neck traumatic neuromas.

NEUROEPITHELIOMA

This neoplasm of the peripheral nerves has been described as "exceedingly rare."[70] There is a rather apparent predilection for the nerves of the brachial plexus, with the neoplasms most often originating from the radial or ulnar nerves or from the plexus itself. Neuroepitheliomas are highly malignant and manifest marked invasive properties. Despite their neuroepithelial derivation, radiosensitivity is not a pronounced feature. The usual course is death after visceral and osseous metastases.

Microscopically, the identification and classification of this lesion with the epithelial-like cells resembling primitive neuroepithelium, as well as the total *absence* of ganglion cells and nerve fibers.[71] Rosettes, pseudorosettes or "clear zones" adjacent to vessels and neurofibrils are not found.

There is either no or minimal stromal reaction to the neoplasm.

GRANULAR CELL TUMOR

This lesion has been surrounded by controversy since 1926 when Abrikosoff[72] considered that it originated from embryonic muscle fibers. Additional confusion, particularly with rhabdomyoma and rhabdomyosarcoma, has been occasioned by the fact that prior to 1955, the term "rhabdomyoma" was used to designate *all* tumors apparently arising from skeletal muscle, whether benign or malignant. The diversity of names used to describe this tumor ("Abrikosoff's tumor," congenital epulis, nonchromaffin paraganglioma, granular cell myoblastoma, granular cell neurofibroma, myoblastic myoma, uniform myoblastoma and embryonal rhabdomyoblastoma) serves to stress the confusion and controversy regarding its nature.

The tumor is now generally recognized as a distinct clinicopathological entity, but, despite the constancy of its histological features, there is no universal agreement as to its nature or histogenesis. Striated muscle, histiocytes, fibroblasts and neural elements have all been considered as possible sources of this tumor. Advocates of a nonneoplastic nature for this tumor consider the probability of inflammatory, degenerative, regenerative or congenital bases as responsible for the development of these tumors.

A myogenic derivation was the earliest proposal and was based on a presumed origin from embryonic muscle and the hypothesis that the granular cells of the tumor and myoblasts were homologous. Histochemical and electron microscopic evidence, however, strongly supports a neurogenic origin (Table 16.4).[73-75] The neural basis of this tumor has been stressed, with the Schwann cell proposed as the source of the "myoblasts."

Evans[76] considers the neurogenic (actually neuroectodermal) theory as a more unifying concept than one based on myogenic sources. A Schwann cell derivation, further, does not detract from the possibility the granular cells may be reactive and/or "histiocytic" and thereby represent a nonneoplastic proliferation to a variety of stimuli.

Very likely no *single* cell type is responsible for all of the forms of granular cell tumors and perhaps various sheath cells with a histiocyte-like potential are the cells of origin. Therefore, granular cell sheath tumor has been proposed as an all encompassing term.[77] In light of the continuing controversy, the World Health Organization (W.H.O.) has proposed the noncommittal name of granular cell tumor. Sobel and Marquet[78] have

Table 16.4
Comparison of Enzyme Reactions—Cells of Granular Cell "Myoblastoma" and Striated Muscle Cells*

Enzyme	Granular Cell "Myoblastoma"	Striated Muscle
Alkaline phosphatase	Negative	Negative
Acid phosphatase	Strongly positive	Negative
Aminopeptidase	Strongly positive	Negative
Cholinesterase (2 substrates)	Equivocal	Moderately positive to strong positive
Succinic dehydrogenase	Equivocal	Strongly positive
Indoxyl acetate esterase	Moderately positive	Negative

reviewed the theories of histogenesis and present light and electron microscopic criteria to distinguish the tumor from other forms of granular cell lesions.

Despite the popularity of the perineural fibroblast theory of genesis, it is difficult to ascribe a neural origin to all granular cell tumors. Thus, the development of granular cell tumors in the cervices of newborn mice after estrogenic stimulation would suggest a myogenic origin in some instances.[78] The growth of a tracheal granular cell tumor during pregnancy has similar pathogenetic implications. Sobel and Marquet's[78] studies indicate the granular cell tumor is derived from an undifferentiated mesenchymal (fibroblast-like) cell.

Regardless of their cell of origin, granular cell tumors present in essentially two clinicopathological forms in the upper aerodigestive tract; those occurring on the gum pads in the newborn and those occurring in later life beneath the mucous membrane of the upper aerodigestive tract. The former, because of unique position and the age of the patients, is considered as a separate diagnostic entity—*congenital epulis*.[79] It is microscopically similar, if not identical to the other forms of granular cell tumor. There is an 8:1 predominance in females and the tumor occurs three times more often on the maxilla than on the mandible, although both sites can be simultaneously involved. In these positions, the congenital epulis is found on the crest of the alveolar ridge in the incisor region.

Objective histological differences between the epulis form of granular cell tumor and the other types are: (1) a relatively high degree of vascularity, not present in other granular cell tumors; (2) a lack of overlying pseudoepitheliomatous hyperplasia; and (3) less differentiated by ultrastructure examination. The lack of pseudoepitheliomatous hyperplasia may be explained on the basis of a more rapid proliferation so that pressure results in a thinning of the overlying epithelium. The granular cell epulis is a benign lesion, does not recur, and has been reported to spontaneously regress.

Table 16.5
Anatomical Distribution: Granular Cell Tumors*

Location	Number	Percent
Subcutaneum	123	32.6
Oral cavity	107	28.1
Tongue	87	23.0
Lip	10	2.6
Buccal	6	1.5
Floor of mouth	2	0.5
Palate	2	0.5
Breast	60	15.9
Larynx	29	7.6
Gastrointestinal tract	16	4.7
Bronchus	13	3.4
Perineum	9	2.4
Hypophysis	9	2.4
Miscellaneous	11	2.9
	377	100.0

* After data collected by Peterson.[79]

The nonepulis form of granular cell tumor is lesion of young adults. The median age of tho presenting in the larynx is 36 years with the ma jority of the tumors occurring in patients betwee the ages of 29 and 42 years. There is a slight fema predominance. Blacks are affected more tha whites.

Since its first description, over 1,200 cases hav been reported in the literature.[79]

Approximately one-third to one-half of all th lesions occur in the tongue and about one-thir present in the skin. The remainder appear in th breast, muscle, larynx, lip, trachea, bronchus, ex ternal auditory canal, mastoid, orbit, common bil duct and neurohypophysis (Table 16.5).

In the upper respiratory system, granular ce tumors occur most frequently in the larynx.[80] Th most common location is the posterior true core but they may occur in the subglottic and supra glottic areas. The bronchus is the next most con mon site in the airway; the trachea is the lea common.[81]

In the aerodigestive tract, the tumors hav ranged in size from 0.3 cm in diameter. They ar sessile or polypoid and only rarely manifest a ulcerated surface. There is no characteristic col and the lesion is usually asymptomatic. In the tongue, the lateral border and tip and dorsum far exceed the posterior third as sites of involvement. In these locations, a flat to slightly raised or button-like configuration is the gross presentation. They also appear rather sharply circumscribed on gross examination. Some tongue lesions may cause slight itching or tickling. The tongue may have as many as three or four discrete lesions. Multiple granular cell tumors may occur simultaneously or progressively and are most often subcutaneous in location.[82]

The majority of granular cell tumors of the upper respiratory tract are intraluminal and are usually solitary. Unlike the congenital epulis, pseudoepitheliomatous hyperplasia of the overlying mucosa is common, ranging from 50 to 65% of the cases. Much has been made of this associated epithelial finding, particularly in reference to the possibility of misdiagnosis as squamous cell carcinoma in shallow biopsies. Compagno et al.[80] found this feature to be a significant diagnostic problem in only 22% of their cases. I know of no example of epithelial malignancy in this mucosal or cutaneous aberration overlying a granular cell tumor.

Microscopic examination discloses a circumscription, but without encapsulation, of the tumor.

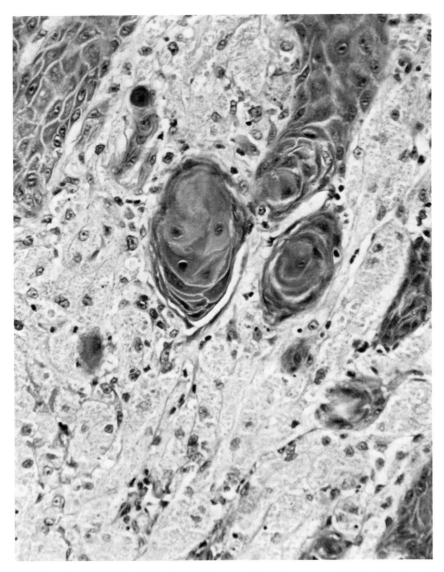

Figure 16.13. Granular cell tumor of the larynx. The granular cells are separated by down-growths of the pseudoepitheliomatous hyperplasia of the surface mucosa.

Tumor cells interdigitate into the adjacent fibrous stroma, striated muscle and surrounding nerves. They are often closely associated with the overlying skin or mucous membrane. In the tongue, striated muscle is almost always intimately associated with the tumor cells. The interposition of cords of cells between strands of striated muscle conveys the appearance of a transition between the granular cells and sarcolemmal syncytium. Nerves may be found in association with the tumors in nearly all cases. A frequent pattern in the lingual granular cell tumors is one in which the tumor cells are concentrically arranged around a myelinated nerve.

The cells of these tumors are distinctive. They are polymorphic, ranging from a definite polyhedral shape to a bizarre spindle form. Characteristically, the cells possess a pale-staining acidophilic and granular cytoplasm. Nuclei are usually small, vesicular or densely chromatic. Mitoses are rare. A central position of the nucleus is the rule and striations are not found (Fig. 16.13). The aggregates of tumor cells are embedded in variable amounts of connective or reticular tissue. Because

of the poor delimitation at the periphery of the lesions, an impression of invasiveness is conveyed to the examiner.

Histochemically, the granular cells of the tumor differ considerably from either normal or degenerating muscle cells. The cytoplasmic granules are periodic acid-Schiff positive (PAS) and also react positively with Sudan black B. The granular cells contain no glycogen. The chemical composition and microscopic appearance of the cells are constant, regardless of the muscular or extramuscular location of the tumor.(Table 16.4).

On occasion, cells with large, strongly PAS-stained acicular bodies (angulate-body cells) may be seen with the light microscope. These cells are usually found in collagenous tissue near fasicles of granular cells. Often they are near vascular channels. The ultrastructural characteristics of forms of granular cell tumors (Fig. 16.14) may be found in the publications by Weiser and Propst,[83] Sobel and Marquet,[78] Chrestian et al.[84] and Garancis et al.[85]

Granular cell tumors, reactive or true neoplasms, are essentially benign processes.[86] In those lesions lacking an apparent circumscription, the

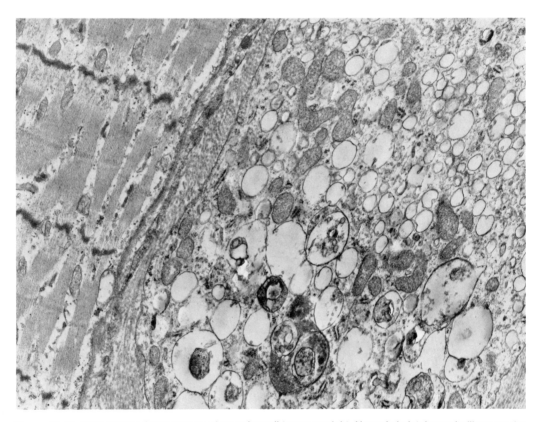

Figure 16.14. Ultrastructural appearance of granular cell tumor on right. Normal skeletal muscle fibers on the left. (Contributed by Joseph A. Regezi, D.D.S.)

microscopic extension cannot be appreciated at the time of surgery and "recurrence" may result. It is also possible that some "recurrences" are actually new primary lesions since approximately 10% of the patients may have multiple lesions in different parts of the body, either synchronously or metachronously.

In that light, I have not been able to accept any of the so-called "malignant granular cell tumors" published in the literature, nor have I seen an example in my practice. Many of the reported lesions are soft-part sarcomas, histiocytomas, or forms of rhabdomyosarcoma. Practically all of these examples have been in the soft tissues or within the smooth muscle of the alimentary or genitourinary tract.[87] All of the laryngeal granular cell tumors have been benign growths. I also question the ability of oral granular cell tumors to undergo malignant transformation. It is true, however, that patients with multiple or multicentric granular cell tumors have a greater tendency to harbor a locally aggressive tumor.

The growth of a granular cell tumor is slow and local excision is the treatment of choice. In the tongue and oral cavity, removal of a wide margin is usually necessary because of the ill-defined borders of many of the lesions. Radiation therapy has proved ineffective since the tumor cells have been demonstrated to be radioresistant.

ACOUSTIC "NEUROMA"

Histologically the acoustic "neuroma" is a schwannoma in the majority of patients. In most, if not all, cases, the tumor arises from the sheath of the vestibular portion of the eighth nerve within the auditory canal.[89] Early clinical diagnosis is essential since the larger the tumor, the fewer are the number of "useful survivors" following surgery and the greater the operative mortality. Recurrences occur after subtotal intracapsular removal (33%) but are unusual if total removal has been effected. Excellent reviews have been presented by Pool et al.,[90] House[91] and Pulec et al.[92]

REFERENCES

1. Abell, M. R., Hart, W. R., and Olson, J. R.: Tumors of the peripheral nervous system. Hum. Pathol. 1:503, 1970.
2. Pineda, A., and Feder, B. H.: Acoustic neuroma: a misnomer. Am. Surg. 33:40, 1967.
3. Masson, N. P.: Experimental and spontaneous schwannomas (peripheral gliomas). Am. J. Pathol. 8:367, 1932.
4. Stout, A. P.: The peripheral manifestations of the specific nerve sheath tumor (neurilemmoma). Am. J. Cancer 24: 751, 1935.
5. Murray, M., and Stout, A. P.: Schwann cell versus fibroblast in origin of specific nerve sheath tumor; observations upon normal nerve sheath and neurilemmomas in vitro. Am. J. Pathol. 16:41, 1940.
6. Rio-Hortega, P. del: Caracteres e interpretacion de las celulas especificas de los neurinomas (schwannomas). Arch. Soc. Argent. Anat. 4:103, 1942.
7. Fisher, E. R., and Vuzevski, V. D.: Cytogenesis of schwannoma (neurilemmoma), neurofibroma, dermatofibroma, and dermatofibrosarcoma, as revealed by electron microscopy. Am. J. Clin. Pathol. 49:141, 1968.
8. Lassmann, H., Jurecka, W., Lassmann, G., Gebhart, W., Matras, H., and Watzek, G.: Different types of benign nerve sheath tumors. Light microscopy, electron microscopy and autoradiography. Virchows Arch. (Pathol. Anat.) 375:197, 1977.
9. Saxen, E.: Tumors of sheaths of peripheral nerves—studies on their structure, histogenesis and symptomatology. Acta Pathol. Microbiol. Scand. 79:1, 1948.
10. Isaccson, P.: Mast cells in benign nerve sheath tumours. J. Pathol. 119:193, 1976.
11. Dahl, I.: Ancient neurilemmoma (schwannoma). Acta Pathol. Microbiol. Scand. (A) 85:812, 1977.
12. Bolande, R. P., and Towler, W. F.: A possible relationship of neuroblastoma to von Recklinghausen's disease. Cancer 26:162, 1970.
13. Fienman, N. L., and Yakovac, W. C.: Neurofibromatosis in childhood. J. Pediatr. 76:339, 1970.
14. O'Driscoll, P. M.: The oral manifestation of multiple neurofibromatosis. Br. J. Oral Surg. 3:22, 1965.
15. Williams, E. D., and Pollack, D. J.: Multiple mucosal neuromata with endocrine tumor: a syndrome allied to von Recklinghausen's disease. J. Pathol. Bacteriol. 91:71, 1966.
16. Heard, G.: Nerve sheath tumours and von Recklinghausen's disease of the nervous system. Ann. R. Coll. Surg. 31:229, 1962.
17. Heard, G.: Malignant disease in von Recklinghausen's neurofibromatosis. Proc. R. Soc. Med. 56:502, 1963.
18. Hunt, J. C., and Pugh, D. G.: Skeletal lesions in neurofibromatoses. Radiology 76:1, 1961.
19. Holt, F. J., and Wright, E. M.: Radiologic features of neurofibromatosis. Radiology 51:647, 1948.
20. Preston, F. W., Walsh, W. S., and Clarke, T. H.: Cutaneous neurofibromatosis (von Recklinghausen's disease): clinical manifestations and incidence of sarcoma in 61 male patients. Arch. Surg. 64:813, 1952.
21. D'Agostino, A. N., Soule, E. H., and Miller, R. H.: Primary malignant neoplasm of nerves (malignant neurilemmoma) in patients without manifestations of multiple neurofibromatosis (von Recklinghausen's disease). Cancer 16:1003, 1963.
22. Stout, A. P.: Tumors of the peripheral nervous system. In Atlas of Tumor Pathology, Section 2, Fascicle 6. Armed Forces Institute of Pathology, Washington, D.C., 1949.
23. D'Agostino, A. N., Soule, E. H., and Miller, R. H.: Sarcomas of the peripheral nerves and somatic soft tissues associated with multiple neurofibromatosis (von Recklinghausen's disease). Cancer 16:1015, 1963.
24. Clairmont, A. A., and Conley, J. J.: Malignant schwannoma of the parapharyngeal space. J. Otolaryngol. 6:28, 1977.
25. Woodruff, J. M., Chernik, N. L., Smith, M. C., Millett, W. B., and Foote, F. W., Jr.: Peripheral nerve tumors with rhabdomyosarcomatous differentiation (malignant "Triton" tumors). Cancer 32:426, 1973.
26. Woodruff, J. M.: Peripheral nerve tumors showing glandular differentiation (glandular schwannomas). Cancer 37:2399, 1976.
27. Alvira, M. M., Mandybur, T. I., and Menefee, M. G.: Light microscopic and ultrastructural observations of a metastasizing malignant epitheliod schwannoma. Cancer 38: 1977, 1976.
28. Karcioglu, Z., Someren, A., and Mathes, S. J.: Ectomesenchymoma. A malignant tumor of migratory neural crest (ectomesenchyme) remnants showing ganglionic, schwannian, melanocytic and rhabdomyoblastic differentiation. Cancer 39:2486, 1977.
29. Katz, A. D., Passy, V., and Kaplan, L.: Neurogenous neo-

plasms of major nerves of face and neck. Arch. Surg. 103: 51, 1971.

30. Mahmoud, N., and Parker, R.: Neurofibrosarcoma of the hypoglossal nerve. J. Laryngol. 89:957, 1975.

31. Daly, J. F., and Roesler, H. K.: Neurilemmoma of the cervical sympathetic chain. Arch. Otolaryngol. 77:262, 1963.

32. DiPietro, J.: Tumors of the peripheral nerves. Tumori 46: 430, 1960.

33. Kragh, L. V., Soule, E. H., and Masson, J. K.: Neurofibromatosis (von Recklinghausen's disease) of the head and neck: cosmetic and reconstructive aspects. Plast. Reconstr. Surg. 25:565, 1960.

34. Oberman, H. A., and Sullenger, G.: Neurogenous tumors of the head and neck. Cancer 20:1992, 1967.

35. Das Gupta, T. K., Brasfield, R. D., Strong, E. W., and Hajdu, S. I.: Benign solitary schwannomas (neurilemmomas). Cancer 24:355, 1969.

36. Davis, W. B., Edgerton, M. T., Jr., and Hoftmeister, F. S.: Neurofibromatosis of the head and neck. Plast. Reconstr. Surg. 14:186, 1954.

37. Kragh, L. V., Soule, E. H., and Masson, J. K.: Benign and malignant neurilemmomas of the head and neck. Surg. Gynecol. Obstet. 111:211, 1960.

38. Rosenfield, L., Graves, H., Jr., and Lawrence, R.: Primary neurogenic tumors of the lateral neck. Ann. Surg. 167:847, 1968.

39. Conley, J. J.: Neurogenous tumors in the neck. Arch. Otolaryngol. 61:167, 1955.

40. Cutler, E. C., and Gross, R. E.: Neurofibroma and neurosarcoma of peripheral nerves, unassociated with von Recklinghausen's disease: a report of 25 cases. Arch. Surg. 33: 733, 1936.

41. Mair, I. W. S., Marhaug, G. O., and Stalsberg, H.: Solitary schwannoma of the cervical vagus nerve. O. R. L. 38:344, 1976.

42. Lavoie, R., Gauthier, G-T., and Lavoie, J. G.: Neurinoma of the facial nerves. Arch. Otolaryngol. 86:374, 1967.

43. Furlow, L. T., and Walsh, T. E.: Neurilemmoma of the facial nerve. Laryngoscope 69:1975, 1959.

44. Hora, J. F., and Brown, A. K., Jr.: Neurilemmoma of the facial nerve. Laryngoscope 24:134, 1964.

45. Conley, J., and Janecka, I.: Schwann cell tumors of the facial nerve. Laryngoscope 84:958, 1974.

46. Conley, J., and Janecka, I.: Neurilemmoma of the head and neck. Trans. Acad. Ophthalmol. Otolaryngol. 80:459, 1975.

47. Helmus, C.: Massive neurilemmoma of the brachial plexus. Arch. Otolaryngol. 93:244, 1971.

48. DeVore, D. T., and Waldron, C. A.: Malignant peripheral nerve tumor of the oral cavity. Oral Surg. 14:56, 1961.

49. Baden, E., Pierce, H. E., and Jackson, W. F.: Multiple neurofibromatosis with oral lesions. Oral Surg. 8:263, 1955.

50. Ayres, W. W., Delaney, A. J., and Bacher, M. H.: Congenital neurofibromatosis macroglossia associated in some cases with von Recklinghausen's disease. Cancer 5:721, 1952.

51. Gallo, W. J., Moss, M., Shapiro, D. N., and Gaul, J. V.: Neurilemmoma: review of the literature and report of five cases. J. Oral. Surg. 35:235, 1977.

52. Robitaille, Y., Seemayer, T. A., and El Deiry, A.: Peripheral nerve tumors involving paranasal sinuses: a case report and review of the literature. Cancer 35:1254, 1975.

53. Iwamura, S., Sugiura, S., and Nomura, Y.: Schwannoma of the nasal cavity. Arch. Otolaryngol. 96:176, 1972.

54. Kaufman, S. M., and Conrad, L. P.: Schwannoma presenting as a nasal polyp. Laryngoscope 86:595, 1976.

55. McIlrath, D. C., ReMine, W. H., Devine, K. D., and Dockerty, M. B.: Tumors of the parapharyngeal region. Surg. Gynecol. Obstet. 116:88, 1967.

56. Putney, F. J., Moran, J. J., and Thomas, G. K.: Neurogenic tumors of the head and neck. Laryngoscope 74:1937, 1964.

57. Gore, D. O., Rankow, R., and Hanford, J. M.: Parapharyngeal neurilemmoma. Surg. Gynecol. Obstet. 103:193, 1956.

58. Horwich, M., and Hawe, P.: Neurilemmoma of the vagus

nerve in the neck; report of two cases. Br. J. Surg. 49:443, 1962.

59. El-Serafy, S.: Rare benign tumors of the larynx. J. Laryngol. Otol. 85:837, 1971.

60. Cummings, C. W., Montgomery, W. W., and Balogh, K., Jr.: Neurogenic tumors of the larynx. Ann. Otol. Rhinol. Laryngol. 78:76, 1969.

61. Chang-Lo, M.: Laryngeal involvement in von Recklinghausen's disease: A case report and review of the literature. Laryngoscope 87:435, 1977.

62. Eversole, L. R.: Central benign and malignant neural neoplasms of the jaws: a review. J. Oral Surg. 27:716, 1969.

63. Prescott, G. H., and White, R. E.: Solitary, central neurofibroma of the mandible: report of case and review of the literature. J. Oral Surg. 28:305, 1970.

64. Shklar, G., and Meyer, I.: Neurogenic tumors of the mouth and jaws. Oral Surg. 16:1075, 1963.

65. Ellis, G. L., Abrams, A. M., and Melrose, R. J.: Intraosseous benign neural sheath neoplasms of the jaws. Report of seven new cases and review of the literature. Oral Surg. 44:731, 1977.

66. Lorson, E. L., DeLong, P. E., Osborn, D. B., and Dolan, K. D.: Neurofibromatosis with central neurofibroma of the mandible: review of the literature and report of case. J. Oral Surg. 35:733, 1977.

67. Eversole, L. R., Schwartz, D., and Sabes, W. R.: Central and peripheral fibrogenic and neurogenic sarcoma of the oral regions. Oral Surg. 36:49, 1973.

68. Huber, C. G., and Lewis, D.: Amputation neuromas. Arch. Surg. 1:85, 1920.

69. Swanson, H. H.: Traumatic neuromas: a review of the literature. Oral Surg. 14:317, 1961.

70. Lagerkvist, B., Ivemark, B., and Sylven, B.: Malignant neuroepithelioma in childhood: report of three cases. Acta Chir. Scand. 135:641, 1969.

71. Stout, A. P., and Murray, M. R.: Neuroepithelioma of the radial nerve with a study of its behavior in vitro. Rev. Can. Biol. 1:651, 1942.

72. Abrikosoff, A.: Uber Myome, ausgehend von der qvergestreiften willkurlichen Muskulatur. Virchows Arch. (Pathol. Anat.) 260:215, 1926.

73. Cracovaner, A. J., and Opler, S. R.: Granular cell myoblastoma of the larynx. Laryngoscope 77:1040, 1967.

74. Garancis, J. C., Komorowski, R. A., and Kuzman, J. F.: Granular cell myoblastoma. Cancer 25:542, 1970.

75. Fisher, E. R., and Wechsler, H.: Granular cell myoblastoma—a misnomer. Electron microscopic and histochemical evidence concerning its Schwann cell derivation and nature (granular cell schwannoma). Cancer 15:936, 1962.

76. Evans, R. W.: Histological appearance of tumors, 2nd Ed., pp. 62–65. Williams & Wilkins Co., Baltimore, 1966.

77. Eversole, L. R.: Granular sheath cell lesions: report of cases. J. Oral Surg. 29:867, 1971.

78. Sobel, H. J., and Marquet, E.: Granular cells and granular cell lesions. Pathol. Annu. 9:43, 1974.

79. Peterson, L. J.: Granular-cell tumor: Review of the literature and report of a case. Oral Surg. 37:728, 1974.

80. Compagno, J., Hyams, V. J., and Ste-Marie, P.: Benign granular cell tumors of the larynx: review of 36 cases with clinicopathologic data. Ann. Otol. 84:308, 1975.

81. Canalis, R. F., Dodson, T. A., Turkell, S. B., and Maenza, R. M.: Granular cell myoblastoma of the cervical trachea. Arch. Otolaryngol. 102:176, 1976.

82. Vance, S. F., and Hudson, R. P., Jr.: Granular cell myoblastoma: clinicopathological study of forty-two patients. Am. J. Clin. Pathol. 52:208, 1969.

83. Weiser, G., and Propst, A.: Elektronenoptische Untersuchung zur Histogenese des Granularen Neurons. Virchows Arch. (Pathol. Anat.) 358:193, 1973.

84. Christian, M. A., Gambarelli, D., Hassoun, J., Gola, R., Toga, M., and Bonerandi, J. J.: Granular cell myoblastoma. J. Cut. Pathol. 4:80, 1977.

85. Garancis, J. G., Komorowski, R. A., and Kuzma, J. F.: Granular cell myoblastoma. Cancer 25:542, 1970.

86. Hagen, J. O., Soule, E. H., and Gores, R. J.: Granular cell

myoblastoma of the oral cavity. Oral Surg. 14:454, 1961.

. Cadotte, M.: Malignant granular-cell myoblastoma. Cancer 33:1417, 1974.

. Allek, D. S., Johnson, W. C., and Graham, J. H.: Granular cell myoblastoma: a histological and enzymatic study. Arch. Dermatol. 98:543, 1968.

. Neely, J. B., Britton, B. H., and Greenberg, S. D.: Microscopic characteristics of the acoustic tumor in relationship of its nerve of origin. Laryngoscope 86:984, 1976.

. Pool, J. L., Pava, A. A., and Greenfield, E. C.: Acoustic Nerve Tumors: Early Diagnosis and Treatment, 2nd Ed. Charles C Thomas, Springfield, Ill., 1970.

. House, W. F. (editor): Acoustic neuroma: monograph II. Arch. Otolaryngol. 88:576, 1968.

. Pulec, J. L., House, W. F., Britton, B. H., Jr., and Hitselberger, W. E.: A system of management of acoustic neuroma

based on 364 cases. Trans. Am. Assoc. Ophthalmol. Otol. 75:48, 1971.

93. Zulch, K. I.: Brain Tumors: Their Biology and Pathology, Springer-Verlag, New York, 1962.

94. Haferkamp, O.: Uber dic Neurome. Z. Krebsforsch. 63:378, 1960.

95. Harkin, J. C., and Reed, R. J.: Tumors of the peripheral nervous system. Atlas Tumor Pathology. Series II, Fascicle 3, Armed Forces Institute of Pathology, Washington, D.C., 1968.

96. Krucke, W.: Pathologie der peripheren Nerven. In Handbuch der Neurochirugie, bearbeitet. V. W. Krucke. Bd 7/3, Springer, Berlin, Heidelberg, 1974.

97. Russell, D. S., and Rubinstein, L. J.: Pathology of Tumours of the Nervous System. 4th ed., Williams & Wilkins Co., Baltimore, 1977.

CHAPTER 17

Other Neuroectodermal Tumors and Related Lesions of the Head and Neck

Exclusive of neurofibromas, schwannomas, their malignant counterparts, and malignant melanomas, which may not be of neuroectodermal origin, tumors taking origin from neuroectoderm are infrequently encountered in an otolaryngological practice. Many, however, are unique to the region of the head and neck, viz., melanotic neuroectodermal tumors of the jaws and esthesioneuroblastomas. Anatomical uniqueness, difficulties in clinical and pathological diagnosis, often paradoxical biological behavior and low incidence sets this group of lesions apart and merits the attention of both the head and neck surgeon and surgical pathologist.

The following entails a clinicopathological evaluation of this group of tumors, specifically: heterotopic brain tissue, melanotic neuroectodermal tumor of the jaws, neuroblastoma and esthesioneuroblastoma. Briefer considerations will be given to more unusual forms of related tumors as they present in the head and neck.

HETEROTOPIC BRAIN TISSUE

Among the most vulnerable events in the development of the human embryo are the formation of the neural tube, its separation from the body coverings and the interposition of mesodermal elements between the two layers. Failure of the normal sequence of embryological events may lead to a variety of defects pertinent to the head and neck surgeon and pathologist. These defects may manifest themselves as tumors and have been recorded in the literature by the following names: encephalocele, encephaloma, choristoma, choristoma-nasofrontalis, nasal glioma, glioma, ganglioblastoma, fibroglioma, ganglioma and astrocytoma.

The neoplastic connotation implied by the last six designations is not justified. Retention of the diagnostic term "glioma" is probably warranted only because of its widespread clinical use (Fig. 17.1). The masses are best considered as developmental anomalies in the form of herniations of the frontal lobes and/or their coverings which exhibit varying degrees of gliosis and/or fibrosis.

The occurrence of extracranial brain tissues is rare. Of the recorded examples in the literature, most have been localized in and around the nose and are seen most frequently in the form of an encephalocele. Encephaloceles may occur at any point, usually the midline over the vertex or at the base of the cranium. Their estimated incidence is one in 4,000 births.[1] Two basic theories of genesis may be entertained: (1) arrested closures of the covering through which meninges and neural tissue herniate; and (2) an initial overgrowth of the neural tube preventing closure of cranial coverings. While as a rule, neuroglial elements as well as meningeal tissue can be identified in the sac or herniation, protrusion may consist only of meninges (meningocele). Variants of meningoceles include the arachnoid cysts, in which there is no demonstrable connection with the cranial cavity, and meningocele in association with an epidermal sinus which may extend for a variable distance inward.

Three anatomical categories of encephalocele exist[2]: occipital, accounting for 75% of the cases; sincipital, situated about the dorsum of the nose, orbits and forehead (15%); and basal, presenting as a herniated sac protruding into the superior meatus of the nasal cavity, epipharynx or sphenomaxillary fossa (10%). Both the occipital and sincipital forms may be visible externally. The basal variant is internal, presenting in the nasal

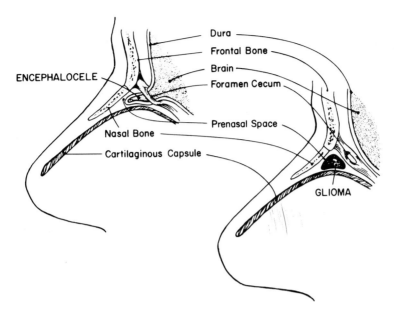

Figure 17.1. Schematic representation of formation of nasal and paranasal herniations of central nervous system tissue. The *completely* sequestered neural tissue is sometimes inappropriately referred to as "glioma."

and pharyngeal spaces. Table 17.1 presents subdivision of the sincipital and basal variants.

Sincipital hernias may produce a tumor visible externally in the midline at the roof of the nose, at the junction of the bony and cartilaginous portion of the nose or near the inner canthus. Basal hernias do not produce a tumor visible on the face, but present in the nasal or nasopharyngeal cavity or even in the mouth or posterior portion of the orbit or sphenomaxillary fossa. The most common and most important type of *basal* encephalocele is the sphenopharyngeal type. Here the hernial sac presents within the nose or pharynx, causing obstruction and deformity of the upper respiratory passages, and constitutes an ever constant threat of spinal fluid rhinorrhea or meningitis.

Encephaloceles with an external manifestation are familiar to the clinician. The tumor presents on either the left or right side of the bridge of the nose. The nasal roof and dorsum may be broadened, with a tendency toward wide-set eyes. The extranasal tumors are smooth, firm, elastic and noncompressible. They are faint red or blue and do not increase in size with straining.

When both intra- and extranasal components are present (10% of cases),[3] there is a communication between the two parts, usually through a defect in the nasal bone or at the lateral margin of the nasal bone. There may or may not be an intracranial communication. When this is present, the connection passes through a defect in the cribriform plate or in the region of the attachment

Table 17.1
Variations of Sincipital and Basal Encephalocele

Sincipital

1. Nasofrontal: protrusion between the nasal and frontal bones
2. Nasoethmoidal: protrusion through foramen caecum, separated from nasal interior by the ethmoid process
3. Naso-orbital: protrusion through medial wall of the orbit, involving frontal, ethmoid and lacrimal bones

Basal

1. Transethmoidal: protrusion through defect in cribriform plate into the superior meatus
2. Sphenoethmoidal: protrusion into epipharynx through a defect between the posterior ethmoid cells and the sphenoid
3. Transphenoidal: protrusion through a patent craniopharyngeal canal into the epipharynx
4. Sphenomaxillary: protrusion through the supraorbital fissure, through the infraorbital tissue and then into the sphenomaxillary fossa; appears as a mass on the medial side of the mandibular ramus

of the frontal bone. Intranasal presentation (30%) is readily mistaken for a nasal polyp, although the lesion is more dense, more glistening and less translucent than the usual polyp. Frequently a cause of nasal obstruction, they may displace the septum, nasal cartilages or bone. The tumors are usually attached by a stalk high within the nasal vault, from the middle turbinate or the lateral wall of the nasal fossa.

Care must be taken to differentiate encephaloceles connecting directly with the subarachnoid or ventricular spaces and those where the pedicle is broken, absorbed or vestigial, leaving an isolated heterotopic mass of brain tissue. Tumors composed of heterotopic neural tissue, predominantly glial, may or may not be connected by a pedicle or stalk to the brain. A central connection may have been lost or may be too small for demonstration. The inappropriate designation of nasal "glioma" has been applied to this form and, even more inappropriately, to the entire group of encephaloceles (Fig. 17.2).

The heterotopias are variants of encephaloceles. They are composed of brain tissue in which there is usually a significant and often dominating gliosis. The nests of glial cells are interlaced with a vascular fibrous tissue network or septae (Fig. 17.2). Secondary changes of fibrogliosis or gemistocytic alteration of glial cells is often seen. Ganglion cells and other neural elements may be present. The gliosis is probably secondary to circulatory impairment, death of cerebral tissue and obliteration of the subarachnoid and perivascular spaces. Any "bizarre" astrocytes that may be present in the lesion are due to hypoxia and compression and should not be confused with neoplastic cells.

The majority of patients present with signs and symptoms during the first year of life, with relative peaks in children between 5 and 10 years of age.[1] Sex incidence is almost equal, and there is no evidence of familial occurrence. Presentation later in life may be due to failure to recognize the lesion in childhood or a herniation through traumatic or acquired bony defects.

Growth of the tumors is usually slow and, in general, commensurate with the general growth of the host. Spontaneous cerebrospinal fluid rhinorrhea may occur, but such a manifestation is generally a complication of a "polypectomy" or biopsy of the nasal mass. X-rays of the sinuses and laminograms aid in the diagnosis. Usually no skull defect can be demonstrated. The incidence of associated anomalies with encephaloceles may be as high as 30% of the cases.[4]

Once diagnosis is established and the threat of meningitis is not deemed serious, there is no great urgency to the removal of these tumors. They are not neoplastic, do not invade surrounding structures and do not retard the growth and development of the child. They may cause no particular difficulty other than excessive tearing or cosmetic deformity. Once treatment is elected, total surgical excision is necessary. Recurrences have been reported, and the lesions are not radiosensitive.

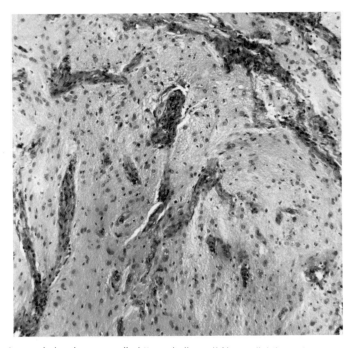

Figure 17.2. Nasal encephalocele or so-called "nasal glioma." Neuroglial tissue is separated by thin vascular septae.

Walker and Resler[5] indicate that a team effort by an ophthalmologist, otolaryngologist and neurosurgeon is desirable for the management of these tumors. The existence of intracranial connections cannot adequately be demonstrated or eliminated by the roentgenographic findings, and they advise a diagnostic craniotomy before any attempt at removal of the tumors.

MELANOTIC NEUROECTODERMAL TUMOR OF JAWS

The plethora of names given to this tumor reflects the confusion, frustration and, sometimes, acrimony attendant to the genesis of the lesion. Rarely has a tumor been given so many designations: neuroectodermal tumor of infancy, congenital melanocarcinoma, melanotic epithelial odontoma, pigmented teratoma, atypical melanoblastoma, melanotic adamantinoma, melanotic (pigmented) ameloblastoma, melanotic (congenital) tumor, pigmented epulis, retinal anlage tumor, retinal or retinoblastic teratoma, retinal choristoma, melanotic progonoma and melanotic anlage tumor.[6]

There have been three principal histogenetic theories: (1) the lesion is a congenital melanocarcinoma; (2) the tumor is odontogenic in origin; (3) the tumor is derived from neuroectoderm. Only the last two have strong proponents. Many authors, particularly oral pathologists, noting the proximity of proliferative odontogenic epithelium in the jaw, have assumed a direct relation and consider the lesions to be melanotic ameloblastomas.[7] They cite association with developing tooth buds or growth in areas of missing teeth as support for an odontogenic origin.

There is, however, little or no microscopic resemblance between the tumor cells and any of those involved in tooth germ formation. It may be further argued that proximity to odontogenic rests, when the lesion occurs in the maxilla or mandible, is not expected or surprising, since the teeth in these areas are undergoing development at this time. Furthermore, the tooth buds are displaced by the expanding mass.

Neural crest derivation, on the other hand, has much to commend it. There is abundant evidence, derived from experiments on the development of lower vertebrates, that the neural crest cells can differentiate into various cell types, i.e., neuroblasts, chromaffin cells, neurolemmal cells and melanoblasts. Electron microscopy tells us the cells appear to be of neural crest origin and are like melanocytes.[8] Biochemical evidence also supports neuroectodermal origin by the observation that the tumor elaborates high levels of vanilmandelic acid (VMA), sharing this property with other neural crest tumors, i.e., neuroblastoma, ganglioneuroblastoma and pheochromocytoma.[9] It appears that neural crest tissue has migrated from its point of origin in a normal fashion, but has been diverted from the usual course and comes to rest in an aberrant location. In that location it functions in the manner it would if it were at its normal destination and induces and stimulates growth in the surrounding tissues. Predilection of this tumor for the cephalic region, especially the anterior maxilla remains unclear. According to Stowens and Lin[10] the pathogenesis of the tumor incorporates the concepts of both choristoma and hamartoma. The hamartomatous element is the pigmented epithelium, for it is basically normal tissue in an abnormal site. The choristomatous element is the tissue induced to grow under the stimulus of the pigmented epithelium. As a consequence, the term "pigmented hamartomatous choristoma of neural crest derivation" may be descriptively accurate.

The histopathological features may be said to be pathognomic. Within a stroma of moderately vascularized fibrous connective tissue, the tumor cells are divided into islands with slit-like alveoli which are irregular in shape and size (Fig. 17.3).

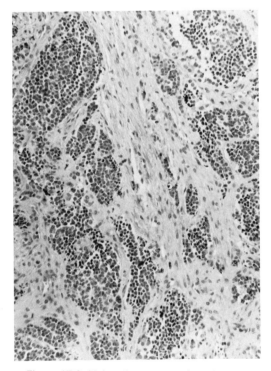

Figure 17.3. Melanotic neuroectodermal tumor.

The cells are of two types; one type is large, with pale abundant cytoplasm and pale nuclei. The cytoplasm contains variable quantities of small brown granules of melanin pigment (Fig. 17.4). These cells line the spaces. The cells within the alveolar spaces are more numerous and often densely packed. They are smaller with scant cytoplasm and dark nuclei. They resemble mature lymphocytes and are supported by a delicate fibrillar network. Mitoses or pleomorphism are not seen.

The lesion is primarily one of the first year of life, with most of the cases occurring in the first 6 months after birth and after a clinical duration of a few weeks to 5 months. Approximately 100 cases have been recorded in the literature.[11] While peculiar to the infant and to the jaws, melanotic neuroectodermal tumor is not restricted to these categories. The lesion has been described, with varying degrees of acceptance, in the anterior fontanel, shoulder, epididymis, cerebellum, scapula and mediastinum. Confusion with a teratoma must account for several of these "examples." The lesion has presented most frequently in the anterior part of the maxilla, i.e., the part formed by the junction of the globular process or lower portion of the frontonasal process with the maxillary process.

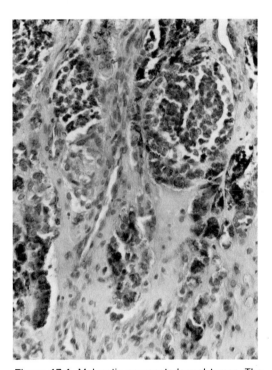

Figure 17.4. Melanotic neuroectodermal tumor. The larger cells contain the melanin pigment. Sometimes elusive, the pigment should be searched for in multiple sections of the tumor.

Maxillary lesions exceed those in the mandible by a 4:1 ratio.

Clinically, an enlargement of the involved site and, in its most usual location (anterior maxilla), and elevation of the lip are the presenting signs. The child is healthy, except for the mass. Overlying mucosa is usually intact. In some instances, due to the pigmentation in the lesion, the mass may be brown or black. Radiologically, the involved bone manifests a circumscribed area of radiolucency and displacement of the tooth germs.

Most authors consider the lesions as benign, albeit occasionally locally aggressive and effectively managed by surgical excision or complete curettage. Brekke and Gorlin,[12] however, caution against too great a therapeutic complacency and regard the 15% recurrence rate as not entirely due to incomplete removal. To my knowledge there have been no instances of metastases. Reports on the response of these tumors to irradiation have been poorly documented and, in general, the tumors have been regarded as radioresistant.

NEUROBLASTOMA

The term "neuroblastoma" is an umbrella covering a spectrum of histological types of neurogenic neoplasms which take their origin from cells derived from embryonic sympathetic neuroblasts, neural crest remnants and the mantle layer of the neural tube. Thus, they may originate in the adrenal gland or sympathetic ganglia of the cervical, posterior mediastinal, retroperitoneal or abdominal regions. That precursor remnants elsewhere may also give rise to these neoplasms is attested to by the rare finding of primary neuroblastomas remote from the above-mentioned sites.

Histological Classification

The neuroblastoma series of neoplasms constitutes a spectrum characterized by varying degrees of maturation of the neoplastic cells toward mature and predominantly mature neural elements. At one end of this histological spectrum, the neoplasms are composed of cells so poorly differentiated that distinction from other small-celled neoplasms may be difficult or even impossible. At the other end (ganglioneuromas), the neoplasms are composed solely of mature cell types (Fig. 17.5). Between these two extremes, these neuroblastic neoplasms may be characterized by: (1) a uniform, partial differentiation; (2) focal partial differentiation; or (3) focal, complete differentiation.

From the foregoing spectrum, a classification may be evolved. The *least* differentiated neoplasm of the neuroblastoma series is the *sympathicogo-*

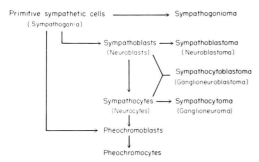

Figure 17.5. Spectrum of neoplasms derived from the primitive sympathetic cells of the neural crest.

nioma. There is no recognizable neurogenesis. The neoplastic cells are roughly the size of mature lymphocytes, possess little cytoplasm and have a dense and hyperchromatic nucleus. The accompanying stroma is fibrillar and glial in appearance. Pseudorosettes may be prominent (Fig. 17.6).

A step up the histological scale is the *sympathicoblastoma*. These cells are differentiating, as manifested by nuclear enlargement and cytoplasmic enlargement, with clear cell borders and an increased affinity for eosin. Ganglion cells of varying maturity may be present. A fibrillar stroma and pseudorosettes may be found, but these features are not as common as in the more immature lesions. Calcification is a finding common to both the sympathicogonioma and sympathicoblastoma.

Ganglioneuromas may be subdivided into mature or partially differentiated types. The partially differentiated forms are termed *ganglioneuroblastomas.* They manifest immature cells of the sympathetic nervous system intermixed with mature ganglion cells and also possess foci of a fibrillar stroma such as are seen in the more primitive neoplasms. The mature *ganglioneuroma* is comprised of clusters of ganglion cells in a mature neurogenous stroma, i.e., nerve fiber, Schwann cells and fibrous connective tissue. On occasion, one encounters a neuroblastomatous neoplasm manifesting two distinctive subtypes, viz., mature ganglioneuroma and a sympathicoblastoma. The biological behavior of this variant is that of its most undifferentiated type.

Some may find the above designations cumbersome and difficult to use. An alternative system is offered by Beckwith and Martin.[13] They grade neuroblastomas in the following manner:

Grade I. Predominantly differentiated: over 50% differentiating elements.
Grade II. Predominantly undifferentiated: 5 to 50% differentiating elements.
Grade III. Slightly differentiated: less than 5% differentiating elements.

Grade IV. Undifferentiated: no recognizable neurogenesis.

Cervical Neuroblastomas

In children, neuroblastoma is surpassed in infancy only by the leukemias and neoplasms of the central nervous system. In children's centers, neuroblastomas account for 10 to 20% of childhood malignancies.[14] Two-thirds of neuroblastomas arise within the abdomen, most frequently from the adrenal glands and neighboring retroperitoneal sympathetic ganglia.

The head and neck surgeon's attention is drawn to neuroblastomas in the form of two clinical presentations: metastases from extracervical primaries or as a primary neoplasm in the cervical region arising from the sympathetic nervous system in the cervical or thoracic areas. The odds are in favor of a neuroblastoma in the head and neck being metastatic, particularly if the metastatic site is within the skull. Skeletal metastases from neuroblastomas may be osteolytic, osteoblastic or a combination of these patterns.

Although there is no consistent metastatic pattern, neuroblastomatous metastases into the orbits and leptomeninges have been categorized as the Hutchinson variety, and the marked hepatomegaly secondary to metastases to the liver from neuro-

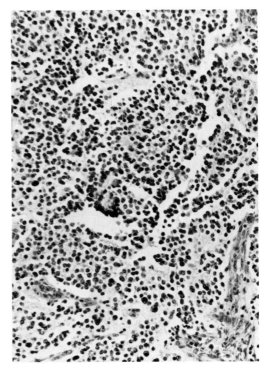

Figure 17.6. Neuroblastoma manifesting a pseudorosette.

blastomas of the adrenals are referred to as the Pepper type. These eponymic designations have implied, in the past, some constancy in metastatic patterns that is not entirely correct. While it is true that there is a propensity on the part of some neuroblastomas to involve bone, particularly the cranium and orbits, involvement of other facial bones, i.e., mandible, is very rare. In the former instance, the metastases may be the first clinical evidence of the neoplasm's existence. By 1976, only nine cases of metastatic neuroblastoma to the jaws had been recorded.[15] All of the secondary jaw deposits occurred in children 2 to 8 years of age. The most commonly affected site has been the molar region and the angle of the mandible. Jaw metastases have been accompanied by widespread metastases in all of the patients. Survival after discovery of the metastasis to the jaws is usually only a matter of weeks.

The extra-adrenal primary, on the basis of its markedly better survival rate, merits distinction from metastatic neuroblastoma.[16] An awareness of extra-adrenal neuroblastoma as an entity in the head and neck region serves as protection against the dangers of mistaking it for a precocious metastasis from a cryptogenic primary lesion elsewhere.[16] This clinical awareness also enables the surgeon to request appropriate roentgenographic investigations and biochemical assays to distinguish other poorly differentiated small-celled neoplasms from neuroblastomas.

In a series of 212 cases of neuroblastomas from the California Tumor Registry, 2% were primary in the cervical area.[14] Dawson[17] has reviewed the case reports in the literature from 1915, indicating that the discrepancies in numbers are due to divergence of views as to the definition of this group of tumors. A safe presumption would be to consider that not more than 5% of all neuroblastomas take their origin from the cervical sympathetic system.

The clinical findings associated with an extra-adrenal neuroblastoma are dependent upon its specific site of origin in the sympathetic nervous system. In the cervical sympathetic area, a mass is usually present in association with symptoms that relate to the pharynx, larynx or esophagus. These include dysphagia, dyspnea, hoarseness, apnea or stridor.

A benign tumor of this group produces a painless, slowly growing mass. The lesion is not attached to the skin but may be relatively fixed to the deep tissues. The carotid artery is usually displaced anteriorly and laterally. The malignant neuroblastoma grows more rapidly and involves local structures, thereby producing otalgia, facial palsy, miosis and other signs and symptoms attendant to invasion. Symptoms occasioned by the hormonal activity of the neoplasms, such as sweating, pyrexia, diarrhea and paroxsymal hypertension, may also occur. These are infrequent and transitory.

Roentgenographic findings may consist of displacement and/or distortion of the laryngopharynx. A stippled calcification within the displacing mass increases the probability that the mass is a neuroblastoma. X-ray findings alone cannot positively distinguish extra-adrenal neuroblastomas from metastatic neuroblastomas. The combined presence or absence of certain findings, however, is highly suggestive of extra-adrenal rather than adrenal gland origin.[16] Specifically, if the roentgenographic work-up of a patient presenting with cervical findings of a neuroblastoma shows no adrenal mass or adrenal calcification and there are normal renal contours without displacement on intravenous pyelography and there are no metastases revealed by skeletal survey, an extra-adrenal origin is most likely.

The clinical course of neuroblastoma is much more accelerated than that of many adult tumors. Hematogenous and lymphogenous metastases may be widespread by the time diagnosis is made. Metastases to bone or to periorbital structures are extremely poor prognostic signs and portend an almost 100% mortality.

Follow-up periods in published series are short, but this is countered by Koop and Hernandez,[18] who state that for practically all childhood neoplasms, 14 months is *equivalent* to a 5-year "cure" period used in adult cancer statistics. The over-all cure rate from several larges series of neuroblastomas has varied from 9.7 to 36%.[14] This rather wide variation is probably related to differences in the distribution of the age of the patients, the site of the primary and the extent of spread of the disease (stage) at first diagnosis. These three factors and others probably play a more important role in determining survival of patients with neuroblastoma than does the mode of treatment.

All studies indicate that *age* at the time of diagnosis is very important in prognosis. It is obvious that children under the age of 1 year have a considerably better chance for "cure." Site of origin ranks second only to age for prognostic purposes. Survival rates of patients with neuroblastoma are considerably greater when the tumor arises from extra-adrenal sites (Table 17.2). The combined experience of 513 cases of retroperitoneal neuroblastoma (including adrenal gland) es-

Table 17.2
Extra-adrenal Neuroblastomas: Survival Rates

Author	No. of Patients	Survival		Duration (years)
		No.	%	
Bodian[20]	51	19	37	1
Fortner et al.[21]	48	8	17	5
King et al.[22]	13	13	100	2
Koop[23]	68	26	38	4
Phillips[24]	20	7	35	3
Young et al.[16]	17	9	53	5

tablishes a survival rate of 19% (2 years)[14] for all age groups. This is to be compared to a survival rate of 50% for mediastinal neuroblastomas, 44% for cervical neuroblastomas and a 53% 2-year rate for sacral neuroblastomas.[14]

Spontaneous regression, a phenomenon occurring more frequently in patients with neuroblastoma than with any other neoplasm, is an additional factor playing on survival figures. Age plays a considerable role in this regression, since, in 25 of 29 reported cases of spontaneous regression, the neoplasm was first noted when the child was less than 1 year old.[14]

A better prognosis has also been associated with increasing maturity of the cells in the neuroblastoma series. Certainly this is true for ganglioneuromas, which usually, if not always, behave in a benign fashion. For the less differentiated variations, it is unclear to what extent the level of maturity influences or modifies the effect of site and age on prognosis. Despite a suggestive tendency for extra-adrenal neuroblastomas occurring in the first year of life to show evidence of maturation, this has been considered insufficient evidence to account for the better prognosis manifested by patients in this age group.[13] Conversely, there is a consistent tendency for adrenal primaries to be less differentiated than extra-adrenal neuroblastomas. Prior to the early 1940's the prognosis for a patient with a neuroblastoma was grave, except for the occasional instance of spontaneous regression.

Besides the possibility of spontaneous regression and maturation of a given neuroblastoma to a less malignant form, the therapist has three basic weapons with which to attack the neoplasm: surgical removal, irradiation of the lesion and chemotherapy.[19] Added to these factors is the commonly accepted observation that the *extra-adrenal* primary lesions behave in a less lethal fashion.

Young et al.[16] have based their treatment of *extra-adrenal* neuroblastomas on staging. *Stage I* is neoplasm localized to primary site, capable of being completely resected and without evidence of regional lymph node involvement. *Stage II* neoplasms are only partially resectable because of local advancement and regional lymph node metastases. *Stage III* types are either those neuroblastomas with distant metastases (skeletal, visceral and distant lymph node involvement) or those with an unknown primary lesion *and* widespread metastases.

Radiotherapists indicate that a positive approach is a requisite for the treatment of the extra-adrenal neuroblastoma, and they indicate a high radiocurability.[16] Stage I neoplasms receive postoperative irradiation to the tumor bed in children older than 1 year of age. A larger radiation dose is applied to Stage II lesions in an effort to affect a cure. Total dose is more important than time, and a variety of fractional schema can be employed. The impact on surrounding normal tissue and its tolerance over-rides the need to adhere to a rigid time-dose schedule. Stage III neoplasms are approached from the standpoint of palliation, but relatively long-term control can be achieved by an aggressive combination of all forms of treatment. Chemotherapy, at best, has only a transient effect and a limited palliative effect. There are indications also that intensive chemotherapy adversely affects survival by impairing host resistance.[19]

ESTHESIONEUROBLASTOMA

Esthesioneuroblastoma is a neurogenic tumor of the olfactory region. The first recording of the neoplasm was by Berger et al.[25] in 1924, when they designated it "l'esthesioneuroepithelioma olfactif." More than 25 years transpired before the first American reports. By 1966 more than 150 cases had been recorded.[26] The number of these neoplasms seen at one institution is small, and, consequently, conclusions reached by various authors are not always congruous. Testimony to the rarity of the lesion may be found in the experience of an active "cancer hospital" (M.D. Anderson Hospital, Houston), where only one example was found in 40,000 surgical specimens over a 13-year period.[27]

The primordia of the olfactory apparatus appear in late somite embryos as two ectodermal thickenings, the olfactory or nasal placodes situated above the stomatodeum and below and lateral to the forebrain. By a proliferation of surrounding mesoderm, these placodes become depressed to form olfactory pits. Further growth of the mesoderm causes the epithelium of each nasal placode to come to lie in the medial and lateral walls of the upper fifth of the corresponding nasal cavity. The neuroblasts in the olfactory epithelium differentiate into nerve cells. These give rise to olfactory nerve fibers which grow toward the apical region of the corresponding cerebral hemisphere. In their course the fibers pierce the roof of the cartilagenous nasal capsule and penetrate into the apical region of the hemisphere (olfactory bulb). During later stages of development, the olfactory nerve fibers are separated into a number of bundles by the developing cribriform plate of the ethmoid. The fibers of the olfactory nerves differ from those of other nerves in that they are entirely of placodal origin and their cell bodies remain in the olfactory epithelium.

The primordial placodes are replaced by olfactory epithelium and become situated in the roof and adjacent parts of each nasal cavity (Fig. 17.7).

In man, the olfactory epithelium (Fig. 17.8) is limited to the upper surface of the superior turbinate, to a corresponding area of the nasal septum and to the undersurface of the cribriform plate in between.[28, 29] In the adult, its size is variable and its margins indistinct. Before the age of 1 or 2 years, the olfactory margin is quite regular. After that time, alterations occur and impart to it a characteristic irregularity. This is greatly exaggerated in later life. Microscopically, however, whether the demarcation line between olfactory and respiratory areas is regular or irregular, the junction between the two territories is always abrupt. Such junctions show no intermingling of cell types except in advanced age of disease.[29]

The olfactory epithelium consists of sensory cells containing bipolar receptor neurons, situated on a lamina propria of varying thickness in which lie the olfactory axons, glands of Bowman, and various connective tissue elements. The nuclei of the sensory cells form several layers surrounded by supporting cells with apically positioned nuclei bordered beneath by a layer of basal cells (Fig. 17.9). In this basal layer resides the reservoir for the differentiation and renewal of the sensory receptors.[30] The olfactory epithelium is similar to certain other renewing cell populations with restricted proliferation sites where products of basal cell division migrate peripherally and replace receptor cells or supporting cells or both. The sensory terminals of the olfactory dendrites bear numerous cilia, the trailing endings of which interweave among the many microvilli which mark the surfaces of the neighboring supporting cells. The olfactory rod is the bulbous enlargement which comprises the only naked region of the entire olfactory neuron. The olfactory nerve then is the only cranial nerve whose first-order neuron cell body resides in a distal epithelium.

Experimental evidence coupled with morphological studies clearly point to the olfactory epithelium as the site of origin of the esthesioneuroblastoma.[28–31] It is also most likely that the human neoplasm originates from the basal cell layer of the olfactory epithelium. The olfactory placode and the olfactory epithelium are generically the same, the former giving rise to the latter with the primordial placode being nonexistent after the embryonal period. No longer tenable for a precursor are the sphenopalatine ganglion and the organ of Jacobson. In accordance with the olfactory epithelial derivation for the neoplasm, esthesioneuroblastomas may take their origin from the

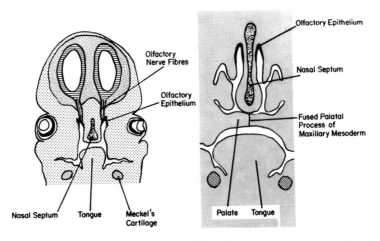

Figure 17.7. Embryological development of the olfactory region of the nasal cavity.

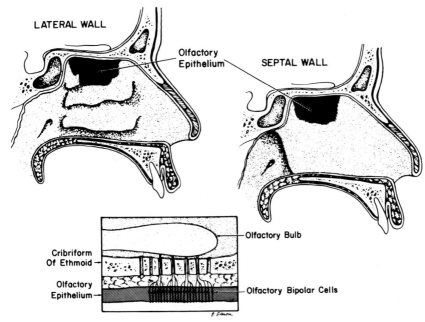

Figure 17.8. Medial and lateral areas of the nasal cavity covered by olfactory epithelium. In the adult these areas are never complete but are interrupted by ingrowths of respiratory epithelium.

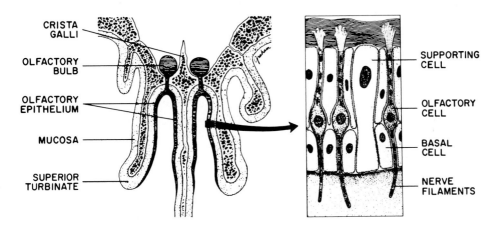

Figure 17.9. Relationships of olfactory epithelium to olfactory bulbs.

upper third of the nasal septum (superior and supreme nasal turbinates of the high nasal cavity and cribriform plate) and the lateral nasal wall.

The neoplasm has occurred over a wide range of ages from the first to the eighth decade of life with an apparent peak incidence in the second decade. Almost two-thirds of all patients have been between 10 and 34 years of age.[32] There is only a slight male dominance.[33]

The symptoms are nonspecific and are those of any intranasal neoplasm. When the disease is still localized, complaints are those of unilateral nasal obstruction, frequent epistaxis, anosomia, head-ache and rhinorrhea. Nasal polypectomy or submucous resection is not infrequent because of these symptoms. Symptoms are usually progressive and may be present for several years before the patient seeks medical care. With local invasion, headaches become severe, diplopia ensues and proptosis or a mass in the malar region is present. The neoplasm is usually fleshy and pinkish gray. As indicated above, it usually involves some area of the nasal olfactory mucosa. When small, it may be seen on a turbinate or it may extend into the paranasal sinuses and cribriform plate.

As both the epithelium and neural portions of

the olfactory mucosa origiante from the same neu-roectodermal thickening, the olfactory placode, the neoplasm is composed of nerve cells, either neurocytes or neuroblasts. Although the neoplasm may vary in pattern, there are certain basic similarities in all. Some authors have subdivided the esthesioneuroblastoma into types according to histological appearance; i.e., those with true rosettes are called neuroepitheliomas, those with pseudorosettes are called neuroblastomas and those with fibril formation and compartmentation, but without rosettes or pseudorosettes, are neurocytomas. This appears overly pedantic, especially since there is no influence of histological type on the biological course of the disease.

Almost all lesions have both neuroblasts and neurocytes, with a predominance of one cell type. Neuroblasts resemble lymphocytes, but are sometimes larger, with a round or oval nucleus, granular chromatin and scanty cytoplasm (Fig. 17.10). Neurocytes possess similar nuclei but have a distinct eosinophilic cytoplasm that may be either tapered, elongated or round. Fibrillar material and pseudorosettes may be found in most of the neoplasms, while true rosette formation is encountered much less often.[33]

The most characteristic growth pattern of these neoplasms consists of an intercellular neurofibril-lary matrix with clusters of small round to ovoid cells grouped by vascular septae (Fig. 17.11). This septate aggregation has been most helpful to the author in differential diagnosis. The presence of prominent nucleoli, considerable cellular pleomorphism, conspicuous numbers of mitoses or an absence of neurofibrillary matrix should caution against the diagnosis.

By light microscopy, a sympathetic neuroblastoma and a typical esthesioneuroblastoma are virtually identical. This histopathological similarity is carried through to the ultrastructural level and indicates that the ultrastructural characteristics of neuroblastomas are similar regardless of location or presumed origin.[34] In the cases studied by electron microscopy secretory-type granules, cytoplasmic fibrils, and microtubules similar to those of neuroblastoma have been found in many of the tumor cells.[34-36] The tumor cells also manifest an argyrophil reaction with the Grimelius technique and formaldehyde-induced fluorescence may demonstrate biogenic amines in the cells.[37] Not all these neoplasms are metabolically active; at least as evidenced by the inconsistent demonstration of intracellular catecholamines. Taxy and Hidvegi[34] point out that although dopamine-beta-hydroxyl-ase, epinephrine and norepinephrine have been documented in an olfactory neuroblastoma, the

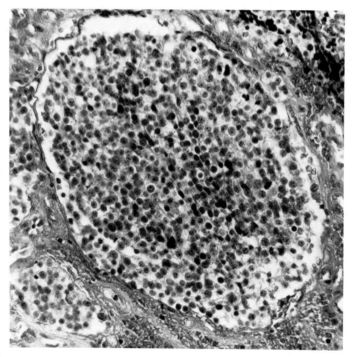

Figure 17.10. Biopsy specimen of an esthesioneuroblastoma. Crushing artefact of this neoplasm may make identification difficult or even impossible.

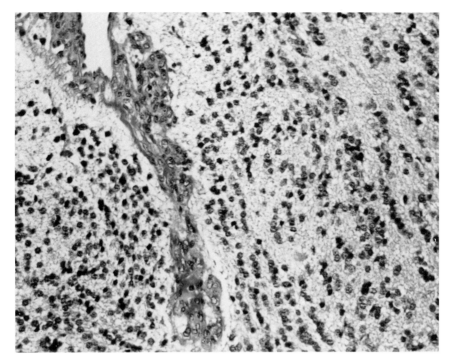

Figure 17.11. Esthesioneuroblastoma manifesting vascular septum and neurofibrillary background.

level of the hydroxylase is 100 times less than that observed in sympathetic neuroblastomas. In addition, I know of no esthesioneuroblastoma that has been associated with systemic manifestations of the catecholamines or with increased urinary or plasma concentrations of the amines or metabolites.

The practical advantage gained by electron microscopy is that the characteristic intracellular findings allow the pathologist to decipher small round cell tumors in the nasal chamber.

Differential diagnosis may be difficult for the pathologist especially if the biopsy specimen is small, nonrepresentative and crushed. Small-celled sarcomas or carcinoma and lymphoma must be ruled out (Fig. 17.10). The course of the disease may extend over many years. *All* of the neoplasms have the potential for local invasion and intracranial extensions as well as systemic metastases, and almost all will invariably recur following inadequate local excision.

Hutter et al.[33] state that neither radical surgery nor irradiation, or a combination of both, has been completely effective in controlling this disease. Further, there is no histological correlation with the clinical course after treatment and the cytological type gives no clue to the expected radiosensitivity or response to treatment. Skolnik et al.,[26]

after reviewing 97 cases, conclude that primary treatment should be surgical resection, with irradiation reserved for persistence, recurrences and metastases. Other prefer a combined initial attack. Data collected by Bailey and Barton[32] point to the latter. These authors relate a 5-year survival rate (cured or with disease) of 45% when treatment was surgery alone or radiation therapy alone. Patients treated by surgical excision of the lesion and irradiation manifested a 67% cure rate. It is to be emphasized that in many cases, the initial response to irradiation and/or surgical resection is excellent. However, after some years, the neoplasm recurs or metastasizes.

Local recurrences have occurred in nearly 50% of the patients. Distant metastases, while not rare, occur uncommonly (20%). Cervical lymph nodes and the lungs are most often the secondary site (Table 17.3, Fig. 17.12). Patients with local recurrences and metastases are noted to be quite susceptible to radiotherapy. Fifty of Skolink's 97 patients were followed-up for 5 years or longer; of these, 26 (52%) survived 5 years.[26] Eleven of these 26 subsequently died. In 45 patients reviewed of Bailey and Barton,[32] the leading cause of death was complications associated with metastases, distant metastases in 11 patients and massive cervical metastases in eight. Of the remaining patients,

Table 17.3
Metastases from Esthesioneuroblastoma*

Location of Metastases	No. of Cases
Cervical lymph nodes	19
Lungs and pleura	13
Long bones	7
Spleen	1
Spinal column	1
Breast	1
Adrenal glands	2
Local extension to brain	24

* Modified from Skolnik et al.[26] and Bailey and Barton[32] and Schenck and Ogura.[38]

nine died as a result of local extension of the neoplasm, often leading to excision of major vessels and nine died of intracranial extension of the tumor. Infections and other non-neoplastic causes accounted for the remainder of deaths.

PITUITARY TUMORS OF THE NASOPHARYNX AND THE NASAL CAVITY

Since the anterior pituitary arises from Rathke's pouch, which is an invagination from the primordium of the nasopharynx, so-called "misplacement" of cells is to be expected. The phenomenon occurs so often, in fact, that pharyngeal hypophysis or pharyngeal pituitary is an acceptable anatomical term.[39, 40] Developing from the proximal part of the hypophyseal duct, the pharyngeal hypophysis is a glandular body containing cells similar to the anterior pituitary or cells not unlike the nests of undifferentiated epithelial cells in the pars tuberalis. Human growth hormone, a prolactin-type factor, and thyrotrophic hormone have been demonstrated in the pharyngeal pituitary.[40]

McGrath,[40] after a survey of 133 pharyngeal hypophyses, stated that the maximum dimensions of the structures were: 9.6 mm long, 1.5 mm wide, 1.0 mm deep and 1.2 mm³ in volume. The pituitary tumor presents as an elongated body in the mucoperiosteum of the roof of the nasopharynx, with its long axis in the midsagittal plane. The anterior oblique part consists of a few columns of cells, which pass posteriorly and deeply from the epithelial surface through the mucous gland layer to expand into the larger horizontal part, which extends posteriorly in the periosteum covering the inferior surface of the body of the sphenoid. The pharyngeal hypophysis is usually asymptomatic. Cysts of the pharyngeal hypophysis are also asymptomatic. An excellent review of the pharyngeal hypophysis and its surgical significance has been presented by Richards and Evans.[41]

Chromophobe tumors found in the nasopharynx *may* be present there by two means: the first and much more likely is that the lesion represents a direct downward extension from the sella turcica; the other *possibility* is that the tumor arose from the pharyngeal pituitary itself. Pituitary adenomas which extend beyond their capsular limits and invade surrounding structures occur infrequently, and the accumulated data concerning their natural history are meager.

Jefferson,[42] in discussing extrasellar extensions of pituitary adenomas, listed the following possible pathways: hypothalamic, frontal, temporal, pharyngeal and posterior fossa. Pharyngeal extension is the most common and is represented by tumor growing downward by absorption of the sellar floor with rupture into the sphenoid sinus. The tumor may also erode into the nasopharynx and eventually into the nasal cavity. Invasion of the nasal cavity is, however, extremely rare.[43] Posterior subtentorial and frontal extension are the rarest forms of growth spread.

Invasion of the nasopharynx and the sinonasal cavities by a primary intracranial pituitary tumor always raises the question of "malignancy"; Jefferson[42] has outlined criteria for malignancy.

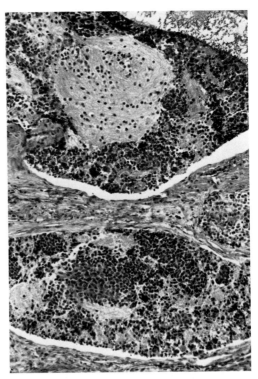

Figure 17.12. Metastatic esthesioneuroblastoma to a cervical lymph node. The microscopic appearance of the metastasis was no different than the primary.

These include: (1) short clinical history; (2) degree of extension and especially invasion of the cavernous sinus; (3) blood-borne metastases; and (4) histological anaplasia. Martins et al.[44] prefer to regard pituitary adenomas more simply as either noninvasive or invasive (extension beyond their capsules and invasion of contiguous structures) or as carcinomas, which are characterized by their ability to metastasize via the blood stream. Since the histological appearances can only rarely be equated with biological behavior, I prefer this characterization over Jefferson's.

Nasopharyngeal presentation of crainopharyngiomas is discussed by Illum et al.[45]

MENINGIOMAS

Meningiomas comprise 14% of all intracranial tumors. Extracranial and extraspinal meningiomas unassociated with a neuraxial lesion are rare; as of 1970, only 40 cases had been reported. This figure is said to be artificially high, since some of the reports concern extension of intracranial tumors and others represent "metastases" from malignant meningiomas. The most frequent sites in which extracranial meningiomas are found are the bones of the skull, the scalp, orbit, nose, paranasal sinuses and middle ear.[46-48] More rarely, extracranial meningiomas have occurred in the cheek and the deep tissues of the neck. One documented case of a meningioma of the parotid gland has been recorded.[49] An intraoral presentation of a meningioma is a medical oddity.

Hoye et al.[50] have classified the possible mechanisms of formation of extracranial meningiomas as follows: (1) primary intracranial meningiomas with direct extension outside of the skull; (2) meningiomas originating from arachnoid cells and accompanying nerve sheaths, such as orbital meningiomas, arising from optic nerve sheaths; (3) meningiomas with no demonstrable connection with a cranial nerve; (4) metastases from intracranial meningiomas.

While the juxtaposition of the nasal cavity and the prosencephalon during embryological development may account for the very rare *primary* intranasal meningiomas, the greatest number of "ectopic meningiomas" are explainable by extracranial arachnoid cell clusters. Schmidt[51] was the first to correct the misconception that the dura mater rather than the arachnoid was the tissue of origin of meningiomas. He described Pacchionian granulations capped by groups of solid cells, which sometimes penetrated the dura, followed blood vessels and pierced the outer dura; this was the route, according to Schmidt,[51] which would account for the occurrence of meningiomas in the skull bones. Cushing[52] next drew attention to the

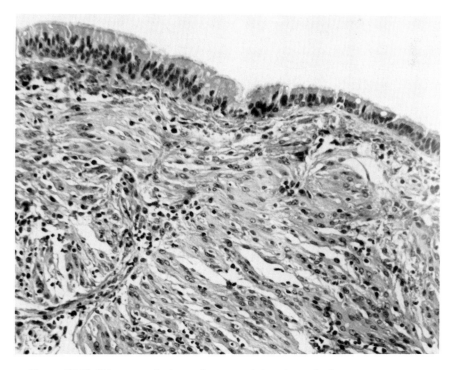

Figure 17.13. Primary meningioma of paranasal sinus beneath sinus mucosa.

fact that arachnoid cells could be found accompanying certain of the cranial nerves and, thus, could be present in the sheaths of the trigeminal nerve, optic nerve in the orbit, the olfactory groove of the ethmoid and the porus acousticus. These were regarded as potential sources of meningiomas. Aoyagi and Kyono[53] have shown that arachnoid cell clusters have a predilection for certain sites, such as the points of penetration of the dura by the third, seventh, ninth, tenth, eleventh and twelfth cranial nerves, and this has been related to the association of meningiomas to these nerves.

Many of the primary extracranial meningiomas relate to the foramina; those unrelated to the foramina still have a similar basic origin, i.e., segregated and displaced arachnoid cells.[54] If the primary orbital meningiomas are excluded, reports of extracranial meningiomas of other sites (not related to an intracranial meningioma) are extremely rare. Most are cutaneous and are confined to the head and neck or to the skin near the vertebral column.[55, 56]

Primary meningiomas of the nasal cavity (Fig. 17.13) and the paranasal sinuses are extremely rare; by 1970, only eight cases had been reported in the literature.[57] Furthermore, extension of an intracranial meningioma into the nasal cavity and paranasal sinuses is also rare. Primary orbital meningiomas may secondarily involve the ethmoid sinuses and nasal cavity.

INVASIVE RETINOBLASTOMA

Retinoblastomas also belong to the family of primitive neuroectodermal tumors. The incidence is high in infants, occurring once in every 23,000 to 34,000 births with a bilateral presentation in 25 to 50% of cases.[58]

Invasion of the extraorbital tissues by a retinoblastoma may require the care of an otolaryngologist, and the head and neck surgeon should be aware of the occasional "suspended viability" of the neoplastic retinoblastoma cells with apparent de novo growth in the antral and nasal vestibular areas.[59]

REFERENCES

1. Blumenfeld, R., and Skolnik, E. M.: Intranasal encephaloceles. Arch. Otolaryngol. 82:527, 1965.
2. New, G. B., and Devine, K. D.: Neurogenic tumors of the nose and throat. Arch. Otolaryngol. 46:163, 1947.
3. Strauss, R. B., Collicott, J. H., Jr., and Hargett, I. R.: Intranasal neuroglial heterotopia. So-called nasal glioma. Am. J. Dis. Child. 111:317, 1966.
4. Orkin, M., and Fisher, I.: Heterotopic brain tissue (heterotopic neural rest): case report with review of related anomalies. Arch Dermatol. 94:699, 1966.

5. Walker, E. A., Jr., and Resler, D. R.: Nasal glioma. Laryngoscope 73:93, 1963.
6. Lurie, H. I.: Congenital melanocarcinoma, melanotic adamatinoma, retinal anlage tumor, progonoma and pigmented epulis of infancy. Cancer 14:1090, 1961.
7. Kerr, D. A., and Pullon, P. A.: A study of the pigmented tumors of jaws of infants (melanotic ameloblastoma, retinal anlage tumor, progonoma). Oral Surg. 18:759, 1964.
8. Misugi, K., Okajima, H., Newton, W. A., Kmetz, D. R., and deLorimier, A. A.: Mediastinal origin of a melanotic progonoma or retinal anlage tumor: ultrastructural evidence for neural crest origin. Cancer 18:477, 1965.
9. Borello, E. D., and Gorlin, R. J.: Melanotic neuroectodermal tumor of infancy—a neoplasm of neural crest origin: report of a case associated with high excretion of vanilmandelic acid. Cancer 19:196, 1966.
10. Stowens, D., and Lin, T.-H.: Melanotic progonoma of the brain. Hum. Pathol. 5:105, 1974.
11. Karma, P., Rasanen, O., and Karja, J.: Melanotic neuroectodermal tumour of infancy. J. Laryngol. 91:973, 1977.
12. Brekke, J. H., and Gorlin, R. J.: Melanotic neuroectodermal tumor of infancy. J. Oral Surg. 33:858, 1975.
13. Beckwith, J. B., and Martin, R. F.: Observation on the histopathology of neuroblastoma (Conference on biology of neuroblastoma). J. Pediatr. Surg. 3:106, 1968.
14. deLorimier, A. A., Bragg, K. U., and Linden, G.: Neuroblastoma in childhood. Am. J. Dis. Child. 118:441, 1969.
15. Snyder, M. B., and Cawson, R. A.: Jaw and pulpal metastasis of an adrenal neuroblastoma. Oral Surg. 40:775, 1975.
16. Young, L. W., Rubin, P., and Hanson, R. E.: The extraadrenal neuroblastoma: high radiocurability and diagnostic accuracy. Am. J. Roentgenol. Radium Ther. Nucl. Med. 108:75, 1970.
17. Dawson, D. A.: Nerve cell tumours of the neck and their secretory activity. J. Laryngol. Otol. 84:203, 1970.
18. Koop, C. E., and Hernandez, R.: Neuroblastoma: experience with 100 cases in children. Surgery 56:726, 1964.
19. Perez, C. A., Vietti, T. J., Ackerman, L. V., Kulapongs, P., and Powers, W. E.: The treatment of malignant sympathetic tumors in children: clinico-pathological correlation. Pediatrics 41:452, 1968.
20. Bodian, M.: Neuroblastoma. Pediatr. Clin. North Am. 6:449, 1959.
21. Fortner, J., Nicastri, A., and Murphey, M. L.: Neuroblastoma: natural history and results of treating 133 cases. Ann. Surg. 167:132, 1968.
22. King, R. L., Stornasli, J. P., and Bolande, R. P.: Neuroblastoma: review of 28 cases and presentation of two cases with metastases and long survival. Am. J. Roentgenol. Radium Ther. Nucl. Med. 85:733, 1961.
23. Koop, C. E.: The role of surgery in resectable, non-resectable and metastatic neuroblastoma. J.A.M.A. 205:157, 1968.
24. Phillips, R.: Neuroblastoma. Ann. R. Coll. Surg. Engl. 12:27, 1953.
25. Berger, L., Luc, and Richard: L'esthesioneuroepitheliome olfactif. Bull. Assoc. Fr. Etude Cancer 13:410, 1924.
26. Skolnik, E. M., Massari, F. S., and Tenta, L. T.: Olfactory neuroepithelioma: review of world literature and presentation of two cases. Arch. Otolaryngol. 84:644, 1966.
27. Aldave, A., and Gallager, H. S.: Olfactory Esthesioneuroepithelioma: report of a case and review of the literature. Arch. Pathol. 67:43, 1959.
28. Naessen, R.: An enquiry on the morphological characteristics and possible changes with age in the olfactory region of man. Acta Otolaryngol. 71:49, 1971.
29. Naessen, R.: The identification and topographical localisation of the olfactory epithelium of man and other mammals. Acta Otolaryngol. 70:51, 1970.
30. Naessen, R.: The "receptor surface" of the olfactory organ (epithelium) of man and guinea-pig. Acta Otolaryngol. 71:335, 1971.
31. Ciges, M., Labella, T., Gayoso, M., and Sanchez, G.: Ultrastructure of the organ of Jacobson and comparative study with olfactory mucosa. Acta Otolaryngol. 71:335, 1971.

32. Bailey, B. J., and Barton, S.: Olfactory neuroblastoma. Management and prognosis. Arch. Otolaryngol. 101:1, 1975.
33. Hutter, R. V. P., Lewis, J. S., Foote, F. W., Jr., and Tollefsen, H. R.: Esthesioneuroblastoma: a clinical and pathological study. Am. J. Surg. 106:748, 1963.
34. Taxy, J. B., and Hidvegi, D. F.: Olfactory neuroblastoma. An ultrastructural study. Cancer 39:131, 1977.
35. Osamura, R. Y., and Fine, G.: Ultrastructure of the esthesioneuroblastoma. Cancer 38:173, 1976.
36. Kahn, L. B.: Esthesioneuroblastoma: a light and electron microscopic study. Hum. Pathol. 5:364, 1974.
37. Wilander, E., Nordlinger, H., Grimelius, L., Larsson, L.-I., and Angelborg, C.: Esthesioneuroblastoma. Histological, histochemical and electron microscopic studies of a case. Virchows Arch. (Pathol. Anat.) 375:123, 1977.
38. Schenk, N. L., and Ogura, J. H.: Esthesioneuroblastoma. An enigma in diagnosis, a dilemma in treatment. Arch. Otolaryngol. 96:322, 1972.
39. Melchionna, R. H., and Moore, R. A.: The pharyngeal pituitary gland. Am. J. Pathol. 14:772, 1938.
40. McGrath, P.: Cysts of sellar and pharyngeal hypophyses. Pathology 3:123, 1972.
41. Richards, S. H., and Evans, I. T. G.: The pharyngeal hypophysis and its surgical significance. J. Laryngol. 88:937, 1974.
42. Jefferson, G.: Extrasellar extensions of pituitary adenomas. Proc. R. Soc. Med. 33:433, 1940.
43. Sadick, M. K., Nagori, M. A., and Jafarey, N. A.: Chromophobe adenoma of the pituitary gland masquerading as bilateral nasal polypi; report of a case. J. Laryngol. 88:169, 1974.
44. Martins, A. N., Hayes, G. J., and Kempe, L. G.: Invasive pituitary adenomas. J. Neurosurg. 22:268, 1965.
45. Illum, P., Elbrond, O., and Nehen, A. M.: Surgical treatment of nasopharyngeal craniopharyngioma. Radical removal by the transpalatal approach. J. Laryngol. 91:227, 1977.
46. Shvangshoti, S., Nesky, M. G., and Fitz-Hugh, G. S.: Parapharyngeal meningioma with special reference to cell of origin. Ann. Otol. 80:464, 1971.
47. Whicker, J. H., Devine, K. D., and MacCarty, C. S.: Diagnostic and therapeutic problems in extracranial meningiomas. Am. J. Surg. 126:452, 1973.
48. Guzowski, J., Paparella, M. M., Rao, K. M., and Hoshino, T.: Meningiomas of the temporal bone. Laryngoscope 86:1141, 1976.
49. Wolff, M., and Rankow, R. M.: Meningioma of the parotid gland: an insight into the pathogenesis of extracranial meningiomas. Hum. Pathol. 2:453, 1971.
50. Hoye, S. J., Hoar, C. S., and Murray, J. E.: Extracranial meningiomas presenting as a tumor of the neck. Am. J. Surg. 100:486, 1960.
51. Schmidt, M. N.: Ueber die Pacchionischen Granulationen und ihr Verhaeltnis zu den Sarcomen und Psammoma der Dura Mater. Virchows Arch. (Pathol. Anat.) 170:429, 1902.
52. Cushing, H.: The meningiomas (dural endothelioma). Their source and favoured seats of origin. Brain 45:282, 1922.
53. Aoyagi, U., and Kyuno, Y.: Ueter die endothelien Zellsapfen in der Dura mater cerebic, and ihre Lokalisation in derselben. Neuroglia 2:1, 1912.
54. Lindstrom, C. G., and Lindstrom, D. W.: On extracranial meningioma: case of primary meningioma of nasal cavity. Acta Otolaryngol. 68:451, 1969.
55. Suzuki, H., Gilbert, E. F., and Zimmerman, B.: Primary extracranial meningioma. Arch. Pathol. 84:202, 1967.
56. Lopez, D. A., Silvers, D. N., and Helwig, E. B.: Cutaneous meningiomas—a clinicopathologic study. Cancer 34:728, 1974.
57. Majoros, M.: Meningioma of the paranasal sinuses. Laryngoscope 80:640, 1970.
58. Reese, A. B.: Tumors of the Eye. Paul B. Hoeber and Sons, Inc., Medical Division, Harper and Rowe Publishers, New York, 1963.
59. Jafek, B. W., Linford, R., and Foos, R. Y.: Late recurrent retinoblastoma in the nasal vestibule. Arch. Otolaryngol. 94:264, 1971.

CHAPTER 18

Soft Tissue Tumors of the Head and Neck: Unusual Forms

The preceding chapters have considered the more commonly encountered supporting tissue tumors in the head and neck. In this chapter I present a clinical and pathological correlation of the unusual forms of soft tissue neoplasms as they present in the head and neck. These include chordomas, neoplasms of smooth muscle, synovial sarcomas, myxomas, tumors of fibroadipose tissue, extraosseous chondromatous and osteogenic neoplasms and alveolar soft part sarcomas.

CHORDOMA

Chordomas are dysontogenetic neoplasms that arise in residual or vestigial remnants of the embryonic notochord. Based on their anatomical predilection, there are three major groups: cranial or spheno-occipital, vertebral and sacrococcygeal. A rarely occurring fourth "dental" subgroup includes maxillary and mandibular chordomas.

More than one-third of chordomas occur at the base of the skull, the majority of these arising from the clivus in the region of the spheno-occipital synchondrosis.[1] Typical ventral extension of these neoplasms is in the direction of the nasopharynx and, occasionally, into the nasal cavity or maxillary antrum.[2] It is this group and those from the cervical region of the vertebrae that hold interest for the head and neck surgeon (Fig. 18.1). The latter appear to have a predilection for the second and third cervical vertebrae. Reference to the topographical relationship between the notochord, the base of the skull and the adjacent parts of the vertebral column in the human embryo assists in an explanation of these unique neoplasms (Fig. 18.2).

Binkhorst et al.[3] have indicated *seven* points of origin of a chordoma in the craniocervical region: dorsum sellae, Blumenbach's clivus, retropharyn-geal notochord vestiges, remnants in the apical ligament of the dens, nuclei pulpose of cervical vertebrae, vestiges in the squama occipitalis and ectopic localizations such as the mandible or frontal sinuses.

Early in the third week of intrauterine life, the notochordal plate develops cranial to the primitive streak. During the fifth week, the notochord becomes enclosed within the bodies of the primitive vertebrae, passing through the mesenchyme which will form the bodies of the atlas and adontoid process, and then enters the basiocciput. Passing through this structure for a short distance, it comes to lie directly in contact with the entoderm of the primitive pharynx. The bar of developing notochord cannot proceed in a cranial direction further than Rathke's pouch, so it comes to lie within the body of the sphenoid, terminating caudal to the pituitary fossa and reaching as far as the dura. As the vertebral column develops, the notochordal bar becomes divided into segments and normally disappears as an integral entity except for its representation as the nucleus pulposus.

During the eighth week of embryonic development, myotomes and sclerotomes undergo descent and fusion to form permanent structures such as the musculature of the tongue and precursors of the basiocciput and basisphenoid. The dermatomes of this region degenerate. At this stage of relative upheaval, it is certainly plausible that small derivatives of the disintegrating notochord become separated from the true notochord to form ectopic rests.[4] In the cervical, thoracic and lumbar regions of the vertebral column, there is not the same degree of developmental activity or degeneration. Thus, chordal ectopia is less likely to be found.

Notochordal remnants or rests have been demonstrated in the region of the clivus, submucosa of the nasopharynx and pharynx, bodies of cervical

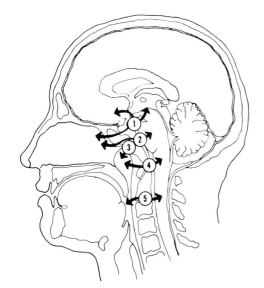

Figure 18.1. Cranial-cervical chordomas. *Arrows* indicate potential directions of growth and eventual clinical presentation.

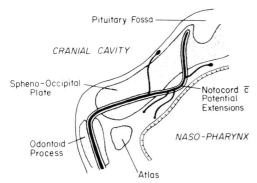

Figure 18.2. Schematic outline of the relations of the primitive notochord to adjacent structures.

vertebrae and elsewhere. This topographical distribution corresponds closely to the sites of occurrence of chordomas. It is most likely that the neoplasms arise from *detached* remnants of the notochord and not from the original rod of notochord or its adult vestiges of the nuclei pulposi.[5]

Chordomas may occur at any age. According to Mabrey,[1] the greatest number of cranial and vertebral chordomas occur in patients between 20 and 40 years of age. This contrasts with a peak age period of 40 to 60 years for the sacrococcygeal neoplasms. The lesions are said to occur more often in males than females. This sex predominance is best seen in the sacrococcygeal group and then declines, in order of frequency, in vertebral and cranial groups.

Most of the craniocervical chordomas described in the literature and in our own series[2] present with a more or less characteristic neuro-ophthalmological and otological symptom pattern with involvement of cranial nerves. Givner,[6] in a review of chordomas of the clivus, stressed the ophthalmological signs and symptoms. In fact, the prominence of such complaints often first leads the patient to seek the aid of an ophthalmologist. Headache, often localized to the fronto-orbital area, is almost constant. Visual disturbances (loss of acuity, diplopia, limitation of visual fields), accomplished by paralysis of eye muscles and ptosis, are commonplace. With progression of the lesion, there is usually involvement of the trigeminal, facial and acoustic nerves. If there is concomitant intracranial extension, hypophyseal and bulbar-pontine signs and symptoms may supervene. There is a tendency for the involvement of cranial nerves to be unilateral and, most often, on the left side. The abducens nerve is involved in at least one-half of cranial cases. Rhino-otological phenomena consist of nasal obstruction, sense of fullness, loss of hearing, aproxia and anosmia, usually in that order of frequency. Secondary infection leads to purulent discharge and rarely epistaxis.

Chordomas presenting in the nasopharynx may have no extension outside this region and may be primary nasopharyngeal tumors, but these are uncommon. It is more likely that they are a downward extension from a cranio-occipital tumor or an upward extension of a high cervical tumor. The clinical presentation of a true cervical chordoma differs somewhat from cranio-occipital growths, as their presence is often overlooked by the patient due to their slow development. Pain is an early symptom, particularly in chordomas developing laterally or posteriorly to the vertebral bodies, giving rise to pressure symptoms from involvement of the spinal cord or nerve roots.

Cervical chordomas that protrude into the pharynx or displace the esophagus or larynx are accompanied by dysphagia or hoarseness and dyspnea. Pharyngeal masses are usually covered with an intact and nonulcerated mucosa.

The outstanding radiographic finding of the anterior and ventrally presenting cervical chordomas are extensive destruction of bone and nasopharyngeal soft tissue masses.[2] These findings, alone or together, are not diagnostic but, when coupled with the clinical history and an otorhinological examination, should lead the examiner toward the proper interpretation. Osseous changes have been observed in as many as 75% of cases.

The amount of destruction of bone produced by the neoplasm is variable and is dependent upon the site of origin and subsequent direction of extension. Stereoscopic submental-vertex (base) projection permits the best evaluation of destruction of bone in the basisphenoid and basioccipital area. Lateral planograms not only aid in the evaluation of bone destruction but also serve to delineate nasopharyngeal extension. Stereoscopic lateral projections show the nasal and nasopharyngeal masses to best advantage and are the most valuable projection for evaluation of the nature and extent of destruction of the sella, dorsum, clinoid processes and clivus. Calcification within the tumor has been described.

Pathological Features

Chordal remnants are rarely missing in the adult, being found in the nuclei pulposi, between the odontoid process of the axis and the occipital bone, in the clivus, dorsum sellae and retropharynx. Congdon[7] classified as benign those "chordomas" found only at the time of necropsy and regarded them as "curiosities" of no clinical importance. Stewart and Morin's[8] designation, "ecchordosis physaliphora," is more appropriate than "benign" chordoma, since it serves to separate these choristomas from the true neoplasm, chordoma.

The typical chordoma is a lobulated, partially translucent, mucoid tumor. The mass is unencapsulated or has a pseudocapsule, and it invades bone and/or dura with facility. Hemorrhagic foci may convert the lobules into currant-jelly masses.

There has not been a case reported of total removal of an intracranial chordoma. The tumor tends to surround nerves and vessels completely rather than push them aside. The softer portions yield to suction easily; other parts, more vascular and solid, are not amenable to this form of removal. Craniocervical tumors are midline and extend up into the base of the brain and/or down into the sphenoid sinus or into the nasopharynx. In the vertebral region, the chordoma infiltrates the vertebral bodies and grows anteriorly into the paraspinal tissues or posteriorly to surround the cord, resembling a metastasis. Once within the spinal canal, growth up or down the canal may occur.

There are no absolute or specific histological features in chordomas. Four findings are, however, fairly constant[9]: (1) an over-all lobular arrangement of cells in the tumor; (2) a tendency of the cells to grow in cords, irregular bands, or in a pseudoacinar form; (3) production of an abundant intercellular mucinous matrix; and, most characteristically, (4) the presence of large physaliphorous and vacuolated cells.

Each tumor is capable of wide structural variation within itself. This is to be emphasized, as it is especially pertinent in the biopsy diagnosis. The least variable morphological finding is the basic architectural pattern of a lobular or nodular aggregation of the neoplastic cells. Incomplete fibrous trabeculae, continuous with compressed peripheral connective tissue, traverse the intercellular matrix and further subdivide the lobules (Fig. 18.3). Cellularity and cytomorphology vary according to the size, age and location of the lobule. Infiltrative or peripheral lobules or nodules have a less mucoid matrix, better formed cells and less intracellular vacuolation than do the cells in the deeper parts of the neoplasm.

The primary cells are oval or polygonal and are often closely apposed to one another, appearing epitheloid. Their cytoplasm is eosinophilic and granular or homogenous. Early vacuolar change may be seen in this cytoplasm (Fig. 18.4). Vacuolation is a continuous process in the life span of the cells and may be equated to an aging process, since stages can be followed from cell to cell until

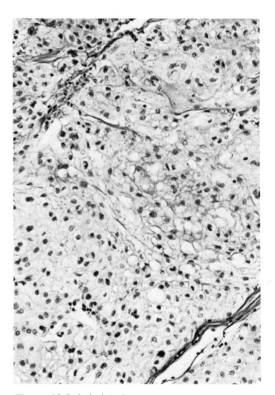

Figure 18.3. Lobulated appearance of the chordoma is imparted by fine connective tissue septae.

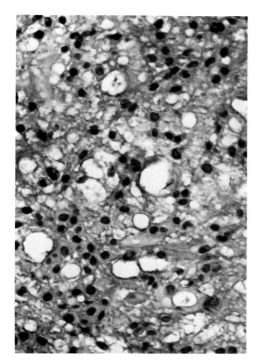

Figure 18.4. Beginning vacuolization in the basic polyhedral and eosinophilic chordoma cell.

the typical physaliphorous cell is achieved. Further progression of vacuolation eventually produces a highly vacuolated syncytium in which cell outlines are destroyed (Fig. 18.5).

The histopathological appearance of the neoplasm is, as can be seen, subject to a variation intrinsic to the neoplasm. This variability is compounded when interpretation of biopsy is attempted. The lesions most often confused with chordoma are the chondromatous neoplasms, mucin-forming carcinoma and benign mucinous processes in the paranasal sinuses such as mucocele. In some areas, principally the older parts of a chordoma, the cells tend to become fusiform or stellate and are often set in a parvicellular matrix. Biopsy from such an area may lead to an erroneous diagnosis of chondrosarcoma. Crawford,[10] in a histochemical study, differentiated chordoma from chondrosarcoma on the basis of *absence* of staining of the ground substance in the former with phosphotungstic acid-hematoxylin and reticulin stains. While my own experience is limited, I have not found these techniques to be very helpful. Other histochemical staining reactions, although of histogenetic importance, offer little assistance. In two personal cases, multiple recurrences have produced tumors indistinguishable from chondrosarcomas. Pena et al.[11] have presented ultrastructural

details of two chordomas, essentially confirming information already deduced by light microscopic and experimental studies.

The ultimate outlook of cases of chordoma is uniformly poor, but many are of slow growth and patients can survive for many years. Their slow, yet obstinately progressive, growth with infiltrative destruction of bone and an almost *inevitable recurrence* after attempted extirpation accounts for the glum prognosis. Even where complete surgical removal of cranial cases appears to have been accomplished or where the disease has been apparently arrested by radiotherapy, there may be a recurrence.

The location and relative inacessibility of the neoplasm in most of the head and neck area makes complete removal almost impossible. The experience of Dahlin and MacCarty[12] is fairly representative. Only two of their 15 patients survived longer than 5 years; one remarkable patient living 18.7 years after subtotal excision and radiation therapy.

The treatment of chrodomas has been unsatisfactory because of the high rate of local recurrence

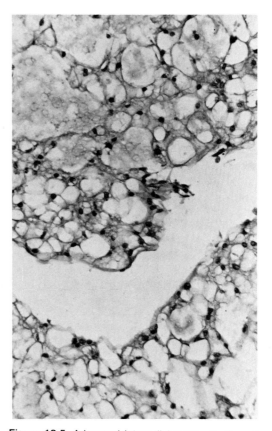

Figure 18.5. Advanced intracellular vacuolization of cells in a chordoma.

after surgical excision. In addition, chordomas are radioresistant and large doses are necessary to achieve tumor control. In the craniocervical region, the surgical treatment hopes to remove as much of the neoplasm as possible. The relative inaccessibility, proximity of the spinal cord, advanced stage of the disease, and possibility of multicentricity make complete removal hazardous and usually impossible. Since it is rare that complete excision of the tumor is achieved, surgery is followed by irradiation of the tumor bed and tumor doses is the range of 7,000 rads in 6 to 7 weeks.[13] Irradiation although not curative, offers the patient significant palliation and regression.

Heffelfinger et al.[14] and Richter et al.,[15] have described a clinicopathological variant termed *chondroid chordoma*. These tumors, occurring at the base of the skull, are associated with a suprisingly better prognosis than the classic nonchondroid chordoma. The chondroid chordoma may contain such an abundant cartilaginous component that a diagnosis of chondroma or chondrosarcoma is suggested or even made (Fig. 18.6). More often there seems to be an admixture of chondroid and chordoma elements that range from small scattered areas of hyaline cartilage in a chordoma background to the reverse in which the chondroid components dominate. Merger between typical chordoma and cartilage should be looked for.

The study by Heffelfinger et al.[14] suggests a considerable difference between the typical spheno-occipital chordomas and the chondroid chordomas; an average survival for 19 patients with chondroid chordomas of 15.8 years as compared to 4.1 years for 36 patients with typical chordoma.

Metastases from craniocervical chordomas are rare.

NEOPLASMS OF SMOOTH MUSCLE

Tumors of smooth muscle origin may occur anywhere in the human body where smooth muscle is present. They occur with a significant frequency in the alimentary tract but are decidedly unusual in the oral cavity, pharynx and upper respiratory tract. Reasons for this low incidence are related to the paucity of significant masses of smooth muscle in these structures.

To account for origin of smooth muscle tumors in areas normally deficient in smooth muscle, three explanations have been given: (1) origin from aberrant undifferentiated mesenchyme; (2) origin from smooth muscle elements in the walls of blood vessels; (3) origin from both sources.

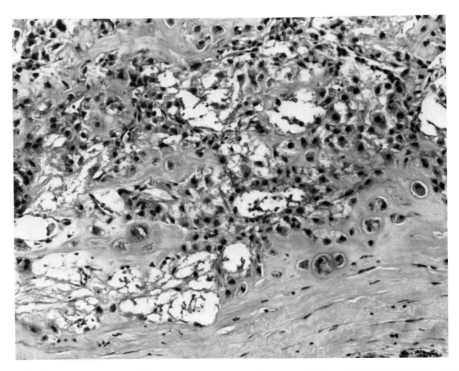

Figure 18.6. Chondroid chordoma. This section presents a mixture of cartilaginous and chordomatous elements.

With respect to the superficial soft tissues, the head and neck area is not an uncommon site for both benign and malignant variants of smooth muscle neoplasms. Approximately 25% of the large series of *superficial soft tissue leiomyosarcomas* reported by Stout and Hill[16] were from this anatomical region (Table 18.1). Leiomyomas of the skin and superficial soft tissues are unlikely to pose any problems to the head and neck surgeons. Almost all superficial soft part leiomyomas are found in the skin. They may extend into the subcutaneum but are rarely confined to it. They are always circumscribed and often encapsulated. They may be multiple or single; if multiple, they are generally small and superficial. Solitary types may involve the mouth secondarily. Sites of origin are the arrectores pilorum muscles and the muscular coats of vessels. Stout[17] considered the musculi cutis diagonales in the cheek as a likely source of some of these tumors.

In contradistinction to the superficial leiomyoma, leiomyosarcomas of the superficial soft tissues develop in the subcutaneum and only secondarily involve the corium. Many of them have the deceptive characteristic of being able to be "shelled out." There is an over-all recurrence rate of 60 to 72%. Stout and Hill's[16] cases manifested either recurrence or metastases or both.

Occasionally a leiomyosarcoma of venous origin (jugular vein) may present in the neck. Unlike leiomyosarcomas of the gastrointestinal tract, those of the superficial soft tissues do not manifest much necrosis or hemorrhage.

Microscopically, leiomyomas are differentiated tumors composed of smooth muscle cells. These cells grow in winding bands or cords that tend to interlace (Fig. 18.7). The nuclei are blunt-ended, and intracellular myofibrils can be found with

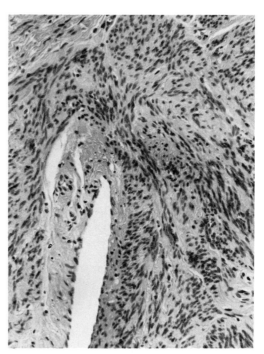

Figure 18.7. Vascular leiomyoma of the oral cavity. Note the palisading of blunt nuclei about the blood vessel.

ease. Nuclei of the cells tend to palisade. Many (approximately one-half) are markedly vascular (vide infra). Bizarre cell forms may be found in random areas.

Leiomyosarcomas resemble the benign version but with very important differences.[16] Features of malignancy are size of the neoplasm and the number of mitoses per high-power field. Malignant smooth muscle neoplasms of the superficial soft parts are usually larger than 2.5 cm in diameter. A smooth muscle neoplasm with no mitoses in 50 or more high-power fields is very likely benign, whereas one with one or more mitoses in every five high-power fields is almost certainly malignant (Fig. 18.8). Certain malignancy is present when there is one or more mitosis per high-power field. Other criteria are anaplasia and bizarre cell forms, less obvious nuclear palisading and inconspicuous myofibrils.

Compared to the superficial soft tissues of the head and neck, the oral cavity and upper respiratory tract are unusual sites of origin for smooth muscle neoplasms. Stout[17, 18] was the first American author to describe a leiomyoma of the oral cavity (five other cases had preceded his report but were in the foreign literature). Since then only occasional reports of benign smooth muscle tu-

Table 18.1
Geographic Distribution of Smooth Muscle Neoplasms of the Superficial Soft Tissues*
Only the lower extremities exceed the head and neck as an area for origin of leiomyosarcomas of the superficial soft tissues.

Anatomical Site	Leiomyoma	Leiomyosarcoma
	no. of cases	
Head and neck	21	9
Scalp	2	3
Neck	8	3
Face	11	3
Trunk	26	6
Upper extremity	35	5
Lower extremity	86	16

* Modified from Stout and Hill.[16]

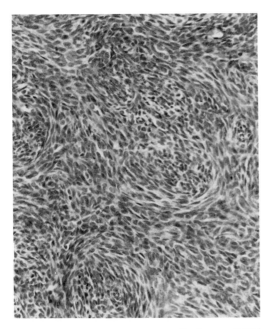

Figure 18.8. Leiomyosarcoma manifesting scattered mitoses and considerable cellularity.

mors in this region have been reported.[19, 20] There is little smooth muscle present in the oral cavity proper. The walls of blood vessels are the largest single source, with the circumvallate papillae and heterotopic smooth muscle representing other potential sources.

Duhig and Ayer[21] have presented an interesting theory of histogenesis. They postulate a progressive development of smooth muscle tumors, beginning with a hemangioma→angioma with much nonstriated muscle→vascular leiomyoma→ leiomyoma with many vessels→solid, relatively avascular leiomyoma. They consider that the vascular leiomyoma may represent only one stage in a continuous process of smooth muscle proliferation and that an appreciable number may not be true neoplasms but merely vascular malformations. If this hypothesis is acceptable, then all "leiomyomas" of the oral cavity proper, but not necessarily of the lips and cheeks, may be of vascular derivation.

By 1977, 51 cases of oral leiomyomas had been reported in the literature.[22, 23] The tongue was the most common site and was followed by the cheeks, palate, lips and gingivae. Their rarity is not due to histological misdiagnosis, but rather to the paucity of smooth muscle in this region. Farman[23] found only five oral cases among 7,748 benign smooth-muscle tumors of the whole body. Most have been superficial, and many have been pedunculated. Lack of pain, unless ulcerated (rare), is an almost constant clinical picture. The leiomyomas of the lips and cheek are generally encapsulated. There is a wide age range, with patients presenting with this tumor in the oral cavity at ages 4½ years to 76 years. There is a slight female predominance.

Leiomyosarcomas have been reported in the cheek, tongue, palate, floor of mouth, gingivae and mandible. Twelve examples had been recorded by 1977.[22] The age range of patients in whom oral leiomyosarcomas were discovered has been 11 months to 88 years. Where information is available, leiomyosarcomas of this region appear to be life-consuming lesions in nearly one-half of the patients. Central (intraosseous) smooth muscle tumors are extremely rare.[24]

The nasal cavity and paranasal sinuses are particularly unusual sites for a leiomyoma. Fu and Perzin[25] added a single case to the other one they could find in the literature.

Leiomyosarcomas are more common but still represent oddities in the upper respiratory tract. Between 1958 and 1976 only 15 cases had been recorded.[26] Of these, nearly three-fourths of the patients manifested recurrences; one-third had evidence of metastases; and approximately one-half of the patients died of their disease. It is to emphasized, however, that the potential of smooth muscle tumors to metastasize cannot always be ascertained histologically. The histological degree of differentiation may be misleading insofar as behavior is concerned. The pharynx shares the low incidence of leiomyosarcomas. Glover and Park[27] reported the third case in 1971.

The great vessels may occasionally be the origin of a leiomyosarcoma in the head and neck. Five such examples have involved the internal jugular vein.[28] To date, none of the large arteries in the head and neck have been the site of a leiomyosarcoma.

Stout's leiomyoblastoma, despite its predilection for the gastrointestinal tract, may very unusually be found in the region of the mouth.[29]

SYNOVIAL SARCOMA (MALIGNANT SYNOVIOMA)

Synovial sarcomas comprise between 8 and 10% of all malignant neoplasms of the somatic soft tissues and are said to be the most common sarcomas of the hands and feet. They are usually found adjacent to articular surfaces or, rarely, in extra-articular sites originating from bursae or tendon sheaths. Primary synovial sarcomas of an area other than the extremities are rare, but they have been reported from the abdominal and chest walls, lower back and the neck.

In 1967, Batsakis et al.,[30] after a review of the literature, accepted only seven cases of primary synovial sarcoma of the neck and added one additional case. Since that time, the lesion has been increasingly recognized so that at this writing over 50 cases have been reported.[31, 32]

In the evolution of synovium, the progenitor mesenchyme differentiates into two compartments, an inner synovial layer and an outer connective tissue layer. Electron microscopy indicates that the cells of both layers are of the same type without a basement membrane separating them. On the basis of tissue culture studies, it has been established that the synovial cell is distinct from the fibroblast *but*, nevertheless, is capable of assuming either cell form. The synovial cell is also capable of assuming diverse shapes; spindle, stellate or "epithelioid" forms. In keeping with the pluripotentiality of mesenchyme, it may then be concluded that the synovial membrane is composed of two interchangeable cell types.

Particularly germane to synovial sarcomas arising in the head and neck is the fact that most synoviomas do not arise from formed adult synovial membranes, and primary involvement of a joint cavity is infrequent. The neoplasm is identifiable as being of synovial origin because of its peculiar mode of differentiation toward that of the non-neoplastic synovial membrane.

Synovioblastic tissue is not plentiful in the head and neck and clearly is not normally present in the retropharyngeal region where many of the head and neck synovial sarcomas appear to have taken their origin. The neck contains synovial tissues not only in the tendinous portions of the cervical muscles but also in the anterior portion of the larynx and pharynx (bursa subhyoidea, bursa laryngaea subcutanea). Clearly these sources cannot be implicated in all cases and it is more likely that most of the sarcomas arise from synovioblastic differentiation of mesenchymal tissues.[33, 34] Recognizing this potential of primitive mesenchyme, Hajdu et al.[35] have proposed a unicellular concept of origin for the tendosynovial sarcomas. (Fig. 18.9).

The exact anatomical site of origin has been difficult to define from a review of reported cases. The parapharyngeal area (retropharynx and hypopharynx) appears to be most often cited. This region is followed by "neck," particularly the anterior neck, around the sternoclavicular and temporomandibular joints, cheeks and tongue. In the latter, the bursa of Boyer and the thyrohyoid ligament have been implicated.

The chief complaint associated with synovial sarcomas of the neck is that of a mass. The neoplasms have been either rather high in the neck, usually palpable beneath the jaws, or lower, near the supraclavicular fossae. Some patients complain of pain or tenderness related to the tumor. This is in accordance with an observed incidence of 40% for these symptoms in synovial sarcomas located elsewhere in the body. Other symptoms relate to the location of the tumor. One-third of the patients in the Armed Forces Institute of Pathology (AFIP) series (retropharyngeal) presented with complaints of hoarseness, dyspnea and dysphagia.[32]

The correct diagnosis preoperatively and at surgery is impossible. Metastasis from a thyroid carcinoma is a very likely preoperative impression and may mislead the pathologist, who, impressed by the acinar arrangement of the epithelial-like components of synovial sarcoma, may consider the lesion also as a metastasis from the thyroid gland. The occasional presence of calcospherite-like bodies in synovial sarcomas does not help matters.

There are no distinctive gross findings. The neoplasm is usually circumscribed and gray or pink. Foci of hemorrhage, necrosis or calcification may be present. Some tumors may have a mucoid or gelatinous consistency in areas. Microcystic areas may be evident. A slightly fibrous, finely whorled pattern, accentuated after formalin fixation, may predominate. The size of the neoplasms has ranged from 1 to 10 cm with a median of 5 cm.

Electron microscopic study clearly supports the synovioblastic origins of these tumors and also indicates there is no difference in the neoplasms regardless of site of origin. All studies identify distinct basal lamina between "epithelial" and stromal components of the tumors, epithelioid type cells with multiple cell attachments (maculae adherens), microvilli, intercellular spaces, free ribosomes, arrays of endoplasmic reticulum a prominent Golgi apparatus, small vesicles, and fibro-

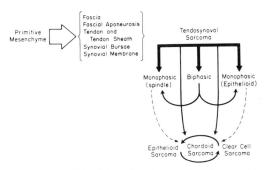

Figure 18.9. Unicellular origin theory of tendosynovial sarcoma as proposed by Hajdu et al.[35] (Modified with permission.)

blast-like cells with variable amounts of extracellular material and mature collagen.

Many of the characteristic histological and cytological features of the synovial membrane are
reproduced in synovial sarcomas. Important
among these features are the coexistence of syn-
ovial-like cells and fibrous connective tissue cells,
the pleomorphism of the former and their tendency to form and line spaces, clefts or crypts. The
"classical" synovial sarcoma manifests two neoplastic cellular components: a spindle cell (fibrosarcoma-like) component and a pseudoepithelioid
component. According to Mackenzie[34] this *biphasic* pattern is the only histological criterion by
which the diagnosis of synovial sarcoma can be
made with certainty (Figs. 18.10 and 18.11). On
occasion, a monophasic (spindle cell) form may be
encountered, and the diagnosis of fibrosarcoma
cannot be excluded. Diligent searching and multiple sections, however, will usually uncover the
cellular duality of the neoplasm.[37] The biphasic
pattern is accentuated by reticulin stains. The
pseudoglandular spaces contain a granular and

acidophilic material. The material is positive with
periodic acid-Schiff (PAS) stains, magenta with
AMP and alcian blue and pink with mucicarmine.
None of these reactions are abolished with pretreatment with testicular hyaluronidase. Hyaluronidase sensitive mucoid material is present in
the stroma surrounding the pseudoglandular
spaces. An ancillary histological feature is an
abundance of mast cells. These are particularly
found in well-differentiated biphasic tumors and
in fibrosarcomatous areas undergoing fibrosis.

A greater therapeutic experience and appropriate follow-up now allows a satisfactory appraisal
of the biological course of synovial sarcomas in
the head and neck. There is no proof that a
synovial sarcoma of the head and neck is less
aggressive than one in the extremity. Roth et al.[32]
report a 47% 5-year survival rate. This is little
different than survivals given by authors for peripheral synovial sarcomas.[38, 39] In the series of
Roth et al.,[32] 12 of 22 followed patients died with
their disease, 11 within a period of 1 to 8 years
after therapy. Ten of these patients had pulmonary

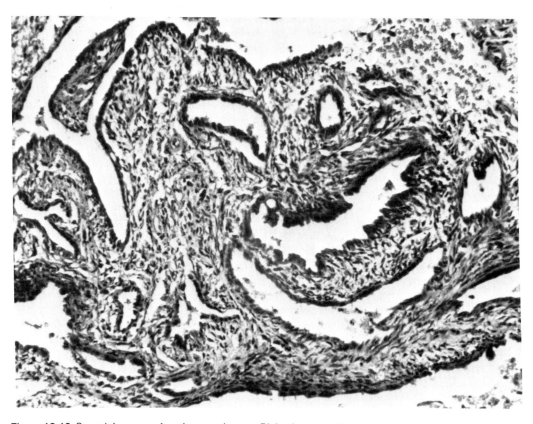

Figure 18.10. Synovial sarcoma from laryngopharynx. Biphasic pattern is apparent but clearly not as developed
as in the sarcoma presented in Figure 18.11.

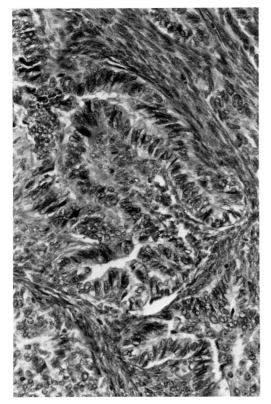

Figure 18.11. Cervical synovial sarcoma manifesting classic biphasic pattern.

metastases at the time of death. Cadman et al.,[38] studying peripheral synovial sarcomas, report that metastases occurred to the lungs in 81% of patients, regional lymph nodes in 23%, and the bones in 20%. Head and neck synovial sarcomas do not appear to share this tendency for regional lymph node and osseous metastases. It has been suggested that a biphasic pattern imparts a better prognosis than a predominantly monophasic or epithelial pattern. I am not of that conviction and consider the size of the tumor to be more pertinent. As far as therapy is concerned, there is no question that *early* radical excision is required. Lockey[31] further considers the best results are obtained by a planned combined surgical-radiotherapy program.

MYXOMA

There is considerable controversy and misunderstanding surrounding this peculiar and rare neoplasm. Because of this, I present, in paraphrase, Stout's criteria[40, 41] for diagnosis before discussing the clinicopathological aspects of this neoplasm: "The myxoma is a tumor composed of sometimes spindle-shaped cells set in a myxoid stroma containing mucopolysaccharide, through which course very delicate reticulin fibers in various directions. The tumor is poorly vascularized and the capillaries do not have the plexiform arrangement of embryonal lipoblastic tissue. Like any other soft tissue tumor, it may become fibrosed in some areas."

The true myxoma deviates from the appearance of the umbilical cord tissue *only* in that it may manifest some areas of secondary fibrosis. There are *no* other recognizable tissue elements in a myxoma, nor does the myxoma differentiate into any other variety of tissues. Any such elements mitigate against the diagnosis (Fig. 18.12).

Myxomas are benign, albeit agressive, neoplasms. The soft tissue myxomas reported to be malignant, in the sense of being capable of metastasis, are unrecognized liposarcomas, rhabdomyosarcomas, leiomyosarcomas, synovial sarcomas or malignant mesenchymomas. Cardiac "myxomas" are the only tumors given the name from which metastases have been reported.

Myxomas in the head and neck occur in the bones of the face and soft tissues and are considered as rare in either. Of the two locations, those in the jaws are the most prevalent. Elsewhere in this anatomical region, myxomas have occurred in the skin and subcutaneum, cheek, deep and aponeurotic tissues, parotid gland, larynx, tonsils and

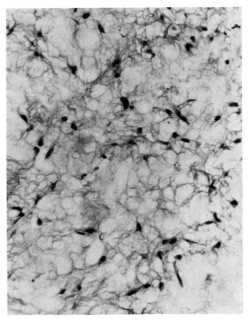

Figure 18.12. Parvicellular myxoma.

ear.[42, 43] The cutaneous myxoid cyst, although related to the myxoma, is considered to be a separate entity.[44]

Soft tissue myxomas may present from birth to old age. They are unusual in children under 16 years, but the behavior of the tumor in children is much like that manifested in the adult patient.[45] The gross appearance of a myxoma is fairly characteristic; slimy, mucoid and pallid, the gelatinous tissue varies from a soft to moderately firm consistency. This characteristic is dependent on the degree of secondary fibrosis in the tumor. They are poorly circumscribed and tend to infiltrate surrounding normal tissues. The aforementioned microscopic description by Stout[40, 41] certainly cannot be bettered and must be adhered to in order to correctly diagnose the lesion.

The usual growth history of a myxoma is slow and with expansive and insidious infiltration. Periods of accelerated growth may occur. It is important to emphasize that while the true myxoma does not metastasize, it can be a very destructive lesion if unchecked. In the head and neck the tumors are usually asymptomatic unless they compress adjacent structures. Recurrences are common except for the variant called "intramuscular myxoma."[46, 47]

Myxomas occurring in muscle (so-called intramuscular myxoma) warrant recognition as a special type of myxoma, according to Enzinger.[46] The head and neck area is a rare site of origin, with the muscles of the thigh being by far the most common single location. Although its basic histological structure is indistinguishable from that of myxomas occurring elsewhere, the tumor is apt to be confused with a "mucoid" sarcoma because of its deep location, infiltrative growth and myxomatous appearance. Distinction from myxoid liposarcoma is primarily based upon the rich vascular network of capillary-sized vessels and small embryonal cells of the liposarcoma (Fig. 18.13). Since liposarcomas are very unusual to rare in the head and neck, a more important differential diagnosis is botryoid embryonal rhabdomyosarcoma.

Radiation therapy is of little value for myxomas, and surgical removal is the accepted manner of treatment for both primary and recurrent lesions.

The interesting association of multiple soft tissue myxomas and fibrous dysplasia of bone has been recognized.[48] While there has been no more than circumstantial evidence to link the two disorders, the possibility of a basic metabolic error is to be considered.

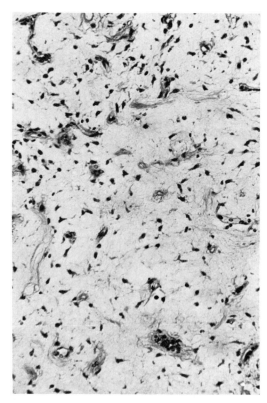

Figure 18.13. Myxoid liposarcoma. Compare the vascularity of the lesion to the relatively avascular myxoma.

TUMORS OF FAT

We have only incomplete knowledge of the histogenesis of normal fat cells. Most likely fat cells are not separate and unalterable cells, but rather their progenitors arose from a multipotential mesenchyme that is capable of simultaneous differentiation into various elements of connective tissue. The finding of fatty tissue from mutable connective tissue cells anywhere in the body and the highly variable cellular components that may constitute liposarcomas lend support to this concept.

Tumorous abnormalities of adipose tissue may occur in a number of forms: (1) lipoma; (2) liposarcoma; (3) lipogranulomatosis; (4) multiple diffuse lipomatosis; (5) multiple, multicentric lipoblastomatosis in association with syndromes, i.e., Gardner's syndrome; and (6) hibernoma.

Lipoma. This designation is used to describe an encapsulated, benign, subcutaneous and submucous tumor that causes little clinical concern. The term is also used to describe certain congenital or acquired lipomatoid masses that do not satisfy the definition of neoplasm. The diffuse "lipomas" in the neck in Madelung's disease can readily be excluded as not representing true neoplasms. In other instances, the distinction between benign neoplasia and malformation and/or hyperplasia may not be clear-cut, and some lipomatoid masses may pass for true neoplasms. Congenital "lipomas" in children may be either, while the majority of the solitary lipomas in adulthood are regarded as neoplasms.

Involvement of the head and neck, despite the general prevalence of lipomas, is relatively low in frequency. In this region, as elsewhere, the lipoma is primarily a neoplasm of the subcutaneum. In the deeper tissues, lipomas may be either inter- or intramuscular. The former is usually the case. Here, the lesion arises from intermuscular fascial septae and only secondarily infiltrates adjacent muscle.

While fat is normally abundant in the submucosa of the tongue, floor of mouth, palate, lip and buccal mucosa, it is of interest that only a fraction of the total numbers of lipomas have been reported from this region, and some of these may have been only lipomatoid masses. Lipomas make up between 1 and 2.2% of all benign neoplasms of the oral cavity. Hatziotis[49] has presented a complete review of lipomas of the oral cavity.

About one-half of the cases occur in the buccal mucosa of the cheek or the buccal sulcus. The tongue, floor of mouth and the lips are the next most frequent sites. In the oral regions lipomas present as painless masses that are soft, smooth and freely movable. They may be attached by a sessile stalk or a pedicle. Less often, deeper lipomas may extend subcutaneously and attain a large size so as to distort the face. The larynx is relatively immune to the presence of lipomas and, when they occur, they are most often in the extrinsic larynx.

In the remainder of the upper aerodigestive tract, the greater portion of all cases of lipomas originate in the hypopharynx with the lower pole of the tonsil, the hypopharyngeal wall and the arytenoepiglottic fold being the main areas of attachment.[50] They are rarely attached to the anterior surface of the epiglottis or the choanal edge. A second group originates submucosally in the retropharyngeal region and postcricoid area. The former are located between the cervical spine and the pharyngeal mucosa, producing a visible intraoral or external mass. Lipomas of the postcricoid area usually drop into the esophagus from their postcricoid location. The nasal cavity and paranasal sinuses are very unusual locations for lipomatous tumor, benign or malignant.[51]

Lipomas are composed of adult fat cells grouped in lobules by vascular connective tissue septae. If the vascularity of the lesion is much greater than that of a simple lipoma, the designation angiolipoma is appropriate (Fig. 18.14). This form is, however, unusual in the head and neck.[52] Lin and Lin[53] indicate there are two types of angiolipoma—noninfiltrating and infiltrating. Noninfiltrating angiolipoma is seen in young individuals and presents as a painful, soft cutaneous nodule. The lesion is well encapsulated and microscopically contains foci of a variable vascular proliferation in a lipoma. They do not recur, even after enucleation. The infiltrating angiolipoma is more deeply located and unencapsulated. Although histologically benign, this lesion, like the infiltrating lipoma, can infiltrate bony, muscular, neural and fibrocollagenous tissue and simulate a malignant neoplasm. As might be expected the recurrence rate is relatively high.[54]

Spindle Cell Lipoma. A lipomatous tumor frequently misinterpreted as a liposarcoma or other soft tissue sarcoma, the spindle cell lipoma has special significance to the head and neck surgeon. The lesion occurs chiefly in middle-aged and elderly males and affects the regions of the shoulder and posterior neck almost exclusively. Other anatomical sites of involvement are unusual. Most of the lesions are painless and many have been present for considerable periods of time before removal. In an AFIP series of 114 cases, the median preoperative duration was 3 years.[55]

In most cases the lesion occurs in the dermis or subcutis as a single, slow-growing mass. Their size varies. An average lesion measures 4.5 cm in major dimension.

The spindle cell lipoma is characterized histologically by a mixture of fat cells and fibroblast-like spindle cells (ultrastructurally similar to fibroblasts) in a matrix with varying amounts of collagen and mucosubstances. There are variations in cellularity; in the amount and distribution of fat cells, spindle cells and collagen both within different areas of the same tumor and from tumor to tumor (Fig. 18.15). A few spindle cell lipomas may show considerable nuclear pleomorphism without mitotic activity. These cellular changes are thought to be regressive in nature and presumed to be analogous with those observed in aging neurilemmonas.[55, 56]

For the pathologist who is unfamiliar with the spindle cell lipoma, the error potential toward

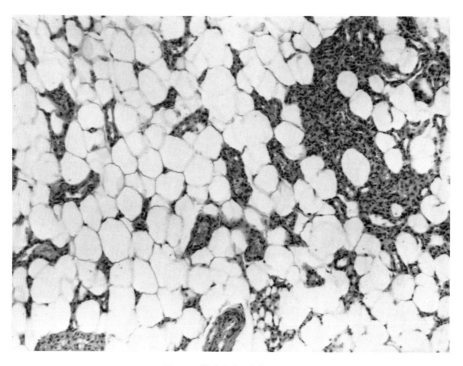

Figure 18.14. Angiolipoma.

malignancy is high. Perhaps one of the most difficult differential diagnoses is the highly differentiated fibrosing liposarcoma. This lesion is also composed of a mixture of fat cells and collagen. However, the sarcoma usually has a more pronounced cellularity and nuclear polymorphism. Multivacuolated lipoblasts are also present while the spindle cell lipoma contains only univacuolated fat cells. The myxoid liposarcoma also has a pooling of the mucoid substance. Of topographic importance, it is to be noted that unlike the spindle cell lipoma, liposarcomas are usually more deeply situated and are larger in size.

Follow-up information in patients with spindle cell lipomas clearly identify the tumor as a benign process and that it is readily curable by local excision.[55, 56]

I am of the opinion that malignant forms of lipomatous tumors arise de novo and not from pre-existing lipomas. Management, then, is conservative. Recurrences occur only in the deeper forms where the intramuscular variant "infiltrative lipomas" present themselves.

Benign Symmetric Lipomatosis. This unusual disorder is characterized by the abnormal deposition of lipomatous tissue in the cervical region, causing massive swelling about the neck. The mass may be so great as to result in a grotesque disfigurement and local pressure symptoms. Lipoma-

tous tissue also accumulates, to a lesser degree, in the axilla and groins of the unfortunate host.

The cause of the disorder is unknown, but a significant number of cases have occurred in patients with an alcoholic history.[57] The clinical presentation of the afflicted person is striking. Often a "horse-collar" cervical appearance is conveyed, with a large posterior cervical hump with extensions into the parotid, supraclavicular, deltoid and pectoral regions. The microscopic appearance of tissue removed from the mass is difficult to distinguish from simple lipomas. There is no predilection for the development of liposarcoma.

Hereditary, multiple lipomatosis differs from benign symmetric lipomatosis in that the former presents with lesions on the arms, legs, lower part of chest and upper abdomen. The alimentary tract and other regions may also be involved. The disorder is hereditary, and multiple members of the afflicted families present with the disorder.

Lipoblastomatosis. Tumors of this disorder occur in the very young, are benign and recur only if incompletely excised. Lipoblastomatosis is a growth of embryonal lipoblasts to form a characteristically lobulated tumor. Despite the myxoid areas and active morphogenesis, the disorder is probably an anomaly of growth rather than a neoplasm.[58] Four of Chung and Enzinger's[59] 34 cases presented in the neck. These authors describe

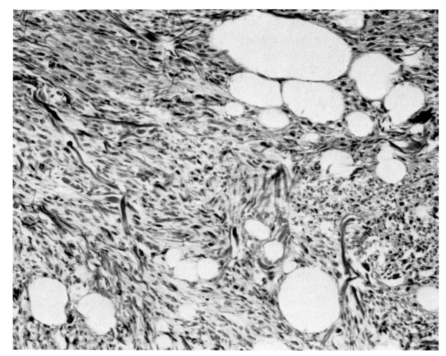

Figure 18.15. Spindle cell lipoma. The characteristic location of the tumor and familiarity with the lesion assists in the diagnosis.

a circumscribed and a diffuse form of the tumor. The former tends to be superficially located and is clinically comparable to a lipoma. The latter is more deeply situated and is analogous to an infantile lipomatosis. Both types exhibit the same histological picture, characterized by lobulated immature adipose tissue consisting of lipoblasts, a plexiform capillary pattern, and a more or less pronounced myxoid stroma. The tumor is cured by local excision. If recurrence appears, it is usually associated with the diffuse type of tumor.

Hibernoma. This uncommon supporting tissue tumor takes its origin from immature or so-called "brown" fat.[60] The majority of these lesions are subcutaneous and are most often reported as arising between the scapulae. Deep seated hibernomas are unusual and benign and are adequately treated by local excision (Fig. 18.16).

Liposarcoma. The liposarcoma is probably the most commonly encountered malignant soft tissue malignancy. The retroperitoneum and peripheral soft tissues are the favorite sites of occurrence. However, like its benign counterpart, the lipoma, it is very rare in the head and neck. The paucity of this neoplasm above the clavicles is exemplified by the fact that only four cases of liposarcoma of the head and neck were encountered in a population of 8.5 million people in Southern England

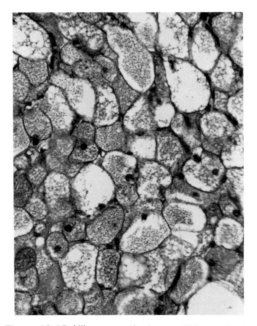

Figure 18.16. Hibernoma, the tumor of "brown fat."

from 1958 to 1965.[61] The neoplasm is rare, also, in patients who are less than 30 years old.

Liposarcomas arise from lipoblasts or totipotential mesenchyme within or adjacent to fascial and intramuscular areas, *not* from a pre-existing li-poma and *rarely* from subcutaneous fibroadipose tissue. Generally, most liposarcomas have reached considerable size before they encroach upon the subcutaneum. Notable exceptions, however, are the rarely occurring liposarcomas of the shoulders, neck and face, where neoplasms of smaller size and short duration may extend into the subcuta-neous fat.[62]

Duration and size of the mass do not correlate closely with prognosis or biological activity. Rapid enlargement and a size of 12 cm or more, however, are associated with a liability to metastasize. The gross appearance of a liposarcoma varies consid-erably and is largely dependent upon its histolog-ical composition, i.e., myxoid components, fibrous elements, vascularization, necrosis, etc. The neo-plasm manifests an apparent circumscription and may convey the impression of encapsulation. These misleading features tempt the surgeon to "shell the neoplasm out" and account for a good many of the recurrences, since satellite nodules about the main mass are very common. After recurrence, the mass is less defined.

The better differentiated liposarcomas often present a jelly-like, moist appearance, the less differentiated varieties with a soft "brain-like" consistency. Hemorrhage and necrosis vary with histological subtypes but are more common with myxoid variants and least conspicuous with the well differentiated types. Unlike the lipoma, cal-cification and ossification are unusual.

Microscopically, liposarcomas recapitulate, in a neoplastic fashion, all stages in the embryogenesis of fatty tissues, from the most primitive lipoblast to the mature lipocyte. Enzinger and Winslow[63] consider liposarcomas as "probably unsurpassed by their wide range in structure and behavior."

Enzinger[64] has rightly pointed out that the mere diagnosis of liposarcoma is of little prognostic value, since histological subdivisions bear greatly on the clinical outcome. It is further my impression that the presence of fibrosarcoma-like elements in the neoplasm increases the malignant potential of a liposarcoma, regardless of the cell type.

A combination of Stout's[65] and Enzinger and Winslow's[63] subdivisions of liposarcomas appears to be most workable. Liposarcomas may be di-vided into four subgroups: (1) myxoid; (2) round cell type; (3) well differentiated or adult type; and (4) pleomorphic type. In many examples, apparent transition from one type to another may compli-cate classification. As a rule of thumb, classifica-tion, then, is dependent upon either a uniform histological pattern or based on the least differ-entiated element.

Electron microscopic and histochemical studies of liposarcomas have been offered by Scarpelli and Greider[66] and Enzinger and Winslow.[63] More than half of *all* liposarcomas recur locally, regard-less of histological subtype. There are, however, significant differences in the survival rates between the four subcategories. The 5-year survival for the myxoid and well differentiated forms exceeds 70%, but this is reduced to only 20% with the pleomorphic and round cell variants.[63]

The propensity for metastasis is also related to histological type. Approximately 30% of patients manifest distant metastases, and these are almost exclusively those patients with pleomorphic and round cell variants.[67,68] Regional lymph node me-tastases are unusual. Radiation appears useful in palliation of the myxoid liposarcoma, but primary management of a liposarcoma is adequate surgical excision. Liposarcomas in children are unusual and are characterized by a more favorable clinical behavior than comparable neoplasms in the adult.[58]

Intraoral liposarcomas are very rare. In an ex-tensive (50-year) review of the literature, Baden and Newman[69] could cull only 40 primary liposar-comas of the head and neck. The scalp, skull, orbit, neck and pharynx were most commonly involved. Principal intraoral sites were the cheek and floor of mouth. Other sites were the larynx, soft palate, upper lip, maxilla and mastoid. The majority of the liposarcomas in the head and neck are myxoid in type, followed distantly by round cell liposarcoma. Survival correlates with histolog-ical type; the best with well differentiated myxoid liposarcomas and lowest in patients with round cell liposarcomas. Sixteen of the 35 patients with sufficient information detailed by Baden and Newman had recurrences, often multiple. Five patients manifested widespread metastases from their head and neck primary lesion.

MESENCHYMOMAS AND EXTRAOSSEOUS CHONDROGENIC AND OSTEOGENIC NEOPLASMS

These three categories of neoplasms are rare in the head and neck. Mesenchymoma is the diag-nostic label given to mixed mesenchymal tumors of varied composition.[70] To be so designated, a neoplasm must be composed of two or more mes-enchymal elements not ordinarily found together in a tumor. Fibrous connective tissue elements are *not* considered as one of the needed components since they are found (in varying proportions) in nearly all mesenchymal tumors.

Benign and malignant variants exist.[71] In the

former, which may be malformations or hamartomas rather than true neoplasms, fat, smooth muscle and vasoformative tissues are most commonly found. Other elements are skeletal muscle, cartilage, lymphoreticular tissue, myxomatous tissue and hematopoietic tissue.

An oddity in the head and neck, benign mesenchymomas are found predominantly in the kidneys and extremities. In a compilation from the literature, the benign mesenchymomas of the head and neck have had the following distribution: skin and/or subcutaneous tissues (eight cases), tongue (four cases), floor of mouth (two cases), trapezius muscle (one case), epiglottis (one case) and trachea (one case). The majority are solitary and circumscribed but not encapsulated. Those found in skeletal muscle always infiltrate. A 20% recurrence rate indicates wide local excision to be the treatment of choice.[72]

Malignant mesenchymomas may be composed of the malignant counterparts of several (two or more) of the tissues found in the benign forms. Rhabdomyosarcomatous and vasoformative malignant elements are the most common. Size and histological composition affect prognosis. The neoplasm is predominantly one of the external soft tissues and of the first quinquennium. Seven of the 42 malignant mesenchymomas reported by Nash and Stout[71] were from the head and neck.

Extraosseous chondrogenic and osteogenic tumors are always controversial wherever they occur. By definition, these soft tissue neoplasms must arise without concomitant involvement of adjacent bone. Care must also be taken to separate metaplastic osteogenesis and chondrogenesis from true extraosseous neoplasms.

Osteomas of the head and neck soft tissues, as elsewhere in the body, are unusual occurrences. Osteomas of the tongue are also rare. All subjects have been in their second or third decades of life, and women predominate. The tumors are characteristically pedunculated and located to either side of the midline approximating the circumvallate papilla.[73] A review of osteomas (osseous choristomas) of the intraoral soft tissues has been presented by Krolls et al.[74]

Osteogenic sarcomas of the extraosseous soft tissues of the head and neck are even more unusual and far fewer in number than cartilaginous neoplasms of the soft or visceral tissues.

Allen and Soule[75] reviewed the Mayo Clinic experience and found none in the head and neck but culled four examples from the literature. They estimated the ratio of extraskeletal to skeletal osteosarcomas to be approximately 1:25. The diagnosis of a primary extraosseous osteogenic sar-

coma rests on three criteria: (1) the presence of a uniform morphological pattern of sarcomatous tissue that excludes the possibility of mixed malignant mesenchymal tumor; (2) the production of sarcomatous tissue of malignant osteoid or bone (or both); and (3) exclusion of a primary osseous origin. A tumor with a mixture of extraosseous malignant chondroid and osteoid tissue, as observed in primary bone sarcomas, is considered to be an osteogenic sarcoma. Their extraosseous location does not impart a better prognosis. A distinct clinical difference lies in the age of onset. While the skeletal variety has a peak incidence in the second decade, unless superimposed on Paget's disease of bone, extraskeletal osteosarcomas rarely occur prior to the fourth decade. In some reported cases therapeutic irradiation has been implicated in the pathogenesis.

A single probable case in larynx has been reported.[76]

Within the oral cavity, "chondromas" usually occur on the palate and the alveolar edges of the upper and lower maxilla.

The head and neck clinician may never encounter a pure cartilaginous lesion of the tongue. By 1977, only 11 acceptable cases of chondroma had been published in the world's literature.[77] In nine of the 11 cases the lesion occurred in the region of the lateral margin of the tongue. In the other two, the lesion was on the dorsal surface. The size of the tumors has varied from 0.3 to 4.5 cm. Chondrosarcoma of the tongue is even more rare.

While trauma *may* be a predisposing factor for the development of the lingual chondroma and osteoma, it is clearly implicated in the osseous and chondromatous metaplastic lesions related to dentures. The anterior jaws are the most common sites for these metaplasias, but any of the denture bearing areas may be predisposed including the hard palate.[78]

Localization in the neck may be a possibility, but, probably in this locale, cartilaginous tumors are best considered as malformations, representing bars associated with branchiogenic remnants.

The distinction between benign and malignant chondromatous neoplasms is a fine one, often impossible to define. Chondrosarcomas have been reported in the tongue, in the submucosa and mucosa of the nasopharynx, in the vicinity of, but not in contact with, the cartilage of the eustachian tube and in the muscles of mastication.[79] Goldman and Perzik[80] reported the only example of an extraosseous chondrosarcoma of the maxilla. Batsakis and Fox[81] have reviewed the cartilaginous tumors of the larynx, citing the cricoid cartilage as the most common site and warning of the danger of underestimating the biological behavior of these neoplasms.

The nasal septum, surprisingly, is not often the site of origin of a chondrosarcoma, most tumors being spurs. By 1970, there were only four examples of chondrosarcoma of the nasal septum in the literature.[82]

ALVEOLAR SOFT PART SARCOMA

This unusual yet distinctive neoplasm occurs chiefly in the extremities of children and young adults. A primary alveolar soft part sarcoma in the head and neck region is a distinct rarity.[83] The third case of an intraoral soft part sarcoma was reported in 1976.[84] All have been in the tongue. The neoplasm, wherever it presents, is slow growing and painless, with a high recurrence rate and a pronounced tendency to metastasize to the lungs, liver, skeleton and, less frequently, to lymph nodes. More than 50% of the entire group are obviously malignant with widespread dissemination. Histological appearances are not reliable indicators of malignancy. Many of those that have spread widely have appeared histologically benign.

The three most common metastatic sites are lungs, bone and brain. Survival rates are 82% in 2 years, 59% in 5 years and 47% in 10 years.[83] No survivors are found at 20 years. Lifetime cures have yet to be described.

Microscopically, the organoid or endocrine-like appearance is uniform and often striking (Fig. 18.17). Individual cells are polyhedral and epithelial-like, often with large, ill-defined cytoplasm. The latter may be relatively clear, ground glass, or coarsely granular and eosinophilic. Nuclei are usually vesicular and large; mitoses are not usually seen. An occasional bizarre cell form may be noted. The cells are arranged in discrete groups, bordered by a delicate and yet distinct collagen that may be emphasized by reticulin stains. A pseudoacinar or tubular arrangement may be a conspicuous feature. Ultrastructural and histochemical studies have not aided in defining histogenesis but do not support a myogenous derivation and favor paraganglionic origin.[85, 86]

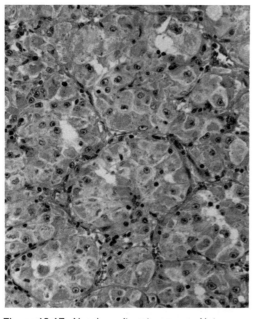

Figure 18.17. Alveolar soft part sarcoma. Note organoid aggregation of large cells resembling an alveolar rhabdomyosarcoma (may be histogenetically the same).

REFERENCES

1. Mabrey, R. E.: Chordoma: a study of 150 cases. Am. J. Cancer 25:501, 1935.
2. Batsakis, J. G., and Kittleson, A. C.: Chordomas: otorhinolaryngologic presentation and diagnosis. Arch. Otolaryngol. 78:168, 1963.
3. Binkhorst, C. D., Schierbeek, P., and Petten, G. J. W.: Neoplasms of the notochord: report of a case of basilar chordoma and bilateral orbital involvement. Acta Otolaryngol. 47:10, 1957.
4. Wright, D.: Nasopharyngeal and cervical chordoma—some aspects of their development and treatment. J. Laryngol. Otol. 82:1337, 1968.
5. Horwitz, T.: Chordal ectopia and its possible relation to chordoma. Arch. Pathol. 31:354, 1941.
6. Givner, I.: Ophthalmologic features of intracranial chordoma and allied tumors of the clivus. Arch. Ophthalmol. 33:397, 1945.
7. Congdon, C. C.: Benign and malignant chordomas: a clinicoanatomical study of 22 cases. Am. J. Pathol. 28:793, 1952.
8. Stewart, M. J., and Morin, J. E.: Chordoma: a review with report of a new sacrococcygeal case. J. Pathol. Bacteriol. 29:41, 1926.
9. Evans, R. W.: Histological Appearance of Tumors, p. 102. E. & S. Livingstone, Ltd., Edinburgh and London, 1956.
10. Crawford, T.: The staining reaction of chordoma. J. Clin. Pathol. 11:110, 1958.
11. Pena, C. E., Horvat, B. L., and Fisher, E. R.: The ultrastructure of chordoma. Am. J. Clin. Pathol. 53:544, 1970.
12. Dahlin, D. C., and MacCarty, C. S.: Chordoma: a study of 59 cases. Cancer 5:1170, 1952.
13. Twefik, H. H., McGinnis, W. L., Nordstrom, D. G., and Latourette, H. B.: Chordoma. Evaluation of clinical behavior and treatment modalities. Int. J. Radiat. Oncol. 2: 959, 1977.
14. Heffelfinger, M. J., Dahlin, D. C., MacCarty, C. S., and Beabout, J. W.: Chordomas and cartilaginous tumors of the skull base. Cancer 32:410, 1973.
15. Richter, H. J., Batsakis, J. G., and Boles, R.: Chordomas: nasopharyngeal presentation and atypical lung survival. Ann. Otol. 84:327, 1975.
16. Stout, A. P., and Hill, W. T.: Leiomyosarcoma of the superficial soft tissues. Cancer 11:844, 1953.
17. Stout, A. P.: Solitary cutaneous and subcutaneous leiomyoma. Am. J. Cancer 29:435, 1937.
18. Stout, A. P.: Leiomyoma of the oral cavity. Am. J. Cancer 34:31, 1938.
19. Hagy, D. M., Halpern, V., and Wood, C.: Leiomyoma of the

oral cavity. Oral Surg. 17:748, 1964.

20. MacDonald, D. G.: Smooth muscle tumors of the mouth. Br. J. Oral. Surg. 6:207, 1969.

21. Duhig, J. T., and Ayer, J. P.: Vascular leiomyoma: a study of 71 cases. Arch. Pathol. 68:424, 1959.

22. Farman, A. G., and Kay, S.: Oral leiomyosarcoma. Report of a case and review of the literature pertaining to smooth-muscle tumors of the oral cavity. Oral Surg. 43:402, 1977.

23. Farman, A. G.: Benign smooth muscle tumors. S. Afr. Med. J. 49:1333, 1975.

24. Goldblatt, L. I., and Edesess, R. B.: Central leiomyoma of the mandible. Report of a case with ultrastructural confirmation. Oral Surg. 43:591, 1977.

25. Fu, Y.-S., and Perzin, K. H.: Nonepithelial tumors of the nasal cavity, paranasal sinuses, and nasopharynx: A clinicopathologic study. IV. Smooth muscle tumors (leiomyoma, leiomyosarcoma). Cancer 35:1300, 1975.

26. Dropkin, L. R., Tang, C. K., and Williams, J. R.: Leiomyosarcoma of the nasal cavity and paranasal sinuses. Ann. Otol. 85:399, 1976.

27. Glover, G. W., and Park, W. W.: Pharyngeal leiomyosarcoma. J. Laryngol. 85:1031, 1971.

28. Kevorkian, J., and Cento, D. P.: Leiomyosarcoma of large arteries and veins. Surgery 73:390, 1973.

29. Appleman, H. D., and Helwig, E. B.: Gastric epitheliod leiomyoma and leiomyosarcoma (leiomyoblastoma). Cancer 38:708, 1976.

30. Batsakis, J. G., Nishiyama, R. H., and Sullinger, G. D.: Synovial sarcomas of the neck. Arch. Otolaryngol. 85:327, 1967.

31. Lockey, M. W.: Rare tumors of the ear, nose and throat: synovial sarcoma of the head and neck. South. Med. J. 69: 316, 1976.

32. Roth, J. A., Enzinger, F. M., and Tannenbaum, M.: Synovial sarcoma of the neck.: A follow-up study of 24 cases. Cancer 35:1243, 1975.

33. Jernstrom, P.: Synovial sarcoma of the pharynx: report of a case. Am. J. Clin. Pathol. 24:957, 1954.

34. Harrison, E. G., Jr., Black, B. M., and Devine, K. D.: Synovial sarcoma primary in the neck. Arch. Pathol. 71: 137, 1961.

35. Hajdu, S. I., Shiu, M. H., and Fortner, J. G.: Tendosynovial sarcoma. A clinicopathological study of 136 cases. Cancer 39:1201, 1977.

36. MacKenzie, D. H.: Synovial sarcoma: a review of 58 cases. Cancer 19:169, 1966.

37. Wright, C. J. E.: Malignant synovioma. J. Pathol. Bacteriol. 64:585, 1952.

38. Cadman, N. L., Soule, E. H., and Kelly, P. J.: Synovial sarcoma. Cancer 18:615, 1965.

39. Murray, J. A.: Synovial sarcoma. Orthop. Clin. North Am. 8:963, 1977.

40. Stout, A. P.: Myxoma: the tumor of primitive mesenchyme. Ann. Surg. 127:706, 1948.

41. Dutz, W., and Stout, A. P.: The myxoma in childhood. Cancer 14:629, 1961.

42. Spengos, M. N., and Schow, C. E.: Myxomas of the soft tissues: report of a case of myxoma in the cheek. J. Oral Surg. 23:140, 1965.

43. Elzay, R. P., and Dutz, W.: Myxomas of the paraoral-oral soft tissues. Oral Surg. 45:246, 1978.

44. Johnson, W. C., Graham, J. H., and Helwig, E. B.: Cutaneous myxoid cyst: a clinicopathological and histochemical study. J. A. M. A. 191:109, 1965.

45. Smith, G. A., Konrad, H. R., and Canalis, R. F.: Childhood myxomas of the head and neck. J. Otolaryngol. 6:423, 1977.

46. Enzinger, F. M.: Intramuscular myxoma: a review and follow-up study of 34 cases. Am. J. Clin. Pathol. 43:104, 1965.

47. Kindblom, L.-G., Stener, B., and Angervall, L.: Intramuscular myxoma. Cancer 34:1737, 1974.

48. Ireland, D. C. R., Soule, E. H., and Ivins, J. C.: Myxoma of somatic soft tissues. A report of 58 patients, three with multiple tumors. Mayo Clin. Proc. 48:401, 1973.

49. Hatziotis, J. C.: Lipoma of the oral cavity. Oral surg. 31:511, 1971.

50. Toppozada, H. H., Shehata, M. A., and Maher, A. I.: Lipoma of the pharynx. J. Laryngol. 87:787, 1973.

51. Fu, Y.-S., and Perzin, K. H.: Non-epithelial tumors of the nasal cavity, paranasal sinuses and nasopharynx. A clinicopathologic study. VII. Adipose tissue tumors (lipoma and liposarcoma). Cancer 40:1314, 1977.

52. Howard, W. R., and Helwig, E. B.: Angiolipoma. Arch. Dermatol. 82:924, 1960.

53. Lin, J. J., and Lin, F.: Two entities in angiolipoma. A study of 459 cases of lipoma with review of literature infiltrating angiolipoma. Cancer 34:720, 1974.

54. Dionne, C. P., and Seemayer, T. A.: Infiltrating lipomas and angiolipomas revisited. Cancer 33:732, 1974.

55. Enzinger, F. M., and Harvey, D. A.: Spindle cell lipoma. Cancer 36:1852, 1975.

56. Angervall, L., Dahl, I., Kindblom, L.-G., and Save-Sodergergh, J.: Spindle cell lipoma. Acta Pathol. Microbiol. Scand. (A) 84:477, 1976.

57. Taylor, L. M., Beahrs, O. H., and Fontana, R. S.: Benign symmetric lipomatosis. Proc. Mayo Clin. 36:96, 1961.

58. Kauffman, S. L., and Stout, A. P.: Lipoblastic tumors of children. Cancer 12:912, 1959.

59. Chung, E. B., and Enzinger, F. M.: Benign lipoblastomatosis. An analysis of 35 cases. Cancer 32:482, 1973.

60. Mesara, B. W., and Batsakis, J. G.: Hibernoma of the neck. Arch. Otolaryngol. 85:199, 1967.

61. Stoller, F. M., and Davis, D. G.: Liposarcoma of the neck. Arch. Otolaryngol. 88:419, 1968.

62. Sauk, J. J., Jr.: Liposarcoma of the head and neck. J. Oral Surg. 29:38, 1971.

63. Enzinger, F. M., and Winslow, D. J.: Liposarcoma: a study of 103 cases. Virchows Arch. (Pathol. Anat.) 335:367, 1962.

64. Enzinger, F. M.: Recent trends in soft tissue pathology. In Tumors of Bone and Soft Tissue, p. 315. Year Book Medical Publishers, Inc., Chicago, 1965.

65. Stout, A. P.: Liposarcoma—the malignant tumor of lipoblasts. Ann. Surg. 119:86, 1944.

66. Scarpelli, D. G., and Greider, M. H.: A correlative cytochemical and electron microscopic study of liposarcoma. Cancer 15:766, 1962.

67. Enterline, H. T., Culberson, J. D., Rochlin, D. B., and Brady, L. W.: Liposarcoma: a clinical and pathological study of 53 cases. Cancer 13:932, 1960.

68. Kindblom, L.-G., Angervall, L., and Svendsen, P.: Liposarcoma. A clinicopathologic, radiographic and prognostic study. Acta Pathol. Microbiol. Scand. Suppl. 253, 1975.

69. Baden, E., and Newman, R.: Liposarcoma of the oropharyngeal region. Review of the literature and report of two cases. Oral Surg. 44:889, 1977.

70. LeBer, M. S., and Stout, A. P.: Benign mesenchymomas in children. Cancer 15:598, 1962.

71. Nash, A., and Stout, A. P.: Malignant mesenchymomas in children. Cancer 14:524, 1961.

72. Bures, C., and Barnes, L.: Benign mesenchymomas of the head and neck. Arch. Pathol. Lab. Med. 102:237, 1978.

73. Cataldo, E., Shklar, C., and Meyer, I.: Osteoma of the tongue. Arch. Otolaryngol. 85:202, 1967.

74. Krolls, S. O., Jacoway, J. R., and Alexander, W. N.: Osseous choristomas (osteomas) of intraoral soft tissue. Oral. Surg. 32:588, 1971.

75. Allen, C. J., and Soule, E. H.: Osteogenic sarcoma of the somatic soft tissues. Clinicopathologic study of 26 cases and review of the literature. Cancer 27:1121, 1971.

76. Morley, A. R., Cameron, D. S., and Watson, A. J.: Osteosarcoma of the larynx. J. Laryngol. 87:997, 1973.

77. Zegarelli, D. J.: Chondroma of the tongue. Oral Surg. 43: 738, 1977.

78. Cutright, D. E.: Osseous and chondromatous metaplasia caused by dentures. Oral Surg. 34:625, 1972.

79. Stout, A. P., and Verner, E. W.: Chondrosarcoma of the extraskeletal soft tissues. Cancer 6:581, 1953.

80. Goldman, R. L., and Perzik, S. L.: Extraosseous chondrosar-

coma of the maxilla. Arch. Surg. 95:30, 1967.

81. Batsakis, J. G., and Fox, J. E.: Supporting tissue neoplasms of the larynx. Surg. Gynecol. Obstet. 131:989, 1970.

82. Aretsky, P. J., Kantu, K., Freund, H. R., and Polisar, I. A.: Chondrosarcoma of the nasal septum. Ann. Otolaryngol. 79:382, 1970.

83. Lieberman, P. H., Foote, F. W., Jr., Stewart, F. W., and Berg, J. W.: Alveolar soft-part sarcoma. J.A.M.A. 198:121, 1966.

84. Olson, R. A. J., and Perkins, K. D.: Alveolar soft-part sarcoma in oral cavity: report of case. J. Oral. Surg. 34:73, 1976.

85. Delaney, W. E.: Non-myogenic tumors involving skeletal muscle. A survey with special reference to alveolar soft part sarcoma. Ann. Clin. Lab. Sci. 5:236, 1975.

86. Unni, K. K., and Soule, E. H.: Alveolar soft part sarcoma. An electron microscopic study. Mayo Clin. Proc. 50:591, 1975.

CHAPTER 19

Paragangliomas of the Head and Neck

The extra-adrenal paraganglia, derived from neural crest cells, make up an extensive and multicentric organ system. According to Glenner and Grimley,[1] the *extra-adrenal* portion of the paraganglion system may be considered as several inter-related "families" which may be grouped quite logically on the basis of anatomical distribution, innervation and microscopic structure. These families include branchiomeric, intravagal, aorticosympathetic, and visceral-autonomic paraganglia.

These paraganglia tend to be distributed symmetrically and segmentally in the para-axial regions of the trunk and in the vicinity of the ontogenetic gill-arches (Fig. 19.1). They may also be found in peripheral portions of the autonomic nervous system. In these locations, they present as very small, macroscopic and microscopic cell groups. Each paraganglion in the head and neck is composed of two cell types: granule storing chief cells and Schwann-like satellite cells. The chief cells contain catecholamines (norepinephrine or a related neurotransmitter substance). According to Glenner and Grimley[1] these cells probably exert a common function in governing local levels of excitation within the autonomic nervous system.

Paraganglia of the head, neck and superior mediastinum closely resemble the carotid bodies (intercarotid paraganglia). These paraganglia are typically related to arterial vasculature and cranial nerves of the ontogenetic gill arches and are designated as *branchiomeric paraganglia*. The branchiomeric paraganglia include jugulotympanic, intercarotid, subclavian, laryngeal, coronary, aorticopulmonary and pulmonary paraganglia. Paraganglia of the orbit and the intravagal paraganglia cannot be distinguished from the branchiomeric class on any microscopic basis, but are not intimately associated with arteries and, therefore, should likely be tentatively considered as a separate group.[1]

Chemosensory reflexes are mediated by certain of the branchiomeric paraganglia (chemoreceptors). They include the carotid bodies and aortic bodies. Studies have shown that the carotid body and aortic body are sensitive to changes in pH and arterial oxygen tension.[2] All of the paraganglia are well vascularized and this suggests a common ability to sense changes in their chemical environment.

There is undeniable evidence of catecholamine storage in the cells of the branchiomeric paraganglia.[1, 3, 4] This occurs in the chief cells and are represented by 0.1 to 0.2 μm granules. The granules have an electron-dense core after fixation with gluteraldehyde and osmium tetroxide. The granules stain with silver or lead hematoxylin preparations but are usually negative after potassium dichromate. A relatively simple demonstration of the catecholamines is achieved by ultraviolet excitation of a blue-green fluorescence after fixation of dried frozen sections with hot formaldehyde vapors.

The carotid body contains two forms of chief cells. The most abundant form has a relatively clear cytoplasm and uniform spherical granules. The other is a dark cell with a condensed cytoplasm and irregular granules. The satellite cells of the paraganglia provide for much of the compartmentalization of the chief cells (organoid pattern). The capillaries of paraganglia are much like those of any endocrine gland. Unmyelinated nerve axons enter the nests of chief cells accompanied by the satellite cells.

Glenner and Grimley[1] advise the elimination of the qualifying designation, nonchromaffin, from any classification. While the presence of a chromaffin reaction in a cell or tissue is highly indicative, it is not absolute proof of the presence of a catecholamine or an indole amine. Further, the absence of the positive reaction, cannot be used as a criterion for determining whether or not such a

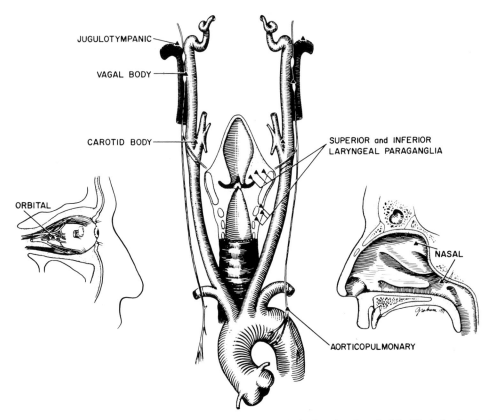

Figure 19.1. Anatomical distribution of paraganglionic tissue in the head and neck. (Modified after Lack et al.[3] by permission.)

reactive substance is absent. Because of the non-specificity of argentaffin or argyrophilic reactions, they too do not provide significant information in these tumors.

The formaldehyde-induced fluorescence method, however, is far more reliable and many authors have demonstrated in carotid body chief cells, the typical fluorescence of formaldehyde conjugated catecholamines. This method should be used in all studies of the normal and abnormal paraganglia to determine the presence of cate-cholamines. A technique suitable for neuroblas-tomas also is one described by Judge et al.[5] The enzyme histochemistry of the human carotid body has been described by Fine et al.[6]

As indicated above, the carotid body behaves as an hypoxia sensor. Carotid bodies appear to serve as initiators of increased ventilation in low oxygen tensions and they can also be seen as suppressors of excess ventilation in high oxygen tensions.[7, 8] Non-neoplastic enlargement of the carotid bodies in subjects living at high altitudes can be reasonably regarded as examples of hyperplasia in response to lowered Po_2. Similar enlargements are

described in chronic hypoxia at sea level. In these instances the patients suffer from emphysema with cor pulmonale or cyanotic heart disease. The histological changes include a hyperplasia of both chief and sustentacular cells and also an increase in size and number of capillaries. A relatively normal cytoarchitecture is maintained within the lobules of the carotid body.

In the following discussion, each of the tumors (Fig. 19.1) of the branchiomeric and related paraganglia is presented separately; *carotid body paraganglioma* (carotid body tumor, carotid body chemodectoma), *jugular paraganglioma* (glomus jugulare and glomus tympanicum tumor, glomus jugulare chemodectoma), *intravagal paraganglioma* (vagal body tumor), *orbital paraganglioma* (orbital chemodectoma) and *laryngeal paraganglioma* (chemodectoma of glomus laryngeum superior and inferior).

Paragangliomas in the head and neck have the following general characteristics: (1) Carotid body tumors are the most often reported lesions. These are followed, in order, by the tumors of the jugu-lotympanic, intravagal, laryngeal, nasal and nasopharyngeal and orbital paraganglia. (2) There is a definite proclivity for multicentric origin (10%) and an association with other malignancies, especially other neural crest tumors (8%).[9, 10] Most synchronous tumors are discovered incidentally. (3) There is a heredofamilial tendency.[9] (4) The estimated incidence of bilaterality of carotid tumors is 2.8%, but increases to 26.0% in hosts showing a familial tendency.[11] These patients may also harbor other extracervical paragangliomas. (5) If sought, nearly all of the branchiomeric and related paragangliomas will demonstrate intracellular catecholamines; a considerably fewer number will manifest systemic evidence of this catecholamine synthesis. (6) Survival and therapeutic morbidity is dependent on the tumor type and extent. The most treacherous lesions occur in the following sequence: jugulare, tympanum, vagale and carotid body. (7) Patients with branchiomeric paragangliomas require a lifelong surveillance. Multicentric tumors can develop at different times, and there is a statistically significant probability that an associated malignancy will develop (particularly with jugular paragangliomas). (8) There is a rather wide clinical variation of response of the paragangliomas to radiotherapy.[12] (9) Microscopically, paragangliomas resemble the tissue from which they arise and in effect, are neoplastic caricatures of that tissue. Noticeable pleomorphism and hyperchromation are common in the tumors, but are not indicative of malignancy. (10) The incidence of true (metastasizing) malignancy varies from 2 to 6% for the entire branchiomeric group of paragangliomas.[13] (11) Carotid and vertebral arteriography is indispensable for diagnosis and selection of therapy. (12) Very likely, surgical removal should be the first line of treatment.

Angiography is a mandatory preoperative assessment of the branchiomeric paragangliomas. Since they are vascular tumors, this technique demonstrates the pattern, vascular supply and extent of the tumors. The carotid paraganglioma is representative. For that tumor, the value of arteriography is as follows:

1. The diagnosis is established.

2. The extent of the tumor and its relationship to the origins of the internal and external carotid arteries is established. The arteries are usually separated by tumors of the carotid body and displaced forward together by the intravagal type. If the tumor is high in the neck, a retrograde jugular venogram may demonstrate invasion of the vein.

3. The collateral circulation can be assessed. It is probably justifiable to perform bilateral carotid angiography to help in this assessment in addition to demonstrating blood supply to the tumor from the opposite side and excluding a contralateral tumor.

There is a significant incidence of cranial nerve paralysis associated with paragangliomas of the head and neck. Spector et al.[14] record an over-all incidence of 37% and an incidence of intracranial extension of 14.6%.

The rarity of paragangliomas from the head and neck region is attested to by the finding of only 69 such tumors at the Sloan-Kettering Memorial Cancer Center from 1937 through 1975.[3] This represents an incidence of 0.012% of over 600,000 cases accessioned in that Center's surgical pathology files.

CAROTID BODY TUMORS

Neoplasia is the only documented pathological condition affecting the paraganglionic tissue, and this change occurs most frequently in the carotid body. The carotid body in man is a small (5 × 5 × 2.5 mm) ovoid structure usually situated at the fork of the common carotid artery. It may also be found upon either the internal carotid or external carotid arteries, or it may be dispersed in small lobules in the immediate vicinity of these arteries. The body is composed of lobules or groups of "epithelioid" cells closely applied to the endothelium of capillaries. These cells are of two types; one has large, pale nuclei with nucleoli and pale vacuolated cytoplasm, and the other has smaller and darker nuclei with a darker cytoplasm. These two types of cells are either chief cells or sustentacular cells. The latter are somewhat less numerous and have long processes which envelop the surface of the chief cells and separate them from the adjacent capillaries.

The lobules of cells are embedded in a richly vascular connective tissue. The capsule and "suspensory" ligament are a condensation of this vascularized connective tissue. Arterioles arising from the bifurcation of the common carotid artery traverse the ligament. Venules at the opposite pole drain into branches of the internal jugular vein. Innervation for the body is derived from the glossopharyngeal, vagus, cervical sympathetic and, occasionally, hypoglossal nerves. Blood flow through the carotid body, per unit of tissue, is greater than in any other organ of the body, being about 40 times that of the heart and four times that of the thyroid gland.

Clinical Features. The average age of 300 patients previously reported was 45 years, with a range of 6 months to 76 years.[15] There is a slight predisposition to women. Very often the time lapse is significant before the patient with a carotid body tumor sees his physician; in one series, the average duration of signs and symptoms before examination was 6.2 years.[16]

In general, signs and symptoms produced by carotid body tumors are nonspecific. The most common complaint or finding is a mass. The typical carotid body tumor is palpable in the neck just inferior to the angle of the mandible, medial and deep to the sternocleidomastoid muscle at the level of the carotid bifurcation. Because the tumor adheres to the carotid sheath, its mobility is restricted in a vertical direction, but it may be moved laterally. A bruit or thrill may be present, and pressure may reduce the bulk of the tumor only to have it recover in size slowly by a series of pulsations after the pressure has been released.

Five to 10% of carotid body tumors may extend into the parapharyngeal region and produce a bulging of the oropharyngeal wall that can be observed by intraoral examination. A few patients have manifested an associated carotid sinus pressure syndrome. Pressure encroachment on the ninth, tenth, and eleventh cranial nerves may produce pain. Very large carotid body tumors may extend to the base of the skull, presenting a solid, fixed mass in the upper lateral part of the neck with external protrusion into the soft palate. According to Conley[17] this variety has the potential to manifest a "dumbbell phenomenon" with intracranial extension via the foramens at the base of the skull.

If the carotid body tumor reaches posteriorly and medially in the neck, there will be no bulge or mass in the palatine area or at the level of the carotid bulb. This exception to the typical pattern of growth exhibited by carotid body tumors is most likely related to separate and distinct, but as yet anatomically undocumented, chemoreceptor tissue in the neck. The lesion may involve the carotid artery system by contiguity rather than by a *de novo* growth pattern in the adventitia of the carotid bulb.[17] There is an apparent higher incidence of multiple carotid body tumors in patients with a demonstrated familial tendency toward the development of these tumors.[18]

Malignant Potential. In attempting to place the problem of malignancy in its proper perspective, the major obstacle that must be overcome is the definition of the criteria that are to be used in determining malignancy. The variations in the percentage of "malignant" carotid body tumors and other paragangliomas undoubtedly rests on the criteria of malignancy accepted by different authors. If one accepts cellular variation, active mitoses and invasion of capsule as *absolute* signs of malignancy, then, in some series, up to 50% of carotid body tumors are malignant.[19] The fallacy of this approach may be judged by follow-up studies in which the survival rate of *histologically* malignant tumors is nearly the same as *histologically* benign tumors. It is my opinion that there is no correlation between the histological appearance of these tumors and their biological behavior. This must be borne in mind by surgeons, especially when they ask for a differentiation between a benign and malignant lesion on frozen section or later.

Monro[20] states that almost all carotid body tumors show some degree of local infiltration and that the most common overt malignant manifestation is local recurrence following local excision. Local infiltration, however, is certainly not an absolute expression of malignancy, particularly when one realizes that tumors that are ordinarily accepted as being benign occasionally demonstrate the ability to infiltrate locally due to the innate growth pattern of the tumor. If one accepts as the *sine qua non* of malignancy histologically proved metastases, less than 10% of *all* paragangliomas are malignant.[3, 13] Even in these instances, the course of the disease may be protracted. The incidence of malignancy in carotid body paragangliomas very likely is no greater than 10%, but has varied widely in given series.[21]

The consensus today is that the majority of the *carotid body tumors* are clinically benign, but a small percentage are malignant (Table 19.1) and capable of metastasizing to regional lymph nodes (Fig. 19.2) or to distant sites.

Diagnosis and Management. Carotid angiography is the most valuable diagnostic aid and is important for the planning of therapy.[17, 22] Arteriography results usually demonstrate a circum-

Table 19.1
Malignant Paragangliomas According to Site of Origin*

Location	No. of Cases	No. of Patients with Metastases	Percentage
Carotid body	approx. 500	32	6
Jugular paraganglion	316	6	2
Vagal body	25	4	20
Mediastinum	20	0	0
Lung	25	0	0
Duodenum	9	0	0
Retroperitoneum	21	6	28

* Modified from Olson and Abell.[67]

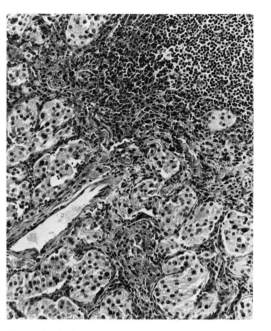

Figure 19.2. Lymph node from neck containing metastatic paraganglioma.

scribed vascular blush at the carotid bifurcation with displacement and separation of the internal and external carotid arteries. The majority of the tumors are fed by the external carotid system, but larger lesions may receive contributions from the thyrocervical trunk. During arteriography it is also important to assess the status of the opposite carotid system and intracerebral circulation if excision is contemplated. The majority of authors indicate that surgical excision is the most effective treatment for carotid body tumors. There have been contrary opinions voiced over the role of radiation in the treatment of these tumors. Some workers claim that radiotherapy has proved ineffective as a cure for *all* of the paragangliomas of the head and neck and that the tumors have been almost universally radioresistant. On the other hand, Grabb and Lampe[23] have concluded that radiotherapy is the preferred form of treatment for glomus jugulare tumors.

Surgical removal of paragangliomas, however, must be predicated upon certain basic precepts, outlined in part by Conley.[17] (1) They are tumors with a slow growth rate and rarely metastasize. (2) The tumors are often associated only with minimal symptoms. (3) Their location is a critical site for surgical removal. (4) The tumors may infiltrate locally and become intimately attached to adjacent structures. (5) Rich vascularity is a feature, and dissection from the carotid artery system makes

dissection both tedious and perilous, a veritable "vast anarchy of arterio-venous connections."[17] (6) Spontaneous regression of carotid body tumors has not been reported.

A formal tissue diagnosis is not usually necessary for proper management of the carotid body tumor. Biopsy, in fact, may be dangerous, particularly if the tumors present in the region of the palate, oral cavity or pharynx, where uncontrolled hemorrhage may interfere with the patient's airway.

The great problem in the treatment of carotid body tumors has been the intimate relation of the tumor to the carotid artery. In many instances, treatment has resulted in the sacrifice of the common, internal or all of the carotid vessels. Rush[24] has pointed out that ligation of the carotid vessels has decreased over the years. This reflects two factors: (1) earlier operations on smaller tumors; and (2) an increasing awareness of the hazards of ligating the common or internal carotid arteries. With this increasing awareness, there has been a corresponding decreased mortality rate associated with the surgery of carotid body tumors. Past reports have established mortality rates of 30 to 50% for ligation of the carotid artery during the surgical removal of carotid body tumors. If the carotid vessels must be ligated, the hazard of the operation far exceeds the risk entailed by the natural biological course of the tumor. However, it has been adequately demonstrated that most of these tumors can be removed by adventitial dissection of the carotid vessels without sacrificing them.

Simple excision of the tumor, before regional growth or size makes it necessary to sacrifice nerves or vessels in removing the tumor, carries with it a mortality rate of only 1.5%. Rush[24] concludes his study by stating that "the only carotid body tumors of which excision must be avoided are those which have encroached so closely upon the base of the skull, that, following excision it is impossible to replace the carotid vessels with a graft." Lack et al.[3] and Irons et al.[13] have outlined therapeutic principles. Because of the possible functional capacity of the tumors, McGuirt and Harker[25] advise preoperative catecholamine determinations. If a functioning tumor is detected preoperatively, the patient should be treated as though he had a pheochromocytoma.

Prognosis. An estimated mortality rate for untreated carotid body tumors is approximately 8%.[24] Local recurrence is enhanced by incomplete resection. Post-treatment tumors have recurred in approximately 12% of the patients 1 to 26 years following operation. Although the neoplasms are slow growing, observation after diagnosis by biopsy may be dangerous, since delay over an extended period of time may make surgical removal hazardous. Early operation is desired and advisable. The indications for surgical intervention demand circumspect judgment and skill in management.

JUGULAR PARAGANGLIOMA (GLOMUS JUGULARE)

The jugular paraganglioma is also known as glomus tympanicum tumor, tympanic body tumor, glomus jugulare, or tumor of the ear of carotid body type. The first documentation of the histological appearance and anatomical location of the glomus jugulare was published by Guild[26] in 1941. He described the glomus jugulare as being composed of one or more "jugular bodies," the average number being about three per ear. The sites of these vary; more than half are in the adventitia of the dome of the jugular bulb and the portion of Jacobson's or Arnold's nerves in the jugular fossa.[27] In one-fourth of patients, glomic bodies are in the mucosa of the cochlear promontory in association with the tympanic plexus of Jacobson's nerve. In one-fifth of patients, jugular bodies are in the tympanic canaliculus and, in other patients, in the descending facial canal.

The normal histological appearance of the jugular paraganglion is similar to that of the carotid body. No physiological function has been proved, but it is assumed that the behavior of the jugular paraganglion is similar to that of the carotid and aortic bodies. The similarity of structure, innervation and neoplasms of this paraganglion to those of other members of the paraganglionic system justifies its inclusion in that system.

Paragangliomas are the most common neoplasms of the middle ear and second to neurilemmomas in frequency of the temporal bone.[28] The term "glomus tympanicum" is used for the tumors originating in the middle ear and jugulare for those arising in the jugulare bulb.

When an otolaryngologist sees a vascular mass in the middle ear he usually makes a diagnosis of or thinks of a paraganglioma. There are, however, two vascular anomalies and an inflammatory condition which lie behind an intact tympanic membrane which may mimic the jugular paraganglioma. The vascular anomalies are a high jugular bulb with or without a bony covering plate and an ectopic intratympanic internal carotid artery. The inflammatory lesion is a solitary cholesterol granuloma which may lie on the promontory behind an intact membrane or be located in the tympanic membrane itself.

Overton and Ritter,[29] after a postmortem temporal bone study concluded that a high placed jugular bulb has an incidence of 6%. Guides to the radiographic and otoscopic recognition of these nonparaganglioma lesions is provided by Valvassori and Buckingham[30] and by Graham.[31]

Clinical Features. The anatomical location of the jugular paraganglioma predisposes to the development of symptoms related to the middle ear or to erosion of the lesion into the cranial vault. Capps[32] has divided cases of jugular paraganglioma into two groups, based on the localization of the neoplasm: a superficial form and a deep form. The majority of patients possess combined forms. In the superficial form, the neoplasm originates from paraganglionic tissue in the floor of the tympanic cavity or in the superior part of the tympanic canaliculus. Symptoms, usually related to the middle ear, are severe subjective noises synchronous with the pulse and a progressive conduction hearing loss. It may be years before the neoplasm causes discoloration of the tympanic membrane, and this is followed by the appearance of a delimited red tumor behind the membrane which eventually penetrates the membrane. A peripheral facial nerve paresis occurs comparatively early, with infiltration into the fallopian canal.

The deep form neoplasms spread primarily under the pars petrosa, thereby giving rise early to central nervous system symptoms. Growth of the neoplasm upward through the floor of the tympanic cavity and eventual visibility behind the tympanic membrane are comparatively late. Deep form tumors are believed to originate from paraganglia situated in the lower part of the canaliculus or in the adventitia of the bulb.

The terminal stages in both superficial and deep forms are characterized by intracranial invasion with neurological signs and symptoms and death. Signs and symptoms may be divided into three major groups: (1) primarily otic; (2) otic and neurological; and (3) primarily neurological; these are further arranged into four clinical groups.[33] Group I: aural symptoms only. This is the most commonly encountered and includes those cases where the only sign of neurological disorder is a seventh nerve palsy. Group II: aural symptoms followed many years later by neurological involvement. Group III: aural and neurological symptoms developing concurrently or within 5 years of each other. This group has a tendency to be associated with a rapid course. Group IV: Neurological manifestations appearing before aural symptoms. This is the least common. A closely related scheme of staging has been offered by Alford and Guilford.[34]

Aural "polyps" and a loss of hearing are the most common presenting features. Approximately one-half of the patients have a mass either in the external canal or behind the tympanic membrane at the time of examination. Ninety-one percent of 277 patients had a hearing loss.[34] Tinnitus of a pulsating nature, facial nerve paralysis, aural discharge, vertigo, hemorrhage and palsy of the ninth, tenth, eleventh and twelfth cranial nerves are other prominent presenting or accompanying symptoms. Typically, the patient is middle aged, and women predominate in a ratio of 4 or 5:1.[34] A familial tendency has been noted.

Roentgen findings have been described in almost all cases.[35] These include evidence of erosion of the petrous portion of the temporal lobe, sclerosis of the mastoid air cells and enlargement of the jugular foramen. Spector et al.[28] have also provided an analysis of the clinical manifestations.

Biological Activity. Characteristically, and like other paragangliomas, jugulare tumors expand slowly. Depending upon their origin, they may grow outward into the external auditory canal or through the petrous pyramid or the internal auditory canal. After extension into the cranial vault, they most often grow extradurally, but they may extend through the dura. In the cranial vault, the lesions may grow forward toward the clinoid process or posteriorly into the posterior fossa. Contiguous structures are encroached upon early; within the middle ear, destruction of adjacent bone permits extension into the mastoid.

Local infiltration is a feature of the jugulare tumors, but true malignancy is rare. While they are regarded as benign in general, they are potentially lethal. Taylor et al.[36] in 1965, accepted 10 cases representing instances of metastatic jugulare tumors. Borsanyi[37] has reported a 4% incidence of metastases in approximately 200 cases. Metastases have occurred in the jugular lymph nodes, liver, lungs and bone.[38]

It is our observation that jugular paragangliomas have a less uniform pattern than carotid body tumors. Like the carotid body paragangliomas, jugular paragangliomas do not contain a significant number of sustentacular cells or nerve endings (Fig. 19.3). Usually the stroma is scant and there is little collagen deposition. Electron microscopy indicates the chief cells contain neurosecretory granules and catecholamines have been demonstrated in the cells.[39, 40] Several of the jugulare tumors have been functional with systemic manifestations. These have been reviewed by Matsuguchi et al.[41]

The treatment of these neoplasms has been sur-

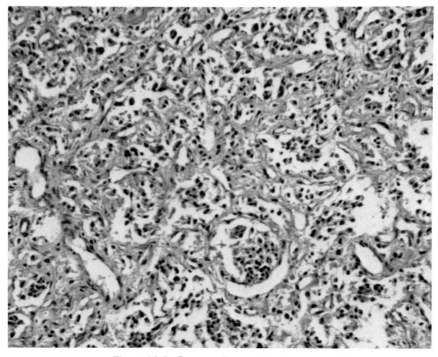

Figure 19.3. Paraganglioma of jugular paraganglion.

gery or radiation and some tumors have merely been observed without treatment. Surgical removal is attempted wherever possible, but Capps[32] states that surgical therapy should be considered only in tumors arising within the tympanic cavity, thus excluding tumors arising in the jugular bulb area. Radical mastoidectomy has been most frequently employed and, in many instances, has been followed by a course of radiation therapy. When neurosurgical procedures have been necessary, the mortality has been high.

Radiation therapy, while having no appreciable affect on the cells of the tumor, has decreased the vascularity of the tumor and, thereby, the over-all size of the lesion. Riemenschneider et al.[42] have expressed pessimism concerning the value of radiation therapy for this disease. Spector et al.[43] come to nearly the same conclusions while Arthur[44] indicates radiotherapy offers an excellent prospect of satisfactory tumor control.

For an authoritative discussion of treatment, the "round table" from the third Workshop in Microsurgery of the Ear should be read.[45, 46]

In general, the prognosis is guarded. Earlier diagnosis may alleviate this poor prognosis. When surgical removal is possible, the prognosis would seem to be best, particularly when the lesion is confined to the middle ear and to the adjacent mastoid. Intracranial extension appears to be a major cause of death.

Referring to the previously mentioned four clinical groups, the over-all prognosis of groups II, III and IV with neurological involvement (other than seventh nerve palsy) is poor, and death usually occurs within 2 years, either from brain stem compression or inhalation bronchopneumonia, and rarely from subarachnoid hemorrhage.

Harrison[47] gives the following survival statistics from his series: 71% alive and well at 5 years; 29% at 10 years; 17% at 15 years; and 10% at 20 years.

INTRAVAGAL PARAGANGLIOMAS (VAGAL BODY TUMORS)

Vagal paragangliomas typically arise from nests of paraganglionic tissue within the perineurium of the vagal nerve just below, or at the ganglion nodosum of the vagus nerve. Characteristically the tumors lie just below the base of the skull near the jugular foramen, are contiguous with the vagus nerve and replace the ganglion nodosum. Intravagal tumors, however, are not restricted to this locale and may be found at various sites along the nerve and may extend to the level of the carotid artery bifurcation. If the tumor lies inferiorly, it may displace the carotid artery anteriorly and laterally and often compresses the jugular vein. There is almost always vagal paralysis in association with an inferiorly placed tumor.

The paraganglioma juxtavagale arises from the middle vagal ganglia and usually displaces the nerve anteromedially. It usually extends along the base of the skull and into the various foramina. As the tumor spreads medially, the arch of the atlas may be destroyed and may complicate resection if spinal cord structures are involved.

Origin from superior vagal paraganglia leads often to a dumbbell type of tumor. Parts of it extend into the posterior cranial fossa and a portion will present into the infratemporal space.

Someren and Karcioglu[48] reported the 48th case of vagal paraganglioma in the literature in 1977. There is a female dominance in the disorder and patients have varied in age from 18 to 65 years.

The tumors are nodular or ovoid and vary from 2.0 to 6.5 cm in greatest dimension. The vagus nerve is often attached at the lower pole of the tumor.

Vagal paragangliomas most commonly manifest as slowly growing and painless masses high in the anterolateral aspect of the neck. On examination, the mass is often noted near the origin of the sternocleidomastoid muscle with a concomitant medial displacement of peritonsillar structures. On occasion, the masses may bulge high in the nasopharynx. Approximately one-half of the patients have had signs or symptoms for more than 3 years before diagnosis. Pharyngeal pain is usually a later sign and indicates irritation of the pharyngeal plexus, often preceding the onset of cranial nerve palsies. Pulsating tinnitus, deafness, syncope and vertigo may also be noted.

Presumptive diagnosis is made by arteriography.[49] Vagal paragangliomas are surrounded by a pharyngeal plexus of veins and consequently tend to appear larger upon arteriography than they really are.[50]

The light microscopic and ultrastructural findings of the vagal tumors do not differ from those of the branchiomeric paragangliomas.[51] The vascular component, while prominent, is said to be less so than in jugular paragangliomas. In addition, hyalinization of the fibrous septae is more marked in the vagal tumors than in carotid tumors. Secretory granules in the cells and even function (catecholamine) have been found.

Although vagal paragangliomas with lymph node and distant metastases have been reported, infiltration into the cranial vault is the usual "malignant" manifestation of these tumors.[52, 53]

Considering distant metastasis as the *only* criterion of malignancy, Druck et al.[53] found seven of 37 reported cases had demonstrated this finding. This 19% incidence is considerably higher than for any other branchiomeric paraganglioma. Regional lymph nodes and lungs are the secondary sites of note.

The primary treatment of vagal body tumors is generally agreed to be surgical resection. Radiotherapy is of value for palliation when surgery is contraindicated, or for intracranial invasion. Spector et al.[54] demonstrated that radiation produces extensive fibrosis and deposition of collagen, but has little effect on the chief cells or vasculature and consequently cannot be expected to eradicate the primary tumor.

PARAGANGLIOMAS OF THE UPPER AIRWAY AND LARYNX

Paragangliomas only rarely present in the nasal cavity, nasopharynx and larynx. In 1975, Scoppa and Tonkin[55] recorded the 13th case of a nasopharyngeal paraganglioma. All of the nasal or nasopharyngeal paragangliomas fall into one of three of the following groups:

1. Tumors arising in nearby structures: jugulare, intravagale, or ciliare paraganglia. This form is the most common.
2. Tumors arising primarily from the mucous membranes of the nasal cavity, paranasal sinuses and nasopharynx. This genesis is one of exclusion.
3. Tumors which have apparently metastasized to the nasal cavities from a remote paraganglioma. This phenomenon is rare.

Scoppa and Tonkin[55] cite evidence showing that paraganglionic tissue is normally present at birth surrounding the terminal part of the maxillary artery in the pterygopalatine fossa ("glomus nasopharyngis"). House et al.,[56] however, consider the nodose ganglia to be the origin of nasopharyngeal paragangliomas.

Two pairs of paraganglia of the larynx have been described which may give rise to paragangliomas.[57, 58] One site is just beneath the epithelium above the anterior end of the vocal cord and in relation to the internal branch of the superior laryngeal nerve; the other is between the thyroid and cricoid cartilages, in relation to the recurrent laryngeal nerve. Minute nests of aberrant paraganglionic tissue are also found anterior to the cricoid cartilage, lateral to it and posteriorly in relation to the transverse arytenoid muscle.

All but two of the 18 reported cases reviewed by Boles[59] occurred in the supraglottic larynx, most commonly in the posterior aspect of the aryepiglottic fold. The size of the tumors has ranged 1 to 7 cm. Symptoms are directly proportional to size.

Males have been involved more often than females and the age range for these tumors has been from 14 to 67 years (mean, 45 years).[60]

Biopsy of the tumors has often been associated with brisk and occasionally severe hemorrhage.

No specific surgical procedure has been consistently used for these tumors. Total laryngectomy should be avoided, if at all possible.

It is my contention that paragangliomas of the larynx are relatively benign lesions. Recurrences are unusual after initial excision. Reports of metastases and even widespread dissemination lack authenticity and are likely misrepresentations of adenocarcinomas.

PARAGANGLIOMAS OF THE ORBIT

The presence of a paraganglion ciliare, according to Thacker and Duckworth,[61] has not been definitely established in man. However, such a structure has been described in the chimpanzee and in monkeys and probably exists in man in the vicinity of the ciliary ganglion within the orbital muscle cone. By mid 1969, only five documented *orbital* paragangliomas had been recorded in the English literature.[62]

GROSS AND MICROSCOPIC APPEARANCE OF PARAGANGLIOMAS

The gross appearance of all paragangliomas is dominated by their vascularity. Carotid body tumors have usually reached the size of 3 × 4 cm before the patient seeks medical attention. They are extremely vascular, lobulated or ovoid and, generally, well encapsulated. They are intimately attached to the carotid vessels and not infrequently surround the arteries.

The jugular paraganglioma tumor is most often polypoid and fills the entire middle ear. There is a marked similarity to granulation tissue, often misleading the observer into considering the mass as an aural inflammatory polyp or hemangioma. In this respect, a histological diagnosis of "hemangioma" rendered on an aural polyp should be looked at with suspicion by the surgeon. Vagal body tumors are ovoid and encapsulated and have measured between 6.5 and 2 cm in major diameter at the time of primary treatment.

All of the tumors, regardless of their site of origin, manifest a decided tendency to mimic the structure of the parent paraganglionic tissue and all are, therefore, similar in their histological appearance. The usual appearance is that of an organoid neoplasm composed of epithelioid cells, divided and surrounded by a richly vascular stroma (Figs. 19.4 and 19.5). If the alveolar nests of cells are closely packed, the indistinct cytoplas-

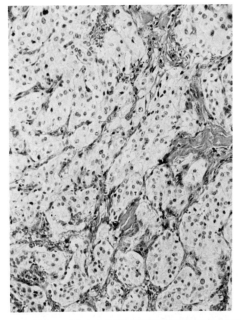

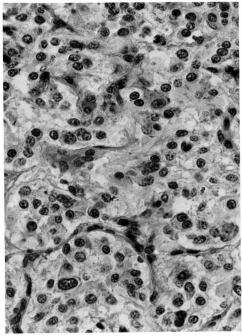

Figure 19.4 (*upper*) and 19.5 (*lower*). Appearance of "classical" carotid body paraganglioma with organoid arrangement of epithelioid cells.

mic boundaries appear to form a syncytium. A peritheliomatous pattern may be presented. In these instances, some of the capillaries have a definite endothelium; in other areas, the neoplastic cells abut directly onto the vascular space. If the latter are abundant, a cavernous hemangiomatous aspect is imparted to the tumor. Accentuation of the alveolar and perivascular arrangement of the cells may be brought about by reticulin preparation.

Variations of the fundamental pattern occur, and most are related to the size and shape of the epithelial cells. The cytoplasm of the cells is typically abundant, clear, and pale staining or finely granular and eosinophilic. Mitotic figures are the exception. The variability of the appearance of the basic or chief cells has been related to postremoval factors such as squeezing or the fixation process. Nerve cells and ganglion cells are not infrequently found in the body of the tumor.

GLOMUS TUMOR

The use of the term *glomus* to designate paraganglionic tissue should be abandoned. The normal glomus is one of several natural transpositions from the arterial to the venous system. It is a specialized arteriovenous anastomosis extending from a preterminal arteriole to an efferent vein. The normal glomus helps to regulate the circulation and blood pressure, temperature, and the interstitial cellular environment. It may also have some secretory function. Two basic cells participate in the glomus; capillary endothelial cells and pericytes. In addition there are smooth muscle cells and nonmyelinated nerve fibrils. There is *no* relation to paraganglionic tissues.

Tumors of the glomic apparatus are benign, organized hamartomas or hyperplasias of the normal structure.[63-66] They occur principally in the subcutaneous tissues, principally of the extremities. At the Mayo Clinic, they comprised 1.6% of 500 soft tissue tumors during a 2½-year period. In the extremities, the tumors are principally subungual.[67] Although they usually occur as single, discrete lesions, the incidence of multiple tumors has been recorded as high as 2.3% in adults and 26.3% of the tumors developed prior to the age of 16 years. Pain is the outstanding symptom of the glomus tumor.

Glomus tumors may also occur in the head and neck and have been reported in the nose, skin of neck, cheek and face.

The tumors may manifest a local infiltration but they are always benign. Because pericytes participate, there is the possibility that an evolution to a hemangiopericytoma may occur. This has never been described. Complete excision is curative.

REFERENCES

1. Glenner, G. G., and Grimley, P. M.: Tumors of the extra-adrenal paraganglion system (including chemoreceptors). In Atlas of Tumor Pathology, Series 2, Fascicle 9., Armed Forces Institute of Pathology, Washington, D.C., 1974.
2. Biscoe, T. J.: Carotid body: structure and function. Physiol. Rev. 51:437, 1971.
3. Lack, E. E., Cubilla, A. L., Woodruff, J. M., and Farr, H. W.: Paragangliomas of the head and neck region. A clinical study of 69 patients. Cancer 39:397, 1977.
4. Kersing, W.: Demonstration of hormonal activity of a glomus jugulare tumour by catecholamine determination. Arch. Otorhinolaryngol. 217:463, 1977.
5. Judge, D. M., McGavran, M. H., and Trapuledi, S.: Fume induced fluorescence in diagnosis of nasal neuroblastoma. Arch. Otolaryngol. 102:97, 1976.
6. Fine, G., Enriquez, P., and Morales, A. R.: Enzyme histochemistry of the human carotid body. Henry Ford Hosp. Med. J. 16:313, 1968.
7. Arias-Stella, J., and Valcarcel, J.: Chief cell hyperplasia in the human carotid body at high altitudes. Physiologic pathologic significance. Hum. Pathol. 7:361, 1976.
8. Lack, E. E.: Carotid body hypertrophy in patients with cystic fibrosis and cyanotic congenital heart disease. Hum. Pathol. 8:39, 1977.
9. Hayes, H. M., Jr., and Fraumeni, J. F., Jr.: Chemodectomas in dogs: epidemiologic comparison with man. J. Natl. Cancer Inst. 52:1455, 1974.
10. Spector, G. J., Ciralsky, R., Maisel, R. H., and Ogura, J. H.: IV. Multiple glomus tumors in the head and neck. Laryngoscope 85:1066, 1975.
11. Cook, R. L.: Bilateral chemodectomas in the neck. J. Laryngol. 91:611, 1977.
12. Handel, S. F., Miller, M. H., Miller, L. S., and Goepfert, H.: Angiographic changes of head and neck chemodectomas following radiotherapy. Arch. Otolaryngol. 103:87, 1977.
13. Irons, G. B., Weiland, L. H., and Brown, W. L.: Paragangliomas of the neck: clinical and pathologic analysis of 116 cases. Surg. Clin. North Am. 57:575, 1977.
14. Spector, G. J., Gado, M., Ciralsky, R., Ogura, J. H., and Maisel, R. H.: Neurologic complications of glomus tumors in the head and neck. Laryngoscope 85:1387, 1975.
15. Fletcher, W. E., and Arnold, J. H.: Carotid body tumor: review of literature and report of unusual case. Am. J. Surg. 87:617, 1954.
16. McIlrath, D. C., and ReMine, W. H.: Carotid body tumors. Surg. Clin. North Am. 43:1135, 1963.
17. Conley, J. J.: The management of carotid body tumors. Surg. Gynecol. Obstet. 117:722, 1963.
18. Resler, D. R., Snow, J. B., Jr., and Williams, G. R.: Multiplicity and familial incidence of carotid body and glomus jugulare tumors. Ann. Otol. Rhinol. Laryngol. 75:114, 1966.
19. Harrington, S. W., Clagett, O. T., and Dockerty, M. B.: Tumors of the carotid body. Ann. Surg. 114:820, 1941.
20. Monro, R. S.: The natural history of the carotid body tumors and their diagnosis and treatment with a report of five cases. Br. J. Surg. 37:445, 1949–1950.
21. Gaylis, H., and Mieny, C. J.: The incidence of malignancy in carotid body tumors. Br. J. Surg. 64:885, 1977.
22. Morris, G. C., Jr., Balas, P. E., Cooley, D. A., Crawford, E. S., and Debakey, M. E.: Surgical treatment of benign and malignant carotid body tumors: clinical experience with 16 tumors in 12 patients. Am. Surg. 29:429, 1963.
23. Grabb, W. B., Jr., and Lampe, I.: The role of radiation therapy in the treatment of chemodectomas of the glomus jugulare. Laryngoscope 75:1861, 1965.
24. Rush, B. F., Jr.: Current concepts in the treatment of carotid body tumors. Surgery 52:697, 1962.
25. McGuirt, W. F., and Harker, L. A.: Carotid body tumors. Arch. Otolaryngol. 101:58, 1975.

26. Guild, S. R.: Hitherto unrecognized structure, glomus jugularis, in man. Anat. Rec. (Suppl. 2) 79:28, 1941.
27. Guild, S. R.: Glomus jugulare, nonchromaffin paraganglion, in man. Ann. Otol. Rhinol. Laryngol. 62:1045, 1953.
28. Spector, G. J., Ciralsky, R. H., and Ogura, J. H.: Glomus tumors in the head and neck. III. Analysis of clinical manifestations. Ann. Otol. 84:73, 1975.
29. Overton, S. B., and Ritter, F. N.: A high placed jugular bulb in the middle ear: a clinical and temporal bone study. Laryngoscope 83:1986, 1973.
30. Valvassori, G. E., and Buckingham, R. A.: Middle ear masses mimicking glomus tumors: radiologic and otoscopic recognition. Ann. Otol. 85:606, 1975.
31. Graham, M. D.: The jugular bulb: its anatomic and clinical considerations in contemporary otology. Laryngoscope 87:105, 1977.
32. Capps, F. C. W.: Tumors of the glomus jugulare or tympanic body. J. Frac. Rad. 7–8:312, 1957.
33. Bickerstaff, E. R., and Howell, J. S.: The neurological importance of tumors of glomus jugulare. Laryngoscope 72:765, 1953.
34. Alford, B. R., and Guilford, F. R.: A comprehensive study of tumors of glomus jugulare. Brain 76:576, 1953.
35. Rice, R. P., and Holman, C. B.: Roentgenographic manifestation of tumors of the glomus jugulare (chemodectoma). Am. J. Roentgenol. Radium Ther. Nucl. Med. 89:1201, 1963.
36. Taylor, D. M., Alford, B. R., and Greenberg, S. D.: Metastases of glomus jugulare tumors. Arch. Otolaryngol. 82:5, 1965.
37. Borsanyi, S. J.: Glomus jugulare tumors. Laryngoscope 72:1336, 1962.
38. Hawk, W. A., and McCormack, L. J.: Nonchromaffin paraganglioma of the glomus jugulare: review of the literature and report of six cases. Cleve. Clin. Q. 26:62, 1959.
39. Kjaergaard, J.: An electron microscopic study of the tympano-jugular glomus. Acta Otolaryngol. 78:84, 1974.
40. Stiller, D., Katenkamp, D., and Kuttner, K.: Jugular body tumors: Hyperplasias or true neoplasms. Light and electron microscopical investigations. Virchows Arch. (Pathol. Anat.) 365:163, 1975.
41. Matsuguchi, H., Tsuneyushi, M., Takeshita, A., Nakamura, M., Kato, T., and Arakawa, E.: Nonadrenaline-secreting glomus jugulare tumor with cyclic change of blood pressure. Arch. Otolaryngol. 135:1111, 1975.
42. Riemenschneider, P. A., Hoople, G. D., Brewer, D., Jones, D., and Ecker, R.: Roentgenographic diagnosis of tumors of glomus jugularis. Am. J. Roentgenol. Radium. Ther. Nucl. Med. 69:59, 1953.
43. Spector, G. J., Maisel, R. H., and Ogura, J. H.: Glomus jugulare tumors. II. A clinicopathologic analysis of the effects of radiotherapy. Ann. Otol. 83:26, 1974.
44. Arthur, K.: Radiotherapy in chemodectoma of the glomus jugulare. Clin. Radiol. 28:415, 1977.
45. McCabe, B., and Fletcher, M.: Selection of therapy of glomus jugulare tumors. From Third Workshop on Microsurgery of the Ear. Arch. Otolaryngol. 89:156, 1969.
46. Rosenwasser, H: Glomus jugulare tumors. From Third Workshop on Microsurgery of the Ear. Arch. Otolaryngol. 89:160, 1969.
47. Harrison, K.: Glomus jugulare tumours: Their clinical behavior and management. Proc. Roy. Soc. Med. 67:264, 1974.
48. Someren, A., and Karcioglu, Z.: Malignant vagal paraganglioma. Report of a case and review of literature. Am. J. Clin. Pathol. 68:400, 1977.
49. Palachios, E.: Chemodectomas of the head and neck. Am. J. Roentgenol. 110:129, 1970.
50. Black, F. O., Myers, E. N., and Barnes, S. M.: Surgical management of vagal chemodectomas. Laryngoscope 87:1259, 1977.
51. Fernandez, B. B., Hernandez, F. J., and Staley, C. J.: Chemodectoma of the vagus nerve. Report of a case with ultrastructural study. Cancer 35:263, 1975.
52. Kahn, L. B.: Vagal body tumor (nonchromaffin paraganglioma, chemodectoma, and carotid body-like tumor) with

cervical node metastasis and familial association. Ultra-structural study and review. Cancer 38:2367, 1976.

53. Druck, N. S., Spector, G. J., Ciralsky, R. H., and Ogura, J. H.: Malignant glomus vagale. Report of a case and review of the literature. Arch. Otolaryngol. 102:634, 1976.

54. Spector, G. J., Compagno, J., Perez, C. A., Maisel, R. H., and Ogura, J. H.: Glomus jugulare tumors: Effects of radiotherapy. Cancer 35:1316, 1975.

55. Scoppa, J., and Tonkin, J. P.: Non-chromaffin paraganglioma of the nasopharynx. J. Laryngol. 89:653, 1975.

56. Hause, J. M., Goodman, M. L., Gacek, R. R., and Green, G. L.: Chemodectomas of the nasopharynx. Arch. Otolaryngol. 96:138, 1972.

57. Lawson, W., and Zak, F. G.: The glomus bodies ("paraganglia") of the human larynx. Laryngoscope 84:98, 1974.

58. Zak, F. G., and Lawson, W.: Glomic (paraganglionic) tissue in the larynx and capsule of the thyroid gland. Mt. Sinai J. Med. N.Y. 39:82, 1972.

59. Boles, R.: Unusual tumors of the larynx. Canad. J. Otolaryngol. 4:328, 1975.

60. Piquet, J. J., Dupont, A., and Houcke, M.: Les paragangliones non chromaffines du larynx. E'tude clinique et em microscopie electronique. Ann. Otolaryngol. 93:255, 1976.

61. Thacker, W. C., and Duckworth, J. K.: Chemodectoma of the orbit. Cancer 23:1233, 1969.

62. Lederer, F. L., Skolnik, E. M., Soboroff, B. J., and Fornatt, E. J.: Nonchromaffin paraganglioma of head and neck. Ann. Otol. Rhinol. Laryngol. 67:305, 1958.

63. Soule, E. H., Ghomley, R. K., and Bulbulian, A. H.: Primary tumors of the soft tissues of the extremities exclusive of epithelial tumors; an analysis of 500 consecutive cases. Arch. Surg. 70:462, 1955.

64. Mollis, W. F., Rosato, F. E., Rosato, E. F., Butler, C. J., and Mayer, L. J.: The glomus tumor. Surg. Gynec. Obstet. 135:705, 1972.

65. Kohout, E., and Stout, A. P.: The glomus tumor in children. Cancer 14:555, 1961.

66. Anagnostou, G. D., Papademetrious, D. G., and Toumazani, M. N.: Subcutaneous glomerus tumors. Surg. Gynec. Obstet. 136:945, 1973.

67. Olson, J. R., and Abell, M. R.: Nonfunctional nonchromaffin paragangliomas of the retroperitoneum. Cancer 23:1358, 1969.

CHAPTER 20

Non-odontogenic Tumors of the Jaws

For convenience of presentation, this chapter is divided into four principal subdivisions: (1) a discussion of chondrogenic and osteogenic neoplasms, including Paget's disease; (2) vascular tumors or lesions of the facial bones and jaws; (3) giant cell lesions and fibro-osseous lesions of the jaws; (4) a presentation of a miscellaneous group of common and uncommon non-odontogenic tumors (Table 20.1).

1. Paget's Disease, Chondrogenic and Osteogenic Neoplasms

PAGET'S DISEASE

Paget's disease (osteitis deformans) is an unusual and idiopathic affliction of the adult skeleton. It is slightly more common in men than in women, and it generally appears between the fourth and sixth decades of life. The disease is extremely common among the elderly, the incidence arising from about 1% in the fifth decade to about 10% in the tenth. Estimations have it that one in every 100 to 150 persons more than 45 years old has Paget's disease, and that 80% of these will have some symptoms referable to the disorder. Subclinical Paget's disease, however, is quite common and is often found when skeletal x-rays are made for other reasons or as an incidental observation at necropsy.

The sacrum, vertebrae, femora, skull, sternum, and pelvis are most commonly involved. The jaws are considered to be less frequently involved than the skull, but this may be due to the infrequency of inspection of oral regions during physical examinations. Stafne and Austin[1] took full mouth radiographs of the jaws in 138 cases in which Paget's disease had involved one or more bones of the skeleton, and in 23 cases there was evidence of jaw involvement. The maxilla was involved in 20 cases and the mandible in three. When the jaws are involved, the skull is almost invariably affected.

The clinical features of this disease when the jaws are involved are related to deformity and prosthetic dental problems and, occasionally, to the hazards that may follow surgical procedures in the region.[2] An ill-defined ache in the affected bone may be a common symptom.

As the disease progresses, there may be growth deformity of the involved bones. Distortions of the weight-bearing portions of the skeleton are common in Paget's disease. Curiously, the mandible may not be strikingly distorted, in spite of the forces of mastication.[3] Gradual enlargement of the jaws results in a spreading of the teeth and an abnormal occlusal pattern. The retroclination of the incisor teeth and the palatoversion of the posterior teeth are constant and most striking features.[2] In the edentulous patient, the changes in the jaws will interfere with the wearing of dentures, and this is often an early complaint. Should a partial denture be worn, it appears to restrain the rate of new bone formation under it, and so appears to form a bed for itself as the surrounding bone expands. Whereas fractures are not uncommon complications in the weight-bearing long bones, they are rare in the jaws.

As a result of extensive arteriovenous communications in the affected bone, the area is characteristically warmer than the unaffected areas. The serum alkaline phosphatase activity reflects the amount and extent of osteoblastic activity in Pa-

Table 20.1
Tumors of the Facial Bones and Skull: A Histological Classification

Type	Benign	Malignant
Hematopoietic and reticulo-endothelial	Histiocytosis	Plasmacytoma Myeloma Malignant lymphoma Histiocytosis

Chondrogenic	Osteochondroma
	Chondroma
	Chondroblastoma
	Chondromyxoid fibroma
		Chondrosarcoma
		  Differentiated
		  Dedifferentiated
		  Mesenchymal

Osteogenic	Osteoma
	Osteoid osteoma
	Osteoblastoma
		Osteogenic sarcoma
		  Endosteal
		  Parosteal
		  Periosteal

Fibrogenic	Fibroma
	  Ossifying
	  Nonossifying
	Desmoplastic fibroma
	? Fibromyxoma
		Fibrosarcoma

Odontogenic	Myxoma	? Myxosarcoma

Notochordal	—	Chordoma
		  Conventional
		  Chondrogenic

Vascular	Hemangioma	Angiosarcoma Hemangiopericytoma
Lipogenic	? Lipoma	? Liposarcoma
Neurogenic	Neurilemmoma Neurofibroma	Neurogenous sarcoma Primary and secondary neuroectodermal tumors
Disputed origin	Giant cell granuloma "Brown" tumor Cherubism Giant cell tumor Benign fibrous histiocytoma	Malignant giant cell tumor Ewing's sarcoma Malignant fibrous histiocytoma

get's disease. If skeletal involvement is minimal, the serum activity is usually normal. For this reason the seum activity, when Paget's disease involves only the jaws, cannot be used for correlation with progression of the jaw lesions.

The radiographic changes vary according to the stage of the disease. Osteoporosis is the initial finding. Later, as a result of a blending of minute areas of radiolucency and increased opacity, the typical "cotton wool" appearance is seen. Radiological evidence is occasionally seen in the jaws before the disorder becomes apparent elsewhere in the skeleton.[4]

Demineralization in the jaws and an increase in the number of trabeculae may give an appearance of ground glass. If teeth are present, there is a gradual loss of the lamina dura. The roots of the teeth may show comparable change. The earliest changes may be a radiolucency around the apices, accompanied by resorption of the latter. Hypercementosis may be diffuse or localized and irregular. The pulp chambers of the teeth frequently calcify.

The microscopic findings also reflect the stage of the disease and are similar to those noted in other parts of the skeleton, except perhaps, that non-cellular calcified masses of bone are more commonly seen. During the early phases, or osteoporotic form of the disease, large quantities of new bone are found in a loose, vascular connective tissue marrow. This new bone does not show a mosaic pattern since there has not been sufficient time for irregular cement lines to form.

In the fully developed stage of Paget's disease, there is coexistent and simultaneous osteoblastic and osteoclastic activity. It is this activity that gives the bone its characteristic mosaic pattern. The latter is the result of the formation of irregular and curved cement lines and depressions on the surface of bone spicules, in turn, the result of osteoclastic resorption (Fig. 20.1). As the disease becomes less active, the marrow becomes less vascular and more fibrotic and may even revert to a fatty marrow. Osteoblasts and osteoclasts are also absent or decreased in the inactive stages.

A presarcomatous stage has been described in transitional areas between fully developed Paget's bone and complicating sarcoma.[5]

The teeth manifest changes in a similar degree. The cementum may show curvilinear markings and a mosaic pattern with resorption of the cementum and dentine and replacement by fibrous tissue and bone typical of Paget's disease.[6]

Although there is no specific treatment of the disease, very careful management is required to avoid complications when the jaws are involved.[7-9] Profuse bleeding may be encountered during alveolectomy when the vascular spaces in the bone are entered. The sclerotic foci of bone also manifest a lowered resistance to infection, and an extraction in a jaw affected with Paget's disease may easily lead to osteomyelitis or to an oral-antral fistula. A late complication, due to pressure on nerves in their bony foramens, is a severe facial neuralgia. The abnormal local circulation in the bones of Paget's disease (multiple arteriovenous shunts), if widespread, predisposes to heart failure. The most serious and important complication is the development of osteogenic sarcoma having its genesis in the abnormal regrowth of bone (Fig. 20.2). Newman reports the incidence of sarcoma to be about 2%.[7]

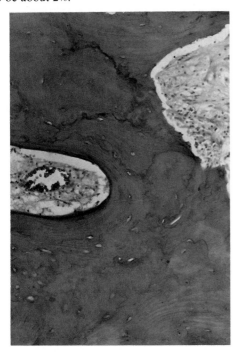

Figure 20.1. Paget's disease in mandible.

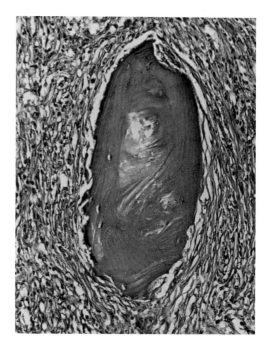

Figure 20.2. Sarcoma arising in Paget's disease.

CARTILAGINOUS NEOPLASMS

Chondromas and chondrosarcomas most frequently affect the pelvis, sternum, scapula, long bones and the bones of the hands and feet. By 1961, 54 cases of chondrogenic neoplasms of the jaws had been reported in the English language literature.[10] Since then, reviews of the subject have been offered by Batsakis and Dito,[11] Kragh et al.,[12] Chaudhry et al.,[13] and Arlen et al.[14]

Apart from the relatively recent emergence of chondrosarcoma as a distinct pathological entity,[15] there exists an inherent complexity in the diagnosis of chondromatous neoplasms. Not only has the degree of malignancy been underestimated in the past, but also the histological analysis is often inadequate. Although the zone between innocent tumors and overt chondrosarcomas may still be incompletely defined and poorly understood, it is certainly evident from clinical experience and published reports that chondrogenic neoplasms are far more often malignant than benign in their clinical or biological course. It is with these aspects in mind that Cahn[16] emphasized that a pathological diagnosis of chondroma in a facial tumor should be viewed with reservation and fairly radical treatment be carried out. Chaudhry et al.,[13] consider chondrogenic neoplasms of the jaws to be more often malignant than benign by a 2:1 ratio. Dahlin[17] records no chondromas of the jaws in his review of 2,276 bone tumors.

When a chondroma is present in the jaws, it manifests slow growth, is locally invasive and difficult to remove and its clinical course is marred by recurrences.[11] In the facial and nose region, chondromas arise from nasal cartilages, ethmoid bones or the maxilla. In the mandible they usually take origin from the coronoid and condyloid processes.[13] Enchondromas are distinctly unusual.

Treatment for chondromas is predicated on their unpredictability of behavior, and wide surgical excision is advisable. Incomplete removal, followed by repeated recurrences, is thought to predispose to the development of chondrosarcoma. In many, if not all, such instances, however, a more probable explanation is misdiagnosis of the primary neoplasm by the pathologist.

Chondrosarcomas occur in the jaws and facial bones far less often than do osteogenic sarcomas, and they are particularly rare in the maxilla. In the mandible, chondrosarcoma has a predilection for the premolar and molar regions. The symphysis and the coronoid process and the condylar processes may also be involved. In the maxilla, the anterior alveolar region is the most common site.

The apparent preference of these tumors for the anterior part of the maxilla and the posterior part of the mandible is of interest. It has been suggested that this is due to the proximity of the anterior maxilla to the cartilaginous nasal capsule and the presence of remnants of Meckel's cartilage in the posterior part of the body of the mandible.[18] This assumption, according to Shira and Bhaskar,[10] has no basis in fact. The mammalian maxilla, a membranous bone, is formed around the nasal capsule and, therefore, has the same association with cartilage in the molar area as it does in the anterior region. The mandible, on the other hand, is formed around Meckel's cartilage, and the remnants of this structure are seen not only in the molar area but also in the anterior region. Therefore, the predilection for certain areas of the jaws has some other basis than the presence of cartilaginous residues.

The temporomandibular joint is a very rare site for primary chondrosarcoma. It is to be distinguished from other benign tumors intrinsic to the joint and particularly synovial chondromatosis.

The peak age of incidence for chondrosarcomas of the jaws is in the third to fifth decade; in 80% of the cases the patients are in the third to the sixth decade. Males and females are about equally affected.

Cartilaginous neoplasms develop out of full-fledged cartilage, and, in contrast to osteogenic sarcomas, the chondrosarcoma never shows neo-plastic osteoid or bone evolving from a sarcomatous stroma. The distinction between the full developed, or obviously benign, chondroma and malignant chondrosarcoma rarely causes interpretive difficulties. Intermediate types are usually underestimated, but this is not necessarily a hazard if the potential biological course of the neoplasm is clearly understood by both the pathologist and the surgeon.

In chondromas, the great majority of cells possess a single nucleus. Their nuclei, even in the rare binucleate cell that may be found, tend to be small in relation to the cell. The chondrosarcoma, on the other hand, is usually richly cellular and manifests either a striking or subtle irregularity of cells and nuclei. There is a plumpness to the cells; multiple nuclei are found, and these may show a pronounced hyperchromatism (Fig. 20.3). Mononuclear giant cells are also present. The nuclear-cytoplasmic ratio is also shifted toward nuclear dominance. Since cell division in chondrosarcomas tends to be amitotic, the scarcity or even absence of mitotic figures should not preclude the diagnosis of malignancy. In the usual case, when mitoses are readily seen, they are not needed to confirm the suspicion of malignancy since other features are also present. Alterations in the matrix are not related to the cell morphology except in terminal stages, where it may not be discernible as chondroid matrix and the cells themselves are primitive and spindle-shaped.

Evans et al.[19] have correlated histological grades

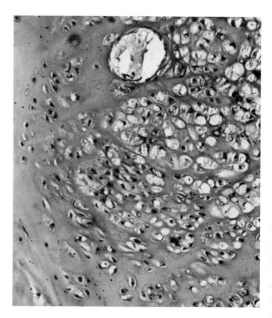

Figure 20.3. Chondrosarcoma of maxilla.

(I to III) with biological course. Marcove and Huvos[20] have done similar correlations. A myxomatous change with cystic alterations in the tumor correlates well with a low or medium histological grade. An absence of cartilagenous lobulation and the presence of spindle cell forms is characteristic of a high grade (III) malignancy and heralds a poor prognosis. There is also some transfer to ultrastructural findings.[21] Many of the latter in low grade chondrosarcoma cells are also found in cells comprising a variety of benign and non-neoplastic lesions of hyaline cartilage and the normal chondrocyte. High grade chondrosarcomas have more ultrastructural features in common with spindle cell sarcomas of the fibroblastic type.

Benign cartilagenous tumors of the nasal cavity, nasopharynx and paranasal sinuses have been reviewed by Kilby and Ambegaokar.[22] There is a strong probability that some of the lesions included by these workers and other investigators in the field do not represent true neoplasms but rather are focal areas of hypertrophy or hyperplasia of nasal septal cartilage or cartilage-capped exostoses.[2] There appears to be an equal sex distribution for the tumors. They have been recorded in patients as young as 8 months and as old as the seventh decade with a relative peak in the third decade. Approximately 50% of the "chondromas" arise from the ethmoids. The nasal septum, antrum, hard palate, nasopharynx and alar cartilages follow. These lesions present usually as slow-growing asymptomatic nodules projecting into the lumen of the nasal cavity or nasopharynx. They are smooth, firm and lobulated, but the consistency may be that of a "ripe pear." Histologically, the chondromas most often demonstrate well differentiated hyaline cartilage without nuclear atypia. Myxochondromatous and fibrochondromatous areas have been described.

It is generally agreed that irradiation is of no value in these lesions and effective management is exclusively surgical.

Chondrosarcomas of facial bones and soft tissues, other than the maxilla and mandible have been reviewed by Coates et al.[24] and Fu and Perzin.[23] Precise localization, because of tumor extension may be difficult, but distribution between the nasal septum, maxilloethmoidal complex, sphenoid sinus and nasopharynx is nearly equal. In the sphenoethmoidal area particularly, the histological differentiation among chondrosarcoma, chondroma, and chordoma may be very difficult, particularly in the light of the hybrid chondroid chordoma (see Chapter 18).

Prognosis for patients with these chondrosarco-

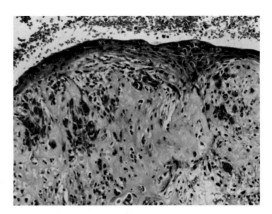

Figure 20.4. Local aggressiveness manifested by a chondrosarcoma of the maxilla. Note the attenuated, metaplastic respiratory epithelium.

mas appears to be directly related to: (1) location; (2) adequacy of primary surgical resection; and (3) histological grade. Tumors growing in the nasopharynx, posterior nasal cavity and sphenoid sinus region have a poor ultimate prognosis although the course of the disease may be prolonged. Death in this group of lesions is almost always due to uncontrolled local growth of the sarcoma. Fu and Perzin[23] claim the only recurrences in their series were in patients who had involvement of the margins of resection. The majority of the chondrosarcomas in this region are well differentiated (grade I) and prognosis is enhanced by that character. In general the course of these lesions is a slow and progressive one. They displace local structures before invading them and terminate, if not checked, with contralateral, orbital or intracranial extension (Fig. 20.4). Metastases are unusual. Fu and Perzin,[23] after review of 25 cases from the literature, indicate that 44% had died of disease; 16% were alive with persistent disease and 32% lived without recurrence after adequate surgical excision. The authors also stressed that death may be late after a relatively prolonged survival. Although regression of chondrosarcoma may occur after radiation therapy, the modality appears limited in its ability to control the disease.

An unusual, yet highly characteristic chondroid neoplasm, the *mesenchymal* chondrosarcoma, has only been recorded in the literature less than 100 times.[25, 26] Yet its uniqueness and predilection for the jaws as well as the ribs warrants inclusion and discussion in this section. Mesenchymal chondrosarcomas arise in extraskeletal as well as skeletal sites. One-third of the reported cases are found in the extraskeletal soft tissues. In contrast with most neoplasms of bone, however, mesenchymal chondrosarcomas rarely involve tubular bones.[25] The ribs and jaws are most commonly involved. I have seen two examples in the maxilla over a 10-year period. Histologically, these neoplasms are highly characteristic.[25, 27] Sheets of undifferentiated small oval or round cells, alternating with zones of easily identifiable cartilaginous tissue, are the hallmarks. In some tumors, the chondroid material is dominant; in others it is not present in every histological section.[25] The cellular regions, however, dominate in the ordinary case. These areas contain undifferentiated cells of slight to rather prominent spindle shape and with small nuclei. Mitoses may be prominent or only occasionally seen. Islands of chondroid differentiation lie in this cellular matrix and, by and large, are innocuous in appearance (Fig. 20.5). Most of the cartilagenous islands appear quite abruptly in the undifferentiated cellular zones, but more gradual transitions are also frequently seen; here, the cartilagenous areas are as mature as and resemble the cartilage seen in ordinary low grade chondrosarcomas.[25]

The histopathological diagnosis, if sampling misses the zones of cartilage, may be difficult. Hemangiopericytoma and synovial sarcoma are the two most frequent misdiagnoses. Ultrastructure studies confirm the presence of two main cell types; poorly differentiated mesenchymal cells and cells showing cartilagenous differentiation.[28] The undifferentiated elements are "precartilage mesenchyme."[29] Jacobson[29] has suggested the developed mesenchymal chondrosarcoma is one form of what he terms "polyhistoma" to designate a neoplasm whose basic cells are small, round and like Ewing's sarcoma, but which differentiate into various mesenchymal structures, most often bone.

The average age of patients with mesenchymal chondrosarcoma is 33 years with more than one-half of the patients in their second or third decades of life when diagnosis is established. This contrasts with a median age of 55 years for chondrosarcomas in general.

For both skeletal and extraskeletal forms, initial wide surgical excision is important. As an aggregate, the lesions manifest recurrences and/or distant metastases in one-third to one-half of the cases.[26] There is considerable variation in the clinical course but in general, the jaw lesions appear to have an accelerated course to death.

To my knowledge, an extraskeletal myxoid chondrosarcoma has not been reported in the head and neck. It is a rare lesion of extraskeletal soft tissues characterized by ill-defined nodular masses of cords and strands of small acidophilic cells separated by abundant mucoid stroma.[30]

High recurrence rates for chondromatous neo-

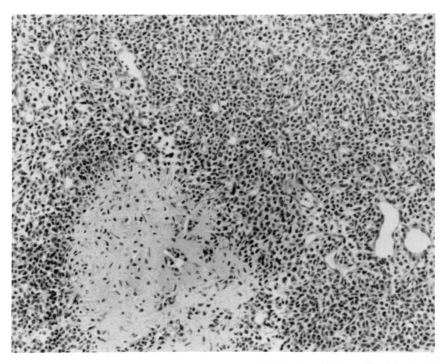

Figure 20.5. Mesenchymal chondrosarcoma with apparent origin in ethmoid sinus. The islands of cartilage serve to distinguish this neoplasm from hemangiopericytoma.

plasms of the facial bones, coupled with an inability to detect the extent of the lesion by x-ray examination, make this group of neoplasms difficult to treat.[11] Thoma and Goldman[31] consider chondrosarcoma very refractory to all methods of treatment, with the only possibility of cure lying in radical surgical excision. Radiation therapy has been used as an adjunct in recurrences or as a form of palliation. Several authors have reported long survival after a combined radiotherapy-surgery approach.[11]

A high recurrence rate, aggressive local extension (Fig. 20.4) and, occasionally, fatal metastases all speak for a poor prognosis. Contrary to the view expressed by Phemister[15] and Lichtenstein and Jaffe,[32] that chondrosarcoma offers a better prognosis than osteogenic sarcoma, all indications are that chondrosarcoma of the jaws carries a more serious prognosis.[13] The 5-year survival rate is lower than that reported for osteogenic sarcoma of the jaws, and the over-all long-term survival is much less.

Death in patients with chondrosarcoma of the jaws is usually related to local extension, with destruction and compromise of vital structures.[11] Since the natural course of a chondrosarcoma may be of long duration, a long period of follow-up is necessary before a "clinical cure" can be justified.[33]

OSTEOGENIC SARCOMA

Osteogenic sarcoma is the most common primary malignant tumor of bone, but it is relatively rare in the oral and facial region. Dahlin found only 20 cases among 469 osteogenic sarcomas of the skeletal system, an incidence of about 4%.[17] McKenna,[34] in a similar survey, reported that among 259 osteogenic sarcomas, one was found in the skull, six in the maxilla and seven in the mandible. His estimates are close to the 6.5% incidence reported by Garrington[35] from data derived from several sources. The incidence of osteogenic sarcoma in the jaws has been very roughly estimated for the United States population as 0.07 per 100,000 per year.

Patients with this neoplasm in the jaws tend to be somewhat older than those with similar lesions elsewhere in the skeletal system. For lesions other than facial, the peak frequency is in male patients between 10 and 25 years old. The average age (at diagnosis) of patients with sarcoma of the jaws is about a decade later. In an Armed Forces series,[35] the ages ranged from 4 to 64 years, with a mean of about 31. An exception to this is noted in the osteogenic sarcoma which occurs in patients with advanced Paget's disease of bone.

As with cases involving other parts of the body, the cases of jaw lesions appear to occur most frequently in male patients, but the magnitude cannot be assessed with certainty. Dehner[36] has reviewed the infrequent occurrence of osteogenic sarcoma in the mandible and maxilla of children.

The mandible is most often the primary site of jaw lesions (Table 20.2). Garrington et al.[35] found the mandible involved in 38 of 56 cases, the remainder being in the maxilla. These authors also noted that, unlike the maxillary cases, the mandibular cases did not reflect a sharp increase in frequency among adult patients as compared with those in younger age groups. They suggested that this might be due to growth centers in the mandible which allow for potential growth and activity throughout life. In the maxilla, the alveolar ridge is a frequent point of origin, whereas the body of the mandible is regarded as the most common site.

As with osteogenic sarcoma of the long bones, circumstantial evidence may occasionally point to predisposing conditions such as irradiation, trauma or pre-existing bone disorders. Yannopoulos et al.[39] recorded 12 cases of osteogenic sarcoma arising in fibrous dysplasia. Four of these patients developed osteogenic sarcomas in facial bones and all four had received irradiation to the area for their fibrous dysplasia. In their series of 44 patients, Kragh et al.[37] found five with previous irradiation and two with pre-existing fibrous dysplasia. Paget's disease, of course, is a known predisposer to the development of osteogenic sarcoma. In the majority of reports, however, there is no antecedent history of trauma or disease. Li-

Table 20.2
Osteogenic Sarcoma of Jaws

Author	Location		Average Age		5-Year Survival (%)	
	Mandible	Maxilla	Mandible	Maxilla	Mandible	Maxilla
Finkelstein[174]	12	12	49	40	50	30
Garrington et al.[35]	38	18	25	28	41	25
Kragh et al.[37]	19	23	33	33	33	19
Caron et al.[38]	17	15	35	37	24	33

Volsi[40] has reviewed pre-existing factors associated with osteogenic sarcoma of the maxilla.

A mass is the most common complaint, but neoplasms of the maxilla may produce early pain. Less common primary complaints are numbness of the lips, loosened teeth, trismus, nasal obstruction and symptoms referable to the eyes. The overall average time between onset and medical attention is 3 to 4 months. Physical examination con-

firms the mass, which may project either buccalward or toward the gingiva. Invasion of the overlying skin is unusual. The alveolar process is generally distended, and the gingiva is reddened or raw and ulcerated.

From a dental viewpoint, symptoms are usually associated with complaints mimicking periapical inflammation. An error in diagnosis may lead to the extraction of teeth involved by neoplasm.

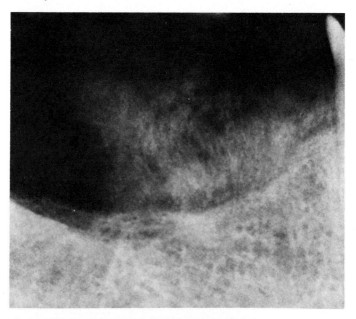

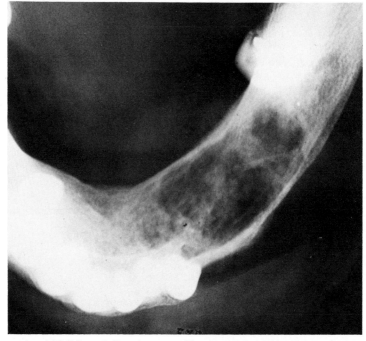

Figures 20.6, (*upper*) and **20.7** (*lower*). Roentgenographic appearances of two types of osteogenic sarcoma of the mandible; the first is the osleoblastic variant, and the second is osteolytic in type.

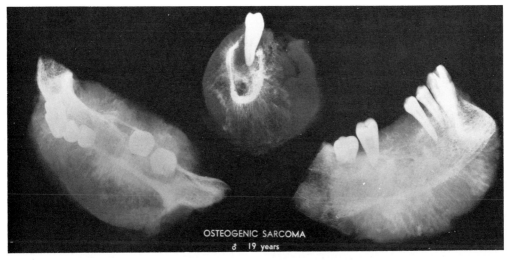

Figure 20.8. Osteogenic sarcoma of the mandible. (Courtesy of D. A. Kerr, D.D.S.)

Richards and Coleman[41] report extractions in the region of the neoplasm 3 weeks to 1 year before diagnosis in 8 of 17 patients.

The radiographic appearances of osteogenic sarcomas are variable, depending on the amount of host bone being destroyed (Figs. 20.6 and 20.7). The "sun-ray" appearance is not consistent and is characteristic only if the neoplasm compromises the cortex where there may be new bone that forms striations which extend perpendicular to the surface (Fig. 20.8). If the lesion is primarily lytic, a specific radiographic appearance is improbable. A sun-ray appearance was present in 25% of the series reported by Garrington et al.[35] A radiological finding said to be almost peculiar to osteogenic sarcoma of the jaws is a symmetrically widened periodontal membrane space about one or more teeth, when seen on a periapical dental view.[35] There is no correlation between the roentgenographic type of osteogenic sarcoma and survival statistics.

Osteogenic sarcoma represents a neoplastic aberrant of the skeletal connective tissue capable of forming bone, and this property is retained to varying degrees in the form of osteoid, bone or osseous intercellular elements within the neoplasm. The microscopic appearance of an osteogenic sarcoma, while characteristic inasmuch as it manifests the presence of a malignant supportive tissue capable of forming osteoid or bone (Fig. 20.9), is, nevertheless, considerably variable. Because of this, histological subclassification is not a rewarding exercise.

Histological variation is manifest not only from lesion to lesion but also from area to area in the same neoplasm. The essential proliferating and

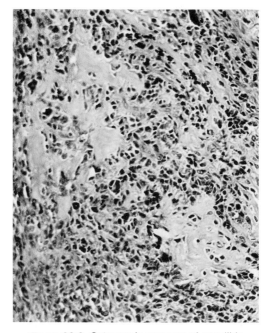

Figure 20.9. Osteogenic sarcoma of mandible.

infiltrative stroma of any osteogenic sarcoma is formed by spindle, oval or polyhedral cells with hyperchromatic nuclei. A highly variegated and anaplastic morphology may be presented. The sarcomatous connective tissue stroma is best seen in the peripheral zones of the neoplasm. In general, the central portions of an osteogenic sarcoma tend to be richer in osteoid or osseous matrix than the peripheral zones which are more cellular and largely unossified. In this regard, Jaffe[42] states that the ossification has a "normalizing" influence on the appearance of the neoplastic cells of the sarcoma. Telangiectatic areas in the neoplasms are not unusual, since the neoplasm is regarded as a relatively vascular lesion.

Individual sarcomas may have abundant cartilage, which arises from a direct transition from sarcomatous spindle cells and not from pre-existing cartilage. When neoplastic changes occur beneath the periosteum, the lesion distends and penetrates it, and when the trabeculae in this subperiosteal neoplastic tissue run at right angles to the longitudinal axis of the bone, a "sunburst" pattern is noted on the x-ray.

The histological appearance of the neoplasm does not bear an apparent relationship to the ultimate course of the disease. On the other hand, the location in the jaws does influence the prognosis, the mandibular neoplasms having a more favorable outlook than those located in the maxilla. Median survival for patients with osteogenic sarcoma of the mandible has been reported as 6.5 years, as compared to 2.9 years for the maxillary osteogenic sarcoma.[35] The prognosis is especially poor with antral neoplasms. In the mandible, a lesion of the symphysis is associated with a more favorable prognosis than are lesions of the body, angle or ramus.

The single most effective therapeutic measure is radical resection, and its effectiveness is directly related to the size and site of the lesion and the amenability to radical surgery. Prophylactic neck dissection does not appear warranted, because the metastases are usually hematogenous.[37] Dissection of the nodes, however, when they are involved by neoplasm, may enhance survival.[35]

While there is a tendency for primary osteogenic sarcomas in the jaws to remain locally invasive for longer periods of time than their counterparts in the skeleton, this attribute has perhaps been overemphasized in the literature. In 24 or the 47 patients followed by Garrington et al.,[35] clinical evidence of metastases developed in time. Caron et al.[38] record distant metastases in 37% of their series of 43 documented cases.

Survival rates associated with osteogenic sarcoma of the jaws, however, do appear to be better than those for extrafacial osteogenic sarcomas. Coventry and Dahlin[43] reported a 5-year survival rate of 19% for osteogenic sarcomas, exclusive of those occurring in the jaws. This is in contrast to 5-year survivals of 21.5%,[34] 31%[34] and 35%[35] reported for osteogenic sarcomas of the jaws.

An unusual, well differentiated, intraosseous osteogenic sarcoma may rarely afflict the jaw bones.[44] This tumor lacks the usual destructive appearance on x-rays and manifests minimal cytological atypia of the supporting tissue spindle cells. Mitoses are also scarce. The lesion may be misdiagnosed as a demoplastic fibroma or contain variable amounts of osteoid, sometimes abundant. The recurrence rate is high but there is a low order of metastasis.

Parosteal osteogenic sarcoma, also called juxtacortical osteogenic sarcoma, is an infrequently encountered variant, especially so in the jaws.[45, 46] The incidence has been reported to range from 1.7% to less than 1% of all bone tumors and less than 4% of osteogenic sarcomas. By 1976, approximately 107 examples had been reported from a variety of primary sites; three from the mandible and one from the maxilla.[46] Unni et al.[45] give the following criteria for diagnosis of parosteal osteogenic sarcoma: (1) no appreciable involvement of the medulla at initial roentgenographic evaluation; (2) the tumors are histologically well differentiated (grade 1 or 2) and characterized by relatively well formed osteoid trabeculae within a spindle cell stroma. The differential diagnosis always considers myositis ossificans.

In the extremities, where the tumors are most often found, the biological course is characterized by recurrence, a tendency to aggressiveness on recurrence and on occasion, metastasis to lung. The presence of histologically active foci in the tumor and medullary involvement affect the prognosis adversely.

II. Vascular Tumors of the Facial Bones and Jaws

Vascular tumors found within bone and in relation to bone range in type from the solitary capillary hemangioma and the multicentric lesions of skeletal angiomatosis to the angiosarcomas. All three of these neoplasms are relatively rare, making up less than 1% of the cases in several large series of bone tumors.[47] The actual incidence of vascular tumors of bone is influenced by the inclusion in this group of angioectasias of either blood

or lymphatic vessels. The asymptomatic vascular lesions found in vertebral bodies may be regarded as being vascular malformations rather than true neoplasms. If these lesions are excluded, benign vascular tumors of bone are reduced to a small group.

Watson and McCarthy,[48] in 1940, carried out the most comprehensive analysis to date of blood and lymph vessel tumors; their study covered 1,363 lesions seen at Memorial Cancer Center in New York City in an 8-year period. Head and neck lesions made up more than one-half of the total number of cases. Hemangiomas of bone, however, were found to be rare and totaled only five cases. These statistics conform to the general over-all incidence of vascular lesions of bone. While hemangiomas are very common outside of bone, their occurrence within the skeletal system is extremely rare.[49]

The clinical importance of the various vascular lesions of the facial bones lies not in their *malignant* potential, since they are almost invariably benign, but in their clinical care and the operative difficulties related to their management. The following discussion will deal with the clinicopathological features of (1) hemangiomas, (2) hemorrhagic bone cysts, (3) aneurysmal bone cysts and (4) malignant vascular neoplasms as they present in the jaws and facial bones.

HEMANGIOMA

The actual incidence of hemangioma of bone, regardless of site, depends upon the interpretation of some of the more common intraosseous vascular lesions by pathologists. Jaffe[42] believes that the more common lesions of the vertebrae represent focal varicosities rather than an intraosseous hemangioma. According to Wyke,[50] the general incidence of hemangioma of bone is 0.7% of osseous neoplasms, and 10% of primary benign neoplasms of the skull are hemangiomas. In this area, the parietal and frontal bones are the most frequently involved. Calvarial hemangiomas have invariably followed a benign course after either irradiation or extirpation.

The nasal bones are uncommon sites for intraosseous hemangiomas.[51] In nearly all reported examples, clinical presentation has been an enlarging mass at the root of the nose. The lesions are slow growing and usually unilateral. Females dominate in a ratio of 4:1. Nearly all cases have been in patients who have been 30 to 60 years of age. While local discomfort is present in all cases, associated nasal symptoms such as epistaxis, rhinorrhea or obstruction are absent. A history of trauma is frequent. The x-ray features are said to be characteristic. An oval or translucent area within the nasal bone is seen in which spicules of bone radiate outward from a central core. The periosteum is intact. Primary surgery has been the method of treatment in all cases. There has not been a problem with intraoperative hemorrhage.

A conservative estimate of primary hemangioma of the jaws would be no more than 60 cases

to date. The zygoma has been reported as the primary site on two occasions.[52] The reviews by Smith,[53] Frankenberg and Panov[54] and Lund and Dahlin[55] emphasize the importance of recognizing these lesions in the jaws. They may not only mimic other tumors of the region, but may represent an unexpected and terrifying experience for the operator when he encounters copious hemorrhage after extraction of teeth or removal of a specimen for biopsy examination.

The peak age incidence is in the second decade of life (one-half of the reported cases have been under 20 years), and the sex ratio is 2:1 with females predominating. Two-thirds of the reported hemangiomas of the jaws have occurred in the mandible. Occasionally there may be a coexistent lesion in the maxilla.

In the mandible, the lesions are usually slow growing and painless. They seldom cause paresthesia. Sixty percent of the patients have had symptoms or a mass for more than 1 year before seeking medical attention. In many patients, the presenting complaint is related to a non-tender swelling that may have slowly enlarged over several months or years.

The teeth associated with a hemangioma may be abnormally spaced and the occlusion correspondingly disturbed. Spontaneous bleeding is uncommon, but hemorrhage around the necks of the teeth in the involved region or severe bleeding after extraction may give clues to the nature of the lesion. Since the lesion is confined to bone, it is not pulsatile. Thrills or bruit are noted only after there has been rapid expansion with arteriovenous fistula formation in the adjacent tissues.

While it has been suggested that diagnosis may be made from roentgenograms,[56] the appearances vary greatly and may be representative of other lesions of the jaws. The principal change is that of an area of rarefaction. In the mandible, this radiolucency is not as sharply defined nor as likely to be round or oval-shaped as it is in other bones (Fig. 20.10). A "honeycomb" or "soap bubble" appearance is the most common roentgenographic feature. This is brought about by expansion of the bone, thinning of the cortex and an irregular fine, lacy, osseous network. The coarsely multilocular regions of rarefaction which expand the cortex to often a paper-like thinness may simulate the roentgenographic appearance of a giant-cell tumor of the jaws. In hemangiomas, however, the loculations are said to be smaller and interspersed with a fine fibrillar network.[55] Viewed in profile, a sunray or sunburst appearance may be presented to the examiner.[57]

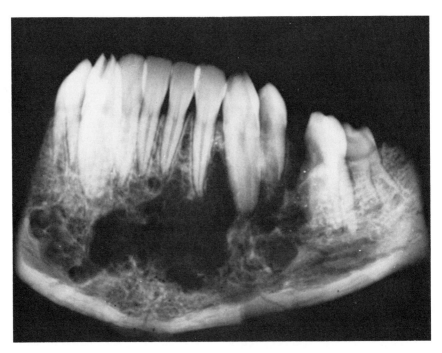

Figure 20.10. Cavernous hemangioma of mandible. Multilocular areas of rarefaction expand the bone. The mandible was resected as a life-saving measure in order to stop hemorrhage.

The histological classification into capillary, cavernous, mixed or hamartomatous is largely academic. For practical purposes, it is best to recognize that the hemangioma may be found in three stages of development: (1) a richly vascular state which bleeds freely at operation; (2) cystic transformation of the lesion accompanied by organizing blood clot; and (3) a sclerotic phase in which ossification occurs. With reference to the latter, Bucy[58] considers ossification to be common to all hemangiomas.

The cavernous variety is made up of large, thin-walled vessels and sinuses which are lined by a single layer of endothelial cells interspersed among bony trabeculae (Fig. 20.11). The capillary hemangioma is made up of fine capillary loops which tend to spread outward in a sunburst fashion. According to Watson and McCarthy[48] the tumors grow independently and do not have an intimate connection with the circulation of the part. Thoma[59] recognizes two varieties, one from the periosteum and the other from the spongiosum.

Because of the penetration of the hemangioma through intertrabecular spaces, the term invasion is often used, with the false suggestion of malignancy being conveyed to the surgeon. The lesions are histologically benign but do possess a potentiality for rapid increase in size and may become locally destructive. Since hemangioma of the jaw is a benign lesion, radical therapy is contraindicated unless forced because of complications such as uncontrollable hemorrhage.[60] Loring[57] also points out that the lesions may be asymptomatic and static, in which instance a policy of noninterference may be the most appropriate.

If teeth are extracted in the region, bleeding is often dramatic and may require hospitalization and extensive surgical intervention. Bleeding is not always such a problem, but several deaths from exsanguination have been reported. Resection, curettage and radiotherapy have been used successfully when treatment has been necessary. Needle aspiration of the lesion and ligation of the artery supplying the affected area have been advised before surgical exploration. Confronted with uncontrollable hemorrhage, marked destruction of local bone, or marked patient discomfort, local segmental mandibular resection is indicated.

HEMORRHAGIC CYSTS

Variously known as a traumatic bone cyst, extravasation cyst, unicameral bone cyst or idiopathic bone cavity, the hemorrhagic bone cyst is an unusual osteolytic lesion which occurs in the jaws and in other bones of the skeleton. Since these intraosseous cavities are not lined by epithelium, the "cyst" designation is a misnomer but,

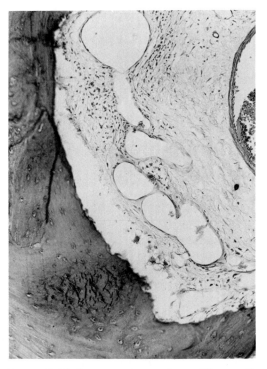

Figure 20.11. Cavernous hemangioma of the mandible. Vessels and sinuses lie in the interstices between bony trabeculae.

nevertheless, is time-honored. Since 1929, the literature has presented only 150 cases in the jaws.[61] The lesion is found usually in young persons (10 to 20 years of age) and is almost never seen in the mandibles of adults over 30 years of age.[62] Males are more commonly involved.

Olech et al.[63] regard trauma as a prime causative factor, with the crucial point in the pathogenesis being a failure of a clot to organize. This is followed by necrosis of many of the bony trabeculae in the spongiosum. The initial cavity is formed and expansion ensues as a result of a progressive local edema.

The posterior part of the mandible is the most common site of involvement, but the lesions are also numerous in the incisor region. Pain is not characteristic, and, in fact, the lesion is often discovered during a routine examination. The patient may give a history of painless enlargement over the affected area of the mandible. The x-ray appearance is not diagnostic. The area of radiolucency may or may not be circumscribed. Scalloping between the teeth has been described as a characteristic feature. The lesion is often above the inferior dental canal, in contrast to the latent bone cavity. The teeth are vital as a rule, and the lamina dura is usually intact.

Surgical exploration demonstrates either a blood-filled cavity or an empty-cavity without a lining membrane. A small quantity of straw-colored fluid may be present in the latter. In a number of cases, the inferior dental neurovascular bundle can be seen lying free in the cavity.[64]

There are no pathognomonic histopathological findings. There is no epithelial lining, areas of osteoclasis and osteoblastic activity are sometimes present and the loose connective tissue lining the bone adjacent to the cavity is of variable thickness and contains numerous blood vessels. Granulation tissue, xanthoma cells and giant cells occasionally are seen.

ANEURYSMAL BONE CYST

The aneurysmal bone cyst was segregated from other solitary cystic lesions of bone by Jaffe and Lichtenstein in 1942.[65] From their clinicopathological[66, 67] studies and that of Dahlin et al.,[68] the lesion may be characterized by the following. (1) Patients are predominantly under 20 years of age. (2) A history of trauma to the area is common. (3) The facial bones and the jaws are infrequently involved. Dominant sites of involvement are the vertebral column and the long bones. (4) A honeycomb or soap-bubble roentgenographic appearance is usual. Destruction of the cortex may be present, and new periosteal bone formation may be apparent. (5) Excessive bleeding or "welling of blood" is manifested on surgical exploration of the lesion. (6) Grossly, the lesion has a spongy appearance with blood-filled spaces. (7) Microscopically, it consists of numerous blood-filled cavernous spaces lined by young connective tissue but devoid of endothelial lining, elastic or muscular elements. Hemosiderin and varying numbers of giant cells are found. (8) The lesion is benign and local curettage is curative.

An aneurysmal bone cyst of the jaws or facial bones is unusual, and, before the report by Bernier and Bhaskar,[69] none of the facial bones were known to have been involved. In 1968, Gruskin and Dahlin[70] reviewed the American literature and found 11 instances of aneurysmal bone cysts that arose in jaw bones. Aneurysmal bone cysts of the jaws comprise less than 2% of these lesions occurring in all bones.[71]

The few cases reported, however, conform, in large part, to the clinicopathological features of the lesion elsewhere in the skeleton. The patients are in their twenties, and females are most often the patients. The mandible is the area of preference, and here it is the body that is most often affected. The lesion in the jaws is usually non-painful and also not tender to palpation. The chief complaint is that of a progressively enlarging mass or deformity with malocclusion. Trauma may be implicated in a significant number of patients.

Roentgenographic features, while perhaps characteristic, are not diagnostic. Roentgenograms show areas of radiolucency which are usually extensive. A honeycomb appearance, because of fine bony septae, is often reported.

Lichtenstein[72] adheres to the view that the lesion results from some persistent local alteration in hemodynamics leading to an increase in venous pressure and the subsequent transformation of the area into a dilated and engorged vascular bed. Two suggested "local" alterations are thrombosis of a large vein or an anomalous arteriovenous communication. Bernier and Bhasker,[69] on the other hand, refute this theory and consider the lesion to represent an unorganized or canalized portion of a hematoma or a false aneurysm.

Recent studies have added a new dimension to the pathogenesis of aneurysmal bone cysts. Biesecker et al.[73] and Buraczewski and Dabska[74] have raised the possibility that aneurysmal bone cysts are secondary lesions following vascular alterations initiated by a definable primary lesion of bone. Thirty-two percent of the series of 66 cases of aneurysmal bone cyst studied by Biesecker et al.[73] had another primary lesion of bone present in the cyst or adjacent to the cyst. They were often present histologically in only one or two sections.

Regardless of the mode of genesis, the affected bone site, wherever its location, is completely transformed with time to resemble an expanded blood-filled sponge. Histological examination of the affected area reveals only meager amounts of tissue. Communicating *pools* of venous blood in a stringy, honeycombed, fibro-osseous meshwork is the typical appearance. The numerous small and large *pools* are usually lined only by flattened spindle-shaped cells with a more or less conspicuous giant cell reaction to inordinate vascularity and hemorrhage (Fig. 20.12). In the intervening tissue, there is a heavy permeation by delicate capillaries. The stroma in other areas may be identical to that of the giant cell granuloma, i.e., giant cells, fibroblasts, capillaries and hemosiderin. Bhaskar et al.[75] deny the presence of smooth muscle in the walls of the blood pools. Osteoid and new bone formation are found in many fields and represent attempted reconstruction.

Thorough curettage or roentgen irradiation in moderate doses or both will usually halt the process of the aneurysmal bone cyst. In the jaws, the

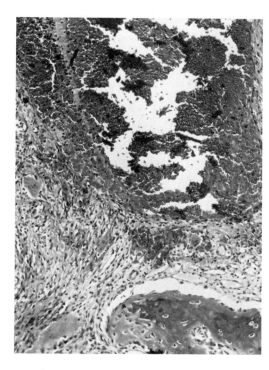

Figure 20.12. Aneurysmal bone cyst of the jaw. Pools of blood lie in a reactive stroma of fibroblasts, hemosiderin and giant cells. New bone formation represents attempts at reconstruction.

lesion is best treated by conservative local curettage.

MALIGNANT VASCULAR TUMORS OF BONE

Primary malignant bone tumors of vascular origin are rare. There is no doubt that the diagnosis is made too frequently when a poorly differentiated sarcoma of bone manifests a prominent vascular pattern. Clinical and pathological criteria for the diagnosis of these tumors have been described in detail.[42, 47, 76]

The variety of diagnostic terms used synonymously for these neoplasms—hemangiosarcoma, angiosarcoma, angioblastic sarcoma, hemangioendothelioma—reflects a state of confusion. The well-differentiated types have been most often labeled as hemangioendothelioma. These manifest a rather indolent behavior. The more poorly differentiated malignant vascular tumors have been usually referred to simply as angiosarcomas.

In both neoplastic types, vascular channels can be identified, but those in the well-differentiated forms more closely resemble the vessels of a reparative process. The vascular spaces are lined by plump endothelial cells showing little atypia and few mitoses. There is often a lobulated pattern, and the intervening septa between the anastomosing vascular spaces often show a lymphocytic infiltration. Peculiarly enough, multicentricity of the well-differentiated neoplasms imparts a better prognosis than do solitary lesions. Poorly differentiated vascular sarcomas show fewer vasoformative features. They are characterized by more irregular anastomosing vascular spaces and a pronounced tendency toward intravascular budding and anaplasia of the endothelial cells.

Involvement of the jaws by this group of primary bone tumors is extremely unusual. This corresponds to their rarity in other parts of the skeleton. Hartman and Stewart[77] reported 10 cases of primary "hemangioendothelioma" of bone, one of which occurred in the mandible of a 10-year-old child. Pindborg and Philipsen[78] reported a single case of malignant angioblastoma in the mandible of a 12-year-old girl. The latter authors considered their case to represent the mandibular counterpart of the so-called tibial adamantinoma.

Whether the neoplasms are called hemangioendothelioma, angiosarcoma, hemangiosarcoma or angioblastoma, it is to be considered that those occurring in bone, although potentially malignant in the biological sense, behave in a more indolent fashion than most lesions designated as angiosarcoma. In bone, they respond well to adequate surgical excision and, in some instances, to x-ray therapy. Radiation therapy alone has resulted in a prolonged survival.

HEMANGIOPERICYTOMAS INVOLVING BONE

Primary intraosseous hemangiopericytomas are very unusual, but some have been recorded in the facial or jaw bones.[47] Distinction should also be made between primary neoplasms and neoplastic involvement by adjacent soft tissue hemangiopericytomas.

MASSIVE OSTEOLYSIS OF BONE

Massive osteolysis (phantom bone, disappearing bone) is very likely a disorder of vascular proliferation. The disorder may affect any bone in the body and are found most frequently around a major joint area, such as the shoulder or pelvis. The disease may be monostotic or polyostotic. Young adults are most frequently affected, although initial diagnosis of the disease often has been made in older individuals. There are no significant biochemical abnormalities in the patients. The mandible and/or maxilla have been involved in approximately 10% of the reported cases.[79, 80]

The disorder begins insidiously and is characterized by progressive massive regional loss of bone with resultant deformity. Bone resorption may be from without or may be completely intraosseous. The resorption may also be generalized in the involved bone. Pain is not common as an initial symptom and is usually secondary to pathological fracture. The resorption often appears to spontaneously arrest. The arrested state may remain stable, but reactivation of the process can occur. Despite a progressive loss of bone, the ultimate disability is often surprisingly mild. In most cases the disease is self-limited.

Radiological findings are striking. The earliest sign is one, or several, clustered intramedullary and subcortical lucent foci of variable sizes. Growth and coalescence of these foci results in an attenuated cortex. This may completely disappear, often resulting in a complete resorption of bone and leaving only periosteum.

The presence of a vascular component in most cases is suggestive that the lesion is a vasoproliferative disorder. Very likely early in the disease process, there is an intraosseous capillary proliferation. Later, the tissues become relatively avascular, and predominantly fibrotic; however, complete avascularity is rare. Active vascularization in the early stages is also held responsible for a disturbance of the osteoclast-osteoblast balance. Adding credence to a vascular basis for the lesion is the finding of angiomatous tissue in the mediastinum and lungs of the rarely occurring fatal cases.

III. Giant Cell and Fibro-osseous Lesions of the Jaws

The presence of multinucleated giant cells (Fig. 20.13) in fibro-osseous lesions of the jaws has led to considerable nosological confusion, and, in fact, too much emphasis has been placed on this histopathological finding. The giant cells in themselves are of little diagnostic importance, and they may be found in a variety of bone lesions affecting the jaws. Most often, they represent osteoclasts and are secondary to the basic underlying process affecting the jaws.

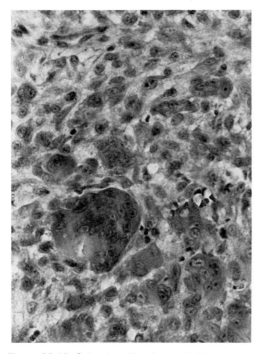

Figure 20.13. Osteoclast-like giant cells lying among spindle stromal cells. They measure from 10 to 100 μm and may contain 10 to over 100 nuclei. The nuclei are distinct and are identical to the nuclei of the stromal cell, suggesting a congeneric origin.

Because there is considerable histological and radiological overlap in appearance of the fibro-osseous lesions of the jaws, with or without giant cells, uncritical interpretation of such lesions must be avoided. This is especially true since most authors believe that the true giant cell tumor of the jawbones is an extremely rare lesion.[75]

GIANT CELL (REPARATIVE) GRANULOMA

This lesion of the jaws presents in two forms: (1) peripheral, involving the gingiva or alveolar mucosa; (2) central, occurring as an endosteal lesion within the jaw bones.[81-83]

A history of trauma is often elicited, but the theory of traumatic etiology is continually challenged. In this regard, many observers are unhappy with the prefix "reparative," as it is not clear what is being repaired. The designation of "giant cell granuloma" seems more appropriate, since it distinguishes the lesion from a neoplasm and avoids contention if infectious granulomas are known to be excluded.

The peripheral giant cell granuloma occurs four times more frequently than the central lesion and makes up less than 1% of surgical pathological accessions.[83, 84] The tissue of both peripheral and central processes is similar, if not identical, and in some cases it is difficult to determine whether the lesion is actually a peripheral lesion or an extension of an intraosseous process.[85]

The peripheral giant cell lesion occurs on the gingiva or alveolar mucosa of endentulous or tooth-bearing areas. Approximately 55% involve the mandibular mucosa. The anterior (incisor or canine) position is the favorite site, followed by the premolar and molar regions, respectively. The size of the lesion rarely exceeds 2 cm. It may be sessile or pedunculated and is usually red to reddish-blue in color. Although, on occasion, the underlying interdental septum is resorbed, the radiographs usually reveal no abnormality.

The surface of the lesion is covered by squamous epithelium, which may be ulcerated. In most instances, the mucosa is intact, and a distinctive connective tissue clear zone is often manifested. The lesion generally known as giant cell epulis is now accepted as being a peripheral giant cell granuloma.

The central lesion is endosteal and involves the mandible more often than the maxilla. The relationship between the peripheral and intraosseous granulomas is uncertain. While it is tempting to speculate that the two are only different anastomical manifestations of the same process, no definite proof has been provided.

At this juncture, it should be known that the giant cell granuloma is *not* restricted to the jawbones. Examples have been reported in the ethmoid, sphenoid and temporal bones.[86]

Age incidence, location and sex susceptibility of the endosteal granuloma are similar to that of aneurysmal bone cyst, from which it should be distinguished. Occurring slightly more often in males, the lesion most often presents in patients between the ages of 10 and 20 years. The peripheral giant cell granuloma shows a wide age distribution, with patients usually past 20 years of age. Nearly two-thirds of the cases have presented in females.

Clinically, the intrabony lesion may be either asymptomatic and discovered incidentally, or it may produce a local deformity of the jaw. In a significant number of patients, the reaction develops after extraction of a tooth.[87] Premolar and molar regions are preferred sites. There may be migration of the teeth in the region of the tumor. The mucosa is usually intact and normal in appearance. Roentgenograms show radiolucent areas of varying size (Fig. 20.14), and, on occasion, the ubiquitous "soap bubble" appearance is presented. Specific diagnosis cannot be made from radiographs alone, but a central giant cell granuloma can usually be excluded if the lesion is posterior to the first molar.

The histopathological appearance of the giant cell granuloma is one of a proliferation of young fibroblastic or mesenchymal connective tissue. The tissue is richly vascular, and a variable number of multinucleated giant cells are always present (Fig. 20.15). The latter are often intimately related with ill-defined vascular spaces. The morphology and distribution of the giant cells manifest considerable variation. Evidence of phagocytic activity is fairly common. Hemosiderin is present in all lesions, as is collagen. Nonspecific calcification, osteoid and bone formation may also be seen. En bloc specimens may manifest a thin peripheral layer of immature trabecular bone.

Injury imposed upon the periodontal membrane, the odontogenic mesenchyma, the dental sac or its ancestral cells is probably the initiating insult. The giant cells are considered a response to hemorrhage, and they assume the characteristics and functions of phagocytes. They are most dense in areas of hemorrhage. The fibrous connective tissue proliferation which forms the basic histopathological lesion is far in excess of that required for repair and reconstruction. It is emphasized again that the stromal elements are the most significant elements of the lesion. With biological time and reduction in the vascularity, the giant cells beome less prominent and more irregular in size and shape.

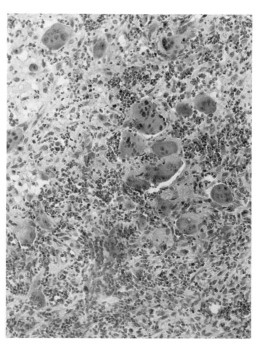

Figure 20.15. Giant cell granuloma of jaw, manifesting fairly typical appearance from a focus where giant cells are evenly distributed.

For both forms of the lesions, simple excision or curettement is the treatment of choice.[87, 88] Irradiation is contraindicated. Recurrence of the peripheral lesion after excision is often described but not well documented. Malignant change in either form has not been convincingly demonstrated.

No central giant cell reparative granuloma has been known to heal completely without surgery.[82] Some of the so-called static lesions at the time of operation appear to contain mostly fibrous tissue with much bone scattered throughout the whole lesion. Curettage is sufficient in most cases, although recurrences have been noted.

THE BONY LESIONS OF HYPERPARATHYROIDISM

An increase in production of parathyroid hormone brings about a release of calcium from the structural or so-called "stable" bone which is not normally exchangeable. Lacunar resorption by osteoclasts is the histological counterpart of this excess hormone action.

Parathyroid hormone administration to an animal is capable of producing a fibroblastic proliferation in the endosteal tissues within 12 hours. Accompanying this reaction is the initiation of a giant cell osteoclasis. In man, when there is a

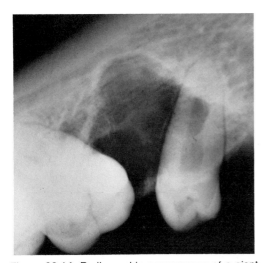

Figure 20.14. Radiographic appearances of a giant cell (reparative) granuloma. There are no diagnostic features.

chronic excess of parathyroid hormone, both fibrous and osteoclastic reactions may be widespread in the skeleton, and in a few foci tumorous areas of giant cells may be produced. These reactions represent the diffuse and focal bone lesions of hyperparathyroidism and are known as osteitis fibrosa, osteitis fibrosa cystica or von Recklinghausen's disease of bone.

In hyperparathyroidism the mandible or maxilla may be the site of a giant cell lesion. In some instances, this localization may actually be the earliest clinical manifestation of the disease. Because the giant cell lesions of hyperparathyroidism cannot be distinguished from other giant cell lesions involving the jaws, the diagnosis of hyperparathyroidism should always be suspected or at least considered if the patient is older, if the maxilla or facial bones or both are the sites of involvement and if recurrences prevail. The importance of a biochemical study (calcium, phosphorus, and alkaline phosphatase) of the patient is underlined by the impossibility of differentiating between giant cell reparative granuloma and the "brown tumor" of hyperparathyroidism.

The pathological process within the bone consists of three principal features: a fibrocellular proliferation in the marrow spaces; numerous osteoclasts, mainly lying within lacunae on the bone surfaces undergoing erosion, but also scattered throughout the fibrous tissue components; and imperfect attempts at regeneration of bone. Resorption of bone starts in the cancellous areas and in the medulla. Extension follow up the Haversian canals and leads to the cancellization of the cortex and, ultimately, to its complete dissolution.

In the diffuse or focal rarefaction of the mandible and maxilla with thinning or even disappearance of the lamina dura, there is no resorption or loss of teeth. The focal or "cystic" lesion is osteolytic and expansive, forming a tumor of brown, yellow or hemorrhagic tissue bulging beyond the normal bone contour. By the time such bone "cysts" appear, there is usually a loss of density of the skeleton as a whole. It is to be recalled that such lesions are cystic only in the radiological sense. Simulating the reparative granuloma, the so-called "brown tumor" is comprised of a spindle cell connective tissue stroma containing numerous osteoclast-like multinucleated cells (Fig. 20.16), free hemorrhage and phagocytes filled with lipid or hemosiderin.

In both the diffuse and focal forms, osteoblastic activity is not impaired, and in many sections there may be seen bone regeneration in the form of discontinuous islands of trabeculae of coarse bone outlined by plump osteoblasts. Resolution of bone

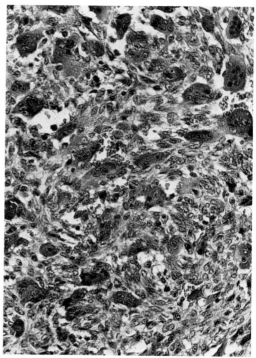

Figure 20.16. So-called "brown tumor" of hyperparathyroidism. There are no diagnostic features, and without the aid of biochemical determinations (calcium and alkaline phosphatase), they may pass for giant cell granulomas and even true giant cell tumors.

lesions after parathyroidectomy has been observed many times. The giant cell foci resolve more slowly than the diffuse lesions. Large focal lesions may even persist as cyst-like translucencies.

A single estimation of the levels of serum calcium, phosphorus and alkaline phosphatase does not exclude the diagnosis of hyperparathyroidism. Repeated analysis are recommended.

Brown tumors are rarely seen in secondary hyperparathyroidism. With the introduction of long-term maintenance hemodialysis, however, there has been increasing note of this association.[89] Patients in end-stage renal disease and on dialysis now appear to manifest the bony changes of hyperparathyroidism more frequently than primary hyperparathyroidism patients. The duration of the hemodialysis seems to correlate with the severity of the disease.

TRUE GIANT CELL TUMOR OF THE JAWS

Most of the lesions "diagnosed" as giant cell tumors are in truth giant cell granulomas. The neoplastic giant cell is extremely rare in the jaws.[75, 84] Waldron and Shafer[85] approach the histogenetic question in another manner and consider the central giant cell reparative granuloma as analogous to, and probably identical with the "benign giant cell tumor" of other bones.

The lesion is characterized by a tendency toward a local aggressiveness, and recurrences are likely. The lesion is seldom seen in patients less than 20 years of age, in contrast to the giant cell reparative granuloma which occurs at an earlier age. According to Bernier,[87] variation in size is not as great as in the reparative granuloma, most being less than 5 cm in diameter. The tumor may involve either the maxilla or the mandible; in the latter, the symphysis and bicuspid regions are primarily involved. Growth of the tumor is intermittent and variable, and pain may be a dominant symptom.

Roentgenograms are not of a diagnostic nature, since the appearance may mimic a number of lesions. When compared to the reparative granuloma, a blurred border of the radiolucent area speaks in favor of a giant cell tumor. The histological pattern in a true giant cell neoplasm is dominated by the giant cells. They are more abundant and slightly larger than in the reparative granuloma (Fig. 20.17). Nuclei of the giant cells may be more numerous, but this is quite variable. The stromal cells manifest a nuclear preponderance in the neoplasm, while there is a stromal cytoplasmic preponderance in the reparative granuloma.

Table 20.3 after Hirschl and Katz[86] presents

suggested histopathological differences between the giant cell tumor and reparative granuloma. The ultrastructure of the true giant cell tumor reveals two distinct types of stromal cells, a mac-

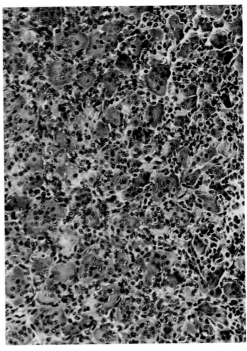

Figure 20.17. True giant cell tumor of jaw bone.

Table 20.3
Giant Cell Reparative Granuloma versus Giant Cell Tumor of Bone*

	Giant Cell Reparative Granulomas of Bone	Giant Cell Tumor of Bone
Age of patient	Usually under 21 years	Usually over 21 years
Clinical behavior	Self-limited; may regress; seldom recurs; never metastasizes	Aggressive; no regression; recurs often; occasionally metastasizes
Histological features	1. Giant cells are grouped around hemorrhagic foci	1. Giant cells are uniformly dispersed and dominate the entire field
	2. Stroma shows oval cells and equally large number of spindled fibroblasts with zones of fibrosis and relatively few giant cells	2. Stroma is richly vascularized and is composed of plump, round and oval cells
	3. Evidence of old and recent hemorrhage with hemosiderin	3. Recent hemorrhage is slight to moderate; hemosiderin is rare
	4. Giant cells are generally smaller; frequently irregular and elongated, and have relatively few nuclei	4. Giant cells are generally larger, more rounded and have a great number of nuclei
	5. Foci of osteoid and new bone function in the center of lesions are frequently present	5. Osteoid or new bone are not characteristically produced
Response to therapy	Usually cured by curettage	Recurs if incomplete excision

* After Hirschl and Katz.[86]

rophage-like cell and fibroblasts. This is not unique and is shared by the reparative granuloma. The giant cells in the giant cell tumor, while having some characteristics of osteoclasts are clearly not identical. While there are also remarkable differences between the stromal cells and the giant cells, the stromal cells have not been excluded as precursors to the giant cells.

To summarize the pertinent differences: (1) true giant cell tumors are seldom seen in the bones of the skull and face; (2) osteoid formation or other evidence of osteogenic activity is not characteristic of true giant cell tumors, except perhaps peripherally at the site of fracture or other injury to adjacent bone; (3) there is a noticeable absence or scantiness of hemorrhage, lipid-laden histiocytes, hemosiderin and inflammatory cells in true giant cell tumors, except in areas of secondary damage or necrosis and fracture[88]; (4) finally, giant cell tumors occur most commonly in the 20- to 40-year-old age group and are rarely seen below the age of 20 years.

Curettage, as in the case of the reparative granuloma, will not usually suffice, but the choice of treatment is more dictated by location and size of the lesion. All available follow-up information emphasizes the benign nature of central giant cell lesions of the jaws. With a single possible exception, I have been unable to find any well-documented evidence of malignant biological behavior of any central giant cell lesion of the jaws. This suggests that the true giant cell tumor of jaws lies intermediate between the rare, frankly malignant, giant cell tumor and the far more numerous and innocuous giant cell reparative granulomas of the jaws.

ANEURYSMAL BONE CYST AND HEMORRHAGIC BONE CYST

Although there may be zones in both of these lesions that overlap with giant cell lesions of the jaws, they are best considered as primarily vascular and have been covered elsewhere in this text.

FIBRO-OSSEOUS LESIONS OF THE JAWS

The term "fibro-osseous lesion" is an acceptable, yet not specific, diagnostic term applied to a *group* of pathological lesions manifesting replacement of normal bony architecture by tissue composed of collagen, fibroblasts and varying amounts of osteoid or calcified tissue. From a clinical perspective, the fibro-osseous lesions may vary from extensive and disfiguring processes to small, localized areas that are discovered only during the course of a routine radiographic study. Radiographically, the picture may vary from a diffuse ground-glass pattern to cystic lesions with relatively little calcification.

Fibrous Dysplasia. The original concept of fibrous dysplasia has been expanded to include a spectrum of diseases, based on histological findings and ranging from a local monostotic form through diffuse polyostotic involvement, to include Albright's syndrome of skeletal lesions, skin pigmentation and precocious puberty. Many general pathologists, regarding fibrous dysplasia as a specific disorder, restrict this diagnosis to lesions which are polyostotic in character and accompanied by abnormal cutaneous pigmentation, disturbances in skeletal growth and an expression of endocrine dysfunction in female patients (Table 20.4).

If restricted to the above, involvement of the oral and jaw regions by polyostotic fibrous dysplasia is uncommon. The majority of patients with jaw lesions diagnosed as fibrous dysplasia do not manifest other skeletal lesions or endocrine changes. Monostotic lesions of the jaws composed of varying amounts of fibrous tissue have been designated as ossifying fibroma, fibrous osteoma, exostosis and osseous dysplasia as well as fibrous dysplasia. The majority probably represent monostotic fibrous dysplasia.

In concurrence with Smith,[90] I would restrict the diagnosis of fibrous dysplasia of the jaws to lesions which are obviously developmental in origin, are first noted relatively early in life, grow actively during childhood and tend to stabilize in adult life. In this sense, dysplasia implies an abnormal tissue development or hamartoma. Smith[90] describes three types of fibrous dysplasia of the jaws according to activity. The first, or active, form is characterized by a richly cellular connective tissue

Table 20.4
Clinical Classification of Fibrous Dysplasia

Classification	Characteristics
Monostotic	Single or multiple lesions confined to one bone. Rarely accompanied by any extraskeletal manifestations.
Polyostotic	Multiple lesions involving more than one bone, but with a tendency toward monomelic or unilateral distribution.
Disseminated	Multiple lesions scattered throughout the skeleton, often unilateral and occasionally accompanied by extraskeletal manifestations.

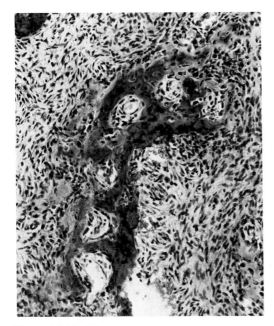

Figure 20.18. Fibrous dysplasia of the jaw in the *active* form, where the stroma is richly cellular, active and contains islands of abnormal and coarse bone.

matrix containing numerous plump fusiform or stellate cells. Mitoses may be numerous, and considerable intercellular collagen is formed. The islands of bone that appear in this matrix demonstrate a characteristic scroll edge and a definite boundary between stroma and the bone island. The bone is coarse and abnormal, and the islands occur in various "jigsaw puzzle" sizes and shapes (Fig. 20.18). The more active the matrix, the fewer the bone islands. The bone does not contain many lacunae and osteoblasts, and there is no resemblance to reparative bone. This active form may be seen at any age through adolescence, but it predominates in the younger patient.

A quiescent, or "potentially active," form of fibrous dysplasia is seen in the older child and adolescent. In this type, the connective tissue matrix is more mature, there are few or no mitoses, and the bone component is more prominent (Fig. 20.19). Osteoblasts, osteoclasts and osteoid are not present. Smith's third form of fibrous dysplasia is the least common and, in effect, represents an inactive state.[90] Characteristic of this form is the degeneration of connective tissue matrix. Bone islands may be completely absent.

The polarization microscope has been used to distinguish true fibrous dysplasia from other fibro-osseous lesions of the jaws.[91] While random birefringence may be present in all such lesions, in fibrous dysplasia only is there persistence of the woven bone pattern and an absence of lamellar bone formation. The oxytalan fiber, so called because of its resistance to acid hydrolysis, has also been used as a marker for differentiating fibro-osseous lesions. This fiber, distinct from collagen, reticulin or elastic fibers, is composed of an amorphous ground substance and is not found or is rare in lesions of hyperparathyroidism, aneurysmal bone cysts or reparative granulomas.

Clinically, the great majority of the lesions of fibrous dysplasia of the jaws appear in the first or second decades of life. In accordance with Smith's[90] histopathological classification, the growth of the lesions is also most active during these decades. Small lesions seldom produce signs or symptoms. Swelling of the affected bone is the most common and constant feature.[92, 93] This may be only minor or so great as to produce a pronounced facial asymmetry. In most instances, the unilaterality of the affliction is striking. Maxillary involvement is more common than mandibular lesions. Lesions in the maxilla not uncommonly lead to a unilateral bulging of the canine fossae and prominence of the zygomatic processes. Extensive involvement may produce proptosis and exophthalmos. Lesions of the mandible most often involve the region of the angle. The overlying

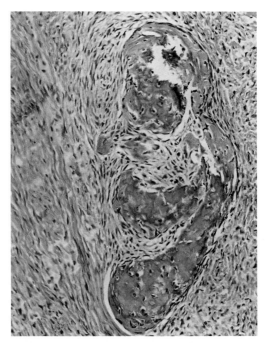

Figure 20.19. Fibrous dysplasia in the "quiescent stage." Stroma is more mature and the bone component is prominent.

mucous membranes are generally normal, and, in most cases, dentition is not affected. Pain is an infrequent complaint. "Pathological" fracture of the mandible secondary to fibrous dysplasia has not been reported. In the experience of some authors, extensive fibrous dysplasia of the facial bones is seen more often in Negroes.

The radiographic appearance of facial fibrous dysplasia is extremely variable, and this is an expression of the ratio of connective tissue to bone islands in the lesions. Sherman and Glauser[94] have classified fibrous dysplasia of the jaws into three main radiographic types. Type I is most often seen in the maxilla and manifests a diffuse, uniform sclerosis that tends to follow the contour of the bone as well as enlarging it. Type II is lytic in character and the most common. Expansion of the cortex and multiloculation and thinning are the essential features. The third type is the uncommon unilocular form of fibrous dysplasia. Large maxillary lesions often manifest obliteration of the maxillary sinus with involvement of the infraorbital margins and malar bones.

The mere presence of fibrous dysplasia of the craniofacial bones is not in itself an indication for treatment. Many small solitary lesions will remain static and asymptomatic. Marked or progressive deformity, pain or interference with function suggest the need for therapy.[93] Complete resection of the involved area is the treatment of choice, but this often results in considerable functional and cosmetic defects demanding extensive reconstruction. Conservatism, therefore, is the basic surgical premise.[93, 95] Partial resection and curettage are followed, in some patients, by progression of residual disease, but this procedure generally results in less deformity. According to Ramsey et al.,[93] complete mandibulectomy or orbital exenteration as part of the *initial* treatment of fibrous dysplasia of the craniofacial bones is not indicated.

Malignant change in fibrous dysplasia deserves consideration. The incidence is difficult to determine, but it is not great. Most reported instances have developed in patients who received previous *radiation therapy* for the fibrous dysplasia.[93, 95] It is clear that radiation treatment of fibrous dysplasia is of no value and is potentially dangerous. In most reported cases, the time interval between the diagnosis of fibrous dysplasia and the development of sarcoma is long. This suggests that a sudden growth phase in a long-standing area of fibrous dysplasia should be viewed with great suspicion and emphasizes the importance of keeping patients with fibrous dysplasia under close observation.

It is quite clear that irradiation plays a significant role in the development of jaw sarcomas. Ten percent of jaw sarcomas arise in irradiated bone and data indicate radiation-induced sarcomas are more frequent in the jaws than elsewhere. The initial lesion, however, that required irradiation appears to be equally important. In a review of the literature, 46% of the cases were found to have had fibrous dysplasia as the initial lesion, whereas 18% of the remaining cases included diverse bone lesions.[96] The jaw bones were assumed to be normal in only 36% of the cases where irradiation was administered to adjacent tissue lesions.

CHERUBISM

Cherubism or familial intraosseous fibrous swelling of the jaws remains, at present, in a clinical category by itself. Like the other clinico-pathological lesions in this discussion, the disorder is characterized by a proliferation of fibrous tissue and variable amounts of giant cells within the jaws.[97, 98]

There does not appear to be sufficient histological justification to "lump" cherubism under the general heading of fibrous dysplasia, since the bone components of the latter are not found in cherubism. Further illustrating the definite value of evaluating the entire clinical, radiological and pathological mosaic before diagnosis is the fact that it may be not only difficult but also impossible to differentiate giant cell reparative granuloma from cherubism by microscopic examination alone.

Although the cause of cherubism is unknown, there is little doubt that the disorder should be classed as a developmental disturbance of the bone-forming mesenchyme. Cherubism is an autosomal dominant disorder with a 100% penetrance in males, a 50% to 70% penetrance in females, and a variable expressivity. Sporadic cases are also reported, but differentiation of these from primary mutations is not always possible. The affected patient is generally described as being normal at birth. The disease usually becomes noticeable during the second to third year of life when a fullness of the cheeks, particularly over the angle of the mandible, becomes apparent.

The mandibular angles are the usual sites of the lesions, and their distribution is symmetrical. Maxillary involvement has been noted in about two-thirds of the reported cases, but the condyles invariably escape. Marked maxillary involvement results in a narrow V-shaped palatal vault. Premature loss of deciduous teeth and a failure of eruption of the permanent teeth are common findings.

The classical appearance of the patient afflicted with the disorder prompted Jones,[99] who first described the disorder, to call the deformity "cherubism," after the angelic cherub of Renaissance art. A "raised-to-heaven" look is imparted to the patient by the diffuse enlargement of the lower half of the face and retraction of the lower eyelids as a result of tightness of facial skin and fullness of the cheeks.

The jaw lesions manifest their greatest expansion during the first and second years after onset. Following this great initial expansion, the disorder tends to remain stationary or progress slowly for the next 5 years. Gradual improvement, or at least cessation of growth, occurs after the age of 10 years, and at puberty there is considerable regression.

In spite of the sometimes extensive involvement of the mandible and maxilla, cherubism seldom causes any functional disability and pain is not a complaint. Enlarged bilateral cervical lymph nodes, while not an essential feature in cherubism, are frequently reported. The lymph nodes are hyperplastic and reactive in nature. Some degree of relationship is indicated by the observations that the bony lesions of cherubism and the cervical adenopathy regress, and may even disappear, at adolescence. A few patients may have other skeletal involvement, but there are no other associated malformations or disease.

Many investigators regard cherubism as a form of hereditary fibrous dysplasia and a variant of polyostotic fibrous dysplasia. Indeed, in rare cases, the presence of skin pigmentation points to a relationship between cherubism and polyostotic fibrous dysplasia or Albright's syndrome, especially since pigmentation occurs in only about one-third of patients with the syndrome.

Multilocular areas of radiolucency in the mandible constitute the most common radiological feature of cherubism. These areas tend to be sharply defined, and the cortex is generally expanded and thinned. As indicated above, the condylar process does not appear to be involved. Developing teeth are often present within the lesions and are markedly displaced.

Long-standing cherubism presents with varying degrees of deformity of the mandible and an irregular sclerosis or diffuse ground-glass appearance. The growth and expansion of the jaw lesions are due to new tissue formed in response to microhemorrhages, which, in turn, are secondary to defective capillaries manifesting an increased fragility and permeability. Surgical exploration of the involved bone reveals the radiolucent areas to be composed of spindle-shaped giant cells, numerous capillaries and varying amounts of collagen (Fig. 20.20).

Some lesions contain abundant hemorrhage and considerable hemosiderin. Giant cell population appears to be related to the foregoing, and, in the more fibrous lesions, giant cells tend to be few in number and individually smaller. Bone formation is not an important histopathological feature, and, when present, it is interpreted as a secondary and reactive phenomenon. Compared with giant cell granuloma, the lesion of cherubism has a looser, less cellular, delicate fibrous tissue component and does not contain new bone formation within the lesion proper. Not everyone, however, agrees that the lesion of cherubism is distinctive.

Thus, in summary, cherubism always has a characteristic giant cell lesion of bone which is frequently in association with: (1) bilateral lesions of the jaws; (2) limitation to the jaws; (3) slowly enlarging and expanding jaw lesions; (4) affected parents or siblings; (5) involution at puberty; (6)

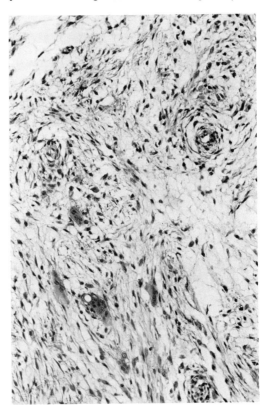

Figure 20.20. Single focus of cherubism with occasional giant cell and a rich vascularity. Elsewhere, the lesion may mimic giant cell granuloma.

bilateral cervical lymphadenopathy; (7) remission after surgery. However, it also may be associated with: (1) a unilateral lesion that may have not become bilateral at the time of the initial examination; (2) involvement of long bones by histologically similar lesions; (3) no cherubic facies unless the orbits are involved; (4) small intact bony (subclinical) lesions; (5) no affected parent; (6) no cervical lymphadenopathy after 7 years of age; (7)

enlargement after surgery; (8) persistence of large lesions into adulthood.

The treatment of each patient suffering from cherubism must be individualized. The lesions can usually be controlled by thorough curettement. Recontouring has also been used with satisfactory results. Hammer and Ketcham[100] review the various surgical modalities. The use of radiation in any form is now universally condemned.

IV. Common and Uncommon Non-odontogenic Tumors

In this fourth and final section of the primary non-odontogenic tumors and tumorous conditions of the jaws, the clinicopathological studies range from the commonplace torus and exostosis, through the unusual myxoma, osteoma and Ewing's sarcoma to the pathological curiosities of central epidermoid carcinoma and mucoepidermoid tumor of the jaws.

TORUS

The torus may be defined as a benign bony growth projecting outward from the surfaces of bone. While it may be difficult at times to separate exostosis from torus, the latter has a distinct racial variation and is probably a heritable trait, at least in some races.

In the jaws, two forms of tori present: torus maxillaris and torus mandibularis. The maxillary form is most common, with an estimated 20% of the population said to have tori of the maxilla. Its favorite site is the palatal midline, where it presents as a bony nodule of variable size and shape. Less often, the maxillary tuberosity is involved. The lesion may be lobulated, and the overlying mucosa may be ulcerated. Tori of the mandible have a lower incidence. In the United States, 8% of the population are said to have the lesion. The lesions are frequently bilateral and present most commonly lingual to the bicuspid teeth. In many subjects they are multiple. A pattern of heredity has also been defined for this lesion.

Both forms are slow-growing processes, and they develop in most patients before the age of 30 years, often in relation to puberty.[101] Histologically, both types manifest the same structure. Adult cortical bone with little stroma or marrow spaces characterizes the majority of tori. Osteogenesis and osteoclasis are rarely observed. Occasionally, especially with a large torus, there may be close resemblance to an osteoma. Removal of a torus is indicated only when there is interference

with speech or mastication, or if a denture is to be fitted over the area.

EXOSTOSIS AND ENOSTOSIS

Exostoses are localized overgrowths of bone of a varied size which may appear as nodular, pedunculated, flat protuberances on the surface of the bone. There is an indistinct borderline between torus, exostosis and osteoma.[101, 102] Enostoses originate from the inner surface of the bone and extend into the medullary portions or spongiosa of the jaws.

Exostoses involving the jaws are common, and many occur in solitary or multiple form. Multiple exostoses of the jaws are less common than maxillary and mandibular tori. Sometimes exostoses are found at the insertion of muscles or tendons. Found most often in the maxilla, exostoses present as hard, well demarcated, submucosal swellings. The canine fossa appears to be a site of predilection.[101] The overlying mucosa is normal. Radiographically, exostoses appear as circumscribed radiopaque masses.

Enostoses are localized growths of a dense bone in the spongiosum. Multiple enostoses, also called chronic sclerosing osteomyelitis or sclerosing osteitis, are considered by Bhaskar and Cutright[103] to be a clinicopathological entity. The disorder is characterized by multiple dense radiopaque lesions in the premolar and molar regions of the jaws. The mandible is involved far more often than the maxilla. There is no correlation between the occurrence of the lesions and the presence or absence of teeth. The greatest number of cases occur in Negroes, particularly in females, and in subjects who are between the ages of 30 and 50 years.

Radiographs have a "pagetoid" appearance with multiple well defined or diffuse dense radiopacities. Solitary and even multiple enostoses may be difficult to distinguish from an endosteal osteoma. The enostosis tends to merge imperceptibly into the surrounding medullary bone, whereas the endosteal osteoma is more likely to be demarcated by a connective tissue capsule.

Microscopically, both exostoses and enostoses are highlighted by the formation of bone. Exostoses generally have a hard, eburnated surface, and the lesions appear to be produced by periosteal apposition of bone lamellae which show a lateral tapering. Most exostoses are composed of compact bone. Large exostoses often become cancellated and are made up of a thick layer of cortical bone containing a spongiosum or medullary area of thin bony trabeculae and fatty marrow. Enostoses are made up of dense cortical bone containing nutrient channels with blood vessels and a scant connective tissue. In some fields, Paget's disease is suggested; in others, the lesion looks like cementum.[103]

Treatment of these "ostoses" consists of surgical removal if they produce masticatory trauma or if a prosthesis is to cover the area.

OSTEOMA

An osteoma may be defined as a benign osteogenic tumor of slow growth containing mature bone. Ringertz[104] noted that osteomas occur almost exclusively on the bones of the skull and face. The tumor in the facial bones may present as either a peripheral or a central (intraosseous) lesion. Peripheral lesions may present externally or internally.

Osteomas are found most frequently in the mandible, especially on the lingual aspect of the horizontal ramus or at the lower border in the region of the angle. Central osteomas are unusual. Large osteomas are unusual. Large osteomas of the ethmofrontal region may fill the entire frontal sinus and extend into the ethmoid labyrinth through the inferior portion of the frontal sinus.[105] Osteomas of the paranasal sinuses occur either in the frontal, ethmoid or maxillary sinuses, in this order of frequency.[106] Osteomas of the sphenoid sinus and bone are very rare[107–112] (Table 20.5).

Although their rate of expansion and growth is very slow, serious complications may ensue, especially with large osteomas of the ethmoidal and frontal sinus regions. Diagnosis is usually made in the age period of 15 to 40 years, after a presenting sign of a painless mass. Duration of symptoms may be as long as 4 years but averages 14 months before the patient seeks medical attention.

Grossly, the lesion presents on the surface of the cortical bone, attached by a pedicle or a sessile stalk (Fig. 20.21). The latter are often so dense that the lesion must be removed with a margin of normal bone around it. Microscopically, there are three variants of osteomas. The osteoma eburneum is composed of lamellae of dense bone with small Haversian spaces. Osteoblasts and connective tissue are inconspicuous. Osteoma spongiosum is composed of mature cancellous bone with a lamellar structure. Many of the trabeculae exhibit osteoblastic activity. A cortical plate may surround the tumor and hematopoiesis may be present within the marrow spaces. With increasing age of the tumor, there is a corresponding decrease in osteogenesis. The osteoma durum lies between the two preceding variants in terms of bone to stroma ratio.

Treatment of osteomas is not generally indicated unless the tumors are symptomatic. Some authors, however, underscore the potentiality for serious

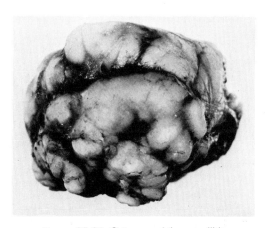

Figure 20.21. Osteoma of the mandible.

Table 20.5
Osteomas of the Paranasal Sinuses

Author	Frontal	Ethmoid	Maxillary	Sphenoid
	%	%	%	%
Malan, quoted by Salinger[106] (458 cases)	38.9	28.8	9.0	23.2
Hallberg and Begley[107] (51 cases)	78.4	19.6	3.9	0
Handousa[108] (35 cases)	57.0	20.0	17.0	2.8
Montgomery[109] (300 cases)	80.0	16.0	4.0	0
Samy and Mostafa[110] (21 cases)	49.0	19.0	28.5	4.5

complications, particularly in the paranasal sinus region, and advise surgical removal of the tumor even before symptoms are produced.[111] There is a low, but ever dangerous, incidence of intracranial complications caused by osteomas of the sinus walls.[112] Recurrences or sarcomatous changes have not been reported.

OSTEOMAS AND GARDNER'S SYNDROME

The classical findings in patients with Gardner's syndrome are a dominant hereditary pattern for hard and soft tissue tumors along with polyposis of the bowel. The prevailing assumption is that there is an inherited systemic defect which has its particular affect on tissues undergoing constant cellular replacement, namely epithelium and collagen.[113] The syndrome is an occasional manifestation of familial polyposis coli, itself a rare condition. The disorder is an autosomal dominant, and it can be predicted that 50% of offspring will be affected.[114] The exact incidence is difficult to estimate, but it is probably lower than one per million population.

All varieties of hard and soft tissue tumors have been reported, but there is a pattern of lesions. Epidermal and/or sebaceous cysts are common, as are subcutaneous fibrous tumors. Long bone lesions are said to be characteristic of melorheostosis. The osseous tumors in the skull and face are usually referred to as osteomas. The greatest number of osteomas occur in the mandible, particularly in the ramus. Patients manifesting the syndrome look surprisingly similar, with masses protruding from the mandibular region and several smaller rounded swellings of the skull.

The head and neck surgeon must be aware of the manifestations of Gardner's syndrome since the initial signs are frequently related to the facial region. The failure to associate multiple soft tissue tumors, osteomas and intestinal polyposis can be a serious error. The incidence of "malignant degeneration" of polyps when gastrointestinal symptoms lead to the diagnosis approaches 40%.[115]

MYXOMA OF BONE

Myxoma of bone, *exclusive of the jaws,* is a controversial entity; many authorities doubt its existence. Such skepticism is well founded and results from confusion of lesions that have myxoid features with true myxoma of bone. A review of 6,000 bone tumors at the Mayo Clinic and an additional 5,000 lesions of bone sent to the Clinic for consultation has led to the acceptance of only

three cases of myxomas of bones other than the jaws.[116]

The myxoma of the jaw bones, on the other hand, while relatively uncommon, is an accepted clinicopathological entity despite the controversy over its histogenesis. Even in the jaws, however, one must exclude the lesion with secondary alterations, the so-called "myxoid imitators."

Histogenetically, the myxoma of jaws has been regarded by various workers as either odontogenic, osteogenic, both, or neither. Those favoring an odontogenic origin cite the virtually exclusive occurrence of this tumor in the jaws, its striking resemblance to dental papillae, and the occasional presence within the tumor of odontogenic rests. It is very likely the *majority* of the central myxomas of jaw bones arise from the mesenchyme of the tooth germ. Ultrastructural findings thus far reported for the tumors are consistent with such an odontogenic origin.[117, 118] They are also not incompatible with an origin from primitive nonodontogenic mesenchymal rests. Histochemical findings are similar and well presented by Harrison.[119]

Although myxomas of the mandible and maxilla are considered rare lesions, they are not as rare as previously described and are found more often than the ameloblastoma.[120] In reviewing 2,276 primary tumors of the bone at the Mayo Clinic, Zimmerman and Dahlin[121] found 26 myxomas, all of which were located in the jaws. This study was extended in 1975 to include 38 cases.[122] Barros et al.[123] published a study of 95 examples of myxoma of the jaws taken from the literature from 1940 to 1966 and presented 21 new cases, spanning a 6-year period from 1961 to 1966.

Myxoma of the jaws is found primarily in young patients. Approximately 67% of the patients are between the ages of 10 and 29 years.[120] The average age of the patient is 30 years, with a range from 10 to 40 years. Age is, however, no limiting factor. There appears to be no sex predilection in the occurrence of this tumor.

A literature review of 213 adequately documented examples of myxomas of the jaws indicates the mandible is a slightly preferred site; 132 from mandible and 91 from maxilla.[124] It is most commonly seen in the ramus, angle of the jaw, molar region and the body of the mandible. The anterior portion of the mandible is rarely affected, and bilateral tumors are oddities. When the maxilla is involved, invasion of the sinus and destruction of the antral walls often occur. In the maxilla, the zygomatic process and alveolar bone are primarily affected.

Although the signs and symptoms vary considerably, most frequently the tumor is noticed because of a slow and progressive swelling of the affected jaw and facial deformity. Very often teeth in the affected region are loosened because of destruction of supporting bone. These teeth remain vital and are frequently displaced away from the expanding mass. The overlying mucosa appears normal or slightly hyperemic and usually bulges outward because of the expansion of the bony cortex beneath it. Pain is inconstant and inconsistent. Symptoms are often present 1 to 3 years before treatment is sought.

The x-ray appearance is that of a multilocular cyst with a dense radiopaque margin. Initially the cortex is intact but thinned and expanded from its normal contour. Progressive growth of the tumor produces perforation and destruction of the cortices and invasion of the soft tissue. In the maxilla, the antrum as well as the alveolar bone is often invaded, giving a dense cloudly appearance to the sinus on a Water's view.

Grossly, the lesion may give the impression of encapsulation, but this is false and incomplete. The most striking gross finding is that of glistening mucus covering the cut surface of the tumor. The mass is soft, shiny, smooth, yellow or whitish-gray and gelatinous (Fig. 20.22). Small shiney filaments can be seen in the cut surface along with occasional coarse, gritty regions indicating calcified regions (Fig. 20.23).

Microscopically, the tumor is characterized by polyhedral or stellate cells embedded in a soft, mucinous matrix. The tumor is parvicellular, and the dominant cell is stellate with long, anastomosing cytoplasmic processes. Nuclei are oval and often hyperchromatic. The loose, weakly basophilic stroma through which course very delicate reticulin fibers resembles both primitive mesenchyme and the stellate reticulum found in developing teeth. Some authors report seeing epithelial strands similar to dental epithelium within the tumor, whereas most workers find no trace of epithelium.[120]

Ultrastructural study has revealed two basic types of tumor cells: secretory and nonsecretory.[117, 118] The former is the principal cell and resembles the fibroblast in many respects. Although the ultrastructural findings indicate an abortive attempt at collagen fibrillogenesis, there is also a prominent secretory activity within the cells, resulting in an excessive production of acid mucopolysaccharide ground substance.

The clinical behavior is not unlike "myxoma" of the soft tissues, i.e., slow progressive growth and a stubborn tendency for resistance or "recurrence" after inadequate removal. This tumor is difficult to eradicate because its boundaries are not well defined. Very often small nests, pockets or loculations of myxoid tumor are hidden behind bony trabeculations and may not be detected.

Although no instances of metastases have been recorded, the tumor is locally aggressive.[120-124] There is a 25% recurrence rate noted in the literature.[120, 125] Colby et al.[126] contend that: "They (myxomas) are nonencapsulated widely infiltrating growths which are difficult to eradicate and may prove fatal by extension to vital structures." Recurrences have been noted as early as 3 months and as late as 10 years after surgery, although usually they are seen in 2 to 3 years.

Myxomas of the jaws should be treated vigorously because of the recurrence rate.[120, 125] Curettage and excision followed by chemical or electrical cautery is acceptable treatment for small le-

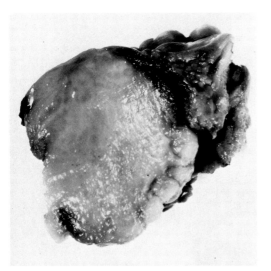
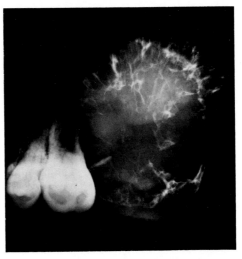

Figures 20.22 (*left*) and **20.23** (*right*). Myxoma of the jaw. (Courtesy of Drs. E. R. Barros and R. Cabrini.)

sions. Resection is reserved for recurrent or extensive lesions. This takes the form of en bloc excision, preserving the continuity of the jaw when possible, local, wide excision, marginal resection or radical resection. Radiation therapy should be avoided.[123]

EWING'S SARCOMA

Ewing's sarcoma of bone is a lesion primarily of the long tubular bones or an innominate bone. The skull and facial bones have the lowest frequency of involvement (9%). Roca et al.[127] found 37 examples involving the jaws in a review of the literature from 1949 to 1967. Potdar[128] and Rapoport et al.[125] have added cases so that approximately 55 cases have been recorded by 1977. Mandibular involvement predominates. Patients are young; the oldest with a Ewing's sarcoma of the jaw has been 38 years old at the time of diagnosis. Males are afflicted more than females. Both of these statistics are in accord with those for Ewing's sarcoma at large. Primary Ewing's sarcoma of the temporal bone is also rare. Only seven cases have been reported in the past 100 years.[130]

Roentgenograms are nebulous and nonspecific and do not provide reliable guides to diagnosis. The findings may simulate those of either infection or other neoplastic diseases. Expansion and an increased density of the cortex, mottled destruction of bone, cystic lobulation and varying degrees of periosteal thickening may be present. The tumor often produces an "onion peel" appearance because of expansive growth and cortical infiltration. An overlying soft tissue mass may be present.

Like its long-bone counterpart, Ewing's sarcoma is often associated with severe pain, tenderness and secondary swelling.

A form of *extraskeletal* sarcoma, resembling Ewing's sarcoma clinically and pathologically, has been described.[131, 132] It is a neoplasm primarily of the lower extremities and the paravertebral region. Angervall and Enzinger[131] include one case originating in the left neck between the carotid sheath and vertebral body in their series. The prognosis of these extraskeletal tumors is like that of osseous Ewing's sarcoma.

Ewing's sarcoma is considered a primary malignant tumor of bone and extraskeletal soft tissues. The mesenchymal cells from which the tumor derives are so undifferentiated that no further classification of the cell of origin seems possible, although attempts continue.[133, 134] Controversy about the existence of the disease as an entity distinct from metastatic neuroblastoma or lymphoma seems to have been resolved. Rather dis-

tinctive histological criteria are now recognized, although some cases still cause anxiety and head-scratching among pathologists.

Microscopically, Ewing's sarcoma is a cellular, usually compact tumor with sheets of rounded or slightly elongated tumor cells. There is little or no intercellular stroma and the cells lack cohesion (Fig. 20.24). The sheets or nests of cells may be outlined by strands of fibrous tissue. The cells are about two or three times the size of a lymphocyte and the nucleus nearly fills the cell. Nuclear membranes are distinct, may be slightly irregular, but not clefted. Nucleoli are not prominent and mitoses are infrequent. Zones of necrosis and hemorrhage may be prominent. In these areas, the viable cells may cluster around blood vessels in a peritheliomatous pattern. Occasionally, the cells are arranged in rosette-like structures (herein the resemblance to neuroblastoma). The pseudorosette pattern is said to be an artefact produced by the collection of cells around foci of granular and necrotic debris. Intracytoplasmic glycogen granules in tumor cells are usually present, but in a minority of cases may be absent. Glycogen is particularly demonstrable if alcoholic fixation or short term exposure to 10% formalin are employed. Strong acid decalcifying agents such as nitric acid may dissolve the glycogen granules. Glycogen is not found in neuroblastoma or primary lymphoma of bone; the two tumors most commonly confused with Ewing's

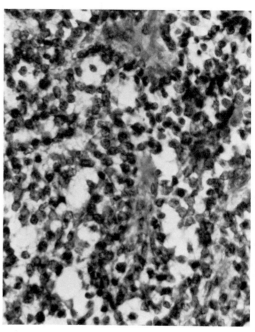

Figure 20.24. Ewing's sarcoma.

sarcoma. This feature cannot be used to distinguish rhabdomyosarcomas from Ewing's tumor since glycogen granules are found in both lesions. It has been suggested that examination of the tumor tissue for monoamine oxidase activity may be of assistance.[135] Imprints are also very helpful in finalizing a diagnosis, particularly when lymphomas need to be excluded.

Ultrastructural studies reveal large amounts of glycogen aggregated in an undifferentiated cytoplasm of cells which show variable amounts of organelles. Intercellular connections of desmosomal type are variably encountered. Apparently membrane specialization is not a constant finding. Despite characterization of the fine-structure of the tumor cells (Table 20.6), the problem of histogenesis remains unresolved.[132-134, 136]

Ewing's sarcoma is a neoplasm that manifests a rapid hematogenous spread. Asymptomatic and often clinically undetected metastasis are quite common. It is estimated that 15% to 30% of patients with the tumors have asymptomatic metastases at diagnosis.[137] In other patients, the metastases usually occur within 6 months after diagnosis. Metastases occur primarily in the lungs and in

Table 20.6
Ewing's Sarcoma—Ultrastructural Features*

Cell shape	Spherical to polygonal with occasional elongated processes
Plasma membrane	Thin (60Å), single layer, ruptures, pinocytotic vesicles
Basement lamina	Absent
Attachment sites	Absent or rudimentary
Ciliary body	Rare
Nucleus	Round to oval, occasionally irregular or indented, fine chromatin, occasional blistering of nuclear membrane
Cytoplasm	Clear, only few organelles
Glycogen	Variable; may be abundant
Mitochondria	5–20/cell, disrupted or degenerated, granules
Phagosomes	Few to rare
Rough endoplasmic reticulum	Sparse
Free ribosome	Moderate
Golgi complex	Rare and usually poorly defined
Intracytoplasmic filaments	Scattered or occasionally in bundles (50–100 Å)
Intercellular spaces	Narrow, amorphous and filamentous matrix

* After Wigger et al.[134]

other bones. The multiple bone involvement occurring in patients with Ewing's sarcoma has led some authors to conclude the disease is multicentric. Against this hypothesis is that one-half of patients do not develop multiple bone lesions and in the majority of instances, a single focus is noted first.

The results of treatment of Ewing's sarcoma, until lately, have been bad, principally because of the frequency of early metastases. Only 8% of 944 patients reviewed in 1967, had survived 5 years.[138] The results from single treatment centers were not much better; the Mayo Clinic achieved a 5-year survival of 16% in 234 patients treated between 1912 and 1968.[139]

There is increasing evidence, accumulated over the past 10 years, of the effectiveness of chemotherapeutic agents in the palliative management of Ewing's sarcoma. At the same time, primary radiation therapy has had a resurgence as the improved tolerance of normal tissues to supervoltage therapy and improved therapeutic techniques have decreased the morbidity following the treatment of the primary lesion with radiation. Surgery is yielding as the usual form of management of the primary bone lesion.[140, 141] Some nonrandomized and retrospective studies, however, support the relative "effectiveness" of control of the primary by surgical resection.[139, 142]

The surgery versus radiotherapy debate has been complicated by the introduction of adjuvant chemotherapy as routine additional treatment. The patient, however, has gained the benefit. In 1975, Pomeroy and Johnson[143] reported a 2-year actuarial survival rate of 56% in a series of 66 consecutive patients treated by combined local irradiation of the primary site and various permutations of cyclophosphamide, vincristine, actinomycin D, methotrexate and whole brain irradiation. Similar enhancement of survival has been reported by others.[144, 145]

There can be little doubt that chemotherapy does prevent some occult metastases from becoming clinically apparent; extension to 5-year survivals indicates this. The patient with Ewing's sarcoma may be said to have a "prognostic risk period" of 36 months. If he suffers no relapse, or if metastases have not occurred for 3 years after treatment of the primary, he may be considered "cured" with a high degree of probability. The "period of risk" is based on the theory that viable tumor cells surviving after definitive therapy grow at more or less the same rate as the original tumor.[146] A recurrent tumor should become clinically manifest within an interval no greater than the longest time that the original primary was present.

The enthusiasm for aggressive combined therapy has to be tempered by severe, acute and late reactions to the combined radio- and chemotherapy. Age and site both influence the radiation morbidity. For the future, the hope is that improved chemotherapy will permit the use of doses of radiation which will control the primary disease without major morbidity.

The low number of Ewing's sarcoma of the jaws and the variety of treatments given preclude any meaningful assessment of effectiveness of treatment and prognosis. It is of interest that long-term survivors have had primary tumors of the maxilla.[147]

MISCELLANEOUS PRIMARY LESIONS

As I have indicated earlier, there is a trend toward consolidation in the classifications of benign fibro-osseous lesions. Many of these non-odontogenic lesions, because of appearance, wide variety of names and confusion, have been placed under the heading of "fibrous dysplasia."

In the first edition of this book, I considered this form of "lumping" as appropriate. In the short time since the publication, I have exercised the prerogative of experience and believe there are sufficient clinicopathological findings to merit separation of this motley group of lesions.

Central "Fibroma" of Jaws

While some authors use the term central fibroma to refer to a presumed specific entity, I use it in the generic sense to signify intraosseous origin of a non-ossifying fibrous lesion. There exist, therefore, at least three basic variants of my central fibroma: nonossifying fibroma, desmoplastic fibroma and the odontogenic fibroma.[148] All are uncommon and the odontogenic fibroma is very imperfectly separated from the others by the presence of odontogenic epithelium in the tumor.[149] The odontogenic fibroma arises from one of the mesenchymal components of the tooth or tooth germ, such as the periodontal membrane, dental papilla, or dental follicle. The central nonodontogenic fibroma is presumably derived from the endosteal mesenchyme of the jaw itself. Conceptually, it is not difficult for me to believe these fibrous lesions are inter-related not only to each other, but also to the true myxoma of bone. The variable degrees of stromal myxoid change and a distinctive vascular pattern of some lesions point to a fibrous variant of the myxoma—*fibromyxoma*. This term is used as a diagnostic one and not merely to signify myxoid change in an otherwise defined soft tissue tumor. Figures 20.25 *A* and *B* and 20.26 present the varying histological appearance of a fibromyxoma as it presents in the facial bones and airways. Figure 20.26 illustrates a fibromyxoma of the laryngeal glottis. Given this myxoid appearance, the tumor departs from the usual slow growing and fairly well demarcated central fibroma of the jaws. This author has been particularly impressed with the local aggressiveness and recurrence rate of the fibromyxoma of the maxilla and paranasal sinuses. These tumors occur principally in patients in their late teens and young adulthood.

The *desmoplastic fibroma* of the jaws may only be a more collagenized form of the spectrum of central non-ossifying fibroma, but it differs in that it has accepted counterparts in the long bones. It is a benign connective tissue tumor that resembles the desmoid tumor of abdominal and extra-abdominal sites. By 1977, there had been approximately 37 cases reported in various bones.[150] It occurs most often in the metaphysis of long bones. Seven cases have been reported in the mandible. No other facial bone appears to have been affected. There is no sex predilection and most of the tumors present in the second decade. Patients usually complain of swelling, intermittent pain and some degree of functional impairment. There is a tendency for the tumor to be quite large when first discovered. Cortical destruction may produce a picture of malignancy. The lesion is radiolucent with a trabelulated or honey-combed background. Grossly the tumor is a dense, tough, rubbery and whorled mass of fibrous connective tissue. The tumor is devoid of bone except at the extreme periphery where there is pre-existing bone. Mitoses are scant or absent in the hypocellular and collagenous tissue. The tumor is benign but manifests a high recurrence rate if not widely excised. Cellular tumors cannot be distinguished from collagenized, hypercellular fibroxyomas and may be confused with fibrosarcomas. The desmoplastic fibroma is over-all much less cellular than the non-osteogenic fibroma. It is to be noted here, that while there may be a resemblance of the non-ossifying fibroma to a fibrous cortical defect, the latter does not appear to have been described in the jaws.

Ossifying Fibroma

A monostotic fibrous lesion of the facial and jaw bones, as well as the long bones, ossifying fibroma is often considered a variant of fibrous dysplasia because of histological similarities.

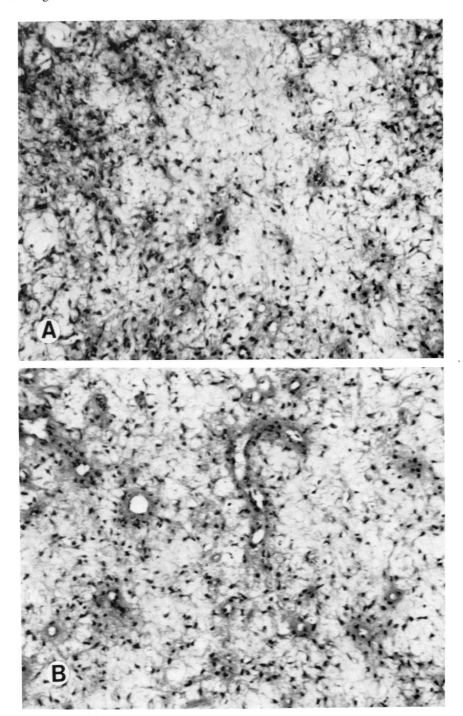

Figure 20.25 A and B. Fibromyxomas (two examples) which presented in the antrum. Both patients with these lesions were in their early teens. Note the distinctive vascularity which is very unlike the odontogenic or nonodontogenic myxoma. Recurrences characterize these lesions.

It clearly belongs in a range of benign fibro-osseous lesions which occur in the jaws and which includes the ossifying fibroma (central and peripheral) cementifying fibroma, benign cementoblas-toma, periapical fibrous dysplasia and true fibrous dysplasia itself.[151]

Hamner et al.[152] provided the impetus to separate fibrous dysplasia from the aforementioned

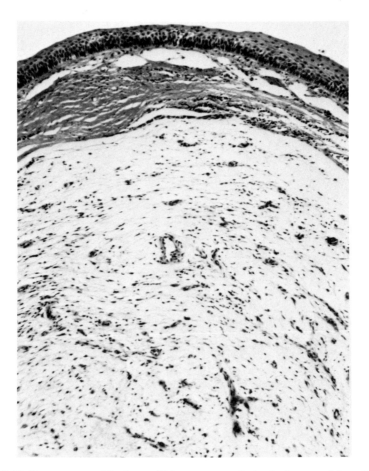

Figure 20.26. Fibromyxoma of the larynx. This nonosseous lesion had recurred three times.

groups. According to these workers fibrous dysplasia is of medullary bone origin with distinctive histological features. The others of the group arise from the fibrous connective tissue of the periodontium which contains mesenchymal blastic cells with the potential to form cementum, alveolar bone and fibrous tissue. Hammer et al.[152] divided these lesions into cementoid, osteoid, cemento-osteoid and fibroid lesions.

Since, in general, the lesions appear to represent a spectrum and since one cannot by any means definitely distinguish between bone and cementum, these lesions have been considered examples of one disease entity.

Both the ossifying and cementifying (cemento-ossifying fibroma) fibromas may occur in the mandible and the maxilla. There is a preference for the former. Both lesions most often present a painless swelling of the involved bone. They appear to occur with nearly equal frequency in both sexes with the greatest incidence of occurence in third and fourth decades of life. The child under 15 is not immune, however.[153]

The radiographic appearance of these lesions varies with the stage of maturity of the lesion. The ossifying fibroma at first appears as a relatively well demarcated radiolucency, but later becomes more mineralized and relatively less well localized. In the mature cementifying fibroma, there is a well defined radiolucency surrounding an area of dense irregular radio-opacity.

Fibrous dysplasia, on the other hand, is often first diagnosed in infancy or childhood. Most authors have shown a predilection for the maxilla. Females are more affected than males. The lesion presents as a painless, slow-growing swelling of the affected part and progresses to deformity. Growth may slow or cease shortly after the onset of puberty. The radiographic appearance varies with maturity and calcification. In general, however, fibrous dysplasia lacks the circumscription of the ossifying fibroma.

The ossifying fibroma presents microscopically as evenly spaced spicules of bone rimmed with osteoblasts and osteoclasts within a fibrous stroma. The spicules are randomly distributed within the fibrous stroma. Most of the spicules are centrally composed of woven bone, but there is evidence of a lamellar transformation at the periphery. Complete maturation to lamellar bone is observed only in isolated spicules. The fibrous stroma shows both loose and dense areas with occasional whorling. A prominent feature is an increased denseness of stroma with rounding of the fibroblasts near the bone spicules. Stromal hemorrhage, inflammation and giant cells are not seen in the unadulterated lesion.

In the uncomplicated case of fibrous dysplasia, the bone is woven without lamellar transformation and there is no appositional rimming of the spicules of bone by osteoblasts or osteoclasts.[154]

The cementifying fibroma may appear inseparable histologically from the ossifying fibroma. There is much more tendency, however, for cementum-like material to be more numerous, ovoid and heavily calcified.

The usually well-circumscribed nature of the ossifying fibroma in the jaws lends itself to relative ease of excision and hence favorable therapeutic results. On occasion, however, particularly in the juvenile, and in the maxilla, the tumor assumes an aggressive behavior and considerable local destruction of bone and recurrences ensue. Attempts at histological identification of this form of the tumor have failed. They do appear, however, to contain more of the cementoid features and are larger than the usually innocuous tumors.[155]

Osteoid Osteoma and Osteoblastoma

These two benign osteoblastic neoplasms of bone are infrequently encountered in the jaws.[156] The two lesions probably constitute only different anatomico-clinical variants of a basic osteoblastic tumor.[156, 157]

While the histological features of both lesions have been well recorded in many publications, no definite histological features have been described by which it is possible to distinguish between them. Resort has been made to a separation based on clinical aspects and size of lesions.[158, 159]

Characterizing both lesions histologically are the presence of small regular trabeculae of woven bone and osteoid lying in a vascular fibrous tissue. A layer of osteoblasts is usually prominent at the trabecular bone surface and osteoclasts are present in the fibrous tissue. These cells sometimes erode the bone, resulting in a remodeling as evidenced by cement lines. Other types of cells are not usual. The degree of mineralization is variable but tends to be greatest in the central regions of the lesions (nidus).

Variations of this basic pattern are mainly in the amount and aggregation of bone and the cellularity of the fibrous tissue. The bony component may be represented by only few, small and scattered trabeculae or may exist as large masses of osteoid (rarely chondroid material may be seen). In the absence of bone, the spindle cell character of the stroma may give way to one where closely packed osteoblasts predominate.

The osteoid trabeculae in benign osteoblastoma are generally broader, longer, and more widely separated than in the osteoid osteoma. It is also usually more vascular. Comparative studies of the ultrastructure of osteoblastoma and osteoid osteoma reveal essentially similar features and appear closely related.[157, 159]

The distinction between the two lesions is mainly one of size and growth potential. While the osteoid osteoma is a lesion of limited growth potential that rarely exceeds 1 cm in greatest dimension, benign osteoblastoma is larger than 1 cm and grows in size. Sclerosis of bone about the osteoid osteoma is a further distinction.

By 1976, 12 osteoid osteomas of the jaws had been reported in the literature.[156] Seven were in the mandible and five in the maxilla. The sexes are equally represented. The age at diagnosis has ranged from 77 years to 4 years. Most of the lesions appear in young adults.

The association of pain that is accentuated at night and relieved by aspirin has been repeatedly emphasized. The significance of these findings as differential diagnostic points remains conjectural. Radiographic findings, however, are more tangible. The osteoid osteoma presents as an eccentric radiolucency with sclerotic borders. The importance of the latter is best expressed by quoting Lichtenstein and Sawyer[160]: "When such a tumor is enveloped by sclerotized bone, we prefer to designate it as osteoid osteoma, rather than a benign osteoblastoma, even though it may be substantially larger than the usual osteoid osteoma."

There is no correlation between the histological appearance of the lesion and the duration of symptoms. This argues against the likelihood of a spontaneous healing of the osteoid osteoma and supports excision en bloc as the proper form of treatment. Curettage is followed by recurrence.

The osteoblastoma is particularly unusual in the facial bones. Nearly 80% of the lesions occur in the vertebrae and bones of the extremities. The calvarium, including the squama of the temporal bone, ranks second as a site of involvement. By 1976, 13 cases of benign osteoblastoma of the jawbones had been recorded in the world literature; 10 in the mandible and three in the maxilla.[156]

Usually the tumor is central, but a periosteal origin has been reported (Fig. 20.27).

There is a slight male predominance for lesions in the facial bones. The age range of the hosts bearing the tumor in the jawbones is 5 to 22 years, narrower than that expressed for osteoid osteoma and for osteoblastomas in the skeleton.

In general, symptoms are not of specific aid in the differential diagnosis of the lesion. Pain may be present, but it is not unusually severe at night.

The radiographic findings are not specific for this radiolucent, solitary lesion, but the broad reactive zone of sclerotic bone which is characteristic of osteoid osteoma is only rarely found in osteoblastoma.

Incomplete excision will yield recurrence and a nonradical en bloc excision is advised.

Synovial Chondromatosis

Synovial chondromatosis is a condition in which foci of cartilage develop in the synovial membrane of a joint, apparently through metaplasia of the sublining connective tissue of the synovial membrane. The knee joint is the most common site of involvement. The temporomandibular joint is an unusual location for the disorder. The importance of the lesion for pathologists is the possibility of misdiagnosing the condition as chondrosarcoma if only histological criteria are used. The usual symptoms in a patient with synovial chondromatosis of the temporomandibular joint are preauricular swelling and limited motion of the joint with deviation of the mandible to the affected side on opening the jaw. Radiographic examinations may often demonstrate no abnormality but occasionally may show various radiopaque masses in the synovium or as loose bodies confined to the area of the joint capsule.[161] Destruction of bone is absent. At the time of surgical exploration, there is an expanded joint capsule which contains either cartilaginous loose bodies or a conglomerate mass of cartilaginous material having a cobblestone surface. In general, the tumor is easily enucleated.

A history and gross operative findings are mandatory for the pathologist. Atypism of cartilage cells may be difficult to distinguish from low-grade chondrosarcoma.

Chondromyxoid Fibroma

The majority of chondromyxoid fibromas occur in the metaphyses of long bones; only a few of the tumors have occurred in the cranial bones and bones of the face.[162] The lesion is generally regarded as benign and recurrences (10%) are attributed to incomplete removal.

Lymphomas of the Facial Bones (Exclusive of Burkitt's Tumor)

Clinically significant involvement of the facial bones by lymphoma, however unusual, is not unexpected. When lymphoma is responsible for an osseous lesion, one of three clinical states may prevail: (1) the lesion may be considered to be primary in the involved bone; (2) similar lesions may be found in regional or distant lymph nodes, in other bones or in any part of the body, and the original lesion may be considered as either a primary or secondary focus; or (3) the osseous lesion may obviously be a secondary lesion in a patient with known diffuse malignant lymphoma.

Criteria for the "primary lymphoma" of bone have been proposed[163]: (1) the primary lesion should originate in a single bone; (2) secondary involvement has been excluded; (3) histological appearance should be identical to that of lymphomas occurring in other tissues; (4) a long history of the disease should exist, during which some of the general symptoms of debility and loss of weight are rarely manifested; (5) metastatic lesions, if present, should be strictly limited to regional lymph nodes, or their appearances should follow the osseous "primary" by not less than 6 months; (6) the lesion should be radiosensitive.

Long tubular bones are preferentially involved over the flat bones of the body. Thirty-one of the 47 cases studied by Shoji and Miller[164] demonstrated the lesions in the long tubular bones with predilection for femur, humerus and tibia, in this order. The flat bones were primary sites in 16 cases, with the most frequent involvement in the pelvic girdle. Our use of the term malignant lymphoma of bone is that suggested by Dahlin and associates,[165, 166] i.e., in a generic sense. This term encompasses the neoplasm ordinarily referred to as reticulum cell sarcoma in the literature on bone tumors. Reimer et al.[167] consider that lymphomas presenting in bone account for approximately 5% of all extranodal lymphomas.

In the head and neck, particularly in those cases where the malignant lymphoma is located in the region of the maxillary antrum or its bony confines, it is often impossible to relate primary origin in the facial bones. Lymphomas in the maxilla vary in their degree of invasion of the involved region. Many present with a major involvement of the antrum with or without prominent maxillary alveolar destruction. Often the walls of the antra are perforated by the lymphoma. In some cases, several of the walls are perforated so that swelling of the maxillary alveolar ridge and the face, obstruction of the nose, or ocular proptosis occurs.

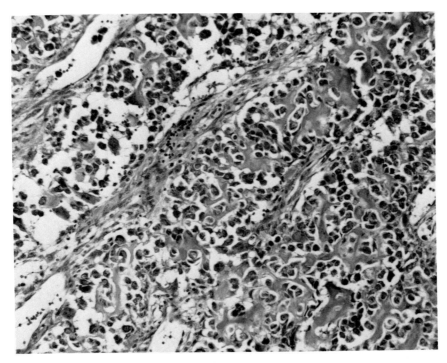

Figure 20.27. Osteoblastoma of the paranasal sinus. Clinical presentation of this lesion was into the nasal cavity.

If we do not exclude the lymphoma of the maxillary antrum from consideration of primary malignant lymphoma of bone, the maxilla is the facial bone most often involved by malignant lymphoma. Excluding this group, the mandible becomes the major site and ranks third in frequency of involvement behind the long tubular bones (humerus, femur and tibia) and the innominate bone.[168]

Men in their fifth, sixth and seventh decades of life constitute the bulk of the patient population. Patients usually seek medical attention because of pain, with or without swelling or a palpable mass. The average duration of signs and symptoms before treatment has been estimated at 10 to 11 months.

There is nothing diagnostic about the x-ray appearance, with the usual picture one of osteolytic destruction often simulating metastatic carcinoma. Diagnosis rests solely on the proper interpretation of an adequate biopsy specimen. Malignant lymphoma of bone presents grossly not unlike lymphomas of other sites. The mass is gray, soft and friable. Necrotic zones may be present and proximal sclerosis is not unusual. Regional lymph nodes are sometimes involved by the same neoplastic process.

Microscopically, the tumor manifests a variety of histological types. Hodgkin's disease is an unusual form, and "giant follicular lymphoma" has not been recorded as occurring primarily in bone. Some of the lesions may be logically classified as histiocytic lymphomas since they are composed of this cell throughout. The majority, however, are classified by Ivins and Dahlin[166] as "mixed lymphomas," indicating that histiocytic cells, lymphoblasts and lymphocytes are present in various proportions. These authors use this variation in cell type as a helpful diagnostic feature, acknowledging at the same time that the reticulum cell is probably the progenitor cell from which the other elements arise. Others, also acknowledging that lymphoma of bone is a heterogenous entity, have subclassified the tumors with histiocytic lymphoma the most common form.[167] This type is followed by diffuse poorly differentiated lymphocytic, diffuse lymphocytic-histiocytic, and undifferentiated lymphomas in that order.

The prognosis in "malignant lymphoma" of bone appears to be significantly better than that in most other primary malignant tumors of bone. The prognosis also compares favorably with primary malignant lymphoma in other sites. Approximately one-quarter of patients can be expected to survive 5 years, and this is increased if the treatment is instituted early.[169] There is, however, a high frequency of disseminated disease in patients with lymphoma presenting in bone. In a National Cancer Institute study, 12 of 14 patients (86%) showed extensive disease (stage IV) after evaluation.[167] In 10 of the 12 patients, the diffuse disease was clinically unsuspected.

A close look at the entire group of "malignant lymphomas" of bone does not form a basis for recommending one method of treatment over another. Because of their reputed radiosensitivity, radiotherapy is the mainstay of therapy.[170]

Tumors of Fat

Tumors allegedly arising in the adipose tissue of marrow are very rare. Johnson[171] has reported an intraosseous lipoma of the mandible. The tumors are benign, but because cortical bone is sometimes destroyed, the radiographic appearance may be that of a malignancy.

Primary Intraosseous Epithelial Tumors

Salivary gland tissue may present within the jaws and may give rise to primary neoplasm. The several possible sources of intraosseous glandular tissue include metaplastic odontogenic cyst lining, ectopic salivary gland tissue or embryologically entrapped retromolar mucous glands.[172]

The mucoepidermoid carcinoma has an apparent proclivity among salivary gland tumors arising centrally within the jaws. Silverglade et al.[173] recorded nine examples. The central mucoepidermoid carcinoma has a predisposition to the posterior part of the mandible, where most of the examples have arisen. The lesion behaves aggressively, with a rapid onset and frequent recurrences. Metastases to cervical lymph nodes have occurred. Wide surgical excision is the treatment of choice.

Central "epidermoid" carcinoma may also arise as an apparent primary in the jaws. Its origin may be from epithelial remnants of (1) the sheath of Hertwig, (2) enamel organ, (3) fusion of facial processes or (4) carcinomatous changes in dental cysts or an ameloblastoma.

REFERENCES

1. Stafne, E. C., and Austin, L. T.: A study of dental roentgenograms in cases of Paget's disease (osteitis deformans), osteitis fibrosa, cystica and osteoma. J. Am. Dent. Assoc. 25:1202, 1938.
2. Cooke, B. E. D.: Paget's disease of the jaws: fifteen cases. Ann. R. Coll. Surg. Engl. 19:223, 1956.
3. Tillman, H. H.: Paget's disease of bone. A clinical, radiographic and histopathologic study of twenty-five cases involving the jaws. Oral Surg. 15:1225, 1962.
4. Lucas, R. B.: Osteitis deformans—jaws and teeth. J. Clin. Pathol. 8:195, 1955.
5. Kelly, P. J., Peterson, L. F., Dahlin, D. C., and Plumge, G. E.: Osteitis deformans (Paget's disease of bone); a morphologic study utilizing microradiography and conventional technics. Radiology 77:368, 1961.
6. Rushton, M. A.: Dental tissues in osteitis deformans. Guy's Hosp. Rep. 88:163, 1938.
7. Newman, F. W.: Paget's disease; statistical study of 82 cases. J. Bone Joint Surg. 28:798, 1946.
8. Annotation: Treatment of Paget's disease. Lancet 1:955, 1971.
9. Bijvoet, O. L. M., Van der Sluys Veer, J., Wildiers, J., and Smeenk, D.: Calcitonin 1969: Proceedings of the Second International Symposium, London, p. 53. Springer-Verlag, New York, 1970.
10. Shira, R. B., and Bhaskar, S. N.: Oral surgery—Oral Pathology Conference No. 6, Walter Reed Army Medical Center, Oral Surg. 16:1255, 1963.
11. Batsakis, J. G., and Dito, W. R.: Chondrosarcoma of the maxilla. Arch. Otolaryngol. 75:55, 1962.
12. Kragh, L. V., Dahlin, D. C., and Erich, J. B.: Cartilaginous tumors of the jaws and facial regions. Am. J. Surg. 99:852, 1960.
13. Chaudhry, A. P., Robinovitch, M. R., Mitchell, D. F., and Vickers, R. A.: Chondrogenic tumors of the jaws. Am. J. Surg. 102:403, 1961.
14. Arlen, M., Tollefsen, H. R., Huvos, A. G., and Marcove, R. C.: Chondrosarcoma of the head and neck. Am. J. Surg. 120:456, 1970.
15. Phemister, D. B.: Chondrosarcoma of bone. Surg. Gynecol. Obstet. 50:216, 1930.
16. Cahn, L. R. (quoted by Blum, T.): Cartilage tumors of the jaws: report of three cases. Oral Surg. 7:1320, 1954.
17. Dahlin, D. C.: Bone Tumors; General Aspects and an Analysis of Cases. Charles C Thomas, Springfield, 1957.
18. Geschickter, C. F.: Tumors of jaws. Am. J. Cancer 24:90, 1935.
19. Evans, H. L., Ayala, A. G., and Romsdahl, M. M.: Prognostic factors in chondrosarcoma of bone. A clinicopathologic analysis with emphasis on histologic grading. Cancer 40:818, 1977.
20. Marcove, R. C., and Huvos, A. G.: Cartilaginous tumors of the sites. Cancer 27:794, 1971.
21. Erlandson, R. A., and Huvos, A. G.: Chondrosarcoma: a light and electron microscopic study. Cancer 34:1642, 1974.
22. Kilby, D., and Ambegaokar, A. G.: The nasal chondroma. Two case reports and a survey of the literature. J. Laryngol. 91:415, 1977.
23. Fu, Y.-S., and Perzin, K. H.: Non-epithelial tumors of the nasal cavity, paranasal sinuses, and nasopharynx: a clinicopathologic study. III. Cartilagenous tumors (chondroma, condrosarcoma). Cancer 34:453, 1974.
24. Coates, H. L., Pearson, B. W., Devine, K. D., and Unni, K. K.: Chondrosarcoma of the nasal cavity, paranasal sinuses, and nasopharynx. Tr. Am. Acad. Ophth. Otol. 84:919, 1977.
25. Salvador, A. H., Beabout, J. W., and Dahlin, D. C.: Mesenchymal chondrosarcoma—observations on 30 new cases. Cancer 28:605, 1971.
26. Guccion, J. G., Font, R. L., Enzinger, F. M., and Zimmerman, L. E.: Extraskeletal mesenchymal chondrosarcoma. Arch. Pathol. 95:336, 1973.
27. Dahlin, D. C., and Henderson, E. D.: Mesenchymal chondrosarcoma: further observations on a new entity. Cancer 15:410, 1962.
28. Fu, Y.-S., and Kay, S.: A comparative ultrastructure study of mesenchymal chondrosarcoma and myxoid chrondrosarcoma. Cancer 33:1531, 1974.
29. Jacobson, S. A.: Polyhistioma. A malignant tumor of bone and extraskeletal tissues. Cancer 40:2116, 1977.
30. Smith, M. T., Farinacci, C. J., Carpenter, H. A., and Bannayan, G. A.: Extraskeletal myxoid chondrosarcoma. A clinicopathological study. Cancer 37:821, 1976.
31. Thoma, K. H., and Goldman, H. M.: Oral Pathology, 5th Ed. C. V. Mosby Co., St. Louis, 1960.

32. Lichtenstein, L., and Jaffe, H. L.: Chondrosarcoma of bone. Am. J. Pathol. 19:553, 1943.

33. Sato, K., Nukaga, H., and Horikoshi, T.: Chondrosarcoma of the jaws and facial skeleton: a review of the Japanese literature. J. Oral Surg. 35:892, 1977.

34. McKenna, R. J. (quoted by M. J. Friedberg, et al.): Osteosarcoma of the maxilla; surgical removal and reconstruction of defect by a dental prosthesis. Oral Surg. 15:883, 1962.

35. Garrington, G. E., Scofield, H. H., Cornyn, J., and Hooker, S. P.: Osteosarcoma of the jaws; analysis of 56 cases. Cancer 20:377, 1967.

36. Dehner, L. P.: Tumors of the mandible and maxilla in children. II. A study of 14 primary and secondary malignant tumors. Cancer 32:112, 1973.

37. Kragh, L. V., Dahlin, D. C., and Erich, J. G.: Osteogenic sarcoma of the jaws and facial bones. Am. J. Surg. 96: 496, 1958.

38. Caron, A. S., Hajdu, S. I., and Strong, E. W.: Osteogenic sarcoma of the facial and cranial bones. Review of forty-three cases. Am. J. Surg. 122:719, 1971.

39. Yannopoulos, K., Bom, A. F., Griffiths, C. O., and Crikelair, G. C.: Osteosarcoma arising in fibrous dysplasia of the facial bones; case report and review of the literature. Am. J. Surg. 107:556, 1964.

40. LiVolsi, V. A.: Osteogenic sarcoma of the maxilla. Arch. Otolaryngol. 103:485, 1977.

41. Richards, W. G., and Coleman, F. C.: Osteogenic sarcoma of jaw. Oral Surg. 10:1156, 1957.

42. Jaffe, H. L.: Tumors and Tumorous Conditions of the Bones and Joints. Lea & Febiger, Philadelphia, 1958.

43. Coventry, M. B., and Dahlin, D. C.: Osteogenic sarcoma: a critical analysis of 430 cases. J. Bone Joint Surg. 39-A: 741, 1957.

44. Unni, K. K., Dahlin, D. C., McLeod, R. A., and Pritchard, D. J.: Intraosseous well differentiated osteosarcoma. Cancer 40:1337, 1977.

45. Unni, K. K., Dahlin, D. C., Beabout, J. W., and Ivins, J. C.: Parosteal osteogenic sarcoma. Cancer 37:2466, 1976.

46. Solomon, M. P., Biernacki, J., Slippen, M., and Rosen, Y.: Parosteal osteogenic sarcoma of the mandible. Arch. Otolaryngol. 101:754, 1975.

47. Dorfman, H. D., Steiner, G. C., and Jaffe, H. L.: Vascular tumors of bone. Hum. Pathol. 2:349, 1971.

48. Watson, W. L., and McCarthy, W. D.: Blood and lymph vessel tumors; report of 1,056 cases. Surg. Gynecol. Obstet. 71:569, 1940.

49. Unni, K. K., Ivins, J. C., Beabout, J. W., and Dahlin, D. C.: Hemangioma, hemangiopericytoma, and hemangioendothelioma (angiosarcoma) of bone. Cancer 27:1403, 1971.

50. Wyke, B. D.: Primary hemangioma of the skull—rare cranial tumor; review of the literature and report of case with special reference to roentgenographic appearance. Am. J. Roentgenol. Radium Ther. Nucl. Med., 61:302, 1949.

51. Bridger, M. W. M.: Haemangioma of the nasal bones. J. Laryngol. 90:191, 1976.

52. Walker, E. A., Jr., and McHenry, L. C.: Primary hemangioma of the zygoma. Arch. Otolaryngol. 81:199, 1965.

53. Smith, H. W.: Hemangioma of jaws; review of literature and report of a case. Arch. Otolaryngol. 70:579, 1960.

54. Frankenberg, B. E., and Panov, V. P.: Germangiomy Litsevogo Cherepa v Rentgenovskom Izobrazhenii. Vopr. Onkol. 5:188, 1959.

55. Lund, B. A., and Dahlin, D. C.: Hemangiomas of the mandible and maxilla. J. Oral Surg. 22:234, 1964.

56. Bucy, P. C., and Capp, C. S.: Primary hemangioma of bone; with special reference to roentgenologic diagnosis. Am. J. Roentgenol. Radium Ther. Nucl. Med. 23:1, 1930.

57. Loring, M. F.: Hemangioma of the mandible; diagnosis and therapy. Arch. Otolaryngol. 85:648, 1967.

58. Bucy, P. C.: The pathology of hemangioma of bone. Am. J. Pathol. 5:381, 1929.

59. Thoma, K. H.: Oral Pathology, 4th Ed., pp. 1313–1317.

C. V. Mosby Co., St. Louis, 1954.

60. Shklar, G., and Meyer, I.: Vascular tumors of the mouth and jaws. Oral Surg. 19:335, 1965.

61. Huebner, G. R., and Turlington, E. G.: So-called traumatic (hemorrhagic) bone cysts of the jaws. Oral Surg. 31:354, 1971.

62. Sharma, J. N.: Hemorrhagic cysts of the mandible. Report of a case. Oral Surg. 24:211, 1967.

63. Olech, E., Sicher, H., and Weinmann, J. P.: Traumatic mandibular bone cysts. Oral Surg. 4:1160, 1951.

64. Howe, G. L.: Haemorrhagic cysts of the mandible. Br. J. Oral Surg. 3:55, 1965.

65. Jaffe, H. L., and Lichtenstein, L.: Solitary unicameral bone cyst with emphasis on the roentgen picture; the pathologic appearance and the pathogenesis. Arch. Surg. 44:1004, 1942.

66. Jaffe, H. L.: Aneurysmal bone cyst. Bull. Hosp. Joint Dis. 11:3, 1950.

67. Lichtenstein, L.: Aneurysmal bone cyst. A pathologic entity commonly mistaken for giant-cell tumor and occasionally for hemangioma and osteogenic sarcoma. Cancer 3:279, 1950.

68. Dahlin, D. C., Besse, B. E., Jr., Pugh, D. G., and Ghormley, R. K.: Aneurysmal bone cysts. Radiology 64:56, 1955.

69. Bernier, J. L., and Bhaskar, S. N.: Aneurysmal bone cysts of the mandible. Oral Surg. 11:1018, 1958.

70. Gruskin, S. F., and Dahlin, D. C.: Aneurysmal bone cysts of the jaws. J. Oral Surg. 26:523, 1968.

71. Daugherty, J. W., and Eversole, L. R.: Aneurysmal bone cyst of the mandible: report of case. J. Oral Surg. 29:737, 1971.

72. Lichtenstein, L.: Aneurysmal bone cyst. Observations of fifty cases. J. Bone Joint Surg. 39-A:873, 1957.

73. Biesecker, J. L., Marcove, R. C., Huvos, A. G., and Mike, V.: Aneurysmal bone cysts: a clinicopathologic study of 66 cases. Cancer 26:615, 1970.

74. Buraczewski, J., and Dabska, M.: Pathogenesis of aneurysmal bone cyst: relationship between the aneurysmal bone cyst and fibrous dysplasia of bone. Cancer 28:597, 1971.

75. Bhaskar, S. N., Bernier, J. L., and Godby, F.: Aneurysmal bone cyst and other giant cell lesions of the jaws; report of 104 cases. J. Oral Surg. 17:30, 1959.

76. Otis, J., Hutter, R. V. P., Foote, F. W., Jr., Marcove, R. C., and Stewart, F. W.: Hemangioendothelioma of bone. Surg. Gynecol. Obstet. 127:295, 1968.

77. Hartmann, W. H., and Stewart, F. W.: Hemangioendothelioma of bone; unusual tumor characterized by indolent course. Cancer 15:846, 1962.

78. Pindborg, J. J., and Philipsen, H. P.: Malignant angioblastoma of the bone; a case occurring in the mandible. Acta Pathol. Microbiol. Scand. 49:408, 1960.

79. Black, M. J., Cassisi, N. J., and Biller, H. F.: Massive mandibular osteolysis. Arch. Otolaryngol. 100:314, 1974.

80. Phillips, R. M., Bush, O. B., and Hall, H. D.: Massive osteolysis (phantom bone, disappearing bone). Report of a case with mandibular involvement. Oral Surg. 34:886, 1972.

81. Jaffe, H. L.: Giant cell reparative granuloma, traumatic bone cyst, and fibrous (fibro-osseous) dysplasia of the jaw bones. Oral Surg. 6:159, 1953.

82. Walker, D. G.: Benign nonodontogenic tumors of the jaws. J. Oral Surg. 28:39, 1970.

83. Giansanti, J. S., and Waldron, C. A.: Peripheral giant cell granuloma: review of 720 cases. J. Oral Surg. 27:787, 1969.

84. Quint, J. H., Lehrman, M., and Loveman, C. E.: Reparative giant cell granuloma. Oral Surg. 17:142, 1964.

85. Waldron, C. A., and Shafer, W. G.: The central giant cell reparative granuloma of the jaws; an analysis of 38 cases. Am. J. Clin. Pathol. 45:437, 1966.

86. Hirschl, S., and Katz, A.: Giant cell reparative granuloma outside the jaw bone: Diagnostic criteria and review of the literature with the first case described in the temporal bone. Hum. Pathol. 5:171, 1974.

87. Bernier, J. L.: The Management of Oral Disease, 2nd Ed.

C. V. Mosby Co., St. Louis, 1959.

88. Hamlin, W. B., and Lund, P. K.: "Giant cell tumors" of the mandible and facial bones. A.M.A. Arch. Otolaryngol. 86:658, 1967.

89. Rao, P., Solomon, M., Avramides, A., Saxena, A., Delano, B. G., Gold, B. M., and Berger, J.: Brown tumors associated with secondary hyperparathyroidism of chronic renal failure. J. Oral Surg. 36:154, 1978.

90. Smith, J. F.: Fibrous dysplasia of the jaws. A.M.A. Arch. Otolaryngol 81:592, 1965.

91. Hamner, J. E., and Fullmer, H. M.: Oxytalan fibers in benign fibro-osseous jaw lesions. A.M.A. Arch. Pathol. 82:35, 1966.

92. Houston, W. O.: Fibrous dysplasia of maxilla and mandible; clinicopathologic study and comparison of facial bone lesions with lesions affecting general skeleton. J. Oral Surg. 23:17, 1965.

93. Ramsey, H. E., Strong, E. W., and Frazell, E. L.: Fibrous dysplasia of the craniofacial bones. Am. J. Surg. 116:542, 1968.

94. Sherman, R. S., and Glauser, O. J.: Radiological identification of fibrous dysplasia of the jaws. Radiology 71:553, 1958.

95. Waldron, C. A.: Fibro-osseous lesions of the jaws. J. Oral Surg. 28:58, 1970.

96. DeLathouwer, C., and Brocheriou, C.: Sarcoma arising in irradiated jawbones. Possible relationship to previous non-malignant bone lesions. Report of six cases and review of the literature. J. Max.-Fac. Surg. 4:8, 1976.

97. Thoma, K. H.: Cherubism and other intraosseous giant cell lesions. Oral Surg. (suppl. 2) 15:1, 1962.

98. Bruce, K. W., Bruwer, A., and Kennedy, R. L. J.: Familial intraosseous fibrous swelling of the jaws ("cherubism"). Oral Surg. 6:995, 1953.

99. Jones, W. A., Gerrie, J., and Pritchard, J.: Cherubism: a familial fibrous dysplasia of the jaws. J. Bone Joint Surg. 32-B:325, 1950.

100. Hamner, J. E., and Ketcham, A. S.: Cherubism: an analysis and treatment. Cancer 23:1133, 1969.

101. Pindborg, J. J.: Tumors of the jaw (benign and malignant). In Oral Pathology, edited by R. W. Tiecke, pp. 287–290. McGraw-Hill, New York, 1965.

102. Rice, D. H., and Batsakis, J. G.: Diseases affecting the jaws. IV. Common and uncommon non-odontogenic tumors. Univ. Mich. Med. Ctr. J. 36:117, 1970.

103. Bhaskar, S. N., and Cutright, D. E.: Multiple enostosis: report of 16 cases. J. Oral Surg. 26:321, 1968.

104. Ringertz, N.: Pathology of malignant tumors arising in the nasal and paranasal sinuses. Acta Otolaryngol. Suppl. 27, 1938.

105. Soboroff, B. J., and Nykiel, F.: Surgical treatment of large osteoma of the ethmo-frontal region. Laryngoscope 76:1068, 1966.

106. Salinger, S.: The paranasal sinuses. Malignant tumors. Arch. Otolaryngol. 30:633, 1939.

107. Hallberg, O. E., and Begley, J. W.: Origin and treatment of osteomas of the paranasal sinuses. Arch. Otolaryngol. 51:750, 1950.

108. Handousa, A.: Primary benign neoplasms of the nose. J. Laryngol. Otol. 66:421, 1952.

109. Montgomery, W. W.: Osteoma of the frontal sinus. Ann. Otol. Rhinol. Laryngol. 69:245, 1960.

110. Samy, L. L., and Mostafa, H.: Osteomata of the nose and paranasal sinuses with a report of twenty-one cases. J. Laryngol. Otol. 85:449, 1971.

111. Brunner, H., and Spiesman, I. G.: Osteoma of the frontal and ethmoid sinuses. Ann. Otol. Rhinol. Laryngol. 57:714, 1948.

112. Teed, R. W., Primary osteoma of the frontal sinus. A.M.A. Arch. Otolaryngol. 33:225, 1941.

113. Rayne, J.: Gardner's syndrome. Br. J. Oral Surg. 6:11, 1968.

114. McKusick, V. A.: Genetic factors in intestinal polyposis. J.A.M.A. 182:271, 1962.

115. Shiffman, M. A.: Familial multiple polyposis associated with soft tissue and hard tissue tumors. J.A.M.A. 182:514, 1962.

116. McClure, D. K., and Dahlin, D. C.: Myxoma of bone: report of three cases. Mayo Clin. Proc. 52:249, 1977.

117. Goldblatt, L. I.: Ultrastructural study of an odontogenic myxoma. Oral Surg. 42:206, 1976.

118. White, D. K., Chen, S.-Y., Mohnac, A. M., and Miller, A. S.: Odontogenic myxoma. A clinical and ultrastructural study. Oral Surg. 39:901, 1975.

119. Harrison, J. D.: Odontogenic myxoma: ultrastructural and histochemical studies. J. Clin. Pathol. 26:570, 1973.

120. Whitman, R. A., Stewart, S., Stoopack, J. G., and Jerrold, T. L.: Myxoma of the mandible: report of case. J. Oral Surg. 29:63, 1971.

121. Zimmerman, D. C., and Dahlin, D. C.: Myxomatous tumors of the jaws. Oral Surg. 11:1069, 1958.

122. Kangur, T. T., Dahlin, D. C., and Turlington, G.: Myxomatous tumors of the jaws. J. Oral Surg. 33:5231, 1975.

123. Barros, E. R., Dominguez, F. V., and Cabrini, R. L.: Myxoma of the jaws. Oral Surg. 27:225, 1969.

124. Farman, A. G., Nortje, C. J., Grotepass, F. W., Farman, F. J., and Van Zyl, J. A.: Myxofibroma of the jaws. Brit. J. Oral Surg. 15:3, 1977–1978.

125. Fu, Y.-S., and Perzin, K. H.: Non-epithelial tumors of the nasal cavity, paranasal sinuses and nasopharynx: a clinicopathologic study. VII. Myxomas. Cancer 39:195, 1977.

126. Colby, R. A., Kerr, D. A., and Robinson, H. B. G.: Color Atlas of Oral Pathology, 2nd Ed., p. 139. J. B. Lippincott Co., Philadelphia, 1961.

127. Roca, A. N., Smith, J. L., Jr., MacComb, W. S., and Jing, B.: Ewing's sarcoma of the maxilla and mandible. Study of six cases. Oral Surg. 25:194, 1968.

128. Potdar, G. G.: Ewing's tumor of the jaws. Oral Surg. 29:505, 1970.

129. Rapoport, A., Sobeinho, J. A., de Carvalho, M. B., Magrin, J., Costa, F. Q., and Quandros, J. V.: Ewing's sarcoma of the mandible. Oral Surg. 44:89, 1977.

130. Naufal, P. M.: Primary sarcomas of the temporal bone. Arch. Otolaryngol. 98:44, 1973.

131. Angervall, L., and Enzinger, F. M.: Extraskeletal neoplasm resembling Ewing's sarcoma. Cancer 36:240, 1975.

132. Szakacs, J. E., Carta, M., and Szakacs, M. R.: Ewing's sarcoma, extraskeletal and of bone. Case report with ultrastructural analysis. Ann. Clin. Lab. Sci. 4:306, 1974.

133. Povysil, C., and Matejovsky, Z.: Ultrastructure of Ewing's tumour. Virchows Arch. (Pathol. Anat.) 374:304, 1977.

134. Wigger, H. J., Salazar, G. H., and Blanc, W. A.: Extraskeletal Ewing's sarcoma. An ultrastructural study. Arch. Pathol. Lab. Med. 101:446, 1977.

135. Jeffree, G. M.: Enzymes of round cell tumours of bone and soft tissue: a histochemical study. J. Pathol. 113:101, 1974.

136. Hou-Jensen, K., Priori, E., and Dmochowski, L.: Studies on ultrastructure of Ewing's sarcoma of bone. Cancer 29:280, 1972.

137. Johnson, R. E., and Pomeroy, T. C.: Evaluation of therapeutic results in Ewing's sarcoma. Am. J. Roentgenol. 123:583, 1975.

138. Falk, S., and Alpert, M.: Five-year survival of patients with Ewing's sarcoma. Surg. Gynecol. Obstet. 124:319, 1967.

139. Pritchard, D. J., Dahlin, D. C., Dauphine, R. T., Taylor, W. F., and Beabout, J. W.: Ewing's sarcoma. J. Bone Joint Surg. (Am.) 57A:10, 1975.

140. Pomeroy, T. C., and Johnson, R. E.: Integrated therapy of Ewing's sarcoma. Front. Radiat. Ther. Oncol. 10:152, 1975.

141. Jenkins, R. D. T.: Radiation treatment of Ewing's sarcoma and osteogenic sarcoma. Can. J. Surg. 20:530, 1977.

142. Kotz, R., Salzer-Kuntschik, M., Zweymuller, K., and Salzer, M.: Therapy and prognosis of the Ewing-sarcoma. Ost. Z. Onkol. 1:15, 1974.

143. Pomeroy, T. C., and Johnson, R. E.: Combined modality therapy of Ewing's sarcoma. Cancer 35:36, 1975.

144. Perez, C. A., Razer, A., Tefft, M., Nesbit, M., Burgert, E. O., Kissane, J., Vietti, T., and Gehan, E. A.: Analysis of local tumor control in Ewing's sarcoma. Preliminary results of a cooperative intergroup study. Cancer 40:2804, 1977.

145. Jaffe, N., Traggis, D., Salian, S., and Cassady, J. R.: Improved outlook for Ewing's sarcoma with combination chemotherapy (vincristine, actinomycin D and cyclophosphamide) and radiation therapy. Cancer 38:1925, 1976.

146. Pearlman, A. W.: Ewing's sarcoma—growth rate and tumor lethal dose. Front. Radiat. Ther. Oncol. 10:48, 1975.

147. Dehner, L. P.: Tumors of the mandible and maxilla in children. II. Study of 14 primary and secondary malignant tumors. Cancer 32:112, 1973.

148. Ferguson, J. W.: Central fibroma of the jaws. Brit. J. Oral Surg. 12:205, 1974.

149. Walker, D. G.: Benign nonodontogenic tumors of the jaws. J. Oral Surg. 28:39, 1970.

150. Nussbaum, G. B., Terz, J. J., and Joy, E. D., Jr.: Desmoplastic fibroma of the mandible in a three-year old child. J. Oral Surg. 34:1117, 1976.

151. Langdon, J. D., Rapidis, A. D., and Patel, M. F.: Ossifying fibroma—one disease or six? An analysis of 39 fibroosseous lesions of the jaws. Br. J. Oral Surg. 14:1, 1976.

152. Hamner, J. E., Scofield, H. H., and Cornyn, J.: Benign fibro-osseous jaw lesions of peridontal membrane origin. An analysis of 249 cases. Cancer 22:861, 1968.

153. Dehner, L. P.: Tumors of the mandible and maxilla in children. I. Clinocopathologic study of 46 histologically benign lesions. Cancer 31:364, 1973.

154. Kempson, R. L.: Ossifying fibroma of the long bones. A light and electron microscopic study. Arch. Pathol. 82:218, 1966.

155. Kennett, S., and Curran, J. B.: Giant cemento-ossifying fibroma: report of case. J. Oral Surg. 30:513, 1972.

156. Farman, A. G., Nortje, C. J., and Grotepass, F.: Periosteal benign osteoblastoma of the mandible. Report of a case and review of the literature pertaining to benign osteoblastic neoplasms of the jaws. Br. J. Oral Surg. 14:12, 1976.

157. Steiner, G. C.: Ultrastructure of osteoblastoma. Cancer 39:2127, 1977.

158. Byers, P. D.: Solitary benign osteoblastic lesions of bone. Osteoid osteoma and benign osteoblastoma. Cancer 22:43, 1968.

159. Steiner, G. C.: Ultrastructure of osteoid osteoma. Hum. Pathol. 7:309, 1976.

160. Lichtenstein, L., and Sawyer, W. R.: Benign osteoblastoma. J. Bone Joint Surg. (Am.) 46:755, 1964.

161. Ballard, R., and Weiland, L. H.: Synovial chondromatosis of the temporomandibular joint. Cancer 30:791, 1972.

162. Grotepass, F. W., Farman, A. G., and Nortje, C. J.: Chondromyxoid fibroma of the mandible. J. Oral Surg. 34:988, 1976.

163. Topolnicki, W., and White, R. J.: Primary reticulum cell sarcoma of the skull: response to irradiation. Cancer 24:569, 1969.

164. Shoji, H., and Miller, T. R.: Primary reticulum cell sarcoma of bone: significance of cllnical features upon the prognosis. Cancer 28:1234, 1971.

165. Steg, R. F., Dahlin, D. C., and Gores, R. J.: Malignant lymphoma of the mandible and maxillary region. Oral Surg. 12:128, 1959.

166. Ivins, J. C., and Dahlin, D. C.: Malignant lymphoma (reticulum cell sarcoma) of bone. Proc. Mayo Clin. 38:375, 1963.

167. Reimer, D. R., Chabner, B. A., Young, R. C., Reddick, K., and Johnson, R. E.: Lymphomas presenting in bone: results of histopathology, staging and therapy. Ann. Intern. Med. 87:50, 1977.

168. Campbell, R. L., Kelly, D. E., and Burkes, E. J.: Primary reticulum-cell sarcoma of the mandible. Review of the literature and report of a case. Oral Surg. 39:918, 1975.

169. Macintosh, D. J., Price, C. H. G., and Jeffree, G. M.: Malignant lymphoma (reticulosarcoma) in bone. Clin. Oncol. 3:287, 1977.

170. Jack, G. A., and Vaeth, J. M.: Radiation therapy of primary reticulum cell sarcoma of bone in adults. Front. Radiat. Ther. Oncol. 10:167, 1975.

171. Johnson, E. C.: Intraosseous lipoma: report of case. J. Oral Surg. 27:868, 1969.

172. Bhaskar, S.: Central mucoepidermoid tumors of the mandible. Cancer 16:721, 1963.

173. Silverglade, L. B., Alvares, O. F., and Olech, E.: Central mucoepidermoid tumor of the jaws. Cancer 22:650, 1968.

174. Finkelstein, J. B.: Osteosarcoma of the jaw bone. Radiol. Clin. North Am. 8:425, 1970.

CHAPTER 21

Epidermal Carcinomas of the Integument of the Nose and Ear

Contributed by JOHN T. HEADINGTON, M.D.

The mortality statistics for skin cancer do not accurately reflect the seriousness of the problem. Although skin cancer accounts for more than 5,000 deaths per year in the United States, about 25% of malignancies of all kinds are skin cancers.[1] Morbidity in terms of recurrence, cosmetic injury and loss of function is substantially greater than mortality and may occur over a much longer period of time (10 to 20 years or longer) than is true for most malignant neoplasms.

The development of skin cancer is the result of a complex interplay between the human environment, the regional topography of the skin, age and genetics. In the sections which follow, some of these elements are discussed in greater detail.

BASAL CELL CARCINOMA OF NASAL SKIN

Basal cell carcinoma of the skin is undoubtedly the most common cancer of the head and neck. Of 840 basal cell carcinomas studied in one large series, 766, or 91.2%, were found in this region.[2] Moreover, slightly more than 25% of these were of nasal skin. The nose is topographically the most common site for basal cell carcinoma and has the greatest density of neoplasms per unit area. The ratio of basal cell carcinoma of the nasal skin to infiltrative squamous cell carcinoma in our series (University of Michigan) is 30:1.[3]

Basal cell carcinoma of the skin of the nose is most frequently encountered in the sixth, seventh and eighth decades of life. Although the incidence is much lower in the second to fourth decades, the high prevalence of this neoplasm results in large numbers of young patients with skin cancer. In a series of 299 patients studied at The University of Michigan, there were 145 females with a mean age of 62.5 years and 154 males with a mean age of 64 years (Fig. 21.1). Eighteen of these patients were younger than 40 years.

The topographical distribution of basal cell carcinoma of nasal skin indicates various sites of predilection. The side, dorsum, tip, ala, including the vestibule, and nasolabial fold are involved with decreasing frequency.

Although several histological types of basal cell carcinoma have been described, most patterns are not significantly related to biological activity. Histologically, it is preferable to designate basal cell carcinomas as either circumscribed or infiltrative. Most basal cell carcinomas grow as discrete or interanastomosing lobules of neoplasm which extend with blunt pushing margins, while the neoplasm, in aggregate, tends to remain circumscribed (Fig. 21.2). Individual tumors are generally characterized by a peripheral nuclear pallisade. Some basal cell carcinomas, however, from the beginning may develop an infiltrative and permeative growth pattern which can microscopically extend a considerable distance beyond clinically detectable margins. These aggressive basal cell carcinomas often lose their tendency to pallisade and, in an isolated sample, can be difficult to characterize (Fig. 21.3).

Microscopically, the differential diagnosis includes trichoepithelioma, squamous cell carcinoma, adenoid cystic carcinoma, some tumors of the eccrine sweat apparatus and some of the incompletely differentiated neoplasms of hair germ.[4]

The clinical appearance of basal cell carcinomas is variable. Most begin as small nodular growths covered by a smooth, hairless, somewhat translucent epidermis. Telangiectatic capillaries over the tumor surface may be prominent. Chronic ulcers, ulceronodular lesions and scaly plaques may be other modes of presentation. Melanin pigmentation may be negligible, spotty or extensive. The

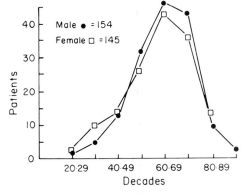

Figure 21.1. Graphic representation of age and sex distribution of 299 patients with basal cell carcinoma of nasal skin. Data presented are from The University of Michigan series.[3]

infiltrative, potentially aggressive lesions are frequently ulcerated even when quite small. The border of an ulcerated neoplasm may be rolled or it may be flat, as with a typical rodent ulcer. The morpheic type is flat or depressed, with an element of increased firmness as a result of the associated fibroplasia.

Recurrence is a frequent problem with basal cell carcinoma of the nasal skin. In Conley's study,[5] 41% of 131 patients in this group experienced recurrence. Microscopically, however, it is often impossible to determine whether a second sample of a neoplasm from a specific area is a persistent neoplasm or represents the growth of a new neoplasm in a closely adjacent field. If new lesions are small and well circumscribed, apparent recurrence is usually not a significant therapeutic problem. However, if the pattern of recurrence is histologically aggressive, it is encumbent upon the therapist to attempt to effect cure with a high degree of certainty while the volume of affected tissue is as small as possible.

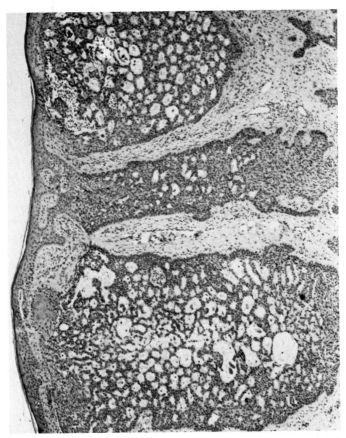

Figure 21.2. Basal cell carcinoma of nasal skin. Although there are several tumor lobules, each is sharply circumscribed from adjacent stroma. The cribriform pattern has no particular prognostic or histogenetic significance.

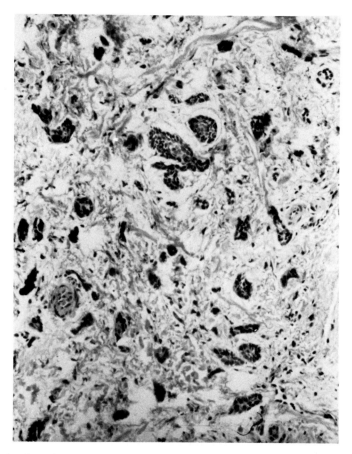

Figure 21.3. Basal cell carcinoma of nasal skin. This is an aggressive, diffusely infiltrative pattern which may infiltrate deeply along fusion planes and neurovascular bundles. The topographical limits of spread are very difficult to determine by clinical examination.

Although distant metastases are rare from basal cell carcinoma, recurrent morbidity and possible death from extension to the base of the brain gives basal cell carcinoma of the nose and central facial area a high priority for successful first attempt therapy.

SQUAMOUS CELL CARCINOMA OF THE NASAL SKIN

Infiltrative squamous cell carcinomas of the skin of the nose, potentially capable of metastasis, are unusual neoplasms. Only 14 of 145 patients with epidermal carcinoma (basal cell and squamous cell carcinoma) in Conley's[5] series had squamous cell neoplasms. Only 11 of 299 epidermal carcinomas of the nose studied at The University of Michigan were classified as infiltrative squamous cell carcinomas.[3] Dysplastic actinic keratoses sufficiently atypical to be called epidermal in situ carcinoma are more common.

The highest incidence of epidermal carcinoma of the nose in men and women in our series is in the sixth, seventh and eighth decades although a wide range is prevalent. The median ages for both sexes and for both basal and squamous cell carcinoma are nearly identical—approximately 65 years. Patients younger than 40 with histologically proved epidermal carcinoma of the skin of the nose should probably be questioned for previous irradiation exposure or for other environmental or hereditary factors.

The topographical distribution in our group of squamous cell carcinomas is varied. Five of 11 neoplasms involved the side of the nose; three appeared on the tip; others occurred on the columella and in the nasolabial fold. Preference for the side and the tip of the nose is consonant with other findings.[5]

The initial clinical configuration of squamous cell carcinoma of the head and neck, including the nose, is generally nodular. With a central irregular keratin mass and rolled borders, the adenoid type may simulate keratoacanthoma. With ulceration and local infiltration, differentiation from basal cell carcinoma is frequently difficult. The differential diagnosis includes chronic infectious granulomas, particularly North American blastomycosis, leprosy and tertiary syphilis.

Although it is true that most squamous cell carcinomas of the head and neck arise in sun-exposed areas, there is little factual evidence that most of metastasizing squamous cell carcinomas of the skin originate in pre-existing actinic keratoses. In our material, a careful study of the margins of infiltrative squamous cell carcinomas did not uniformly reflect the morphology of focal actinic dysplasia. This is in contrast to those concurrent changes frequently observed with infiltrative basal cell carcinomas. Moreover, in Conley's[5] series, as well as in our own, a number of patients had received irradiation therapy for nonmalignant cutaneous conditions such as acne. Therefore, to incriminate actinic keratoses post hoc as the probable precursors of most infiltrative squamous cell carcinoma of the skin is, at best, an over simplification.

The histological types of squamous cell carcinoma of the skin are: adenoid (acantholytic), Bowen's type, verrucous, spindle-pleomorphic and generic. Generic squamous cell carcinoma usually begins as a noduloulcerative lesion. Local growth is often highly infiltrative and is characterized by small angular islands and nests of atypical cells usually without much keratinization. In any large series of squamous cell carcinomas, other unclassifiable variants also occur.

In 20% of our patients who had squamous cell carcinoma, both squamous cell carcinoma and basal cell carcinoma were found in contiguity.

One of the most troublesome problems in differential diagnosis is the occasional difficulty in distinguishing a slightly keratinizing basal cell carcinoma from a poorly keratinizing squamous cell carcinoma, for both may have somewhat similar histological patterns. There is a tendency for the microscopist to "over diagnose" keratinizing basal cell carcinoma as squamous cell carcinoma. The differential microscopic features are best summarized as follows. Angular keratinizing islands with large pleomorphic peripheral nuclei containing coarse chromatin and prominent nucleoli associated with negligible or slight stromal reaction (generic squamous cell carcinomas) tend to behave as squamous cell carcinomas capable of metastasis; angular keratinizing neoplastic islands with relatively small uniform nuclei associated with a moderate to marked fibroproliferative stromal reaction and abundant stromal acid mucosubstance tend to behave as basal cell carcinoma and very rarely metastasize.

Few conclusions about biological behavior can be drawn from the small number of reported cases of squamous cell carcinoma of the skin of the nose. In Conley's small series,[5] three patients (21%) had metastases to the neck, and two died from their disease. Among our few cases, two patients (20%) developed distant metastases. These small series are undoubtably biased by institutional and other factors.

BASAL CELL CARCINOMA OF THE PINNA

If superficial multicentric basal cell carcinoma is excluded, basal cell carcinoma of the skin is predominately a neoplasm of the head and neck. In the study by Brodkin et al.[2] of 840 lesions from all sites, 766 or 91.2%, were located on the head and neck. Of these 766 basal cell carcinomas only 12 occurred on the external ear.

Compared with the central area of the face, basal cell carcinoma of the pinna is relatively uncommon. Also, on the pinna itself, the topographical distribution of basal cell carcinoma is not uniform. In a series reported by Huriez et al.,[6] 72% of 48 basal cell carcinomas occurring on and around the external ear were found on the postauricular, retroauricular and preauricular areas. In contrast with squamous cell carcinoma, there is significant sparing of the helix and anterior surface of the pinna. This has also been confirmed by Fabian and Thomitzek,[7] who found 11 of 21 basal cell carcinomas of the pinna confined to the tragus and concha.

Basal cell carcinoma of the pinna is more commonly a lesion of males. One series reports an incidence of 66% in males,[6] but 90% of 53 basal cell carcinomas of the pinna treated at The University of Michigan were found in males. When a basal cell carcinoma develops on the pinna of a female, she is likely to be older than a male with an equivalent lesion. The median age for females in our material is 77.8 years; the median age for males is 66.1 years. However, as Robertson[8] has shown, with similar genetic and activity patterns, individuals will develop more skin cancer at an earlier age under high ultraviolet exposure as compared with areas where ultraviolet is less intense. It is not clear whether a specific correlation exists between the occurrence of basal cell carcinoma and ultraviolet exposure or whether these data primarily reflect an increase in squamous cell carcinoma and solar keratoses. The development of elastosis as an indirect measure of the intensity of ultraviolet exposure does not correlate well with either the prevalence or distribution of basal cell carcinoma of the pinna, particularly of the helix where there is virtually an inverse topographical relationship.[2]

The clinical appearance of basal cell carcinoma of the pinna does not differ from basal cell carcinoma arising elsewhere. Individual lesions may develop as nodules or as plaques, with varying degrees of thickening and induration. If the epidermis remains intact, it may be thinned; the resulting semitransparent epidermis over the subjacent neoplasm produces a whitish or pearly appearance. Epidermal thinning is often accompanied by capillary telangectasia. Erosion of epidermis with crusting and bleeding may also occur. None of these changes, however, may be regarded as diagnostic for basal cell carcinoma. As pointed out by Lightstone et al.,[9] the clinical diagnosis of basal cell carcinoma may be incorrect as often as one time in four even in the hands of experienced dermatologists alert to cutaneous oncology.

A number of different histological patterns have been described for basal cell carcinoma. Among them are adenoid, trichoid and solid or primordial types. Most of these patterns, which vaguely resemble grandular or pilar structures, are relatively meaningless to the natural history of the neoplasm. The pattern of growth (circumscribed or permeative) is the most important prognostic feature.

There are few distinctive cytological features of the individual cells of basal cell carcinoma. The small amount of cytoplasm, the compact nucleus with a bland chromatin pattern, and the small nucleolus are by no means characteristic. In very aggressive, highly infiltrative variants, the nucleus and nucleolus are often large and the chromatin pattern coarser. These changes occasionally approximate the appearance of a small cell variant of poorly differentiated squamous cell carcinoma although the latter is an extremely uncommon primary neoplasm of skin. The presence of foci of postmitotic keratinizing cells may be seen in both aggressive and nonaggressive histological types of basal cell carcinoma. These foci by themselves have little influence on biological behavior and do not justify the designation of basosquamous or metatypical carcinoma. Melanin is usually found in well circumscribed basal cell carcinomas, especially in the primordial pattern, but is rarely encountered in aggressive histological types. Foci of dystrophic calcification may be common.

Some basal cell carcinomas evoke a striking stromal fibroplasia, commonly seen with aggressive infiltrating neoplasms, although, on occasion, stromal fibrosis may be seen with almost any pattern. Retraction spaces developing at the tumor-stromal interface help differentiate basal cell carcinoma from trichoepithelioma. There is little or no evidence of a stromal inductive effect as is seen in some neoplasms of hair germ.[4]

There are few published reports of the natural history of basal cell carcinoma of the external ear. Fabian and Thomitzek,[7] reporting the short term results of surgical treatment, recorded one recurrence and one patient with metastases in 6 months to 1.5 years after treatment. In the series by Huriez et al.,[6] nine of 46 patients with basal cell carcinoma of the external ear and juxta-auricular skin experienced recurrent neoplasm. There were two deaths, one in a patient judged incurable.

Aggressive basal cell carcinomas of the external ear, like those of the central facial area, deserve to be regarded with considerable respect for their infiltrative potential. Because almost half of basal cell carcinomas of the pinna will be found in the area of the tragus and concha, early extension may involve the parotid gland and/or the soft tissue anterior to the external canal.

Although metastases from basal cell carcinomas are rare, the aggressive and infiltrative lesion can readily extend along soft tissue pathways of least resistance, particularly embryonic fusion planes and neurovascular adventitia so that the true extension of the infiltrating neoplasm may be far beyond the ability of the clinician to determine the limits of spread. Under such circumstances, which are not at all unusual with recurrent basal cell carcinoma, wide surgical excision and extensive x-ray therapy may remain blind procedures. Within these constraints, topographic surgery ("chemosurgery"), with area-by-area frozen section control, offers the greatest chance for cure.

SQUAMOUS CELL CARCINOMA OF THE PINNA

Considerable circumstantial evidence favors an etiological role for ultraviolet light in the development of squamous cell carcinoma of the head and neck. The spectral wavelengths which produce sunburn and presumably some cancers in human skin are approximately between 290 and 325 mm. This fraction, which is only a small part of total sunlight, varies considerably with the angle of the sun. Other variables, such as season, time of day, latitude, and reflected light affect the quantity (energy per unit area) of ultraviolet. Urbach,[1] in a comprehensive study, found that there are certain areas of the human head which receive many times more ultraviolet radiation than do others. The orbits, the upper lip, the anterior area of the neck and the nasolabial folds are somewhat protected; by contrast, the tops of the ears, the nose, the scalp and the lower posterior neck receive maximum amounts of ultraviolet light.

In a large series reported from the Skin and Cancer Hospital (Philadelphia),[1] 88% of 548 basal cell carcinomas and 68% of 60 squamous cell carcinomas occurred on the head and neck. The percentage of distribution on the head and neck agrees very closely with that given by Brodkin et al.[2] and with a large series by Magnusson.[10]

There is a distinctly different distribution for squamous cell carcinoma and basal cell carcinoma of the pinna. In a series of 123 cases reported from France, 55% of squamous cell carcinomas occurred on the rim of the pinna compared to only 14% of basal cell carcinomas.[6] By contrast, 72% of basal cell carcinomas were located in the postauricular, retroauricular, and preauricular areas compared to only 26% of squamous cell carcinomas. Other large series also suggest significant topographical differences in the distribution of squamous cell carcinoma and basal cell carcinoma of the pinna, but only in a few of these studies have squamous cell carcinoma and basal cell carcinoma been considered as separate entities.

In Lederman's series[11] the distribution of squamous cell carcinoma of the pinna (101 cases) was: helix, 34; antihelix, 13; tragus, 8; antitragus, 1; concha, 8; lobule, 3; retroauricular sulcus and posterior surface, 27; and unspecified, 7. Very similar findings were recorded by Shiffman.[12]

Squamous cell carcinoma of the pinna is almost exclusively a disease of Caucasians. Examples of squamous cell carcinoma of the pinna in Negroes have not been reported, and squamous cell carcinoma is only rarely cited as occurring in Negroes in various large general series of skin cancer of the head and neck. In a study of adenoid squamous cell carcinoma of the skin from the Armed Forces Institute of Pathology,[13] 85% of 96 patients had blue, gray or green eyes, 50% had blonde, red, auburn, or sandy hair and 94% had a fair or ruddy skin. These phenotypic data emphasize an important genetic component in the epidemiology of squamous cell carcinoma of the skin.

Squamous cell carcinoma of the pinna is predominantly a disease of the fifth and sixth decades and beyond. The mean age, however, will vary with the genetic character of the population at risk

and the degree of exposure to ultraviolet light.[8] There is also evidence[6, 11] that the risk for squamous cell carcinoma of the pinna increases with age, the greatest prevalence being found in men 70 or older. The mean age of 68 male patients with squamous cell carcinoma of the pinna seen at the University of Michigan was 68 years.[3] While carcinoma of the skin of the head and neck predominates in males, this tendency is greatly emphasized in studies of squamous cell carcinoma of the pinna. Sixty-eight of 71 squamous cell carcinomas of the pinna evaluated at The University of Michigan[3] occurred in men, and of Shiffman's 52 patients,[12] only two were women.

The clinical characteristics of squamous cell carcinoma of the pinna are not diagnostic. Although the clinical accuracy of the diagnosis of squamous cell carcinoma of the skin has not been studied, there is no reason to believe that the accuracy of clinical diagnosis would be superior for this histological type as compared to basal cell carcinoma.[9] Basal cell carcinoma and keratoacanthoma are the most important additions to a clinical differential diagnosis of carcinoma of the external ear. Other tumors, such as melanoma, and atypical fibroxanthoma are uncommon.

Infiltrative lesions are frequently somewhat nodular with irregular margins. Fixation to underlying dermis or to cartilage is an early indication of aggressive growth. Ulceration with crusting and bleeding is not unusual in more advanced lesions. In terms of gross configuration, it is worth noting that adenoid squamous cell carcinoma[13] may closely simulate keratoacanthoma, a discrete nodular lesion with elevated rolled borders and a central keratinous mass (Fig. 21.4).

Actinic keratoses of the pinna are very common. Microscopic study of such lesions will reveal a histological and cytological spectrum of changes which vary from epidermal dysplasia to carcinoma in situ. An arbitrary dividing line between dysplasia and carcinoma in situ is the presence of full-thickness dysplasia. The latter finding justifies a diagnosis of carcinoma in situ. In general, it is our bias to allow considerable latitude within what may be called dysplastic epithelium and to be conservative with the diagnosis of epidermal carcinoma in situ. On strictly morphological grounds it is our conviction that most infiltrative squamous cell carcinoma of the pinna capable of metastasizing probably do not arise from pre-existing actinic keratoses but arise de novo.

Some general understanding of the behavior and prognosis of squamous cell carcinoma of the pinna is beginning to emerge from contemporary

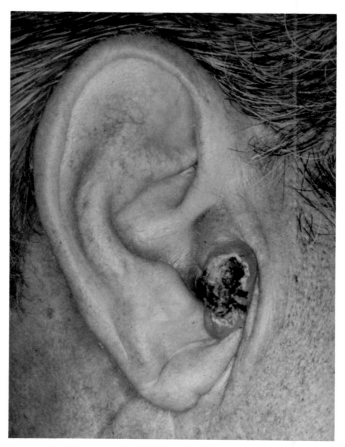

Figure 21.4. Adenoid squamous cell carcinoma of the pinna. Differentiation of this variant of squamous cell carcinoma from keratoacanthoma may be impossible on clinical grounds alone. Note rolled discrete margins and central keratinous mass, not a central ulcer.

studies by Huriez et al.,[6] Blake and Wilson,[14] and Shiffman.[12]

Histological evaluation of squamous cell carcinoma of the pinna should include some estimate of tumor size (volume), notations as to the extent of growth (intradermal, to or into cartilage), perineural invasion, angiolymphatic spread, a semiquantitation of host response, and most importantly, discrimination of the histological type. Seventy-one squamous cell carcinomas of the pinna collected from the files of The University of Michigan were so evaluated.[3] This series contained all lesions encountered as nonreferral cases presented to the Department of Dermatology out-patient clinic and thus includes a nonselected sample of early lesions. In situ lesions represented 14%, infiltrative tumors 86%. Infiltrative squamous cell carcinomas were histologically classified as generic, adenoid (acantholytic), spindle/pleomorphic (including desmoplastic) and unclassified. Bowen's and verrucous types were not encountered on the pinna. Three patients with infiltrative lesions developed metastatic disease. In each of these, tumor type was generic and either infiltrated to the cartilage (2) or spread to paraauricular soft tissue (1).

Undoubtably, no single factor determines prognosis. As Shiffman[12] indicates, in contrast to earlier reports, tumor size (volume) is probably not a dominant element. At present, no single histological finding is, by statistical analysis, significantly associated with a poor prognosis. The University of Michigan study suggests but does not yet prove that the generic type is the histological type most likely to metastasize. Tumor volume and depth of tissue penetration may also play a role but these are likewise unmeasured parameters. Angiolymphatic invasion and perineural spread did not occur often enough to permit a meaningful histological analysis.

Simple clinical staging is probably useful. If regional lymph nodes are clinically negative for metastatic disease, prophylactic node dissection probably need not be done—there being no clear-cut histological guidelines as yet. No statement has yet been made about the value of therapeutic node dissection for management of advance disease metastatic to regional lymph nodes.

At first glance there appears to be increasing data to support the long-held notion that squamous cell carcinoma of the pinna has a worse prognosis than other nonaural sites of the skin of the head and neck. The cumulated death rate from four aggregated series (250 cases) is an impressive 17%. In general, however, these series undoubtedly represent an important degree of patient selection for specialty clinics. The University of Michigan series,[3] in addition to early nonselected cases seen by dermatologists also included some advanced referral cases. In the latter series, metastases were found in but three patients, only one of whom died from metastatic disease. The accumulated 17% death rate is undoubtedly artificially high. A statement whether this is greater than for other areas of the skin cannot be made because there are no series which match age, sex, histological type of tumor, and size or extent of growth when first biopsied. Until the latter information is available, the presumptive aggressive character of squamous cell carcinoma of the pinna will remain biologically unclear and pragmatically academic.

SQUAMOUS CELL CARCINOMA OF THE EXTERNAL AUDITORY CANAL

Most of the information about carcinoma of the external auditory canal has been derived from clinical studies which are not morphologically clean, i.e., clinicopathological correlation has not been related to specific histological types of neoplasms. To date, no prospective study for evaluation of clinical staging and uniform therapeutic methods with long term follow-up has been reported.

The most common malignant neoplasm arising from the skin of the external ear canal is undoubtedly squamous cell carcinoma. Primary melanomas and adenoid cystic carcinomas are rare. Although a great variety of benign and malignant neoplasms exotic for this location has been described in various case reports,[15] these lesions will not be reviewed here.

The true incidence of squamous cell carcinoma of the external auditory canal is unknown. Most published data reflect the numbers of neoplasms seen as a fraction of all clinic or hospital visits. The total number of reported cases, estimated at about 300, cannot be taken as an accurate measure of prevalence. Although Lederman[11] believes that the incidence is increasing, there is no epidemiological evidence that this is so.

The etiology of squamous cell carcinoma of the external auditory canal is obscure. Ultraviolet light would appear to be of minimal significance. There is a temptation to point to the high incidence of a coexisting ear disease, chronic otitis externa and otitis media, as playing a causative role. The homology is made between carcinoma of the external canal, with chronic draining otitis media, and squamous cell carcinoma of the skin around a chronic osteomyelitis sinus (Marjolin's ulcer). But the implied role of chronic inflammation is not yet proved. Other possibilities, such as selective sequestration and concentration of carcinogens within cerumen and aflatoxin production by otherwise innocuous Aspergillus species resident within the canal, need to be considered.

Several previous studies have indicated that there is little difference between the incidence of squamous cell carcinoma of the ear canal in men and women. In our material at The University of Michigan, however, there is a striking incidence of primary neoplasms in females (16 of 17 cases) when the histological type is squamous cell carcinoma.[16] We have carefully excluded all tumors which might have arisen in the skin of the external meatus and secondarily involved the canal. In 105 cases recorded by Lewis,[17] 40 occurred in males and 65 in females. The reason for female preponderance is unknown.

Most cancers clinically described as early are found within the membranous canal.[17] This finding is probably synonymous with early detectability. There are few important anatomical barriers to restrict carcinomas which may arise from the cartilagenous portion of the canal, because the cartilagenous walls are easily infiltrated and spread may occur anteriorly to the parotid gland. The posterior wall is even a less effective barrier to spread than the anterior wall and the neoplasms may present as swellings in the posterior auricular sulcus. By contrast, carcinomas arising in the bony portion of the canal are surrounded by dense bone which proves a more effective barrier to spread than does cartilage. In these circumstances the spread of tumor is more likely along the longitudinal axis of the canal with eventual invasion of the middle ear and the cartilagenous part of the canal.

Chronic pruritus and pain are common to almost all patients with squamous cell carcinoma of the external auditory canal. Many patients also describe chronic discharge. Swelling behind ear, decreased hearing and facial paralysis are occasionally noted. Neoplastic involvement of epithelium results in superficial friability, excessive keratinization, fissuring, oozing or bleeding. Nodular, plaque-like, polypoid, ulcerative, and even annular modes of clinical presentation have been observed.

The microscopic features of primary squamous cell carcinoma of the ear canal have not been described in detail. Much of our material, as well as that of others, is in the form of biopsies which represent samples too small for adequate evaluation of larger lesions. Nevertheless, within these limitations, only three of 20 cases were judged well differentiated. The remaining were considered histologically either moderately or poorly differentiated.[16] Where the periphery of a neoplasm could be observed, the pattern most commonly was one of aggressive, poorly delineated infiltrative strands and nests of cells. Lobular patterns with pushing margins were also occasionally seen. Islands of postmitotic cornifying cells, a feature of most well-differentiated squamous cell carcinomas, were uncommon. Individual cells frequently were small and polyhedral, but in none of our cases was an undifferentiated spindle cell or pleomorphic component observed. Stromal and inflammatory responses were not remarkable.

Clinicopathological staging of squamous cell carcinoma of the external canal has not yet evolved, but advanced lesions with evidence for involvement of tissue outside the canal with or without lymph node metastases have an ominous prognostic implication—one of 10 patients treated at The University of Michigan survived 18 months. Early lesions in which there is no evidence for spread beyond the canal or involvement of the temporal bone do much better[18] although follow-up data for periods of 10 years or longer are not available.

The only large series of patients receiving more or less uniform management was reported by Lewis.[17] A summary of contemporary therapeutic attitudes might be made as follows: (1) Early squamous cell carcinomas of the external auditory canal probably do not require subtotal temporal bone resection for cure. It is uncertain whether surgery alone or radiotherapy alone is superior or whether they are about equally effective. (2) Subtotal temporal bone resection is the current treatment of choice for advanced squamous cancer of the external auditory canal. It is uncertain whether radiotherapy either preceding or following surgery significantly improves survival although the effec-

tiveness of radiotherapy is implied in retrospective studies.

Survival, based on Lederman's[11] data, is about 25% at 3, 5, and 10 years. Lewis[17] gives a 5-year salvage rate for advanced cases of 25% (20 of 81 cases). These data suggest that if initial therapy is successful, late recurrence is not a significant problem. This is in marked contrast with the outlook for adenoid cystic carcinoma of the external canal.

ADENOID CYSTIC CARCINOMA OF THE EXTERNAL AUDITORY CANAL

Adenoid cystic carcinoma (cylindroma) having primary origin in the external ear canal is an uncommon but well-recognized neoplasm. Undoubtedly in the past, neoplasms arising in adjacent parotid gland and secondarily infiltrating the ear canal have been included in case reports, but Pulec et al.,[19] in a review of the literature, found 17 cases as acceptable primary neoplasms and added 21 new cases.

Adenoid cystic carcinomas arising in salivary glands, parabronchial glands, uterine cervix, skin and breast have been regarded as duct cell neoplasms of distinctive histological type. Pulec et al.[19] believes that the adenoid cystic carcinomas of the external ear canal arise from ceruminous secretory coils or ducts. Origin from the secretory coil would, however, be contrary to the presumed ductal origin of cells of this neoplasm originating in other sites. Early cases were reported singly or were contained in mixed series and many were often labeled as ceruminous gland carcinomas or basal cell carcinoma.

Nineteen of 21 patients of Pulec et al.[19] presented with a mass in the ear canal, but these were not considered characteristic for adenoid cystic carcinoma. The microscopic pattern of primary adenoid cystic carcinomas of the external canal does not significantly deviate from that described in other sites. Both solid and microcystic patterns are frequently represented. The proclivity for neural extension, often seen in other neoplasms of this type, was also evident in these cases. The microscopic differential diagnosis should include basal cell carcinoma and a poorly differentiated squamous cell carcinoma of small cell type. In the Pulec et al.[19] series, the average age of patients at the onset of symptoms was 42; the oldest was 61 and the youngest 21.

The prognosis of adenoid cystic carcinoma of the ear canal does not substantially differ from similar carcinomas arising in deep structures elsewhere. The course is often long but usually relentless. Of the 21 patients of Pulec et al.,[19] 10 were alive with metastasis when the study was completed. Therapeutically, Pulec[20] recommends: "(1) wide excision of the entire external auditory canal, surrounding bone and part of the pinna; (2) extensive radical mastoidectomy; (3) total parotidectomy and mandibular condylectomy."

GLAND CELL TUMORS OF THE EXTERNAL CANAL

The integument of the external ear canal contains both eccrine and modified apocrine glands (ceruminous glands) as well as sebaceous glands. By homology with nonaural skin, a bewildering array of gland cell neoplasms is theoretically possible. The following simplified classification includes most of the gland cell tumors of importance which occur in the external auditory canal:

Apocrine Adenoma (Ceruminoma): A benign adenomatous tumor showing apocrine secretory differentiation.

Apocrine Carcinoma (Ceruminous Gland Adenocarcinoma): A malignant gland cell tumor showing apocrine secretory differentiation.

Adenoid Cystic Carcinoma: A malignant duct cell tumor (eccrine or apocrine) indistinguishable from similar neoplasms arising elsewhere.

The benign tumors of the external canal showing eccrine secretory or ductal differentiation and sebaceous differentiation are similar to those found in other areas.

Benign mixed tumors of the external canal are well known and the malignant mixed tumor may be encountered. Mucoepidermoid tumors have been described.[20] Primary mucinous carcinomas and malignant variants of acrospiroma are also possible but have not yet been reported. Unclassifiable adenocarcinomas primary in the external canal also are encountered.

There is no advantage, as suggested by Michel et al.,[22] in retaining "ceruminoma" as a generic term with limited clinical value having once established that numerous past references to cerumi-

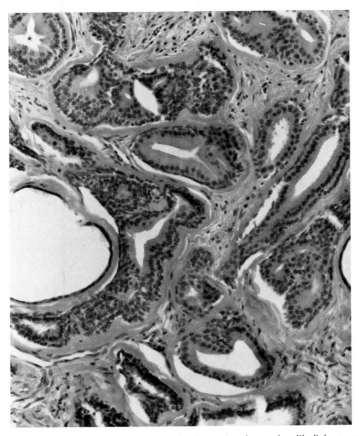

Figure 21.5. Ceruminoma composed of glands manifesting a two-layered epithelial composition—an inner columnar, eosinophilic layer and a closely applied myoepithelial layer.

noma clearly represent a heterogenous group of neoplasms. If therapeutic strategies are to be refined on the basis of histological specificity, then only a specific clinical pathological correlation should be implied. We prefer to limit ceruminoma to a benign adenoma of ceruminous gland origin showing secretory differentiation which can be defined using light microscopic, histochemical and ultrastructural criteria.

The histological appearance of ceruminoma (apocrine adenoma) includes evidence for "capitate" secretion by cuboidal or columnar cells forming distinct glandular spaces. The secretory cells may be backed by a reserve cell layer to produce a double-layered epithelium. Such glandular units while circumscribed may not be encapsulated (Fig. 21.5). Frozen section histochemical demonstrations for hydrolytic enzymes should be strongly positive although these have not yet been reported. Paraffin embedded sections may show the presence of lipochrome and/or iron common to apocrine secretory units elsewhere. Ultrastructural features have been described.[23]

The clinical characteristics of ceruminoma as defined above are not diagnostic. Such tumors may result in symptoms related to obstruction of the ear canal. Pain is uncommon unless there is associated inflammation. Pruritis and otorrhea may occur. Complete local excision is curative.

REFERENCES

1. Urbach, F.: Geographic pathology of skin cancer. In The Biologic Effects of Ultraviolet Radiation, edited by F. Urbach, p. 635. Pergamon Press, Oxford, England, 1969.
2. Brodkin, R. H., Kopf, A. W., and Andrade, R.: Basal-cell epithelioma and elastosis: A comparison of distribution. In The Biologic Effects of Ultraviolet Radiation, edited by F. Urbach, p. 581. Pergamon Press, Oxford, England, 1969.
3. Headington, J. T.: Unpublished observations.
4. Headington, J. T.: Tumors of the hair follicle. A Review. Am. J. Pathol. 85:480, 1976.
5. Conley, J.: Cancer of the skin of the nose. Arch. Otolaryngol. 85:55, 1966.
6. Huriez, C., Lebeurre, R., and Lepere, B.: Etude de 126 tumeurs auriculaires malignes observees en 9 ans a la clinique dermatologique universitaire de Lille. Bull. Soc. Fr. Dermatol. Syphiligr. 69:886, 1962.
7. Fabian, G., and Thomitzek, C. K.: Basaliome des aussern ohres. H. N. O. 11:321, 1963.
8. Robertson, D. F.: Correlation of observed ultraviolet exposure and skin cancer incidence in the population in Queensland and New Guinea. In The Biological Effects of Ultraviolet Radiation, edited by F. Urbach, p. 619. Pergamon Press, Oxford, England, 1969.
9. Lightstone, A. C., Kopf, A. W., and Garfinkel, L.: Diagnostic accuracy—a new approach to its evaluation. Arch. Dermatol. 91:497, 1965.
10. Magnusson, A. H. W.: Skin cancer. Acta Radiol. Suppl. 22: 1, 1935.
11. Lederman, M.: Malignant tumors of the ear. J. Laryngol. Otol. 79:885, 1965.
12. Shiffman, N. J.: Squamous cell carcinomas of the skin of the pinna. Can. J. Surg. 18:279, 1975.
13. Johnson, W. C., and Helwig, E. B.: Adenoid squamous cell carcinoma. Cancer 19:1939, 1966.
14. Blake, G. B., and Wilson, J. S.: Malignant tumours of ear and their treatment. Br. J. Plast. Surg. 27:67, 1974.
15. Nelms, R. C., and Paparella, M. M.: Early external auditory canal tumors. Laryngoscope 78:986, 1968.
16. Johns, M. E., and Headington, J. T.: Squamous cell carcinoma of the external auditory canal. A clinicopathologic study of 20 cases. Arch. Otolaryngol. 100:45, 1974.
17. Lewis, J. S.: Carcinoma of the ear. Arch. Otolaryngol. 97:41, 1973.
18. Crabtree, J. A., Britton, B. H., and Pierce, M. K.: Carcinoma of the external auditory canal. Laryngoscope 86:405, 1976.
19. Pulec, J. L., Parkhill, E. M., and Devine, K. J.: Adenoid cystic carcinoma (cylindroma) of the external auditory canal. Trans. Am. Acad. Ophthalmol. Otolaryngol. 67: 673, 1963.
20. Pulec, J. L.: Glandular tumors of the external auditory canal. Laryngoscope 87:1601, 1977.
21. Mandour, M. A., El-Ghazzaevi, E. F., Toppozada, H. H., and Nalaty, H. A.: Histological and histochemical study of the activity of ceruminous glands in normal and excessive wax accumulation. J. Laryngol. 88:1075, 1974.
22. Michel, R. C., Woodward, B. H., Shelburne, J. D., and Bossen, E. H.: Ceruminous gland adenocarcinoma. A light and electron microscopic study. Cancer 41:545, 1978.
23. Welti, C. V., Pardo, V., Millard, M., and Gerston, K.: Tumors of ceruminous glands. Cancer 29:1169, 1972.

CHAPTER 22

Melanomas (Cutaneous and Mucosal) of the Head and Neck

It has been estimated that there are about 2,000 million melanocytes in the human epidermis. These cells are distributed with considerable regional variation; there are two or three times as many melanocytes per unit area in the epidermis of the *cheek* and *forehead* as in other skin areas.[1] These melanocytic densities fall with age of the host but manifest neither racial nor sex variability. Variation in skin pigmentation is dependent not upon the number of melanocytes, but rather on their physiological activity. Areas of the head and neck normally devoid of pigment (e.g., the intraoral and intranasal surfaces) in Caucasians are nevertheless abundantly supplied with melanocytes. The same pertains to the epidermis of the albino and surfaces of the palms, soles and penis. The ubiquitous melanocyte is thus available everywhere in the epidermis and in some mucous membranes, with those at certain sites especially liable to produce malignant melanomas. This risk is independent of the risk of squamous cell carcinoma arising at the same sites.

A Caucasian manifests an average of 15 pigmented lesions over his body. The likelihood that one of these will lead into a malignant melanoma is one to 1 million. Ten thousand surgeons, excising a nevus every 15 minutes for 8 hours a day would take 25 years to eradicate all the nevi in the present population.[2] The uncertainty of which pigmented lesion is benign, however, dictates that those lesions in areas of especial liability or those subject to trauma be surgically excised. A black cutaneous lesion, particularly if there has been recent growth, is usually viewed with alarm. This prompts the usual response of wide and deep excision. While this management cannot be criticized too severely, Epstein[3] relates that many individuals have disfiguring scars as a result of the "enthusiasm of a concerned operator in handling a black benign growth." In his personal series of 599 patients with black lesions of the skin, only 2% had malignant melanomas.

Melanomas comprise 1.2% of all malignancies and are responsible for 0.74% of all deaths from cancer. Over 90% of these malignancies occur in the skin.[4] Their frequency appears to be increasing. Epidemiological aspects of melanoma are reviewed by McGovern[5] and Cochran.[6]

Once melanoma is present in a patient, he is at increased risk for the simultaneous or sequential development of another melanoma. The incidence of this phenomenon is estimated at 1.3% to 3.8% of all cases. The risk is age and sex dependant. Data from Milan, Italy, indicate that a malignant melanoma patient is about 900 times more likely to have a second primary lesion than an individual in the general population.[7]

Whether or not there had been an antecedent nevus, melanoma develops along one of three clinically and histologically distinct ways. The delineation of these types and apparent differences in behavior and prognosis have led to a practical classification consisting of three subtypes: (1) melanoma arising in Hutchinson's melanocytic freckle (associated with lentigo maligna); (2) melanoma arising as a premalignant melanosis (superficial spreading melanoma or "pagetoid melanoma"); (3) nodular melanoma (including melanoma arising de novo). Each of these types represents a distinct clinicopathological entity. Nodular melanoma is the most malignant, and that arising in Hutchinson's melanotic freckle is the least malignant. The greater malignancy of the nodular melanoma is associated with the higher proportion with deep invasion and a higher proportion of histological anaplastic features. An abridgement of the clinical and pathological features of each type follows.

1. Melanoma Arising in Hutchinson's Melanotic Freckle. Hutchinson's melanotic freckle (malignant lentigo) is a spreading macular pigmentation occurring most commonly in the skin of the temple and malar regions of elderly patients. It occurs also on the other exposed areas of the face and neck and, on occasion, on the dorsum of the wrists and forearms.

It is usually present in skin manifesting rather severe solar changes. The lesion is characterized by an irregularity in shape, as well as variations in the distribution and intensity of the pigmentation. The latter may vary from a dirty grayish-brown to a bluish-black. In general it is distinctly macular and not elevated above the surface of the skin, but especially in the darker, central parts there may gradually develop slightly elevated, fairly flat areas that have been considered as signs of initial malignant degeneration. The growth is, in general, slow, progressing for years and years. It regresses and advances in a manner likened to an infection and may even disappear completely. Its reappearance, however, can be safely predicted. Eventually, after a period of years, as long as 40 or more, an invasive nodule of melanoma appears.

Histologically, the lesion is a lentigenous proliferation of atypical melanocytes with elongation of the rete pegs, an increase in pigmentation, especially in the basal layer, and enlarged and atypical melanocytes. Clustering of the melanocytes as in junctional nevi is not common unless malignancy is developing. In some portions of the lesion, no junctional melanocytes are found, but there may be large amounts of pigmentation in the dermis. The histological structure in the initial phase corresponds to a benign nevoid lentigo, and all intermediate phases between this or senile lentigo and malignant melanoma may occur, even simultaneously within the same tumor. A fairly dense lymphocytic infiltrate is in the dermis beneath the lesion, and phagocytes containing pigment are easily found among the inflammatory cells. With the supervention of malignancy, the cells are similar to those of other forms of melanoma, but usually have a lower degree of anaplasia. The frequency with which the lesion involves the skin of the head and neck is seen in Table 22.1.

Since the change from benignity to malignancy is gradual and slowly progressive, it is natural that the interpretation of the degree of malignancy is highly dependent on the individual pathologist's criteria. Because of the rather uniform clinical presentations, the diagnosis is more often clinical than histological. Figure 22.1, taken from McGovern's[8] study, emphasizes the better prognosis associated with melanomas arising in Hutchinson's melanotic freckle and stresses the difference

Table 22.1
Site of Origin of Primary Melanomas*

Site	Melanoma in Hutchinson's Freckle	Melanoma in Premalignant Melanosis	Nodular Melanoma
Head and neck	18	20	31
Arm		9	8
Hand and forearm	2	6	3
Thorax and abdomen		12	12
Lower extremity		39	36
Mucosae			4
Site unknown			2

* Reproduced from McGovern[8] by permission.

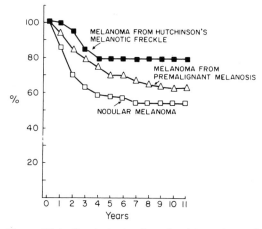

Figure 22.1. Survival rates based solely on type of melanoma (after McGovern[8]).

from melanomas arising as premalignant melanosis. This confirms what has already been well demonstrated by electron microscopy.[9]

2. Melanoma Arising as a Premalignant Melanosis (pagetoid melanoma, superficial spreading melanoma). This neoplasm is usually more circumscribed than Hutchinson's melanotic freckle and starts as a superficial spreading pigmentation that is seldom larger than 2 cm in diameter before ulceration and bleeding are presented. These two additional features indicate that invasion of the dermis has occurred. Invasion of the dermis occurs much earlier than in Hutchinson's melanotic freckle, and a history of months is more common than one of years. The skin of the head and neck is a region of predilection, but the lesion occurs on other exposed regions of the skin as well as unexposed surfaces. It also affects mucous membranes such as the conjunctiva, vulva and mouth.

Microscopically, there is what is best described as a pagetoid invasion of the epidermis by malignant melanocytes from the junctional region. These clusters of melanocytes are found in all parts of the junctional zone and not predominantly on the ridges as in junctional nevi. According to McGovern,[8] the pagetoid pattern is often helpful in deciding whether a lesion is a melanoma or a compound nevus. It must be remembered however, that rapidly growing nevi in children may also manifest individual melanocytes carried up in the epidermis to the surface. The pagetoid invasion persists even after there has been dermal invasion and may be seen both in the epidermis overlying the nodule of melanoma and in the adjacent pigmented skin.

3. Nodular Melanoma. This type of melanoma is invasive from the beginning; even when it originates from a pre-existent junctional nevus, there is no preliminary stage or peripheral spreading pigmentation. Both exposed and unexposed skin are affected, and the majority of mucosal melanomas are of this variety. Nodular melanomas also exhibit more cellular anaplasia than melanomas commencing as premalignant melanosis or Hutchinson's melanotic freckle.

Based on histological stages of invasion the nodular melanomas have a considerably higher proportion of tumors with deep invasion than the other two varieties. Survival rates are inversely proportional to the depth of invasion (Fig. 22.2). Nodular melanoma is associated with nevi less frequently than melanoma commencing as premalignant melanosis, but solar changes in the skin are more common.

CLASSIFICATION OF MALIGNANT MELANOMA AND ITS HISTOLOGICAL REPORTING

In recent years there has been considerable advance in the evaluation of *histological* factors affecting choice of therapy and prognosis of malignant melanoma. The fruits of these investigations have led to proposed standardization of nomenclature and histological reporting by surgical pathologists. Before considering these aspects, several points need to be made. Classification schemes have been successfully applied only to cutaneous melanomas (Table 22.2). Very little similar work has been done with mucosal melanomas of the head and neck. The presence of muscle bundles and lack of true subcutis in the oral and nasal areas make determinations of the level of invasion difficult or impossible. While some of the histological factors exhibit rather strong correlation with prognosis, a complete prognostic index must in-

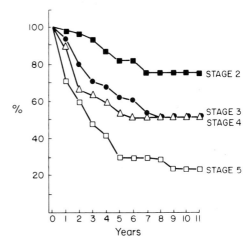

Figure 22.2. Survival rates for melanoma based on the depth of invasion of the primary neoplasm (after McGovern[8]).

clude sex, site, size, duration of symptoms and stage of the disease.[10, 11] Finally, much of the survival data and morbidity of melanomas presented later in this chapter have been extracted from studies usually dealing with head and neck melanomas as an aggregate or by clinical stage and have not included the prognostic refinements afforded by histological evaluation.

Apart from the rare malignant melanoma occurring in blue nevi, primary cutaneous melanomas arise in one of three ways, regardless of the presence or absence of a pre-existing nevus.[12] These three types have been mentioned above and are: (1) malignant melanoma, invasive with adjacent intraepidermal component of Hutchinson's melanotic freckle type; (2) malignant melanoma, invasive, with adjacent intraepidermal component of superficial spreading type; and (3) malignant melanoma, invasive, with adjacent intraepidermal component. In cases where this type of characterization is not possible, a fourth reporting mode— malignant melanoma, invasive, without classifiable adjacent intraepidermal component—is suggested.[12]

Added to this form of histological typing (lentigo-maligna-melanoma, superficial spreading melanoma, nodular melanoma) is the determination of the depth of invasion of the melanomas. For this purpose, the method of Clark et al.[13] has been widely used (Fig. 22.3). The levels are: (1) tumor confined to the epidermis (intraepidermal level); (2) tumor invading the papillary area but not extending to the reticular layer (papillary-dermis level); (3) tumor filling and expanding the papillary zone and impinging upon, but not invad-

Table 22.2
Malignant Melanoma[20]

Type of Malignant Melanoma	Levels of Invasion	Clinical Staging
1. Superficial-spreading 2. Lentigo-maligna 3. Melanoma with unclassified radial growth phase	Levels II–V according to depth	Appropriate clinical stage
4. Melanoma, nodular 5. Melanoma with origin in a giant hairy nevus 6. Volar-subungual melanoma* 7. Mucosal melanoma (oral, nasal, vaginal, anus, etc.)*		
8. Melanoma without detectable primary	Invasion levels not applicable	
9. Melanoma with origin in blue nevus 10. Visceral melanoma 11. Other melanomas (childhood and origin in dermal nevi)	Invasion levels other than those with origin in giant hairy nevi	

* The majority of volar-subungual melanomas and the mucosal melanomas have been considered as specific biological forms of the disease. They are characterized by a distinctive radial growth phase, followed by a vertical growth phase. Superficial-spreading and nodular types also occur.

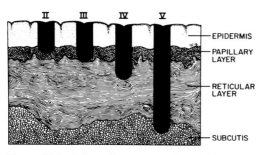

Figure 22.3. Schematic representation of the system used to register depth of invasion by melanomas.

ing the reticular zone (papillary-reticular-interface level); (4) tumor with penetration into the reticular layer of the dermis (reticular-dermis level); and (5) tumor invading the hypoderm (subcutaneous-fat level). For demonstration of the papillary-reticular interface of the dermis, the use of trichrome stains is suggested. The papillary layer is composed of fine collagen fibers, whereas the reticular layer is composed of coarse collagen fibers, organized into bundles, many of which interlace.

There appear to be correlations between the type of melanoma and the depth of invasion as assessed by the foregoing scheme.[14, 15] Whether the *depth* of invasion or the *type* of melanoma is decisive for prognosis or whether *both* have to be considered has been recently clarified. Among tumors of equal depth of invasion, the type of melanoma has little prognostic impact. The depth is clearly more important.[15]

Evaluation of depth of invasion and horizontal growth, however, considers only two dimensions of a melanoma. Two melanomas can have the same diameter but differ greatly in thickness because of variation in either depth of invasion or degree of protrusion from the surface of the skin or both. Although studies have shown that prognosis correlates well with staging of depth of invasion, there is clearly an enhancement by objective measurements of tumor volume.[16, 17] The relative merits of this technique are, in fact, so great that measurement is considered by some to be preferable to subjective evaluation of depth of invasion.[16]

The thickness and level of invasion of cutaneous melanoma are *independent* variables. They are relatively congruent in levels II and V, but not in levels III and IV.[16] This is due to the great variation in thickness for levels III and IV. Since the chance of developing recurrent disease appears to be directly proportional to tumor thickness and mean survival following surgery appears to inversely proportional to tumor thickness, the heterogeneity within level III and IV melanomas is a serious weakness if the level of invasion is to be used to guide therapy.[16, 18]

Dealing with stage I melanomas, Breslow[16] regards tumor thickness rather than level of invasion as an index for selection of patients for prophylactic node dissection. He considers that patients with lesions less than 0.76 mm thick should not be subjected to dissection of lymph nodes, while those with lesions greater than 1.50 mm should be so treated. Indications for dissection for the group of patients with lesions 0.76 to 1.50 mm thick are obscure. Cohen et al.[19] have performed a retrospective study correlating thickness and depth, among other findings as functions of prognostic factors. They found the *site* of the melanoma and the lymph node status to be more strongly correlated with prognosis than the level of invasion or the thickness of the primary lesion. With regard to the prognostic implications of Clark's levels of invasion, there appears to be a difference between the 5- and 10-year results. Cohen et al.[19] report a substantial difference in survival according to differences in the original Clark level of invasion at 5 years. These differences were not as pronounced at 10 years following the lymph node dissection. The division of melanoma thickness into <1.50 mm and >1.50 mm provided some prognostic discrimination at 5 years, but again, these differences were not pronounced at 10 years after the node dissection.

The 10-year survival of their patients with one to three histologically positive nodes was 55%. This is relatively high when compared to reports in which survival is not measured as a function of the *number* of positive nodes. Patients with four or more positive nodes had an 8-year survival of only 25%. In patients with clinically negative, histologically positive nodes the 10-year survival was 70%. Patients with clinically positive, histologically positive nodes manifested a 10-year survival of 50%.

What are some of the conclusions that can be made from the foregoing? Histopathological staging of the depth of invasion has limitations, not only in its subjectivity but also from its two-dimensional perspective. Objective measurements of tumor size or volume remove these defects, but still are capable of suffering from sampling error. Since a sampling error may affect both depth and

volume evaluation; this may be moot. Given *prospective* studies, the micrometric method of volume sizing may replace depth evaluation as a prognostic and therapeutic indicator. The hazards of using data from nonrandomized retrospective studies for the selection of patients for prophylactic lymphadenectomy appear too great to make a judgment at this time. Given prospective study information, the primary value of such pretherapeutic factors would seem to be the identification of patients with poor or favorable prognosis, rather than in a selection of patients who would benefit from prophylactic node dissection.

Other histological factors such as type of melanoma play either little or negligible roles in prognostication. Evaluation of the quantitative and qualitative aspects of the chronic inflammatory reaction at the advancing edge of the tumor, and vascular (lymphatic and blood) invasion remain as histological features requiring more study.[20]

The prognostic significance of clinical stage and lymph node metastases is well recognized and will not be replaced by any refinement of histological assessment. The complete prognostic index must include all of the above as well as patient and clinical factors. Given this multivariate index, some 90% of cutaneous melanomas may be predicted as to outcome. This predictability, however, degrades after 5 years postoperatively.[11]

MELANOMAS OF THE SKIN OF THE HEAD AND NECK

In approximately 50% of all cases, malignancy *apparently* results from the transformation of a seemingly benign melanocytic lesion (nevus) of the skin to one of aggressive character. As we have already indicated, nevi are so very common that such a change actually represents an infrequent occurrence. No area of the skin is exempt. The skin of the head, face and neck is second only to the skin of the extremities in total incidence of malignant melanoma (20%).[21]

Figure 22.4 illustrates the relative frequency of site of involvement of malignant melanoma in the *skin* of the head and neck (549 cases).[21-23] The cheeks, scalp and skin of the neck, in accordance with melanocytic density, are most often involved by a primary malignant melanoma. The skin of the nose and that of the chin are two areas of low involvement. In a like manner, the anatomical sites associated with the most favorable prognosis are the skin of the cheeks and the neck. In the instance of melanoma of the ear, the *exact* location also appears to directly influence prognosis. Le-

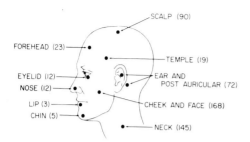

Figure 22.4. Geographic localization of 549 cutaneous melanomas in the head and neck region. Data presented represent information derived from the studies of Catlin,[22] Simmons[23] and Conley and Pack.[21]

sions of the central ear (canal, concha, tragus and antitragus) and the retroauricular zone have a grave prognosis.[24]

Gross features of the neoplasm (i.e., clinical size, ulceration and satellitosis) do not appear to significantly alter prognosis, and such positive findings should not deter an aggressive treatment of the primary lesion. In this respect, it is noteworthy that many of the melanomas of the head and neck are less than 2.0 cm in diameter at their discovery. This is undoubtedly due to a combination of their pigmentation and location on an exposed part of the body. Amelanotic and achromatic melanomas of this area of skin are the rare exception.

Adding to the belief that malignant melanomas frequently arise in *existing* pigmented nevi which were dismissed as "harmless and benign" are the observations that a considerable percentage of patients are known to have had their pigmented lesion for 10 years or longer. Sylven and Hamberger[25] report that one-half of their patients with melanoma of the ear had a pre-existing nevus.

Approximately three-quarters of the patients manifesting cutaneous melanomas of the head and neck are between the ages of 30 and 70 years, with a peak at 40 years. In Ballantyne's[26] series of 397 cases, 16 patients were under the age of 20 years at the time of diagnosis and 24 were over 80 years of age. Males dominate in a ratio of 2:1.

Current studies of melanoma of the skin of the head and neck indicate that, in an over-all perspective, it has a very respectable 5-year survival rate. Catlin[22] reports an absolute 5-year cure rate of 40.7% (73 of 179 patients). Seventy-one of his patients were without evidence of disease at 5 years after treatment. The capricious character of melanoma is demonstrated, however, by the observation that an additional nine patients were dead at 10 years follow-up. Ballantyne's[26] statistics are even more encouraging. He reports a 65.7% 5-year survival for patients with localized mela-

noma. These data compare favorably with most of the more common squamous cell carcinomas of the mouth, pharynx and larynx. Huvos et al.[27] in a retrospective study of 119 patients evaluated the various prognostic factors in cutaneous melanoma of the head and neck. The 10-year actuarial survival rates for clinical stage I patients when grouped according to dermal penetration level in their study were: level II, 80%; level III, 60%; level IV, 57%; and level V, 44%. Correlations of importance were noted between ulceration and depth of invasion, cellular pigment production and clinical pigmentation, as well as size of the primary tumor and depth of dermal invasion. The pattern of tumor cells, whether spindle, epithelioid, or mixed offered no prognostic significance. Additional factors were described by Hansen and McCarten.[17] They found Clark's classification, using histological landmarks to correlate well with survival in their cases of head and neck melanomas. However, finer distinction within levels was achieved by measurement of tumor thickness and grading according to the presence or absence of significant lymphocytic infiltration.

The influence of metastases to regional lymph nodes, as expected, is an adverse one with respect to survival (Fig. 22.5). Kragh and Erich[28] report a 75% and a 65.9% 3- and 5-year survival rate in their patients without metastases at the time of treatment. For the same time periods, patients with metastases manifested a 39.4% and a 23.1% survivorship. Ballantyne's[26] data are similar. His patients with regional node metastases manifested a 29% 5-year survival as compared to a 76.9% and 60.8% survival rate for patients with localized cutaneous melanoma of the skin of the head and neck, treated with and without prophylactic neck dissection, respectively. The skin of the external ear does not appear to share this optimistic outlook for prognosis. In a review published in 1968, only 16 of 79 patients survived 5 years (Table 22.3).

In a study of *stage I head and neck cutaneous melanomas*, Ames et al.[35] report the M. D. Anderson Hospital (Houston) experience as a 5-year determinate survival of 61% and 5- and 10-year actuarial survivals of 65% and 55% respectively. In an identical analysis of stage I invasive melanoma of the trunk and extremities at the same hospital, the 5- and 10-year actuarial survivals were 65% and 56% for the trunk and 88% and 84% for the extremities respectively. The determinate survivals at 5 years for trunk and extremities were 59% and 83% respectively. In all groups the depth of invasion was at least level III. In their patients with neck dissection, more than 80% of the local recur-

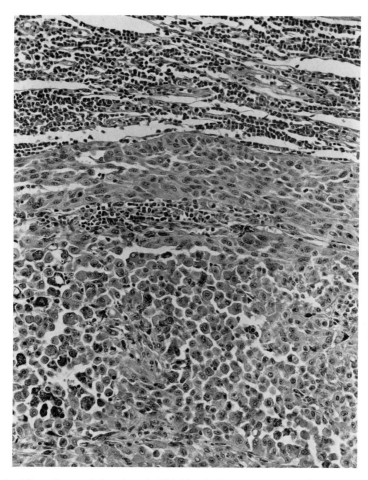

Figure 22.5. Metastatic melanoma in lymph node. This histological finding adversely affects survival, regardless of treatment.

Table 22.3
Malignant Melanoma of External Ear

The low 5-year survival rate for melanomas of the external ear places this cutaneous region of the head and neck near the bottom for prognosis.

Authors	No. of Cases	5-Year Survivors
Broders[29]	3	0
Affleck[30]	1	0
Sylven and Hamberger[25]	34	11
Friedman and Radcliffe[31]	1	0
Daland[32]	8	?
Lewis[33]	2	0
Pack and Ariel[34]	5	0
Conley and Pack[21]	18	3
Ward and Acquarelli[24]	4	2

rences developed within the first 24 months. Similarly, in patients not sustaining initial neck dissection, 80% of those who subsequently had clinically positive regional nodes did so within 24 months.

Patients with elective neck dissections having histologically negative nodes had a survival rate of 76% and 67% at 5 and 10 years; patients with histologically positive nodes had a 33.5% survival at 5 and 10 years. Of interest in the M. D. Anderson Hospital series is the observation that all of the initial treatment failures were among patients who did not have nodal dissection. Each of these patients were subsequently treated with therapeutic neck dissection. Of this group only 24% were alive at the conclusion of the study; the remainder all subsequently had systemic metastasis. Over-all, nearly 22% of 166 patients had systemic metastases (lungs, brain, skin, extraregional nodes, liver and bone).

MELANOMAS OF THE ORAL CAVITY

In the skin, malignant melanoma is the third most frequently encountered malignancy, representing 4.1 to 7.0% of all skin cancers. By comparison, melanomas of the oral mucous membranes are rare (Table 22.4). Between 0.4 and 1.4% of all melanomas are estimated to arise in the oral cavity and its structures.[36] Their relative incidence among mucosal neoplasms of the head and neck may be roughly deduced from the review by Hormia and Vuori.[37] These authors encountered 11 mucosal melanomas of the head and neck in 7,253 cases of malignancies of the mucous membranes of the upper respiratory and gastrointestinal tracts between 1953 and 1964. Five melanomas were in the nasal cavity, four arose in the palate, one in the tongue and one in the larynx.

Benign forms of pigmentation are not uncommon within the oral cavity. Melanosis of portions of the mucosa in Negroes is a racial characteristic and is considered physiological. This scattered melanosis is present in over 50% of Negroes and may be found in varying degrees in other racial stocks, notably Latins, as well as in some whites.[38] The Japanese are relatively common hosts for melanomas arising from the oral mucosa. The tumors make up 7.5% of all malignant melanomas and 35% of all mucosal melanomas.[39] Nearly two-thirds of the cases can be found to be associated with some form of pre-existing, concurrent or later developing melanoses. The biological behavior and histological patterns of these melanoses are similar to those of lentigo maligna of the skin.

The pigmentation of the human gingiva is due to the presence of pigment granules in cells of the basal layer where it is stored. The melanin itself is elaborated by specific clear cells (melanoblasts) morphologically and histochemically analogous to melanocytes of the skin.[40] These cells manifest long dendritic processes. The cells are normal inhabitants of the basal layer regardless of whether or not there is clinical pigmentation. Despite the presence of the pigment-formative and pigment-storing cells, focal lesions arising from proliferation of cells or increased production of pigment are apparently rare.

The morphology of the oral melanocyte is similar to that reported in full-thickness preparations of the epidermis of human skin. In Caucasians there are no major differences in the distribution of dopa-positive melanocytes in different parts of the gingivae of the jaws in either sex.[41] In view of this distribution, the findings of Chaudhry et al.[36] that primary intraoral melanomas are twice as common in the male as in the female and that in 80% of cases, the melanoma arises in the maxilla, remain unexplained.

Based on reported cases, it is assumed that malignant melanocytic lesions of the oral mucosa far exceed the number of benign pigmented lesions. An indication that this represents a reporting artefact is to be found in the report by Trodahl and Sprague,[42] who have had the largest single experience to date. Of 135 acceptable cases, they classified 93 as benign and 42 as malignant. Lentigo, ephelis, and blue nevi represented 30% of the benign lesions, and the remainder were cellular nevi. Nearly two-thirds of all benign melanocytic lesions are said to occur on the vermilion and lining mucosa of the lips. The remainder are scattered among other intraoral sites, with the palate and the gingival and buccal mucosa being next in order of frequency. Table 22.5, modified from the study by Page et al.[43] compares the clinical features of the oral and labial melanotic macule (ephelis, focal melanosis), the oral cellular nevi, and oral melanoma.

Malignant melanoma of the oral mucosa may take its origin from apparently healthy mucosa and nevi or from the unusual malignant lentigo (Hutchinson's melanotic freckle).[44] Greene et al.[45] have proposed three criteria for acceptance of a melanoma as primary in the oral cavity: (1) demonstration of clinical and microscopic tumor; (2) presence of intraepithelial (junctional) activity; and (3) inability to demonstrate any other primary lesion. Some degree of assurance may be taken from the observation that secondary melanomas are unusual and exceptional in this location. With only minor variations, the sites of malignant involvement, in descending order, are: the palate, alveolar ridge, buccal mucosa, mandibular mucosa, lips, tongue and floor of mouth. Over 80% of the malignant melanomas of the oral cavity are maxillary in location.

Primary intraoral melanomas far out-number metastatic melanomas to that region; at least as judged by the literature. In a 60-year period (1912

Table 22.4
Relative Frequency of Malignant Melanomas of the Skin and Mucous Membranes (Oral and Upper Respiratory Tract)
The rarity of mucosal melanomas of the head and neck is evidenced by these statistics from major "cancer" institutions.

Author	Period of Study	No. of Cases	
		Skin	Mucous Membranes
Ballantyne[26]	1944–1966	405	13
Conley and Pack[21]	1935–1961	142	11
Kragh and Erich[28]	1945–1954	109	20
Moore and Martin[54]	1930–1948	274	27

Table 22.5
Oral Melanocytic Lesions: Clinical Comparison*

Clinical Feature	Oral Melanotic Macule	Labial Melanotic Macule	Oral Nevus	Oral Melanoma
Age (years) (mean)	5–72 (43)	16–69 (27.5)	3–78 (38)	22–90 (50.5)
Sex	No predilection	No predilection	No predilection	3:1 male
Race	90+% Caucasian	100% Caucasian	88% Caucasian	80% Caucasian
Site (%)	Gingiva, 36 Buccal, 31 Palate, 26 Other, 6	All lip	Palate, 46 Lips, 22 Buccal, 13 Gingiva, 11 Others, 7	Maxilla, 80 Other, 20

* Modified from Page et al.[43]

to 1971) only seven cases of metastatic melanomas to the tongue had been reported.[46] Other intraoral sites of metastasis with a lesser incidence are the tonsils, hypopharynx, palate and gingiva.

Some general characteristics of malignant melanoma in this anatomical region are as follows. There is an apparent male predominance. The highest incidence is in patients between the ages of 50 and 70 years; from this it is inferred that oral melanomas appear at a more advanced age than those of the skin. Malignant melanoma in the mouth has not been reported in persons under 20 years of age. Racial incidence data are, perhaps, slanted because of the type of patients reported in the literature, which indicates that the majority of malignant melanomas occur in Caucasians. A more probable ratio would appear to be 2:1 in favor of whites. Intraoral melanomas, for example, are found with greater frequency in Uganda than in the temperate areas of the world. Garrington et al.[47] have reported a case of intraoral melanoma in a human albino.

The lesions are rarely achromatic, presenting as tan to black lesions. Variable in size, they may measure up to several centimeters at the time of treatment. They are usually soft and painless and, at times, hemorrhagic. While they do not often present with an indurated base, the neoplasm may cause loosening of the teeth or become adherent to deeper planes and destroy adjacent bone. It is of significance to note that when the malignancy has appeared to develop on a pre-existing nevus, the patient has been aware of the lesion from childhood.[48]

As Trodahl and Sprague[42] point out, "purely focal brown, blue or bluish-black pigmentations are not infrequently noted by the clinician who routinely and carefully examines the oral cavity."

Racial pigmentation is generally symmetrical in a bilateral fashion and is usually limited to the buccal and labial surfaces of the gingiva. Exogenous and often iatrogenic focal pigmentation, particularly that known as the "amalgam tattoo," may manifest metallic fragments in the oral roentgenograms of the area and may be deduced by careful history. Hemoglobin breakdown products, in a localized area, may also present a difficult diagnostic problem.

Benign melanocytic lesions differ from malignant melanoma in being relatively smaller and more regular in shape and not as prone to secondary ulceration or hemorrhage. Nevertheless, differentiation from malignant melanoma by clinical inspection alone is difficult. A significant number (25%) of intraoral melanomas may be considered as innocuous on original inspection.

With the foregoing in mind, there is little to deny that prophylactic excisional biopsy is always indicated for any focal pigmented lesion of the oral mucosa that does not have "an indisputably innocuous" etiology. A fatal outcome is practically certain in all cases of intraoral malignant melanomas, although there is a suggestion that those lesions classified as arising from Hutchinson's melanotic freckle and superficial melanomas may have a better prognosis. Chaudhry et al.[36] record only three of 93 patients surviving more than 5 years after diagnosis and treatment, and Allen[49] gives a 5.9% 5-year survival rate. The majority of patients die within 1 or 2 years of the onset of the disease, with recurrent, often destructive local lesions and regional lymph node metastases, followed by visceral spread, especially to the brain, lungs, spine, skin and liver. Chaudhry et al.[36] found regional lymph node involvement in more than 50% of their group of patients and visceral dissemination in 20%. This adverse biological behavior is shared by all areas within the oral cavity, including the tongue.[50]

MELANOMAS OF THE UPPER RESPIRATORY TRACT

The incidence of malignant melanoma in the whole body is approximately two new cases per 100,000 population per year. Most authors, regarding the oral, nasal, paranasal and pharyngeal cavities as a unit, put the incidence in the area at approximately 2% of all malignant neoplasms.[51] The majority of these are intraoral, with the nasal and paranasal sites comprising less than 1% of *all* malignant melanomas.[52]

Testimony to the relative rarity of mucosal melanomas in the head and neck may be found in the Sloan-Kettering Memorial Cancer Center experience where 74 patients with this malignancy were recorded in a 30-year period.[53]

The exact site of origin of many of the cases from the upper respiratory tract is difficult to determine.[55] Many patients manifest neoplasm both in the nose and in the paranasal sinuses at the time the diagnosis is established. Where the site of origin has been definable, the majority of upper respiratory tract melanomas arise in the nasal cavity (Fig. 22.6). Between 0.5 and 0.85% of *all* malignant melanomas are said to arise in the nose.[51] The mucous membranes of the nose and paranasal sinuses are only rarely involved by metastatic melanoma (Table 22.6).

Melanocytes in the nasal cavities of both Caucasians and Negroes can be found in the respiratory epithelium, nasal glands and commonly in the superficial and deep stroma of the septum and middle and interior turbinates[57] (sites of apparent predilection for melanoma). These cells are present in the stroma of most Caucasians and all Negro adults. Intraepithelial melanocytes occur focally and are observed only in adult negroes. No melanocytes are found in young Negro children.[57] Melanocytes are also found in the masseter and temporalis muscles of human fetuses and neonates,[58] larynx[59, 60] and middle ear.[61] It is of considerable histogenetic interest that although the olfactory epithelium of the high nasal cavity is relatively rich in melanin pigment, no melanomas have arisen from this epithelium.

Malignant melanoma of the upper respiratory tract appears to arise de novo without a precursor lesion. As late as 1966, there had been no reports of benign melanocytic lesions in this mucosal region.[62] The majority of the neoplasms are in either the anterior part of the nasal septum or the middle and inferior turbinates.[63, 64] Paradoxically, these two areas are devoid of visible pigmentation, and the olfactory area that contains pigment within the epithelium has not been cited as a point of origin. The assumption is that, much like oral melanomas, the neoplasms originate from melanocytes in the mucosa of the upper respiratory tract. Junctional changes in mucosa are rarely observed because of the bulky replacement produced by the neoplasm.[65]

There is no significant sex difference pertinent to melanomas of the upper respiratory tract. The patients' age distribution coincides with that for melanoma elsewhere in the head and neck. Over two-thirds of published cases give the peak age incidence in the fourth to sixth decades of life. The disease is predominantly one of Caucasians.

Clinical symptoms are of little assistance in prebiopsy diagnosis. Unilateral nasal obstruction or epistaxis is most often the initial complaint. Pain is uncommon. While it has been written that nasal melanomas tend to present with a more "sudden onset" than other types of nasal cavity malignancies, the duration of signs and symptoms before medical attention is sought is variable. Inspection of the nasal cavity may disclose a sessile mass, polyp or large obstructing tumor. The neoplasm is frequently pigmented (Fig. 22.6), but the presence of pigment may change throughout the course of the disease and this variation has no bearing on prognosis.

Vagueness over the site of origin does not apply to the oropharynx or larynx. In the oropharynx, reported melanomas have been restricted to the palatine tonsils. The extremely rare laryngeal melanomas take their origin in the extrinsic larynx in the region of the ventricular fossa and false cords. By 1970, Shanon et al.[66] reported the larynx had been affected by melanoma 15 times; of these, 10 were considered primary and five as metastatic melanomas. Three were epiglottic. It is interesting to note that, of the metastases to the larynx from remote primary lesions, only renal cell carcinoma and melanoma have been implicated. As one progresses down the respiratory tract, the frequency of melanoma declines. Reid and Mehta[67] tabulated nine examples of lower respiratory tract melanoma by 1966.

There is a decided tendency for melanoma of the upper respiratory tract to be more pleomorphic than its cutaneous counterparts. The finding of intracytoplasmic melanin aids in confirming a diagnosis, even if a prolonged search of multiple sections is necessary. Gallagher[65] lists three strin-

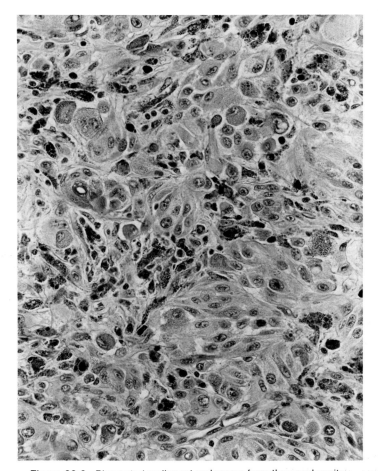

Figure 22.6. Pigmented malignant melanoma from the nasal cavity.

Table 22.6
Mucosal Melanoma: Upper Airway Sites

	Shah et al.[53]	Conley and Pack[54]	Freed-man et al.[56]
Nasal cavity	39	12	29
Paranasal sinuses	6	6	18
Larynx-laryngopharynx	4	8	—
Combined (nasal and sinuses)	—	—	9

gent criteria for the intracytoplasmic pigment: (1) the Fontana stain for melanin should be positive; (2) the pigment should be capable of being bleached by the permanganate-oxidase method; (3) a stain for iron pigment should be negative.

The biological course of upper respiratory tract melanomas is marked by early local recurrences and extension and frequent metastases to lymph nodes and viscera. Fifty-five percent of Gallagher's[65] series had either local or regional lymph node involvement or distant metastases within 1 year of the diagnosis. Predicting prognosis for patients is subject to the site of origin and certainly to the delay before diagnosis is made. Melanomas of the oral cavity have an impressive delay time before diagnosis, but the culpability must be shared by both the surgeon and the patient. Very early lymph node involvement is also present for melanomas of the nasal fossa where regional nodes and deep cervical and posterior pharyngeal nodes contain metastases. Melanomas of the oropharyngeal region are particularly vicious, with a short duration of symptoms and early metastases. Melanoma of the tonsil is the most discouraging of all.[68]

Survival statistics for upper respiratory tract melanomas are poor, rated only next to anorectal melanomas for the lowest survivorship. Gallagher[65] cites a mean survival after biopsy diagnosis of 2.3 years for nasal and paranasal melanomas. Eleven percent survived 5 years, and 0.5%

survived 10 years. Ravid and Esteves[69] record only a 6% survival for 5 or more years. Harrison's[70] series had a 5-year survivorship of 16%; this offers some small note of optimism, in that patients who survive the first 2 post-treatment years tend to have a more reasonable outlook.

At the Karolinska Sjukhuset, mucosal melanomas of the head and neck had a 17% 5-year survival and a 10-year survival rate of 7%.[71] It is to be stressed, however, that there is a never ceasing death risk. Apparently quiescent disease is temporarily held in check by a competent immunological system only to consume the patient later. Surgery is the treatment of choice. Radiotherapy appears to have little effect on the majority of mucosal melanomas.[72] It may play a role in the management of inoperable recurrences and help to prolong life.[56]

Emphasizing once again the greater mortality of the head and neck mucosal melanoma versus head and neck cutaneous melanoma is the experience by Conley and Hamaker.[73] They analyzed the absolute 5-year or greater cure rate in 556 cases of melanoma of the head and neck. The rate was 25.6% for mucosal and cutaneous lesions combined, an 8% rate for mucosal alone and 27.8% for cutaneous melanoma. Elective versus no elective neck dissection in stage I disease demonstrated a 5-year or greater absolute cure of 55% as compared to 38.5%. Distant metastases occurred in 30% of patients with elective neck dissection but in 70% of patients with therapeutic neck dissection.

MELANOMA OF THE MAJOR SALIVARY GLANDS

The major salivary glands are extremely unusual sites for primary melanoma, despite the fact that melanoblasts and dopa-positive cells are a normal and constant feature of parotid ductal and acinar cells. Greene and Bernier[74] report five cases from files of the Armed Forces Institute of Pathology and make mention of other isolated case reports.

The neoplasms arise directly from melanoblasts in salivary gland (parotid) tissue and may be differentiated from metastatic foci of melanoma by history or by their histological appearance. Melanoma metastatic to the parotid gland appears in the intraparotid lymph nodes or as a well delineated lesion in the parotid gland. Primary melanomas are, by contrast, infiltrative and poorly demarcated, or they completely replace the involved salivary glands. Since experience with melanomas of salivary glands is small, precise knowledge of

their biological behavior is unknown, but should not be markedly different from melanomas of the skin. This is indicated by recurrence or distant spread within months or a few years in three of the five patients reported by Greene and Bernier.[74]

MELANOMAS WITHOUT A KNOWN PRIMARY SITE

Approximately 4% of patients with malignant melanoma present with melanomas in lymph nodes in the absence of an apparent cutaneous or mucosal primary lesion.[75] In over one-half of these cases the disease is clinically confined to lymph nodes. Spontaneous regression of the primary is thought to account for some cases of this type, but the etiology in many remains obscure. A possible explanation for some of these cryptogenic melanomas is a de novo origin within a lymph node bearing area or in lymph nodes. The M. D. Anderson Hospital experience supports a spontaneous regression of the primary.[75] The pattern of their stage III B category followed the known primary distribution of head and neck melanomas. A peak age incidence in the fifth decade, is also consistent with what is known of primary cutaneous or mucosal sites. According to McGovern,[76] spontaneous regression of cutaneous melanomas occurs only with melanomas having a component of the superficial spreading type. Histologically the active phase of the regression is characterized by a dense infiltrate of lymphocytes similar to that seen in spontaneously disappearing nevi. The regression process may continue until the tumor has been completely destroyed, or it may stop when only a part of the tumor has been destroyed. The lymphocytes disappear when the process halts, leaving vascular scar tissues with a variable number of pigment-containing phagocytes.

The possibility of origin of some of these melanomas from nevus cell aggregates in lymph nodes themselves cannot be dismissed.[77, 78] Although seemingly rare, these nodal lesions may occur more often than the literature indicates. These benign cellular foci are arranged in either a band-like or nodular fashion within the capsule of the lymph nodes.

Patients with melanoma involving lymph nodes without an evident primary who are treated with lymph node dissections have a 5-year survival that is somewhat better than comparable groups of patients with nodal metastases from known primaries.[78, 79] This observation is again consistent with either regression of the primary lesion or nodal origin from nevus cell aggregates.

MALIGNANT MELANOMA OF THE HEAD AND NECK IN CHILDREN

In the recent past, melanomas presenting in children were considered to carry a good prognosis. This erroneous concept was due to the inclusion in survival data of certain benign nevi, simulating malignancy in their histological appearance.[80] The term "juvenile melanoma" has since been applied to this type of atypical nevus (Fig. 22.7). This designation does not seem to be appropriate for any reason since its biological behavior, after removal, is that of a benign lesion. Malignant melanoma is a rarity before puberty, and the adjective "juvenile" is falsely restrictive since similar lesions occur in adults, albeit much less frequently. Perhaps Helwig's term "spindle cell nevus," adopted by Kernen and Ackerman,[81] is more appropriate. I have encouraged the diagnostic appellation "atypical juvenile nevus."

The common locations of this benign lesion are the cheeks, forehead, ear, nose, trunk, buttocks and extremities. Most often it presents on the skin of the face, especially the cheeks, and has been noticed only for a few weeks or months. Nearly all are small and superficial (2 to 3 cm). They are most often pink, circumscribed and manifest a smooth, non-ulcerated surface without hair.

The cells of the lesion are plump and larger than ordinary nevus cells. They are disposed in a variety of patterns and often appear loosely arranged because of stromal edema. Combinations or intermixtures of spindle and epthelioid cells occur in a variable proportion. While some evidence of junctional activity is present, the lesion is primarily intradermal. The epidermis is attenuated, frequently hyperkeratotic, and occasionally presents with pseudoepitheliomatous hyperplasia. The lower border of the lesion is sharply demarcated and may have an associated lymphocytic and plasma cell infiltrate. Pigmentation is variable and commonly sparse. Giant cells may be present, and the nucleoli of the cells, although conspicuous, are never disproportionately large as in malignant melanoma. The degree of mitotic activity is of little assistance because of its variability. In this lesion, however, they are seldom atypical. The nuclear chromatin pattern—absence of a significant upward epidermal spread, absence of atypical mitoses, and the presence of some nevus cell maturity at the base—help Weedon and Little[82] to distinguish the atypical nevi from melanomas.

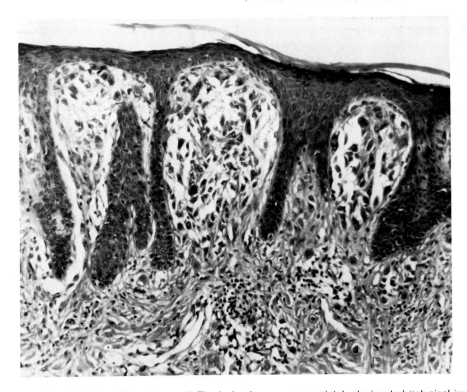

Figure 22.7. So-called "juvenile melanoma." The lesion is more appropriately designated "atypical juvenile nevus."

Even with these criteria, however, it may not be possible to always distinguish with certainty between malignant melanoma and atypical nevus. Skov-Jensen et al.[83] consider malignant melanoma in children to be divisible into three categories: (1) congenital; (2) malignant melanoma developing before puberty; and (3) malignant melanoma developing before puberty in a nevus pigmentosus gianticus. Only the last two concern the head and neck surgeon. Of 41 cases of malignant melanoma in children (under 14 years of age) recorded in the literature up to 1966,[83] 11 arose from the skin of the head and neck (four from nevus pigmentosus gianticus). In all cases, metatases were present predominantly to regional lymph nodes, with the lesions arising from the nevus gianticus also manifesting generalized metastases. The 3-year survival rate in children compares with the 5-year survival rate in adults at a similar stage of the disease.[84]

TREATMENT

Surgical resection remains the primary treatment of choice. Although an occasional melanoma is radiosensitive, it is doubtful whether any is ever "radiocurable." If radiation therapy is used, it is usually in conjunction with surgical removal of the neoplasm. Regional perfusion of cytotoxic drugs in cases of recurrent melanomas of the extremities has been encouraging, but an effective "vascular isolation" of the nasal and paranasal passages is difficult to achieve and the role of systemic or other forms of local chemotherapy has yet to be established for melanomas of the head and neck.

Biopsy diagnosis is essential, especially for those doubtful melanocytic lesions of the oral cavity and upper respiratory tract. As I have earlier stated, there is no evidence that preliminary biopsy of the primary lesion increases the risk of metastatic dissemination or unfavorably affects prognosis.

The axiom that the initial attack on a primary melanoma should be the most effective possible is well illustrated in patients manifesting melanomas of the head and neck. McNeer et al.[85] consider the high recurrence rate exhibited by melanomas of the head and neck to be partially explained by an operator's reluctance to disfigure his patient. Follow-up operative procedures are usually compromised by ensuing scars and distortion of regional tissues. Catlin,[22] for example, records a higher 5-year "cure" rate in patients who *did not* have some form of preliminary surgical treatment. Paradoxically, he also admits the best over-all results were

obtained in patients who came to his clinic free of melanoma and a history of recent local excision.

The mode of treatment and its extent, while definitely a key to the improving statistics concerning survival of patients with melanomas, is but one factor influencing the prognosis of patients. Early diagnosis is very important, especially for the mucosal melanomas of the head and neck. Anatomical site bears considerably not only on effective management but also with respect to diagnostic accessibility and lymphatic drainage. Lesions near the midline where drainage is unpredictable or multiple carry a lower survivorship. Effective surgical management by the first surgeon to see the patient contributes strongly to an enhanced prognosis. "Femaleness," although having no influence on the initiation or prevalence of melanoma in the head and neck, tends to improve the prognosis, especially in the premenopausal period. Although not as clearly defined, genetic, immunological and endocrine factors also play a role in the final outcome of the patient. Spontaneous regression of the neoplasm, often of the primary rather than the secondary sites, must also be considered.

Since malignant melanomas, in general, are noted for their unpredictable biological behavior, the *stage* of the disease at primary diagnosis is the best objective prognostic guide. Stage of the lesion is not concerned with the size or histological features of the primary lesion, but is based on the extent of spread of the disease. Various institutions have created their own clinical stages, but these represent modifications of the Memorial Hospital for Cancer and Allied Diseases scheme.[86] Stage I is local disease only with the primary melanoma being present, previously excised or locally recurrent; stage II consists of palpable regional lymph nodes; stage III indicates widespread metastatic melanoma (Table 22.7).

Based on the foregoing factors and clinical stages, five major categories of surgical attack exist, but individualization of patient care, particularly in the head and neck, is always indicated: (1) wide local excision as primary treatment; (2) wide local excision with dissection of the regional, *clinically involved* lymph nodes (therapeutic neck dissection); (3) dissection of the regional, *clinically positive* lymph nodes without excision of the primary (primary either under control or occult); (4) wide local excision with prophylactic (elective) lymph node dissection *at the time* of primary excision; (5) wide local excision with "late" nodal dissection *after* the development of clinically positive regional lymph nodes (therapeutic). Ade-

Table 22.7
Clinical Staging of Malignant Melanoma*

Stage	Characteristics
I.	Localized melanoma (no evidence of metastasis)
1.	Primary untreated or removed by excisional biopsy
2.	Local recurrence of melanoma within 4 cm of primary site
3.	Multiple primary melanomas
II.	Metastases limited to regional lymph nodes
1.	Primary present or excised with simultaneous metastasis
2.	Primary controlled with subsequent metastasis
3.	Local recurrence with metastasis
4.	In-transit metastasis beyond 4 cm from primary site
5.	Occult or unknown primary with metastasis
III.	Disseminated melanoma
1.	Visceral and/or multiple lymph node metastases
2.	Multiple cutaneous and/or subcutaneous metastases

* Reproduced from Goldsmith et al.[26] by permission. Clinical staging based on the above or variants thereof constitutes the most reliable single criterion for prognostication.

quate local excision and the amount of margin varies with the size, nature and site of the lesion. It appears that the inclusion of the underlying fascia does not improve "cure" or recurrence rates as long as wide local excision has been done initially.

Earlier in this chapter we discussed the additive preoperative contributions of histological staging (levels of invasion and tumor thickness) and presented some statistical data in support. Huvos et al.,[87] Ironside et al.,[88] and Franklin et al.,[89] provide further support. There is good correlation between the microscopic assessment and the incidence of lymph node metastases. Franklin et al.[89] relate the following in that respect: level II, 7.5% positive nodes; level III, 42% positive nodes; level IV, 53% positive nodes; and level V, 94% positive nodes.

There is little disagreement among surgeons that a patient with melanoma of the head and neck and *clinically involved* regional lymph nodes should have a regional lymph node dissection. This may be considered a "therapeutic lymph node dissection," indicating the objective to eradicate all grossly involved tissue. There is a trend, particularly with melanomas of the extremities, to perform the regional lymph node dissection "in continuity" with the excision of the primary melanoma. In practice, in-continuity dissection for head and neck melanomas seems applicable only when the primary lesions lend themselves to such

an operative procedure, i.e., skin of neck, lower part of cheek, posterior auricular scalp, etc. Shah and Goldsmith,[90] in a well-studied and large series, concluded that, for melanomas situated at a distance from the regional lymph nodes, a discontinuous lymph node dissection is equally satisfactory, since the survival statistics are comparable for both in-continuity and discontinuous lymph node dissection.

Prophylactic node dissection, in contrast to therapeutic resection, has been and continues to be a controversial technique of surgical management for malignant melanoma. Arguments for prophylactic dissection seem simple and straightforward. Lymphogenous spread is characteristic of melanoma, and the regional lymph nodes are commonly involved early in the biological course of the disease. Furthermore, clinical palpation, particularly of cervical lymph nodes, is a crudely inaccurate method of discerning the presence or absence of metastases.

Opponents of prophylactic neck dissection argue that the incidence of occult metastases is insufficient to warrant prophylactic removal of nodes. Furthermore, it is said to encourage the appearance of diffuse metastases between the sites of the primary and lymph node resection—the "in-transit metastasis."[91] The use of prophylactic, in-continuity resection reduces the incidence of in-transit metastases. Finally, even though lymph node metastases may not have taken place, the disease may be "incurable" because of hematogenous spread of the neoplasm.

Mundth et al.,[92] discussing 427 cases of malignant melanoma from multiple areas including the head and neck, present strong clinical and statistical support for prophylactic node dissection. The 5-year survival of all patients with *negative* nodes was 76%, and the 10-year survival was 62%. Positive (with metastases) nodes reduced the 5- and 10-year survivals to 22% and 5%, respectively. Incorporation of prophylactic lymph node dissection for patients with clinically uninvolved nodes but histologically positive nodes yielded a 5-year survival that was significantly better (59%) than the 5-year survival of all patients with nodal metastases treated by various means. The survival rate, however, was not significantly different from that of patients having a prophylactic node dissection and histologically negative lymph nodes. The same authors claim that prophylactic node dissection in six patients who had microscopically positive lymph nodes resulted in a "cure." They indicate that delay of the neck dissection until the onset of clinical involvement would have reduced the chance for cure to less than 10%. Donnellan et al.[93] report a 10-year actuarial survival rate of 86% in level II and 44% in level V melanomas of the head and neck. Ballantyne[26] reports a 5-year survival of 77% with no evidence of disease in patients who had an elective neck dissection and a survival rate of 26% of those patients who had a therapeutic neck dissection. In the Mayo Clinic[94] experience, the over-all survival for head and neck melanomas was 45%; this dropped to 22% when nodes were clinically positive. When prophylactic neck dissection was performed, there was a 73% 5-year survival; 79% if the nodes were histologically negative.

In the upper respiratory tract group of melanomas, inaccessibility, extent of disease and recurrences have promoted some clinical experience with irradiation. In general, irradiation alone has not controlled the disease, and some form of surgical procedure has been required later in the course of the disease. In the Armed Forces Institute of Pathology files there are records of three patients who were treated solely with irradiation, and all three died within 1 year.[64] Combination therapy (surgical and radiation) has not enhanced survival rates.

REFERENCES

1. Leading article: Malignant melanomas. Lancet 1:76, 1968.
2. Hugo, N. E.: Malignant melanoma: brief review of current therapy. Milit. Med. 134:52, 1969.
3. Epstein, E., Bragg, K., and Linden, G.: Biopsy and prognosis of malignant melanoma. J. A. M. A. 208:1369, 1969.
4. Franklin, J. D., Reynolds, V. H., Bowers, D. G., Jr., and Lynch, J. B.: Cutaneous melanoma of the head and neck. Clin. Plast. Surg. 3:413, 1976.
5. McGovern, V. J.: Epidemiological aspects of melanoma. Pathology 9:233, 1977.
6. Cochran, A. J.: The biology and treatment of malignant melanoma. Eur. J. Cancer 12:585, 1976.
7. Veronesi, U., Cascinelli, N., and Bufalino, R.: Evaluation of the risk of multiple primaries in malignant cutaneous melanoma. Tumori 62:127, 1976.
8. McGovern, V. J.: The classification of melanoma and its relationship with prognosis. Pathology 2:85, 1970.
9. McGovern, V. J., and LaneBrown, M. M.: The Nature of the Melanoma, pp. 100–106. Charles C Thomas, Springfield, Ill., 1969.
10. Magnus, K.: Prognosis in malignant melanoma of the skin. Significance of stage of disease, anatomical site, sex, age and period of diagnosis. Cancer 40:389, 1977.
11. Barclay, T. L., Crockett, D. J., Eastwood, D. S., and Eastwood, J.: Assessment of prognosis in cutaneous malignant melanoma. Br. J. Surg. 64:54, 1977.
12. McGovern, V. J., Mihm, M. C., Jr., and Bailly, C.: The classification of malignant melanoma and its histologic reporting. Cancer 32:1446, 1973.
13. Clark, W. H., Jr., From, L., Bernadino, E. A., and Mihm, M. C., Jr.: The histogenesis and histologic behavior of primary human malignant melanoma of the skin. Cancer Res. 29:707, 1969.
14. Wanebo, H. J., Woodruff, J., and Fortner, J. G.: Malignant melanoma of the extremities: a clinicopathologic study using levels of invasion (microstage). Cancer 35:666, 1975.
15. Hermanek, P., Hornstein, O. P., Tonak, J., and Weidner, F.: Malignes Melanom. Invasion stiefe und Melanomtyp. Beitr. Path. Bd. 157:269, 1976.
16. Breslow, A.: Tumor thickness, level of invasion and node dissection in Stage I cutaneous melanomas. Ann. Surg. 182:572, 1975.
17. Hansen, M. G., and McCarten, A. B.: Tumor thickness and lymphocytic infiltration in malignant melanoma of the head and neck. Am. J. Surg. 128:557, 1974.
18. Breslow, A.: Thickness, cross-sectional areas and depth of invasion in the prognosis of cutaneous melanoma. Ann. Surg. 172:902, 1970.
19. Cohen, M. H., Ketcham, A. S., Felix, E. J., Li, S. -H., Tomaszewski, M., Costa, J., Rabson, A. S., Simon, R. M., and Rosenberg, S. A.: Prognostic factors in patients undergoing lymphadenectomy for malignant melanoma. Ann. Surg. 186:635, 1977.
20. Clark, W. H., Ainsworth, A. M., Bernardino, E. A., Yang, C. -H., Mihm, M. C., Jr., and Reed, R. J.: The developmental biology of primary human malignant melanomas. Sem. Oncol. 2:83, 1975.
21. Conley, J. J., and Pack, G. T.: Melanoma of head and neck. Surg. Gynecol. Obstet. 116:15, 1963.
22. Catlin, D.: Cutaneous melanoma of head and neck. Am J. Surg. 112:512, 1966.
23. Simmons, J. N.: Malignant melanoma of head and neck. Am J. Surg. 116:494, 1968.
24. Ward, N. O., and Acquarelli, M. J.: Malignant melanoma of external ear. Cancer 21:226, 1968.
25. Sylven, B., and Hamberger, C. A.: Malignant melanoma of external ear. Ann. Otol. Rhinol. Laryngol. 59:631, 1950.
26. Ballantyne, A. J.: Malignant melanoma of skin of head and neck: analysis of 405 cases. Am. J. Surg. 120:425, 1970.
27. Huvos, A. G., Mike, V., Donnellan, M. J., Seemayer, T., and Strong, E. W.: Prognostic factors in cutaneous melanoma of the head and neck. Am. J. Pathol. 71:33, 1973.
28. Kragh, L. V., and Erich, J. B.: Malignant melanoma of head and neck. Ann. Surg. 151:91, 1960.
29. Broders, A. C.: Epithelioma of ear: study of 63 cases. Surg. Clin. North Am. 1:1401, 1921.
30. Affleck, D. H.: Melanomas. Am. J. Cancer 27:120, 1936.
31. Friedman, I., and Radcliffe, A.: Otosclerosis associated with malignant melanoma of ear. J. Laryngol. Otol. 68:114, 1954.
32. Daland, E. M.: Malignant melanoma. N. Engl. J. Med 260:453, 1959.
33. Lewis, J. S.: Cancer of ear. Laryngoscope 70:551, 1960.
34. Pack, T. G., and Ariel, I. M.: Treatment of Cancer and Allied Diseases, 2nd Ed. P. B. Hoeber, New York, 1962.
35. Ames, F. C., Sugarbaker, E. V., and Ballantyne, A. J.: Analysis of survival and disease control in Stage I melanoma of the head and neck. Am. J. Surg. 132:484, 1976.
36. Chaudhry, A. P., Hampel, A., and Gorlin, R. J.: Primary malignant melanoma of oral cavity. Review of 105 cases. Cancer 11:923, 1958.
37. Hormia, M., and Vuori, E. E. J.: Mucosal melanoma of head and neck. J. Laryngol. Otol. 83:349, 1969.
38. Dummett, C. O., and Bolden, T. E.: Melanoblasts in gingival irritation. Milit. Med. 129:1191, 1964.
39. Takagi, M., Ishikawa, G., and Mori, W.: Primary malignant melanoma of the oral cavity in Japan. With special reference to mucosal melanomas. Cancer 34:358, 1974.
40. Laidlaw, G. F., and Cahn, L. R.: Melanoblasts in gum. J. Dent. Res. 12:534, 1932.
41. Soames, J. V.: The morphology and quantitative distribution of dopa-positive melanocytes in the gingival epithelium of Caucasians. Oral Surg. 38:254, 1974.
42. Trodahl, J. N., and Sprague, W. G.: Benign and malignant melanocytic lesions of oral mucosa: analysis of 135 cases. Cancer 25:812, 1970.
43. Page, L. R., Corio, R. L., Crawford, B. E., Giansanti, J. S., and Weathers, D. R.: The oral melanotic macule. Oral Surg. 44:219, 1977.
44. Robinson, L., and Hukill, P. B.: Hutchinson's melanotic freckle in oral mucous membrane. Cancer 26:297, 1970.

45. Greene, G. W., Haynes, J. W., Dozier, M., Blumberg, J. M., and Bernier, J. L.: Primary malignant melanoma of oral mucosa. Oral Surg. 6:1435, 1953.

46. Miller, A. S., and Pullon, P. A.: Metastatic malignant melanoma of the tongue. Arch. Dermatol. 103:201, 1971.

47. Garrington, G. E., Scofield, H. H., Coryn, J., and Lacy, G. R.: Intraoral malignant melanoma in human albino. Oral Surg. 24:224, 1967.

48. Grinspan, D., Abulfia, J., Diaz, J., and Berdichesky, R.: Melanoma of oral mucosa. Oral Surg. 28:1, 1969.

49. Allen, A. C.: The Skin, 2nd Ed., p. 967. C. V. Mosby Co., St. Louis, 1967.

50. Principato, J. J., Sika, J. V., and Sandler, H. C.: Primary malignant melanoma of tongue: case report and review of literature. Cancer 18:1641, 1965.

51. Moore, E. S., and Martin, H.: Melanoma of upper respiratory tract and oral cavity. Cancer 8:1167, 1955.

52. Mesara, B. W., and Burton, W. D.: Primary malignant melanoma of upper respiratory tract. Cancer 21:217, 1968.

53. Shah, J. P., Huvos, A. G., and Strong, E. W.: Mucosal melanomas of the head and neck. Am J. Surg. 134:531, 1977.

54. Conley, J., and Pack, G. T.: Melanoma of the mucous membranes of the head and neck. Arch. Otolaryngol. 99: 315, 1974.

55. Barton, R. T.: Mucosal melanomas of the head and neck. Laryngoscope 85:93, 1975.

56. Freedman, H. M., DeSanto, L. W., Devine, K. D., and Weiland, L. H.: Malignant melanoma of the nasal cavity and paranasal sinuses. Arch. Otolaryngol. 97:322, 1973.

57. Zak, F. G., and Lawson, W.: The presence of melanocytes in the nasal cavity. Ann. Otol. 83:515, 1974.

58. Zak, F. G., and Lawson, W.: Studies on melanocytes III. Melanocytes in muscles of mastication. Mt. Sinai J. Med. 42:591, 1975.

59. Busuttil, A.: Dendritic pigmented cells within human laryngeal mucosa. Arch. Otolaryngol. 102:43, 1976.

60. Goldman, J. L., Lawson, W., and Zak, F. G.: The presence of melanocytes in the human larynx. Laryngoscope 82: 824, 1972.

61. Reed, W. B., and Sugarman, G. I.: Unilateral nevus of Ota with sensorineural deafness. Arch. Dermatol. 109:881, 1974.

62. Crone, R. P.: Malignant amelanotic melanomas of nasal septum and maxillary sinus. Laryngoscope 76:1826, 1966.

63. Walker, E. A., and Snow, J. B., Jr.: Management of melanoma of nose and paranasal sinuses. A.M.A. Arch. Otolaryngol. 89:652, 1969.

64. Holdcraft, J., and Gallagher, J. C.: Malignant melanomas of nasal and paranasal sinus mucosa. Ann. Otol. Rhinol. Laryngol. 78:5, 1969.

65. Gallagher, J. C.: Upper respiratory melanoma: pathology and growth rate. Ann. Otol. Rhinol. Laryngol. 79:551, 1970.

66. Shanon, E., Covo, J., and Loeventhal, M.: Neoplasm of epiglottis: case treated by supraglottic laryngectomy. A.M.A. Arch. Otolaryngol. 91:304, 1970.

67. Reid, J. D., and Mehta, V. T.: Melanoma of lower respiratory tract. Cancer 19:627, 1966.

68. Svane-Knudsen, V.: Primary malignant melanoma of tonsil. Acta Otolaryng. (Stockh.) 47:364, 1957.

69. Ravid, R. M., and Esteves, J. A.: Malignant melanoma of nose and paranasal sinuses and juvenile melanoma of nose. A.M.A. Arch. Otolaryngol. 72:431, 1960.

70. Harrison, D. F. N.: Malignant melanomata of nasal cavity. Proc. R. Soc. Med. 61:13, 1968.

71. Eneroth, C. -M., and Lundberg, C.: Mucosal malignant melanomas of the head and neck. With special reference to cases having a prolonged clinical course. Acta Otolaryngol. 80:452, 1975.

72. Harrison, D. F.: Malignant melanomata arising in the nasal mucous membrane. J. Laryngol. 90:993, 1976.

73. Conley, J., and Hamaker, R. C.: Melanoma of the head and neck. Laryngoscope 87:760, 1977.

74. Greene, G. W., Jr., and Bernier, J. L.: Primary malignant melanomas of parotid gland. Oral Surg. 14:108, 1961.

75. Baab, G. H., and McBride, C. M.: Malignant melanoma. The patient with an unknown site of primary origin. Arch. Surg. 110:896, 1975.

76. McGovern, V. J.: Spontaneous regression of melanoma. Pathology 7:91, 1975.

77. Hart, W. R.: Primary nevus of a lymph node. Am. J. Clin. Pathol. 55:88, 1971.

78. Ridolfi, R. L., Rosen, P. P., and Thaler, H.: Nevus cell aggregates associated with lymph nodes: estimated frequency and clinical significance. Cancer 39:164, 1977.

79. DasGupta, T., Bowden, L., and Berg, J. W.: Malignant melanoma of unknown primary origin. Surg. Gynecol. Obstet. 117:341, 1963.

80. Allen, A. C., and Spitz, S.: Malignant melanoma: clinicopathological analysis of criteria for diagnosis and prognosis. Cancer 6:1, 1953.

81. Kernen, J. A., and Ackerman, L. V.: Spindle cell nevi and epithelioid cell nevi (so-called juvenile melanomas) in children and adults. Cancer 13:612, 1960.

82. Weedon, D., and Little, J. H.: Spindle and epitheliod cell nevi in children and adults. A review of 211 cases of the Spitz nevus. Cancer 40:217, 1977.

83. Skov-Jensen, T., Hastrup, J., and Lambrethsen, E.: Malignant melanoma in children. Cancer 19:620, 1966.

84. Shanon, E., Samuel, Y., and Adler, A.: Malignant melanoma of the head and neck in children. Review of the literature and report of a case. Arch. Otolaryngol. 102:244, 1976.

85. McNeer, G., Das Gupta, T., and Stillbolt, D.: Local recurrences of melanomas after treatment: possible causes and suggested corrections. Plast. Reconstr. Surg. 37:204, 1966.

86. Goldsmith, H. S., Shah, J. P., and Kim, D. H.: Prognostic significance of lymph node dissection in treatment of malignant melanoma. Cancer 26:606, 1970.

87. Huvos, A. G., Shah, J. P., and Mike, V.: Prognostic factors in cutaneous malignant melanoma. A comparative study of long term and short term survivors. Hum. Pathol. 5:347, 1974.

88. Ironside, P., Pitt, T. T. E., and Rank, B. K.: Malignant melanoma: some aspects of pathology and prognosis. Aust. N. Z. J. Surg. 47:70, 1977.

89. Franklin, J. D., Reynolds, V. H., Bowers, D. G., Jr., and Lynch, J. B.: Cutaneous melanoma of the head and neck. Clin. Plast. Surg. 3:413, 1976.

90. Shah, J. P., and Goldsmith, H. S.: Dissection for malignant melanoma. Cancer 26:610, 1970.

91. Annotation: Regional lymph nodes in malignant melanoma. Lancet 1:1412, 1966.

92. Mundth, E. D., Guralnick, E. A., and Raker, J. W.: Malignant melanoma: clinical study of 427 cases. Ann. Surg. 162:15, 1965.

93. Donnellan, M. J., Seemayer, T., and Huvos, A. G.: Clinicopathologic study of cutaneous melanoma of the head and neck. Am. J. Surg. 124:150, 1972.

94. Simons, J. N.: Malignant melanoma of the head and neck. In Symposium on Malignancies of the Head and Neck. C. V. Mosby Co., St. Louis, 1975.

CHAPTER 23

Lymphoreticular Disorders

Contributed by BERTRAM SCHNITZER, M.D. and
DON K. WEAVER, M.D.

In many patients the presence of a lymphoretic-ular disorder above the clavicles is only one clinical manifestation, albeit often the presenting one, of a systemic disease. In practice, however, it is very difficult to assess the frequency of primary versus secondary lymphomas in the head and neck. Rosenberg et al.[1] found in 1,269 cases of malignant lymphoma that 8.9% of the lesions were first noted in this area of the body. Although difficulty with identifying primary involvement is a source of confusion, it is more than matched by the general misunderstanding and confusion that has "bedeviled the entire lymphoreticular system."[2] Studies continue to be hampered by a lack of agreement on such fundamental issues as terminology and definition of component tissues and cells.

CLASSIFICATION OF LYMPHOMAS

Malignant lymphomas may be defined as neo-plastic proliferations of the cells of the lymphoreticular system. They are divided into non-Hodgkin's lymphomas and Hodgkin's disease. The non-Hodgkin's lymphomas are classified both cytologically and according to their histological pattern.[3, 4] Cytologically, these lymphomas are classified as lymphocytic, well or poorly differentiated; as histiocytic (reticulum cell sarcoma); as mixed lymphocytic-histiocytic; or as undifferentiated, either of the Burkitt's type or of the non-Burkitt's type (Table 23.1). The histological pattern may be either diffuse (Fig. 23.1) or nodular (follicular) (Fig. 23.2). The importance of including the histological pattern in the diagnosis lies in the fact that a nodular lymphoma of a certain cytological type has a better prognosis than its diffuse counterpart. Three types of lymphomas may have a nodular pattern: poorly differentiated lymphocytic type, the histiocytic type, and the mixed lympho-cytic-histiocytic type. The poorly differentiated lymphocytic lymphoma and the mixed types are much more frequently seen with a nodular pattern than the histiocytic lymphoma. Although some lymphomas have a nodular growth pattern in the original lymph node biopsy, the pattern usually changes to the diffuse type during the course of the disease. This pattern change is often gradual and may not be complete for many years.[3, 5] The transition to the diffuse pattern is accompanied by a worsening of the prognosis.

Nodular lymphomas which are predominantly of the poorly differentiated lymphocytic and mixed types are seen slightly more often in females than in males[6] and are seen more often in patients over the age of 40. We have never seen a patient with nodular lymphoma under the age of 25 and only rarely below age 35. Clinically, nodular and diffuse non-Hodgkin's lymphomas are often disseminated at the time of diagnosis despite relatively mild or no symptoms.[7]

One of the most important and difficult differential diagnoses in lymph node pathology is between benign reactive follicular hyperplasia and nodular lymphoma. The criteria which aid in this differential diagnosis have been listed by Rappaport et al.[3] The most reliable distinguishing feature is the presence of phagocytic macrophages (tingible bodies) in the follicle center which characteristically lends a "starry sky" appearance to the reactive follicles. Other features characteristic of a benign reactive follicle include the sharp demarcation of the follicle center from the surrounding mantle of mature lymphocytes and the presence of many normal mitotic figures in reactive centers. In nodular lymphomas, phagocytic macrophages are absent, the delineation between cells of the neoplastic nodules and internodular cells may not be

Table 23.1
Classification of Non-Hodgkin's Lymphomas*

1. Lymphocytic, well differentiated
2. Lymphocytic, poorly differentiated†
3. Histiocytic†
4. Mixed (lymphocytic-histiocytic)†
5. Undifferentiated, Burkitt's type
6. Undifferentiated, non-Burkitt's type

* Modified from Rappaport.[4]
† Diffuse or nodular.

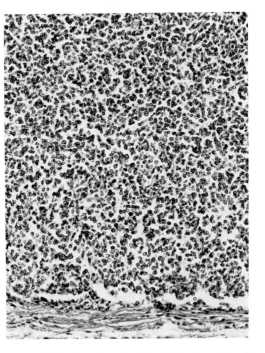

Figure 23.1. Lymph node with a *diffuse* type of malignant lymphoma. The normal architecture of the node is effaced by a uniform cellular proliferation.

as distinct, and fading of cells of the nodules into the internodular areas may be present. The number of mitotic figures in neoplastic nodules is usually smaller than in reactive follicles. The identification of cytologically malignant cells in the nodular aggregates is the most reliable way to diagnose nodular lymphomas. Although severe follicular hyperplasias which may resemble nodular lymphomas microscopically are commonly seen in lymph node biopsies in children, they are rarely seen in nodes of adults with the exception of two disorders; rheumatoid arthritis[8] and secondary syphilis.[9] In both these disorders, the microscopic picture may be identical. The feature distinguishing these two diseases from nodular lymphoma is the presence of many plasma cells between the large reactive follicles seen throughout both cortex and medulla of the nodes.

All cytological types of lymphomas may have a diffuse histological pattern. Some of the diffuse lymphomas may have evolved from nodular types. Histiocytic lymphomas are much more frequently seen with the diffuse than with the nodular pattern, in contrast to the poorly differentiated lymphocytic lymphoma, which, in the older age group, is seen with approximately equal frequency with the nodular and diffuse growth pattern.

Lymphomas may also be classified as lymph nodal or extranodal. Although most malignant lymphomas first present in lymph nodes, especially in lymph nodes of the neck, some, especially diffuse lymphomas, may be found in other lymphoreticular organs such as the spleen, Waldeyer's ring, gastrointestinal tract, bone marrow or thymus. Lymphomas occasionally present in tissue outside these major lymphoreticular organs and may be found in almost any site, attesting to the widespread distribution of the precursor cells of the lymphoreticular system. The undifferentiated lymphoma of Burkitt's type often presents and proliferates outside the lymphoreticular organs.[10]

Considerable overlap exists between some malignant lymphomas and leukemias. This is especially true of well differentiated lymphocytic lymphoma and chronic lymphocytic leukemia which are probably the same disease[11, 12] (vide infra). In contrast, poorly differentiated lymphocytic lymphoma becomes leukemic comparatively infrequently,[5] while the leukemic phase of histiocytic and undifferentiated lymphomas is rare.[13, 14] The poorly differentiated lymphocytic lymphomas of childhood, in contrast to the poorly differentiated lymphomas of adults, frequently terminate in leukemia.[15]

Recently, a number of new classifications of lymphomas based on immunological and functional studies have been proposed.[16–19] Although such studies have shown that some of our current concepts about the lymphoreticular system, about the terminology we use, and about our classifications of malignant lymphomas may be erroneous, at the time of this writing pathologists continue to use the current classifications because of their established clinical and prognostic value.

Well Differentiated Lymphocytic Lymphoma, Diffuse

Well differentiated lymphocytic lymphomas are comparatively rare. The well differentiated lymphocytes are cytologically indistinguishable from normal lymphocytes seen in tissue (Fig. 23.3). They are small to medium-sized with round or oval nuclei containing aggregated chromatin. Since these cells do not appear to be cytologically

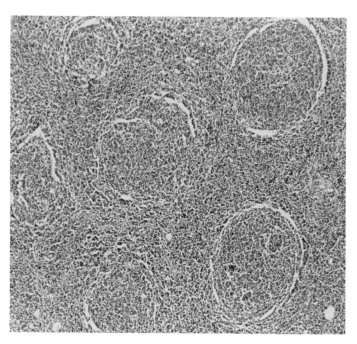

Figure 23.2. Lymph node with obliteration of the normal architecture and replacement by a *nodular* (follicular) type of lymphoma.

abnormal, a diagnosis of this lymphoma is made on the basis of the obliteration of the normal nodal architecture by a proliferation of uniform mature-appearing lymphocytes. The cells of this lymphoma do not aggregate into nodules.

Although often considered to be distinct entities, well differentiated lymphocytic lymphoma and chronic lymphocytic leukemia are closely related and probably represent the same disease.[10–12] When an enlarged lymph node is biopsied during the course of chronic lymphocytic leukemia, the histological appearance is that of a diffuse type of well differentiated lymphocytic lymphoma. At times, the diagnosis of lymphoma is made when lymph nodes are involved before lymphocytosis is present in the peripheral blood. Bone marrow and peripheral blood involvement (leukemia) usually ensue in the following months.

Thus, the leukemic phase of well differentiated lymphocytic lymphoma is the rule rather than the exception. The lymphocytes in the blood and bone marrow, as might be expected, are normal, mature-appearing cells. Well differentiated lymphocytic lymphoma, like chronic lymphocytic leukemia, is rare before the age of 40 and most frequently occurs after the age of 55.

Other disorders of lymphoproliferation which may closely resemble well differentiated lymphocytic lymphoma cytologically include Walden-strom's macroglobulinemia and related immu-nosecretory processes.[20, 21] These disorders should be thought of when the histological picture in a lymph node consists of a diffuse proliferation of uniform lymphoid cells and the patient does not have chronic lymphocytic leukemia, or when on careful microscopic examination, plasma cells and plasmocytoid cells are noted among mature-appearing lymphoid cells. A periodic acid-Schiff (PAS) reaction may reveal intranuclear and/or intracytoplasmic inclusions of PAS-positive im-munoglobulin which is produced by these cells.[21] A definitive diagnosis of Waldenstrom's macro-globulinemia, however, rests on the demonstration of a monoclonal increase of IgM immunoglobulin in the patient's serum.

Poorly Differentiated Lymphocytic Lymphoma

Poorly differentiated lymphocytic lymphomas are the most common of all non-Hodgkin's lym-phomas. The cells of this lymphoma are larger than those of the well differentiated lymphocytic type; the nuclei are pleomorphic, irregular and angulated, and commonly have nuclear clefts and indentations (Fig. 23.4). The nuclear chromatin is not conspicuously clumped, and nucleoli are seen in many of the cells. The histological pattern may be diffuse or nodular. At the time of the initial lymph node biopsy, this lymphoma is seen in its

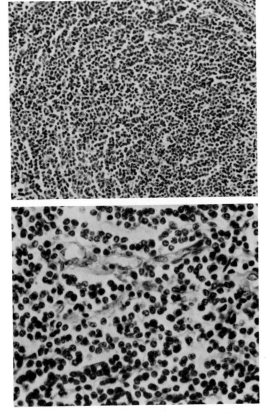

Figure 23.3. Lymphocytic lymphoma, well differentiated, diffuse. There is a diffuse monotonous proliferation of mature lymphocytes with round and regular nuclei which have coarse nuclear chromatin.

nodular form slightly more frequently than in its diffuse form. During the course of the disease, however, the nodular histological pattern often changes to a diffuse pattern, a change accompanied by a worsening of the prognosis.

In contrast to the frequent bone marrow and peripheral blood involvement by well differentiated lymphocytic lymphoma, the poorly differentiated lymphocytic lymphoma is infrequently leukemic. The bone marrow is more often infiltrated by lymphoma cells than is the peripheral blood. Bone marrow involvement is especially seen with the nodular pattern. When the lymphoma cells are found in considerable numbers in the peripheral blood, however, the term "lymphosarcoma cell leukemia" has been applied.[5] The leukemic phase of this lymphoma may be associated with either the nodular or diffuse histological pattern in the lymph node.[5]

In Wright's stained material, the nuclear chromatin of the lymphosarcoma cell or the poorly differentiated lymphocyte has a relatively coarse structure, a single, well defined nucleolus is frequently present, and the nucleus may be indented or clefted. This cell differs morphologically from the lymphoblast, whose nucleus is usually round or convoluted and whose chromatin structure is not clumped but rather finely reticulated. The poorly differentiated lymphocyte is not a typical blast cell, mature lymphocyte or prolymphocyte, but represents a neoplastic lymphocytic cell.[5]

Poorly differentiated lymphocytic lymphomas of childhood behave differently from these lymphomas in adults. In children, they tend to progress to leukemia and in the leukemic phase are indistinguishable from acute (lymphocytic) leukemia of childhood.[15]

Histiocytic Lymphoma

Histiocytic lymphomas are seen predominantly in adults, particularly in the older age group. Although they morphologically resemble normal tissue histiocytes, their derivation from histiocytes is doubtful. Recent immunological studies suggest that in many instances these cells are derived from B lymphocytes.[22, 23] Morphologically, the cells are larger than the cells in lymphocytic lymphomas.

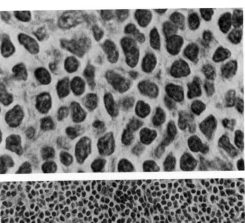

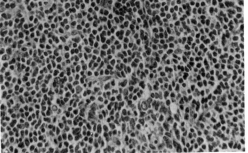

Figure 23.4. Lymphocytic lymphoma, poorly differentiated, diffuse. The neoplastic lymphocytes have pleomorphic, irregular and angular nuclei and scanty cytoplasm. Nucleoli are frequently seen.

Their nuclei are round or oval and vesicular, containing little aggregated chromatin, which is located beneath the nuclear membrane (Fig. 23.5). One or several large nucleoli are seen in most of these cells. The diffuse pattern is much more common than its nodular counterpart. Clinically, histiocytic lymphomas are aggressive and patient survivals are usually short.[15] Some of these neoplasms have very pleomorphic, bizarre and multinucleated giant tumor cells which occasionally resemble Reed-Sternberg cells. They may, therefore, be confused with Hodgkin's disease. Rarely, histiocytic lymphomas become leukemic, and when they do, they may resemble histiomonocytic leukemias.[13, 14]

Histiocytic lymphomas must be differentiated from cases of malignant histiocytosis[24] (histiocytic medullary reticulosis[25]). While histiocytic lymphomas grow in discrete masses, the cells in cases of malignant histiocytosis usually proliferate in sinuses of lymph nodes, splenic red pulp, bone marrow and liver. Evidence of erythrophagocytosis by the histiocytes is often seen in malignant histiocytosis but is not observed in histiocytic lymphoma.

Mixed (Lymphocytic-Histiocytic) Lymphoma

Mixed lymphocytic-histiocytic lymphoma is less frequent than the poorly differentiated lymphocytic and histiocytic lymphomas. It is composed of approximately equal numbers of poorly differentiated lymphocytes and histiocytes (Fig. 23.6). This lymphoma is seen more often in its nodular than in its diffuse pattern, which is rare. During the course of the disease, progression to the histiocytic type of lymphoma may be seen.

Undifferentiated Lymphoma, Burkitt's Type

Undifferentiated lymphomas of Burkitt's type are frequently seen in children (vide infra) and have distinctive cytological features.[10] They are termed undifferentiated because of the absence of cytological or cytochemical evidence of differentiation toward either lymphocytes or histiocytes. The cells are uniform, have a diameter ranging from 10 to 25 μm, and contain round to oval nuclei with coarsely clumped chromatin and clearly defined parachromatin (Fig. 23.7). One to four prominent nucleoli are present, and mitotic figures are frequently seen. The cytoplasm is strongly pyroninophilic and contains many small vacuoles which are best seen on Wright's stained imprints. These vacuoles contain neutral lipid. A so-called "starry sky" pattern due to the presence of benign macrophages scattered among the malignant cells is characteristic of Burkitt's tumor, but occasionally this pattern is absent. The starry sky pattern is not

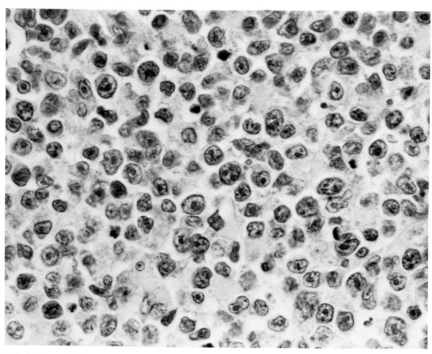

Figure 23.5. Histiocytic lymphoma, diffuse. The histiocytes are larger than poorly differentiated lymphocytes. The nuclei are round or oval and vesicular and contain one or more prominent nucleoli.

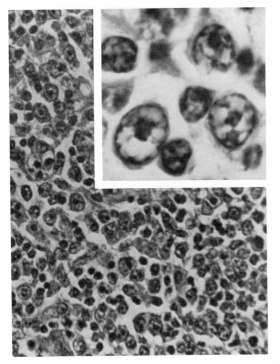

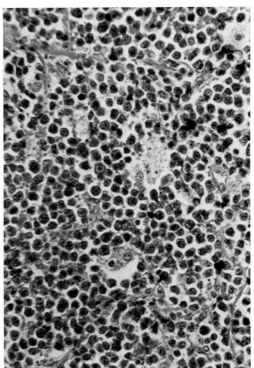

Figure 23.6. Mixed lymphocytic-histiocytic lymphoma. This lymphoma consists of approximately equal numbers of poorly differentiated lymphocytes and histiocytes.

Figure 23.7. Undifferentiated lymphoma, Burkitt's type. Two cell types are seen: the predominant cells with uniform nuclei and the benign macrophages. The combination produces a "starry sky" appearance.

restricted to Burkitt's tumor but may be seen in other rapidly proliferating lymphomas in children and adults. Extranodal involvement of this lymphoma is frequent (vide infra). Ultrastructural features of the Burkitt's cells include a cytoplasm containing many ribosomes which account for the pyroninophilia, as well as lipid inclusions in some of the cells (Fig. 23.8).

Undifferentiated, Non-Burkitt's Lymphoma

Lymphomas of the undifferentiated non-Burkitt's type are rare. Like the cells in Burkitt's lymphoma, the cells of the non-Burkitt's type do not show features of either lymphocytes or of histiocytes; in contrast to Burkitt's tumor, the cells are not monomorphic but show considerable pleomorphism of their nuclei.[15] Nucleoli are usually larger than those in the cells in Burkitt's lymphoma. This lymphoma, which is seen only in the diffuse form and most often in adults with nodal disease, has an unfavorable prognosis.

Staging of Non-Hodgkin's Lymphomas

Staging of malignant lymphomas is important in: (1) defining the extent of the disease; and (2)

determining the best course of therapy. Clinical and pathological staging classifications known as the Ann Arbor Staging Classification were established for Hodgkin's disease in 1971[26] (see Hodgkin's disease). The staging classifications take into account the presence of both nodal as well as extranodal involvement by the lymphoma. In contrast to Hodgkin's disease, extranodal involvement is much more frequent in non-Hodgkin's lymphomas at the time of the initial diagnosis, whereas in Hodgkin's disease, the process is usually limited to lymph nodes.[27] Involvement of Waldeyer's ring and the gastrointestinal tract is also more common in non-Hodgkin's lymphomas.

Although the value of staging laparotomy (pathological staging) has been proved for Hodgkin's disease, and a number of studies[28–31] have shown that the same staging classifications may be useful in disclosing occult sites of disease in non-Hodgkin's lymphomas, the clinical value of staging laparotomies in non-Hodgkin's lymphomas is uncertain at the time of this writing. Despite the fact that laparotomies have led to the discovery of a more advanced stage in many patients, it should

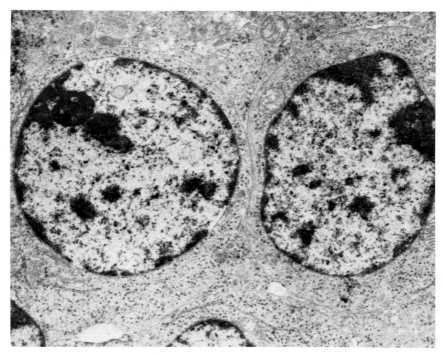

Figure 23.8. Electron micrograph of a Burkitt's lymphoma cell. The nucleus contains a prominent nucleolus and the cytoplasm is studded with many ribosomes.

be recognized that in many of these cases, the more advanced stage of the disease has not led to a change in the type or extent of therapy. A recent report by Johnson et al.[7] does not agree that the Ann Arbor Staging Classification is a "satisfactory guide to the management and prognosis of the non-Hodgkin's lymphomas"[29] and Chabner et al.[32] reported that the presence of disseminated non-Hodgkin's lymphoma can be detected in the majority of patients without the use of staging laparotomy.

Prognosis of Non-Hodgkin's Lymphomas

The factors important in influencing the prognosis of non-Hodgkin's lymphomas include: (1) the cytological classification; (2) the histological pattern (diffuse or nodular); and (3) the stage of the disease. In general, improved survival is seen for each cell type with the nodular rather than the diffuse pattern with the possible exception of the histiocytic type. The well differentiated lymphocytic lymphomas, even in their widespread leukemic stage (chronic lymphocytic leukemia), and the nodular, poorly differentiated lymphocytic lymphomas have the best prognosis among the lymphomas. Also, in contrast to the diffuse lymphomas, the prognosis of the nodular, poorly differentiated lymphocytic lymphoma is not poor despite the comparatively frequent involvement of

the bone marrow (stage IV) at the time of diagnosis. Prognosis of the diffuse lymphomas, the nodular histiocytic, and the nodular mixed lymphocytic-histiocytic lymphomas appears to be worse than that of the well differentiated and nodular, poorly differentiated lymphocytic lymphomas, their prognosis generally being less favorable in the more advanced stages.

Hodgkin's Disease

Hodgkin's disease was described by Thomas Hodgkin in 1832.[33] Although the cause of the disease is still not known there have been in recent years many advances in our understanding of the nature, diagnostic evaluation, clinical staging, histopathological classification, epidemiology, prognosis and therapy of Hodgkin's disease.

Hodgkin's disease affects individuals of all age groups. The age-specific incidence curves are generally bimodal, with one peak occurring in young adult life (15 to 35 years) and the other in old age.[34] Males are affected more often than females in all age groups. The disease is first detected primarily in the neck, especially in the supraclavicular or midcervical lymph nodes, although enlargement of nodes from the mastoid process to the clavicle may be seen. Extranodal origin of Hodgkin's disease appears to be much less frequent than such origin in other lymphomas.

The question of whether Hodgkin's disease is unicentric or multicentric in origin has not been answered, although Rosenberg and Kaplan[35] have provided evidence that most cases are unicentric in origin and that the pattern of spread of Hodgkin's disease is predictable. Smithers,[36] however, taking issue with this concept, hypothesizes that in early Hodgkin's disease a random pattern of involvement may exist, based on a varying lymph node susceptibility to an agent or agents which cause the disease. The origin might, therefore, be either unifocal or multifocal. In its later stages, Hodgkin's disease might spread like other tumors by metastases to nonlymphoid organs.[37, 38]

There is also a controversy about whether Hodgkin's disease is a single disease or whether it represents more than one disorder, perhaps with different potential etiological factors involved.[39, 40]

The proliferation of a single cell type, which is characteristic of other types of lymphomas, does not hold true for Hodgkin's disease. In addition to malignant cells, which are often in the minority and sometimes difficult to find in Hodgkin's disease, other apparently benign inflammatory cells, such as lymphocytes, eosinophils, plasma cells and benign-appearing histiocytes, make up the majority of the proliferating cells.

Staging of Hodgkin's Disease

New diagnostic and therapeutic measures during the past decade have drastically changed the prognosis of the disease. To determine whether a case of Hodgkin's disease is curable, it is imperative to determine accurately the extent of tumor involvement throughout the body. After a histological diagnosis of lymphoma is made, but before treatment is begun, a thorough search for occult neoplasm must be undertaken, particularly for occult tumor involvement of lymph nodes below the diaphragm, in the spleen, in the liver and in the bone marrow. After the extent of dissemination of Hodgkin's disease is thus established, the stage of the patient's disease is determined as a guide to the type and extent of therapy to be used.

The stage of the disease is also important in determining the prognosis.[41] Generally, stages I and II of Hodgkin's disease have a better prognosis than stages III and IV (vide infra). In addition to the stage, the histological subtype of Hodgkin's disease can have an important prognostic influence on survival, even within the same clinical stage.[42] The prognosis of Hodgkin's disease also appears to be related to the age and sex of the patient.

There have been many attempts at clinical classification of Hodgkin's disease. A significant modification of pre-existing classifications of Hodgkin's disease occurred in 1965 at the conference held in Rye, New York.[43] Further changes in the Rye Staging Classification were effected at the Symposium of Staging in Hodgkin's Disease held in Ann Arbor, Michigan (Table 23.2).[26] Two systems of classification were proposed at the latter conference: (1) clinical staging; and (2) pathological staging.

Clinical staging procedures include initial biopsy, history and physical examination, laboratory tests and radiographic studies.[26] The pathological stage adds histological diagnoses obtained at staging laparotomy. These staging procedures, thus, permit more precise comparison of data between various medical centers. They take into account both lymph nodal and extranodal involvement and, by means of subscripted symbols, indicate the tissue sampled and the results of the histological examination as either positive or negative for Hodgkin's disease (Table 23.2).

The Reed-Sternberg Cell

The Reed-Sternberg cell is a peculiar, giant, malignant-appearing cell which must be present for a diagnosis of Hodgkin's disease to be made. There are a number of variants of Reed-Sternberg cells, and at least one of these variants is essential for a diagnosis of Hodgkin's disease (Fig. 23.9). The Reed-Sternberg cells are large, with abundant cytoplasm which stains slightly eosinophilic or amphophilic. The nucleus is vesicular, the chromatin is condensed at the periphery beneath the nuclear membrane, and fine strands of chromatin may be seen radiating out from the nucleolus.[44] The nucleus may be bilobate, each lobe containing a large inclusion-like nucleolus, or there may be two nuclei within the cytoplasm, each nucleus again containing a large nucleolus. In addition, there are multinucleated Reed-Sternberg cells with two or more nuclei containing nucleoli. Mononuclear cells with the same cytological features are often present in Hodgkin's disease but are not diagnostic of the disease. These mononuclear cells may be related to or may actually represent early Reed-Sternberg cells. The diagnostic Reed-Sternberg cells may in fact be dead-end cells, incapable of dividing, whereas the mononuclear cells are known to be capable of further division.[45] Because morphologically similar or identical mononuclear cells may be seen in lymph nodes of patients with a number of different viral diseases, a diagnosis of Hodgkin's disease should never be made unless either bilobate, binucleate or multinucleate Reed-Sternberg cells are present.

Although Reed-Sternberg cells are essential for

Table 23.2
Pathological Staging Classification (Ann Arbor)*

Stage I

Involvement of a single lymph node region (I) or of a single extralymphatic organ or site (I_E).

Stage II

Involvement of two or more lymph node regions on the same side of the diaphragm (II) or localized involvement of extralymphatic organ or site and of one or more lymph node regions on the same side of the diaphragm (II_E). An optional recommendation is that the numbers of node regions involved be indicated by a subscript (e.g., II_3).

Stage III

Involvement of lymph node regions on both sides of the diaphragm (III), which may also be accompanied by localized involvement of extralymphatic organ or site (III_E) or by involvement of the spleen (III_S) or both (III_{SE}).

Stage IV

Diffuse or disseminated involvement of one or more extralymphatic organs or tissues with or without associated lymph node enlargement. The reason for classifying the patient as stage IV should be identified further by defining site by symbols.

Symbols for tissue sampled and results of histopathological examination:

N+ or N−

For another lymph node positive for disease or negative to biopsy

H+ or H−

For liver positive or negative by liver biopsy.

S+ or S−

For spleen positive or negative following splenectomy.

L+ or L−

For lung positive or negative by biopsy.

M+ or M−

For marrow positive or negative by biopsy or smear.

P+ or P−

For pleura involved or negative by biopsy or cytological examination.

D+ or D−

For skin involved or negative by biopsy.

Each stage will be subdivided into A and B categories, B for those with defined general symptoms and A for those without. The B classification will be given to those patients with: (1) unexplained weight loss of more than 10% of body weight in the 6 months previous to admission; (2) unexplained fever with temperature above 38°; and (3) night sweats.

* Applies only to patients at the time of disease presentation and before therapy is undertaken.

a diagnosis of Hodgkin's disease, Reed-Sternberg cells by themselves are not pathognomonic of Hodgkin's disease. Cells which are cytologically indistinguishable from the Reed-Sternberg cells in

Hodgkin's disease (Reed-Sternberg-like cells) have been reported in lymph nodes of patients with infectious mononucleosis,[46] with treated lymphocytic lymphoma and treated chronic lymphocytic leukemia,[47] with Burkitt's lymphoma,[48] and with other benign and malignant conditions.[49] Therefore, a diagnosis of Hodgkin's disease should be made only when Reed-Sternberg cells are found in an environment of cells characteristic of one of the histological types of Hodgkin's disease.

Histological Classification of Hodgkin's Disease

The diversity of the histological picture of Hodgkin's disease has led to numerous terms and unsatisfactory attempts at classification. In 1963 Lukes[50] and in 1966 Lukes et al.[51] published a morphological classification of Hodgkin's disease which was based on the predominant histological features and the relative frequency of the presence of lymphocytes, Reed-Sternberg cells and characteristic types of fibrosis. In their classification, which superceded that of Jackson and Parker,[52] Lukes and Butler[53] correlated the relationship between the histological type of Hodgkin's disease, the clinical stage of the disease and its prognosis. The most important contribution of this new classification was the emergence of the nodular sclerosis type of Hodgkin's disease as one of the three histological types into which the older heterogeneous "granuloma" group was split (Table 23.3). Nodular sclerosis is today the most frequent type of Hodgkin's disease. Mixed cellularity is next in frequency of incidence, while the third type separated from the old granuloma group, namely, the diffuse fibrosis type, is comparatively rare and belongs in the lymphocyte depletion type of the Rye Classification. The old paragranuloma group received the more descriptive name of lymphocytic and/or histiocytic Hodgkin's disease, and because of the predominance of lymphocytes in this type, it was named lymphocyte predominance at the Rye Conference. The old Hodgkin's sarcoma was called reticular Hodgkin's in the Lukes and Butler classification, and because of the paucity of lymphocytes, it is the lymphocyte depletion type in the Rye Classification. Nodular sclerosis and mixed cellularity retained their names in the Rye scheme.

Although the classification of Lukes and Butler[53] and its modification, the Rye classification,[54] have succeeded in subdividing the old granuloma group, they have also increased the difficulty in accurately diagnosing the histological types of this classification.[42] This is especially true of the Rye classification.

The general histological features of malignant

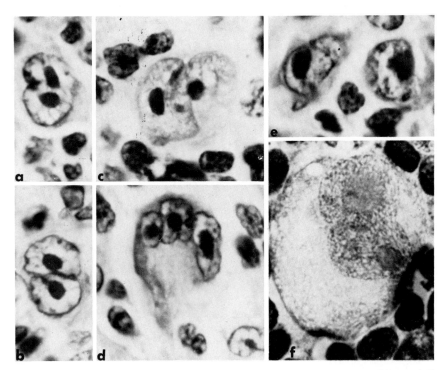

Figure 23.9. Reed-Sternberg cells. a, the nucleus consists of two lobes separated by a cleft, each lobe containing a prominent nucleolus; b and c, cells with two nuclei, each with a nucleolus; d, a multinucleated Reed-Sternberg cell; e, two reticular cells (these are not Reed-Sternberg cells); f, binucleated Reed-Sternberg cell.

Table 23.3
Histological Classification of Hodgkin's Disease

Jackson and Parker, 1947[52]	Lukes and Butler, 1966[50]	Rye, 1966[51]
Paragranuloma	Lymphocytic and/or histiocytic 1. Nodular 2. Diffuse	Lymphocyte pre-dominance
Granuloma	Nodular sclerosis Mixed	Nodular sclerosis Mixed cellularity
Sarcoma	{ Diffuse fibrosis Reticular }	Lymphocyte deple-tion

lymphomas, such as effacement of the normal architecture of the lymph node, also hold true for Hodgkin's disease. Less frequently, partial involvement of the node may be observed. The pertinent histological features of the different histological types of Hodgkin's disease are summarized in Table 23.4.

Lymphocytic and/or Histiocytic or Lymphocyte Predominance

The most common cell in lymphocyte predominance Hodgkin's disease is a mature-appearing lymphocyte. Varying numbers of benign histio-cytes may be scattered among the lymphocytes. These histiocytes are often seen in clusters and may resemble the aggregates of histiocytes of sarcoid. In some cases, histiocytes are rare or absent and the proliferation is purely lymphocytic. The lymphocytic cells have the appearance of normal, small, mature lymphocytes. The histiocytes have abundant, pale-staining cytoplasm and cytologically benign nuclei which may be folded or lobulated. Various mixtures of lymphocytes and histiocytes are seen in different cases. Eosinophils and plasma cells are rare or absent. The malignant cells (Reed-Sternberg cells) are usually rare and

Table 23.4
Histological Features of Hodgkin's Disease

Rye Classification	Pertinent Histological Features	Relative Prognosis
Lymphocyte pre-dominance	1. Many lymphocytes or a mixture of lympho-cytes and histiocytes 2. Few typical Reed-Sternberg cells 3. Absence of necrosis and fibrosis	Most favorable
Nodular sclerosis	1. Nodules of lymphoreticular cells partially or completely separated by bands of collagen 2. Many "lacunar cell" variants of Reed-Stern-berg cells	Favorable
Mixed cellularity	1. Mixture of cells including lymphocytes, eosin-ophils, plasma cells, and histiocytes 2. Many Reed-Sternberg cells 3. Foci of necrosis and fibrosis	Guarded
Lymphocyte deple-tion	1. Many Reed-Sternberg cells and malignant histiocytes or abundant fibrosis and hypocel-lularity 2. Few lymphocytes	Least favorable

difficult to find, and, at times, many sections must be examined before characteristic Reed-Sternberg cells are seen. A Reed-Sternberg cell variant with large, convoluted, twisted, overlapping nuclei with small nucleoli and a small amount of pale-staining cytoplasm is seen more frequently than the classical Reed-Sternberg cell. The histological pattern may be diffuse or less frequently nodular. In the latter form, the nodules are often poorly defined and the cellular proliferation is predominantly lymphocytic. Lymphocyte predominance is strongly associated with clinical stages I and II. It leads all other types of Hodgkin's disease in the number of patients surviving for periods of 5 to 10 years.[55, 56] This type of Hodgkin's disease may be histologically confused with well differentiated lymphocytic lymphoma. This is especially true when few Reed-Sternberg cells are present, and the proliferation is purely lymphocytic. A careful search for Reed-Sternberg cells should be carried out when the histological picture suggests well differentiated lymphocytic lymphoma in the absence of chronic lymphocyte leukemia. It should also be noted that well differentiated lymphocytic lymphomas or chronic lymphocytic leukemia are usually not seen in children or young adults, and a diagnosis of Hodgkin's disease in these young patients would be more likely. Lymphocyte predominance Hodgkin's disease must also be differentiated from Lennert's lymphoma (vide infra) and from toxoplasmosis lymphadenopathy.

Nodular Sclerosis

The typical histological picture of nodular sclerosis is characterized by bands of collagen which extend from the capsule into the lymph node and partially or entirely subdivide the node into cellular nodules of abnormal lymphoreticular tissue (Fig. 23.10). The second distinctive feature is the presence of large "reticular" cells with hyperlobulated nuclei surrounded by clear spaces or lacunae which are the result of fixation artefact. These cells are thought to be variants of Reed-Sternberg cells and are known as "lacunar" cells. The amount of collagen tissue may vary greatly from case to case and even in the same biopsy specimen. The collagen nature of the fibrous bands is confirmed by its birefringence in polarized light. In contrast, the fibrous tissue in the diffuse fibrosis type of Hodgkin's disease is not birefringent. Typical Reed-Sternberg cells may be difficult to find, but the variants of these cells are often numerous. The cellular proliferation within the nodules may be identical to that seen in the other types of Hodgkin's disease. There appears to be no relationship between the prognosis and the type of cellular proliferation in the nodules. The so-called "cellular phase" of nodular sclerosing Hodgkin's disease which was first described by Lukes et al.[51] and more recently publicized,[44, 57] may, in contrast to the typical nodular sclerosis, contain neither prominent nodules nor sclerosis (Fig. 23.11). It may represent the early form of nodular sclerosis and may consist only of clusters of lacunar cells, while the bands of collagen may be sparse or absent and the nodules, therefore, indistinct or lacking.

Nodular sclerosis is the most frequent type of Hodgkin's disease in most of the published series of cases using the new classifications of Hodgkin's disease. Nodular sclerosis is also the most frequent type of Hodgkin's disease in children.[58, 59] It is the only type of Hodgkin's disease which is seen more frequently in females, and it is the subtype with a distinctive pattern of anatomical distribution, often involving the lower cervical nodes and the

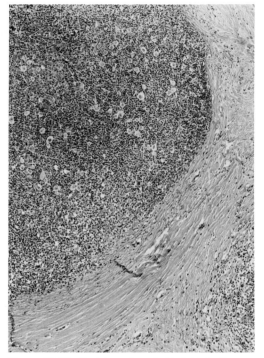

Figure 23.10. Nodular sclerosis Hodgkin's disease. The lymph node is divided into cellular nodules by bands of collagen. "Lacunar" variants of Reed-Sternberg cells are readily seen.

mediastinum.[60] It is most frequently in clinical stage II at the time of initial biopsy. In clinical stages I and II, the prognosis of the nodular sclerosis is the second best of all types of Hodgkin's disease.

Mixed Cellularity

As the name implies, this type of Hodgkin's disease is characterized by a mixture of cell types which include a variable number of lymphocytes, eosinophils, plasma cells, neutrophils and benign-appearing histiocytes (Fig. 23.12). Foci of necrosis and fibrosis may be present, but bands of collagen are absent. Reed-Sternberg cells and abnormal, malignant-appearing histiocytes are usually numerous and are readily found.

The mixed cellularity type of Hodgkin's disease is found in both males and females in all clinical stages without predilection for any one stage at the time of lymph node biopsy. Involvement below the diaphragm is noted to be more frequent with the mixed type than with the lymphocyte predominance or nodular sclerosis types when staging laparotomy is performed. Mixed cellularity type of Hodgkin's disease has the third best prognosis, generally falling between nodular sclerosis and lymphocytic depletion.

Mixed cellularity Hodgkin's disease must be differentiated from a recently described entity called immunoblastic[61] or angioimmunoblastic lymphadenopathy[62, 63] (vide infra). This latter disorder may closely resemble Hodgkin's disease histologically, but characteristic Reed-Sternberg cells are lacking.

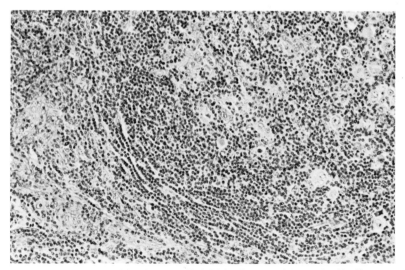

Figure 23.11. Cellular phase of nodular sclerosing Hodgkin's disease, characterized by lacunar cells, a scanty amount of vascular fibrous tissue and indistinct nodules. The lacunar cells are characteristic of nodular sclerosis.

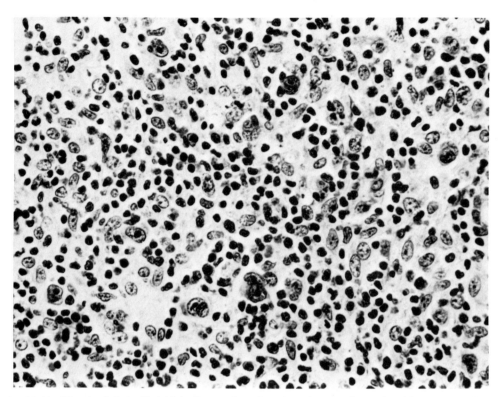

Figure 23.12. Mixed cellularity Hodgkin's disease. Lymphocytes, plasma cells, eosinophils, malignant histiocytes and Reed-Sternberg cells are seen.

Diffuse Fibrosis, Reticular Type or Lymphocyte Depletion

The diffuse fibrosis and reticular types (Fig. 23.13) have in common a depletion of lymphocytes and a proliferation of malignant histiocytes (reticular cells) and Reed-Sternberg cells. A disorderly fibrosis is the prominent feature in the diffuse fibrosis type, while a proliferation of reticular cells and Reed-Sternberg cells is characteristic of the reticular type. The diffuse fibrosis type may be composed mainly of a hypocellular amorphous material which is not birefringent, or there may be cellular fibroblastic areas. Focal cellular areas composed of malignant histiocytes and Reed-Sternberg cells are usually found. The reticular type has many bizarre large giant cells with prominent nucleoli, and fibrosis is either not prominent or is entirely absent. Focal areas of necrosis may be seen in both histological types. The lymphocytic depletion type of Hodgkin's disease is most often seen in stages III and IV at the time of initial lymph node biopsy and has the worst prognosis.

Malignant Lymphoma with a High Content of Epithelioid Histiocytes (Lennert's Lymphoma)

Malignant lymphoma with a high content of epithelioid histiocytes, also known as Lennert's lymphoma does not fit into any of the current lymphoma classifications. It was first described in 1968 by Lennert and Mestagh[64] who originally thought it represented a type of Hodgkin's disease in which Reed-Sternberg cells were absent or hard to find. Later, Lennert et al.[65] renamed this lymphoma "lymphoepithelioid cellular lymphoma" and no longer considered it to be a form of Hodgkin's disease. Clinically, this lymphoma is seen in elderly patients, and involvement of cervical lymph nodes and tonsils is often found. An allergic history is frequently noted.[66]

Histologically, the lymph node architecture is effaced by a proliferation of a mixture of cells, similar to that seen in Hodgkin's disease (Fig. 23.14). Characteristically, there is a prominent infiltration by epithelioid histiocytes in poorly circumscribed clusters or groups which vary in size

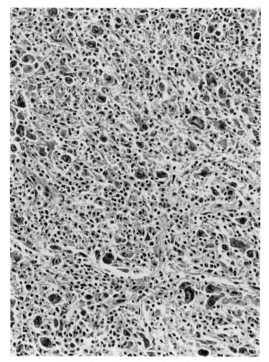

Figure 23.13. Lymphocyte depletion (reticular) Hodgkin's disease. Bizarre malignant histiocytes and Reed-Sternberg cells predominate. Relatively few lymphocytes are present.

from two to 20 cells (Fig. 23.14). In addition, there are lymphocytes with nuclei varying considerably in shape and containing aggregated chromatin. In some cases, varying numbers of plasma cells, immunoblasts, and eosinophils may be scattered among the lymphocytes and histiocytes. Occasional Langhans-type giant cells may be seen. Vascular proliferation is not a prominent feature, and mitoses are rare. Occasional cells resembling Reed-Sternberg cells may be found in some cases.

Although few cases of Lennert's lymphoma have been reported, it is quite likely that many cases of this disorder have been diagnosed as other lymphomas or as benign reactive lesions. The disorder histologically most closely resembling Lennert's lymphoma is Hodgkin's disease, especially lymphocytic and/or histiocytic (lymphocyte predominance) type. In the latter disorder, however, the nuclei of the lymphocyte are round or oval and do not vary in shape as much as do lymphocytes in Lennert's lymphoma. Clusters of histiocytes, however, may be seen in both disorders, and Reed-Sternberg cells may be very hard to find in lymphocyte predominance Hodgkin's

disease. When eosinophils and plasma cells are present, Lennert's lymphoma may resemble the mixed cellularity type of Hodgkin's disease. Reed-Sternberg cells, however, are readily found in this type of Hodgkin's disease. Lennert's lymphoma must also be differentiated from two non-neoplastic disorders, namely, from immunoblastic[61] or angioimmunoblastic[62, 63] lymphadenopathy and from toxoplasmosis lymphadenopathy.[67] In most instances, the numbers of immunoblasts, plasma and plasmacytoid cells are considerably smaller in Lennert's lymphoma than in immunoblastic disorders. Also, the prominent vascular proliferation and the deposits of interstitial PAS-positive amorphous material characteristic of immunoblastic lymphadenopathy are not seen in Lennert's lymphoma. In toxoplasmosis lymphadenopathy, the nodal architecture is maintained, follicle centers are often prominent, and ill-defined collections of epithelioid histiocytes encroach upon and are seen within some follicle centers as well as scattered throughout the node. Follicle centers are usually not seen in Lennert's lymphoma but when present, they are compressed and small.

Prognosis of Lennert's lymphoma is difficult to judge from the small series of cases observed. The 15 patients studied by Burke and Butler[66] fell into two groups: one had a limited response to treatment in which the time of survival ranged from 1 to 18 months, while the other group responded well to therapy. Whether Lennert's lymphoma is a variant of another disease, such as Hodgkin's disease or immunoblastic lymphadenopathy, or whether it is a separate and distinct entity awaits the results of investigation of additional cases.[66]

Immunoblastic or Angioimmunoblastic Lymphadenopathy

Immunoblastic[61] or angioimmunoblastic[62, 63] lymphadenopathy are closely related non-neoplastic lymphoproliferative or immunoproliferative disorders which may both clinically as well as histologically simulate malignant lymphomas, especially Hodgkin's disease. These disorders are seen most often in adults over the age of 50, but they have also been described in two patients under age 30. Clinically, there is often generalized or sometimes regional lymphadenopathy, fever, weight loss, rash, polyclonal hyperglobulinemia, and a Coombs-positive hemolytic anemia. When regional lymphadenopathy is the presenting sign, the cervical and supraclavicular lymph nodes are most frequently involved.

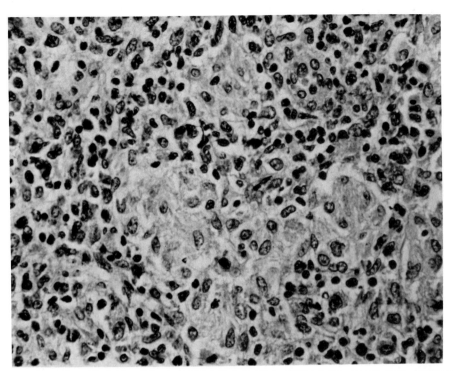

Figure 23.14. Lymphoepithelioid cellular lymphoma (Lennert's lymphoma). The lymph node architecture is effaced by a proliferation of a mixture of lymphocytes and benign-appearing histiocytes. The histiocytes are often arranged in clusters.

Morphologically, the disorders are characterized by: (1) proliferation of arborized vessels; (2) proliferation of immune-reactive cells (B lymphocytes) including lymphocytes, plasma cells, plasmacytoid cells, and immunoblasts (blastically transformed lymphocytes); and (3) deposits of acidophilic interstitial material (Figs. 23.15 and 23.16). Histiocytes and eosinophils are often present in variable numbers, imparting a mixed cellular proliferation which may closely resemble Hodgkin's disease, especially, the mixed cellularity type. It has been proposed that this abnormal cellular proliferation is triggered by a hypersensitivity reaction to therapeutic agents.[61] The disorders often become systemic, and histological evidence of involvement of a number of sites including spleen, liver, bone marrow, skin and lung has been noted.[61-63, 68]

Prognosis of these immune disorders is variable. The median survival of 18 fatal cases reported by Lukes and Tindle[61] was 15 months, while Frizzera et al.[63] were able to show two patterns of evolution of angioimmunoblastic lymphadenopathy: (1) long survival (24 to 67 months) with or without treatment; and (2) rapid progression (1 to 19 months) regardless of treatment.

In three cases of immunoblastic lymphadenopathy described by Lukes and Tindle[61] and in one of the cases observed by Schnitzer et al.,[68] transformation of the non-neoplastic immunoblastic lymphadenopathy into a malignancy of immunoblasts, namely, immunoblastic sarcoma, occurred. In our case, immunoblastic sarcoma was found only in the skin, while at necropsy, multiple sites of immunoblastic lymphadenopathy were also found. In contrast to the mixed cellular proliferation of immunoblastic lymphadenopathy, a monomorphous proliferation of immunoblasts which may focally, partially or completely replace the lymph node is seen in immunoblastic sarcoma.[61]

LYMPHOMAS OF THE HEAD AND NECK

It is difficult to determine the actual frequency of primary lymphoma in extranodal sites in the head and neck. The terms "primary" lymphomas or lymphomas "arising in" certain extranodal structures are usually not warranted because of insufficient evidence of the absence of nodal or extranodal involvement elsewhere with secondary spread to structures of the head and neck. In most of the reports of lymphoma of the head and neck,

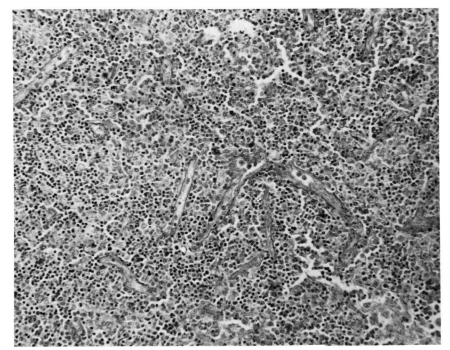

Figure 23.15. Paracortical region of lymph node from a patient with immunoblastic lymphadenopathy showing proliferation of branching vessels.

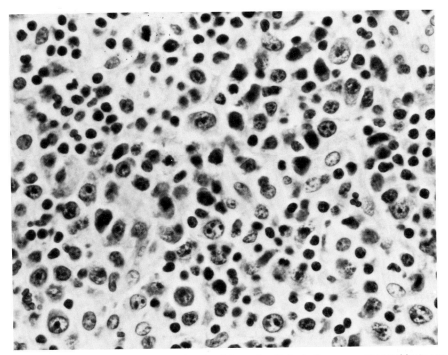

Figure 23.16. Immunoblastic lymphadenopathy. A mixture of cells including many immunoblasts are present between branching vessels in the cortical region of the lymph node.

modern methods of detection of occult disease below the diaphragm (lymphangiography and laparotomy) have not been used; thus, the extent of the tumor has not been adequately assessed. Banfi et al.,[69] who evaluated 225 patients with lymphoma and "primary" involvement of Waldeyer's ring, were able to demonstrate in 151 cases (without lymphangiography) that 22.5% of cases of lymphoma were apparently confined to Waldeyer's ring; in 62.3%, the tumor involved also the cervical nodes; and distant nodes were involved in addition to Waldeyer's ring in 15.2%. In the 74 cases in which lower limb lymphangiography was performed, cases in which lymphoma was apparently confined to Waldeyer's ring fell to 13.5%; 41.9% also had cervical node involvement, and 44.6% had involvement of distant nodes. It is possible that additional cases had occult nodal and extranodal involvement which were not seen on lymphangiography.

One should be aware of certain difficulties encountered in the diagnosis of lymphomas of the head and neck region, especially in the area of Waldeyer's ring where considerable and variable amounts of lymphoid tissue are normally present. As with submandibular lymph nodes, which we recommend not biopsying when other nodes are enlarged because they drain regions of frequent infections and, therefore, often show an atypical hyperplasia which may simulate lymphoma, the lymphoreticular tissue of Waldeyer's ring may also undergo similar atypical lymphoma-like reactive changes possibly leading to a misdiagnosis of lymphoma. One should use extreme caution in diagnosing lymphomas in these extranodal sites (as well as in other parts of the body, such as the gastrointestinal tract, orbit and lung) when regional lymph nodes are not enlarged and involved.

Another difficulty we have encountered in evaluating extranodal biopsies, especially from Waldeyer's ring, is related to the nature of the biopsy. Biopsies from tonsils or nasopharynx are often small and sometimes partly crushed and, thus, become extremely difficult to evaluate. On several occasions we have seen small tonsillar biopsies which were histologically indistinguishable from lymphocytic lymphomas, but because of the size of the biopsy we did not feel justified in making a diagnosis of malignancy. Subsequent removal of these tonsils revealed a typical picture of reactive hyperplasia. The biopsy had been taken from an interfollicular region in which there was a diffuse proliferation of lymphocytes. Tonsillectomy rather than a punch biopsy is preferred in middle-aged or elderly individuals with unilateral enlargement

of the tonsil. Biopsies inadequate for proper evaluation, therefore, constitute a major hazard in the diagnosis of lymphomas from this region. Because of the frequent minor infections of the upper respiratory tract which result in repeated stimuli to and reactive hyperplasias in the lymphoid tissue in this region, it should be remembered that atypical reactive changes, particularly when seen in small tissue biopsies, should be interpreted carefully. The presence of a mixture of cells, including plasma cells which are often seen in the region of Waldeyer's ring, usually points toward a benign reactive process.

After lymph nodes, the most frequent sites of involvement by lymphoma of the head and neck are the structures of Waldeyer's ring. The tonsils are most often involved, followed by the nasopharynx and the lymphoid tissue of the base of the tongue, which is the least frequent site of primary involvement by lymphoma. Grossly, these lesions most commonly appear as exophytic, smooth, submucosal and nonulcerative.[70] The exact site of origin from Waldeyer's ring is often difficult to determine because of the large size and the extent of involvement of the lesions, especially in the tonsil and tongue areas. In contrast to these two zones where the lesions may remain asymptomatic and permit larger growths of tumor, in the nasopharynx symptoms generally related to the ear usually lead to early detection of the tumor when it is still fairly small. Most of the patients with lymphoma involving the pharynx are in the fifth to eighth decade of life.

Lymphoma in Waldeyer's ring is, in most cases, not confined to that one area. The majority of patients have involvement of cervical lymph nodes, and, as in other lymphomas, occult disease below the diaphragm is not infrequently found. In a considerable number of cases, extranodal lymphoma, especially lymphoma of the gastrointestinal tract, is associated with "primary" involvement of Waldeyer's ring. Less frequent sites of lymphoma of the head and neck include the soft palate, oropharynx, pharyngeal wall, larynx, major and minor salivary glands, oral cavity, jaws and muscles of the head and neck, orbit, paranasal sinuses, nasal cavity, thyroid, scalp and lips. Generalized lymphomas involving the ear and temporal bones,[71] the facial nerve, the hypotympanum and the mastoid air cells[72] have been reported.

The majority of cases of extranodal lymphomas of the head and neck are histiocytic lymphomas and lymphocytic lymphomas of the diffuse type. Involvement of extranodal sites of the head and neck by Hodgkin's disease is rare, which is in keeping with lymphomas in other regions where the non-Hodgkin's lymphomas are much more frequently extranodal than are those of Hodgkin's disease type. Kadin et al.[73] found Hodgkin's disease involving Waldeyer's ring in only one of 117 patients studied. In contrast, Todd et al.[74] reported 16 patients with Hodgkin's disease involving Waldeyer's ring. Eight had disease of the nasopharynx, seven of the tonsil and one of the posterior pharyngeal wall. Four of the cases in which the tonsils were involved, however, appear to be examples of a non-Hodgkin's lymphoma, namely, Lennert's lymphoma (see page 460).

Nodular lymphomas are also comparatively rare in extranodal sites of the head and neck. In a study of 153 cases of lymphomas of the head and neck, 100% of cases of Hodgkin's disease and 91% of cases of nodular lymphoma were found to be within cervical lymph nodes but not in extranodal sites.[75] In contrast, lymphocytic lymphoma and histiocytic lymphoma were found in extranodal sites of the head and neck in 67 and 58% of cases.

Most of the patients with lymphoma limited to the head and neck can be treated with radiotherapy, usually megavoltage radiotherapy. Details of radiation therapy are reported by Fuller[76] and Wang.[70] Chemotherapy is the treatment of choice in patients with disseminated lymphoma. Surgery is reserved for carefully selected situations and often only as an adjunct to radiation therapy. Catlin[77] reported that operations were performed upon 36% of 249 of his patients for either curative, palliative or diagnostic purposes. Catlin[77] lists five of the more common and important indications for surgery of head and neck lymphomas: (1) bulky nodes limited to one side of the neck; (2) multiple localized thyroid and parotid gland tumors; (3) infection and/or obstruction caused by tumors involving the nasal cavity and paranasal sinuses; (4) residual lymphoma which failed to respond to radiation therapy; (5) inability to establish a diagnosis despite previous biopsies.

EVOLVING CLASSIFICATIONS OF LYMPHOMAS

The morphological classification of non-Hodgkin's lymphomas proposed by Rappaport et al.[3, 4] which was discussed earlier in this chapter, is based on the cytological characteristics of the neoplastic cells and on their architectural arrangement. The nuclear size and configuration are the criteria used to separate these cells into the various cytological groups. Despite the fact that Rappaport's classification is the only one at the present

time that is known to correlate with prognosis and to work in clinicopathological studies,[29] it was proposed before the rapid advances in experimental immunology and it has been shown to be scientifically incorrect.[19, 23, 29, 65, 78, 79] In addition to objections to terminology in this classification scheme, such as the use of the term "histiocytic" for cells of lymphoid rather than of "true" histiocytic (macrophage) origin, there are more important criticisms, namely, that most of the cytological types in Rappaport's scheme are heterogeneous and consist of a number of distinctive cell types when classified according to the new functional classification of Lukes and Collins[19] (vide infra). Thus, included within the category of poorly differentiated lymphocytic lymphoma of Rappaport's[3, 4] scheme are two immunomorphological types of lymphoma with widely different behavior, response to therapy and prognosis. These are the small cleaved follicle center cell lymphoma, which is generally associated with a good prognosis, and the convoluted cell lymphoma (both from the classification of Lukes and Collins),[19] which has a poor prognosis. At least five different lymphomas in the classification of Lukes and Collins (large cleaved and noncleaved follicle center cell lymphomas, immunoblastic sarcoma of B- or T-cell type, and a lymphoma of true histiocytes)[19] might be included within the histiocytic group of Rappaport's scheme. Some of the insufficiencies of Rappaport's classification, however, have been corrected by the addition of four new categories[80]: namely, (1) malignant lymphoma, lymphoblastic; (2) Burkitt's lymphoma; (3) mycosis fungoides; and (4) malignant lymphoma, immunoblastic (Table 23.5). Lymphoblastic lymphoma, which corresponds to the convoluted cell lymphoma of Lukes and Collins, therefore, has been taken out of the category of poorly differentiated lymphocytic lymphoma, and Burkitt's tumor, which is known to be a B-cell neoplasm with distinctive clinicopathological features, is categorized all by itself. Mycosis fungoides is recognized as a T-cell lymphoma which originates in the skin, and the term "immunoblastic lymphoma" is reserved for a neoplasm of large lymphoid cells with plasmacytoid features arising in pre-existing immunoproliferative processes.

Although one or the other of these "modern" classification schemes may in the future supplant the morphological scheme of Rappaport, at the time of this writing, there have been no comprehensive clinicopathological studies of any of the newly proposed classifications, and it has not been determined whether any of these classifications

Table 23.5
New Classifications of Lymphomas

Lukes and Collins[19,82] (1974; 1977)	Kiel[18] (1974)	Dorfman[17] (1974)	Bennett, Farrer-Brown, Henry, and Jelliffe[16] (1974)	W.H.O.[81] (1976)	Rappoport[80] (1977)
U-cell (undefined) T-cell 　Small lymphocyte 　Convoluted lympho-cyte 　Sezary cell—mycosis fungoides 　Immunoblastic sar-coma 　Lennert's lymphoma B-cell 　Small lymphocyte 　Plasmacytoid lympho-cyte 　Follicular center cell (follicular or diffuse with or without sclerosis) 　　Small cleaved 　　Large cleaved 　　Small transformed (noncleaved) 　　Large transformed (noncleaved) 　Immunoblastic sar-coma 　Hairy cell leukemia Histiocytic	Low-grade malignancy 　Malignant lymphoma (ML)—lymphocytic (CLL and others) 　ML—lymphoplasmacy-toid (immunocytic) 　ML—centrocytic 　ML—centroblastic-cen-trocytic: follicular* follicular* and diffuse diffuse* High-grade malignancy 　ML—centroblastic 　ML—lymphoblastic Burkitt's type Convoluted-cell type Others 　ML—immunoblastic	Follicular lymphomas† (Follicular or follicular and diffuse) 　Small lymphoid 　Mixed small and large lymphoid 　Large lymphoid Diffuse lymphomas† 　Small lymphocytic 　Atypical small lymphoid 　Lymphoblastic Convoluted Nonconvoluted 　Large lymphoid 　Mixed small and large lymphoid 　Histiocytic 　Burkitt's lymphoma 　Mycosis fungoides 　Undefined	Follicular lymphomas 　*Grade 1* 　Follicle cell, predomi-nantly small 　Follicle cell, mixed small and large 　Follicle cell, predomi-nantly large Diffuse lymphomas 　Lymphocytic, well differ-entiated (small round lymphocyte) 　Lymphocytic, intermedi-ate differentiation (small follicle cell) 　*Grade 2* 　Lymphocytic, poorly dif-ferentiated 　Mixed small lymphoid and undifferentiated large cell 　Undifferentiated large cell 　Plasma cell 　True histiocyte 　Unclassified Plasmacytoid differentia-tion in lymphocytic tumors and banded or line sclerosis are recorded.	Lymphosarcomas 　Nodular lymphosar-coma 　Prolymphocytic 　Prolymphocytic, lym-phoblastic 　Diffuse lymphosarcoma 　Lymphocytic 　Lymphoplasmacytic 　Prolymphocytic 　Lymphoblastic 　Immunoblastic 　Burkitt's tumor Mycosis fungoides Plasmacytoma Reticulosarcoma Unclassified malignant lymphomas	Malignant lymphomas　Well differentiated lymphocytic Poorly differentiated lymphocytic‡ Mixed cell‡ Histiocytic lym-phoma‡ Undifferentiated lymphoma Burkitt's lymphoma Lymphoblastic lym-phoma Mycosis fungoides Immunoblastic lym-phoma

* With or without sclerosis.

† Composite lymphomas, comprising two well defined and apparently different types of lymphoma within the same tissue; lymphomas associated with sclerosis; lymphomas showing plasmacytoid differentiation; and those diffuse lymphomas associated with epithelioid cells are suitably designated.

‡ Nodular and diffuse.

will be useful or as useful as its predecessor in predicting the course and prognosis of non-Hodgkin's lymphomas. It is important, however, for physicians to keep abreast of the new terminologies and classifications and to understand the basis for these classifications. Therefore, we will briefly discuss some of the new classifications, concentrating on the scheme of Lukes and Collins.[19]

New Classifications

In recent years, there has been a rash of publications proposing new classification schemes for non-Hodgkin's lymphomas (Table 23.5). These include: (1) the Kiel classification in Germany[18]; (2) the classification of Bennett et al.[16] in Great Britain; and (3) in the United States, the classifications of Lukes and Collins[19] as well as (4) that of Dorfman.[17] Another scheme has more recently been published by the World Health Organization,[81] and Rappaport has expanded his classification scheme.[80]

Lukes and Collins Classification[19, 82] (Table 23.5). This revolutionary functional classification is based on the relationship of malignant lymphomas to the T and B systems of lymphocytes and on the alterations observed in lymphocyte transformation.[19] Thus, lymphomas are classified on the basis of immunological markers, and the B and T nature of these neoplasms can be recognized on morphological grounds.[82, 83]

Although small lymphocytes are morphologically homogeneous, they are functionally heterogeneous; i.e., they are made up of two functionally separate cell types, namely, the T lymphocytes which are responsible for cell-mediated immunity, or the B lymphocytes, the precursors of plasma cells, which provide humoral immunity.[84, 85] The localization and traffic of these two groups of lymphocytes also differ.[86, 87] T-cells are found chiefly in the paracortical area of lymph nodes and in the periarterial lymphoid sheath of the spleen, while B-cells populate predominantly the follicle centers and medullary cords of lymph nodes and the follicle centers of the white pulp of the spleen.[87] These lymphocytes, which also circulate in the blood, "home" to these anatomical regions in the lymph nodes and spleen, and their circulatory pathways may be mimicked by the cells of some of the lymphomas, thereby giving an insight into the manner in which these disorders spread.[88]

Most lymphomas are B-cell neoplasms, and the majority arise in follicle centers.[89, 90] These follicle center cell (FCC) lymphomas mimic their normal counterparts in the follicle center and are classified, like them, into small and large cleaved and noncleaved (transformed) FCC types.[19] Each of these cytological types may have a diffuse, follicular or diffuse and follicular pattern. In general, the cleaved FCC lymphomas are slow growing, have a follicular or partly follicular pattern, and have a better prognosis than lymphomas of the noncleaved cells. The latter tend to be diffuse, rapidly growing, aggressive neoplasms associated with a poor prognosis. The cleaved cells correspond to the poorly differentiated lymphocytic lymphoma of the traditional classification, while the small noncleaved or transformed FCC lymphomas correspond to the undifferentiated type of Burkitt's or non-Burkitt's lymphoma of the modified Rappaport scheme.[80] The large noncleaved FCC lymphomas correspond to the histiocytic lymphomas of the traditional classification. The small lymphocyte lymphoma, which may arise from the lymphocytes surrounding the follicle center (Table 23.6), corresponds to the well differentiated lymphocytic lymphoma or chronic lymphocytic leukemia of Rappaport's scheme, while the plasmacytoid lymphocyte lymphoma corresponds

Table 23.6
Transformation of B Lymphocytes (Modified from Lukes and Collins[19])

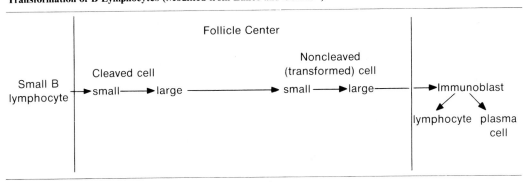

to Waldenstrom's macroglobulinemia or to lymphomas with Ig monoclonal gammopathies. Immunoblastic sarcoma of B-cells is a neoplasm of transformed follicle centers cells (Table 23.6). It is usually diffuse and the cells often exhibit plasmacytoid features.[19, 82] This is an aggressive neoplasm in which mitotic figures are numerous, and it is often seen in chronic abnormal immune states such as in immunosuppressed patients, in patients with Hashimoto's disease, Sjögren's syndrome, Waldenstrom's macroglobulinemia, rheumatoid arthritis, lupus erythematosus, and in patients with immune deficiency diseases. These neoplasms were often included with histiocytic lymphomas in Rappaport's classification. Lukes and Collins[82] have also included hairy cell leukemia among B-cell lymphomas, since the weight of evidence is now in favor of a lymphocytic origin rather than a monocytic-histiocytic origin of this disorder.

Classified under the T-cell lymphomas is the convoluted lymphocytic type described by Barcos and Lukes.[91] The same or a closely related disorder is called lymphoblastic lymphoma by Nathwani et al.[92] This neoplasm is believed to arise from immature lymphocytes of the thymus and is characteristically seen in children and young adults. Patients often present with a rapidly enlarging neoplasm of the mediastinum. Initially, the tumor is highly responsive to radiation and corticosteroid therapy. After several weeks or months a leukemic phase develops. Central nervous system relapse may occur. This lymphoma was usually classified as a poorly differentiated lymphocytic lymphoma in Rappaport's scheme. Mycosis fungoides and Sezary's syndrome, which may be considered to be the leukemic phase of mycosis fungoides, are cutaneous T-cell lymphomas.[24] The cells of these disorders characteristically have highly convoluted nuclei, and involve the papillary dermis and the epidermis. Pautrier abscesses are characteristic of this disease.[92, 93] In addition, spread to lymph nodes and viscera occurs. Early nodal involvement may be detected in the paracortical (T-cell) region. Sezary's syndrome has been shown to be a neoplasm of helper T lymphocytes.[94] The small lymphocyte lymphoma of T-cells is cytologically similar to its B-cell counterpart, although the nuclei of the cells may be more irregular. Immunoblastic sarcomas of T-cells exist but are difficult to diagnose on morphological grounds alone. The nuclei of these cells show a wide range of sizes, and the abundant cytoplasm exhibits less pyroninophilia than does the immunoblastic sarcoma of B-cells. The cells also do not show the plasmacytoid features of the B-cell neoplasm. Finally, Lennert's lymphoma (malignant lymphoma with a high content of epithelioid histiocytes) which is characterized by lymphocytes which have irregularly shaped but noncleaved nuclei and are associated with a large epithelioid component has been shown to be a T-cell neoplasm.[82, 90, 95]

Undefined cell lymphoma is a term reserved for those lymphomas which, with our present techniques show no surface markers. Many cases of acute lymphoblastic leukemia are placed into this category.[82]

Histiocytic lymphomas are neoplasms of true histiocytes and are very rare. They may be identified cytochemically by their positive alpha-naphthylbutyrate esterase reaction, and they fail to form E rosettes (T-cell marker) or produce surface immunoglobulin (B-cell property).[82]

Other Classifications. The Kiel classification[18] like that of Lukes and Collins[19] also used a functional approach. Although the classifications of these two schemes are similar, the terminologies of each differ. The centrocytic cells correspond to the cleaved cells, and the centroblasts are called noncleaved cells in the Lukes and Collins' classification.[19] The lymphomas of the Kiel scheme are divided into low- and high-grade malignancies (Table 23.5).

The terminology of both the Bennett et al.[16] classification and that of Dorfman,[17] is descriptive and, therefore, easier for pathologists to understand and apply to their diagnostic work.

The International Histological Classification (WHO)[81] resurrects such terms as "lymphosarcoma" and "reticulosarcoma" and also uses some of the new terms. Confusion will undoubtedly arise over the term "prolymphocytic" which is used for a recently described leukemia[31] different from the leukemic phase of nodular, poorly differentiated lymphocytic leukemia.

BURKITT'S TUMOR

In 1968 Burkitt[96] first called attention to the large number of malignant lymphomas in African children who presented with a lesion in the jaw and later progressed to a generalized, yet aleukemic, disease. Since then, a surfeit of information has confused as well as clarified this unusual neoplasm.

It is now abundantly clear that Burkitt's lymphoma cannot be regarded as an exclusively African disease but is indeed worldwide. Burkitt[97] himself has summarized the evidence on the occurrence and prevalence of the disease outside Africa. Nevertheless, it is still reasonable to distinguish geographic areas where the disease is endemic from those in which only sporadic cases occur. In this regard, "the lesion stands like a Colossus among tumors of the jaw in tropical Africa" and is the most common tumor in childhood in Uganda.[92]

A memorandum from the World Health Organization[99] has summarized the important clinical and gross pathological features of this neoplasm. Although many of the clinical features of Burkitt's tumor, particularly the anatomical presentation and distribution, tend to be characteristic, none is pathognomonic. The principal clinical and gross anatomical features characterizing the lesions are as follows. (1) Although predominantly a tumor of childhood, the disease may occur in any age group, and this aspect is manifested most often in non-African cases. (2) If untreated, the disease runs a rapidly fatal course. (3) The disease is usually multifocal and predominantly extralymphnodal with involvement of one or more of the following sites: abdominal and/or pelvic viscera, retroperitoneal soft tissues, facial bones and/or long bones, thyroid gland, salivary glands and central nervous system.

Retroperitoneal masses and nodular involvement of the viscera are found in virtually all cases, even when the jaw lesions are the dominant manifestation. The frequency of jaw tumors as indicated above is definitely related to the age of the host. The apparent lower incidence of jaw tumors in the reports from North America may reflect either this age difference or may possibly be related to a greater susceptibility of the jaws of Africans to tumor growths. A comparison of African and American Burkitt's lymphoma is presented in Table 23.7.[100, 101]

The kidneys, liver, endocrine glands and gonads are frequently involved. Bilateral ovarian tumors in females at all ages are a particularly characteristic feature of the disease, as are massive bilateral breast tumors in premenopausal women. Gonadal involvement is always bilateral, symmetrical and diffuse, and it obliterates the normal architecture. Nodular deposits in the epicardium and myocardium are not infrequent.

There is a conspicuous sparing of the peripheral lymph nodes in most cases, and splenic involvement is uncommon. Generalized peripheral lymphadenopathy is rare, and mediastinal node involvement is likewise uncommon. Involvement of Waldeyer's ring is rare in cases of Burkitt's tumor in Africa but has been reported in the United States and England.

Paraplegia may be a presenting sign of Burkitt's tumor. This is the result of either meningeal involvement with cord compression or infarction of the lower thoracic cord secondary to neoplastic obstruction of the blood supply. Involvement of the meninges, base of brain, cranial nerves and

Table 23.7
Burkitt's Lymphoma: American versus African Types

	American Cases	African Cases
Age (years)	12.2 (mean)	9.1 (mean)
Sites of involvement	Abdominal predominance; jaw relatively uncommon	Jaw predominance in young; abdominal predominance in older patients
Epidemiology		
1. Time-space cluster	Yes	Yes
2. Absence of high altitude cases	Yes	Yes
3. Relation to EBV* antibody titer	Higher than controls; not as high as African	Elevated
4. EBV genome in tumor	Not detected with certainty. Some tumors contain EBV.	Detected in most cases
Therapeutic response	Good response to early high dose of cyclophosphamide	Same
Relapse patterns	Late relapse not yet observed	Two patterns 1. Early, resistant to further treatment 2. Late, response to further treatment comparable to previously untreated patients

* EBV, Epstein-Barr virus.

even central nervous system tissue has been recognized with increasing frequency. Although nodular marrow involvement is frequently seen in bones, diffuse infiltration or replacement is uncommon except as a terminal or preterminal event. The process appears to be aleukemic in most cases.

All reports clearly indicate that the neoplasm affects the jaws in a high proportion of cases, and it is the jaw lesion that has been most characteristic. The frequency ranges from 50% of cases in highly endemic regions (such as tropical Africa) to 15% in areas where it is rarely encountered (such as the United States). Involvement of the jaws may follow or be succeeded by the clinical appearance of tumors elsewhere. Involvement of other bones is never as frequent as the jaws. This tumor affinity for the jaws and facial bones is unusual in view of the paucity of marrow in these bones relative to the cranium, which is rarely involved. The incidence of jaw involvement is highest at age 3 years and thereafter drops steadily. It is distinctly uncommon in subjects over 15 years of age.

According to Adatia,[102] involvement of the jaws in Uganda is almost invariably posterior at the onset and is more often in the maxilla than the mandible in about a 2:1 ratio. When more than one quadrant is affected, simultaneous deposits in all four quadrants are the most common clinical finding. The next most common combination is a tumor in the ipsilateral maxilla and mandible.

In the majority of patients with jaw lesions, the initial features are intraoral. Loosening of the deciduous molar and premolar teeth is followed by expansion of the gingiva and displacement and distortion of the teeth which have been dislodged from their sockets. Although the teeth may lose their bony support, pain is minimal and tenderness, anesthesia or paresthesia is slight to absent. Maxillary tumors may invade the orbit before invading the mouth. Thus, proptosis becomes the presenting clinical feature. The neoplasm eventually bursts through bone into the facial soft tissues and produces an external swelling which increases rapidly in size. Ulceration through the skin is rare.

Since the lesion is osteolytic, one of the earliest radiographic signs is a loss of or break in the lamina dura around erupted or developing teeth. Small discrete radiolucencies may also be seen at this stage. These later coalesce to produce larger radiolucent defects in the jaws. In the maxilla, the earliest sign may be blurring of the shadow of the antrum. All these early signs may antedate clinical signs or symptoms. According to Adatia,[102] over 80% of patients with jaw tumors have neoplastic involvement in more than one quadrant of the jaws, whereas only one-third to one-half of the patients have a *clinically* obvious tumor in more than one quadrant.

Subperiosteal new bone formation is not an uncommon later finding and is most clearly demonstrable in radiographs of the mandible. The new bone is deposited as spicules at right angles to the jaw, giving a sunray appearance. While the microscopic appearance of the lesion is considered elsewhere, it is pertinent to note here that there are few examples in which the dental pulp is as commonly invaded by a malignant tumor as in Burkitt's tumor.

Untreated growth of the lymphoma is exceedingly rapid and most of the children die within 4 to 6 months of the onset of the disease. In some of the older children, survival may extend for 1 year or more. Spontaneous remissions have been observed. From a therapeutic standpoint, this particular lymphoma appears to be one of the most "therapy-sensitive" of all neoplasms. It manifests a high degree of sensitivity to a wide variety of therapeutic agents.[103]

The growth pattern of Burkitt's tumor tends toward an expanding nodular mass rather than to a diffuse infiltration of cells. This leads to an encasement of organs and viscera with a secondary extension from capsules or surfaces. Sections of the tumor present a rather monotonous overgrowth of undifferentiated lymphoreticular cells. There is little variation in size and shape of cells or their nuclei. The over-all monotomy is broken by a "starry sky" pattern produced by a uniform scattering of macrophages with abundant, clear cytoplasm containing tumor cells or cellular debris (Figure 23.7). Mitotic activity may be high, and nucleoli are prominent.

In both imprint preparations and well fixed tissue sections, the neoplastic cells manifest a marked cytoplasmic pyroninophilia. This can be destroyed by prior digestion with ribonuclease. Lipid droplets within the cytoplasm can be demonstrated, and a minority of cells may contain coarse PAS-positive cytoplasmic granules.

Kinetic studies have defined Burkitt's lymphoma as the fastest growing neoplasm in man.[104] Potential doubling time approaches 24 hours, and the growth fraction approaches 100%. This rapid proliferation has important clinical implications: (1) the rapid increase in size may obstruct or compress vital structures; (2) profound metabolic abnormalities can result from this rapid cell turnover or from tumor lysis after chemotherapy; and (3) the rapid proliferation accounts in part for the extreme sensitivity of Burkitt's lymphoma to alkylating cell-cycle specific agents.

Studies have demonstrated by surface markers and histochemical analysis that African cases are indistinguishable from sporadic cases occurring elsewhere in the world.[104] The tumor cells have the characteristics of B lymphocytes and probably arise from germinal follicles. Genetic marker studies suggest that lymphomas arise from single clones. The multicentric pattern of growth and spread may be determined by the "homing" characteristics of the B lymphocyte as well as by local tissue and immunological factors.

Based on light and electron microscopic findings, Burkitt's tumor is an undifferentiated malignant lymphoma. The typical African cases show more primitive lymphoreticular cells with frequent deep nuclear indentations and very little ergastoplasm. Non-African forms show an extent of lymphoid differentiation characterized by longer profiles of ergastoplasm, more mitochondria and a lesser tendency to deep indentation of the nuclear membrane. Notwithstanding the spectrum of possible differentiation observed in Burkitt's lymphoma, the ultrastructure of the tumor is considered nearly diagnostic.[105]

Before we depart from the pathological consideration of Burkitt's tumor, a short consideration of "starry sky" appearance seems appropriate. This picturesquely described appearance is due to the presence of large, clear, mature phagocytic cells amid a background of swollen darker and immature lymphoid cells. While the cells in Burkitt's lymphoma are poorly differentiated lymphocytes (lymphoblasts), the phagocytic macrophages are benign and reactive cells. Whether they represent a reaction to the breakdown products of the neoplastic cells or to some other structures or represent a type of host response to the neoplasm is unknown.

Two further points need to be emphasized. In the past, histiophagocytosis has been considered a hallmark of benign hyperplasia in lymph nodes. However, it is now well known that considerable phagocytosis may also be seen in malignant lymphomas, intra- or extranodal. The "starry sky" is not restricted to Burkitt's-type lesions but may be found in lymphomas in children and adults and in lymphomas of the lymphoblastic and histiocytic cell types in cats, dogs and cattle.

What Burkitt started as a nosogeographic adventure has evolved into a complex and fascinating assessment and approach to the study of lymphoproliferative disorders. Witness the intense and diverse epidemiological activity relating to Burkitt's lymphoma.

Tissue culture and histochemical studies have supported the view that these tumors develop from the cells of the reticuloendothelial system. The tissue culture growth pattern, however, is quite distinct from that of the more common malignancies of the reticuloendothelial system. Several cell-line cultures have been established from the tumor cells. From these a clear *association* of the Epstein-Barr virus (EBV) and Burkitt's lymphoma has been established. This association is so strong that Burkitt's lymphoma has been considered a malignant proliferation of a clone carrying the EBV. Seroepidemiology indicates that patients have significantly higher titers of antibody to the virus capsid than controls. Biochemical studies have also established the presence of the EBV genome in the tumor cells in up to 97% of patients examined.[104] It has been noted, however, that in contrast to African Burkitt's lymphoma, there is an absence of nucleotide sequence homologous to the virus in the American forms.[106] As it is with the association of EBV and nasopharyngeal carcinoma, the biological significance of the virus to the relationship in Burkitt's lymphoma remains unsolved at present.

Dramatic remissions occur in over 90% of patients following high-dose alkylating agent therapy. Relapse occurs in approximately two-thirds of these patients, most often in patients with advanced stages.[104] The response to therapy in endemic and nonendemic types is identical.[107] The important determinants of successful remission induction include judicious surgical "debulking," high-dose alkylating agent chemotherapy, appropriate supportive care and an awareness of the metabolic consequences of rapid tumor lysis. Once remission is achieved, the major determinants of relapse appear to be clinical stage and adequacy of induction therapy. Early escape from remission is usually associated with advanced stage of disease and responds poorly to reinduction (Table 23.7). Late relapse on the other hand, often appears in new previously uninvolved areas and responds well to chemotherapy.

When more is learned of normal B-cell regulation and blocking factors, immunotherapy may find a role in the treatment of these disorders.[108]

The place of radiotherapy in the management of Burkitt's lymphoma is unknown. It may have a role in the acute, nonsurgical reduction of localized bulk of tumor.

Plasma Cell Neoplasms in the Head and Neck

Plasma cell neoplasms presenting in the head and neck region may be solitary or of multifocal origin. They have been categorized in the following manner: (1) a manifestation of multiple myeloma; (2) a manifestation of plasma cell myelomatosis; (3) solitary plasmacytoma of bone; and (4) extramedullary plasmacytoma ("primary" plasmacytoma of soft tissues).

The frequency of the extramedullary form in a large population study is seen in Figure 23.17 adopted from Pahor's[109] evaluation of the Birmingham Regional Cancer Registry. Expressed in a different way, the incidence of extramedullary tumors as compared to multiple myeloma is 1:40.

The enigmatic relationship between these lesions themselves and the latter three collectively with multiple myeloma has generated a plethora of clinical and pathological reports. The note of exasperation expressed by Stout and Kenney[100] is representative of the experience of others in their efforts to resolve the clinicopathological status of this group of plasma cell disorders. It is our contention that attempts to subdivide the primary plasmacytic dyscrasias into separate and rigid nosological entities are not consistent with their ultimate biological behavior; indeed, such efforts ignore the capricious and protean characteristics of this group of disorders.[111]

Extramedullary Plasmacytoma. Approximately 80% of all extramedullary plasmacytomas have been seen in the head and neck.[112] No portion of the upper respiratory tract is immune to the development of the tumor. There is, however, a predilection for the nasopharynx, nasal cavity, paranasal sinuses and tonsils. Exact delimitation, as with other neoplasms of this region, is difficult. Primary involvement of the major salivary glands is very unusual (Table 23.8).[113] In the upper air passages, the majority of extramedullary plasma cell tumors occur in single form. Rarely have they been met in the form of multiple lesions (10%). The most common sites are the nose and sinuses. Male patients exceed women by a ratio of 4:1, and three-fourths of the patients present between the ages of 40 and 70 years.

The gross appearance is nonspecific and varies considerably from polypoid to sessile, becoming

Table 23.8
Extramedullary Plasmacytomas—Head and Neck*

Location	No. of Cases
Nasopharynx	45
Nose	45
Antrum and paranasal sinuses	36
Tonsils and pharynx	32
Palate, gum and maxilla	13
Oropharynx	16
Larynx	11
Combined	6
Floor of mouth and tongue	5
Cervical lymph nodes	1
Parotid gland	1
Submandibular gland	1
Unspecified	9

* Collected data from Poole and Marchetta,[114] Pahor,[109] Noorani,[115] Touma,[116] Booth et al.[117] and Gorenstein et al.[118]

lobulated with increasing size. Most often the mass is gray-red to deep red; color perhaps is related to the capillary network of the stroma of the tumor. Ulceration is rare and, when it occurs, is probably due to previous interference. The polypoid form appears to behave in a less aggressive manner and is usually confined to the soft tissues. The more aggressive tumors are usually soft and friable. Superficial mucosal spread is common. Invasion of underlying bone is a feature of the more malignant types.

Despite the ubiquitousness of the plasma cell in inflammatory reactions in the upper respiratory tract, there is general agreement that there should be no difficulty in differentiating plasma cell neoplasms (plasmacytomas) from reactive plasma cell "granulomas." Plasmacytomas are virtually monomorphic and are composed of a nearly "pure culture" of plasma cells arranged in relatively broad sheets on a delicate reticular stroma, the latter consisting primarily of a capillary network (Figure 23.18). Plasmacytomas replace tissue, unlike inflammatory reactions which infiltrate by a disposition of plasma cells through involved tissues. Cataldo and Meyer[119] state that the only plasma cell neoplasms containing inflammatory cells are those in which the surface epithelium is ulcerated. Even in these instances, the reaction is minimal and does not extend throughout the neoplastic tissues. A histological finding, which we regard as important in the differentiation of these tumors from inflammatory lesions, is the relative scarcity, or even absence, of Russell bodies in the plasmacytomas. The so-called plasma cell granulomas of the oral cavity, upper airway and lung

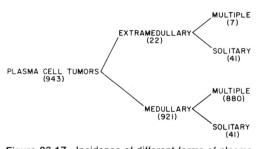

Figure 23.17. Incidence of different forms of plasma cell tumors.

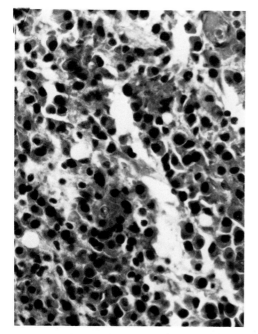

Figure 23.18. Nasopharyngeal plasmacytoma in which the cell is readily recognized as being of plasmacytic origin. Note the eccentric nuclei and the loose reticular stroma.

are uncommon lesions.[120, 121] In the oral cavity, the lesion is usually exophytic and affects the gingiva most often. Maxillary and mandibular gingivae are equally involved. The lesions are seen on the marginal, interdental, and attached gingiva. Bone loss may or may not be present. There is no sex predilection and the lesion can occur at any age. Multiple lesions are rare.

Morphological features of the plasma cells are variable also and appear related to the maturity of the cell. There is not a close relationship between the level of maturity of the cell and the ultimate behavior of the neoplasm. In a given lesion, cellular maturity may be so varied that identification may rest upon the finding and recognition of the more mature plasma cells. These appear similar to the normal plasma cell, possessing an eccentrically placed, dark-staining nucleus. The so-called wheel-spoke arrangement of nuclear chromatin is not commonly seen. In tissue sections stained with hematoxylin, the cytoplasm is eosinophilic or exhibits a pale basophilia. With increasing immaturity, the cells become larger, there is frequently a notable increase in nuclear size, and the position of the nucleus becomes more central. The chromatin in young cells is less clumped and in the least mature cells is reticular. Bi- or trinucleation

may be present, but binucleation is not restricted to young cells. Mitotic figures are rarely seen. Amyloid may be observed in about 15% of the cases.

Absence of the usual cytological indices for malignancy is not evidence of the benignancy of plasma cell tumors and, unfortunately, the microscopic appearance is not a guide to the potential aggressiveness of the tumor. Our histopathological analysis and those of others confirm Hellwig's[122] opinion that "localization and gross appearance are more reliable criteria than histological appearances in prognostication."

Solitary Plasmacytoma of the Jaws. Solitary osseous myeloma or plasmacytoma has a peak age incidence in the sixth decade, and few patients are less than 30 years of age. Sites of involvement in decreasing frequency are: ilium, femur, humerus, thoracic vertebrae and skull. The apparently solitary plasmacytoma of the jaw is rare. Webb et al.,[123] after a search of the literature, could uncover only nine cases; five were in males. The majority of lesions presented at the posterior portion of the mandible, often at the angle.

The most common clinical findings are a palpable tumor and a history of progressively increasing pain.[124] Regional lymph node involvement has not been associated with this form of plasmacytic dyscrasia. Two different x-ray characteristics have been described: (1) a sharply demarcated, osteolytic, multicystic lesion located in the medulla; (2) a destructive, trabeculated lesion occasionally manifesting cortical expansion.

Clinical Course and Ultimate Outcome. Figure 23.19 illustrates the interrelationship of the four principal plasmacytic dyscrasias. All are united by one pathological change: an abnormal proliferation of plasma cells derived from progenitor cells (primitive and pleuripotential reticulum cells) in or outside the bone marrow. Since there is considerable clinical overlap, the individual plasmacytic dyscrasias are best considered as parts of a continuous spectrum of disease, rather than as separate distinct clinical or pathological entities.

Reliance upon clinical, biochemical and hematological findings to differentiate the variants is fraught with pitfalls. Osserman[125] doubts that a "typical" case of multiple myeloma exists, indicating the considerable overlaps of clinical and pathological variants. Waldenström[126] and others have shown that a proliferation of plasma cells may exist for months or years before there are clinically recognizable symptoms, radiographic changes or hematological abnormalities.

Although abnormal laboratory findings are usu-

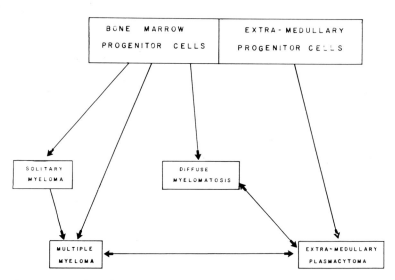

Figure 23.19. Inter-relationship of the main plasma cell dyscrasias, emphasizing that they most likely represent a spectrum rather than isolated entities.

ally not associated with extramedullary plasma cell tumors, the so-called solitary myeloma of the jaws is commonly associated with abnormal serum protein configurations which, interestingly, manifest a decrease in gamma globulin concentration after removal of the tumor.[127] This may only reflect poor selection and scanty follow-up of this latter group. The need for complete investigation of any patient who has a "primary" plasmacytoma of the upper respiratory tract or of the jaws is highlighted by: (1) the number of lesions which eventuate into more diffuse forms of the plasmacytic dyscrasias; and (2) clinical recordings that from 30 to 70% of patients are actually suffering from the multiple form of the disease.

Involvement of the jaws is certainly not uncommon in multiple myeloma. The majority of these lesions occur in the mandible, where they may be the initial manifestation of the disease. There may be a spotty distribution of lesions throughout the maxilla and the mandible, but in most instances, the mandible alone is affected. Here the initial lesion tends to appear in the posterior region where marrow spaces are largest, extending forward along and below the mandibular canal. There is also a tendency toward extension up into the marrow spaces of edentulous regions and into the ramus.

There thus appears to be no sharp line of demarcation between these two forms of apparently localized plasmacytoma and other plasmacytic dyscrasias. The extramedullary upper respiratory tract plasmacytoma and "solitary" myeloma of the

jaw bones are best considered as components of a continuous spectrum of plasma cell disorders, each capable of rendering a variety of clinical expressions, from a localized lesion to a progressive disseminated and lethal disease. They may assume the following clinical characteristics: (1) be the initial clinical evidence of a recognized diffuse myeloma; (2) evolve into systemic myeloma after a variable latent period; (3) remain localized and persistent, causing death by expansile growth; or (4) respond satisfactorily to local treatment without evidence of recurrence or dissemination, over long periods of follow-up.

In the extramedullary form, two clinicopathological findings appear to have an adverse effect on the clinical course of the disease: (1) recurrence and/or persistence of the upper respiratory tract plasmacytoma after initial treatment; and (2) invasion of underlying or contiguous bone. Cervical lymph node involvement (approximately 25% of cases) does not necessarily portend a bad prognosis nor does it indicate involvement of bone as a prerequisite. The presence of amyloid in the lesion (15% of cases) does not preclude long survival.

A sense of watchful expectancy must be employed in all patients manifesting apparently solitary plasmacytoma (osseous or extramedullary), acknowledging at the same time that even as in the more diffuse myelomas, the disorder is compatible with long if not natural survival after treatment. Treatment of these solitary lesions, particularly the aggressive upper respiratory tract ones, must be carried out. Batsakis et al.[111] have concluded that radiosensitivity is not a uniform characteristic of these tumors, whereas others indicate a favorable response to irradiation, even when there is involvement of underlying bone.

There certainly is no overwhelming treatment method of choice. The majority of the extramedullary forms are treated by electrocoagulation or surgical excision, or radiation, either alone or in combination. There is no clear indication that one form of treatment is superior to the other. For lesions presenting in the jaws, treatment may involve either surgical resection of the affected portion or irradiation. If curettage is the only form of surgical intervention, it must be followed by irradiation.

IDIOPATHIC HISTIOCYTOSIS

The idiopathic histiocytoses are a group of diseases presenting as a diverse clinical tapestry stitched together by the thread of their morphological similarities which are predominated by the proliferated mature histiocyte. Their etiologies are unknown and the nosologic state of the art may be likened to a histological classification of infectious granulomas without the benefit of cultures or special microbiological stains.

Almost all investigators agree that subjects with idiopathic histiocytosis may present in one of three ways: (1) as an acute, rapidly progressive illness, usually in an infant or young child, manifest by an exfoliative dermatitis, hepatosplenomegaly, lymphadenopathy, anemia and thrombocytopenia (acute disseminated histiocytosis, acute differentiated hystiocytosis, nonlipid reticuloendotheliosis, Letterer-Siwe disease); (2) as a chronic disseminated disease usually initially discovered in young children, but also occurring in adults, with signs and symptoms of focal osseous, visceral or osseous and visceral lesions which may produce intractable otitis media, osseous defects especially in the skull, lymphadenopathy, hepatosplenomegaly, exophthalmus, eczematoid skin lesions, chronic gingival or palatal ulcers, diabetes insipidus, or symptoms of pituitary insufficiency (multifocal eosinophilic granuloma, chronic disseminated histiocytosis, chronic differentiated histiocytosis, Hand-Schüler-Christian disease); (3) as a unifocal eosinophilic granuloma which presents as a lytic lesion in the bone or as a single infiltrative lesion in the viscera.

The presence of the same clinical and morphological manifestations in acute disseminated histiocytosis and multicentric eosinophilic granuloma has resulted in divergent opinions about the classification of these diseases. One group of investigators feels that acute disseminated histiocytosis is a neoplastic disease nosologically unrelated to multifocal and unifocal eosinophilic granuloma.[128-130] Lieberman et al.[128] argue that the original description of Letterer and Siwe was imprecise and that the syndrome described represents a potpourri of infectious and neoplastic diseases. Other authors, equally authoritative and persuasive, argue that acute disseminated histiocytosis, multifocal eosinophilic granuloma and unifocal eosinophilic granuloma represent different clinical expressions of the same disease which may begin as one clinical syndrome and terminate as another.[131-133]

The differences in classification may be more apparent than real. A recent study of histiocytosis in childhood disclosed two distinct morphological lesions. One lesion consisted of proliferated, mature histiocytes, usually with distinct cell borders, which diffusely infiltrated the reticuloendothelial system. Neither eosinophils, giant cells, necrosis nor fibrosis accompanied the histiocytic infiltrates; evidence of phagocytosis was scant or absent. Subjects with these histological findings presented clinically as the Letterer-Siwe syndrome and died of their disease after a short illness. Excluding the cytological benignity of the infiltrate, the anatomical distribution and clinical course mimicked a malignant neoplasm.

A second morphological lesion proliferated as sheets of histiocytes with indistinct cell borders, often appearing in syncytia, always attended by eosinophils and giant cells and frequently associated with necrosis and fibrosis. The infiltrate involved a single viscera or bone or disseminated in several viscera or bone, but in either instance the lesions were always morphologically focal. These patients manifested the symptoms of multifocal eosinophilic granuloma and acute disseminated histiocytosis but evinced a more protracted benign course and did not die as a direct result of their disease. Adhering to these strict morphological criteria, Newton and Hamoudi[134] found no convincing evidence that the disease manifest by pure histiocytic infiltrates ever transformed into disseminated multifocal eosinophilic granuloma. These findings correlate with the interpretations of Cline and Golde[130] who felt that histiocytes in acute disseminated histiocytosis were immature and that they bore no definite relationship to multifocal eosinophilic granuloma or unifocal eosinophilic granuloma.

The infiltrate in acute disseminated histiocytosis involves the liver sinusoids, red pulp of the spleen, mucosa of the colon, medullary cavities of bone, interstitium of the lung, skin and lymph nodes. Of special interest is the propensity for infiltration of the anterior cervical lymph nodes.[135] Moderately enlarged, pink-tan, soft lymph nodes contain proliferated histiocytes which distend the sinusoids of the node obscuring, but not effacing the architecture. The capsule and paranodal adipose tissue are free of histiocytes.

Multifocal eosinophilic granuloma frequently involves the head and neck. The skull, especially the temporal bone, is a favored site of circumscribed lytic lesions, often presenting as intractable otitis media.[136] The most dramatic presentation occurs when histiocytes and eosinophils infiltrate the orbital bone, soft tissues, or both, resulting in exophthalmus which occurs in up to 19% of patients.[137] Lytic infiltrates in the mandible and alveolar ridge and periodontal infiltrates composed of histiocytes and eosinophils can produce gingival swellings, pain, necrosis and ulcers and displace fully or partially formed teeth or result in the loss of permanent teeth.[138] Lymph node involvement occurs in multicentric lesions or as an isolated finding. The infiltrate in the lymph node differs from that of acute disseminated histiocytosis only in composition, harboring eosinophils, giant cells, areas of necrosis and fibrosis. The polymorphous reaction usually distorts the architecture of the lymph node more than in acute disseminated histiocytosis, but cortical and paracortical lymphoid structures are usually discernible.

The mortality in idiopathic histiocytosis depends upon the age of onset, on the number of organs involved, and the composition of the infiltrate. When the disease begins in neonates, the mortality may be as high as 77%.[139] Numerous studies have confirmed that the greater the extent of the disease at the time of diagnosis, the poorer the prognosis.[136, 139] Those patients with bone and more than three different visceral lesions or with more than four visceral lesions without bone involvement have an especially poor prognosis. Correlation of survival data with age suggests that the disease is more disseminated in younger subjects at the time of diagnosis. Poor prognostic signs include skin infiltrates and pancytopenia. On the other hand, subjects with involvement of one or more bones and the absence of visceral lesions almost never die of their disease.[140] Dissemination of an initial solitary lesion usually occurs before 5 years of age, and within the first 6 months of the illness. If new bone lesions fail to appear after 12 months, one may anticipate cure with conservative therapy.[133]

The cellular composition of the infiltrate also influences prognosis. Subjects with pure histiocytic infiltrates or with only meager eosinophils in the infiltrate fare less well than those with abundant eosinophilic infiltrates. Patients with multifocal eosinophilic granuloma often suffer recurrent osseous or visceral lesions resulting in prolonged morbidity, but they fail to demonstrate the mortality associated with acute disseminated histiocytosis. Thus a child less than 2 years of age with purely histiocytic proliferation diffusely infiltrating the reticuloendothelial system has an extremely guarded prognosis, whereas a child of the same age with multifocal eosinophilic granuloma may suffer prolonged morbidity and recurrences, but his death lacks the certainty associated with acute disseminated histiocytosis. Prolonged survival in acute disseminating histiocytosis, while distinctly unusual, has been reported.[141]

The etiology of idiopathic histiocytosis remains unknown. Based upon reports of Letterer-Siwe disease and other morphologically related syndromes in siblings[142] and twins,[143] genetic predisposition has been suggested for acute disseminated histiocytosis; however, no pattern of inheritance emerges for multifocal eosinophilic granuloma.[144] Acute disseminated histiocytosis behaves clinically as a malignant neoplasm. The diffuse infiltrates of the reticuloendothelial system mimicks lymphoma or leukemia. Some have suggested that acute disseminated histiocytosis is the childhood counterpart of histiocytic medullary reticulosis or reticulum cell sarcoma.[128, 130] Others find it most difficult to reconcile the cytologically benign occurrence of the histiocytes in acute disseminated histiocytosis with a malignant neoplasm.[145, 146]

The ubiquity of histiocytes in inflammatory lesions, the clinical coincidence of fever with the occurrence of pathological lesions, and the dramatic response of lesions to cortical steroids and to noncancerocidal therapy suggests that an infectious agent is responsible for idiopathic histiocytosis. This suggestion is periodically reinforced by reports of histiocytosis occurring in still and live born infants of mothers given virus vaccine[147] or suffering rubella[148] early in pregnancy.

An infectious etiology received impetus because of the discovery of granules within the cytoplasm of histiocytes from patients with histiocytosis. The granules, approximately 40 nm wide, contain a central filament and the walls of the organelles were continuous with a vesicular terminal extension.[149] The granules occur only in cytoplasm of histiocytes and are not extracytoplasmic or found in other cells. They are not specific for idiopathic histiocytosis occurring in numerous other diseases and in Langhan cells in the normal dermis.[150] Their reconstruction suggests a disc or plate-like structure unlike any known group of viruses. Not a typical organelle of histiocytes, the granules may represent a specific type of histiocyte possibly deployed in response to antigens.

Although children with disseminated histiocytosis have responded normally to antigenic challenges of cell-mediated and humoral immune responses,[151] subjects have been reported with combined immunodeficiency disease and disseminated histiocytosis.[152, 153] These patients manifest clinical findings of Letterer-Siwe syndrome, histiocytosis and thymic dysplasia. In view of the widespread histiocytic proliferations in inflammatory diseases, any association between idiopathic histiocytosis and other diseases must be interpreted with caution.

Acute disseminated histiocytosis must be differentiated from malignant histiocytosis and lymphoma. Although clinically the diseases may be similar, the benign appearance of cells in acute disseminated histiocytosis should differentiate it from the malignant histiocytic disorders. In addition, the architecture of the lymph node is preserved in acute disseminated histiocytosis and effaced when infiltrated by cytologically malignant histiocytes. Skin infiltrations occur in the papillary dermis in acute disseminated histiocytosis or multicentric eosinophilic granuloma, whereas malignant lymphomas typically infiltrate the perivascular areas of the reticular dermis, sparing the subepithelial portion of the papillary dermis.[154]

Other diseases of uncertain etiology which may clinically mimic acute disseminated histiocytosis and in which proliferated histiocytes comprise a prominent part include familial reticuloendotheliosis, familial and congenital hemophagocytic reticulosis[155–157] and combined immunodeficiency disease. The first two diseases are polymorphous infiltrates of lymphocytes, lymphoblasts, plasma cells and phagocytic histiocytes which efface lymph node architecture. The last disease has the typical histological alterations of thymic dysplasia, in addition to a disseminated histiocytosis. Sinus histiocytosis with massive lymphadenopathy may be confused with acute disseminated histiocytosis. The massive lymph node enlargement is usually cervical but the prominence of histiocytic phagocytosis serve to differentiate it from acute disseminated histiocytosis on the one hand and the absence of eosinophils and necrosis serve to differentiate it from multicentric eosinophilic granuloma on the other.[158]

Multicentric eosinophilic granuloma presents a distinct histological finding, but the presence of eosinophils may alert the morphologist to a diagnosis of Hodgkin's disease. Such an error should be avoided if one adheres to rigid criteria for the Reed-Sternberg cells.

Unifocal eosinophilic granuloma has been successfully treated with curettage and low voltage radiation. Multifocal eosinophilic granuloma and acute disseminated histiocytosis usually require chemotherapy which has included cortical steroids, alkylating agents, antifols, Vinca alkaloids and cytotoxic forms of antibiotics. Results of combined studies of children's cancer therapy disclose that the disease is unlikely to respond to other chemotherapeutic agents if it is resistant to the combination of prednisone and 6-mercaptopurine, prednisone and vinblastine or vinbastine alone.

CHEDIAK-HIGASHI SYNDROME (CHS)

CHS is a rare disorder of lysosomal origin inherited as an autosomal recessive gene. The disease becomes manifest in early childhood with diminished pigmentation in the skin, hair and eyes, in only one or in any combination of these organs, followed by neutropenia and recurrent infections of the skin and upper and lower respiratory tracts usually caused by *Staphylococcus aureus* or beta-hemolytic streptococci. Months or years after the onset of symptoms, the patients usually either die of overwhelming infections or their disease terminates in a fulminating lymphoproliferative disorder characterized by one or more of the following: anemia, neutropenia, thrombocytopenia, lymphadenopathy, hepatomegaly, splenomegaly, pulmonary infiltrates. The mean age at death in 37 fatal cases was 4.1 years.[159]

Examination of Wright-stained films of the peripheral blood shows distinctive large slate-gray intracytoplasmic granules in neutrophils, and large azurophilic granules in the cytoplasm of lymphocytes and monocytes. Bone marrow aspiration usually yields a hypercellular specimen with a granulocytic,[160] or more rarely, erythrocytic hyperplasia.[161] Granulocytic precursors contain cytoplasmic vacuoles and acidophilic inclusions occupy the cytoplasm of many promyelocytes and myelocytes.[160] Lymphocytic infiltrates in the marrow vary with the stage of the disease becoming abundant during the accelerated phase.

Biopsy of an enlarged lymph node reveals morphological alterations similar to that observed in lymphomas. The architecture of the node is obscured, germinal centers are reduced or absent and the cellular infiltrate consists of large and small lymphocytes, plasma cells and histiocytes. Although the pattern of the infiltrate in lymph nodes, spleen, liver and kidney resembles lymphomas, the cellular composition does not. The polymorphous infiltrate in CHS is dissimilar to the monomorphic infiltrate present in non-Hodgkin's lymphomas. The polymorphous infiltrate may suggest Hodgkin's disease, but the absence of Reed-Sternberg cells and knowledge of the clinical and hemological manifestations eliminate this consideration.

Studies of host defense in patients with CHS disclose defects in neither the production of antibodies nor in cell-mediated immunity.[162] Chinks in the armor of host defense occur in the granulocytes, not the lymphocytes. Neutrophils display impaired chemotactic activity to different chemotactic stimuli while the viability, passive motility and adhesiveness of the CHS neutrophils are normal.[162] The CHS neutrophils readily phagocytize bacteria but destroy bacteria, especially Gram-positive cocci, at a delayed rate.[163] The failure of prompt bacteriocidal activity resides not in the metabolism of the granulocyte because the respiratory burst, oxygen consumption, hexosemonophosphate-shunt activity, nitro-blue tetrazolium reduction, formate oxidation and iodination of bacteria are either normal or increased in CHS granulocytes.[163]

Defective lysosomes cripple the killing power of the CHS neutrophil. Although the maturation of secondary lysosomes in neutrophils proceeds normally, the primary lysosomes in promyelocytes fuse producing few large lysosomes that become the slate-gray inclusions of mature neutrophils.[164] In man, primary lysosomes production is also abnormal in the eosinophils, lymphocytes and melanocytes.[164] The defective granulation of the latter cell produces the partial albinism. The origin of abnormal lysosomes in monocytes remains uncertain. These large pleomorphic lysosomes fail to release their full complement of enzymes, especially beta-glucuronidase and peroxidase, into the phagocytic vacuoles. Failure of prompt degranulation and release of peroxidase into the phagosome correlates with the reduced prompt bacteriocidal activity observed in cells from patients with CHS. The cause of defective lysosomal function remains unknown, and the search for an etiology delves ever deeper into cellular function. Relatively increased quantities of cyclic adenosine 3',5'-monophosphate or decreased quantities of cyclic guanosine 3',5'-monophosphate and their opposing action on microtubular function, which may

regulate degranulation in human leukocytes, could be responsible for the defect in CHS.[165] These theoretical considerations extend beyond the research laboratory for ascorbic acid, which reduces cyclic adenosine 3',5'-monophosphate levels in granulocytes, has corrected the functional defects in cells from patients with CHS.[165]

HYDANTOIN LYMPHADENOPATHY

Lymphadenopathy associated with hydantoin medication is a rare, but well established, disorder. Although subjects of any age may be affected, about one-half of reported cases occur in children or in young adults.[166] The typical patient has fever, an erythematous cutaneous rash and eosinophilia. Generalized lymphadenopathy or, rarely, localized lymphadenopathy[167] almost always accompanies these symptoms. Hepatomegaly and splenomegaly occur sufficiently often to be considered part of the syndrome. The clinical manifestations subside when the drug is stopped only to reappear on reinstituting the medication. Mephenytoin and phenytoin most frequently precipitate this perplexing disorder.

Excised lymph nodes are large, but otherwise grossly unremarkable. The lymph nodes display varied histological patterns ranging from hyperplasia to proliferations that mimic lymphoma. In the latter instance, a polymorphous infiltrate consisting predominantly of lymphocytes and immunoblasts with scattered eosinophils and plasma cells obscures or obliterates the architecture of the lymph node. Necrotic neutrophilic foci and fibrosis may punctuate the lymph node. A prominent vascular scaffold supports these proliferated lymphoid cells. When numerous pleomorphic immunoblasts accompanied by immature, clefted lymphocytes obscure nodal architecture, the epitaph pseudolymphoma is applied. Unfortunately, a diagnosis of pseudolymphoma fails to absolve one of the specter of malignancy, for several cases have been reported where an initial lymph node biopsy revealed atypical hyperplasia followed by regression of lymphadenopathy with cessation of anticonvulsant therapy only to find lymphoma in a subsequent biopsy.[168]

The association of lymphoma and hydantoin therapy occurs 2 to 4 times as frequently as in controlled populations, but the absolute risk of a recipient of hydantoin developing lymphoma is less than one per thousand per year.[169] Reports of suppressed immune activity in selected subjects taking phenytoin[170] suggest a similar pathogenesis for the development of non-Hodgkin's lymphoma in these patients and in therapeutically immuno-depressed subjects.[169] Selected animal studies support this concept for phenytoin has produced immunosuppression, immunostimulation and lymphomas in mice.[171, 172]

The differentiation of hydantoin lymphadenopathy from monomorphic histiocytic and lymphocytic lymphomas should present no difficulties since the infiltrate in hydantoin lymphadenopathy almost always contains more than one cell type. Greater difficulties ensue in differentiating the polymorphous infiltrate, necrosis and pleomorphic immunoblasts of anticonvulsant lymphadenopathy from mixed Hodgkin's disease. Here, differentiation hinges upon stringent criteria for the Reed-Sternberg cells which fortunately are easily found in mixed Hodgkin's disease and do not occur in hydantoin lymphadenopathy.

Differentiating hydantoin lymphadenopathy from mixed histiocytic-lymphocytic lymphoma may prove especially taxing if the former contains a predominance of pleomorphic immunoblasts and immature lymphocytes and the nodal architecture is obscured. The increased vascularity in hydantoin lymphadenopathy may avert one from a diagnosis of mixed histiocytic-lymphocytic lymphoma. A history of taking hydantoin provides a helpful adjuvant in differentiating atypical hyperplasia from lymphoma; however, the increased incidence of lymphoma occurring in subjects treated with hydantoin makes too great a reliance upon the history hazardous. When the buffer zone between atypical hyperplasia and lymphoma is reached, the pathologist should diagnose the former, suggest cessation of hydantoin therapy and careful follow-up of the subject to confirm that the lymphadenopathy disappears. Failure of shrinkage of enlarged nodes or reappearance of lymphadenopathy or the appearance of splenomegaly, mediastinal widening or hemological abnormalities should sound a tocsin and more tissue should be removed.

VIRAL LYMPHADENOPATHY

Cervical lymph node enlargement is no stranger to viral infections. Vaccinia inoculations,[173] herpes zoster[174] and infectious mononucleosis[174, 175] have been associated with enlarged, movable, usually tender lymphadenopathy. The size of the nodes, a failure to inquire about vaccination or the paucity of signs and symptoms accompanying the adenopathy may induce the clinician to remove the gland for biopsy.

The lymph nodes are large and pale. Histologically, the hyperplastic lymphoid tissue may proliferate diffusely through the paracortical portion of the gland, form well defined or confluent follicles or exhibit a diffuse and follicular pattern. Exuberant cellular proliferations to varying degrees obscure the medullary sinuses, fill the peripheral sinuses and infiltrate the capsule, spilling into the perinodal tissues. Although the infiltrations are extensive, the basic lymph node architecture, especially when stained for reticulum, remains.

Small and large lymphocytes, plasma cells, histiocytes, pyronophilic lymphoid cells and immunoblasts constitute the polymorphous infiltrate associated with viral lymphadenopathy. The most striking cell, the immunoblast, is 15 to 20 μm in diameter and usually contains a single oval, reniform or lobulated nucleus cradling a prominent basophilic nucleolus near the nuclear membrane. Binucleate and multinucleated cells occur more rarely. An amphophilic, strongly pyronophilic cytoplasm surrounds the nucleus. The proliferation of immunoblasts within the lymph node imparts a mottled texture to the fabric of the node. Attention to the scaffolding of the node discloses an increased number of small vessels lined by hyperplastic endothelial cells within the medulla and cortex.

Even though an exuberant cellular proliferation obscures the lymph node architecture, several features serve to differentiate the lymph nodes of viral lymphadenopathy from the lymph nodes of lymphomas. The mottled appearance of the lymph node sections, the rich vascular endothelial proliferation and the polymorphous cellular infiltrate should serve to differentiate a viral lymphadenopathy from lymphocytic lymphomas, mixed lymphocytic-histiocytic lymphomas, histiocytic lymphomas and Burkitt's lymphoma.

The histological differentiation from Hodgkin's disease proves more difficult since both conditions contain polymorphous infiltrates. Although an interfollicular cellular influx widens and distorts the medulla and cortex of the node, the basic nodal structure is discernible in viral lymphadenopathies. Hodgkin's disease may affect only part of the lymph node; however, where it is present, effacement of architecture tends to be absolute even with reticulum stains. Viral lymphadenopathies, unlike Hodgkin's disease, contain abundant immunoblasts and in the case of infectious mononucleosis large, atypical lymphocytes stuff the sinuses. Immunoblasts with multiple and bilobed nuclei may mimic Reed-Sternberg cells so closely that experienced morphologists cannot distinguish them,[176] therefore, attention to architectural differences between viral lymphadenopathies and Hodgkin's disease becomes necessary. Differentiation of viral lymphadenopathies from immunoblastic sarcoma should present no problem if the polymorphous infiltrate in the former is recognized.

The differentiation of viral lymphadenopathies from immunoblastic lymphadenopathy[177, 178] proves challenging and on morphological grounds alone may be impossible. Distortion of lymph node structure, polymorphous cellular infiltrates, abundant immunoblastic cells and endothelial vascular proliferations are common to both diseases although the arborizing venule-sized vessels in immunoblastic lymphadenopathy are more profuse than in viral lymphadenopathies. Also, intercellular PAS positive eosinophilic amorphous material occurs more constantly in immunoblastic lymphadenopathy. Since these are quantitative criteria, clinical information may be the only means of differentiating immunoblastic lymphadenopathy from viral lymphadenopathies.

Lymphadenopathy following vaccination, and herpes zoster infections are clearly related to viral infections. Until this decade infectious mononucleosis was only presumed to be a virus infection. Since 1968 evidence has accumulated linking infectious mononucleosis to Epstein-Barr virus (EBV) infection.[179-181] The virus has been isolated in saliva and in the oropharynx explaining its prevalence in ages where salivary exchange occurs.[182] The EBV preferentially infects bursa derived (B) lymphocytes; however, infected cells are rare in the blood, and the predominant atypical lymphocyte is a thymus dependent (T) cell.[183] The abundance of T lymphocytes correlates with paracortical hyperplasia observed in lymph nodes. T lymphocytes serve as the effector cells and are thought to destroy the infected B lymphocytes.[183, 184]

Whether by accident or design, numerous autoantibodies, anti-i,[185] anti-N,[186] Donath-Landsteiner cold hemolysins,[187] form transiently during the acute phase of the disease. Numerous specific antibodies to EBV also form; the most clinically useful include EB viral capsid antibodies, EB nuclear antibodies and antibodies to a diffuse component of EBV induced early antigen.[188] The characteristic heterophile antibody, although well known, remains an enigma, for neither its mode of origin nor its role in limiting the disease are understood. It does not appear in Burkitt's lymphoma as in other self-limiting EBV infections.

Infectious mononucleosis may present in children, in the elderly[189] and in young adults; the majority of cases occur in the latter. Clinical manifestations are protean and include malaise, fatigue, adenopathy, fever, pharyngitis, headache, palatal enanthm, splenomegaly and jaundice. Confronted with such an array of nonspecific signs and symptoms, laboratory work is necessary to confirm the diagnosis. White cell counts usually range between 10,000 and 20,000 with an absolute lymphocytosis. The atypical lymphocyte constitutes the predominant cell. Since atypical lymphocytosis occurs in other virus diseases that may manifest signs and symptoms similar to infectious mononucleosis, the diagnosis relies upon serological criteria.

Heterophile antibodies produced with EBV infection agglutinate sheep red blood cells as do antibodies to Forssman antigen. To differentiate these antibodies, differential absorption is employed. The heterophile antibody of infectious mononucleosis agglutinates sheep red blood cells after absorption of sera on guinea pig kidney but not after absorption on beef red cell stroma. Original tests have been simplified by substituting the more sensitive citrate preserved horse erythrocytes for sheep red blood cells and performing the differential absorption as a slide test. An even simpler one step test using aldehyde-treated horse erythrocytes is said to be as accurate as the differential absorption spot test.[190] Heterophile agglutinins appear in the first week of the illness in 75% of cases and most become positive by the third week. When the signs and symptoms of infectious mononucleosis are accompanied by a persistently negative heterophile agglutination (10% of subjects), or if one wishes to determine the immunity or susceptibility of an individual to infectious mononucleosis, titers of antibodies to EBV capsid antigen, EBV diffuse component of early antigen and EBV nuclear antigen are appropriate.

The viral capsid antibodies develop with the onset of clinical symptoms, peak in about 2 weeks and gradually fall to levels observed in subjects with past infections. Antibodies to the diffuse component of the EBV induced early antigen exhibit a brief transient rise in 80% of infected patients[191] and reflect current or recent disease. Antibodies to the EBV-associated nuclear antigen begin to appear in a minority of patients after 3 to 4 weeks, but by 6 months all convalescent sera carry this antibody.[191]

Although complications of infectious mononucleosis occur in less than 1% of patients, they can be serious and include splenic rupture, meningitis, encephalitis, Guillain-Barré syndrome, pneumonia, hemolytic anemia, thrombocytopenia, myocarditis and liver necrosis.

TOXOPLASMOSIS

Toxoplasmosis is a prevalent infection affecting an estimated 75 million persons in the United States alone.[192] Most acquired toxoplasmosis presents clinically in the child or the adult as a generalized lymphadenopathy inconsistently accompanied by chills, fever or both.[193] Although the lymphoid enlargement can include even hilar lymph nodes, the posterior cervical lymph nodes are most frequently affected.[192] Involved nodes are occasionally tender to palpation, but are usually painless. Fluctuation in nodal size often occurs during the illness, and the spleen may be transiently palpable.

Toxoplasma gondii is an obligate intracellular coccidia that reproduces by schizogony and gametogony in the intestinal epithelium of the cat and by endodyogeny within host tissues.[194] Ingestion of either the oocyst excreted in the cat feces or the form present in fresh undercooked meat (pork, beef or mutton) produce infections in humans.[194] Within human tissues, *T. gondii* may exist as a rapidly proliferating tachyzoite contained within a cellular cytoplasmic vacuole or as a slowly proliferating bradyzoite encircled by a true cyst wall.[194]

The histological appearance of the lymph node is characteristic.[192, 193, 195, 196] Nodal architecture persists. Hyperplastic lymphoid follicles and germinal centers of variable size occupy the cortex and extend into the medullary cords of the node. Mitotic figures within germinal centers may abound and macrophages containing tingible bodies are often prominent and may be mistaken for the organisms. Histocytes with pale eosinophilic cytoplasm proliferate in sinuses and spread into the cortical and paracortical tissue. Aggregates of these histiocytes produce loosely constructed, irregularly outlined granulomas composed of 4 to 5 cells (Fig. 23.20). Langhan's giant cells, necrosis or fibrosis are rarely found. The medullary sinuses may contain scattered plasma cells and eosinophils, but often contain immunoblasts with large irregular nuclei and scant basophilic cytoplasm that extend into the subcapsular sinuses.

The morphological appearance of toxoplasmosis in lymph nodes is sufficiently characteristic that the diagnosis can be made upon histological grounds.[196] The proliferated immunoblasts and

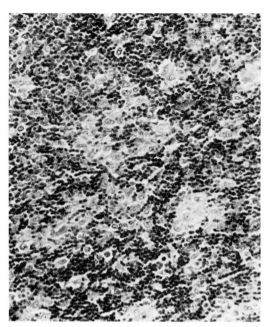

Figure 23.20. Toxoplasmosis lymphadenitis. Small collections of histiocytes and "microgranulomas" within and around germinal centers and follicles are characteristic.

epithelial histiocytes may suggest Hodgkin's disease or Lennart's lymphoma, but the topographical preservation of the lymph node, the prominent lymphoid and germinal follicles and the absence of Reed-Sternberg cells should prevent such mistakes. Confusion of toxoplasmosis with acute disseminated idiopathic histiocytosis may occur especially in a young child. Although the infiltrate in lymph nodes in acute disseminated histiocytosis consists of numerous benign appearing histiocytes, the proliferation is within the sinuses failing to spread into the cortical and paracortical areas and microgranulomas fail to form. Sarcoidosis and infectious granulomas should present no problems in differential diagnosis since their granulomas are composed of a tight regular proliferation of histiocytes with giant cells, and in the latter instance are often accompanied by central necrosis.

Confirmation of the diagnosis of toxoplasmosis is only rarely accomplished by histological identification of either the pseudocyst or true cyst in lymphoid tissue. The true cyst has a wall 1 μm thick surrounding numerous thin crescentic shaped organism 2 by 6 μm in diameter. These organisms contain glycogen granules 1 to 2 μm in diameter. PAS reagent stains the cyst pale red.

Rupture of these cysts may be responsible for focal necrosis sometimes observed in the lymph nodes.

Presence of the parasite can be confirmed by injecting blood or a saline suspension of pulverized tissue into the peritoneum of albino mice. In the presence of *T. gondii* a peritoneal exudate forms 10 to 14 days after innoculation. Smears of the peritoneal exudate treated with Romanoski stains yield crescent shaped trophozoites 2 to 4 μm by 5 to 7 μm with a rounded and pointed end.[197]

Since many laboratories do not have animals for innoculation, serological procedures must suffice to confirm a diagnosis of toxoplasmosis. The Sabin-Feldmen dye test, a pioneer in serological diagnosis, utilizes live organisms for the detection of antitoxoplasma antibodies and has been supplanted as a routine test by the hemagglutination inhibition test and the indirect fluorescent antibody test, each of which uses an antigen of killed organisms. The former test becomes positive 14 to 21 days after infection and remains positive for life. Like the Sabin-Feldmen dye test, antibodies detected by the indirect fluorescent antibody technique rise 7 to 14 days after infection, reach titers comparable to the Sabin-Feldmen dye test and remain elevated for life. False positive results using the indirect fluorescent antibody technique occur in patients with elevated antinuclear antibody levels. To differentiate acute from chronic infection, an indirect fluorescent antibody test for IgM and a complement fixation test are available. Antibodies composed of IgM rise early in infection and usually disappear after 3 to 5 months. Complement fixing antibody becomes positive later than any other serological test and often reverts to normal within 1 year.[197]

ANGIOFOLLICULAR LYMPH NODE MALFORMATION

The neck is the second most common site for the peculiar lymphoid masses, which manifest a strong predilection for the anterior or posterior mediastinum or hilum of the lung, known by various appellations including giant lymph node hyperplasia,[198] lymphoid hamartoma,[199] angiomatous lymphoid hamartoma,[200] and angiofollicular lymph node hyperplasia.[201] Since existing terms commit one to an etiological stance, we have used the noncommittal descriptive term of angiofollicular lymph node malformation.

Clinically and pathologically these tumors may be divided into hyaline-vascular and plasma cell lesions.[198] The hyaline-vascular tumor presents as a single, circumscribed collection of lymphoid tissue studded by diffuse, prominent follicles with indeterminate subcapsular and medullary sinuses. The follicles are smaller than reactive follicles and typically consist of small pale centers, composed of an arteriole lined by plump endothelial cells often surrounded by large, pale, squamoid cells and concentric layers of small lymphocytes. Proliferated vessels, frequently hyalinized, also perforate the follicle, branch within the interfollicular tissues and extend to the capsule of the node.[201] The rich interfollicular vascularity obscures the lymphoid sinuses. Nodules of fibrous tissue may disrupt an interfollicular area that contains prominent numbers of small lymphocytes and scattered plasma cells, eosinophils and immunoblasts. A remnant of normal lymph node can be identified in about 60% of lesions indicating that the alterations occurred within a previously normal structure.[198] Characteristically, subjects with hyaline-vascular malformation are asymptomatic unless their enlarged lymph node compresses adjacent hilar or mediastinal structures.

A second localized enlargement of lymphoid tissue usually involving several nodes within a group has been described in the mediastinum, hilum and abdominal cavity. This lesion consists of lymphoid tissue containing large germinal centers throughout the node with partial effacement of the subcapsular and medullary sinuses by proliferated, tortuous vessels and sheets of plasma cells. The prominent vascularity and the presence of scattered angiofollicular centers in some of these nodes suggests a relationship to the angiofollicular lymph node malformation. Patients with this lesion also present with localized lymph node enlargement but may also experience fever, sweating, fatigue, splenomegaly and adenopathy in other locations. They also manifest numerous hematological and chemical abnormalities such as anemia, diminished serum iron and iron binding capacity, elevated sedimentation rate, low serum albumin, elevated serum globulins, leukocytosis, thrombocytosis and increased alkaline phosphatase activity.[198] Extirpation of the enlarged lymph nodes produces prompt remission of symptoms and the return of laboratory test values to normal.

A differential diagnosis of angiofollicular malformation from follicular lymphoma should present no problems if the vascular component is identified. Although prominent interfollicular fibrosis, bizarre immunoblasts, plasma cells and eosinophils could trap the unwary into diagnosing Hodgkin's disease, attention to the prominent vascular component and the presence of diffuse small follicles in angiofollicular malformation should avoid this mistake. The plasma cell lesion is morphologically so similar to lymph nodes from patients with rheumatoid arthritis[202] that differentiation using histological criteria alone may not be possible.

The essence of angiofollicular malformations remains unknown. Most authors feel these localized tumors represent either localized hyperplasias or hamartomas, and each advocate presents persuasive arguments for their concepts. At present, the major importance of this small class of tumors is that they are recognized as benign, that they are easily managed and that radical operations or radiation therapy should be avoided.

MISCELLANEOUS ATYPICAL LYMPHADENOPATHIES

Sinus Histiocytosis with Massive Lymphadenopathy (SHML). Typically, SHML presents as bilateral cervical lymphadenopathy, often of startling proportions, in a subject less than 20 years old.[203, 204] The patient usually has fever, leukocytosis, hypergammaglobulinemia and an elevated sedimentation rate. Lymph nodes in other sites, the tonsils and extranodal tissue including the orbit, eyelid, testicle, epidural space and bone may be affected.[205, 206] Hepatosplenomegaly rarely occurs. Histological examination of excised nodal tissue discloses massively dilated medullary and peripheral sinuses filled with proliferated histiocytes which have abundant, granular or vacuolated cytoplasms, oval or round nuclei and prominent nucleoli. The cytoplasm of the histiocytes often contains lymphocytes and, more rarely, plasma cells and red blood cells. Lymphoid follicles are usually absent, but distinct islands of medullary cords persevere and contain abundant numbers of plasma cells. The exuberance of the histiocytic proliferation may efface the architecture of the node; however, the banal appearance of the cells should differentiate this lesion from histiocytic lymphoma or malignant histiocytosis. Acute disseminated histiocytosis may morphologically resemble SHML, but the nuclei of the cells in acute disseminated histiocytosis tend to be folded and their nucleoli are inconspicuous; furthermore, the extent of the histiocytic infiltrate in acute disseminated histiocytosis is less than that in SHML. Also, acute disseminated histiocytosis is relentlessly progressive with hepatosplenomegaly and skin involvement. Isolated eosinophilic granuloma and multifocal eosinophilic granuloma are differentiated from SHML by the presence of eosinophils and necrosis in the former diseases

and their absence in SHML. The cause of SHML is unknown. Bacterial cultures, tests for bacterial antibodies and antibodies to EBV and tests of immune function have yielded inconsistent results.[204] The disease usually follows a leisurely, benign course with resolution of adenopathy after weeks or months and requires no treatment unless the anatomical location of the infiltrate produces distressing signs or symptoms.

Kawasaki Disease (Mucocutaneous Lymph Node Syndrome). Kawasaki disease is an acute febrile illness of unknown etiology. The disease occurs most frequently in infants and children below 5 years of age and the principal clinical manifestations, which occur in over 75% of subjects, consist of: fever of over 5 days duration unresponsive to antibiotics; bilateral ocular conjunctival congestion; dryness, fissuring and diffuse redness of lips and mouth; palmar and plantar erythema, peripheral edema and membranous desquamation of digital skin; truncal polymorphous exanthema without vesicles or crusts; and acute nonpurulent swelling of cervical lymph nodes to greater than 1.5 cm in diameter.[207, 208] Arthralgia or arthritis and diarrhea occur less constantly. Commonly encountered laboratory abnormalities include a polymorphonuclear leukocytosis, an elevated sedimentation rate, elevated alpha-2-globulins and a positive C-reactive protein. The disease is generally self-limited, but carditis and death can intervene. Autopsies of victims of Kawasaki disease have disclosed aneurysms, panarteritis and scarring in the coronary arteries morphologically resembling the findings observed in infantile polyarteritis nodosa.[208] Lymph nodes are seldom removed in this disorder, but when they are removed punctate necrosis, proliferated immunoblasts and perivascular fibrosis are disclosed.[208, 209] The disease is endemic in Japan and has been reported in the United States.[209, 210] Quests for a constant infectious agent have so far been unrewarding. An elevated IgE discovered in patients with Kawasaki disease raises the spectrum of an allergic etiology and would correlate with the notion that an allergic vasculitis plays a part in this disease.[211]

Dermatopathic Lymphadenitis. Skin disease associated with regional adenopathy can produce the entity dermatopathic lymphadenitis.[212] The skin eruption may begin as a localized exudative, exfoliative, lichenous or pigmented dermatitis and progress to a generalized dermatitis. The lymph nodes are usually superficial, discrete, firm, nontender and movable. Histologically, histiocytes with abundant pale vacuolated cytoplasm and oval or elongated nuclei containing one or two small nucleoli fill the sinusoids and compress the cortical and paracortical areas. The profligate histiocytic proliferation may obscure, but not destroy the nodal architecture, respects the capsule, but leaves few lymphoid follicles. Intracytoplasmic melanin pigment is often a conspicuous, but an inconstant, feature. Patients with chronic lymphatic leukemia, poorly differentiated lymphocytic lymphoma and mycosis fungoides can experience an exfoliative dermatitis. A lymph node removed for biopsy may disclose the underlying disease, may be a typical example of dermatopathic lymphadenitis or may evince the alterations of both benign and malignant infiltrations. Little difficulty should be encountered in recognizing the infiltrate of lymphocytic leukemia or poorly differentiated lymphocytic lymphoma, but since the nodal infiltrate in mycosis fungoides is typically patchy preserving normal foci, its differentiation from dermatopathic lymphadenopathy may pose problems.[213] These problems can be lessened if one observes the cytological details of the large cells in mycosis fungoides which with their amphophilic, often pyrinophilic cytoplasm and large nuclei containing coarsely, irregularly clumped chromatin should provide a striking contrast to the abundant, foamy, often pigmented cytoplasm and regular vesicular nucleus found in histiocytes in dermatopathic lymphadenitis.[213]

SUBCUTANEOUS ANGIOBLASTIC LYMPHOID HYPERPLASIA WITH EOSINOPHILIA (KIMURA'S DISEASE)

This lesion has a predilection for the *subcutaneous* tissues of the head and neck, although cases have been reported on the trunk and extremities. The lesions usually present as a solitary nodule but are occasionally multiple. Most of the reported cases have occurred in young adults, but the range has been from 10 to 42 years at first presentation.[214]

Peripheral blood eosinophilia is often present during the course of the lesion.

Histologically, the lesion is composed of an irregular proliferation of vascular spaces and channels lined by plump endothelial cells. Intracytoplasmic vacuoles are frequent in the latter. A hyperplastic lymphoid infiltrate and prominent tissue eosinophilia complete the picture.

Very likely, the lesions undergo a maturation process. Initially, there is an angioblastic phase accompanied by a diffuse lymphoid infiltrate. Later the vascular activity diminishes and varying degrees of fibrosis develop. It is in this phase that the hyperplastic lymphoid tissue assumes dominance with follicle and germinal center formation.

There is considerable variation in the amount of fibrosis and circumscription.

Histological similarity exists with the granulomatous reaction of insect bites, granuloma faciale and on occasion, angiosarcoma.

The etiology is unknown. Therapy consists of surgical excision of the mass.

EFFECTS OF RADIATION ON LYMPHORETICULAR TISSUES

Histopathology of Lymph Nodes after Lymphangiography

Lymphangiography (lymphangioadenography) is the radiographic visualization of lymph vessels and lymph nodes following intralymphatic injection of radiopaque material. Applications of the technique and its role in the definition of normal and abnormal patterns of the cervical lymphatic system have been masterfully presented by Fisch.[215]

The contrast medium is usually an organic iodine in combination with a base, viz., ethyl esters of poppy seed oil. The histological appearance of lymph nodes filled with the contrast medium has been studied in surgical specimens obtained by radical neck dissection and in biopsy samples taken at various time intervals following lymphangiography.[215, 216] There are three over-all changes associated with the postlymphangiographic state in lymph nodes. These are: an apparent hypoplasia or disappearance of germinal centers; sinus histiocytosis; and, particularly characteristic, the presence of the contrast oil itself.

Depending on the time interval, varying appearances are present within the involved nodes. Early, there is only oil in the sinuses. Neutrophilic leukocytes exude into the sinuses in the time span of 24 hours to 3 days postinjection, and, after a time, this initial acute inflammatory response (which is inconstant) is shifted to a foreign body giant cell reaction. The giant cells are invariably of the multinucleated foreign body type and are formed primarily from sinus histiocytes contiguous to the oil droplets.

The giant cell reaction is seen most often 4 days after angiography and once established tends to persist unchanged for several months. The cells are also observed in areas where contrast oil is present longer. The foreign body reaction ceases after the elimination of the oily contrast material from the lymph nodes. Radiologically, the elimination of the injected contrast material is normally completed after 1 year.[215] Extravasated contrast material is visible even longer.

Thorium Dioxide (Thorotrast) and Neoplasms of the Head and Neck

Thorotrast, a colloidal suspension of thorium dioxide, was introduced into the radiological armamentarium of contrast media in 1929. For some years afterward (1930 to 1945), it was widely used in a variety of diagnostic procedures, including visualization of the spleen, liver, kidneys, breast, sinuses, brain and vascular systems by intracavitary, interstitial and intravascular administration. This rather extensive use was done in the face of a warning by the Council of Pharmacy and Chemistry of the American Medical Association,[217] who warned against and disapproved of the use of thorium dioxide as a diagnostic agent because of its radioactive properties.

Thorium is a naturally occurring radioactive substance which emits alpha and beta particles and gamma rays. The major emission is that of alpha particles with a long half-life of 1.4×10^{10} years. The beta particles and gamma rays emitted are too feeble to be of physiological significance. The parent element, thorium, decays to mesothorium and radiothorium, which are also powerful alpha emitters. During the decay process, the radioactivity of *thorium* decreases to 50% in 5 years, but then the activity actually increases as radiothorium breaks down to form its alpha-emitting daughters. After 10 years, the residual radioactivity is 54%, increasing to a peak in the next 15 years.

Injected into the blood vessels, thorotrast is retained mostly in the reticuloendothelial system and, therefore, in organs where reticuloendothelial cells are the most numerous such as the spleen, lymph nodes, bone marrow and liver (Figure 23.21). Excretion studies indicate that only minute amounts of thorium dioxide are eliminated after injection. The major portion remains in the body *permanently*, where, as indicated above, it is distributed principally in the reticuloendothelial system.

Adverse effects of thorotrast injections are late in appearing and consist of (1) fibrosis, (2) so-called "thorotrastomas" and (3) development of malignant neoplasms.[218-220] The late lesion most frequently observed after thorotrast injection is fibrosis, both local, due to extravasation at the site of injection, and diffuse, in the tissues where the medium is deposited (liver, spleen, lymph nodes and bone marrow).

Thorotrastomas are distinctive forms of fibrosis produced by the extravascular deposition of thorium dioxide. The local formation of fibrous tissue around thorotrast deposits is called a thorotras-

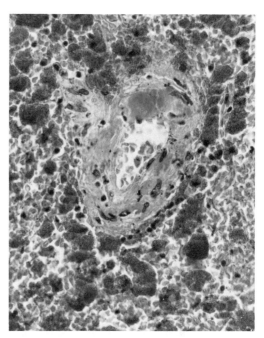

Figure 23.21. Characteristic blue-gray granular contrast material (thorotrast) in reticuloendothelial cells of the spleen.

toma or thorotrast granuloma. Most cases are located in the cervical region, as cerebral angiography was by far the most frequent diagnostic procedure involved. The granulomas are very hard, partly calcified and adherent to contiguous structures. On cut section, they are chalky white, sometimes with areas of softening. Large soft areas are very likely the result of ischemia from radiation-induced obliteration of the blood supply. Histologically, the granuloma is composed of very dense, hyalinized connective tissue in which thorotrast is either present within histiocytes or found free.

The development of malignancy constitutes the most serious after-effect of thorotrast injection. Criteria generally accepted in order to ascribe a neoplasm to thorotrast are as follows.[220] Thorium dioxide granules should be found in the immediate vicinity of the tumor, the latency period should be sufficiently long and the radiation dose should be sufficiently high.

The carcinogenic property of thorotrast had been repeatedly demonstrated in experimental animals *before* the first malignant tumor in man could be attributed to the substance. Since then, a significant number of examples of neoplastic induction have been reported. Approximately 200 pathologically confirmed cases are by now reported in the literature, and the number is steadily increasing.[220] The majority of the neoplasms appear in the main reticuloendothelial organs of the body, the liver and spleen, and particularly in the liver, but local tumor induction is becoming increasingly recognized and may increase after the relatively long latent period of 10 to 20 years has passed.

A second group of malignant neoplasms develops after local deposition of thorotrast used for the visualization of body cavities and tubular structures. It is this group and the thorotrast granulomas that are of primary interest to the head and neck surgeon.

Grove and Cooke,[221] in 1940, described the use of thorotrast in the roentgenographic examination of the sinuses in 117 cases. In the short time span of their study, they found no harmful effect from the radioactivity. Hofer,[222] in 1952, first described the probable relationship between intrasinus injection of thorotrast and carcinoma of the maxillary antrum. Since then, reviews have appeared in the otolaryngological literature.[219, 223-225] From these reviews, the following conclusions can be made: (1) thorotrast, retained in any body cavity or organ, is carcinogenic; (2) in those patients in whom thorotrast has been instilled in a body cavity, such as a paranasal sinus, an attempt should be made to remove it; (3) every otolaryngologist should review his records and try to locate those patients in whom thorotrast has been instilled into the sinuses or who have had extravasation of thorotrast into the soft tissues of the neck during angiographic studies; (4) the latent period of 10 to 20 years between thorotrast instillation and the development of a sinus neoplasm usually obtains.

Aside from the ever present danger of carcinogenesis, however, the fibrosis and granulomatous response to extravascular thorotrast constitutes a considerable hazard and morbidity. Levowitz et al.[226] describe the findings in 45 cases of cervical, perivascular granuloma. The foreign material promotes a severe desmoplastic response in which the musculofascial structures are replaced by contracting connective tissue. This process gave rise to a fixed, hard neck mass in 60% of the patients under study. Specific lesions noted were destruction of the cervical segments of the ninth through twelfth cranial nerves and sympathetic nerves. These structures were eventually replaced by fibrous connective tissue. Disturbances in deglutition, paralysis of the vocal cords, atrophy of the tongue and Horner's syndrome occurred.

Clinical diagnosis is readily made by observing an irregular and densely opacified mass within the visceral compartment of the neck. A possible confusion with other calcified lesions may be readily resolved by the demonstration of significant radioactivity over the mass.

Lymph Nodes and Irradiation

The effect of ionizing irradiation in normal lymph nodes and lymphatic vessels has largely been derived from observations of clinical material. Notable exceptions do, however, exist.[227] Experimental studies have yielded two divergent views concerning *functional* impairment following exposure of lymph nodes to ionizing irradiation: (1) irradiation may *increase* the resistance of lymph nodes to metastatic spread; and (2) irradiation increases the incidence of metastases to the lymph nodes by impairing the function of the lymphatics and lymph nodes. Other reports suggest radiation produces an obstruction of the lymphatic vessels by a perivascular fibrosis.

The experiments of Sherman and O'Brien[228] and Shina and Goldenberg[229] are representative of the current uncertainty over the effects of ionizing irradiation on function. The former investigators, using dogs as their experimental animal, concluded that the physical agent had little effect on lymph node and lymphatic function. Although there is a reduction in size and a replacement fibrosis after exposure, the lymph flow appears unaffected. Shina and Goldenberg,[229] on the other hand, presented evidence that the filtration capacity of lymph nodes is decreased after radiation therapy.

Histomorphological alterations in the postirradiated lymph node are well defined. They fall into three phases. The early phase is one of cellular destruction. This is followed by an intermediate phase of repopulation which may begin as soon as 24 hours after the irradiation. The late phase is one dominated by regressive alterations. During the first day after irradiation there is a severe degeneration of lymphocytes and disappearance of follicles. Repopulation, however, is prompt, with the lymph nodes almost completely restored after 24 hours. There are, however, fewer mitoses, fewer mast cells and no germinal centers. Germinal centers reappear a few days after the irradiation, and after 8 weeks the granulated mast cells are again numerous. Repopulation is usually so effective that during the first weeks after irradiation, it is difficult, on the basis of a single lymph node examination, to determine whether or not the node has been irradiated.

The progressive atrophy of the lymph node is observed after about 2 weeks. This is manifested by a secondary depletion or disappearance of the lymphocytes, follicles and germinal centers and an almost simultaneous increase in connective tissue. This leads to almost complete eradication of the lymph node structure after 9 to 12 months. Even then, however, most of the sinuses are open and clearly defined with a well presented reticulin network.

REFERENCES

1. Rosenberg, S. A., Diamond, H. D., Jaslowitz, B., and Craver, L. F.: Lymphosarcoma; a review of 1,269 cases. Medicine 40:31, 1961.
2. Symmers, W. St. C.: The lymphoreticular system. In Systemic Pathology, edited by G. P. Wright and W. St. C. Symmers. Longmans, Green and Co., Ltd., London, 1966.
3. Rappaport, J., Winter, W. J., and Hicks, E. B.: Follicular lymphoma: re-evaluation of its position in the scheme of malignant lymphoma; based on a survey of 253 cases. Cancer 9:792, 1956.
4. Rappaport, H.: Tumors of hematopoietic system. In Atlas of Tumor Pathology, Section II, Fascicle 8. Armed Forces Institute of Pathology, Washington, D.C., 1966.
5. Schnitzer, B., Loesel, L. S., and Reed, R. E.: Lymphosarcoma cell leukemia. A clinicopathologic study. Cancer 26:1082, 1970.
6. Lotz, M. I., Chabner, B., De Vita, V. T. Jr., Johnson, R. E., and Berard, C. W.: Pathological staging of 100 consecutive untreated patients with non Hodgkin's lymphomas. Cancer 37:266, 1976.
7. Johnson, R. E., De Vita, V. T. Jr., Kun, L. E., Chabner, B. R., Chretien, P. B., Berard, C. W., and Johnson, S. K.: Patterns of involvement with malignant lymphoma and implications for treatment decision making. Brit. J. Cancer 31 (suppl. II): 237, 1975.
8. Nosanchuk, J. S., and Schnitzer, B.: Follicular hyperplasia in lymph nodes from patients with rheumatoid arthritis. Cancer 24:343, 1969.
9. Hartsock, R. J., Halling, L. W., and King, F. M.: Luetic lymphadenitis. A clinical and histologic study of 20 cases. Am. J. Clin. Pathol. 53:304, 1970.
10. Histopathological definition of Burkitt's tumor. Memorandum Review. Bull. W. H. O. 40:601, 1969.
11. Schnitzer, B.: Malignant lymphomas. Univ. Mich. Med. Ctr. J. 36:32, 1970.
12. Sheehan, W. W.: The relationship between lymphocytic leukemias and lymphomas. In Recent Results in Cancer Research, vol. 36, p. 24, edited by J. E. Ultman, M. L. Griem, W. H. Kirsten, and R. W. Wissler. Current Concepts in the Management of Leukemia and Lymphoma, Springer-Verlag, Berlin, 1971.
13. Schnitzer, B., and Kass, L.: Leukemic phase of reticulum cell sarcoma (histiocytic lymphoma). Cancer 31:547, 1973.
14. Belding, H. W., Daland, G. A., and Parker, F., Jr.: Histiocytic and monocytic leukemia: a clinical, hematological and pathological differentiation. Cancer 8:237, 1955.
15. Braylan, R. C., Jaffe, E. S., and Berard, C. W.: Malignant lymphomas: current classification and new observations. In Pathology Annual, p. 213, edited by S. C. Sommers. Appleton-Century-Crofts, New York, 1975.
16. Bennett, M. H., Farrer-Brown, G., Henry, K., and Jelliffe, A. M.: Classification of non-Hodgkin's lymphomas. Lancet 2:405, 1974.
17. Dorfman, R. F.: Classification of non-Hodgkin's lymphomas. Lancet 2:261, 1974.
18. Gerard-Marchant, R., Hamlin, I., Lennert, K., Rilke, F., Stansfeld, A. G., and van Unnik, J. A. M.: Classification of non-Hodgkin's lymphomas. Lancet 2:406, 1974.
19. Lukes, R. J., and Collins, R. D.: Immunologic characteri-

zation of human malignant lymphomas. Cancer 34:1488, 1974.
20. Dutcher, T. F., and Fahey, J. L.: The histopathology of macroglobulinemia of Waldenström. J. Natl. Cancer Inst. 22:887, 1959.
21. Kim, H., Heller, P., and Rappaport, H.: Monoclonal gammopathies associated with lymphoproliferative disorders. Am. J. Clin. Pathol. 59:282, 1973.
22. Stein, H., Lennert, K., and Parwaresch, M. R.: Malignant lymphomas of B cell type. Lancet 2:855, 1972.
23. Brouet, J. C., Preudhomme, J. L., Flandrin, G., Chelloul, N., and Seligman, M.: Brief communication: membrane markers in "histiocytic" lymphomas (reticulum cell sarcomas). J. Natl. Cancer Inst. 56:631, 1976.
24. Byrne, G. E., Jr., and Rappaport, H.: Malignant histiocytosis. In Malignant Diseases of the Hematopoietic System, p. 145. Gann Monograph on Cancer Research 15. Univ. Tokyo Press, Tokyo, 1973.
25. Scott, R. B., and Robb-Smith, A. H. T.: Histiocytic medullary reticulosis. Lancet 2:194, 1939.
26. Carbone, P. P., Kaplan, H. S., Musshoff, K., Smithers, D. W., and Tubiana, M.: Report on the committee on Hodgkin's disease staging classification. Cancer Res. 31:1860, 1971.
27. Ultman, J. E., and Stein, R. S.: Non-Hodgkin's lymphoma. An approach to staging and therapy. CA. 25:320, 1975.
28. Ferguson, D., Allen, L., Griem, M., Moran, M., Rappaport, H., and Ultman, J.: Surgical experience with staging laparotomy in 125 patients with lymphoma. Arch. Intern. Med. 131:356, 1973.
29. Jones, S., Fuks, Z., Bull, M., Kadin, M., Dorfman, R., Kaplan, H., Rosenberg, S., and Kim, H.: Non-Hodgkin's lymphomas. IV. Clinico-pathologic correlation in 405 cases. Cancer 31:806, 1973.
30. Veronesi, U., Musumeci, R., Pizzetti, F., Gennari, L., and Bonadonna, G.: The value of staging laparotomy in non-Hodgkin's lymphoma. Cancer 33:446, 1974.
31. Moran, E. M., Ultman, J. E., Ferguson, D. J., Hoffer, P. B., Ranniger, K., and Rapparport, H.: Staging laparotomy in non-Hodgkin's lymphoma. Brit. J. Cancer 31 (suppl. II):228, 1975.
32. Chabner, B. A., Johnson, R. E., Young, R. E., Canellos, G. P., Hubbard, S. P., Johnson, S. K., and DeVita, V. T., Jr.: Sequential nonsurgical and surgical staging of non-Hodgkin's lymphoma. Ann. Intern. Med. 85:149, 1976.
33. Hodgkin, T.: On some morbid appearances of the absorbent glands and spleen. Med.-Chir. Trans. 17:68, 1832.
34. MacMahon, B.: Epidemiology of Hodgkin's disease. Cancer Res. 26:1189, 1966.
35. Rosenberg, S. A., and Kaplan, H. S.: Evidence for an orderly progression in the spread of Hodgkin's disease. Cancer Res. 26:1225, 1966.
36. Smithers, D. W.: Spread of Hodgkin's disease. Lancet 1: 1262, 1970.
37. Rappaport, H., and Strum, S. B.: Vascular invasion in Hodgkin's disease; its incidence and relationship to the spread of the disease. Cancer 25:1304, 1970.
38. Strum, S. B., Hutchison, G. B., Park, J. K., and Rappaport, H.: Further observations on the biologic significance of vascular invasion in Hodgkin's disease. Cancer 27:1, 1971.
39. Davidson, J. W., and Clarke, E. A.: The Hodgkin maze. Lancet 1:1051, 1970.
40. MacMahon, B., Cole, P., and Newell, G. R.: Hodgkin's disease: one entity or two? Lancet 2:1285, 1970.
41. Glatstein, E., Guernsey, J. M., Rosenberg, S. A., and Kaplan, H. S.: The value of laparotomy and splenectomy in the staging of Hodgkin's disease. Cancer 24:709, 1969.
42. Keller, A. R., Kaplan, H. S., Lukes, R. J., and Rappaport, H.: Correlation of histopathology with other prognostic indicators. Cancer 22:487, 1968.
43. Rosenberg, S. A.: Report of the committee on staging of Hodgkin's disease. Cancer Res. 26:1310, 1966.
44. Lukes, R. J.: Criteria for involvement of lymph node, bone marrow, spleen and liver in Hodgkin's disease. Cancer

Res. 31:1755, 1971.

45. Peckham, M. J., and Cooper, E. H.: Proliferation characteristics of the various classes of cells in Hodgkin's disease. Cancer 24:135, 1969.

46. Lukes, R. J., Tindle, B. H., and Parker, J. W.: Reed-Sternberg-like cells in infectious mononucleosis. Lancet 2:1003, 1969.

47. Schnitzer, B.: Reed-Sternberg-like cells in lymphocytic lymphoma and chronic lymphocytic leukemia. Lancet 1: 1399, 1970.

48. Wright, D. H.: Reed-Sternberg-like cells in recurrent Burkitt lymphomas. Lancet 1:1052, 1970.

49. Strum, S. B., Park, J. K., and Rappaport, H.: Observation of cells resembling Sternberg-Reed cells in conditions other than Hodgkin's disease. Cancer 26:176, 1970.

50. Lukes, R. J.: Relationship of histologic features to clinical stages in Hodgkin's disease. Am. J. Roentgenol. Radium Ther. Nucl. Med. 90:944, 1963.

51. Lukes, R. J., Butler, J. J., and Hicks, E. B.: The natural history of Hodgkin's disease as related to its pathologic picture. Symposium on clinical aspects of Hodgkin's disease. Cancer 19:317, 1966.

52. Jackson, H., Jr., and Parker, F., Jr.: Hodgkin's disease. II. Pathology. New Engl. J. Med. 231:35, 1944.

53. Lukes, R. J., and Butler, J. J.: The pathology and nomenclature of Hodgkin's disease. Cancer Res. 26:1063, 1966.

54. Lukes, R. J., Craver, L. L., Hall, T. C., Rappaport, H., and Ruben, P.: Hodgkin's disease; report of nomenclature committee. Cancer Res. 26:1311, 1966.

55. Hamann, W., Oehlert, W., Musshoff, K., Nufs, A., and Schnelbacher, B.: Histologic classification of Hodgkin's disease and its relevance to prognosis. Ger. Med. Mon. 15:509, 1970.

56. Fuller, L. M., Gamble, J. F., and Butler, J. J.: Influence in localized Hodgkin's disease treated with intensive large volume radiotherapy. J. Radiol. 98:641, 1971.

57. Strum, S. B., and Rappaport, H.: Interrelations of the histologic types of Hodgkin's disease. Arch. Pathol. 91: 127, 1971.

58. Strum, S. B., and Rappaport, H.: Hodgkin's disease in the first decade. Pediatrics 46:748, 1970.

59. Schnitzer, B., Nishiyama, R. H., Heidelberger, K. P., and Weaver, D. K.: Hodgkin's disease in children. Cancer 31: 560, 1973.

60. Berard, C. W., Thomas, L. B., Axtell, L. M., Kruse, M., Newell, G., and Kagan, R.: The relationship of histopathologic subtype to clinical stage of Hodgkin's disease at diagnosis. Cancer Res. 31:1776, 1971.

61. Lukes, R. J., and Tindle, B. H.: Immunoblastic lymphadenopathy: a hyperimmune entity resembling Hodgkin's disease. New Engl. J. Med. 291:1, 1975.

62. Frizzera, G., Moran, E. M., and Rappaport, H.: Angio-immunoblastic lymphadenopathy with dysproteinemia. Lancet 1:1070, 1974.

63. Frizzera, G., Moran, E. M., and Rappaport, H.: Angio-immunoblastic lymphadenopathy. Diagnosis and clinical course. Am. J. Med. 59:803, 1975.

64. Lennert, K., and Mestagh, J.: Lymphogranulomatosen mit konstant hohem epitheliodzellgehalt. Virchows Arch. (Pathol. Anat.) 344:1, 1968.

65. Lennert, K., More, N., Stein, H., and Kaiserling, E.: The histopathology of malignant lymphoma. Br. J. Haemat. 31 (suppl.):193, 1975.

66. Burke, J. S., and Butler, J. J.: Malignant lymphoma with a high content of epithelioid histiocytes (Lennert's lymphoma). Am. J. Clin. Pathol. 66:1, 1976.

67. Saxen, E., and Saxen, L.: The histologic diagnosis of glandular toxoplasmosis. Lab. Invest. 8:386, 1959.

68. Schnitzer, B., Meadows, T. R., Gehrke, C. F., and Jackson, W. L.: Immunoblastic lymphadenopathy. Light and electron microscopic observations. Lab. Invest. 34:332, 1976.

69. Banfi, A., Bonadonna, G., Carnevali, G., Molinari, R., and Monfardini, S.: Lymphoreticular sarcoma with primary involvement of Waldeyer's ring. Cancer 26:341, 1970.

70. Wang, C. C.: Malignant lymphoma of Waldeyer's ring. Radiology 92:1335, 1969.

71. Paparella, M. M., and El Fiky, F. M.: Ear involvement in malignant lymphoma. Ann. Otol. 81:352, 1972.

72. Palva, T., Palva, A., Dammert, K., and Karma, P.: Malignant lymphoma invading the facial nerve. Arch. Otolaryngol. 99:433, 1974.

73. Kadin, M. E., Glatstein, E., and Dorfman, R. F.: Clinicopathologic studies of 117 untreated patients subjected to laparotomy for the staging of Hodgkin's disease. Cancer 27:1277, 1971.

74. Todd, G. B., Chir, M. B., and Michaels, L.: Hodgkin's disease involving Waldeyer's lymphoid ring. Cancer 34: 1769, 1974.

75. McNelis, F. L., and Pai, V. T.: Malignant lymphoma of head and neck. Laryngoscope 79:1076, 1969.

76. Fuller, L. M.: Results of intensive regional radiation therapy in the treatment of Hodgkin's disease and the malignant lymphomas of the head and neck. Am. J. Roentgenol. Radium Ther. Nucl. Med. 99:340, 1967.

77. Catlin, D.: Surgery for head and neck lymphomas. Surgery 60:1160, 1966.

78. Butler, J. J., Stryker, J. A., and Schullenberger, C. C.: A clinicopathologic study of stages I and II non-Hodgkin's lymphoma using the Lukes-Collins classification. Br. J. Cancer 31 (suppl. II):208, 1975.

79. Hansen, J. A., and Good, R. A.: Malignant disease of the lymphoid system in immunological perspective. Hum. Pathol. 5:567, 1974.

80. Rappaport, H.: In Discussion II: Round Table discussion of histopathologic classification. C. W. Berard, Chairman. Cancer Treat. Rep. 61:1037, 1977.

81. Mathe, G., Rappaport, H., O'Conor, G. T., and Torloni, H.: Histological and cytological typing of neoplastic diseases of hematopoietic and lymphoid tissues. In W. H. O. International Histological Classification of Tumors, No. 14 Geneva, W. H. O., 1976.

82. Lukes, R. J., and Collins, R. D.: Lukes-Collins classification and its significance. Cancer Treat. Rep. 61:971, 1977.

83. Parker, J. W., Taylor, C. R., Pattengale, P. K., Royston, I., Tindle, B. H., Cain, M. J., and Lukes, R. J.: Morphologic and cytochemical comparison of human lymphoblastoid T-cell and B-cell lines. J. Natl. Cancer Inst. 60:59, 1978.

84. Raff, M. C.: Two distinct populations of peripheral lymphocytes in mice distinguishable by immunofluorescence. Immunology 19:637, 1970.

85. Unanue, E. R., Grey, H. M., Rabellino, E., Campbell, P., and Schmidtke, J.: Immunoglobulins on the surface of lymphocytes. II. The bone marrow as the main source of lymphocytes with detectable surface-bound immunoglobulins. J. Exp. Med. 133:1188, 1971.

86. Ford, W. L., and Gowans, J. L.: The traffic of lymphocytes. Semin. Hematol. 6:67, 1969.

87. Craddock, G. G., Longmire, R., and McMillan, R.: Lymphocytes and the immune response. N. Engl. J. Med. 285: 324, 1971.

88. Pilgrim, H. E.: Relationship of the selective metastatic behavior of reticular tissues to the migration patterns of their normal cells of origin. J. Natl. Cancer Inst. 49:3, 1972.

89. Jaffe, E. S., Shevach, E. M., Frank, M. M., Berard, C. W., and Green, I.: Nodular lymphoma. Evidence for origin from follicular B lymphocytes. N. Engl. J. Med. 290:813, 1974.

90. Lukes, R. J., Taylor, C. R., Parker, J. W., Lincoln, T. L., Pattengale, P. K., and Tindle, B. H.: A morphologic and immunologic surface marker study of 299 cases of non-Hodgkin lymphomas and related leukemias. Am. J. Pathol. 90:461, 1978.

91. Barcos, M. P., and Lukes, R. J.: Malignant lymphoma of convoluted lymphocytes. A new entity of possible T-cell type. In Conflicts of Childhood Cancer. An evaluation of current management, vol. 4, edited by I. F. Sinks and J. O. Godden. A.R. Liss, Inc., New York, 1975.

92. Nathwani, B., Kim, H., and Rappaport, H.: Malignant lymphoma, lymphoblastic. Cancer 38:964, 1976.

93. Schein, P. S., MacDonald, J. S., and Edelson, R.: Cutaneous T-cell lymphoma. Cancer 38:1859, 1976.

94. Broder, S., Edelson, R., Lutzner, M. A., Nelson, D. L., MacDermott, R. P., Durm, M. E., Goldman, C. K., Meade, B., and Waldmann, T. A.: The Sezary syndrome. A malignant proliferation of helper T-cells. J. Clin. Invest. 58:1297, 1976.

95. Kim, H., Jacobs, C., Warnke, R. A., and Dorfman, R. A.: Malignant lymphoma with a high content of epithelioid histiocytes. A distinct clinicopathologic entity and a form of so-called Lennert's lymphoma. Cancer 41:620, 1978.

96. Burkitt, D.: A sarcoma involving jaws in African children. Br. J. Surg. 46:218, 1958.

97. Burkitt, D.: Burkitt's lymphoma outside the known endemic area of Africa and New Guinea. Int. J. Cancer 2:562, 1967.

98. Anand, S. V., Davey, W. W., and Cohen, B.: Tumors of the jaw in West Africa: a review of 256 patients. Br. J. Surg. 54:901, 1967.

99. Histopathological definition of Burkitt's tumor, Memorandum Review. Bull. W. H. O. 40:601, 1969.

100. Terrill, D. G., Lee, A., LeDonne, M. A., and Nusbaum, T.: American Burkitt's lymphoma in Pittsburgh, Pennsylvania. Oral Surg. 44:411, 1977.

101. Judson, S. C., Henle, W., and Henle, G.: A cluster of Epstein-Barr-virus-associated American Burkitt's lymphoma. N. Engl. J. Med. 297:464, 1977.

102. Adatia, A. K.: Dental tissues and Burkitt's tumor. Oral Surg. 25:221, 1968.

103. Carbone, P. P., Berard, C. W., Bennett, J. M., Ziegler, J. L., Cohen, M. H., and Gerber, P.: Burkitt's tumor. Ann. Intern. Med. 70:817, 1969.

104. Ziegler, J. L.: Burkitt's lymphoma. Med. Clin. North Am. 61:1073, 1977.

105. Katayama, I., Uehara, H., Gleser, R. A., and Weintraub, L.: The value of electron microscopy in the diagnosis of Burkitt's lymphoma. Am. J. Clin. Pathol. 61:540, 1974.

106. Pagano, J. S., Huang, C. H., and Levine, P.: Absence of Epstein-Barr viral DNA in American Burkitt's lymphoma. N. Engl. J. Med. 284:1395, 1973.

107. Ziegler, J. L.: Treatment results of 54 American patients with Burkitt's lymphoma are similar to the African experience. N. Engl. J. Med. 297:75, 1977.

108. Purlito, D. T., DeFlorio, D., Hutt, L. M., Bhawan, J., Yang, J. P. S., Otto, R., and Edwards, W.: Variable phenotypic expression of an x-linked recessive lymphoproliferative syndrome. N. Engl. J. Med. 297:1077, 1977.

109. Pahor, A. L.: Extramedullary plasmacytoma of the head and neck, parotid and submandibular salivary glands. J. Laryngol. 91:241, 1977.

110. Stout, A. P., and Kenney, F. R.: Primary plasma-cell tumors of the upper air passages and oral cavity. Cancer 2:261, 1949.

111. Batsakis, J. G., Fries, G. T., Goldman, R. T., and Karlsberg, R. C.: Upper respiratory tract plasmacytoma: extramedullary myeloma. Arch. Otolaryngol. 79:613, 1964.

112. Dolin, S., and Dewar, J. P.: Extramedullary plasmacytoma. Am. J. Pathol. 32:83, 1956.

113. Pascoe, H. R., and Dorfman, R. F.: Extramedullary plasmacytoma of the submaxillary gland. Am. J. Clin. Pathol. 51:501, 1969.

114. Poole, A. G., and Marchetta, F. C.: Extramedullary plasmacytoma of the head and neck. Cancer 22:141, 1968.

115. Noorani, M. A.: Plasmacytoma of middle ear and upper respiratory tract. J. Laryngol. 89:105, 1975.

116. Touma, Y. B.: Extramedullary plasmacytoma of the head and neck. J. Laryngol. 85:125, 1971.

117. Booth, J. B., Cheesman, A. D., and Vincenti, N. H.: Extramedullary plasmacytoma of the upper respiratory tract. Ann. Otol. 82:709, 1973.

118. Gorenstein, A., Neel, H. B., III, Devine, K. D., and Weiland, L. H.: Solitary extramedullary plasmacytoma of the larynx. Arch. Otolaryngol. 103:159, 1977.

119. Cataldo, E., and Meyer, I.: Solitary and multiple plasmacell tumors of the jaws and oral cavity. Oral Surg. 22:628, 1966.

120. Acevedo, A., and Buhler, J. E.: Plasma cell granuloma of the gingiva. Oral Surg. 43:196, 1977.

121. Bahadori, M., and Liebow, A. A.: Plasma cell granulomas of the lung. Cancer 31:191, 1973.

122. Hellwig, C. A.: Extramedullary plasma cell tumors as observed in various locations. Arch. Pathol. 36:95, 1943.

123. Webb, H. E., Devine, K. N., and Harrison, E. G., Jr.: Solitary myeloma of the mandible. Oral Surg. 22:1, 1966.

124. Raley, L. L., and Granite, E. L.: Plasmacytoma of the maxilla: report of case. J. Oral Surg. 35:497, 1977.

125. Osserman, E. F.: Plasma cell myeloma. II. Clinical aspects. N. Engl. J. Med. 261:952, 1959.

126. Waldenström, J.: Changing concepts of multiple myeloma. Acta Paediatr. (suppl. 100) 53:87, 1954.

127. Ewing, M. R., and Foote, F. W., Jr.: Plasma-cell tumors of mouth and upper air passages. Cancer 5:499, 1952.

128. Lieberman, P. H., Jones, C. R., Dargeon, H. W. K., and Begg, C. F.: Reappraisal of eosinophilic granuloma of bone, Hand-Schüller-Christian syndrome and Letterer-Siwe syndrome. Medicine 48:375, 1969.

129. Otani, S.: Discussion of eosinophilic granuloma of bone, Letterer-Siwe disease and Hand-Schüller-Christian disease. J. Mt. Sinai Hosp. N.Y. 24:1079, 1957.

130. Cline, M. J., and Golde, D. W.: A review and re-evaluation of the histiocytic disorders. Am. J. Med. 55:49, 1973.

131. Lichtenstein, L.: Histiocytosis X (eosinophilic granuloma of bone, Letterer-Siwe disease and Schüller-Christian disease). Further observations of pathologic and clinical importance. J. Bone Joint Surg. 48A:76, 1964.

132. Oberman, H. A.: Idiopathic histiocytosis, clinicopathologic study of 40 cases and review of the literature on eosinophilic granuloma of bone, Hand-Schüller-Christian disease and Letterer-Siwe disease. Pediatrics 28:307, 1961.

133. Schajowicz, F., and Stullitel, J.: Eosinophilic granuloma of bone and its relationship to Hand-Schüller-Christian and Letterer-Siwe syndromes. J. Bone Joint Surg. (Br.) 55:545, 1973.

134. Newton, W. A., and Hamoudi, A. B.: Histiocytosis: Histologic classification with clinical correlation. In Perspectives in Pediatric Pathology, edited by H. S. Rosenberg and R. P. Bolande, vol. 1, pp. 251–283. Year Book Medical Publishers, Inc., Chicago, 1973.

135. Vogel, J. M., and Vogel, P.: Idiopathic histiocytosis: A discussion of eosinophilic granuloma, Hand-Schüller-Christian and Letterer-Siwe syndromes. Semin. Hematol. 9:349, 1972.

136. Tors, M.: A survey of Hand-Schüller-Christian disease in otolaryngology. Acta Otolaryng. 62:217, 1966.

137. Enriquez, P., Dahlin, D. C., Hayles, A. B., and Henderson, E. D.: Histiocytosis X, a clinical study. Mayo Clin. Proc. 42:88, 1967.

138. Moskow, R., Levine, L. J., and Marin, A.: Multifocal eosinophilic granuloma simulating periodontal disease. N.Y. State Dent. J. 37:607, 1971.

139. Lucaya, J.: Histiocytosis X. Am. J. Dis. Child. 121:289, 1971.

140. Daneshbod, K., and Kissane, J. M.: Histiocytosis. The prognosis of polycystic eosinophilic granuloma. Am. J. Clin. Pathol. 65:601, 1976.

141. Doede, K. G., and Rappaport, H.: Long-term survival of patients with acute differentiated histiocytosis (Letterer-Siwe disease). Cancer 20:1782, 1967.

142. Miller, D. R.: Familial reticuloendotheliosis: concurrence of disease in five siblings. Pediatrics 38:986, 1966.

143. Juberg, R. C., Kloepter, H. W., and Oberman, H. A.: Genetic determination of acute disseminated histiocytosis X (Letterer-Siwe syndrome) Pediatrics 45:753, 1970.

144. Zinkham, W. H.: Multifocal eosinophilic granuloma: natural history, etiology and management. Am. J. Med. 60:457, 1976.

145. Dorfman, R. F., and Warnke, R.: Lymphadenopathy simulating the malignant lymphomas. Hum. Pathol. 5:519, 1974.

146. Rappaport, H.: Tumors of the hematopoietic system. In Atlas of Tumor Pathology, Section II, Fascicle 8. Armed Forces Institute of Pathology, Washington, D.C., 1966.

147. Ahnquist, G., and Holyoke, J. B.: Congenital Letterer-Siwe disease (reticuloendotheliosis) in a term stillborn infant.

J. Pediat. 57:897, 1960.

148. Claman, H. N., Suva, H. V., Githens, H. H., and Hathaway, W. E.: Histiocytic reaction in dysgammaglobulinemia and congenital rubella. Pediatrics 46:89, 1970.

149. deMan, J. C. H.: Rod-like tubular structures in the cytoplasm of histiocytes in "histiocytosis X." J. Pathol. Bacteriol. 95:123, 1968.

150. Vernon, M. L., Fountain, L., Krelo, H. M., Horta-Barbosa, L., Fuccillo, D. A., and Sever, H. K.: Birbeck's granules (Langhans' cell granules) in human lymph nodes. Am. J. Clin. Pathol. 60:771, 1973.

151. Leikins, S., Puruganan, G., Frankel, A., Steerman, R., and Chandra, R.: Immunologic parameters in histiocytosis X. Cancer 32:796, 1973.

152. Cederbaum, S. D., Niwayama, G., Stiehm, E. R., Neerhout, R. C., Ammann, A. J., and Berman, W.: Combined immunodeficiency presenting as the Letterer-Siwe syndrome. J. Pediatr. 85:466, 1974.

153. Ochs, H. D., Davis, S. D., Mickelson, E., Lerner, K. G., and Wedgwood, R. S.: Combined immunodeficiency and reticuloendotheliosis with eosinophilia. J. Pediatr. 85:463, 1974.

154. Long, J. C., Mihm, M. C., and Qazi, R.: Malignant lymphoma of the skin. A clinicopathologic study of lymphoma other than mycosis fungoides diagnosed by skin biopsy. Cancer 38:1282, 1976.

155. Nelson, P., Santamaria, A., Olson, R. L., and Nayak, N. C.: Generalized lymphohistiocytic infiltration. A familial disease not previously described and different from Letterer-Siwe disease and Chediak-Higaski syndrome. Pediatrics 27:931, 1961.

156. Bell, R. J. M., Brafield, A. J. E., Barnes, N. D., and France, N. E.: Familial hemophagocytic reticulosis. Arch. Dis. Child. 43:601, 1968.

157. Koto, A., Morecki, R., and Santorneou, M.: Congenital hemophagocytic reticulosis. Am. J. Clin. Pathol. 65:495, 1976.

158. Rosai, J., and Dorfman, R. F.: Sinus histiocytosis with massive lymphadenopathy. Arch. Pathol. 87:63, 1969.

159. Blume, R. S., and Wolff, S.: The Chediak-Higashi syndrome: studies in four patients and a review of the literature. Medicine 54:247, 1972.

160. Blume, R. S., Bennett, J. M., Yankee, R. A., and Wolff, S. M.: Defective granulation in the Chediak-Higashi syndrome. N. Engl. J. Med. 279:1009, 1968.

161. Valenzuela, R., Aikawa, M., O'Regan, S., and Makker, S.: Chediak-Higashi syndrome in a black infant. Am. J. Clin. Pathol. 65:483, 1976.

162. Wolff, S. M., Dale, D. C., Clark, R. A., Root, R. K., Kimball, H. R.: The Chediak-Higashi syndrome: studies of host defenses. Ann. Int. Med. 76:293, 1972.

163. Root, R. K., Rosenthal, A. S., and Balestra, D. J.: Abnormal bacteriocidal, metabolic and lysosomal functions of Chediak-Higashi syndrome leukocytes. J. Clin. Invest. 51: 649, 1972.

164. Davis, W. C., and Douglas, S. D.: Defective granule formation and function in the Chediak-Higashi syndrome in man and animals. Semin. Hematol. 9:431, 1972.

165. Boxer, L. A., Watanabe, A. M., Rister, M., Besch, H. R., Allen, J., and Baehner, R. L.: Correction of leukocytic function in Chediak-Higashi syndrome by ascorbate. N. Engl. J. Med. 295:1041, 1976.

166. Saltzstein, S. L., and Ackerman, L. V.: Lymphadenopathy induced by anticonvulsant drugs and mimicking clinically and pathologically malignant lymphomas. Cancer 12:164, 1959.

167. Greene, D. A.: Localized cervical lymphadenopathy induced by diphenylhydantoin sodium. Arch. Otolaryngol. 101:446, 1975.

168. Gams, R. A., Neal, J. A., and Conrad, F. G.: Hydantoin-induced pseudo-pseudolymphoma. Ann. Int. Med. 69: 557, 1968.

169. Li, F. P., Willard, D. R., Goodman, and Vawter, G.: Malignant lymphoma after diphenylhydantoin (Dilantin) therapy. Cancer 36:1359, 1975.

170. Sorrell, T. C., Forbes, I. J., Burness, F. R., and Rischbieth,

R. H. C.: Depression of immunological function in patients treated with phenytoin sodium(sodium diphenylhydantoin). Lancet 2:1233, 1971.

171. Kruger, G., Harris, D., and Sussman, E.: Effect of dilantin in mice. II. Lymphoreticular tissue atypia and neoplasia after chronic exposure. Z. Krebsforsch. 78:290, 1972.

172. Kruger, G. R. F., and Harris, D.: Is phenytoin carcinogenic? Lancet 1:323, 1972.

173. Hartsock, R. J.: Postvaccinial lymphadenitis:hyperplasia of lymphoid tissue that simulates malignant lymphomas. Cancer 21:632, 1968.

174. Dorfman, R. F., and Warnke, R.: Lymphadenopathy simulating malignant lymphomas. Hum. Pathol. 5:519, 1974.

175. Salvador, A. H., Harrison, E. G., and Kyle, R. A.: Lymphadenopathy due to infectious mononucleosis: its confusion with malignant lymphoma. Cancer 27:1029, 1971.

176. Tindle, B. H., Parker, J. W., and Lukes, R. J.: "Reed-Sternberg cells" in infectious mononucleosis? Am. J. Clin. Pathol. 58:607, 1972.

177. Frizzera, G., Moran, E. M., and Rappaport, H.: Angioimmunoblastic lymphadenopathy. Am. J. Med. 59:803, 1975.

178. Lukes, R. J., and Tindle, B. H.: Immunoblastic lymphadenopathy. N. Engl. J. Med. 292:1, 1975.

179. Henle, G., Henle, W., and Diehl, V.: Relation of Burkitt's tumor-associated herpes-type virus to infectious mononucleosis. Proc. Natl. Acad. Sci. 59:94, 1968.

180. Niederman, J. C., Evans, A. S., Subrahamanyan, M. S., and McCollum, R. W.: Prevalence, incidence and persistence of EB virus antibody in young adults. N. Engl. J. Med. 282:361, 1970.

181. Sutton, R. N.: The EB virus in relation to infectious mononucleosis. J. Clin. Pathol. (suppl.) 6:58, 1972.

182. Niederman, J. C., Miller, G., Pearson, H. A., Pagano, J. S., and Dowaliby, J. M.: Infectious mononucleosis: Epstein-Barr virus shedding in saliva and the oropharynx. N. Engl. J. Med. 294:1355, 1976.

183. Carter, R. L.: Infectious mononucleosis: model for self-limiting lymphoproliferation. Lancet 1:846, 1975.

184. Rocchi, G., Felici, A., Ragona, G., and Heinz, A.: Quantitative evaluation of Epstein-Barr-virus-infected mononuclear peripheral blood leukocytes in infectious mononucleosis. N. Engl. J. Med. 296:132, 1977.

185. Troxel, D. B., Innella, F., and Cohen, R. J.: Infectious mononucleosis complicated by hemolytic anemia due to anti-i. Am. J. Clin. Pathol. 46:625, 1966.

186. Bowman, H. S., Marsh, W. L., Schumacher, H. R., Oyen, R., and Reihart, J.: Auto anti-N immunohemolytic anemia in infectious mononucleosis. Am. J. Clin. Pathol. 61: 465, 1974.

187. Wishart, M. M., and Davey, M. G.: Infectious mononucleosis complicated by acute hemolytic anemia with a positive Donath-Landsteiner reaction. J. Clin. Pathol. 26:332, 1973.

188. Ginsburg, C. M., Henle, W., Henle, G., and Horwitz, C. A.: Infectious mononucleosis in children. Evaluation of Epstein-Barr virus-specific serologic data. J.A.M.A. 237:781, 1977.

189. Horwitz, C. A., Henle, W., Henle, G., Segal, M., Arnold, T., Lewis, F. B., Zanick, D., and Ward, P. C. J.: Clinical and laboratory evaluation of elderly patients with heterophile antibody positive infectious mononucleosis. Am. J. Med. 61:333, 1976.

190. Myhre, B. A., and Nakayama, V.: Serologic evaluation of the Mono-Chek test. Am. J. Clin. Pathol. 65:987, 1976.

191. Andiman, W. A., and Miller, G.: Epstein-Barr virus. In Manual of Clinical Immunology, edited by N. R. Rose and H. Friedman, p. 428. American Society for Microbiology, Washington, D. C., 1976.

192. Gray, G. F., Jr., Kimball, A. C., and Kean, B. H.: The posterior cervical lymph node in toxoplasmosis. Am. J. Pathol. 69:349, 1972.

193. Jacobs, L.: Toxoplasma and toxoplasmosis. Ann. Rev. Microbiol. 17:429, 1963.

194. Jacobs, L.: New knowledge of toxoplasma and toxoplasmosis. Adv. Parasitol. 11:631, 1973.

195. Saxen, E., and Saxen, L.: The histologic diagnosis of glandular toxoplasmosis. Lab. Invest. 8:326, 1959.
196. Dorfman, R. F., and Remington, J. S.: Value of lymph node biopsy of acute acquired toxoplasmosis. N. Engl. J. Med. 289:878, 1973.
197. Lunde, M. N.: Laboratory methods in the diagnosis of toxoplasmosis. Health Lab. Sci. 10:319, 1973.
198. Keller, A. R., Hochholzer, L., and Castleman, B.: Hyaline-vascular and plasma-cell types of giant lymph node hyperplasia of the mediastinum and other locations. Cancer 29:670, 1972.
199. Abell, M. R.: Lymph nodal hamartoma versus thymic choristoma of pulmonary hilum. Arch. Pathol. 64:584, 1957.
200. Tung, K. S. K., and McCormack, L. J.: Angiomatous lymphoid hamartoma. Report of five cases with a review of the literature. Cancer 20:525, 1967.
201. Anagnostou, D., and Harrison, C. V.: Angiofollicular lymph node hyperplasia. J. Clin. Pathol. 25:306, 1972.
202. Nosanchuk, J. S., and Schnitzer, B.: Follicular hyperplasia in lymph nodes from patients with rheumatoid arthritis. Cancer 24:343, 1969.
203. Rosai, J., and Dorfman, R. F.: Sinus histiocytosis with massive lymphadenopathy: a pseudolymphomatous benign disorder. Cancer 30:1174, 1972.
204. Lampert, F., and Lennert, K.: Sinus histiocytosis with massive lymphadenopathy: fifteen new cases. Cancer 37:783, 1976.
205. Kessler, E., Srulijes, C., Toledo, E., and Shalit, M.: Sinus histiocytosis with massive lymphadenopathy and spinal epidural involvement. Cancer 38:1614, 1976.
206. Ramos, C. V.: Widespread bone involvement in sinus histiocytosis. Arch. Pathol. Lab. Med. 100:606, 1976.
207. Kawasaki, T., Kosaki, F., Okawa, S., Shigematsu, I. and Yanagawa, H.: A new infantile acute febrile mucocutaneous lymph node syndrome (MLNS) prevailing in Japan. Pediatrics 54:273, 1974.
208. Tanaka, N., Sekimoto, K., and Naoe, S.: Kawasaki disease relationship with infantile periarteritis nodosa. Arch. Pathol. Lab. Med. 100:81, 1976.
209. Brown, J. S., Billmeier, G. J., Cox, F., Ibrahim, M., Stepp, W. P., and Gibson, R.: Mucocutaneous lymph node syndrome in the continental United States. J. Pediatr. 88:81, 1976.
210. Bergeson, P. S., and Schoenike, S. L.: Mucocutaneous lymph node syndrome: a case masquerading as Rocky Mountain spotted fever. J. A. M. A. 237:2299, 1977.
211. Kusakawa, S., and Heiner, D. C.: Elevated levels of immunoglobulin E in the acute febrile mucocutaneous lymph node syndrome. Pediatr. Res. 10:108, 1976.
212. Lymon, C. W., and Jackson, R.: Lipomelanotic reticulosis.
Arch. Dermatol. 71:303, 1955.
213. Rappaport, H., and Thomas, L. B.: Mycosis fungoides: the pathology of extracutaneous involvement. Cancer 34:1198, 1974.
214. Reed, R. J., and Terazakis, N.: Subcutaneous angioblastic lymphoid hyperplasia with eosinophilia (Kimura's disease). Cancer 29:489, 1972.
215. Fisch, U.: Lymphography of the Cervical Lymphatic System. W. B. Saunders, Philadelphia, 1968.
216. Ravel, R.: Histopathology of lymph nodes after lymphangiography. Am. J. Clin. Pathol. 46:335, 1966.
217. Council on Pharmacy and Chemistry: Thorotrast. J. A. M. A. 99:183, 1932.
218. Wegener, K., Wesch, H., and Kampmann, H.: Investigations into human thorotrastosis. Tissue concentrations of 232-Th and late effects in 13 autopsy cases. Virch. Arch. (Pathol. Anat.) 371:131, 1976.
219. Trible, W. M., and Small, A.: Thorium dioxide granuloma of the neck: a case report of four cases. Laryngoscope 86:1633, 1976.
220. Grampa, G.: Radiation injury with particular reference to thorotrast. In Pathology Annual, edited by S. C. Sommers, vol. 6, pp. 147–169. Appleton-Century-Crofts, New York, 1971.
221. Grove, R. C., and Cooke, R. A.: The use of thorium dioxide in roentgenography of the sinuses. Am. J. Roentgenol. Radium Ther. Nucl. Med. 44:680, 1940.
222. Hofer, O.: Kieferhohlen karzinom durch radium haltiges kontrastomitte herovgerufen. Dtsch. Zahnaerztl. Z. 7:736, 1952.
223. Muzaffar, K., and Nichols, R. D.: Thorotrast (thorium dioxide) granuloma of the neck: surgical considerations. Ann. Otol. 84:245, 1975.
224. Johnsen, N. J., Prytz, S., and Albrechtsen, R.: Facial paralysis caused of carcinoma developed in thorotrastoma in the parotid gland. J. Laryngol. 90:571, 1976.
225. Hasson, J., Hartman, K. S., Milikow, E., and Mittelman, J. A.: Thorotrast-induced extraskeletal osteosarcoma of the cervical region. Report of a case. Cancer 36:1827, 1975.
226. Levowitz, B. S., Huges, R. E., and Alford, T. C.: Treatment of thorium dioxide granuloma of the neck. N. Engl. J. Med. 268:340, 1963.
227. Engeset, A.: Irradiation of lymph nodes and vessels. Acta Radiol. suppl. 229, 1964.
228. Sherman, J. O., and O'Brien, P. H.: Effect of ionizing irradiation on normal lymphatic vessels and lymph nodes. Cancer 20:185, 1967.
229. Shina, B. K., and Goldenberg, G. J.: Effect of irradiation on lymph flow and filtration function of lymph nodes. Cancer 26:1239, 1970.

CHAPTER 24

Wegener's Granulomatosis and Midline (Nonhealing) ''Granuloma''

The two terms which form the title of this chapter were once synonymous with at least 23 others in use as diagnoses for a heterogeneous group of entities, whose only common feature was a slowly progressive ulceration and destruction of the nose and paranasal sinuses. Wegener's granulomatosis has been rescued from being a nearly meaningless term to one signifying a specific, albeit clinically diverse disease. It has survived an ambiance of ill-judged therapeutic complacency to the present time when its correct diagnosis yields a marked improvement in patient survival. True Wegener's granulomatosis is exquisitively sensitive to *cyclophosphamide* therapy. Reports indicate that in most cases, long-term remissions and even cures can be achieved with the use of that drug.[1]

Therapeutic advances have also been made with the lesions encompassed by the term midline (nonhealing) "granuloma" which like Wegener's granulomatosis present a spectrum of clinical manifestations. Histological definition is less precise, in part due to transition forms within the group.

The reader may justifiably object to the use of midline "granuloma" as a generic heading. I use it for the lack of a better one but fully appreciate the heterogeneity of both clinical and pathological manifestations. Used appropriately by the pathologist it should always shake the head and neck physician from complacency in the management of the patient and instill caution in prognosis.

It should be obvious that not all necrotizing lesions of the upper airway fall into either Wegener's granulomatosis or midline "granuloma." Across the world, these two disorders likely make up the least frequent causes of that disability. Table 24.1 presents a listing of the other more often encountered causes. In most instances, evidence of underlying systemic disease, identification of causal organism, characteristic morphology and careful history will clarify the pathogenesis.

The degree of destruction of facial structures varies with the pathogenesis. Few, however, approximate the destruction produced by idiopathic midline "granuloma" and polymorphic reticulosis.

Before a detailed consideration of Wegener's granulomatosis and the midline "granuloma" spectrum, a brief consideration of two of the noninfective granulomas (sarcoidosis; steroidal) is in order to emphasize that granulomas occur in many disorders.

Gordon *et al.*[2] relate that the diagnosis of intranasal sarcoid was first made in 1937 and in the 40 years since that publication 64 cases have been reported in the literature. The incidence of this form of involvement is very likely greater. The detection of a nasal sarcoid lesion may provide a lead to the discovery of lesions elsewhere in the head and neck: tonsil, tongue, salivary glands, lacrimal glands, bronchial mucosa, paranasal sinuses, larynx, cranial nerves and skin.[3] Intranasal sarcoidosis appears to have a predilection for the nasal septum or inferior turbinates. Nasal bone involvement is rarely seen and is usually secondary to extension from the diseased skin or mucosa. The nasal mucosal lesions may appear as tiny, 1-mm yellow nodules surrounded by a hyperemic mucosa or be larger because of coalescence of the granulomas. Later there may be a rhinitis with mucopurulent discharge and erosion and crusting of the mucosa. In the fibrotic stages, thickening of the septum and turbinates is noted, with an occasional polypoid mass that may cause nasal obstruction. Synechiae may form between the inferior turbinate and septum causing a stenosis of the airway. Nasal septal perforation may occur.

Wolff[4] has called attention to distinctive granulomatous lesions of the nasal mucous membranes following local steroid injection. These granulomatous foci bear a striking resemblance to rheumatoid nodules but contain a crystalline foreign material.

Table 24.1.
Differential Diagnosis of Wegener's Granulomatosis and the Spectrum of Midline (Nonhealing) Granuloma*

I. Vasculitic diseases
    Periarteritis nodosa
    Systemic lupus erythematosus
    Scleroderma
    Sjögren's—Sicca syndromes
    Henoch-Schonlein purpura
    Hypersensitivity angiitis
    Goodpasture's syndrome
II. A. Specific granulomatous and B. Granulomatous diseases
    A. Tuberculosis
        Lues-Yaws
        Leprosy
        Actinomycosis
        Blastomycosis
        Moniliasis
        Rhinosporidiosis
        Histoplasmosis
        Cryptococcosis
        Mucormycosis
        Sporotrichosis
    B. Rhinosclerosis
        Sarcoidosis
        Foreign body and factitial
        Berylliosis and other chemical
III. Bacterial and protozoal
    Staphylococcus
    Streptococcus
    Anthrax
    Glanders
    Rhinoscleroma
    Tulraemia
    Noma
    Leishmaniasis
IV. Neoplastic
    Histiocytoses
    Lymphoma
    Mycosis fungoides
    Nonkeratinizing squamous cell carcinoma (lymphoepithelioma)
V. Neoplasm-simulation
    Necrotizing sialometaplasia
    Pyogenic granuloma

* From *Head and Neck Surgery*, *1*:213, 1979, Houghton Mifflin Co., Boston.

Wegener's Granulomatosis

Described by Wegener[5] in 1939 under the term "rhinogenic granulomatosis," the disorder bearing his name was characterized by three criteria: (1) necrotizing granulomas with vasculitis of upper and lower respiratory tracts; (2) a systemic vasculitis; and (3) focal necrotizing glomerulitis. Early therapeutic experiences indicated the disease to be rapidly fatal and ending in death within only a few months. That limited forms of the disease with a relatively more benign course compared with the classic or generalized form existed, became recognized in 1966.[6] This was further expanded conceptually in 1976.[7] Wegener's granulomatosis is now best regarded as a clinical continuum or spectrum. Necrotizing granulomas *with* vasculitis form the common pathological basis for diagnosis. Each of the major sites of involvement in Wegener's granulomatosis—upper respiratory tract, lungs and kidneys—may be involved alone or in any combination except the kidney which cannot be involved alone because focal necrotizing glomerulitis is nonspecific. Patients may evolve from a single focus through the complete system complex or their disease may remain stationary in the upper or lower respiratory tract without renal disease. This phenomenon likely represents a different tempo of the disease in different patients or a halt to progression brought about by therapy. It may also be that patients without manifestations of renal involvement have subclinical glomerulonephritis and that some eventuate into generalized Wegener's granulomatosis.[8] It is rare, however, for patients to present with renal failure in the absence of significant and easily detectable disease in other organ systems.[9]

Since all, or nearly all patients with Wegener's granulomatosis manifest some form of respiratory tract involvement, the head and neck physician interacts with nearly every patient. The upper or lower respiratory tract, or in most cases, both, attract one's attention, but a few patients present with oral, ear or pharyngeal symptoms (vide infra). It is unusual for patients to present with pulmonary disease without any evidence of upper airway disease.[9] The nasal and paranasal clinical findings are by no means specific. A history of chronic sinusitis with purulent rhinorrhea is obtained from some patients. Pansinusitis is quite common. In descending order of frequency, the maxillary, ethmoid, frontal, and sphenoid sinuses are involved.[11] With secondary bacterial infection, the organism most often encountered is *Staphylococcus aureus*. As testimony to the frequency of nasal and paranasal involvement, McDonald *et al.*[11] found that 31 of 52 of their patients with known Wegener's granulomatosis had the disease in their nose, either alone or in conjunction with other sites during some course of their illness. In nine of these subjects the nasal involvement was the only manifestation of the disease. In five of the patients there was evidence of subglottic stenosis of the airway, very likely a result of mucosal granulomatous inflammation. At any rate, nasal involvement is a useful early sign and is of diagnostic significance.

The intranasal lesions range from mucosal swelling and obstruction to advanced intranasal or extranasal deformity, or both. Over-all, a mucosal crusting is the most common finding. This typically consists of large, green, foul-smelling crusts, which, when removed, leave a raw and friable surface. This has an important histopathological corrollary. According to McDonald et al.[11] the gross appearance is reminiscent of atrophic rhinitis. The granulation tissue response favors the turbinates bilaterally or universally. There may be concomitant septal mucosal involvement. Seven of the 31 patients described by McDonald et al.[11] also *presented* with saddle deformity in addition to the mucosal crusting. Not all such patients had a perforation of the septum. Systemic symptoms and signs are usually out of proportion to the nasal involvement.

Given adequate and representative tissue from biopsy, Wegener's granulomatosis in the upper airway presents with the following histological features: (1) a rather characteristic gangrenous-like crust overlying active pyogenic granulation tissue that contains an abundance of fibrin, fibrinoid material and acute inflammatory cells; (2) beneath these two layers (if the crust is intact) lies a subacute inflammatory zone wherein the majority of vascular changes and granulomas reside; (3) an outer more chronic zone manifesting fewer, yet identifiable granulomas and vasculitis. The granulomas are of epithelioid type and may be non-necrotic, possess zones of fibrinoid necrosis or contain microabscesses (necrotizing and suppurative granulomas). A microscopic vasculitis is a *requirement* for the histopathological diagnosis (Fig. 24.1). It can be identified as a variable degree of transmural infiltration of the wall of the vessel and is often obscured by the generalized tissue reaction. Fibrinoid vascular necrosis is prominent.[12] Focal vasculitis, healing vasculitis with thrombosis, and fibrous obliteration are common observations. Eosinophils often make up a significant percentage of the inflammatory cells. Giant cells are usually readily found (Fig. 24.2). In the absence of firm histological evidence, one must rely on the presence or absence of the typical clinical and pathological findings in other organs to establish the diagnosis. Fauci and Wolff[9] consider it unreasonable to exclude the diagnosis in the presence of clear-cut sinus disease when a single biopsy specimen fails to reveal a granulomatous vasculitis in the presence of clinicopathological findings typical of Wegener's granulomatosis in other organs.

Involvement of the oral tissues in Wegener's granulomatosis is fairly common: oropharyngeal,

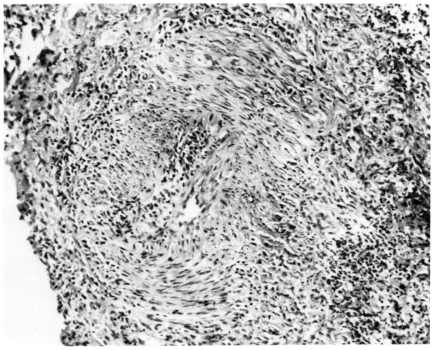

Figure 24.1. Vasculitis of artery in lamina propria of nasal mucosa from a patient with Wegener's granulomatosis.

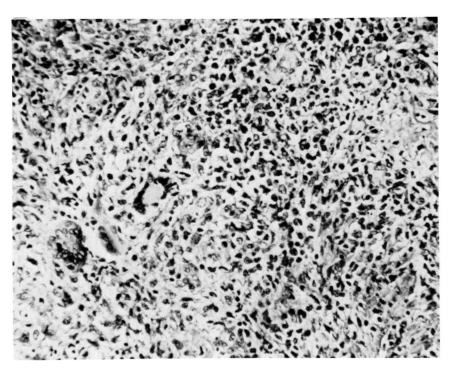

Figure 24.2. Wegener's granulomatosis of nose. Two giant cells are surrounded by inflammatory cells.

lingual and gingival. In unusual cases, the oral manifestations may be among the initial complaints.[13] Destruction of the hard palate or alveolar bone by spread of contiguous lesions in the nose and sinuses is only *rarely* seen in *true* Wegener's granulomatosis, where the nasal lesions are known to be less destructive than the disorders masquerading as or misdiagnosed as Wegener's granulomatosis.[8, 10] In the latter condition, palatal ulceration may be independent of nasal lesions, may occur in multiple form, or may result from an oropharyngeal granuloma involving the fauces, uvula and soft palate. A peculiar and likely specific, gingivitis starting in the interductal papillae and spreading to the remainder of the gingiva and periodontium has been described by Scott and Finch.[13]

Accompanying sinus and oral disease in Wegener's granulomatosis is secondary bacterial infection resulting from damaged mucosal surfaces. In the paranasal sinuses, *S. aureus* is the microbe most frequently responsible for such infections. Fauci and Wolff[9] point out that in an apparent flare-up of disease activity confined to the paranasal sinuses in a patient otherwise in complete remission on or following therapy, secondary infection must be ruled out before such a condition is considered to be a manifestation of a true relapse.

Systemic involvement by Wegener's granulom-

atosis hardly spares any organ system.[14] The eyes may be involved in up to 40% of cases. This involvement may be primary (vascular) or by contiguity from adjacent upper airway lesions. Ocular lesions include corneoscleral ulceration, necro-granulomatous keratitis, granulomatous sclerouveitis and conjunctivitis with occasional proptosis and pseudotumor of the orbit. Retinal artery and vein involvement have also been recorded. About one-third of patients have involvement of the ear, usually manifested by recurrent middle ear inflammation and pain. Hearing loss may indeed be a presenting complaint. Cutaneous involvement is said to occur in up to 50% of patients but muscle involvement is uncommon. Joint symptoms, while they may be present, do not usually play a major role in the presenting symptoms or in the over-all course of the disease. Vasculitis of the coronary vasculature, valvulitis and pericarditis are the cardiac manifestations. The nervous system is involved in a significant proportion of cases: between 25% and 50%. A mononeuritis complex is not an infrequent finding. The lungs are almost invariably involved and changes range from small, sometimes subclinical lesions to multiple nodular infiltrates and cavitation. In severe cases, there may be a fulminant respiratory failure. The pulmonary infiltrates may be fleeting and transient. Mediastinal or hilar lymph node enlargement is extremely unusual and should be regarded as suggestive of another diagnosis. Renal involvement is the feared complication for once there is functional impairment, the renal disease does not spontaneously arrest or regress. The most frequent finding is a focal necrotizing glomerulitis not unlike that seen in subacute bacterial endocarditis and certain forms of periarteritis nodosa. Long term survival is directly contingent on the degree of kidney impairment. Hypertension is not a significant problem in these patients. Prior to the use of cytotoxic agents as therapy in this disorder, most patients died of their renal disease, with a mean survival of 5 months from the onset of clinically evident renal involvement.[9] Table 24.2 presents some of the systemic involvement in the patients studied by Wolff et al.[10]

In summary, Wegener's granulomatosis is a distinct clinical entity that exists in a clinical spectrum that ranges from a mitigated or limited form to an overwhelmingly fulminate vasculitis with death from uremia. It is important also to underscore that malignancy in the neoplastic sense has not been a feature of the disease. The extent of the upper airway destruction in Wegener's granulomatosis, when compared to other so-called midline granulomas, is less and the lesions rarely, if ever, erode through the skin, facial bones or palate. The hallmark of the inflammatory reaction is a granulomatous vasculitis.

Midline (Nonhealing) "Granuloma"

The extraction of Wegener's granulomatosis from the group of disorders formerly called "lethal midline granuloma" leaves a cluster of lesions that once led Edgerton and DesPrez[15] to state " . . . it is still an unresolved question whether lethal midline granuloma represents a tumor unlike all other tumors, an infection unlike other infections, or a defect in the immune system." We are coming closer to the answer to this question and are at a point where the clinician should no longer accept a clinical diagnosis of lethal midline granuloma, or a histological diagnosis of "consistent with lethal midline granuloma."[16] Recent investigations have shown that separate clinicopathological entities exist in the formerly lumped classification. Not all are lethal and clearly not all are granulomatous. Since they share clinical signs and symptoms referrable to the nasal cavity and midfacial tissues, a *temporarily* acceptable *clinical* diagnostic designation is midline (nonhealing) "granuloma."

Under midline (nonhealing) granuloma there are at least three histologically definable lesions: (1) a localized destructive lesion of the upper airway characterized by *nonspecific* acute and chronic inflammation and necrosis; (2) a pseudo-lymphomatous tissue reaction called polymorphic reticulosis by some and lymphomatoid granulomatosis by others; and (3) extranodal lymphoma. While destructive midfacial lesions may arise from a de novo lymphoma without evidence (clinical or pathological) of a pre-existing lesion, the scarcity of primary extranodal lymphomas in this region point to the strong probability that the three aforementioned lesions are inter-related and form an evolutionary spectrum. Transition forms clearly exist and these along with difficulties in histopathological interpretation make this group of lesions some of the most difficult in all of surgical pathology. At one time Harrison[17] was so unim-

Table 24.2
Wegener's Granulomatosis—Clinicopathological Aspects*

Anatomical Region	Percent of Patients	Features
Nose and nasopharynx	91	Ulcers, necrotizing granulomas, saddle-nose
Paranasal sinuses	95	Sinusitis, necrotizing granulomas, secondary infection
Ears	38	Otitis media
Lungs	100	Pulmonary infiltrates and necrotizing granulomatous vasculitis
Kidneys	81	Focal and fulminant glomerulonephritis
Heart	29	Coronary vasculitis, pericarditis
Nervous system	24	Mononeuritis complex; vascular disease
Skin	48	Cutaneous vasculitis and ulcers
Joints	57	Fleeting polyarthralgias

* Modified from Wolff et al.[10]

pressed by the pathologist's guidance, that he carried out therapy only by consideration of the clinical aspects of the case.

Evidence for a hypersensitivity basis for midline granuloma is incomplete, but there are increasing suggestions of an impairment of delayed hypersensitivity. This is in contrast to Wegener's granulomatosis where cell-mediated reactions are said to be normal.[8] The tissue reactions are those of an immunoproliferative process and one is struck by the nearly completely analogous sequence of morphological events occurring in the development of the salivary lesions of Sjögren's syndrome; even to the advent of lymphoreticular neoplasms. The offending antigen is unidentified.

Admitting the difficulties in histopathological diagnosis and in securing representative biopsy material, there are three tissue phases in the spectrum of midline (nonhealing) granuloma. The first is true *idiopathic midline granuloma*, a localized disorder not characterized by visceral lesions.[7, 8] It is a locally destructive process in the upper airway and manifests a relatively nondescript and nonspecific inflammatory reaction and acute and chronic inflammation and necrosis. Vasculitis (usually secondary), granulomas and giant cells are only infrequently found. Despite this undistinctive tissue reaction, the upper airway lesions are relentlessly destructive and often erode through facial tissues and bone. Most patients have a pansinusitis with destructive lesions of the nasal septum or soft and hard palate or both. Superinfection is common. This is in contrast to the far less destructive character of Wegener's granulomatosis. Also in contrast, is the relative freedom of systemic signs despite the locally destructive lesions in patients with midline granuloma. Therapy is mandatory because of the uniformly fatal outcome of the midline granuloma.[8] Dramatic long-term remissions can be achieved with high-dose, local irradiation.[8]

The fulminant inflammatory response to unknown antigens seen in *idiopathic* midline granuloma may exist alone or be in transition to the second of our recognizable tissue phases of midline granuloma. Fauci et al.[8] are adamant, however, that evolution to a pseudolymphomatous reaction is not a requirement for the localized destruction in *idiopathic* midline granuloma. Our own experience supports this.

The pseudolymphomatous reaction mentioned above is a necrotizing, atypical lymphoproliferative lesion best considered for the time being as *polymorphic reticulosis*.[18, 19] Histologically, the lesions of polymorphic reticulosis are separable from Wegener's granulomatosis by the absence of necrotizing epithelioid granulomas, a tendency toward a necrotizing angioinfiltrative growth pattern and abundant atypical lymphoproliferative cellular component. There has also never been an associated glomerulitis. The lack of an atypical cellular infiltrate further distinguishes Wegener's granulomatosis. Polymorphic reticulosis usually presents as a necrotizing lymphoreticular infiltration of the submucosa that surrounds the submucosal glands and has a predilection for angiocentric or angioinfiltrative growth patterns.[19] Surface ulceration invariably occurs and this extends down into the underlying angular zones of necrosis. The process is destructive with erosion through the mucosa, bone and cartilage. The frequent angiocentric infiltration is held responsible for the necrosis due to the involvement of small veins and arteries. This perivascular and intravascular extension of the cells leads to thrombosis and what is misinterpreted as a specific vasculitis but there is no fibrinoid necrosis, and giant cells and granulomas are absent.[12, 16, 19] It is, however, the cellular infiltrate that is key to the diagnosis of polymorphic reticulosis. Its polymorphic character distinguishes the lesion from the monomorphic lymphomas, but imperfectly from histiocytic lymphoma.[20] The infiltrate is indeed polymorphic and consists of variable zones of small lymphocytes, scattered immunoblastic forms, histiocytes, plasma cells and occasional eosinophils. Interspersed are malignant-appearing cells (sheets of larger lymphocytes and immunoblasts with scattered mitoses). Superimposed and often integral to these cells are an admixture of acute and chronic inflammatory cells. In the absence of the atypical cells, there is a resemblance of the tissue response to luetic infection.

Clinically the lesions may be preceded by a long nasal prodrome and the nasal lesions can be locally ulcerative and destructive as well as diffuse. In the upper aerodigestive tract polymorphic reticulosis involves the nasal cavity and paranasal sinuses, larynx, tracheobronchial tree, palate, pharynx and nasopharynx. The nasal lesions are often bilateral. The most common symptom of upper airway involvement is progressive nasal obstruction. Purulent or bloody nasal discharge is a prominent feature. Like Wegener's granulomatosis, but unlike idiopathic midline granuloma, the systemic complaints are often out of proportion to the nasal systems.[17] These include malaise, fatigue, night sweats and pyrexia.

There is no question that polymorphic reticulosis is closely linked to lymphoma. There is abundant evidence, clinically and histologically to confirm this.[18–20] Were it not that pathologists become prisoners of their own nomenclature and frustrated by the seemingly endless proliferation of reclassifications of the lymphomas, polymorphic reticulosis would be called a lymphoma. Michaels and Gregory[20] have provided such evidence in their consideration that the lesion is a histiocytic lymphoma.

The protean clinical features of polymorphic reticulosis also links it with lymphoma. Although it commonly presents in the head and neck, other sites such as the lungs, kidneys, skin and gastrointestinal tract may be involved either alone or in conjunction with head and neck lesions. Conversely, "spread" or multifocal involvement in these structures and lymph nodes and spleen may follow a formerly localized airway lesion. It is, therefore, always a *potentially* sytemic disease and bears similarity, if not identity, with lymphomatoid granulomatosis.[21, 22] In the Mayo Clinic series of 32 patients with polymorphic reticulosis, the upper airway was involved either alone or in conjunction with other sites in 24 patients.[19] These sites were palate, larynx, pharynx, trachea, lungs, skin, stomach, spleen, liver, gastrointestinal tract, kidneys and orbit. In eight patients, the upper airway was not involved. It is important to recognize that the renal lesions were nodular masses, like a metastasis and in no way like the renal lesions of Wegener's granulomatosis. Three patients showed changes of lymphoma at necropsy and in one patient, a second biopsy from the nose showed a "tendency" to lymphoma when compared to tissue from an earlier biopsy. There is a response to radiation for localized lesions of the upper airway treated early. A poor outcome is associated with multifocal involvement which necessitates systemic therapy.

The third recognizable lesion presenting as a locally destructive and nonhealing midline granuloma is lymphoma of the readily classifiable type, although Hodgkin's disease is very unusual in this location (Fig. 24.3). These lymphomas are extra-

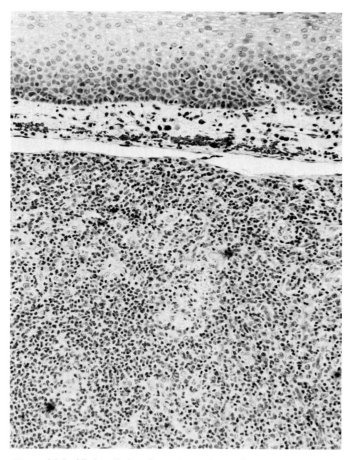

Figure 24.3. Histiocytic lymphoma beneath nasal mucous membrane.

Table 24.3
Differential Features: Wegener's Granulomatosis and Midline (Nonhealing) "Granuloma"*

Wegener's Granulomatosis	Midline (nonhealing) "Granuloma" Idiopathic Midline Granuloma	Polymorphic Reticulosis
1. Diffuse, inflammatory disease of upper airway; predominantly sinuses and nose. Rarely, if ever erodes palate and facial soft tissues.	1. Destructive, localized or diffuse lesions with characteristic extension through palate and facial soft tissue.	1. Destructive, localized or diffuse lesions with destruction of bone and extension through facial soft tissues.
2. Systemic disease a. Lungs b. Kidneys c. Small vessel vasculitis d. May not have airway involvement.	2. Localized to airway and upper aerodigestive tract. 3. May remain histologically benign or evolve into polymorphic reticulosis.	2. Localized or systemic: a. Related to lymphomatoid granulomatosis b. No vasculitis or glomerulitis c. May not have airway lesions.
3. No known association with lymphoreticular malignancy.	4. In the pure form, the inflammatory reaction is perplexingly nonspecific. Granulomas and giant cells are infrequent. No atpyical cellular infiltrate unless in transition to polymorphic reticulosis.	3. May remain as polymorphic reticulosis or evolve into lymphoma (extranodal) or disseminated.
4. Basic histological lesion: Necrotizing vasculitis with epithelioid granulomas, giant cells, and fibrinoid necrosis. No atypical lymphoreticular infiltrate.	5. Treatment is radiation.	4. Characteristic atypical and polymorphic lymphoreticular cellular infiltrate. Angiocentric growth patterns may simulate vasculitis, but fibrinoid necrosis is absent in vessel walls.
5. Treatment is cyclophosphamide with or without steroids.		5. Treatment is radiation for localized lesions.

* From Head and Neck Surgery, 1:213, 1979, Houghton Mifflin Co., Boston.

nodal, but may be only a harbinger of systemic disease. The lymphoma may have evolved through a midline granuloma sequence or may have arisen de novo.

Table 24.3 presents clinicopathological features that may assist to distinguish between Wegener's granulomatosis, idiopathic midline "granuloma" and polymorphic reticulosis. This form of tabulation should not be considered the denouement of these lesions. Studies by Israel et al.[23] and Saldana et al.[21] raise the possibility, once again, of an interrelationship between the disorders. Figure 24.4 conceptualizes the responses of the upper airway and lungs to a postulated antigen. The terms in parenthesis are the histopathological equivalents as rendered by Saldana et al.[21] in their study of pulmonary lesions. The benign lymphocytic angiitis and granulomatosis and idiopathic nonhealing "granuloma" do not have equivalents and at the present time do not appear to be related. Furthermore, the only extra pulmonary lesions with benign lymphocytic angiitis have been in the skin. This lesion has responded to therapy used with success in patients having classic localized or systemic Wegener's granulomatosis and whether it represents an early form of the latter is not known.

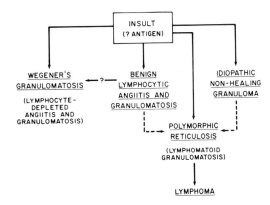

Figure 24.4. Postulated inter-relationship of nonhealing midline facial lesions. (From Head and Neck Surgery, 1:213, 1979, Houghton Mifflin Co., Boston.)

More likely the lesion represents an early form of lymphomatoid granulomatosis.[23]

REFERENCES

1. Fauci, A. S.: Granulomatous vasculitides: distinct but related. Ann. Intern. Med. 87:782, 1977.
2. Gordon, W. W., Cohn, A. M., and Greenberg, S. D.: Nasal sarcoidosis. Arch. Otolaryngol. 102:11, 1976.
3. Miglets, A. W., Viall, J. H., and Kataria,Y.P.: Sarcoidosis of the head and neck. Laryngoscope 87:2038, 1977.

4. Wolff, M.: Granulomas in nasal mucous membranes following local steroid injections. Am. J. Clin. Pathol. 62:775, 1974.

5. Wegener, F.: Über eine eigenartige rhinogene Granulomatose mit besonderer Beteilgung des Arteriensystems und der Nieren. Beitr. Pathol. 102:36, 1939.

6. Carrington, C. B., and Liebow, A. A.: Limited forms of angiitis and granulomatosis of Wegener's type. A. J. Med. 41:497, 1966.

7. DeRemee, R. D., McDonald, T. J., Harrison, E. G., Jr., and Coles, D. T.: Wegener's granulomatosis. Anatomic correlates, a proposed classification. Mayo Clin. Proc. 51:777, 1976.

8. Fauci, A. S., Johnson, R. E., and Wolff, S. M.: Radiation therapy of midline granuloma. Ann. Intern. Med. 84:140, 1976.

9. Fauci, A. S., and Wolff, S. M.: Wegener's granulomatosis and related diseases. D.M. 23:5, 1977.

10. Wolff, S. M., Fauci, A. S., Horn, R. G., and Bale, D. C.: Wegener's granulomatosis. Ann. Intern. Med. 81:513, 1974.

11. McDonald, T. J., DeRemee, R. A., Kern, E. B., and Harrison, E. G., Jr.: Nasal manifestations of Wegener's granulomatosis. Laryngoscope 84:2101, 1974.

12. Fechner, R. E., and Lamppin, D. W.: Midline malignant reticulosis: a clinicopathologic entity. Arch. Otolaryngol. 95:467, 1972.

13. Scott, J., and Finch, L. D.: Wegener's granulomatosis presenting as gingivitis. Review of the clinical and pathologic features. Report of a case. Oral Surg. 34:920, 1972.

14. Medical Staff Conference, University of California, San Francisco: Wegener's granulomatosis. West. J. Med. 121:123, 1974.

15. Edgerton, M. T., and DesPrez, J. D.: Lethal midline granuloma of the face. Br. J. Plast. Surg. 9:200, 1956.

16. McGuirt, W. F., and Rose, E. F.: Lethal midline granuloma: A pathological spectrum. J. Laryngol. 90:459, 1976.

17. Harrison, D. N.: Non-healing granulomata of the upper respiratory tract. Br. Med. J. 4:205, 1974.

18. Eichel, B. S., Harrison, E. G., Jr., Devine, K. D., Scanlon, P. W., and Brown, H. A.: Primary lymphoma of the nose including a relationship to lethal midline granuloma. Am. J. Surg. 112:597, 1966.

19. McDonald, T. J., DeRemee, R. D., Harrison, E. C., Jr., Facer, G. W., and Devine, K. D.: The protean clinical features of polymorphic reticulosis (lethal midline granuloma). Laryngoscope 86:936, 1976.

20. Michaels, L., and Gregory, M.: Pathology of "non-healing (midline) granuloma." J. Clin, Pathol. 30:317, 1977.

21. Saldana, M. J., Patchefsky, A. S., Israel, H. I., and Atkinson, G. W.: Pulmonary angiitis and granulomatosis. The relationship between histological features, organ involvement, and response to treatment. Hum. Pathol. 4:391, 1977.

22. Liebow, A. A.: The J. Burns Amerson Lecture. Pulmonary angiitis and granulomatosis. Am. Rev. Resp. Dis. 108:1, 1973.

23. Israel, H. L., Patchefsky, A. S., and Saldana, M. J.: Wegener's granulomatosis, and benign lymphocytic angiitis and granulomatosis of the lung. Recognition and treatment. Ann. Intern. Med. 87:691, 1977.

CHAPTER 25

Immunological Considerations in Head and Neck Cancer

Contributed by MICHAEL E. JOHNS, M.D.

The study of immune mechanisms in patients with cancer is being actively pursued in medical centers around the world. Researchers are investigating the belief that the cancer cell is immunologically unique. If the specific immunological characteristics of the cancer cell can be identified, tests of these markers could lead to the early detection of a cancer while it is still in a microscopic phase. Hopefully this would lead to an ultimate triumph over cancer, possibly in the form of a vaccine as used today in infectious diseases.

In this direction there are many questions to be addressed along the way. These include questions such as: Why do cancers occur in the face of an active immunological defense surveillance system which destroys "foreign" cells? What are the specific impacts of the tumor on the immune mechanism? What are the differences of local effects such as the lymph node versus systemic mechanisms? Are there immunological markers which can be identified which will lead to diagnosis and detection of recurrence and which may have prognostic significance? Do the conventionally used treatments have a significant impact on the immune mechanisms? Will we be able to manipulate the immune system to treat cancer?

The answers to these and many other questions are not complete but many parts of the puzzle are now being put in place and an answer will soon evolve which will let us know whether there is a role for immune manipulation in cancer therapy.

The impairment of cell mediated immunity is particularly seen in melanoma, squamous cell carcinoma and sarcomas.[1-6] Squamous cell carcinomas of the head and neck result in a greater than expected impairment of the immune system. The reason for this has not been clarified.

In this chapter, I review those principles of immunology which provide a background to allow an understanding of the immunological problems seen in patients with head and neck cancer. The effects of extrinsic factors which affect the immune system of these patients will be studied. In addition, the status of immunotherapy for these cancers will be surveyed with a view to future plans.

BASIC PRINCIPLES

The immune system can be divided into two components: (1) the gut associated (bursa equivalent), lymphoid tissue primarily responsible for humoral and secretory immunity; and (2) the thymus dependent lymphoid tissue responsible for cell mediated immunity (Fig. 25.1). The lymphocytes are the fundamental cellular component of the immune system. They can be divided into two categories: B lymphocytes (bone marrow derived) or bursa equivalent and T lymphocytes (thymus derived). To simply look at these cells under the light microscope one is not able to tell a B-cell from a T-cell. They look alike and both are motile, nonphagocytic cells. However, these cells are different from a standpoint of specific function and mechanisms of effecting these functions (Table 25.1). The other cell which plays an adjunctive role in tumor immunology is the macrophage.

B-cells comprise 15% of all blood lymphocytes. They are found in the follicles around germinal centers of lymph nodes where they account for 15% of all lymphocytes. The B-cell is primarily responsible for humoral immunity. This is accomplished by the synthesis and secretion of immunoglobulins after it has matured into a plasma cell. The ultimate role then is the synthesis and secretion of antibody in response to antigens. B lymphocytes can be identified by cell surface markers

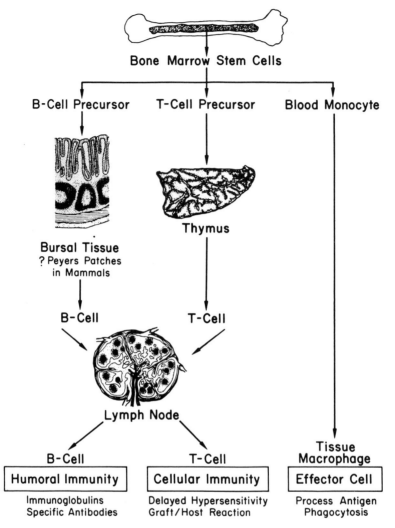

Figure 25.1.   Immune system development.

including: (1) receptor for the Fc portion of the immunoglobulin molecule; (2) cell surface immunoglobulins (1,000-fold greater than T-cells); and (3) receptor for the third component of complement (C3).

The *T-cells* comprise 85% of the circulating blood lymphocytes. In addition, they are found in the periarterial and deep cortical areas of the lymph nodes, making up 85% of the lymphocyte population of the lymph node. They are also found in Peyer's patches, the bone marrow and the white pulp of the spleen. The T-cell system is primarily responsible for the cell mediated immune processes and is that portion of the immune system which plays the major role in the immune response to tumor. In addition, T-cells initiate graft-host reactions, participate in the cancer immunosur-

veillance system, and are a major portion of the body's defense against certain viruses, fungi, and intracellular bacterial pathogens. These cells may be identified by the ability of surface receptors on T-cells to react with unsensitized sheep red blood cells to form rosettes. These T lymphocytes may be divided into subpopulations depending on the effector mechanism which they assume. They may develop into "killer T-cells" capable of destroying other cells (e.g., tumor cells) when sensitized to a particular antigen. Other T-cells may function in the production of lymphokines when they are antigenically stimulated.

Lymphokines are secreted cell products of low molecular weight which include the following: (1) chemotactic factor—a factor which attracts macrophages to aid in destroying the foreign antigen;

Table 25.1
Some Properties of T and B Lymphocytes

Property	T-cell	B-cell
Site of origin	Thymus	Bursa of fabricius (birds), gastrointestinal tract, fetal liver (mammals)
Distribution in lymph nodes and spleen	Interfollicular (paracortical)	Follicular (cortical)
Frequency		
Blood	85	15
Lymph	90	10
Lymph node	85	15
Spleen	65	35
Helper	Releases Lymphokines Stimulators for B-cells	No
Secretes antibodies	No	Yes
Inactivated by		
Radiation	+	++++
Steroids	+	++

(2) transfer factor—a regulatory agent which is capable of transferring cell mediated immunity from a sensitized to a nonsensitized individual; (3) macrophage arming factors—these include macrophage inhibiting factor (MIF) which prevents the migration of macrophages from the site of injury and macrophage activating factor (MAF) which "turns on" the macrophage to destroy the tumor cell; (4) antiviral agents such as interferon which have been documented to have a small amount of antitumor effect as well; (5) cytotoxic factor—the lymphocytotoxic factors which have a direct toxic effect on the tumor or foreign cell.

Other subpopulations of T-cells include the "helper cells" which facilitate B-cell antibody production and suppressor cells which can suppress antibody production by B-cells.

Monocytes

The third cell population which plays a role in tumor immunology is the circulating monocyte which further differentiates into macrophages in tissues undergoing an antigenic challenge. These are large mononuclear cells capable of highly active phagocytosis. It is also felt, although not yet fully delineated, that the macrophage will process antigens so that it may subsequently be presented to lymphocytes with a resultant enhanced lymphocyte response to the antigen. In addition, these cells are sensitive to certain of the above mentioned lymphokines which, when stimulated by them, greatly enhances their phagocytic activity with resultant destruction of the stimulating anti-

gen-bearing cell. This is carried out through the action of the cytoplasmic enzymes. In vitro studies have also shown that macrophages can kill tumor cells by nonphagocytic mechanisms.

The Immune Response to Tumor

We can now look at the immune response to a tumor cell or cells which presents itself to the host. This is the response which provides for the "immunologic surveillance" as coined by Burnet.[7] This system of immune monitoring is based on the tenant that tumors possess, on their cell surfaces, antigens which allow the host body to recognize them as other than "self." With the knowledge of the above mentioned cellular components of the immune system, we can study the interaction of the tumor cells, the antigen released by the tumor, these effector cells and antibody.

The initial sensitization which elicits the primary immune response occurs as a tumor cell with its tumor associated antigen (TAA) is attacked by the macrophage. The macrophage can then act in two roles: (1) the tumor antigen is phagocytized and is processed, perhaps by being coupled with macrophage RNA, and then exteriorized to be taken up by the T lymphocyte; or (2) becomes an aggressive activated macrophage which has a direct cytotoxic effect on the tumor cell.

The T-cells can become sensitized effector cells by the macrophage processed antigen or directly by nonprocessed TAA or can interact with a B lymphocyte which can itself become an effector cell with direct effect on the tumor. The B-cell also can differentiate into plasma cells which can produce antibody to act on the tumor target cell. The sensitized T lymphocyte can act by the release of lymphokines or by becoming a killer cell itself (see Fig. 25.2).

The fact that tumors develop in the face of such immune surveillance indicates that the system is not "fail safe" and that some neoplasms have the ability to either sneak by or disguise themselves. Other alternative theories would be that the immune system is suppressed or not at full strength due to such factors as aging, underlying systemic disease or drugs.[8-10] There is no single explanation for the success of tumor growth in the face of an intact immune response. The sneaking through theory, aluded to above, proposes that cancer starting as individual cells may not excite an immunological recognition early in its growth, and that by the time the immune system becomes alert to this new tumor the cancer is established and has reached proportions too large for the host immune system to deal with.

Another potential explanation is that of antigenic modulation; that is, the ability of cancer cells to lose their antigen or to mask it in the face of an impending immunological attack. This has been shown to occur in mice leukemia cells.

A third alternative by which cancers may escape the immunological surveillance system is by flooding of the host with tumor antigens. The tumor antigens will then bind specific antibodies or receptor surfaces on the lymphocytes and prevent them from recognizing and destroying the tumor cells. This is a form of blocking antigen.

Of course, any factors affecting the host by a suppression of immune response such as treatment with immunosuppressive agents or immunodeficiency states would not allow the host to mount an adequate immune response to an invading cancer cell antigen. And it has been observed that an increased frequency of malignancy occurs in patients on chronic immunosuppressive therapy.

MEASUREMENTS OF IMMUNORESPONSIVENESS

Humoral antibodies have been quantifiable for some time. The cell mediated immune reactivity has been much more difficult to identify and quantify. With new laboratory techniques we can now evaluate the cellular component of the immune reaction. Keeping in mind the previously described mechanisms of the immune response to tumor antigens, one can see that the viability of the immune response can be determined by measuring the magnitude or quality of response at any

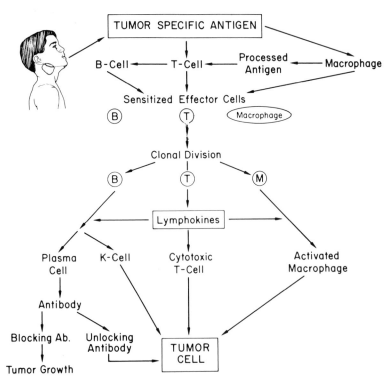

Figure 25.2.   In vivo tumor/host immune reaction.

of the steps of the immunosurveillance mechanism. These tests might include such nonspecific measures as the host response to recall antigens or more direct and specific measures of individual components of the immmune response such as B- or T-cell counts, lymphocyte blastogenesis, macrophage inhibition factor, immunoglobulins or lymphocyte cytotoxicity.

Recall Antigens

The standard practice in determining the strength of cell mediated immunity (CMI) has been to administer skin tests to patients looking for existing sensitivities to antigens such as tuberculosis, mumps, Candida, trichophyton, histoplasmosis, or streptokinase-streptodornase. These tests have the disadvantage in reliance on a previous exposure to the antigen. Thus, if there is no response, it is possible that the patient has not been exposed to the antigen and a firm conclusion as to the absence of CMI cannot be firmly gained.

The use of dinitrochlorobenzene (DNCB) as a contact sensitizing agent has advantages over the above mentioned reactions. This test does not require previous exposure to the allergen as both the sensitization and the challenge are an integrated part of the test itself. Thus, both the afferent and efferent limb of the immune response can be measured. Ninety-five to ninety-eight percent of normal patients can be sensitized to this chemical. DNCB is a hapten which by binding with lysine in epidermoid protein forms an antigen to elicit the immune response. This test does not require prior sensitization to DNCB and such a prior sensitization is extremely rare. The major disadvantage of this test is that a 14-day lapse is required between sensitization and challenge and then another 2 days are required to read the challenge response. Thus, in the head and neck cancer patient, a total of 16 days would be lost if one is being careful that no factor other than the patient's interaction with his tumor is to the evaluated. Starting radiotherapy, general anesthesia or surgery all may have an affect on the immune response. Bleumink et al.[6] have reported another disadvantage in that the possibility of a future cutaneous reaction may occur should the patient come in contact with dinitrophenol, dinitroanisole or dinitro-orthocresol (these chemicals may be used in laboratories, the chemical industry, and as insecticides or fungicides). This possibility is quite remote but must be kept in mind. There are various techniques of administering DNCB.[6] Two such techniques have been clearly delineated by Bleumink et al.[6] and Catalona et al.[11] Although these two techniques are different, they each can

be quantified. These seem to be the most reliable. Other techniques described are not clearly quantifiable.[6] The technique described by Bleumink et al.[6] is easily reproducible and is described here. The patient is sensitized by topically applying 2 mg of DNCB (0.1 ml of 2% solution in acetone) within the area of a 2-cm polyethylene ring on the volar aspect of the arm. Fourteen days later the patient receives challenge doses of 30 μg and 3 μg and the patient is examined for a delayed cutaneous hypersensitivity response at 48 hours. Bleumink et al.[6] then grades each challenge dose site using a grading system as follows: 1, erythema; 2, erythema and induration; 3, erythema, induration and vesiculation; and 4, erythema, induration, vesiculation and ulceration. This then allows for 12 points to be given for maximum response at all three challenge sites. The technique by Catalona et al.[11] is somewhat more involved and requires biopsy of the challenge site if erythema only is noted at 14 days. In addition, they use a challenge dose of 50 μg which Bleumink et al.[6] feel can in itself result in an erythematous response and, in fact, in Catalona et al's.[11] series 27% of normal controls developed a flare response. The main advantage of this test is that it does not have to be performed in a sophisticated laboratory. Bleumink et al.[6] found that a normal DNCB score was 8 ± 3. In melanoma patients the average DNCB score was 4.5 ± 3 and patients with Hodgkin's disease had an average DNCB score of 2.5 ± 2.5. In addition, they found in *both* the normal controls and the tumor patients a lower DNCB score for persons over 50 years of age. This points up two facts: first, that the minimum response decreases with aging is perhaps an explanation for tumors occurring with greater frequency in the greater than 50-year-old population; and second, that before one draws conclusions from DNCB testing the results must be compared to age matched controls.

Other measures of CMI are more rapid, do not require a delay in treatment and are somewhat more specific but they do require more sophisticated laboratory personnel and facilities available to perform them. In addition, as will be pointed out in the head and neck cancer patient, these tests do not seem to be any more reliable prognostically (or unreliable depending on one's outlook) as recall antigens or DNCB skin testing.

T Lymphocyte Cell Counts

The T lymphocytes or thymus-derived lymphocytes present in the peripheral blood can be counted using special techniques and provide an indicator of immune competence in patients with malignant tumors. The method of counting T-cells is that of the spontaneous rosette formation. The method used to quantify T-cells was originally described by Wybran and Fudenberg[12] and has been modified by various authors. The basic technique involves the separation of lymphocytes from the other cellular elements of peripheral venous blood. A measured aliquot of the lymphocyte cell suspension is incubated with sheep red blood cells and then resuspended. Then using a hemocytometer 200 mononuclear cells are counted keeping track of the number of these cells which form rosettes with red blood cells. A lymphocyte can be called a T-cell if it forms rosettes with three or more sheep red blood cells. This test has been used as a marker of immune reactivity in patients with head and neck cancer in a number of studies that we will discuss later. It should be mentioned that this is a quantitative test which is not specific for a given antigen but merely gives an estimate of the percentage of T lymphocytes circulating in the patient's peripheral blood which can be compared to normal controls. Absolute T-cell levels can be determined by calculating the corresponding total and differential white blood cell counts.

B-cell

B lymphocytes may be identified by incubating these monocytes with fluorescein labeled immunoglobulin antibodies. Since the B-cell has specific antibodies and specific receptor sites for immunoglobulins, the cells will take up the fluorescein labeled antibodies and can be detected by using fluorescent microscopy. B-cell counts have not been used as a marker of immunological competence in cancer patients.

Lymphocyte Reactivity

The capability of lymphocytes to respond to stimulation in vitro by a nonspecific mitogen such as phytohemagglutinin (PHA) or concanavalin A (Con A) is another means of assessing the competence of the cellular mediated immune system. In this method, lymphocytes are cultured in an incubator with the previously mentioned mitogens. These mitogens result in the blastic transformation of lymphocytes. After incubation of the lymphocytes for a predetermined period of time, tritiated thymidine is added to the cell culture suspensions 24 hours before harvest of these cells. At the completion of this incubation period, the cell suspensions from each culture are filtered and the amount of labeled DNA incubated into the lymphocytes is determined by measuring the labeled DNA in a scintillation counter. The lymphocyte reactivity may then be compared to that of normal control lymphocytes which have not been stimulated. This then is a measure of the lymphocyte's ability to respond to an antigen.

Tumor Associated Antigens

DNCB testing, T-cell counts and lymphocyte reactivity are the most common parameters utilized to measure the competence of the immunological response. These measures, however, are all nonspecific indicators of the immune system. The search for tumor associated or tumor specific antigens would be most valuable in the diagnosis and possibly treatment of cancers. Antigens can be isolated from tumors which differ from normally occurring tissue antigens and these will elicit an immune response in the host. In the head and neck, to date, there have been no tumor associated or tumor specific antigen consistently identified for squamous cell carcinomas. However, their value in diagnosis is obvious. If a specific antigen could be identified for squamous cell carcinoma of the head and neck region, a sensitive radioimmunoassay could be developed to detect this specific antigen in small quantities. This would allow mass screening for early detection. In addition the evaluation of the completeness of the chosen treatment modality in the eradication of tumor could be evaluated by the presence or absence of the tumor specific antigen.

An example of a tumor associated antigen which has been found to occur with adenocarcinomas of the colon is the carcinoembryonic antigen (CEA). This is a tumor associated antigen, in that it is not specific for adenocarcinoma of the colon but has also been identified in other cancers derived from the endoderm of the gastrointestinal tract. This antigen has been found to be present in some patients with squamous cell carcinoma of the oral cavity, pharynx and larynx but not to occur with a frequent enough incidence to make it clinically useful for diagnosis or managements.[13] The major use of CEA is the serial testing in follow-up of colon cancer patients after curative therapy.[14]

Viral-Induced Antibodies

Evidence of virus-induced antigens in human tumors such as nasopharyngeal carcinoma and other squamous cell malignancies of the head and neck have been described. Nasopharyngeal carcinoma has been associated with antibodies directed against the viral capsule antigen of the Epstein-Barr virus (EBV).[15] Patients with nasopharyngeal carcinoma have elevated titers of Epstein-Barr antibodies and the degree of elevation has been correlated with the extent of the neoplasm. After successful therapy, the titers of Epstein-Barr antibodies will fall.[16] Antibodies to the EBV have also been associated with Burkitt's lymphoma and infectious mononucleosis.

Recently the use of the EBV antigen to identify occult nasopharyngeal carcinomas has been described.[17] In this report of 11 patients with occult primary carcinomas one patient had positive EBV antibodies in serum IgA and subsequently developed a nasopharyngeal carcinoma. Coates et al.[17] found that viral capsid antibodies to EBV in the serum IgA fraction were highly specific for nasopharyngeal carcinomas whereas viral capsid antigens in the IgG serum fraction were positive in 77% of normal controls and only indicated that an individual had a previous infection with EBV at some time in his life.

Antibodies to herpes virus TAA have been isolated from human squamous carcinomas of the head and neck. Hollinshead et al.[18] showed a 90% incidence of herpes simplex virus nonvirion antibodies in patients with laryngeal cancer and in 62% of a series of patients with squamous cell carcinoma of other head and neck sites. By contrast, they found these antibodies to be present in only 6% of normal and 8% of patients with nonsquamous malignancies. In 1976 Silverman et al.[19] reported a similar high incidence of herpes virus TAA in 89% of patients with squamous cell carcinoma and also found that 90% of the patients who were cured of their squamous cell carcinoma still persisted in carrying the herpes virus TAA antibodies. They also demonstrated that the immune defects as measured by lymphocyte reactivity persisted in the postreatment stages of the patient's follow-up. These authors suggest that these data support an etiological role for herpes simplex virus in cancers of the head and neck.

Smith et al.,[20, 21] in two publications in 1976, however, reported that the percentage of positive sera was significantly lower in patients more than 3 years tumor free than in untreated patients or patients less than 3 years since treatment. In addition they suggested a high frequency of these antibodies in heavy smokers and patients using alcohol as compared to control groups. This population is at high risk for developing head and neck cancers and a possible correlation with the elevated titers seen in patients with head and neck cancer is suggested.

Conclusions concerning this possible etiology for head and neck cancer are not warranted at this time.

FACTORS INFLUENCING IMMUNE REACTIVITY

Pretreatment Factors

Smoking, alcohol and poor nutrition are characteristic of the patient with head and neck cancer. They are cofactors in the etiology of these malignancies and as expected all have an effect on the immune response.

Chretien[22] reports that studies of immune response in mice exposed to tobacco smoke show an increase in lymphocyte reactivity to PHA in the first 4 to 10 weeks. When exposed to tobacco smoke for prolonged periods, however, a reversal occurs with a decline in the immune reactivity. He has noted similar findings in human subjects. He found that normal adults who have a history of less than a 20-pack year smoking history and are under 40 years in age have higher lymphocyte response to PHA and higher T-cell levels than nonsmoking age matched controls. Patients with a higher consumption of tobacco or smokers over age 40 have depressed lymphocyte reactivity to PHA which continues to decline with age and continued cigarette consumption. T-cell blood levels, however, remain elevated.

Severe alcoholism has been associated with immunological abnormalities. Recall antigens and DNCB testing have been found to be defective in cirrhotic patients.[23] A later study confirmed the same defects in alcoholics with or without liver disease. In addition the patients demonstrated a responsiveness to croton oil (a nonspecific inflammatory agent) which further substantiates this defect. A defect of lymphocyte reactivity to PHA was not found in either group.[24] Lundy et al.[25] in another study of alcoholic patients with varying degrees of liver damage found a normal response to recall antigens and DNCB but a depressed response to PHA and a low T-cell count. In this study the patients were in a normal nutritional state, hence the findings were felt to not be contaminated by the effects of malnutrition. Rehabilitated alcoholics had completely normal immune function tests suggesting that the defects seen in alcoholics are reversible.

Malnutrition secondary to depressed caloric and protein intake is a particular problem for the head and neck cancer patient. The anatomical location in the aerodigestive tract and the associated pain exacerbate this problem in these patients.

Evidence suggests that malnutrition is associated with impairment of both B- and T-cell mediated immune functions.[26] This is another factor which can contribute to the immune suppression of the head and neck cancer patient.

The head and neck cancer patient who is usually a heavy smoker, often an alcoholic, and frequently malnourished has all three of these factors contributing to his immunosuppressed state to say nothing of the tumor burden itself. It would be interesting to know whether there would be such a high frequency of immune depression in head and neck cancer patients without these predisposing factors.

Treatment Factors

The treatment of cancer mandates the employment of radical measures. All of these have the theoretic potential to depress the host immune response. Radical surgery accompanied by a long anesthetic exposure, radical radiotherapy, and radical chemotherapy may cause such a depression.[27] If this is so perhaps these modalities of treatment may enhance distant metastases by suppressing the host immunosurveillance against microscopically metastatic tumor cells even while a primary tumor mass is responding to the local therapy.

It is extremely difficult to separate the effects of surgery and anesthesia on immunoresponsiveness. Jubert et al.[27] used lymphocyte blastogenic reactivity in response to a variety of mitogens to study the effects of anesthetic agents and surgery. They found that halothane, ether, cyclopropamide, and nitrous oxide all suppressed immunoresponsiveness during the intraoperative period. But halothane and nitrous oxide anesthetized patients had completely normal lymphocyte response 7 days postoperatively. Patients given ether and cyclopropamide had continued depression of lymphocyte response 7 to 10 days postoperatively; the former having a greater depressive effect on B-cells and the latter depressing both B- and T-cells responsiveness.

Jubert et al.[27] were also able to correlate depressed lymphocyte reactivity with the amount of blood loss. Patients losing greater than 500 cc of blood had decreased reactivity. This was then used as a measure of surgical effect on immune response.

It must be kept in mind that these are *in vitro* tests of immune function. This becomes more important when Slade et al.'s[28] findings in 12 normal renal transplant donors are reviewed. They studied both in vitro and in vivo measures of immune response. They found that in vitro tests of immune response fell with the induction of general anesthesia and reached a nadir on the first postoperative evening (postnephrectomy) with a complete return to normal by the fifth postoperative day. In vivo testing (using recall antigens to SK/SD, mumps, Candida) had a more gradual decline falling slowly for 5 days. The SK/SD response returned to normal by 10 to 14 days and took up to 3 weeks for a return to normal for mumps and Candida. This suggests poor correlation of in vivo and in vitro tests.

Lundy et al.[29] using a mouse model, have shown impairment of cell mediated cytotoxicity when halothane anesthesia was combined with surgery. They used a biological in vivo marker of immune activity by studying the frequency of pulmonary metastasis occurring when 5×10^4 fibrosarcoma cells were injected into the mouse tail vein just prior to halothane anesthesia and hind limb amputation surgery. Pulmonary metastasis in the halothane/surgery group had a greater than 2-fold increase in pulmonary metastasis when compared to the halothane group alone. When thiabendazol (TBZ), a nonspecific immunopotentiator, was given intraperitoneally in the perioperative period the number of pulmonary metastasis returned to control levels.

The finding of an immunologically reversible anesthesia/surgery induced tumor-specific immune deficit manifested by the significant biological result of pulmonary metastasis demonstrates the potential of our standard therapeutic approaches to contribute to distant metastasis while eradicating local disease. One must, of course, keep in perspective that this is animal data and the mice had no local tumor burden which the immune system had already failed to cope with.

Radiation therapy, a frequently employed modality in the treatment of head and neck cancer, has been shown to result in a depressed lymphocyte count.[30] There is, however, conflicting data regarding the effect of radiotherapy on in vivo and in vitro markers of immune function. It has been reported that radiotherapy decreases the in vitro lymphocyte reactivity to PHA.[31-33] Other investigators, however, when using in vivo tests such as DNCB and other standard recall antigens have found no defect of cell mediated immunity.[34-36] Ghossien et al.[36] studied a large group of cancer patients with both in vivo and in vitro tests. They found normal in vivo tests and depressed in vitro tests. This led them to the just conclusion that the evaluation of the effect of radiotherapy on the immune system depends on the test used.

Recently trials of adjuvant chemotherapy in advanced head and neck cancers which are amenable to surgery have begun in an attempt to reduce the incidence of distant metastasis and improve survival. The use of such regimens requires that patients clinically free of disease undergo prolonged treatment with potentially immunosuppressive agents. Methotrexate is the most commonly employed drug and recently has been used in high doses up to 7.5 g/m². Other drugs used in head and neck cancer include: bleomycin, cis-platinum and adriomycin. Chemotherapeutic agents vary in their degree of immunosuppressiveness. Suppression of the host immune response could result in a detrimental effect on the host-tumor relationship. Roth et al.[37] recently have looked at both in vivo (DNCB) and in vitro (lymphocyte reactivity) tests of immune function in patients undergoing long term adjuvant chemotherapy with high dose methotrexate and adriomycin. In vivo tests were not changed during therapy. In vitro tests were depressed at 24 hours but returned to pretreatment levels at 48 hours. It appears that, for methotrexate and adriomycin, long-term adjuvant therapy does not alter in vivo and in vitro CMI. Similar information is needed for other drug combinations now being used in the treatment of head and neck cancers.

It is apparent then that our treatment modalities have the ability to promote immunosuppression and hence distant metastasis. The variability of response of CMI to different modalities and lack of correlation with in vivo and in vitro tests indicates a need for more careful evaluations. It is possible that immune manipulation should be employed to offset the immunosuppressive effects of our conventional therapy. However, there will be great difficulty to prove effectiveness of such immune therapy as there are so many variables which play a role in the survival of the cancer patient. More specific testing methods of tumor induced CMI must be developed so we can be sure we are manipulating that portion of the immune system which is "interested" in the tumor itself.

Immunoprognosis

As the head and neck surgeon draws up a treatment program for his cancer patient he has come to rely on the tumor-node-metastases (TNM) clinical staging system to estimate the prognosis for that individual patient. Within each stage, however, there are treatment failures and treatment cures even through the TNM staging may be the same and the cancer located in the identical site. It has been suggested that defects in CMI might explain this and thus provide a new prognostic marker to allow a more aggressive conventional therapeutic program and perhaps adjuvant chemoimmunotherapy.

This correlation has been looked for through

the use of DNCB testing and also in vitro tests. Unfortunately, the hope of correlating a negative DNCB test with poor prognosis has yielded varying results from investigator to investigator. The best correlation was made by Eilber et al.[38] who found: (1) alterations in cellular immunity correlated with the extent of the primary in that patients with inoperable cancer had an 80% incidence of anergy; and (2) the immunological reactivity, or lack of it, correlated with the clinical course; 90% of anergic patients developed recurrent disease within 1 year. These findings gave great hope. Unfortunately staging head and neck cancer patients into operable and inoperable groups is not enough stratification to allow confidence in their conclusions. In addition no investigator has been able to confirm such a high frequency of accurate prognostication. Lundy et al.[39] also showed that in a group of patients with head and neck cancer studied by stage, but not by site, a correlation of a negative DNCB test to early recurrence and shortened survival occurred. They also found that once the disease involved the lymph nodes this correlation could not be made. This latter finding is in contrast to Stefani et al.[40] who noted in their series that there was no correlation between DNCB testing and stage of disease, but a definite correlation with the extent of lymph node involvement. Maisel and Ogura[41] had the oportunity of a longer follow-up time of 2 years and found that 91% of their DNCB positive patients were tumor free but only 55% of DNCB negative patients were tumor free.

In a study of 63 head and neck cancer patients treated by radiation therapy, of those with "early disease", 16 of 18 were DNCB reactive and had disease control.[42, 43] One of the two nonreactors had short term disease control. Thirty-three of 45 patients with advanced disease were DNCB reactive. Nineteen of the 33 (58%) were controlled by radiation therapy. Of the 12 nonreactors, only two were controlled. Once again if one is looking for a prognostic indicator that would suggest the need for more aggressive therapy, 42% of DNCB positive patients with "advanced disease" would have been missed. Gilbert et al.[44] in a recent review of the value of pretreatment DNCB response concluded that the DNCB test does not provide an adequate prognostic indicator of treatment success or failure.

There have been a number of reports attempting to correlate T-cell counts and lymphocyte reactivity with prognosis but each of the investigators conclude that they could not correlate survival with T lymphocyte levels or lymphocyte reactivity.[45–48] In a study of 183 patients by Hilal et al.[5] in which DNCB, lymphocyte count, and mixed lymphocyte cultures in response to a number of common mitogens was studied, only lymphocyte reactivity to PHA correlated with increasing tumor burden. The DNCB test results did not correlate with increasing stages of disease. They did find a statistically significant correlation with tumor recurrence in stages I and II but not in stages III and IV. None of the in vitro tests were found to correlate with tumor control.

It appears that the data available so far is more confusing than helpful in using the currently available tests of immune responsiveness to predict prognosis. Certainly the clinical staging systems are more accurate in predicting prognosis than these tests alone. It may be that the DNCB test will be of some value as an additional prognostic sign in stages I and II disease.

The problem with most studies to date is their lack of homogeneity and assessment of all factors affecting CMI. The patients are not stratified by site, treatment modality, age by decade or nutritional status. All these factors will affect either immune response or prognosis. A more specific test for the immune response to the tumor itself along with a stratified study considering all factors is necessary in order to find a test which will help predict prognosis.

A question we must ask ourselves is whether the tumor (primary or recurrence) is a result of a failure of CMI or if the depressed immune state is a result of the tumor burden itself. Perhaps both are involved.

IMMUNOTHERAPY

It has been demonstrated in animal models and suggested by trials in man that manipulation by specific or nonspecific stimulation of the immune system can destroy tumor cells. The tenant on which this form of therapy rests is that a tumor contains specific antigens which, when immune agents are administered, allows an immune response directed against the cancer cells containing these antigens and these cells destroyed. In man most attempts have been in the form of a nonspecific stimulation of the immune mechanism with the assumption that this will benefit the host.

In head and neck cancer Donaldson[49] first proposed a role for immunotherapy in 1972. He reported a 62% response rate in 32 patients with recurrent or advanced cancers and a mean duration of response greater than 46 weeks. He utilized a chemoimmunotherapy regimen of methotrexate 45 to 60 mg/M^2, BCG, and isoniazid.[50] Such results when compared to previously reported responses to methotrexate alone are remarkable. This prompted studies by three other teams of investigators who attempted to duplicate Donaldson's results.[51–53] In addition Suen et al.[53] investigated different chemotherapeutic regimens with and without immunotherapy in the form of BCG and isoniazid. None of these investigators were able to show any improved tumor responsiveness or prolonged duration of response of chemoimmunotherapy over chemotherapy alone. However, it should be noted that these trials involved patients with advanced disease. Experimental animal models have shown that tumor burdens of 10^6 cells or less can be handled immunologically but when this is exceeded the immune response may be overwhelmed.[54] Thus patients with advanced disease and hence massive tumor burdens would be the least likely to respond. In man this has been suggested in a BCG immune therapy trial for cancer of the lung. In patients with stage I lung cancer treated by surgical resection and a single inoculation of BCG into the pleural space postoperatively, fewer recurrences were noted than a randomized group of control patients treated with surgical resection alone.[55] This was not true in patients with a more advanced tumor burden of stage II and III lung cancer. Those treated with intrapleural BCG in the advanced tumors had the same number of metastases on follow up as the control group.

It would seem that using BCG and other nonspecific immune stimulants, e.g., *Corynebacterium parvum*, should be applied when there is minimal tumor burden.

Another factor to be considered in the use of immune therapy is that the host must be able to respond to the immune agent. As previously pointed out, patients with head and neck cancer frequently are anergic or undergo treatments which suppress the host immune response. In these patients, reconstituting the immune system is necessary prior to any attempts to stimulate it. Levamisole, an antihelmenthic, has been shown to stimulate depressed immune systems. Experimental data shows that Levamisole restores immune reactivity toward normal but not to a hyperimmune level.[56] Results of clinical trials have been few. An increased disease free interval and prolonged survival have been reported in stage III breast cancer treated with radiation therapy and Levamisole.[57] There has been one study of the use of Levamisole in surgically resectable (although not staged by TNM) squamous cell carcinomas of the head and neck.[58] All of the patients were anergic to recall antigens following surgery. They were started on Levamisol 1 to 2 weeks following surgery and after 6 to 8 weeks of therapy, three of the six patients developed positive skin tests. Of the six patients only one was without recurrence at the time of the report. This is, of course, only a preliminary study and there were many uncontrolled factors.

Other agents which can reconstitute defects of cellular immunity are thymosin[59] and transfer factor. These have not been adequately evaluated.

A third factor to consider in the search for an immunotherapeutic regimen is the identification of a tumor specific antigen. If such an antigen could be found, a directed stimulation of the immune system to produce a specific antibody could be carried out. This would result in the destruction of the tumor cells which contain the specific antigen and hence microscopic deposits of cells not removed by conventional therapy could be eliminated. To date no such treatment trial in head and neck cancers has begun. It is possible that such a treatment program for nasopharyngeal carcinoma may be available in the future. For other head and neck sites, a search for such a tumor specific antigen must continue.

A fourth factor to be considered in an immune therapy program is the development of tests which will allow the identification of tumor protective factors such as blocking antibodies and might be hiding a tumor specific antigen from the host's immune response. Such blocking factors reduce the effectiveness of immune therapy. The development of a method to remove such factors is not currently in view.

Browder and Chretien[60] have made suggestions for immunotherapy trials which encompass the above mentioned principles. They suggest immunoreconstitution be carried out prior to and throughout conventional therapy and immunostimulation combined with chemotherapy be continued upon completion of the conventional therapy.

It is apparent then that as of this writing there is no immunotherapy regimen of proven efficacy. In fact, there is no evidence, as yet, that immunotherapy will prolong survival, increase the disease free interval, or increase cure rates in head and neck cancer. Future immunotherapy trials must be carefully controlled with the consideration of all factors which effect the immune response. Immunodepressive factors should be corrected or controlled. Improved markers of immune competence must be developed which are quantitative and accurately measure immune competence as it relates to the host's tumor. These markers should also be immunoprognostic and tell the oncologist when he must be more aggressive in his management. In addition, if specific tumor antigens can be identified, we could have a "fingerprinting" method to announce that the tumor is present, or not allowing for prophylactic scanning of the "healthy" population and/or detection of recurrence, when the tumor burden is still microscopic.

At the present time it would seem that *routine* monitoring of the immune response by other than recall antigens and/or DNCB testing is of little value to the patient. Other tests should be considered experimental and the costs not be borne by the patient. They should be done only as a part controlled study designed to study the multiple facets of the host-tumor response. Immunotherapy regimens must be considered in the same light.

REFERENCES

1. Eilber, F. R., and Maton, D. L.: Impaired immunologic reactivity and recurrence following cancer surgery. Cancer 25:362, 1970.
2. Chretien, P. B., Chowder, W. L., Gertner, H. R., Sample, W. F., and Catalona, W. J.: Correlation of preoperative lymphocyte reactivity with the clinical course of cancer patients. Surg. Gynecol. Obstet. 136:380, 1973.
3. Olkowski, Z. L., and Wilkins, S. A.: T-lymphocyte levels in the peripheral blood of patients with cancer of the head and neck. Am. J. Surg. 130:440, 1975.
4. Potvin, C., Tarpley, J. L., and Chretien, P. B.: Thymus-derived lymphocytes in patients with solid malignancies. Clin. Immunol. Immunopathol. 3:476, 1975.
5. Hilal, E. Y., Wanebo, H. J., and Pinsky, C. M.: Immunologic evaluation and prognosis in patients with head and neck cancer. Am. J. Surg. 134:469, 1977.
6. Bleumink, E., Nater, J. P., Koops, H. S., and Tite, T. H.: A standard method for DNCB sensitization testing in patients with neoplasms. Cancer 33:911, 1974.
7. Burnet, F. M.: Immunologic aspects of malignant disease. Lancet 1:1171, 1967.
8. Penn, I., and Starzl, T. E.: Malignant tumors arising de novo in immunosuppressed organ transplant recipients. Transplantation 14:407, 1972.
9. Walde, B. K., Robertson, M. R., and Jeremy, D.: Skin cancer and immunosuppression. Lancet 2:1282, 1973.
10. Gatti, R. A., and Good, R. A.: Occurrence of malignancy in immunodeficiency diseases. Cancer 28:89, 1971.
11. Catalona, W. J., Taylor, P. T., Rabson, A. S., and Chretien, P. B.: A method for dinitrochlorobenzene contact sensitization—clinicopathologic study. N. Engl. J. Med. 286:399, 1972.
12. Wybran, J., and Fudenberg, H. H.: Rosette formation: A test for cellular immunity. Trans. Assoc. Am. Physicians. 84:239, 1971.
13. Silverman, N. A., Alexander, J. C., and Chretien, P. B.: CEA levels in head and neck cancer. Cancer 37:2204, 1976.
14. Meeker, W. R.: The use and abuse of CEA testing in clinical practice. Cancer 41:854, 1978.
15. Sako, K., Manowada, J., and Marchetta, F. C.: Epstein-Barr virus antibodies in patients with carcinoma of the nasopharynx and carcinoma of other sites in the head and

neck. Am. J. Surg. 130:437, 1975.

16. Henle, G., and Henle, W.: Epstein-Barr virus-specific IgA serum antibodies as an outstanding feature of nasopharyngeal carcinoma. Int. J. Cancer 17:1, 1976.

17. Coates, H. L., Pearson, G. R., Neel, H. B. Weiland, L. H., and Devine, K. D.: An immunologic base for detection of occult primary malignancies of the head and neck. Cancer 41:912, 1978.

18. Hollinshead, A. C., Lee, O., Chretien, P. B., Tarpley, J. L., Rawls, W. E., and Adam, E.: Antibodies to herpes virus-nonunion antigens in squamous carcinomas. Science 182: 713, 1973.

19. Silverman, N. A., Alexander, J. C., Hollinshead, A. S., and Chretien, P. B.: Correlations of tumor burden with in vitro lymphocyte reactivity and antibodies to herpes virus tumor-associated antigens in head and neck squamous carcinoma. Cancer 37:135, 1976.

20. Smith, H. G., Horowitz, N., Silverman, N. A., Henson, D. E., and Chretien, P. B.: Humoral immunity to herpes simplex viral-induced antigens in smokers. Cancer 38: 1155, 1976.

21. Smith, H. G., Chretien, P. B. and Henson, D. E.: Viral-specific humoral immunity to herpes-simplex-induced antigens in patients with squamous carcinoma of the head and neck. Am. J. Surg. 132:541, 1976.

22. Chretien, P. B.: The effects of smoking on immunocompetence. Laryngoscope 88 (suppl. 8):11, 1978.

23. Straus, B., Berenyi, M. R., Haun, J., and Straus, E.: Delayed hypersensitivity in alcoholic cirrhosis. Am. J. Dig. Dis. 16: 509, 1971.

24. Berenyi, M. R., Straus, B., and Cruz, D.: In vivo and in vitro studies of cellular immunity in alcoholic cirrhosis. Am. J. Dig. Dis. 19:199, 1974.

25. Lundy, J., Raaf, J. H., Deakins, S., Jacobs, D. A., Tsung-dao, L., Jacobowitz, D., Spear, C., Wanebo, H., and Old, L. J.: The acute and chronic effects of alcohol on the human immune system. Surg. Gynecol. Obstet. 141:212, 1975.

26. Law, D. K., Dudrick, S. J., and Abdon, N. I.: The effects of protein calorie malnutrition on immune competence of the surgical patient. Surg. Gynecol. Obstet. 139:257, 1974.

27. Jubert, A. V., Lee, E. T., Hersh, E. M., and McBride, C. M.: Effects of surgery, anesthesia, and intraoperative blood loss on immunocompetence. J. Surg. Res. 15:399, 1973.

28. Slade, M. S., Simmons, R. L., Yunis, E., and Greenberg, L. J.: Immunodepression after major surgery in normal patients. Surgery 78:363, 1975.

29. Lundy, J., Lovett, E. J., Hamilton, S., and Contran, P.: Halothane, surgery, immunosuppression, and artificial pulmonary metastasis. Cancer 41:827, 1978.

30. Goswitz, F. A., Andrew, G. A., and Kriseley, R. M. P.: Effects of local irradiation on the peripheral blood and bone marrow. Blood 21:605, 1963.

31. Thomas, J. W., Cory, P., Lewis, H. S., and Yuen, A.: Effect of therapeutic irradiation on lymphocyte transformation in lung cancer. Cancer 27:1046, 1971.

32. Stjernsward, J., Yondal, M., Vanky, F., Wigzell, H., and Sealy, R.: Lymphopenia and change in distribution of human B and T lymphocytes in peripheral blood induced by irradiation for mammary carcinoma. Lancet 1:1352, 1972.

33. Cosimi, A.B., Brunstetter, F. H., and Hemmerer, W. T.: Cellular immune competence of breast cancer patients receiving immunotherapy. Arch. Surg. 107:531, 1973.

34. Clement, J. A., and Kramer, S.: Immunocompetence in patients with solid tumors undergoing cobalt 60 irradiation. Cancer 34:193, 1974.

35. Gross, L., Mantredi, G. L., and Protos, A.: Effect of cobalt 60 irradiation upon cell mediated immunity. Radiology 106:653, 1973.

36. Ghossein, N. A., Bosworth, J. L., and Bases, R. E.: The effect of radical radiotherapy on delayed hypersensitivity and the inflammatory response. Cancer 35:1616, 1975.

37. Roth, J. A., Eilber, F. R., and Morton, D. L.: Effect of Adriamycin and high dose methotrexate on in vivo and in

vitro cell mediated immunity in cancer patients. Cancer 41:814, 1978.

38. Eilber, R. R., Morton, D. L., and Ketcham, A. S.: Immunologic abnormalities in head and neck cancer. Am. J. Surg. 128:534, 1974.

39. Lundy, J., Wanebo, H., Pinsky, C., Strong, E., and Oeltgen, H.: Delayed hypersensitivity reactions in patients with squamous cell cancer of the head and neck. Am. J. Surg. 128:530, 1974.

40. Stefani, S., Kerman, R., and Abbati, J.: Serial studies of immunocompetence in head and neck cancer patients undergoing radiation therapy. Am. J. Roentgenol. Radium Ther. Nucl. Med. 126:880, 1976.

41. Maisel, R. H., and Ogura, H. H.: Dinitrochlorobenzene skin sensitization and peripheral lymphocyte count: predictors of survival in head and neck cancer. Ann. Otol. Rhinol. Laryngol. 85:517, 1976.

42. Bosworth, J. L., Thaler, S., and Ghossein, N. A.: Delayed hypersensitivity and local control of patients treated by radiotherapy for head and neck cancer. Am. J. Surg. 132: 46, 1976.

43. Bosworth, J. L., Ghossein, N. A., and Brooks, T. L.: Delayed hypersensitivity in patients treated by curative radiotherapy. Cancer 36:353, 1975.

44. Gilbert, H. A., Kagan, A. R., Miles, J., Flores, L., Nussbaum, H., Rao, A. R., and Chan, P.: The usefulness of pretreatment DNCB in 85 patients with squamous cell carcinoma of the upper aerodigestive tract. J. Surg. Oncol. 10:73, 1978.

45. Jenkins, V. K., Pranab, R., Ellis, H. N., Griffiths, C. M., Perry, R. R., and Olson, M. H.: Lymphocyte response in patients with head and neck cancer. Arch. Otolaryngol. 102:596, 1976.

46. Wanebo, H. J., Jun, M. Y., Strong, E. W., and Oettgen, H. F.: T cell deficiency in patients with squamous cell cancer of the head and neck. Am. J. Surg. 130:445, 1975.

47. Eastham, R. J., Mason, J. M., Jennings, B. R., Belew, P. W., and Maguda, T. A.: T cell rosette test in squamous cell carcinoma of the head and neck. Arch. Otolaryngol. 102: 171, 1976.

48. Mason, J. M., Kitchens, G. G., Eastham, R. J., and Jennings, B. R.: T lymphocytes and survival of head and neck squamous cell carcinoma. Arch. Otolaryngol. 103:223, 1977.

49. Donaldson, R. C.: Methotrexate plus bacillus Calmette-Guerin (BCG) and Isoniazid in the treatment of cancer of the head and neck. Am. J. Surg. 124:527, 1972.

50. Donaldson, R. C.: Chemoimmunotherapy for cancer of the head and neck. Am. J. Surg. 126:507, 1973.

51. Eilber, F. R., and Morton, D. L.: Adjuvant chemoimmunotherapy in advanced lesions of the head and neck. Am. J. Roentgenol. 126:1082, 1976.

52. Woods, J. E., DeSanto, L. W., and Ritts, R. E.: A controlled study of combined methotrexate, BCG, and INH therapy for squamous cell carcinoma of the head and neck. Surg. Clin. North Am. 57:769, 1977.

53. Suen, Y. Y., Richman, S. P., Livingston, R. B., Hersh, E. M., Craig, R., and Tonymon, K.: Results of BCG adjuvant immunotherapy in 100 patients with epidermoid carcinoma of the head and neck. Am. J. Surg. 134:474, 1977.

54. Shin, H. S., Pasternack, G. R., Economou, J. S., Johnson, R. J., and Hayden, M. L.: Immunotherapy of cancer with antibody. Science 194:327, 1976.

55. Amery, W. K.: A placebo-controlled levamisole study in resectable lung cancer. In Immunotherapy of Cancer: Present Status of Trials in Man; edited by D. Windorst and W. D. Terry, Raven Press New York (in press); as quoted in Browder, J. P., and Chretien, P. B.: Immune reactivity in head and neck squamous carcinoma and relevance to the design of immunotherapy trials. Semin. Oncol. 4:431, 1977.

56. Symoens, J.: Levamisole, an antianergic chemotherapeutic agent: an overview. In Control of Neoplasia by Modulation of the Immune System, edited by M. A. Chingos.

57. Rojas, A. F., Mickiewicz, E., Fierstein, J. N., Glait, H., and

Raven Press, New York, 1977.

Olivari, A. J.: Levamisole in advanced human breast cancer. Lancet 1:211, 1976.

58. Wilkins, S. A., and Olkowski, Z. L.: Immunocompetence of cancer patients treated with levamisole. Cancer 39:487, 1977.

59. Kenady, D. E., Chretien, P. B., Potvin, C., and Simon, R.

M.: Thymosin reconstitution of T cell deficits *in vitro* in cancer patients. Cancer 39:575, 1977.

60. Browder, J. P., and Chretien, P. B.: Immune reactivity in head and neck squamous carcinoma and relevance to the design of immunotherapy trials. Semin. Oncol., 4:431, 1977.

CHAPTER 26

Cysts, Sinuses and "Coeles"

In other chapters, discussions of a variety of benign cystic lesions of the head and neck have been presented. These have included the odontogenic and fissural cysts and parenchymal cysts, among others.

The present chapter considers a "pot pourri" of congenital or acquired lesions. These are: abnormalities of the branchial apparatus; mucoceles, mucous cysts and related lesions; cysts of the larynx and laryngoceles; and diverticula of the trachea and pharynx.

ABNORMALITIES OF THE BRANCHIAL APPARATUS

One of the most controversial cysts of the head and neck, principally concerning the tissue and mode of origin, is the lateral cervical cyst or branchial cyst. Despite their rather infrequent occurrence, the congenital cysts and sinuses of the neck continue to arouse interest. This is primarily due to the complicated and as yet imperfectly understood developmental history of the structures in and near the neck and the changing relationships that occur in this region during embryological life.[1-5]

There are three major theories proposed to explain the origins of most lateral cervical cysts: (1) the branchial apparatus hypothesis; (2) the thymic duct hypothesis; and (3) origin from parotid gland inclusions. I favor the first of these hypotheses.

The branchial apparatus begins to develop at about the 15th day of gestation. It consists of five transverse mesodermal bars, the branchial arches, which are separated by grooves or clefts (Fig. 26.1). These structures are covered externally by a flat epithelium and lined internally by columnar epithelium. Each cleft is in contact with an outpouching of the pharynx, the pharyngeal pouch, and the two are separated by a thin membrane. Each branchial arch contains a central cartilage, a blood vessel and a nerve.

The first arch gives rise to the maxilla and mandible; its vessel becomes the facial artery, and its nerve the maxillary and mandibular branches of the trigeminal nerve. The first cleft gives rise to the external auditory meatus, and its closing membrane persists as the tympanic membrane. The eustachian tube, middle ear and inner part of the tympanic membrane arise from the first pouch.

The second arch forms the lesser cornu of the hyoid bone and the styloid process. The second arch vessel persists as the lingual branch of the external carotid artery, and the nerve as the facial nerve.

The fate of the second cleft is not definitely known, but it is this second cleft that is believed to be responsible for most of the lateral branchial anomalies (95%). The ventral part of the second branchial pouch gives rise to the palatine tonsil and tonsillar fossa. The dorsal part is incorporated into the pharyngotympanic tube. With further growth, the second arch extends caudally to overlap the third and fourth arches, with the result that the second, third and fourth clefts open into a common passage called the cervical sinus.

Other structures originating from the second arch are part of the auricle, skin of the upper anterior neck, stapes, posterior tympanic wall, stylohyoid ligament, lesser horn of the hyoid, anterior base of tongue and the palatoglossus, and posterior belly of the digastric, stylohyoid, platysma, facial, auricular, occipital and stapedius muscles.

Structures originating from the third arch are body and greater horns of the hyoid bone, posterior portion of the base of the tongue, palatopharyngeus and stylopharyngeus muscles, skin over the carotid triangle of the neck, glossopharyngeal nerve and caudal third of the internal carotid artery. The third pouch gives rise to the thymus and lower parathyroid glands.

Structures having origin from the fourth arch are upper portions of the thyroid cartilage, cricothyroid and some pharyngeal muscles, superior

514

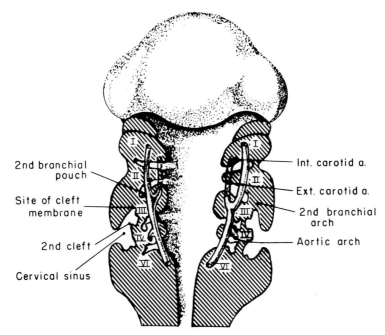

Figure 26.1. Coronal section through branchial arches of a 5-week embryo.

laryngeal branch of the vagus nerve, arch of the aorta on the left and subclavian artery on the right.

Originating from the fifth and sixth arches are part of the skin of the neck, lower portion of the thyroid cartilage, cricoid cartilage, laryngeal muscles, recurrent laryngeal branch of the vagus nerve and pulmonary artery.

The ear is formed by the coalescence of a number of tubercles about the opening of the first cleft. These tubercles arise from both the first and second arches. The helix and tragus originate from the first arch, and the antihelix and antitragus develop from the second arch.

The tongue arises chiefly from the first arch, originally from paired lateral swellings in the 4- to 5-week old embryo. An unpaired eminence, the tuberculum impar is also present.

There is little to recommend the thymic duct hypothesis. Wenglowski[6] felt that the lateral cervical cysts took their origin along the course of the thymic duct because he found it difficult to explain the appearance of cysts below the hyoid bone with a branchial arch theory of origin. However, since there is no unequivocal thymic tissue in the walls of the majority of branchial cysts and since there is a considerably wider anatomical distribution of the cysts than one could consider plausible if the thymus were the origin, this theory is not widely accepted. Amr[2] has pointed out, in addition, that at no stage in its development does the thymic duct have any connection with the ectoderm.

The parotid gland inclusion hypothesis[3, 7] cannot be so readily dismissed but nevertheless is an unlikely explanation for the majority of the lateral cervical cysts.[4, 8] When one attempts to correlate the incidence of branchial cysts with the areas of greatest concentrations of two types of epithelial remnants which would give rise to the cysts—parotid versus branchial—it would appear that the branchial apparatus is the more likely source (yet not exclusive) of these unique cysts.

Branchiogenic Anomalies. Congenital anomalies resulting from abnormalities of the first cleft are relatively rare when compared with those of second-cleft origin.

Anomalous growth of the first branchial arch results in a wide spectrum of congenital disorders. The syndromes of the first branchial arch are reviewed by Brownstein et al.[9]

Accessory tragi, while usually presenting as an isolated anomaly, may occasionally be associated with such lesions as cleft lip, cleft palate and hypoplasia of the mandible. Accessory tragi, appearing at birth as solitary or multiple, unilateral or bilateral, sessile, pedunculated or acuminate papules or nodules, may be located between the pretragal and sternoclavicular areas. They usually occur in the preauricular region, often slightly above or below the level of the tragus.

They may be soft or cartilaginous in consistency and usually measure less than 1 cm in length. Ulceration is unusual.

The lesions are easily excised and have been described under a variety of dispositions. Pathologists have usually dismissed them as "fibroepithelial papillomas," without appreciating their histological similarity to the normal anatomy of the external ear.[9] In lesions without cartilage, the precise nature of the lesion has rarely been recognized on objective histological grounds. Those lesions containing cartilage have often been called ectopic cartilage or chondroma or skin tag with cartilage.

Accessory tragi should be considered in the clinical differential diagnosis of papules or nodules located along the course of migration of the first pharyngeal arches (between the pretragal and supraclavicular regions). If a lesion has been present since birth and has a cartilaginous consistency, an accessory tragus is a most likely diagnosis.[9]

The histopathological appearance, while characteristic, is not diagnostic. The over-all configuration is that a sessile or pedunculated polyp. Aside from the location and configuration of the lesion, the histopathological features are similar to the external ear of fetuses and adults.[9]

Brownstein et al.[9] point out that although a cutaneous tag and an accessory tragus may both have a similar configuration and consist of an epithelial lining enclosing fibrovascular and adipose tissue, the former lacks epidermal adenexa, whereas the latter contains eccrine sweat glands and pilosebaceous units.

Considerably more important lesions are those related to anomalies of the first branchial groove.[10, 11] First and second embryological arch structures of the developing pinna are concerned with formation of pretragal sinuses and cysts, and not with the anomalies of the first groove.

The true incidence of anomalies of the first branchial groove is difficult to determine, but it is quite low. They probably constitute less than 1% of all branchial arch anomalies. Because of this rarity, there is (1) failure to recognize these lesions clinically, (2) inadequate removal that leads to surgical failure, infection, and recurrence, (3) danger of harm to the facial nerve during surgical treatment, and (4) general unawareness of the histopathological appearances of the lesions by pathologists.

There are two distinct anomalies of the first branchial groove (Fig. 26.2). Type I (ectodermal) is a lesion of the first cleft only. Type II (ectodermal and mesodermal) has contributions from the first cleft and from portions of the first and second branchial arches as well. Both may be regarded as duplication anomalies of either the membranous (type I) or membranous and cartiligenous portions

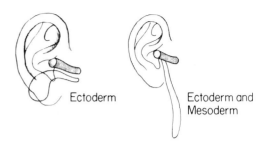

Ectoderm   Ectoderm and Mesoderm

TYPE I   **TYPE II**

Figure 26.2.   Two types of first branchial groove lesions.

(type II) of the external ear canal. Neither type is associated with pretragal cysts or sinuses.

The type I lesions are histologically epidermoid cysts and possess no cartilage or adenexal structures (Fig. 26.3). Typically, type I lesions course medially, inferiorly, and posteriorly to the pinna and the concha of the ear. Drainage may occur from a cyst or sinus at any of these sites. Extensions may occur anterior to the earlobe. These are superior to the main trunk of the facial nerve, usually are parallel to the external ear canal, and end in a cul-de-sac on or near a bony plate at the level of the mesotympanum. Parotid tissue may be intimately associated with the sinus tract and may completely surround it.

Type II lesions are more numerous, more intimately associated with the parotid gland and since they are duplication abnormalities of the membranous *and* cartilaginous portions of the ear canal, contain skin (usually with adenexal structures) and cartilage (Fig. 26.4). They are most often diagnosed after infection and incision and drainage of an abscess at a point below the angle of the mandible. The upward extensions of this lesion pass over the angle or the horizontal ramus of the mandible. They continue upward, through the parotid gland, passing lateral or medial to the VIIth nerve, and in rare instances, actually split its trunk. An ending may present as a sinus, inferior to the canal, that drains at the bony-cartilaginous junction. The middle ear is normal.

Based on clinical and anatomical findings, both types of first-groove anomalies can and should be distinguished from congenital aural sinuses and auricular tags. The congenital sinus characteristically has an inconspicuous opening at the anterior margin of the ascending limb of the helix. These sinuses are usually short, but may arborize and follow a tortuous course in the vicinity of the external ear. They are lateral, superior and posterior to the parotid gland and the facial nerve, and

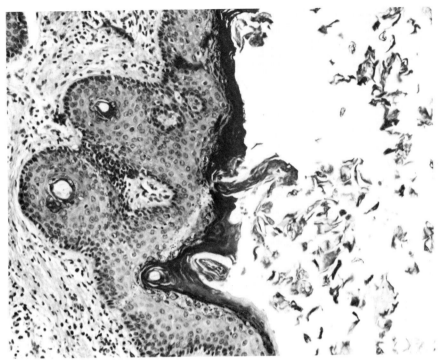

Figure 26.3.   Type I first branchial groove lesion. Histologically the lesion appears as an epidermal inclusion cyst.

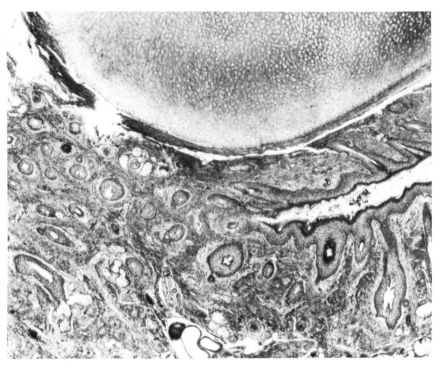

Figure 26.4.   Type II first branchial groove lesion. While both types I and II are duplication anomalies of the external auditory canal, type II lesions most closely parallel the canal histologically.

end blindly along the external auditory canal. They arise from inclusions of ectodermal elements within the rapidly proliferating mesenchymal hillocks (auricular tubercles) and are located on the cephalic and caudal edges of the second and first branchial arches. The sinuses are indistinguishable from first-cleft anomalies by microscopic examinations and resemble the so-called dermoid cysts in other areas of facial fusion. Hyaline cartilage is not found.

Auricular tags are present at birth and are pedunculated, firm nodules located anywhere between the pretragal and sternoclavicular areas. Vellus hairs often protrude from the surface. Infection is rare. The auricular tag is often associated with other anomalies of the first branchial arch, while first groove anomalies are usually free of other congenital aberrations.

In addition to the gross distinctions, the auricular tags are easy to distinguish from first-cleft lesions. Frequently the epidermis is corrugated and is in contact with a dermis that contains pilosebaceous elements and eccrine sweat glands. A central plate of hyaline cartilage is located in the center of the connective tissue core of the tag.

Aronsohn et al.[12] have outlined the principles to be followed in the management of the first cleft lesion.

The majority of branchial cysts arise from the second branchial cleft or from the cervical sinus, or branchial pouch. If the membrane separating the second cleft and pouch breaks down, a complete fistulous tract may persist, extending from the surface of the neck to the pharynx. Incomplete sinus tracts may occur, which open externally or internally. Because the sternomastoid muscle develops in mesoderm behind the last branchial cleft, external sinuses and fistulas open along its anterior border.

ReMine[8] reminds us that the proximal portion of the internal carotid artery is of third-arch origin and that a second-cleft fistula necessarily must pass ventral to this vessel. It courses between the internal and external carotid arteries, entering the pharynx in the region of the supratonsillar fossa. This is the situation that prevails in practically all instances of branchial-cleft cyst and sinus that occur in the neck. As mentioned above, cysts, sinuses and fistulae at other locations may be noted rarely; but a great majority of these developmental anomalies appear at this site. For this reason, most investigators agree that these anomalies originate from the second cleft and pouch.[13]

Branchial cysts from the second branchial cleft are found deep to the sternomastoid muscle or along its anterior border, most commonly at the level of the angle of the mandible.

The external opening of a branchial cleft fistula is usually along the lower anterior border of the sternomastoid muscle, just above the clavicle. A well developed tract runs upward and from the opening along the muscle and through the deep fascia toward the carotid sheath. It then passes between the external and internal carotid arteries. At the level of the hyoid bone the fistula passes medially, superficial to the hypoglossal (XII) nerve and deep to the stylohyoid muscle and the posterior belly of the digastric, to end in the pharynx. The internal orifice is located in the base of the tonsillar fossa.

Himalstein[1] has offered a classification of second pouch branchial cysts and fistulae. It incorporates some features of Bailey's[14] subdivision and is based on seven units. Singly or combined, his seven units encompass most, if not all, second pouch anomalies. From the skin inward, in the direction of dissection for a complete fistula, the seven units are as follows:

1. An external skin opening anywhere along the anterior border of the sternomastoid from the hyoid to the sternum.

2. A segment along the sternomastoid just deep to the cervical fascia. If isolated as a cyst, it conforms to Bailey's type I cyst.[14]

3. A segment lying on the carotid sheath. If isolated, it is the most common cyst type, Bailey's type II.[14]

4. A segment in or ventral to the carotid bifurcation.

5. A segment near the pharyngeal wall or the faucial tonsil region, i.e., Bailey's type IV cyst.

6. A pharyngeal opening in the tonsillar fossa region.

7. A nasopharyngeal segment which extends from the tonsillar fossa to the eustachian orifice region or to the base of the skull.

Most branchial cysts present as painless, fluctuant and smooth swellings just below the angle of the mandible along the anterior border of the sternomastoid muscle. The usual age of record is between 10 and 40 years, but the range is from birth to over 80 years. A sudden appearance or the sudden enlargement of a pre-existing mass is usually associated with an upper respiratory infection.

The most common symptom of a branchial cleft sinus is a small opening just above the clavicle through which a serum-like fluid exudes.

The cysts are typically thin-walled and only rarely attached to contiguous structures (Fig. 26.5). They are usually filled with a turbid, yellowish

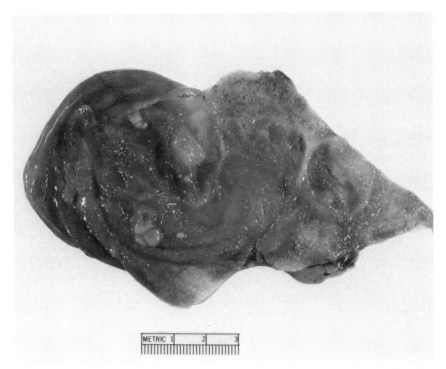

Figure 26.5. Second branchial cleft (pouch) cyst. The nodular excresences represent focally prominent accumulations of lymphoid tissue.

fluid which may contain cholesterol crystals. Microscopically, the cysts are usually lined with a stratified squamous epithelium with lymphoid tissue deep to the lining membrane (Fig. 26.6). Occasional areas of columnar epithelium are seen and about 4% of the cysts will have their lining composed entirely of columnar (respiratory type) epithelium.

Fistulae are most often lined by a stratified squamous epithelium in the external portions and by a columnar type epithelium in their internal parts.

The preferred treatment is complete surgical excision. Although branchial cysts may fluctuate in size, they never spontaneously regress. Newman[15] contends that irradiation is contraindicated and that sclerosing agents are unsatisfactory.

Guidelines to surgical management and technique may be found in several reports.[8, 13, 15–17]

Third branchial cleft defects are rare. There are, however, approximately 15 reported cases of third branchial cleft-pharyngeal pouch remnants in the literature.[19, 20] Cysts occur in the region of the ventricle of the larynx and are lined with a stratified squamous epithelium. To my knowledge, a *complete* branchial pouch fistula has not been recorded. A fistula should open into the plane of the thyrohyoid membrane. An internal fistula may open into the trachea or larynx and give rise to air sacs. The external opening of a fistula opens anterior to the lower third of the sternocleidomastoid muscle. The tract then passes between the common carotid artery and vagus nerve with the internal opening in the pyriform sinus. The third cleft defect also passes posterior and inferior to the glossopharyngeal nerve that runs in the third arch.

Fourth branchial cleft (pharyngeal pouch) remnants are so rare that a case presentation is always noteworthy. Tucker and Skolnick[21] have done just that after their careful search of the literature failed to disclose any documented examples. A complete fistula of the fourth cleft is thought to be only a theoretical possibility inasmuch as the tract would have to course below the fourth branchial artery (aorta on the left and subclavian artery on the right), emptying into the upper esophagus. In favor of Tucker and Skolnick's[21] case being a legitimate fourth branchial remnant was the lesion's relationship to the pyriform sinus and its passage external to the recurrent laryngeal nerve.

Another rare, but related anomaly is the fourth and/or sixth pouch branchial cyst of the mediastinum.

Midline branchiogenic anomalies and syn-

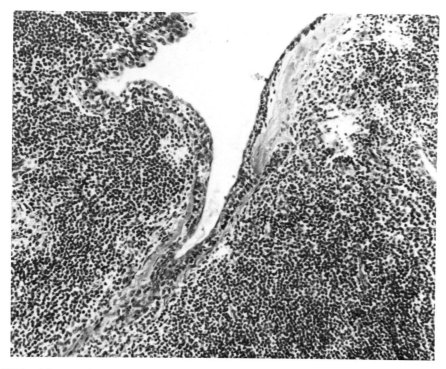

Figure 26.6.   Microscopic appearance of a typical second branchial cleft cyst showing the usual relationship of the lining epithelium and accompanying lymphoid tissue.

dromes are far less frequent than those in the lateral necks and the defects of the medial or ventral portions of the branchial systems are not well recognized. Cosman and Crikelair[18] have presented a brief review.

A discussion of the controversial and ill defined branchiogenic carcinoma is found in Chapter 12.

MUCOCELES OF THE ORAL CAVITY

These commonly occurring benign lesions of the oral mucous membranes have had a modest controversy centered about their pathogenesis. In the past, oral mucoceles were thought to arise from obstruction of an excretory duct causing a back pressure of mucous and the development of an epithelial lined cyst. Studies by Chaudhry et al.[22] and Bhaskar et al.[23] indicate that the lesion is most often produced as a result of trauma with injury or disruption of the excretory duct of a minor salivary gland and the subsequent escape of mucus into the adjacent tissue. It has also been shown that most mucoceles of the oral cavity are not lined by epithelium but rather are mucous pools surrounded by connective tissue and a variety of tissue reactions.

The present author, like Cohen[24] considers there are two types of "mucoceles"—one in which mu-

cus has extravasated into the tissue and may or may not be enclosed by granulation tissue (a mucous extravasation cyst) and a much less common one which in effect is a mucous retention cyst and is lined with epithelium.

Mucoceles occur most commonly in the lower lip. The remainder occur in the cheek, palate, floor of the mouth, tongue and retromolar fossa, which are the regions where mucous glands are normally found. Although mucous glands are also present in the upper lip, mucoceles in this area are rare (Table 26.1).[25, 26]

Discussions of mucoceles of the floor of the mouth and ranulae have been presented elsewhere (Chapter 3).

As indicated above, the majority of mucoceles of the oral regions occur in the lower lip and away from the midline. Cataldo and Mosadomi,[26] in their study of 348 cases on the lips, did not find a single example in the midline.

The lesions are consistently described as painless, freely movable, smooth, soft or firm masses varying in size from a few millimeters to several centimeters.

The ease and reliability of clinical diagnosis is readily apparent from reports considering large numbers of clinical cases.

Mucoceles of the oral cavity occur most often in

children and young adults. Nearly half of the reported cases have presented in patients less than 21 years of age and more than 25% have occurred between the ages of 11 and 20 years.[26]

Two histological appearances are observed. The first in which the lesion is characterized by extravasation of mucous is considerably more numerous than the mucous retention cyst type of mucocele.

The extravasation mucocele usually has its walls poorly defined and composed of granulation tissue of varying degrees of maturity. The age of the granulation tissue and its character may not cor-

Table 26.1
Anatomical Location of Mucoceles

Site	No. of Cases	Percent of Total
Lower lip	607	61.1
Buccal mucosa	157	15.8
Floor of mouth	126	12.7
Palate	37	3.7
Tongue	24	2.4
Upper lip	19	1.9
Other sites	24	2.4
	994	100.0

Statistical data derived from the studies by Cataldo and Mosadomi[26] and Harrison.[25]

relate with the clinical age of the lesions. The "cyst" area consists of mucin or mucoid material containing scattered inflammatory cells with a predominance of histiocytes. These cells are often at the margins of the pool of fluid (Fig. 26.7). In instances where a definable "cystic" structure is lacking, the mucinous material is dispersed into the surrounding connective tissue, where it may induce an inflammatory reaction. At times only aggregates of histiocytes characterize the lesion. In some cases, it may be possible to see a breach in the duct of a mucous gland from which mucus has leaked into the tissue.

The mucous retention cyst variant of mucocele is a true cyst with an epithelial lining that is in continuity with the lining of a duct. The epithelium may be a flattened columnar type or be squamous cell in character as a result of metaplasia due to obstruction and inflammation.

The mucous gland tissue in relation to a mucocele is often the site of ductal distention and atrophy of acini with an accompanying chronic inflammatory infiltrate and fibrosis.

Treatment is surgical removal of the mucocele and the associated mucous gland. Recurrence is minimal.

Lymphoepithelial Cysts. Benign lymphoepithe-

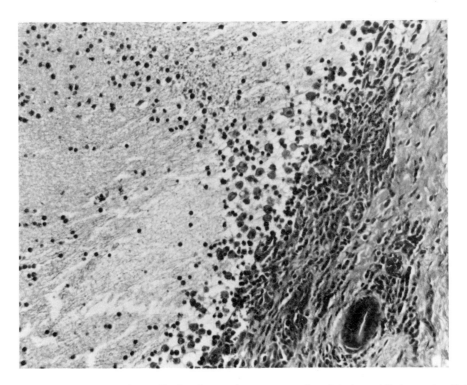

Figure 26.7. Mucocele from lip manifesting the usual appearance of such lesions at their margins. Note the absence of a definable epithelial lining and the numerous histiocytic cells.

lial cysts of the oral cavity are unusual and have been recorded in the literature as branchial cysts, branchiogenic cysts and pseudocysts.[27]

The floor of the mouth is almost exclusively the site of location of these lesions although a number have also been reported as arising from the tongue.

Males in their thirties or forties are most often the subjects presenting with the lesions.

These entities usually appear as small, soft, pink to yellow, elevated, submucosal tumors. When traumatized or irritated, they may become symptomatic.

Microscopically, the cysts are well circumscribed and located beneath the epithelium. The lining of the cysts is almost uniformly parakeratotic squamous epithelium. Surrounding the cyst lining, in varying thickness are accumulations of lymphocytes, often arranged in a follicular pattern. A communication or continuity with the mucosal epithelium is usually not observed. The cyst cavities contain keratin debris, lymphocytes and an amorphous, slightly eosinophilic fluid.

It is postulated that these lesions arise from epithelium which during embryogenesis, becomes included within the lymphoid aggregations in the mucosa of the oral cavity.

Treatment consists of local and conservative excision.

MUCOUS RETENTION CYSTS AND MUCOCELES OF THE PARANASAL SINUSES

Mucous retention cysts and mucoceles of the sinuses have obstruction as the principal factor in their pathogenesis. The former arise after blockage of secretion in ducts and are forms of secretory retention cysts. The blockage may be either allergic or inflammatory in nature. They commonly involve the maxillary sinuses, but are occasionally found in the frontal or sphenoid sinuses. Paparella[28] noted an incidence of nearly 10% in 500 consecutive sinus x-rays taken over a 1½-year period and considered the mucosal cyst as the most common solitary benign lesion of the maxillary sinus.

While the mucous retention cyst is in effect a mucocele, the latter term when applied to the paranasal sinuses carries a somewhat different connotation. All sinus mucoceles are cysts since they are lined by epithelium and while some paranasal sinus mucoceles may pass through a retention cyst phase, the majority result from the accumulation of mucinous secretions within a blocked or obstructed sinus cavity.

A mucocele may therefore be produced by an outlet obstruction to a sinus ostium or compartmental ostium or by progressive dilatation of an obstructed gland (retention cyst). The ostia may be occluded by an inflammatory process, new growths (osseous or epithelial) or after trauma. The theory that obstruction may be due to a congenital absence of the nasofrontal duct is, however, untenable.

From a radiographic point of view, the term mucocele is used when any encapsulated fluid mass within a sinus becomes sufficiently distended to fill the sinus or the sinus compartment. The term "retention cyst" is applied to a fluid mass (mucoid or serous) which remains distinctly separate from bone and is still surrounded by air within the sinus, except at its base.

The mucous retention cysts are not often symptomatic and their importance lies in differentiating them from other space occupying lesions in the sinus.[28, 29] Most are radiologically dome-shaped homogenous masses sharply defined and profiled by sinus air. Their favorite site is along the floor of the antrum. The sinus may be free of other abnormalities or the cyst may be associated with a thickened membrane or secondary infection. A large cyst may completely fill the sinus, giving no clue to its cystic nature.

Cannulation and drainage through the inferior meatus establishes the diagnosis and is curative in many cases. Caldwell-Luc surgery is reserved for very large cysts or recurrent symptomatic cysts.

Mucoceles are most often found in the frontal and ethmoid sinuses, possibly because of the dependent position of their ostia. The frequency statistics from the Manhattan Eye, Ear and Throat Hospital is representative of the sites of involvement.[30] Of 100 patients with mucoceles seen at that institution, 64 had frontal and 30 had ethmoidal mucoceles; five were in the maxillary antrum and only one was in the sphenoid sinus.

The clinical picture varies according to the site of the lesion and the direction and extent of expansion of the mucocele.

The first manifestation of a frontal sinus mucocele may be pain (intermittent). There is a gradual thinning of the walls of the frontal sinus. Expansion of the mucocele is in the direction of least resistance (usually the floor of the frontal sinus). A soft tissue swelling may appear above the medial canthus and occasionally at the superomedial aspect of the orbit. The mass is cystic and may impart an "egg shell" sensation on palpation.

The mucocele may erode through the interfrontal septum to involve the contralateral sinus or may extend through the anterior wall of the frontal sinus causing an external deformity, or through the posterior wall into the anterior cranial fossa. Displacement of the ocular globe is also noted in both frontal and ethmoid sinus mucoceles. The relative constancy of proptosis is highlighted by the lesion being the most common cause of unilateral proptosis.[30] A frontal mucocele may displace the globe inferiorly and laterally, as well as anteriorly. Mucoceles of the ethmoid sinuses produce proptosis with a forward and lateral displacement of the globe.

The pathogenesis of mucoceles and pyoceles of the ethmoid sinus is similar to that outlined for the frontal sinus mucoceles. The direction of expansion in these instances is usually through the lamina papyracea.

Mucoceles of the maxillary and particularly the sphenoid sinus are rare.[31] Those of the maxillary sinus frequently mimic carcinomas with signs and symptoms dependent upon the direction the mucocele expands the sinus cavity. There may be swelling of the cheek, alterations in dentition, deformity of the lateral nasal wall, or erosion of the floor of the orbit with proptosis, enophthalmus and diplopia.

Mucoceles of the sphenoid sinus[30] are much less common than mucoceles of the frontal sinus or any other sinus. The etiology is the same as for mucoceles elsewhere in the sinuses—obstruction, usually secondary to chronic sinusitis. This process precludes drainage and leads to a dilated epithelial lined cavity filled with tenacious fluid.

Clinical symptoms are most commonly headaches and ophthalmological abnormalities ("sphenoid fissure syndrome" or "ophthalmoplegic migraine") and usually arise from pressure of the expanding mass. Because the posterior ethmoidal cells offer the least barrier, pressure from the expanding mucocele is primarily transmitted to this area and, thus, to the orbital apices causing visual symptoms. Intranasal extension causes rhinorrhea and nasal obstruction. Parasellar and intraorbital expansion is accompanied by ophthalmoplegia, optic atrophy or proptosis. Extension into the cranium produces increased intracranial pressure and may lead to meningitis and/or brain abscess.

Any mucocele can become infected (pyocele) and then the additional signs and symptoms of acute sinusitis are superimposed.

Mucoceles are often recognized on the basis of their x-ray appearances. The involved sinus is opacified by the entrapped mucus which has displaced all intrasinus air. With time, pressure produces a gradual erosion of the sinus walls so that the mucoperiosteal margin decalcifies and the normally scalloped borders disappear. Further progression and continuation of the process makes the sinus appear more radiolucent since the loss of bone more than cancels out the replacement of air. At this point, the "classical" appearance is at hand with an abnormal radiolucency involving the frontal or ethmoid sinuses.[30] The affected adjacent bone (osteolysis or osteomyelitis) frequently has a zone of sclerosis about the margin of the lesion. About 5% manifest macroscopic calcification in the walls.[30]

Caldwell, Waters', optic foramen and basal views are all required for complete assessment.[30] Laminagrams are also helpful. Since the usual path of extension of frontal and ethmoidal mucoceles is into the orbit, the radiographic demonstration of a smooth oval erosion in the frontoethmoidal areas offers a clue to the diagnosis in patients with unilateral proptosis.

The pathological features, while not specific, are sufficiently distinctive to be diagnostic. The contents vary from thick but otherwise normal mucoid secretions to a tenacious gelatinous type. The color may be yellow, brown, gray or streaked with red and black. Desquamated epithelial cells and lipid containing macrophages may be found in the fluid. Purulent exudate is seen in the pyocele. The contents of the mucocele are usually sterile.

Histological examination of the wall of a mucocele usually indicates it is the distended mucoperiosteal lining of the sinus. The sac is usually thin-walled and consists of a fibrous tissue stroma with a lining of low cuboidal or stratified columnar epithelium. Long-standing chronic inflammation may induce a squamous metaplasia.

When the lining of a maxillary cyst is nearly or completely squamous in character, the lesion has been called a "cholesteatoma."[32, 33] These are very rare in the sinuses and closely mimic a mucocele radiologically. The two most acceptable theories of origin are: (1) squamous metaplasia after chronic inflammation; or (2) extension of squamous epithelium into the sinus cavity via a fistula (e.g., buccal epithelium via an oroantral fistula).

A *pseudocyst* is a fairly common lesion that occurs in the paranasal sinuses. Pseudocysts represent loculated fluid or exudate in the loose subepithelial connective tissue of the maxillary sinus. They are symptomatic only when they are large, producing local symptoms as well as fatigue, lassitude and headache.

The differential diagnosis and the management of mucoceles are well presented in the papers by

Wigh,[29] Schuknecht and Lindsay,[34] and Zizmor and Noyek.[30]

CYSTS OF THE LARYNX

There are many classifications for "cysts" of the larynx. They range in complexity from very elaborate ones based on flimsy embryological evidence to a simple grouping proposed by DeSanto et al.[35]

The majority of the benign cystic lesions of the larynx are *acquired* and are most often easily categorized by their location.

Epiglottic cysts are the most common and arise after obstruction of the mucous-gland ducts with consequent retention of secretions and dilation of the duct and its associated gland. Chronic inflammation is usually cited as the cause of the primary obstruction. A similar genesis pertains to cysts of the vallecula, aryepiglottic fold, arytenoids and the false cords.

Many epiglottic or vallecular cysts are asymptomatic. The latter are often multiple and when symptoms are produced, they are usually those of having a foreign body in the throat.

Epiglottic cysts are predominantly an adult lesion. Their size varies and may reach 3 cm in greatest diameter. Retention cysts of the vocal cords produce hoarseness early in their development and consequently are usually less than 5 mm in size when treated.

The epithelial linings of the epiglottic, vocal cord and other acquired or retention cysts are usually stratified squamous in type.

Transoral removal of these retention cysts is usually all that is required in their management.

The so-called "congenital cyst" of the larynx is surrounded by confusion, both clinically and pathologically. Nevertheless, a feature common to *all* forms of "congenital cysts" is their location. All sites are lateral-supraglottic and beneath normal laryngeal mucosa. Depending on the size of the cyst, distortion of the aryepiglottic fold, false cord, or ventricle occurs, either separately or in combination. Large cysts can also bulge laterally into the pyriform sinus or superiorly into the vallecula. They often overlie the true cords and may obscure the glottis. Extralaryngeal extension of these cysts into the upper portion of the anterior cervical triangle also occurs.

For many years, the diagnosis of "congenital cyst" was reserved for those lesions found in infants, but similar lesions—also considered as congenital—may occur in patients whose ages range from the newborn to over 70 years.

Symptoms vary with age of the patient, size of the cyst and whether or not there is clinical presentation of the cyst into the neck.

The size of the reported cysts has varied from a few millimeters to 7.5 cm.

In adults the symptoms are those of any space-occupying lesion of the larynx. Hoarseness or weakness of the voice are usual findings. Because of their smaller larynges, the primary symptoms in infants are dyspnea and difficult respiration.

A number of hypotheses have been proposed to explain the pathogenesis of the *congenital cyst* of the larynx. None, however, have withstood the test of either clinical or embryological study. The consideration that the cysts represent visceral-pouch anomalies, i.e., branchial cleft cysts within the larynx, is opposed to the usually accepted location of the visceral pouches which is *lateral* to the embryonic larynx. Identity with isolated laryngoceles or cysts arising from obstruction of ducts may be closer to the truth but not completely acceptable.

Whatever their genesis, it is certain that the histological character of the cyst cannot be used in defining which cysts are congenital. More than one-half the number are said to be lined by a respiratory epithelium. Others have a stratified squamous epithelial lining. Still others manifest combinations of the two epithelia or are devoid of an epithelial lining.

Treatment for the symptomatic forms is that outlined for the acquired cysts and is dependent largely on their size.

Classification of cysts of the larynx beyond that of acquired and congenital and in relation to site may be superfluous. This is particularly so since the congenital category is difficult to define and there are no good histological means of separating the various cysts from one another or from a laryngocele. The classification proposed by DeSanto et al.,[35] however, is attractive because of its simplicity and therapeutic practicality. Their classification is based on clinical findings, the most pertinent being: (1) site in the larynx; (2) size and content of the cyst; and (3) the cyst's relation to the laryngeal mucosa. The histological nature of the cyst lining is not sufficiently constant to aid in the classification of the cyst.

The classification (saccular, ductal and thyroid-cartilage foraminal cysts) with description follows.

Saccular Cysts. These laryngeal cysts are submucosal and are covered with mucous membrane. They are supraglottic and may develop anywhere in the plane of the saccule. In this position, they may distort the aryepiglottic fold, false cord, ventricle, or the vallecula singly or in various combinations. A *laryngocele* (vide infra) differs from a saccular cyst only in that it contains air, whereas the saccular cyst contains mucus. Figure 26.8 from Scott's[36] study of the laryngeal saccule and sinus illustrates the position of the saccule in man.

Anterior and lateral types are the two subcategories of saccular cysts. Anterior saccular cysts are found near the saccular orifice at the anterior ventricle. They may bulge deeply into the ventricle and usually overhang the anterior glottis. Because of their location, the cysts have also been called "ventricular-area cysts." According to DeSanto et al.,[35] many lesions called "eversion of the saccule" may be this form of saccular cyst.

The *lateral* saccular cyst of this classification is the "congenital cyst" of other reports. The cyst bulges the false cord, aryepiglottic fold, or ventricle, or if very large, the entire supraglottic larynx. Some large cysts may extend to or through the thyrohyoid membrane into the neck.

As a rule all cysts in the saccular category are the largest laryngeal cysts. They are rarely less than 1 cm in diameter.

Ductal Cysts. These laryngeal cysts may be found at any site within the larynx and are the result of the retention of secretions in the collecting ducts of glands. In contrast to the saccular forms, these cysts are more superficially located and smaller. Most of the cysts are less than 1 cm in diameter.

Thyroid-cartilage Foraminal Cysts. Retention of mucus in herniated laryngeal mucosa is believed to be the basis of development for this very rare type of laryngeal cyst.[35]

Obstruction forms the etiological basis for the development of both saccular and ductal type cysts of the larynx.

The normal anatomical variations between the various appendages of the saccule, considered with its embryological development, may reasonably explain how saccular obstruction may be held responsible for the saccular cysts. This obstruction may be either developmental or acquired.

Obstruction is also responsible for the development of ductal cysts. The actual causes of the obstruction and cyst formation are manifold and include infection, neoplasms, leukoplakia and trauma. Oxyphilia in the cyst epithelium is a histological variant and is not pathogenetically important.

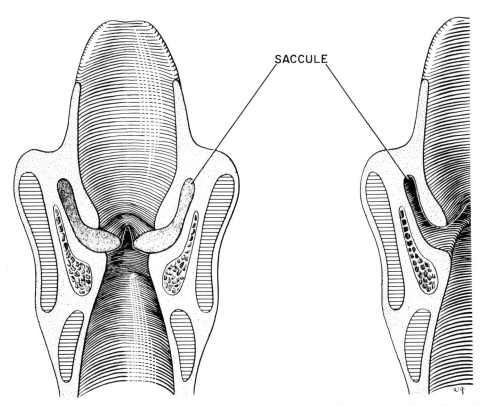

Figure 26.8. Saccule of the larynx in man schematically exaggerated to show regional relationships. (From G. B. D. Scott.[36])

LARYNGOCELE

The laryngeal ventricle is a normal finding in man and is found only in mammals. It is definable as a small recess located between the false vocal cords above and the true vocal cords below and is elliptical in shape. Anteriorly, in the roof, this recess ends blindly in a pouch, the appendix or sacculus.

Embryologically, the laryngeal ventricle is formed by the splitting of the thyroarytenoid sphincter, forming the lower internal true cords and upper false cords.[37] The sacculus has taken form by the second month of intrauterine development and by the time of birth is of relatively large size. Regression of size begins at the end of the sixth year.[38] Sacculi are said to be more common in men than women, the ratio being 7:1. Caucasian sacculi are said to be larger than those in the Negro. Almost 90% of the reported cases are in Caucasians.

Laryngeal air sacs are also normal anatomical findings in many animals and the development of laryngoceles in man has been considered an atavistic phenomenon. In the chimpanzee and orangutan, these air sacs serve as part of the breathing apparatus and extend out into the neck or, at times, over onto the anterior chest.[39]

Tucker and Smith[40] have demonstrated enlargement of the sacculus in a significant number of asymptomatic patients after sectioning of the entire larynx. The connective tissue layer in the laryngeal ventricle is thinner than that found elsewhere in the larynx and represents therefore, only a minimal barrier separating the ventricle from the supraglottic space and the pyriform fossa.

Dilation or herniation of the sacculus or the appendix beyond the range associated with various stages of development and age represents a laryngocele. The term dates back to Virchow, who described a simple enlargement of the saccule of the ventricle. An occupational predilection was mentioned by Larrey, Napoleon's Surgeon-in-Chief during the Egyptian campaign, who commented on the bilateral air-containing masses in the necks of the muezzins who shouted the Koran from the roofs of the mosques.

In contemporary use, laryngocele is an air-filled anomalous air sac communicating with the laryngeal ventricle. The term is synonomous with aerocele or pneumatocele of the larynx. Progression in enlargement is furthered by anything which increases intralaryngeal pressure, such as coughing and the playing of wind instruments. A laryngocele becomes clinically perceptible when it is filled

with air through a rise in pressure within the larynx, or when it becomes infected and filled with pus. The latter is then designated a laryngopyocele, which can present as an acute emergency and which, if untreated, may prove fatal.

Several factors contribute to the formation of a laryngocele. The two most common factors seem to be a prolonged or chronic increase in intraglottic pressure and an associated long sacculus. The former is the most important and the disorder is unusual in children, presenting clinically at middle age. Other lesions associated with laryngoceles are chronic granulomatous diseases such as tuberculosis and laryngeal neoplasms. With respect to the latter, it is good otolaryngological practice to exclude the concurrence of carcinoma in patients manifesting laryngoceles.

Many laryngoceles are asymptomatic and the occurrence of the disorder is more common than tabulation in the literature would indicate.[41]

Laryngoceles may be unilateral or bilateral and may be internal (lying within the confines of the larynx); external (presenting in the neck), or have a combined mode of presentation (Fig. 26.9). The internal variety is confined within the larynx, causing the ventricular band and the aryepiglottic fold to bulge and obscure the true fold (Fig. 26.10). The external type appears as a swelling in the neck, usually at or about the level of the hyoid bone and just anterior to the sternomastoid muscle, but they have been reported almost anywhere in the neck. According to Harrison[42] a large laryngocele works its way between the perichondrium lining the medial side of the thyroid ala, and the ventricular band, and then enlarges upward, reaching the upper border of the thyroid cartilages deep to the thyrohyoid membrane. It then passes deep to the lateral border of this membrane, and emerges in the neck through the gaps between the middle and inferior constrictus of the pharynx. In the mixed or combined form, internal and external portions are joined by an isthmus at the thyrohyoid membrane, imparting an hourglass appearance.[43]

DeRosario et al.[44] reported that in their review they found 70% internal type, 25% external type, and 5% combined or mixed type. Canalis et al.,[45] however, after a review of 115 cases, conclude the mixed type is most common (44%). In 23% of their cases the laryngocele was bilateral.

The diagnosis of laryngocele is a clinical one, based principally on history and physical signs. Small internal laryngoceles are symptomless, but with enlargement they may give rise to hoarseness, breathlessness and stridor and appear as a bulge

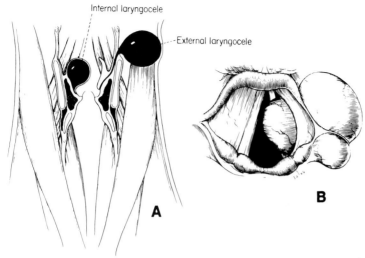

Figure 26.9. Coronal section of neck. *A*, illustrates forms of external and internal laryngoceles. *B*, a diagrammatic appearance of a combined (internal and external) laryngocele.

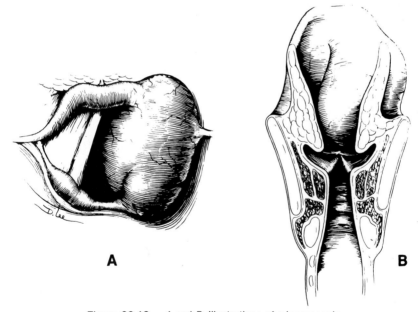

Figure 26.10. *A* and *B*. Illustrations of a laryngocele.

above the vocal cord. External laryngoceles are tympanitic on percussion, and the bulge increases in size with coughing or with a Valsalva maneuver. Occasionally, after reduction of the swelling, air may be heard escaping back into the larynx with a hissing sound. Plain x-ray of the neck will show unilateral or bilateral cystic air-containing spaces connected with the larynx. Tomograms of the larynx may be of assistance in diagnosis by revealing continuity between the internal and external portions of the laryngocele.

The clinical features of a laryngopyocele are those of a laryngocele with super-added infection (Table 26.2). This complication is unusual, but despite its rarity, is worthy of note because of the high mortality rate, death occurring from asphyxia or from discharge of the saccular contents into the bronchial tree.

All laryngoceles large enough to produce symptoms should be excised. Consensus is almost universal that the surgical approach should be through an external incision for both internal and

Table 26.2
Signs and Symptoms of a Combined Laryngocele-
Pyocele

Laryngoceles	Pyocele
Cough	Pain
Hoarseness	Tenderness
Compressible neck mass	Purulent intralaryngeal discharge
Dyspnea	Bad taste
Dysphagia	Foul breath
	Asphyxia

external types. The acute inflammatory reaction associated with a laryngopyocele usually necessitates incision and drainage and excision later, during quiescence.

Laryngoceles are generally lined by respiratory (ciliated, pseudostratified columnar) epithleium. Focal areas of squamous metaplasia may be present and in chronically infected laryngoceles, the entire epithelium may be of this type. The wall of the usual, noninfected laryngocele is devoid of inflammatory cells.

TRACHEAL DIVERTICULA OR TRACHEOCELES

Tracheoceles are recorded in the literature only rarely and are of two pathogenetic types: congenital and acquired. They may, on occasion, be of clinical significance, i.e., pressure on the recurrent laryngeal nerve or because of secondary infection. Postmortem discovery, however, is the usual event.

Unlike the pouching of the whole or the greater part of the posterior wall of the trachea seen in association with emphysema, both congenital and acquired tracheal outpouchings arise from the anterior wall of the trachea in the median line, close to the thyroid gland. The majority are right-sided. Goldman and Wilson[46] have presented a summary of reported cases.

Duct obstruction and chronic inflammatory weakening of the tracheal wall are held responsible for the cystic ductal dilation that produces the acquired tracheocele. Unlike its congenital counterpart, there are no cartilage or muscle in the wall of the outpouching.

The pathogenesis of the congenital tracheocele, is related to an aberration of tracheal budding in the embryo. In its more developed form the abnormal bud becomes a tracheal bronchus or supplies an accessory lung. If this development is abortive, a tracheal diverticulum results. Should the abnormal bud end blindly and also lose its tracheal connective, a mediastinal tracheobronchial cyst may result.

Tracheocutaneous fistula is a very unusual and late complication of tracheostomy.[47] The incidence is estimated at 0.3 to 0.5%. The fistula results after respiratory epithelium spreads from the trachea along the cannula and reaches the skin. There is no apparent relationship to the method of tracheostomy. A pretracheal cyst may develop if the cutaneous opening is obliterated.

PHARYNGEAL POUCHES

The simplest classification of pharyngeal pouches relates to their anatomical location and accepts the probability that both congenital and acquired forms occur.[48] Based on location, these lesions can be designated as posterier and lateral pouches. The rarely occurring and asymptomatic anteriorly located "pouches" are now recognized as well developed vallecular fossae.

The most common pharyngeal pouch is the posterior hypopharyngeal pouch (pharyngoesophageal diverticulum, Zenker's pulsion diverticulum and esophageal diverticulum). These pouches represent herniations of the mucosa and submucosa through the space between the oblique and circular fibers of the inferior pharyngeal constrictor muscle. They have a strikingly constant localization "in the hypopharynx, in the midline, or the posterior wall, exactly opposite the orifice of the esophagus and are entirely pharyngeal in origin"[47] (Fig. 26.11).

At the onset of development there is a single

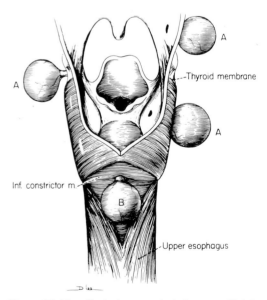

Figure 26.11. Posterior aspect of pharynx with lateral pharyngeal pouches, *A*, and posterior hypopharyngeal pouch, *B*. (Modified from Ward et al.[47])

outpouching. This is followed by sac formation, and eventually gravitational dependency. The posterior wall of the sac comes to lie in direct continuity with the posterior pharyngeal wall. Thus food or instruments tend to enter the pouch rather than into the esophagus. The principal symptoms are presented in Table 26.3, and are compared to those associated with lateral pharyngeal pouches.

Lateral pharyngeal pouches are considerably more rare and have been reviewed by Fowler.[49] While the majority of posterior pouches are presumed to be of acquired nature, lateral pharyngeal pouches have been the cause of considerable controversy as to their congenital versus acquired origin. Their location in the tonsillar fossae, valleculae and pyriform fossae has been related to persistent vestiges of the second, third and fourth embryological pharyngeal pouches.

The first clinical abnormality is usually a soft cystic mass in the lateral portion of the neck which can be increased by a Valsalva maneuver.

Radiographic techniques to diagnose and localize the pharyngeal pouches are described by Ward et al.[47] and include cinefluorography, postinjection radiography and laminagraphy.

The evolution of the surgical management for pharyngeal pouches has been reviewed by Ward et al.[47] and Warren.[50]

LARYNGEAL WEBS AND CLEFTS

Laryngeal webs constitute about 5% of the congenital anomalies of larynx (exceeded by laryngomalacia, neurogenic anomalies and subglottic stenosis).[51, 52] Seventy-five percent of the webs are at the level of the vocal cords; the remainder are supraglottic, i.e. connecting ventricular bands, or subglottic and associated with anomalies of the cricoid cartilage. The majority of the glottic webs lie anteriorly between the cords; only 1 to 2% are posterior.

Table 26.3
Signs and Symptoms of Pharyngeal Pouches*

Posterior Hypopharyngeal (In usual order of presentation)	Lateral Pharyngeal
Dysphagia	Dysphagia
Regurgitation	Intermittent neck mass
Bad taste	Hoarseness
Foul breath	Regurgitation
Gurgling noises	Bad taste
Coughing-choking	Foul breath
Weight loss	
Hoarseness	
Compressible neck mass	

* Modified from Ward et al.[45]

Symptoms and signs of extensive laryngeal webs usually date from birth with stridor, weak phonation and feeding problems being salient. Webs are also found as coincidental findings in adults.

A few of the laryngeal webs consist only of a thin membrane but the majority have a considerable mesodermal element of connective tissue, skeletal muscle, fibroadipose tissue and even cartilage. Mucous glands are also commonly found in the webs. A thick and occasionally papillary squamous epithelium covers the upper surface and respiratory epithelium, the under surface of glottic webs.

Hardingham and Walsh-Waring[52] have reviewed the management of these lesions.

Congenital posterior clefts between the laryngotrachea and esophagus follow failure of rostral advancement in the formation of the tracheoesophageal septum and a resultant failure of dorsal fusion of the cricoid cartilage. The severity of the laryngotracheoesophageal cleft is dependent upon the gestational age at which fusion is arrested. Most cases have involved only the cricoid and upper tracheal rings, but some defects extend to the carina. Interarytenoid clefts involving only the cricoid very likely represent isolated defects independent of tracheoesophageal fusion.

Diagnosis is suggested by a triad of husky voice, feeding difficulties, and aspiration pneumonia, but laryngoscopy is essential to the correct diagnosis. Radiographic studies should be deferred until after the endoscopy. The radiologist should also be alerted to the possibility of multiple tracheoesophageal fistulas in connection with the laryngotracheal cleft. Pillsbury and Fischer[53] have outlined the diagnostic measures and management of these disorders. Montgomery and Smith[54] have considered the adult presentation of laryngeal clefts.

REFERENCES

1. Himalstein, M. R.: Correlation of surgical anatomy and embryology in lateral cervical anomalies. Trans. Am. Acad. Ophthal. Otolaryngol. 75:974, 1971.
2. Amr, M.: Cervical cysts, sinuses, and fistulae of branchial, pharyngothymic duct, and thyroglossal duct origin. Br. J. Plast. Surg. 17:148, 1964.
3. Bhaskar, S. N., and Bernier, J. L.: Histogenesis of branchial cysts: A report of 468 cases. Am. J. Pathol. 35:407, 1959.
4. Little, J. W., and Rickles, N. H.: The histogenesis of the branchial cyst. Am. J. Pathol. 50:533, 1967.
5. Albers, C. D.: Branchial anomalies. J. A. M. A. 183:309, 1963.
6. Wenglowski, R.: Ueber die Halsfistein und Cysten. Arch. Klin. Chir. 100:789, 1913.
7. Bernier, J. L., and Bhaskar, S. N.: Lymphoepithelial lesions of the salivary glands; histogenesis and classification based on 186 cases. Cancer 11:1159, 1958.
8. ReMine, W. H.: Branchial-cleft cysts and sinuses: Their embryologic development and surgical management. Surg. Clin. North Am. 43:1033, 1963.

9. Brownstein, M. H., Wagner, N., and Helwig, E. B.: Accessory tragi. Arch. Derm. 104:625, 1971.

10. Work, W. P., and Proctor, C. A.: The otologist and first branchial cleft anomalies. Ann. Otol. 72:548, 1963.

11. Crymble, B., and Braithwaite, F.: Anomalies of the first branchial cleft. Brit. J. Surg. 51:420, 1964.

12. Aronsohn, R. S., Batsakis, J. G., Rice, D. H., and Work, W. P.: Anomalies of the first branchial cleft. Arch. Otolaryngol. 102:737, 1976.

13. McPhail, N., and Mustard, R. A.: Branchial cleft anomalies: A review of 87 cases treated at The Toronto General Hospital. Can. Med. Assoc. J. 94:174, 1966.

14. Bailey, H.: Branchial Cysts, and Other Essays on Surgical Subjects in the Facio-cervical Region. H. K. Lewis, London, 1929.

15. Newman, J.: Diagnosis and treatment of congenital cysts of the neck. Eye Ear Nose Throat Mon. 45:43, 1966.

16. Simpson, R. A.: Lateral cervical cysts and fistulas. Laryngoscope 79:30, 1969.

17. Rudberg, R. D.: Congenital fistulas of the neck: with particular reference to the causes of post-operative recurrences. Acta Otolaryng. Suppl. 116:271, 1954.

18. Cosman, B., and Crikelair, G. F.: Midline branchiogenic syndromes. Plast. Reconstr. Surg. 44:41, 1969.

19. Lyall, D.: Congenital cyst of third branchial cleft. Arch. Otolaryngol. 64:540, 1956.

20. Proctor, B., and Proctor, C.: Congenital lesions of the head and neck. Otolaryngol. Clin. North Am. 3:221, 1970.

21. Tucker, H. M., and Skolnick, M. L.: Fourth branchial cleft (pharyngeal pouch) remnant. Trans. Am. Acad. Ophthal. Otolaryngol. 77:368, 1973.

22. Chaudhry, A. P., Reynolds, D. H., LaChapelle, C. F., and Vickers, R. A.: A clinical and experimental study of mucocele (retention cyst). J. Dent. Res. 39:1253, 1960.

23. Bhaskar, S. N., Bolden, T. E., and Weinmann, J. P.: Experimental obstructive adenitis in the mouse. J. Dis. Res. 35:852, 1956.

24. Cohen, L.: Mucoceles of the oral cavity. Oral Surg. 19:365, 1965.

25. Harrison, J. D.: Salivary mucoceles. Oral Surg. 39:268, 1965.

26. Cataldo, E., and Mosadomi, A.: Mucoceles of the oral mucous membrane. Arch. Otolaryngol. 91:360, 1970.

27. Bhaskar, S. N.: Lymphoepithelial cysts of the oral cavity. Oral Surg. 21:120, 1966.

28. Paparella, M.: Mucosal cyst of the maxillary sinus. Arch. Otolaryngol. 77:650, 1963.

29. Wigh, R.: Mucoceles of the fronto-ethmoidal sinuses. Analysis of roentgen criteria. Relation of frontal bone mucoceles to ethmoidal sinuses. Radiology 54:579, 1950.

30. Zizmor, J., and Noyek, A. M.: Cysts and benign tumors of the paranasal sinuses. Semin. Roentgenol. 3:172, 1968.

31. Ghosh, P., and Desmond, A. F.: Sphenoidal mucocele. J. Laryngol. 84:1073, 1970.

32. Baxter, J. S. R.: Cholesteatoma of the maxillary sinus. J. Laryngol. 80:1059, 1966.

33. Pegerel, B. S., and Budd, E. G.: Cholesteatoma of the maxillary sinus. Arch. Otolaryngol. 82:532, 1965.

34. Schuknecht, H. F., and Lindsay, J. R.: Benign cysts of the paranasal sinuses. Arch. Otolaryngol. 49:609, 1949.

35. DeSanto, L. W., Devine, K. D., and Weiland, L. H.: Cysts of the larynx—classification. Laryngoscope 80:145, 1970.

36. Scott, G. B. D.: A morphometric study of the laryngeal saccule and sinus. Clin. Otolaryngol. 1:115, 1976.

37. Lane, S. L., Cohen, B., and Ippolito, C.: Coexisting internal and external laryngoceles. Am. J. Surg. 96:810, 1958.

38. Broyles, E. N.: Anatomical observations concerning the laryngeal appendix. Ann. Otol. 68:461, 1959.

39. Negus, V. E.: The Mechanism of the Larynx, Chapter V. C.V. Mosby Co., St. Louis, 1929.

40. Tucker, G. F., Jr., and Smith, H. R., Jr.: A histological demonstration of the development of laryngeal connective tissue compartments. Trans. Am. Acad. Ophthal. and Otolaryngol. 66:308, 1962.

41. Fredrickson, J. M., and Ward, P. H.: Laryngocele ventricularis. Arch. Otolaryng. 76:568, 1962.

42. Harrison, K.: Laryngoceles in the human. J. Laryngol. 64:777, 1950.

43. Wright, L. D., and Magunda, T. A.: Laryngocele: Case report and review of the literature. Laryngoscope 74:396, 1964.

44. DeRosario, J., and Nelson, P. A., Nash, H. T., and Schmitz, R. L.: External Laryngocele. Arch. Surg. 78:422, 1959.

45. Canalis, R. F., Maxwell, D. S., and Hemenway, W. C.: Laryngocele—an updated review. J. Otolaryngol. 6:191, 1977.

46. Goldman, L., and Wilson, J. G.: Tracheal diverticulosis. Arch. Otolaryng. 65:554, 1957.

47. Lotan, A. N., Eliacher, I., and Joachims, H. Z.: Pretracheal air cyst: late complication of tracheostomy. Arch. Otolaryngol. 103:596, 1977.

48. Ward, P. H., Fredrickson, J. M., Strandjord, N. M., and Valvassori, G. E.: Laryngeal and pharyngeal pouches: surgical approach and the use of cinefluorographic and other radiologic techniques as diagnostic aid. Laryngoscope 73:564, 1963.

49. Fowler, W. G.: Lateral pharyngeal diverticula. Ann. Surg. 155:161, 1962.

50. Warren, K. W.: Some technical consideration in the management of pharyngoesophageal diverticulus. Surg. Clin. North Am. 40:633, 1960.

51. Holinger, L. D., Wong, H. W., and Hemenway, W. G.: Simultaneous glottic and supraglottic laryngeal webs. Report of a case. Arch. Otolaryngol. 101:496, 1975.

52. Hardingham, M., and Walsh-Waring, G. P.: The treatment of congenital laryngeal web. J. Laryngol. 89:273, 1975.

53. Pillsbury, H. C., and Fischer, N. D.: Laryngotracheoesophageal cleft: diagnosis, management and presentation of a new diagnostic device. Arch. Otolaryngol. 103:735, 1977.

54. Montgomery, W. W., and Smith, S. A.: Congenital laryngeal defects in the adult. Ann. Otol. 85:491, 1976.

CHAPTER 27

Odontogenic Lesions—Tumors and Cysts

Contributed by KENNETH D. McCLATCHEY, D.D.S., M.S., M.D.

Odontogenesis, as noted by Eversole et al.,[1] is the most intricate display of somatic differentiation in the vertebrate organism. The processes of histodifferentiation and morphodifferentiation in odontogenesis require an elaborate interplay between epithelial and mesenchymal tissues.:

Ameloblastic epithelium → differentiation of fibroblasts of the dental papilla into → odontoblasts → dentin matrix differentiation into functional ameloblasts → enamel matrix → calcified dentin and enamel → formed tooth (Fig. 27.1)

The entire process of histodifferentiation through maturation lasts several years and considering the complexity of the process it is amazing that so few odontogenic cysts and tumors are identified.

Classifications of odontogenic tumors have varied as much as the theories of odontogenesis. They have been based upon circumstantial evidence depending upon morphological, histochemical and physiological resemblances. Broca[2] first classified odontogenic tumors in 1868. Since that first notation they have evolved to a classification by Gorlin et al.[3, 4] which is founded primarily on the embryonal inductive influence that cells of one dental tissue exert upon the cells of another dental tissue. The classification used in the following discussion is that of Gorlin, with modifications (Table 27.1).

A variety of other classifications have been proposed; some are based on the degree of differentiation of the odontogenic tumor, others emphasize biological behavior even attempting to separate odontogenic neoplasms from neoplastic-like or hamartomatous lesions[5–9] (Table 27.2).

Whatever classification one uses, the important point to remember is the separation of hamartoma from true neoplasm. For example, rather extensive clinical and histological evidence indicates that odontomas cannot be considered true neoplasms but rather tumor-like developmental malformations involving tissues with an odontogenic potential. A new entity, squamous odontogenic tumor,[10] is debatable as to whether it is hamartoma or a true neoplasm. Ameloblastoma, on the other hand, is a true neoplasm of bone and sometimes of soft tissue.

According to Bhaskar,[11] odontogenic tumors comprise about 9.0% of all tumors of the oral cavity and about 2.4% of all lesions biopsied by dentists. These statistics apply to the United States and are *not* applicable in other countries since there is considerable geographic variation. In Africa, for example, the ameloblastoma alone constitutes more than 25% of all tumors of the jaw.[11]

An indication of the few occasions a general pathologist will have to examine an odontogenic tumor is the conservative estimate offered by Baden[7]: 0.002 to 0.003% of all surgical specimens received in large medical centers.

EPITHELIAL ODONTOGENIC TUMORS WITH MINIMAL INDUCTION OF THE MESENCHYME

Ameloblastoma

Ameloblastomas constitute only a small percentage of all jaw tumors; about 1% of all tumors and cysts in the jaws. The tumor has also gone under the name of adamantinoma. Despite the inaccuracy of this synonym (enamel is not pro-

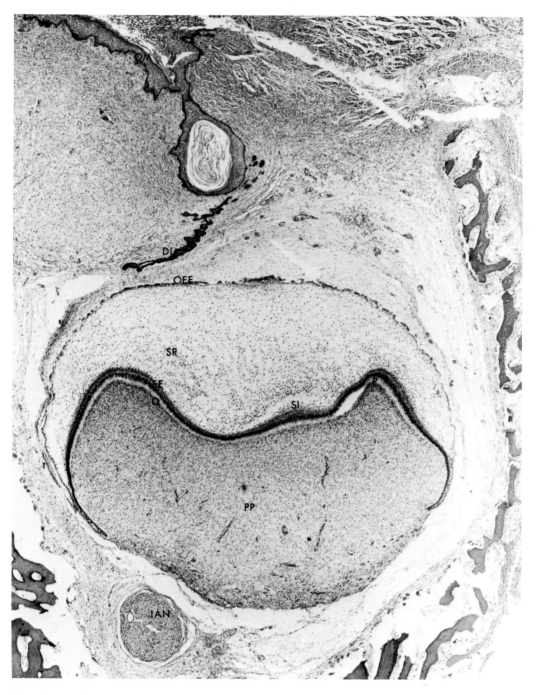

Figure 27.1.   Developing molar tooth. *OM,* oral mucosa; *DL,* dental lamina; *OEE,* outer enamel epithelium; *SI,* stratum intermedium; *SR,* stellate reticulum; *IEE,* inner enamel epithelium (preameloblasts); *O,* odontoblast; *P,* predentin; *PP,* primitive pulp; *IAN,* inferior alveolar nerve.

duced), it still is used but should die a natural death.

Peripheral ameloblastoma is a soft tissue variant of ameloblastoma occurring in soft tissue overlying

a tooth-bearing region of the jaws. Lee et al.[15], Wesley et al.[17] and Gardner[18] have reviewed the subject and concluded that unlike the aggressive growth pattern of central ameloblastoma, the peripheral ameloblastoma is a less aggressive neoplasm that can be treated by a more conservative surgical approach. Gardner also noted a tendency of the tumor to histologically resemble the acanthomatous variant of ameloblastoma.[17]

Despite reports to the contrary, we consider that ameloblastomas only rarely arise from a non-neoplastic cyst (dentigerous cyst). Recently Robinson and Martinez[19] stated that the hypothesis that ameloblastoma arises in a dentigenous cyst is defensible only when it can be demonstrated that a non-neoplastic cyst existed prior to the appearance of ameloblastoma or when both the lining epithelium seen normally in odontogenic non-neoplastic cysts and ameloblastic epithelium are present side by side. They proposed the term "unicystic ameloblastoma" for those unicystic lesions associated or unassociated with an unerupted tooth which demonstrates ameloblastic epithelium throughout. They reported less aggressive growth and suggest enucleation rather than partial or complete jaw resection.

The theories of pathogenesis of simple ameloblastoma have included origin from the basal layer of oral mucous membrane, remants of dental lamina and the enamel organ. The various theories of pathogenesis have been reviewed by Hertz.[12, 13] Classically, the average age at diagnosis of simple ameloblastoma is 39 years, yet it does occur in octogenarians as well as children. Young and Robinson[14] reporting on ameloblastoma in children noted that the lesion in children is not aggressive and surgical conservatism should be practiced.

Eighty percent of ameloblastomas arise in the mandible with the molar-ramus region the most frequent site of involvement. This area of anatomical predilection enhances the "dental lamina theory" of origin since this is the site where the posterior prolongation of the lamina proliferates continuously for a period of at least 4 years after birth in order to maintain its position and to compensate for the forward growth of the jaws

TABLE 27.1
The Odontogenic Tumors*

I. Epithelial odontogenic tumors
   A. Minimal or no inductive change in connective tissue
      1. Ameloblastoma
      2. Adenomatoid odontogenic tumor
      3. Calcifying epithelial odontogenic tumor
      4. Squamous odontogenic tumor
   B. Marked inductive change in connective tissue
      1. Ameloblastic fibroma
      2. Ameloblastic fibrosarcoma
      3. Odontoma
         a. Compound and complex odontoma
         b. Ameloblastic odontoma
         c. Ameloblastic fibro-odontoma
II. Mesodermal odontogenic tumors
   A. Myxoma and/or myxofibroma (of questionable odontogenic origin)
   B. Odontogenic fibroma
   C. Cementoma
      1. Periapical cemental (fibrous) dysplasia
      2. Benign (true) cementoblastoma
      3. Cementifying fibroma
      4. Familial multiple (gigantiform) cementoma

* Modified after Gorlin et al.[3, 4]

TABLE 27.2
Baden's[6] Classification of Odontogenic Tumors

Neoplasms	Hamartomas		Dysplasia
	Epithelial	Mixed	
1. Benign epithelial Ameloblastoma	Odontogenic gingival epithelial hamartoma	Ameloblastic myxoma	Periapical cemental dysplasia
2. Calcifying epithelial Odontogenic tumor	Ameloblastic adenomatoid tumor (adenoameloblastoma)	Ameloblastic fibroma Dentinoma	Familial gigantiform cementoma
3. Benign mesodermal Odontogenic myxoma Odontogenic fibroma Benign (true) cementoma Cementifying fibroma	Epulis of newborn (?)	Ameloblastic odontoma	
		Complex odontoma	
4. Malignant Squamous cell carcinoma arising in an ameloblastoma Ameloblastic fibrosarcoma Ameloblastic dentino- or odontosarcoma		Compound odontoma	

prior to the formation of the third molar teeth. In the maxilla, also, the third molar region is the favorite site. When present in the maxilla (20%), the tumors may extend into the maxillary sinus, nose, orbit, or even the base of the skull. Complete excision in this area is extremely difficult once the tumor breaks through the maxillary antrum to invade ethmoid air cells, pterygomaxillary fossa, temporal fossa and base of brain.[15]

The roentgenographic appearance of any ameloblastoma is nonspecific, yet very suggestive. The classic appearance of an ameloblastoma is that of a multilocular radiolucency (Fig. 27.2).

The gross appearance of an early ameloblastoma is one of a relatively circumscribed cystic or solid lesion, gray-white to gray-yellow. Large tumors demonstrate necrotic foci and cystic degeneration.

Microscopically the tumor is composed of two basic histological patterns: follicular, in which islands of epithelium are found in a fibrous stroma; and plexiform, in which islands of mature fibrous stroma are found intermingled with strands and cords of epithelium. Both patterns may be present in the same tumor but usually one predominates. Histological variations within the epithelial islands, some of which have occasioned histological subclassifications, include cystic, basal cell, acanthomatous, granular cell, hemangiomatous and neuromatous.

The ultimate histomorphological "clue" necessary for the diagnosis of ameloblastoma is the tendency of the tumor to mimic the enamel organ. In both patterns, follicular and plexiform, the outermost cells resemble those of the ameloblastic layer or inner enamel epithelium.

The "ameloblastic" cells at the periphery are columnar with their nuclei polarized away from the basal membrane. The central parts of the epithelial islands are composed of a loose stellate reticulum-like network of cells[20] (Fig. 27. 3 A. and B.). Squamous metaplasia is common in these areas (so-called acanthomatous ameloblastoma). Baden[7] claims that squamous metaplasia occurs in

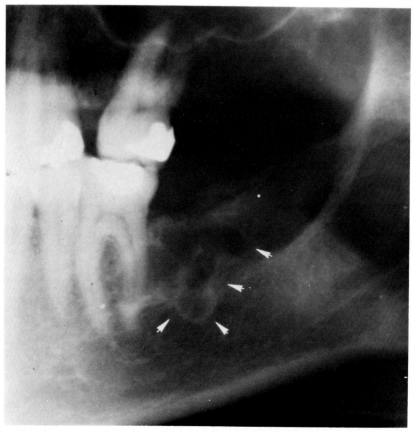

Figure 27.2.   Roentgenogram of small ameloblastoma of mandible demonstrating typical multiloculated radiolucency.

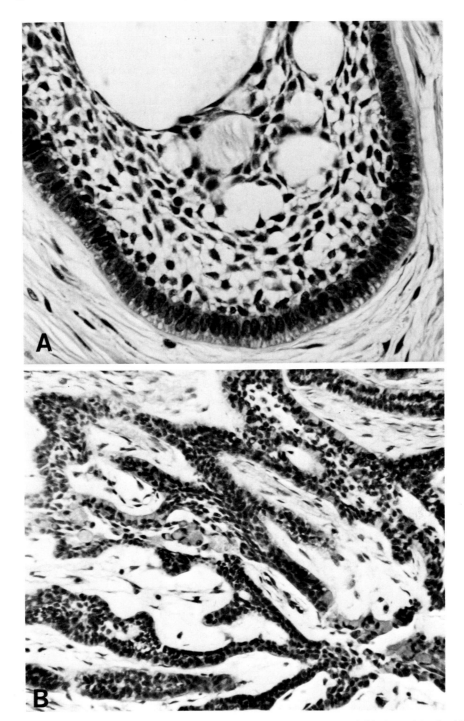

Figure 27.3. *A,* ameloblastoma. Note the peripheral palisading. *B,* plexiform ameloblastoma. Islands of fibrous stroma intermingle with strands and cords of ameloblastic epithelium.

8 to 45% of all cases of ameloblastoma. Keratinization is not marked in most cases. Rarely the entire tumor is replaced by squamous cells and even "keratin pearls." Calcification may occur but never as prominently as in craniopharyngioma or other odontogenic tumors noted below.[21–23] Cystic degeneration may be evident in both the stellate areas of the epithelium and in the stroma.

The stroma of ameloblastomas is usually a passive participant in the tumor. Two alterations of the stroma, however, are worthy of mention. Stromal vascularity, may at times, be very marked and has occasioned the subclassification, hemangioameloblastoma. Since the vessels are not neoplastic, this form should not be separated from the parent group. Kerr[24] has seen a prominent vascular component *only* in previously operated ameloblastomas and regards the vessels as reactive to operative injury. A second stromal feature may be the result of periepithelial induction; i.e., a narrow, hyalinized zone in proximity to the ameloblastic layer.

Because ameloblastoma occurs at any age and manifests a relative radioinsensitivity, surgical intervention is the treatment of choice. Attempts have been made to correlate gross and microscopic features with response to treatment. Solid ameloblastomas have been thought to have a higher recurrence rate. A similar association has been thought to exist with squamous metaplasia and increased cellularity of the tumor. To date such postulates have not proven to be true. It is safe to say at this time that there is no way to predict clinical outcomes using just histological findings.

Despite the lack of cellular malignant characteristics, simple ameloblastoma has a tendency to continually grow and invade surrounding tissues.[4] The neoplasm has the capacity for continued growth and surgical removal is made difficult by the likelihood of extension beyond the supposed margins of the tumor. Because of this tendency, recurrence is likely if too conservative a removal is attempted. In the study of Becker and Pertl,[25] patients treated by radiotherapy exhibited a 41.6% recurrence rate. Patients treated conservatively manifested a 60% recurrence rate and patients who underwent more radical surgery for their ameloblastoma had the lowest (4.5%) recurrence rate. Mehlisch et al.[20] record a recurrence of 50% or more in almost all situations where "conservative" treatment was used.

While the foregoing discussion points out the disadvantages and failings of conservative forms of management—excision, cautery and curettage—the use of these forms of treatment, in combination with each other, or other therapeutic modes, decidely increases effectiveness.[20]

No one form of therapy is always indicated just as no one form is never indicated. The plan of treatment must be individualized for each patient, always keeping in mind the likelihood of recurrence, based on age, location, radiographic appearance and histomorphology.

The ability of an ameloblastoma to metastasize is often a topic of discussion in the literature and among medical and dental professionals. The actual number of acceptable cases is small and the occurrence of metastases is rare. Metastasis is more likely to occur in patients who have had a tumor of long duration, with multiple surgical procedures or radiation therapy. In the cases reported, the interval between histological diagnosis and verified lung metastases has been very long.[4, 26, 27]

Metastases may arise via lymphatic, blood vascular or aerogenous spread (Table 27.3).

ADENOMATOID ODONTOGENIC TUMOR (ADENOMELOBLASTOMA)

Original suggestions that the adenomatoid odontogenic tumor is a variant of the simple ameloblastoma have been proven invalid.[4, 28, 29] The tumor is most likely not neoplastic, but represents a developmental overgrowth of odontogenic tissue or a hamartoma. It is important to make a distinction between this tumor and ameloblastoma in order to avoid serious errors in treatment (Table 27.4).

Over 100 cases of this benign, slow-growing lesion with an excellent prognosis have been reported. About 70% of patients present in the second decade with an age range from 5 to nearly 50 years. There is a modest female predominance. Localized painless swelling is the most common form of presentation.

The adenomatoid odontogenic tumor occurs exclusively in the anterior tooth-bearing area with 40% being found in intimate association with an impacted tooth. Sixty percent occur in the maxilla, where the incisior-cuspid area is most frequently involved.

TABLE 27.3
Summary of Malignant (with Metastases) Ameloblastoma*

Total number of cases (1972)	19
Age range of patients	9–44 years
Time lapse, primary to metastasis	3–40 years
Site of primary lesion	Mandible (19 cases)
Sites of metastases	Lymph nodes, 6 cases
	Lungs, 13 cases
	Bones, 4 cases
	Misc. sites: kidney, brain, heart, spleen, lip and parotid, 4 cases

* Abstracted from data presented by Herceg and Harding.[27]

TABLE 27.4
Differential Features—Ameloblastoma and Adenomatoid Odontogenic Tumor*

	Ameloblastoma	Adenomatoid Odontogenic Tumor
Age	Usually in 4th decade	Usually in 2nd decade
Sex	Predominantly males	2:1 in favor of females
Location	Mandible—ramus, angle molar region	Anterior jaws
Clinical course	Local aggressiveness; recurrences are common and removal is often difficult	Commonly associated with an impacted tooth, recurrences are unusual to rare. Removal is easy.
Histological appearances	1. Follicular or plexiform variants	1. Numerous "tubular or ductal" areas
	2. Frequent areas of stellate reticulum	2. Stellate areas are scant to absent
	3. Frequent epithelial metaplasia	3. Metaplasia is unusual
	4. Calcification is rare	4. Calcification is common
	5. Nuclei of cells lining follicles are polarized toward lumen	5. Nuclei of cells lining "ducts" are polarized away from lumen
	6. No elaboration of "hyaline" eosinophilic material	6. Elaboration of "hyaline" eosinophilic material is common

* Modified from Gorlin et al.[3]

Radiographs generally display a well demarcated unilocular radiolucency, frequently associated with an unerupted or impacted tooth. The radiograph may also reveal, as noted by Courtney and Kerr,[30] peripheral condensing osteitis and the presence of small radiopacities in the central radiolucency.

Encapsulation, obvious calcification, and gross cystic alteration characterize the prototypic gross appearance.

Microscopically the tumor is well encapsulated with a central proliferation of epithelium. The central area of the tumor is characterized by rosettes, duct-like tubular structures and even trabecular or cribiform proliferation of cuboidal or columnar epithelium (Fig. 27.4).

Certain of the tumor cells, in the various configurations, appear to be actively secreting. A pink sometimes fibrillar, sometimes amorphous material is found within and between tumor cells as well as within the lumen of duct-like structures. The tumor cells are rich in glycogen and the material elaborated by the cells appears to be an acid mucopolysaccharide. An excellent discussion of the histogenesis of the eosinophilic material by Courtney and Kerr,[30] convinces this author that the material is the result of continued basement membrane production by preameloblasts due to the lack of mesenchymal induction of the epithelium to produce enamel.

Varying amounts of calcification of the dys-

trophic type, are noted in the epithelium and occasionally in the scant connective tissue stroma or capsule peripherally. Small calcified spheres or larger calcifying amorphous eosinophilic masses may be seen.

Correct therapy is conservative, but the surgical treatment must be based on a correct histological interpretation and differentiation from ameloblastoma. Recurrences have *not* been reported after simple enucleation and even after incomplete removal.[31] The majority of reported cases have been followed for less than 7 years.[30]

CALCIFYING EPITHELIAL ODONTOGENIC TUMOR (PINDBORG TUMOR)

Less than 50 cases of this tumor have been reported.[7] It is to be distinguished from the calcifying odontogenic cyst and appears to arise often from reduced enamel or dental epithelium. The Pindborg tumor, as it is also called, behaves clinically much like an ameloblastoma, i.e., invasive and locally recurrent, and presenting in essentially the same age groups.[32–35] Also, like the ameloblastoma, there are rare extraosseous examples.[33]

There is a distinct mandibular predilection (75%) and most of the tumors are encountered in the premolar region. The tumor is found often in association with an unerupted tooth.

Radiographic examination reveals a unilocular or multilocular cystic lesion with numerous scat-

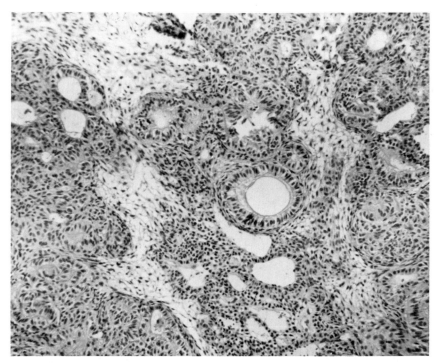

Figure 27.4.   Adenomatoid odontogenic tumor. Rosettes and duct-like tubular structures in a proliferation of cuboidal odontogenic epithelium.

tered islands of irregular calcification. Early in development, however, the tumor is characterized by a well defined radiolucent area around the coronal aspect of a fully formed unerupted tooth. The appearance is not unlike that of a dentigerous cyst.[34]

The striking features of this neoplasm are the cellular pleomorphism, a curious extracellular matrix and calcification.[7] Although a variable picture may be presented, the tumor most often appears as sheets of relatively large, polyhedral epithelial cells separated by a scant connective tissue stroma (Fig. 27.5). There is a "tight packing" of the epithelial cells, each of which has a distinct cytoplasmic border. The cytoplasm is finely granular and acidophilic. Intercellular bridges are found. A fairly constant finding is a gradual disintegration of cell membranes. Binucleate, trinucleate and markedly pleomorphic cells may be seen. The nuclei are usually vesicular and nucleoli are distinct. Mitoses are rare.

A particularly distinctive feature is the presence of homogeneous, eosinophilic, often spherical, "amyloid-like" bodies in and among the epithelial masses or in the stroma.[34, 35] Dystrophic calcification is also a distinctive feature and may be within the epithelium or the stroma. If the calcification occurs in the amyloid bodies, calcospherites or "psammoma bodies" are produced and are not

unlike those found in carcinomas of the thyroid and meningiomas. If the calcification is extensive, the true nature of the neoplasm may be obscured. The calcification appears to increase with age of the tumor.

An electron microscopic study has been presented by Mainwaring et al.[36] who indicate the ultrastructural features of the cells are comparable to the cells of the stratum intermedium of the enamel organ.

The tumor manifests a variable local aggressiveness; some examples are markedly aggressive, others only after a long dormant period. Krolls and Pindborg[37] postulated that the two products within the Pindborg tumor, namely calcifications and an amorphous amyloid-like material, indicate greater tumor differentiation and account for its low recurrence rate. Metastases have not been reported to date.[7] The tumor should be treated like an ameloblastoma.

EPITHELIAL ODONTOGENIC TUMORS WITH MARKED INDUCTION OF THE MESENCHYMA

Ameloblastic Fibroma

The characteristics of the epithelium seen in this rarely occurring tumor would appear to equate it most closely to the root sheath of Hertwig.[5] Gorlin

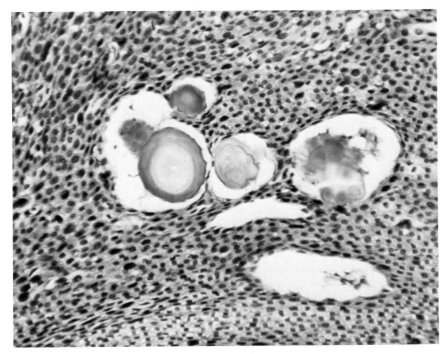

Figure 27.5. Pindborg tumor. A proliferation of relatively large polyhedral odontogenic epithelial cells containing "psammoma bodies."

et al.[3] point out that this lesion has been reported in the literature most often as a "soft-mixed odontoma" because of the apparent epithelial and mesenchymal components. The tumors have also been misdiagnosed as simple ameloblastomas in children.

Clinically, the lesion is completely benign. It often occurs in the younger age group during the period of tooth formation, raising the possibility of a hamartomatous overgrowth. The vast majority of patients are between 5 and 20 years of age. There is no sex preference.

The clinical presentation is usually that of a painless and asymptomatic swelling of the premolar-molar area of the mandible or less often of the premolar-molar area of the maxilla. Its x-ray appearance cannot be distinguished from an ameloblastoma. The tumor expands the cortical plates but does not invade.[3]

Microscopically, an ameloblastic fibroma appears encapsulated and is composed of cords, buds and islands of epithelial cells in a mesenchymal connective tissue stroma. The latter resembles the fibromyxoid tissue of the dental papilla and differs from the mature stroma observed in ameloblastomas (Fig. 27.6).

The epithelial elements of the tumor form two patterns of growth. The first consists of small follicles, which, unlike those of the ameloblastoma, show little tendency for stellate reticulum arrangement or for macrocystic degeneration. The second characteristic pattern is that of strands of epithelium produced by double layers of cuboidal cells occasionally widened and exhibiting a small amount of stellate reticulum. Both patterns may be present throughout the same tumor. Nuclear orientation is not marked, but when present, tends to be away from the basement membrane. It is, however, the mesodermal stromal component which permits separation of the ameloblastoma from the ameloblastic fibroma. The stroma strongly resembles the embryonal connective tissue of the primitive dental pulp (Fig. 27.6). At times there is a pronounced cellularity of the stroma and this has occasioned the histological diagnosis of ameloblastic sarcoma or fibrosarcoma. In general, however, the cellularity of the stroma bears no relationship to clinical behavior. There is a "maturational theory" that proposes that ameloblastic fibroma is the soft tissue anlage of the odontoma, and that the ameloblastic odontoma or ameloblastic fibro-odontoma are intermediate maturational phases of such fibromatous growths.

Ameloblastic sarcoma is the malignant counterpart of the ameloblastic fibroma. The lesion is very rare and considered by some a doubtful entity.[4] The epithelium is indistinguishable from that seen

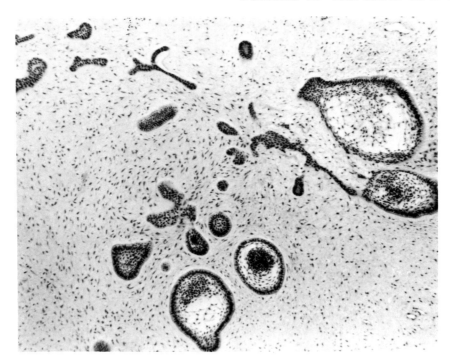

Figure 27.6. Ameloblastic fibroma. Cords, buds and islands of ameloblastic epithelium in a fibromyxoid tissue stroma. Stellate reticulum formation is noted in the larger islands.

in an ameloblastic fibroma or ameloblastoma but it is set in a cellular mesodermal stroma, whose cells manifest the histological features of a fibrosarcoma. There is a high mitotic index, often with mitotic atypia in the stromal cells.

The majority of the tumors occur in the mandible and in patients who are significantly older than patients with ameloblastic fibromas. Rapid growth and pain highlight the clinical presentation and this clinical aggressiveness is carried over to the x-ray appearance where extensive and poorly defined destruction of bone is portrayed.

Recurrences are frequent and local destruction may lead to death of the host. To date, there have been no cases with metastases.[4]

Squamous Odontogenic Tumor

Recently Pullon et al.[10] described a previously unnamed benign oral lesion. The lesion presents as a painless mass, loose teeth, or asymptomatic radiolucency involving alveolar bone adjacent to a tooth. There is no apparent predilection for mandible or maxilla. There is no sex predilection. The mean age of occurrence is 26 years with a range from 11 to 42 years.

On the basis of the few reported cases (six) the tumor appears to originate from nests of Malassez in the periodontal ligament or from gingival mucosa. The tumor appears as benign squamous is-

lands in a dense collagen connective tissue stroma. The squamous islands are purely squamous in appearance and lack the peripheral columnar polarized layer of cells which is typically present in "acanthomatous" ameloblastoma. Prekeratin and keratin surrounding calcified islands can be found within the squamous epithelium (Fig. 27.7).

The lesion should be treated by complete surgical excision.

ODONTOMAS

In Gorlin's[3, 4] classification and in this discussion, the term odontoma is used to denote a tumor in which induction has resulted in the development of both enamel and dentin. Dentin and enamel are found in all odontomas, cementum only in the mature complex and compound ondontomas.

In order of decreasing frequency, the three subcategories of odontoma may be ranked as follows: (1) compound odontoma, and complex odontoma; (2) ameloblastic odontoma; (3) ameloblastic fibroodontoma.

The epithelial cells of these tumors are fully differentiated with respect to their secretory and inductive properties and, as such, are fully capable of producing adult tooth tissue.

Morphologically the odontomas contain the tissue elements seen in adult tooth structures. In

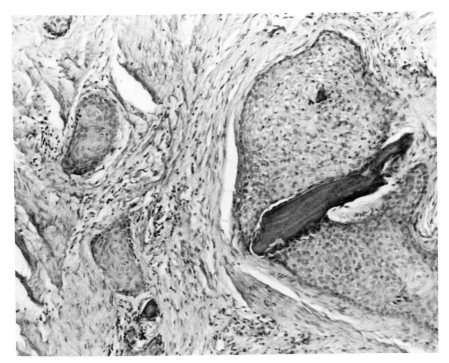

Figure 27.7. Squamous odontogenic tumor. Pure squamous odontogenic epithelial islands in a mature fibrous connective tissue stroma. A calcified island is noted in a large squamous epithelial island.

complex odontomas these elements are randomly distributed, whereas in compound odontomas, the relative position of the dental tissues are normal, but the "teeth" which result are dwarfed and multiple. The majority of the odontomas are hamartomas.

Compound Odontoma

The high degree of morpho- and histodifferentiation of tissues in this tumor separates it from the complex odontoma. However, this separation may be difficult in any given lesion because of the histological overlap. When calcified structures manifest sufficient anatomical similarity to normal teeth, even though they be small and deformed, the term, compound, is justified (Fig. 27.8).

The only significant difference in clinical behavior and clinical presentation from the complex odontoma is the predilection of the compound odontoma for the incisor-cuspid region.

The dental roentgenogram may be quite characteristic—a mass of diminutive tooth-like structures, surrounded by a narrow, radiolucent band.[4, 7, 38] Not infrequently, these tumors occur between the roots of the deciduous anterior teeth and prevent the eruption of permanent teeth.

The teeth are usually distorted and dwarfed. Microscopically, there is normal tooth tissue arrangement. The number of teeth has ranged from 3 to 4 to about 2,000 tiny teeth.[4]

No recurrence follows conservative surgical removal.

Complex Odontoma

Essentially, this hamartomatous lesion with limited growth potential, differs from the ameloblastic odontoma by the absence of ameloblastic tissue. While less common than the compound odontoma, it is far more prevalent than the ameloblastic odontoma.

The biological course of a complex odontoma is one of a slow and nonaggressive growth. There is a 2:1 sex preference for females with the majority of the tumors diagnosed in the second and third decades of life.[4, 7] Over two-thirds of the reported examples have occurred in the second and third molar areas and they are slightly more common in the mandible.

The complex odontoma is not uncommonly associated with an unerupted tooth and may be related to a dentigenous cyst.

Roentgenograms reveal irregular radiopacities separated by a narrow radiolucent band from the surrounding bone, or within a cystic lesion.

Gross examination discloses a stony hard mass, measuring one to several centimeters in size, and

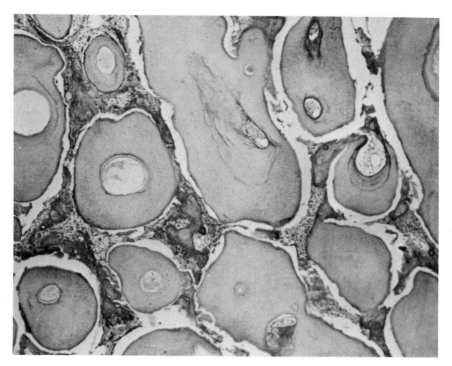

Figure 27.8.   Complex odontoma. Dentin is the prominent component.

surrounded by a fibrous capsule or a cyst wall.[7] The surface is smooth and lobulated with enamel areas adjacent to coarser ivory-like tissue.

Microscopically, histodifferentiation is well developed with enamel, enamel matrix, dentin, dentinoid, pulp tissue and cementum all present in a variable relationship to one another. Decalcified preparations indicate dentin is the most plentiful component with enamel and cementum being present only in moderate amounts. Morphodifferentiation, in contrast to the developed histodifferentiation is highly variable. Most of the tumors manifest an appearance intermediate between a haphazard arrangement of tissue and lesions differing only slightly from the normal tooth.

Multiple sections of a seemingly nonepithelial tumor will occasionally reveal ameloblastic epithelium thus making the lesion an ameloblastic odontoma.

Conservative surgery usually results in a complete cure.

Ameloblastic Odontoma

According to Spouge,[5] this odontogenic hamartoma seems to mean different things to different observers and consequently its characteristics have been poorly defined. Gorlin,[4] on the other hand, has defined the tumor as "the simultaneous occurrence of ameloblastic tissue and a complex or compound odontoma within the same tumor."

Spouge[5] considers it very likely that the lesions are merely complex or compound odontomas in which the formative enamel organ elements have failed to degenerate and are still histologically prominent or even actively proliferating.

The tumors are found, with few exceptions, in children and are somewhat more common in the maxilla. Growth is slow as would be expected in a highly differentiated benign lesion. Roentgenograms manifest areas of cyst-like destruction.

A variety of tissues are present in ameloblastic odontomas: ameloblastic epithelium, stellate reticulum, enamel matrix, enamel, dentin, osteodentin, bone and pulpal tissue. Most often these tissues are randomly arranged, but evidence of small tooth formation may be seen. The "odontomatous" zones are centrally placed in the tumors while the ameloblastoma-like areas are usually found in the peripheral and more immature areas.

Simple curettage may be curative, but the presence of ameloblastic epithelium in these tumors is held accountable for the recurrences that occasionally take place after curettage. There is some indication that maturation of these lesions to ameloblastic fibro-odontoma and even complex odontomas may occur.

Ameloblastic Fibro-odontoma

Hooker,[39] in 1967 separated a distinct group of lesions which he called ameloblastic fibro-odontoma from those that had been previously described as ameloblastic odontomas. Subsequently, Tsagaris[40] in 1972 reviewed 77 cases including Hooker's cases and noted a median age of 13 years with approximately 73% occurring in patients younger than 20 years. Of the 29 patients Tsagaris was able to follow, only one tumor recurred and that case demonstrated inadequate primary surgical removal. Miller et al.,[41] after reviewing seven additional cases, noted that there is no recurrence after adequate surgical curettage.

Histologically the tumor is composed of both hard and soft tissues. The hard tissue elements, as in the odontoma and ameloblastic odontoma, are composed of dentin with foci of enamel matrix, cementum and immature pulp tissue. The adherent contiguous soft tissue component, the component that actually differentiates the ameloblastic fibro-odontoma from the ameloblastic fibroma, is composed of ovoid and spindle shaped fibroblasts in which are scattered islands of ameloblastic epithelium arranged in a follicular or plexiform pattern as in the ameloblastic fibroma (Fig. 27.9).

Malignant transformation of the stroma has been reported and the lesion is then called an ameloblastic dentinosarcoma.[7] Rapid growth, often to a great size, and bizarre stromal cells characterize this variant. The histopathology is that of a fibrosarcoma or osteogenic sarcoma. (It must be emphasized that this adverse change in an ameloblastic odontoma is very rare and questionable.)[7] The age of these patients is significantly older than patients with ameloblastic fibromas or ameloblastic fibro-odontomas.

CEMENTOMA

The diagnostic term, *cementoma,* has encompassed several unrelated lesions: periapical cemental dysplasia, benign (true) cementoblastoma (true cementoma), cementifying fibroma and familial multiple (gigantiform) cementoma.[4, 7, 42]

The lesions are derived from the periodontal membrane. The periodontal membrane is composed of collagen fibers, mucopolysaccharides and oxytalan fibers possessing the ability to produce cementum, alveolar bone and fibrous tissue. Under pathological conditions blastic cells from the periodontal membrane can produce tumors composed of either cementum, lamellar bone, fibrous tissue or any combination of these three tissues.

Periapical cemental dysplasia is the most frequently encountered lesion of the group.[38] A neoplastic or traumatic genesis for the lesion has been largely disproved and it is likely that periapical cemental dysplasia is comparable to fibrous dysplasia of bone.[7] There is, however, no association between this lesion and systemic disease.

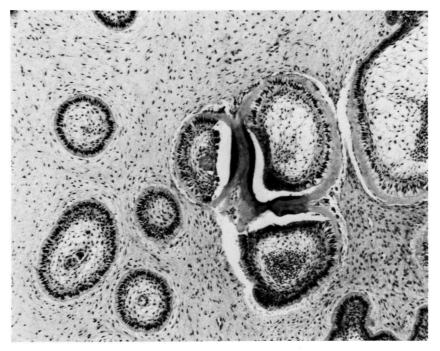

Figure 27.9. Ameloblastic fibro-odontoma. Ameloblastic epithelium in a fibromyxoid stroma focally producing dentin and cementum.

Blacks appear to be particularly subject to the disorder. There is a very heavy predominence of females and the lesions are only rarely seen in subjects who are under 25 years of age.

The teeth involved are nearly always mandibular (incisors) and the lesions are often multiple (60 to 70% of cases).[38, 42] Periapical cemental dysplasia rarely involves the maxillary teeth. (Table 27.5) The teeth are always vital.

Primarily asymptomatic, the lesions are most often found on routine dental x-rays. The radiographic appearance of the lesions depends on the stage of development of the lesions. A periapical radiolucency continuous with the periodontal membrane and attached to the apex of the tooth is seen in early stages. A periapical cyst or granuloma may be simulated.

The lesion may radiographically stay in the so-called first stage of development for an indefinite period of time or progress to a second stage—a partly radiolucent and partly radiopaque lesion. Increased amounts of cementum may be deposited on the root and calcification may be initiated in the lesion, principally in the center.[7]

The "third" stage is roentgenographically represented by an irregular or regular radiopaque mass of uniform density surrounded by a thin radiolucency representing the periodontal ligament and separating the mass from the apex of the tooth.[7]

The microscopic appearance also depends upon the stage of development of the lesions thereby producing considerable variations in different examples.

Fibroblasts, collagen and moderate vascularity make up the predominant findings in the early stages. The appearance of periapical cemental dys-plasia at this stage of development is "osteolytic" and has been likened to that of a young periodontal ligament at the apex of a tooth.[6, 38] With progression of the disease, there is a transition from the loose, edematous vascular connective tissue to a cellular stroma with scattered small foci of immature cementum. Fibroblasts differentiate into cementoblasts or osteoblasts in this stage (Fig. 27.10). The cementoblastic stage of development is characterized by a progressive enlargement of cementicles and a coalescence of the cementum to form large solid masses of cementum. If osteoblastic activity is prominent, the histological appearance of fibrous dysplasia is conveyed to the microscopist. A pagetoid appearance may also be presented. Chronic sclerosing osteitis may be indistinguishable from the correct diagnoses if only calcified osteocementum and avascular necrosis dominate the light microscopic appearance.[7] The third stage of development is known as the "mature inactive stage."[7]

There is a tendency for periapical cemental dysplasia to clinically "burn" itself out.[7] This tendency is mirrored in the fully calcified osteocementum of the "mature inactive stage." According to Baden,[7] surgery is indicated only if ulceration of the gingiva and a chronic secondary infection do not respond to conservative therapy.

The *cementifying fibroma* is considered a variant of periapical cemental dysplasia presenting usually in older persons and in the mandibular molar or premolar region. Microscopically it is composed of small round to ovoid islands of acellular cementum (sometimes surrounded by a prominent precementum layer) within an immature fibrous connective tissue stroma.

Benign (true) cementoblastomas are rare tumors and are most likely neoplastic in contrast to periapical cemental dysplasia and cementifying fibroma. The tumor is apparently self-limiting and does not recur after enucleation.[6]

The tumor is attached to the tooth root and may actually involve the root canal. A mandibular premolar or molar tooth is most frequently involved (Fig. 27.11).

There is no apparent race or sex predilection. Most patients have been under 25 years of age.

Fused globules of cementum or separate areas of cementogenesis are seen on microscopic examination.

Inherited probably as an autosomal dominant, *familial multiple (gigantiform) cementoma* is a large deforming tumor seen most often in middle-aged black women.[7]

Large sheets of avascular and acellular osteo-

TABLE 27.5
Localization of Periapical "Cementomas"—N = 636*

Radiographic Location	Mandibular (N = 595)		Maxillary (N = 41)	
	Single	Multiple	Single	Multiple
Incisors				
Central	100	126	10	2
Lateral	85	89	13	2
Cuspids	27	33	2	0
Premolars				
First	25	9	0	0
Second	13	10	1	0
Molars				
First	27	15	6	0
Second	18	12	4	0
Third	5	1	1	0
Totals	300	295	37	4

* Data presented is that of Zegarelli et al.[42]

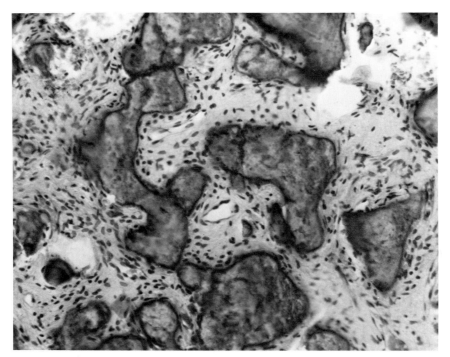

Figure 27.10. Cementoma. Foci of immature cementum in a vascular immature fibrous connective tissue stroma.

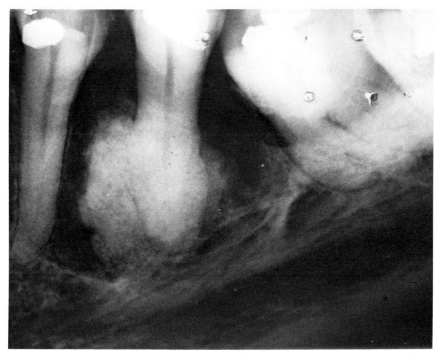

Figure 27.11. Cementoblastoma. Roentogram demonstrates radiopaque cementum attached to premolar tooth root.

cementum with little fibrovascular stroma make up the histological features. Ischemic necrosis is common.

Table 27.6 graphically compares the clinicopathological features of "cementomas"[43] noted above.

ODONTOGENIC MYXOMA AND FIBROMA

The histogenesis of odontogenic myxoma is poorly understood and it may well take origin from either dental tissues, nondental mesenchyma, or even represent a dysplastic bone lesion. Baden[7] reviews the evidence for and against odontogenic origin. It is pertinent to emphasize that there are distinctive criteria for the diagnosis of a myxoma and the pathologist should not over-diagnose as a myxoma, myxomatous degeneration in fibro-osseous lesions of the jaws or retained pulp of a tooth following extraction (Fig. 27.12).

Radiographically the odontogenic myxoma cannot be differentiated from numerous other odontogenic cysts and tumors when it is small, although when the tumor enlarges it presents as a multiloculated radiolucency that may perforate the cortex. The posterior mandible is more often affected than the maxilla.[44]

Microscopic examination reveals loosely arranged stellate shaped cells within an intercellular substance rich in hyaluronic acid. Occasionally islands of inactive odontogenic epithelium and even fragments of calcification are noted within the neoplasm. Recurrences are common, up to 25%. The primary reason for the high recurrence rate is inadequate primary surgical therapy. The tumor is not radiosensitive.

Classically the odontogenic fibroma consists of a fibrous connective tissue stroma containing various numbers of odontogenic rest-like epithelial islands. It is important to note that the epithelial islands are smaller than those found in ameloblastic fibroma or simple ameloblastoma. The epithelial islands must not demonstrate the peripheral pallisade or stellate reticulum characteristic of ameloblastoma. Various types of calcification, including dentin, cementum or bone, are found in varying amounts within the neoplasm.

The tumor is treated by enucleation.

The odontogenic fibroma "soft odontoma" is a debatable diagnosis and a rare lesion. This is also the opinion of Kerr and Courtney[45] and contrasts sharply with Bhaskar's[11] statistics (23% of all odontogenic tumors). The tumor most often occurs centrally although it may be peripheral.

CYSTS (INCLUDING FISSURAL CYSTS)

Epithelial cysts or cystic lesions in the midfacial and oral regions are predominately of odontogenic

TABLE 27.6
"Cementoma"*

Subclassification	Location	Sex/Age	Radiographic Features	Histological Features	Clinical Course
Periapical cemental dysplasia	Root apices of anterior mandibular teeth	F/25	Radiolucent to mottled radiopaque mass at apex of tooth roots	Cementicles, osteocementum, and woven bone in vascular fibrous connective tissue	Do not recur after simple excision—*if* excision is necessary
Cementifying fibroma	Mandibular molar	No predilection/middle age	Radiolucent defect with central mottled radiopaque mass	Cementicles within fibrous connective tissue	No recurrence after simple excision
Benign cementoblastoma	Attached to mandibular molar or premolar tooth root	M/25	Radiopaque mass attached to tooth root	Mass of osteocementum attached to tooth root	No recurrence after simple excision
"Gigantiform" cementoma	Multiple lesions of mandible and/or maxilla	F (black)/middle age	Ill-defined radiolucent to radiopaque lesions	Cementum admixed with lamellar bone within fibrous connective tissue adjacent to active bone resorption	If symptomatic or complicated by osteomyelitis may require aggressive treatment

* Modified after Krausen et al.[43]

There has existed a multiplicity of suggested classifications for benign cystic lesions of the jaws. Even those in contemporary use require revisions as newer concepts challenge the embryological basis for classification.[47] Killey and Kay[46] have reviewed the evolution of these schema from 1945 to the present day.

A conventional classification of epithelial jaw cysts is presented in Table 27.7.

It has been considered that most midfacial and maxillary cysts arise from defects in embryogenesis, either in the fusion of the facial processes, or from an abnormal development of the dental follicle.[48]

Fissural cysts are said to form at points of junction of developing structures within the head and neck. Either incomplete resorption of epithelial tissue (enclaving) or a delay in the development of growth centers are held responsible for the development of the lesions. Such cysts, therefore, may be midline (medial fissural cyst) or lateral, i.e., at the junction of the premaxillary and maxillary processes (Fig. 27.13).

Both medial and lateral fissural cysts may be present in soft tissue or within bone or both. While it is theoretically possible for a medial fissural cyst to occur in the upper lip, no examples have been reported.[47]

With regard to the so-called category of cysts, the entire mechanism of epithelial entrapment between fusing embryonic processes is being seriously questioned; the revised proposition holds

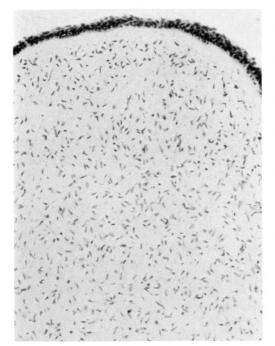

Figure 27.12. Retained pulp. Circumscribed fibromyxoid connective tissue partially surfaced by degenerated odontoblasts.

origin or arise from "accidents" in the embryological development of the region.

Well known to oral surgeons and oral pathologists, these benign cysts are also important to the head and neck surgeon and general pathologist. This is true not only from a differential diagnostic standpoint, but also from the aspect of the selection of appropriate therapy.

High quality radiographic examinations, precise localization and accurate history are necessary prerequisites for clinical diagnosis and histopathological interpretation. The common similarities of the epithelial linings of the various cysts makes pathological diagnosis "fool-hardy" without this preliminary information.

Cysts of the maxilla and mandible are by no means rare and although small cysts can only be detected radiographically (usually on routine dental examinations), larger cysts can be diagnosed by careful clinical examination.

Many benign cystic lesions of the jaw tend to increase in size if left unattended, and this may eventually lead to serious complications. Surgical intervention is indicated in most instances. There are two main types of operations—enucleation and marsupialization. Results are usually quite satisfactory and recurrences are exceptional *if* the operation has been adequately performed.[46]

TABLE 27.7
Epithelial Cysts of the Jaws: A Classification

I. Odontogenic
  A. Periodontal
    1. Apical
    2. Lateral
    3. Residual
  B. Dentigerous
    1. Eruption
  C. Gingival
  D. Odontogenic keratocyst (primordial)
    1. Nevoid basal cell carcinoma syndrome
  E. Keratinizing and calcifying odontogenic cyst
II. Fissural
  A. Lateral
    1. Nasolabial (nasoalveolar)
    2. Globulomaxillary
  B. Medial
    1. Nasopalatine duct
      a. Incisive canal cyst
      b. Cyst of palatine papilla
    2. Median palatal
  C. Median mandibular

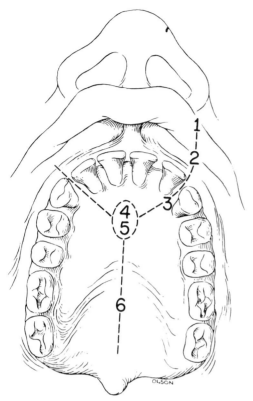

Figure 27.13. Distribution of fissural cysts: *1*, nasolabial; *2*, nasoalveolar; *3*, globulomaxillary; *4*, nasopalatine; *5*, cyst of palatine papilla; *6*, median palatal.

that centers of proliferating mesoderm enlarge, thus smoothing out intervening ectodermal furrows. "Accordingly, since mesenchymal protrusions at no stage coalesce, epithelium is never liable to sequestration."[48]

If our classical histogenetic explanations are found to be untenable, classification and diagnostic nomenclature will have to be seriously revised. Anticipating this change, Main[48] considers that of all the nonodontogenic cysts, only the nasopalatine is of undoubted histogenesis, i.e., from vestigial bilateral oronasal ducts.

Lateral Fissural Cysts of Maxilla

Cysts in the region of fusion between the maxillary and globular process have been reported under a variety of names. The three most common designations have been nasoalveolar, nasolabial and globulomaxillary, often used synonymously. Kerr,[49] citing defective fusion of the nasoglobular process as the primary involvement, considers all cystic lesions occurring in the line of fusion as nasoglobular. He further categorizes the cysts ac-

cording to locations. Bernier[50] questions the practicality of separating the nasolabial cyst apart from the globulomaxillary cyst.

Nasolabial Cysts (Nasoalveolar Cysts). If reports in the world literature are an indication, nasolabial cysts are uncommon lesions.[51] Nonetheless their importance lies in the fact that they are more often misdiagnosed or unrecognized than by their consideration as a clinical entity.

Since the cysts are located in the soft tissues of the upper lip and the lateral aspect of the nose, and not in the alveolar process, nasolabial is preferred to nasoalveolar. Kerr[49] reserves "nasoalveolar" for those cysts with erosion of the maxillary labial cortical bone.

The usual clinical presentation is that of a patient who seeks advice because of an increasing facial deformity. Speculum examination demonstrates a painless swelling behind the ala nasi, in front of the inferior turbinate and in the lateral half of the nasal floor. Oral examination discloses a swelling that fills the labial vestibule sulcus and pushes the lip forward. Fluctuance may be elicited between the oral and nasal swellings. Lateral extension into the cheek behind the ala nasi splays the anterior nares and reduces the nasofacial sulcus.

Intranasal extension is into the inferior meatus. Subsequent enlargement displaces the tip of the inferior turbinate medially to abut against the nasal septum, producing unilateral nasal obstruction.[52]

Despite their developmental origin, clinical manifestations are usually deferred until adulthood. Occasionally bilateral, they usually occur with equal frequency on either side of the nasal vestibule. There is a definite racial predilection for blacks and a less well established dominance among women (4:1).

The cysts are prone to infection. A "furuncle" of the floor of the nasal vestibule should always raise the suspicion of an infected nasoalveolar cyst. Infection produces a rapid enlargement of the cyst and may be the occasion for the first appreciation of the cyst by the patient. Pericystic inflammation may extend into the cheek and the upper lip.

So-called "malignant degeneration" is an oddity; only one example has been reported.[52]

Diagnosis is made through a combination of the rather characteristic clinical presentation, routine intraoral radiography and dental vitality tests. Aspiration of the cyst is not diagnostically helpful and may be contraindicated.

Figure 27.13 illustrates the location of some developmental cysts that may figure in a differential diagnosis. These premaxillary cysts can be divided into medial and lateral groups.[52] Cysts of dental origin, it must be remembered, can occur in either site. Only the lateral group of cysts should really present any diagnostic problems, as the nasoalveolar cyst rarely extends to the midline.

Globulomaxillary Cysts. These cysts present in the same region as the nasoalveolar cysts. The globulomaxillary cysts are typical embryological inclusion cysts at the point of union of the maxillary and globular process and like the median cysts can produce a complete dehiscence of the palate and separation of the cuspid and lateral incisor teeth. They comprise fewer than 3% of all cysts of the jaws.

Globulomaxillary cysts are usually asymptomatic unless they are secondarily infected. When they are infected they are capable of distorting the maxillary sinus.

Radiographs of a globulomaxillary cyst demonstrate a well defined, often pear shaped radiolucency between the roots of the maxillary lateral incisor and the cuspid, causing a divergence of the tooth roots.[53] Uninfected cysts are lined by a ciliated columnar or stratified squamous epithelium.

Confusion may ensue in distinguishing the nasolabial cyst and globulomaxillary cyst from an acute abscess arising from a maxillary anterior tooth, or a radicular cyst associated with a maxillary anterior tooth. These can be identified by appropriate history and radiographs.

Unless the nasolabial cyst is exceptionally large (usually 1 to 4 cm) and of long duration, there will be *no* radiographic evidence of the lesion. Longstanding cysts may thin the bony nasal floor and produce deepening of the nasal notch of the maxilla.[52]

The constant anatomical position of the lateral fissural cysts and their relation to the point of fusion of the maxillary, globular and lateral nasal processes support origin from either enclaved respiratory or oral mucous membrane. Therefore, there is nothing pathognomonic about the histopathological appearance of lateral fissural cysts. They may be lined by a variety of epithelia, probably related to metaplasia from pressure and/or infection. On occasion, the cyst may be denuded. Ten of 12 nasoalveolar cysts reported by Bull et al.[54] manifested a respiratory epithelial lining. A fairly constant feature of nasoalveolar cysts, except in instances of extensive squamous metaplasia, is the great numbers of goblet cells. These present in all stages of secretion but without tubular gland formation. The wall is made up of fibrous connective tissue and is nonspecific. As a general rule,

inflammatory cells are absent or widely dispersed unless there has been recurrent infection.

Because of the potential of facial deformation, risk of infection and their sequelae, the lateral fissural cyst should be surgically excised (sublabial incision).[52]

Median Fissural Cysts of Maxilla

Median cysts include nasopalatine cyst, cyst of the palatine papilla and median palatal cyst.

Nasopalatine Cysts. The nasopalatine ducts in man are inconsistently developed structures possessing no utility, but providing the basis for development of cystic lesions.[55]

The ducts may, in essence, be considered as "unconnected masses of epithelium" representing the early fetal epithelium used to cover developing structures of the region. The incisive canal is a passageway through the bone of the hard palate connecting the oral and nasal cavities. These structures are formed when the maxillary palatine processes join with and partly overgrow the premaxilla on either side of the nasal septum, resulting in an inconstant pair of ducts in canals traversing downward and forward from the floor of the anterior nasal cavity to just posterior to the incisive papilla.

In most mammals, the ducts remain patent, functioning together with Jacobson's organ as an accessory olfactory organ. The ducts can be found as late as the fifth month in the human fetus and may even be present in the newborn.[55] Normally, the lower parts become obliterated in utero and only the upper (nasal) ends remain, terminating blindly behind the central incisors.[55]

The cysts are generally considered to arise from the nasopalatine duct or its remnants and may occur at any age. Their clinical discovery, however, occurs most often in the fourth to sixth decades of life. They are the *most common fissural cysts.*

Symptoms may relate to swelling and drainage, but almost 40% are asymptomatic.[55] Pain is uncommon.

There are really two types of nasopalatine cysts—incisive canal cysts and cysts of the papilla palatina. Arising in the incisive canal, variants remain in the bony canal and by definition are situated within the bony canal. The cysts of the papilla palatina are not intraosseous and this is the sole difference. Radiographs will manifest bony erosion of the incisive canal only with incisive canal cysts, *not* from cysts of the papilla palatina.

Abrams et al.[55] consider that a radiolucency of the incisive canal greater than 0.6 cm in diameter must be present before the adjective "cystic" can be appropriately applied. Round lesions with sharp, defined and condensed outlines are more likely to be cystic than the oval or irregularly outlined radiolucencies which usually represent enlarged incisive fossae. Heart-shaped lesions and particularly lesions which separate the central incisors are most likely incisive canal cysts. Occlusal x-ray projections are helpful to locate the cyst lingual to the central incision.

Squamous epithelium is the most common lining of the cyst. Cuboidal and pseudostratified columnar cells with or without cilia are also frequently found. The type of epithelium is largely dependent on the site of origin in relation to the nasal or oral end of the canal. Within the connective tissue wall of the cyst can be found a prominent neurovascular bundle as well as occasional islands of cartilage.

Median Palatine Cysts. This nonodontogenic cyst is formed from the epithelial remnants in the median palatine fissure of the maxilla. Presumably enclaved at the time of fusion of the two palatine processes, the epithelium apparently proliferates late in life. They bear no relation to the incisive canal.

The cysts present in the midline suture of the hard palate behind the incisive canal and in the palatine papilla. As a rule the lesions are asymptomatic, discovered most often during routine oral examinations.[56]

Palatal radiographs demonstrate a well circumscribed, radiolucent area opposite the bicuspid and molar region, frequently bordered by a sclerotic layer of bone.

If the origin is from the oral mucosa, the lining is squamous cell in type; if from respiratory or nasal mucosa, the epithelium is columnar or cuboidal.

The prefered treatment is enucleation.

Fissural Cyst of Mandible

Median Mandibular Cyst. Very rare (6 cases reported by 1970) and of disputed origin, the median mandibular cyst occurs in the symphysis.[57] The lesion is asymptomatic unless there is secondary infection. The teeth in the area must be vital if the possibility of a radicular cyst is to be completely ruled out.

Intraoral, periapical radiographs manifest divergence of tooth roots and a well circumscribed, unilocular radiolucent lesion that may or may not extend to the alveolar crest. The teeth in the involved area react normally to thermal and electrical stimuli.

A squamous epithelial lining is usually present. Treatment is by surgical enucleation.

Odontogenic Cysts

It is not the intent of the author to consider odontogenic cysts in great detail. Nevertheless, the head and neck surgeon and pathologist must be cognizant of their general characteristics in order to include or exclude them in a differential diagnosis (Fig. 27.14).

The epithelium associated with an odontogenic cyst is derived from tooth germ, reduced enamel epithelium of a crown, epithelial rests of Malassez, remnants of Hertwig's sheath, or remnants of dental lamina.

Periodontal Cysts

Periapical Cysts (Radicular Cysts). These are the most common of all cystic lesions in the jaw. Their incidence is highest in the anterior maxilla and posterior mandible.

Periapical inflammation associated with severe pulpal inflammation or pulpal death secondary to dental caries or trauma is believed to be the initiating factor in the development of the periapical cyst. Subsequently, stimulated by the pulpal inflammation or death, remnants of the odontogenic epithelium ("the Rests of Malassez") proliferate in a periapical granuloma to form a epithelial lined space (Fig. 27.15).

The teeth most often involved with this type of cyst formation are the maxillary central incisors. Periapical cysts rarely involve deciduous teeth. They most commonly involve the permanent dentition in the fourth decade.

While periapical cysts are most often solitary and related to a single tooth, it is not unusual to find two or three concurrent cysts on the root apices of a multirooted molar tooth. These several cysts may merge, often with the destruction of their walls, to form a monolocular cavity.

The discovery of a periapical cyst is often by chance, the result of routine radiographic examination. Symptoms may be minimal until suppuration is superimposed, or an obvious deformity is produced by expansion of the cyst. An associated intraoral sinus "parulus" may form and occasionally a chronic sinus track may be established which leads externally to the face or neck.

A temporary pressure neuropathy may follow suppuration associated with a cyst.[46]

A small or moderate-sized apical periodontal cyst appears as a spheroidal, pear or flask shaped zone of radiolucency surrounded by a rather prominent radio-opaque margin (condensing osteitis) which merges with the lamina dura of the involved tooth. The trabeculae of the surrounding bone is normal.

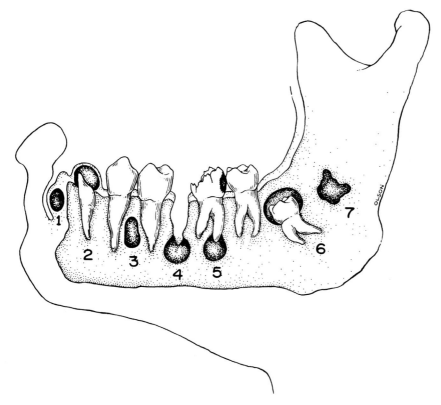

Figure 27.14. Odontogenic cysts: *1,* gingival; *2,* eruption; *3,* lateral periodontal; *4,* residual; *5,* periapical (radicular); *6,* dentigerous; *7,* primordial.

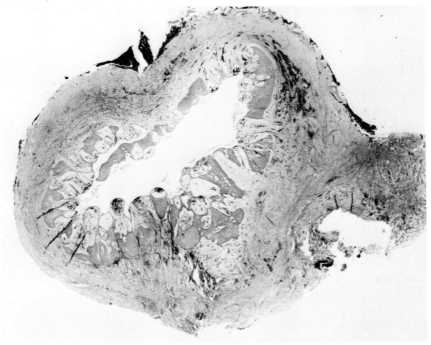

Figure 27.15. Periapical cyst. Fibrous connective tissue containing a space lined by hyperplastic stratified squamous epithelium.

The histological appearance varies with the age of the cyst and the cyst's contents vary with the presence or absence of infection.

Young cysts are lined by a thick, hyperplastic stratified squamous epithelium. There may be microcyst formation. The connective tissue is diffusely infiltrated by chronic inflammatory cells. In the mature cyst, focal keratinization may be present, goblet cells, and even hyaline bodies (Rushton bodies) may be found within the cyst lining. The vascularity and inflammatory reaction are also decreased in the mature cyst. Cholesterol crystal clefts and foreign body giant cell reaction can be seen in the wall.

The most commonly applied treatment is enucleation. Marsupialization carries disadvantages but may be necessary for larger cysts.

Lateral Periodontal Cyst. Relatively uncommon, the small lateral periodontal cyst is usually found in adults along the roots of the mandibular cuspid or premolars.[58] In order to be so designated, the lateral periodontal cyst must be located in bone and have no communication with the oral cavity.[46] Lateral "inflammatory" cysts are to be distinguished from lateral "developmental" cysts which are also located alongside the tooth and which correspond in formative pattern to the primordial cyst to be discussed later.[46] The lateral "inflammatory" periodontal cyst is probably caused by an extension of an inflammatory process through an accessory root canal, not unlike the genesis of a periapical cyst discussed above.

Treatment of choice for the developmental type of lateral periodontal cyst is enucleation with preservation of adjoining teeth. An "inflammatory" lateral cyst is removed together with the involved tooth if root canal therapy cannot be accomplished.

Residual Cyst

This is the name given to a periapical cyst which has been overlooked after the extraction of the causative tooth or root.

Alternative processes which can result in the occurrence of a residual cyst are: (1) incomplete removal of a periapical cyst or granuloma; (2) persistence and enlargement of a dentigerous cyst; and (3) exfoliation of a small cyst after extraction of a deciduous tooth or retained root.[46]

Dentigerous Cysts

A dentigerous cyst probably arises from the enamel organ after amelogenesis has been completed. The cyst surrounds the crown of an unerupted tooth. It forms as the result of fluid collection within the cell layers of the reduced enamel epithelium or between the crown and the reduced enamel epithelium. Since the expanding cyst space is enveloped by a dental follicle, the term follicular cyst is sometimes substituted for its more common "dentigerous"[46] designation.

A dentigerous cyst is formed in association with a normal permanent tooth; rarely it may be associated with a supernumerary tooth.

Three positional variants exist, of academic interest only: central, lateral and circumferential. The most common type is central with the cyst encompassing the coronal aspect of the tooth.

Dentigerous cysts occur in the mandible more frequently than in the maxilla. Late erupting teeth are those most frequently associated with dentigerous cyst formation, and in order of importance these are: the mandibular third molar, upper canine, maxillary third molar and lower second molar.

Most dentigerous cysts are solitary with the commonest age periods for diagnosis being childhood and adolescence. The rate of growth in the bone of a child is rapid—measurements of 4 to 5 cm in diameter in a time span of 3 to 4 years. In adults, dentigerous cyst enlargement is much slower.

Many of the clinical features are similar to those seen in patients with periodontal cysts. Often, however, a tooth will be missing from the permanent dentition, submerged by the overlying cyst. An unsuspected supernumerary tooth or odontoma can also be responsible for such clinical signs.

If the cyst remains clinically asymptomatic or dormant, its presence may only be recognized on routine radiography. The radiographic presentation is essentially that of a unilocular radiolucency associated with an unerupted tooth (Fig. 27.16). Killey and Kay[46] state that occasionally an ostensible multilocularity is seen, but the appearance is not attributable to true septal loculation and merely represents ridging of the bony wall of the cavity. Uninfected cysts manifest a sharp, well defined cortical margin. With suppuration, loss of the marginal cortex will take place and the infection may be accompanied by the deposition of a surface layer of identifiable subperiostral new bone.

The dentigerous cyst may become the most destructive of all benign odontogenic cysts and may cause expansion of bone with subsequent facial asymmetry, extreme displacement of teeth, and pain (Figs. 27.16 and 27.17).

Microscopically there is considerable variability. In general, the cyst is composed of a thin

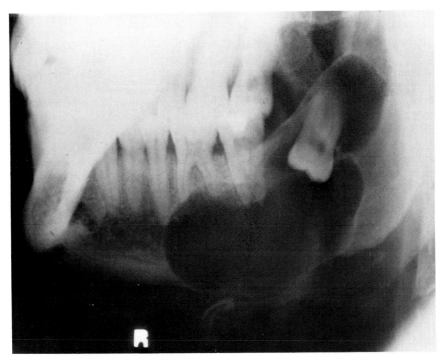

Figure 27.16. Dentigerous cyst. Large radiolucency associated with an unerupted mandibular third molar.

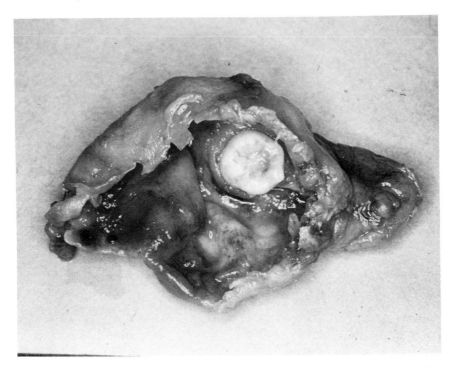

Figure 27.17. Dentigerous cyst. Cyst membrane associated with the crown of a tooth.

connective tissue wall lined by a stratified squamous epithelium that is continuous with the reduced enamel epithelium covering the crown of the tooth.

Acanthosis and infiltration of inflammatory cells into the adjacent tissue are a result of secondary infection. The capsule is usually composed of dense connective tissue in which there may be found scattered inflammatory cells, cholesterol clefts and a few foreign body giant cells.

The epithelial lining of dentigerous cysts has a wide potential. Occasionally, the cysts may be lined by respiratory epithelium, or at least, mucus-producing cells. About 3% are said to be associated with a thin layer of keratin. The dentigerous cyst, as previously stated, has the potential to develop ameloblastoma.

Marsupialization or, alternatively, careful enucleation *with* the tooth of origin is the treatment of choice.

Eruption Cyst

The eruption cyst commonly occurs in childhood as a bluish, translucent dome shaped lesion of the alveolar ridge overlying an erupting tooth. A study by Seward[59] showed that eruption cysts occurred in 11% of infants during eruption of the deciduous incisors and in 30% of infants during eruption of deciduous canines and molars. The cyst occurs more frequently in females than males in a ratio of 2:1.

The eruption cyst is generally considered a form of deciduous cyst found only in children. The origin of the cyst is attributed to degenerative cystic changes in the reduced enamel epithelium after completion of amelogenesis. Another theory proposes that the cyst originates from remnants of the dental lamina overlying the erupting tooth. Because hemorrhage often occurs into the cyst, such a cyst is referred to clinically as an eruption hematoma. The cyst is lined by nonkeratinizing stratified squamous epithelium.

Reasons for treatment of the cyst are superimposed infection and/or failure or delay in eruption of a deciduous or permanent tooth. The most common method of treatment is removal of a portion of the cyst overlying the crown of the tooth to permit unhindered eruption.

Gingival Cysts

Gingival cysts occur in both newborn infants and adults. The gingival cyst of the newborn occurs more often than the adult cyst. Gingival cysts of the newborn are also referred to as Epstein's pearls or Bohn's nodules. Gingival cysts of the newborn present as small white nodules on the alveolar ridge. The cysts are actually the result of cystic degeneration of the rests of the dental lamina. There really is no need for treatment, as the small cysts are gradually exfoliated into the oral cavity.

The cysts are lined by stratified squamous epithelium which occasionally may demonstrate ker-

atinization. The cysts, although exhibiting a keratinized epithelium, do not meet the other characteristics, to be discussed later, necessary to define an odontogenic keratocyst.

The adult form of gingival cyst, like the gingival cyst of the newborn, results from cystic degeneration of remnants of the dental lamina. The cyst presents as a swelling of the gingiva, occasionally a bluish translucent swelling similar to the clinical appearance of a small mucous retention cyst. The cyst occurs most often in the mandibular premolar and cuspid region[60] and in the experience of this author, more often in females and black individuals.

Histologically, this form of the cyst, like the cyst of the newborn, is lined by stratified squamous epithelium. Treatment is simple excision.

Odontogenic Keratocyst (Primordial Cyst)

The term "primordial" means of the simplest and most underdeveloped character. A primordial cyst occurs in the enamel organ before dental hard tissues are formed. As noted by Gardner et al.[61] and Robinson,[62] confusion and controversy have enveloped the diagnosis of "primordial cyst" versus "odontogenic keratocyst." Gardner et al.[61] offer the best solution and that is "to consider the term primordial cyst as being purely conceptual and to discontinue its use to identify a specific entity. The term odontogenic keratocyst should be retained to designate a specific entity having a characteristic histological appearance and a specific clinical behavior, namely an aggressive growth potential and a tendency to recur after removal."

Eversole et al.,[63] after reviewing the British and American literature, drew the conclusion that the keratocyst may occur in association with dentigerous, lateral periodontal and residual cysts as well as the entity called "primordial" cyst.

Differences of opinion exist concerning the incidence of the primordial (keratocyst) cyst. These range from a high of 10% of all epithelial-lined cysts of the jaws to statements contending the primordial cysts (keratocysts) are most frequently found (80% of the time) in the mandibular third molar region. The cysts, according to Gorlin,[53] must not come in contact with a crown or root apex of a tooth. While this developmental lesion may take the place of a missing tooth, it is on occasion diagnosed in the presence of a complete dentition. This anomalous occurrence is explained by the supposition that the cyst has developed from the primordial cells of a supernumerary tooth!

Radiologically, the cysts appear as well defined

radiolucent areas with a distinct margin of condensing osteitis. True multiloculation is seen.

When a tooth is absent from an otherwise normal dental arch with no history of previous extraction, an area of rarefaction in that position is suggestive of a replacement by a primordial cyst (keratocyst).[46]

The histological features of the odontogenic keratocyst (primordial cyst) are quite characteristic (Fig. 27.18). They are: (1) a thin stratified squamous epithelium, usually six to eight cells thick, and ortho- or parakeratotic; the epithelium seldom manifests rete ridges and a corrugated appearance is fairly characteristic; (2) the cyst wall is thin when compared with other odontogenic cysts, and there is a paucity of inflammatory cells (unless there has been infection); (3) "daughter cysts" may be noted in the wall (these represent either satellite cysts or a folding of the lining epithelium); (4) orthokeratotic, or parakeratotic layers on the surface often accompanied by keratin within the cavity of the cyst; and (5) variable cyst contents ranging from a clear fluid with a protein content of less than 3.5 g/100 ml to one that is murky and filled with keratin or squames.[64]

It is imperative to remember that keratinization is not specific for the odontogenic keratocyst. The other characteristics cited above must be identified. The frequency of keratinization in other cysts of the jaws, including dentigerous, residual, lateral

periodontal and even fissural cysts, varies from 3.3 to 5.5%. Additional characteristics have been cited by Toller[64] and include completeness of the epithelial lining and the absence of cholesterol in the wall of the cyst or in the cyst contents.

The benign microscopic appearance of the odontogenic keratocyst (primordial cyst) should not lull one into complacency and forget its well known locally aggressive behavior. Eversole et al.[63] noted a 35% recurrence rate over a 5-year period and suggested that the 35% figure may be a low estimate. The 35% figure is put in perspective when one notes that other odontogenic cysts have a recurrence rate only as *high* as 6%.

The reasons for the locally aggressive behavior of the odontogenic keratocyst are based upon the pathogenesis of the lesion and the cellular characteristics of the keratocyst. The predilection of the keratocyst for the posterior mandible lends support to the theory that the keratocyst takes origin from the distal extension of the dental lamina. Main[65] has noted that the mitotic activity of the primordial cyst (keratocyst) is comparable to that of the ameloblastoma and the dental lamina. In addition, Toller[66] using autoradiographic methods noted that the epithelium of the primordial cyst (keratocyst) has a higher mitotic activity than the epithelia of the buccal mucosa or the nonkeratinizing epithelium of periapical cysts. Using the scanning electron microscope, Wysocki and Sapp[67]

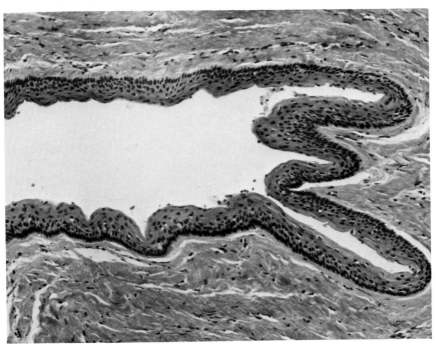

Figure 27.18. Keratocyst displaying its deceptively innocuous lining.

noted the greater cellularity in the epithelium of parakeratinized cysts (Fig. 27.19). They noted that the increased cellularity correlated with the increased mitotic activity in keratocysts.

In addition to, and probably more important than, the inherent cell potential of the cyst epithelium for recurrence, is the existence of daughter or satellite cysts peripheral to the primary cyst. The daughter cysts are postulated as remnants of the dental lamina. Surgical difficulties, including friability of the lining, size and shape of the lesion, and restricted access, are postulated as further causes of recurrence.

Attenborough[68] claims that the only definitive aid to prebiopsy diagnosis of a keratocyst is aspiration. The finding of a much lower soluble protein content in the case of an odontogenic keratocyst as compared with simple cysts and the presence of squames in the fluid are useful aids to preoperative diagnosis.

Methods of treatment of the odontogenic keratocyst have included enucleation, enucleation with chemical fixation, marsupialization, marsupialization followed by enucleation, resection and, by a few, radiotherapy. Selection of a method, however, is largely dictated by the size, extent and localization of the lesion.

Nevoid Basal Cell Carcinoma Syndrome

It has been over a quarter of a century since Philipsen[69] noted an association of odontogenic cysts with multiple basal cell carcinomas. Delineation of a syndrome, by Gorlin and Goltz,[70] with jaw cysts and basal cell carcinomas as major components subsequently evolved in 1960.

Originally based on a clinical misinterpretation, the first designation of the syndrome was "basal cell nevus syndrome." Although still in use, "nevoid basal cell carcinoma syndrome" is the preferred terminology. The principal cutaneous lesions are basal cell carcinomas, which are "nevoid" only by virtue of their relatively early clinical onset.

The syndrome is conditioned by an autosomal dominant gene with variable and usually high penetrance and expressivity. There is no racial exclusion and no sex predilection.

The principal characteristics of the syndrome are cysts of the jaws, multiple, early appearing, basal cell carcinomas of the skin, developmental anomalies of the skeleton, a peculiar dyskeratotic pitting of the hands and feet, and ectopic soft tissue calcifications. These and other non-basal-cell carcinoma components of the syndrome are shown in Figure 27.20.

The keratocysts in patients with the nevoid basal cell carcinoma syndrome commonly appear a decade earlier than those in the "solitary keratocyst" patient. The jaw cysts are further characterized by their multiplicity, bilateralism and continuous development. This feature is important from a surgical viewpoint and results not only from persist-

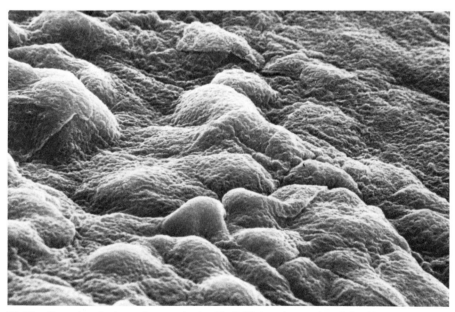

Figure 27.19. Scanning electron micrograph of epithelial lining of a parakeratinized keratocyst. The surface corrugations are easily identified and the irregular surface of the epithelial cells is evident. (Contributed by George P. Wysocki and J. Philip Sapp.)

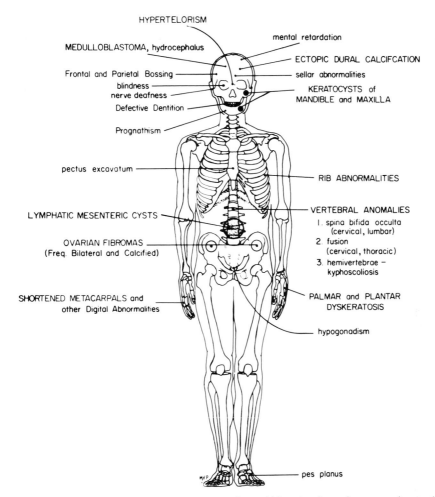

Figure 27.20. Non-basal-cell carcinoma components of nevoid basal cell carcinoma syndrome. (Bold type indicates prominent components.)

ence after incomplete enucleation, but also from multiple daughter cysts or satellite cysts.

The cuspid-to-first molar region and maxillary second molar region with extension of the maxillary cysts into the sinuses are the most commonly involved sites.

Cyst size varies from microscopic lesions to those of several centimeters in diameter. Large cysts may reach sufficient size to cause "pathological" fractures.

Invasion of the maxillary sinuses may produce signs and symptoms of a chronic sinusitis. Displacement of the anterior wall of the maxilla and elevation of the infraorbital vessels may occur.

If few in number, the cysts may be mistaken for more conventional cysts or even ameloblastoma. A small number have developed in or are associated with ameloblastoma.

The histogenesis and microscopic appearance of the jaw cysts of patients with the syndrome are those of the odontogenic keratocyst. However, not all keratocysts are related to the syndrome.

The jaw cysts or other osseous abnormalities, or both, may precede the cutaneous lesions by several or more years, but occurrences of multiple basal cell carcinomas in childhood should arouse suspicions of the syndrome.

The onset of the basal cell carcinomas is early, often between the ages of 7 and 14 years. They are multiple, and patients may have several thousands of them.[71] The carcinomas may or may not be pigmented (Fig. 27.21). They develop from multiple or multicentric foci in any region of the body throughout life.

Even in the child, the lesions are histologically basal cell carcinomas, but they defer their malignant or locally destructive behavior until after the first decade of life. Nevi are actually few in number and are not essential for definitions of the syndrome.

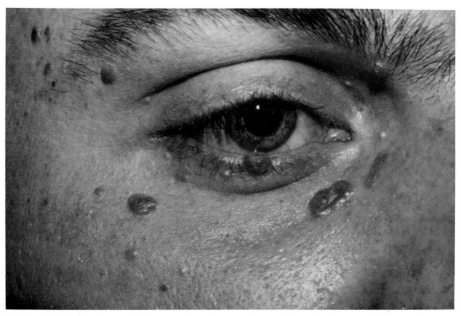

Figure 27.21. Multiple, pigmented basal cell carcinomas in a patient with the nevoid basal cell carcinoma. (Contributed by G. E. Kakascik, M.D.).

A major (50 to 70% of cases) cutaneous manifestation is dyskeratotic plugging of the palms and soles.[71]

There is no way in which a pathologist can diagnose the nevoid basal cell carcinoma syndrome solely by examination of a histological preparation of the basal cell carcinomas. However, he may suspect the syndrome when: (1) the patient is young (below the age of 30 years); (2) several basal cell carcinomas are present or have been previously removed; (3) the carcinoma is from an unexposed part of the body; (4) there is a multicentric pattern; and (5) recognizable osteoid is present within the neoplasm.

In a large series of 340 cutaneous lesions, only 22 true nevus cell tumors were present in 13 patients.[71] Four of these were intimately associated with basal cell carcinomas. This frequency of nevi is no greater than would be expected in the general population.

Keratinizing and Calcifying Odontogenic Cysts

The keratinizing and calcifying odontogenic cyst was first described in 1962 by Gorlin et al.[72] As noted by Chen and Miller,[73] the keratinizing and calcifying odontogenic cyst refers to a cyst, yet many cases have occurred as solid masses. Freidman et al.[74] noted 11.5% of the cases they examined were described as solid tumors. There is an equal sex distribution of the cysts and an equal distribution between the maxilla and the mandible. Two thirds of the cysts have been intraosseous and one third, extraosseous.

The cysts occur in all age groups with most cases presenting in the 10- to 19-year age range.

Radiographically, the cyst appears as a well circumscribed radiolucency with intraluminal radiopacities occasionally noted.

Histologically the cyst is lined by stratified squamous epithelium, which in some areas, may exhibit a prominent basal cell layer of cuboidal to columnar cells. Within the epithelium are found the characteristic cells of the keratinizing and calcifying odontogenic cyst, "ghost cells" (Fig. 27.22). Ghost cells appear as ovoid deeply eosinophilic granular cells. They are also occasionally found in the adjacent connective tissue. Osteoid and dentinoid materials have been found in 40% of reported cases and calcified deposits in 70%. Gorlin et al.[75] attribute the pathogenesis of calcification to the disintegration of the basal layer of the cyst epithelium with subsequent ingrowth of granulation tissue which engulfs the ghost cells and treats them as foreign bodies. They then may undergo subsequent calcification.

Similar calcification and keratinization have been noted in the craniopharyngioma and in the cutaneous epithelioma of Malherbe. In addition, four types of odontogenic tumor are known to occur in combination with keratinizing and calci-

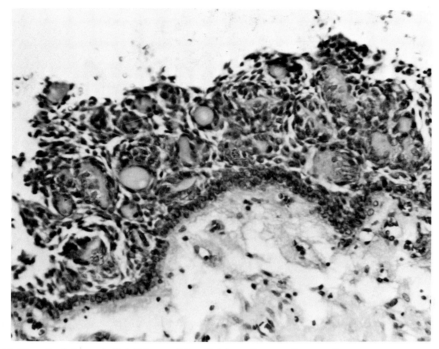

Figure 27.22. Gorlin's cyst. Calcifying and keratinizing odontogenic cyst. Prominent basal cell layer and stellate reticulum-like epithelium as well as calcification and keratinization.

fying cysts. These include ameloblastoma, ameloblastic odontoma, ameloblastic fibro-odontoma and complex odontoma.

Treatment of keratinizing and calcifying odontogenic cysts, as with any odontogenic cyst, is total excision. The cysts have no tendency to recur, but because of the association with other odontogenic tumors, the pathologist must sample the specimen adequately to ensure there is no other pathological lesion.

Multiple Cysts of the Jaws

The occurrence of multiple jaw cysts in an individual at the same time is rare.

Multiple periodontal (periapical) cysts may arise in patients with poor dental hygiene and if inadequately treated or ignored at the time of extractions, numerous residual cysts will remain.

Multiple dentigerous cysts tend to be located in different sections of the mouth and are usually present in both the upper and lower jaws. Numerous dentigerous cysts can be seen in association with cleidocranial dysostosis and in a rare type of hypoplastic amelogenesis imperfecta in which numerous teeth are unerupted.[53]

As already noted, the association of multiple keratocysts of the jaws (primordial cysts) with multiple cutaneous "nevoid" basal cell, carcinomas and numerous skeletal anomalies has been recognized since 1959.[71]

Malignant Transformation of the Epithelial Lining of Odontogenic Cysts

The epithelial lining of odontogenic cysts may, on rare occasions, undergo malignant changes. This complication has been reported in *all* types of odontogenic cysts.[76] Few of the cases have been sufficiently well documented for a critical evaluation, Faulkner et al.,[77] in a survey of the literature in 1957, found that only 8 of 48 cases were acceptable. Killey and Kay[46] quote Bernier who had commented that he had not observed any malignant changes in the histological examination of 2,000 odontogenic cysts.

When malignant change supervenes in an odontogenic cyst it probably does so under the influence of a prolonged and chronic inflammation. All accepted cases have been of squamous cell carcinoma type.

Origin in an odontogenic cyst is difficult or impossible to prove unless a *direct* transition from normal to neoplastic tissue is seen. Proven cases which involve dentigerous cysts are of particular interest, since the presence of a tooth and its anatomical relation to neoplasm in an odontogenic cyst offer added suggestive evidence that this transformation took place in an odontogenic cyst and not, for example, in a fissural cyst.[76]

Kay and Kramer[78] have provided a resumé of the arguments and criteria by which malignancy can be presumed to have occurred in relationship to the wall of an odontogenic cyst. The mandible is involved almost twice as often as the maxilla.

Eversole et al.,[63] in reviewing the literature, noted that from a total of 32 acceptable instances of central epidermoid carcinoma, 75% were associated with an odontogenic cyst. Mucoepidermoid carcinoma central in bone (27 instances) was associated with a cyst or impacted tooth in 48% of the cases.

Following neoplastic transformation, the carcinoma is usually of a low grade malignancy. Lymph node metastases and dissemination by bloodstream are late events, even though osseous extension and invasion of adjacent soft tissues may be extensive.[46]

Morrison and Deeley[79] indicate that primary central squamous cell carcinoma of the jaws, which include those arising from odontogenic cysts, appear to be more sensitive to irradiation than similar tumors arising from the alveolar mucosa, even when the latter do not involve bone. Despite this radiosensitivity, the recommended treatment is wide surgical resection and in the lower jaw; this entails a hemimandibulectomy. Regional lymph nodes should also be excised and examined.

Finally, in reference to neoplastic change, Bhaskar[80] claims that 82% of follicular cysts (primordial and dentigerous) contain remnants of odontogenic epithelium within their connective tissue walls; 5% to 6% of these cysts show evidence of ameloblastic proliferation.

REFERENCES

1. Eversole, L. R., Tomich, E. E., and Cherrick, H. M.: Histogenesis of odontogenic tumors. Oral Surg. 32:569, 1971.
2. Broca, P.: Traite des Tumeurs, vol. I, p. 350. P. Asselin, Paris, 1866.
3. Gorlin, R. J., Meskin, L. H., and Brodey, R.: Odontogenic tumors in man and animals: pathological classification and clinical behavior. A review. Ann. N. Y. Acad. Sci. 108:722, 1963.
4. Gorlin, R. J.: Odontogenic tumors. In Thomas' Oral Pathology, 6th Ed., pp. 481–515, edited by R. J. Gorlin and H. M. Goldman. C. V. Mosby Co., St. Louis, 1970.
5. Spouge, J. D.: Odontogenic tumors. Oral Surg. 24:392, 1967.
6. Pindborg, J. J., and Clausen, F.: Classification of odontogenic tumors; suggestion. Acta Odont. Scand. 16:293, 1958.
7. Baden, E.: Odontogenic tumors. Pathol. Annu. vol. 6:475, 1971.
8. Shear, M.: Unity of tumours of odontogenic epithelium. Br. J. Oral Surg. 2:212, 1965.
9. Meyer, I., and Shklar, G.: Odontogenic tumors. In Textbook of Oral Surgery, pp. 465–484, edited by W. C. Guralnick, Little Brown & Co., Boston, 1968.
10. Pullon, P. A., Shafer, W. G., Elzay, R. P., Kerr, D. A., and

11. Bhaskar, S. N.: Synopsis of Oral Pathology, 3rd Ed. C. V. Mosby Co., St. Louis, 1969.
12. Hertz, J.: Adamantinoma: Studies in histopathology and prognosis. Acta Med. Scand. 142:(suppl.)529, 1952.
13. Hertz, J.: Adamantinoma: Histo-pathologic and prognostic studies. Acta Chir. Scand. 102:405, 1952.
14. Young, D. R., and Robinson, M.: Ameloblastoma in children: Report of a case. Oral Surg. 15:1155, 1962.
15. Sehdev, M. K., Huuos, A. G., Strong, E. W., Gerold, F. P., and Willis, G. W.: Ameloblastoma of maxilla and mandible. Cancer 33:324, 1974.
16. Lee, K. W., Chin, T. C., and Paul, G.: Peripheral ameloblastoma. Br. J. Oral Surg. 8:150, 1970.
17. Wesley, R. K., Borninski, E. R., Mintz, S.: Peripheral ameloblastoma: report of case and review of the literature. J. Oral Surg. 35:670, 1977.
18. Gardner, D. G.: Peripheral ameloblastoma. Cancer 39:1625, 1977.
19. Robinson, L., and Martinez, M. G.: Unicystic ameloblastoma. Cancer 40:2278, 1977.
20. Mehlisch, D. R., Dahlin, D. C., and Masson, J. K.: Ameloblastoma: a clinicopathologic report. J. Oral Surg. 30:9, 1972.
21. Ghatak, N. R., Hirano, A., and Zimmerman, H. M.: Ultrastructure of a craniopharyngioma. Cancer 27:1465, 1971.
22. Moe, H., Clausen, F., and Philipsen, H. P.: The ultrastructure of the simple ameloblastoma. Acta Pathol. Microbiol. Scand. 2:140, 1961.
23. Seemayer, T. A., Blundell, J. S., and Wiglesworth: Pituitary craniopharyngioma with tooth formation. Cancer 29:423, 1972.
24. Kerr, D. A.: Personal communication.
25. Becker, R., and Pertl, A.: Zur therapie des Ameloblastoms. Dtsch. Zahn Mund Kieferheilkd. 49:423, 1967.
26. Dahlgren, S. E., Ekstrom, C., and Mossberg, B.: Mandibular amelobastoma with pulmonary and mediastinal lymph node metastases. Acta Otolaryng. 72:220, 1971.
27. Herceg, S. J., and Harding, R. L.: Malignant ameloblastoma with pulmonary metastases: Report of a case and review of the literature. Plast. Reconstr. Surg. 49:456, 1972.
28. Philipsen, H. P., and Birn, H.: The adenomatoid odontogenic tumor: Ameloblastic adenomatoid tumor or adenoameloblastoma. Acta Pathol. Microbiol. Scand. 75:375, 1969.
29. Cina, M. T., Dahlin, D. C., and Gores, R. J.: Ameloblastic adenomatoid tumors: A report of four new cases. Am. J. Clin. Pathol. 39:59, 1963.
30. Courtnery, R. M., and Kerr, D. A.: The odontogenic adenomatoid tumor. Oral Surg. 39:424, 1975.
31. Abrams, A. M., Melrose, R. J., and Howell, F. V.: Adenoameloblastoma: a clinical pathologic study of ten new cases. Cancer 22:175, 1968.
32. Pindborg, J. J.: Calcifying epithelial odontogenic tumor. Cancer 11:838, 1958.
33. Pindborg, J. J.: The calcifying epithelial odontogenic tumor: Review of literature and report of an extra-osseous case. Acta Odontol. Scand. 24:419, 1966.
34. Gargiulo, E. A., Ziter, W. D., and Mastrocola, R.: Calcifying epithelial odontogenic tumor: report of case and review of literature. J. Oral Surg. 29:862, 1971.
35. Vap, D. R., Dahlin, D. C., and Turlington, E. G.: Pindborg tumour: the so-called calcifying epithelial odontogenic tumour. Cancer 25:629, 1970.
36. Mainwaring, A. R., Ahmed, A., Hopkinson, J. M., and Anderson, P.: A clinical and electron microscopic study of a calcifying epithelial odontogenic tumour. J. Clin. Pathol. 24:152, 1971.
37. Krolls, S. O., and Pindborg, J. J.: Calcifying epithelial odontogenic tumor: A survey of 23 cases and discussions of histomorphologic variations. Arch. Pathol. 98:206, 1974.
38. Hamner, J. E., Scofield, H. H., and Coryn, J.: Benign fibroosseous jaw lesions of periodontal membrane origin: An analysis of 249 cases. Cancer 22:861, 1968.
39. Hooker, S. P.: Ameloblastic odontoma: An analysis of twenty-six cases. Oral Surg. 24:375, 1967.

Corio, R. L.: Squamous odontogenic tumor. Oral Surg. 40:616, 1975.

40. Tsagaris, G. T.: A review of the ameloblastic fibro-odontoma. M.S. Thesis, George Washington University, Washington, D. C., 1972.
41. Miller, A. S., Lopez, C. F., Pullon, P. A., and Elzay, R. P.: Ameloblastic fibro-odontoma. Oral Surg. 41:354, 1976.
42. Zegarelli, E. V., Kutscher, A. H., Napoli, N., Iurono, F., and Hoffman, P.: The cementoma: a study of 230 patients with 435 cementomas. Oral Surg. 17:219, 1964.
43. Krausen, A. S., Pullon, P. A., Gulmen, S., Schenck, N. L., and Ogura, J.: Cementomas—aggressive or innocuous neoplasms. Arch. Otolaryngol. 103:349, 1977.
44. White, D. K., Chen, S., Mohnac, A. M., and Miller, A. S.: Odontogenic myxoma. Oral Surg. 39:901, 1975.
45. Kerr, D. A., and Courtney, R.: Personal communication.
46. Killey, H. C., and Kay, L. W.: Benign lesions of the jaws: their diagnosis and treatment. E. & S. Livingstone, Ltd., Edinburgh, 1966.
47. Beekhuis, G. J., and Watson, T. H.: Midfacial cysts. Arch. Otolaryng. 85:62, 1967.
48. Main, D. M. G.: Epithelial jaw cysts: a clinicopathological reappraisal. Br. J. Oral Surg. 8:114, 1970.
49. Kerr, D. A.: Personal communication. Cited by Waldrop, A. C., Jr., and Capadanno, J. A.: Bilateral nasolabial cysts: report of a case. J. Oral Surg. 24:347, 1966.
50. Bernier, J. L.: Management of oral disease: a treatise on the recognition, identification and treatment of diseases of the oral region, 2nd Ed., p. 534. C. V. Mosby Co., St. Louis, 1959.
51. Santora, E., Ballantyne, A. J., and Hinds, E. C.: Nasoalveolar cyst: report of case. J. Oral Surg. 28:117, 1970.
52. Walsh-Waring, G. P.: Nasoalveolar cysts: aetiology, presentation and treatment. J. Laryngol. 81:263, 1967.
53. Gorlin, R. J.: Cysts of the jaws, oral floor, and neck. In Thoma's Oral Pathology, 6th Ed., edited by R. J. Gorlin and H. M. Goldman. C. V. Mosby Co., St. Louis, 1970.
54. Bull, T. R., McNeill, K. A., Milner, G., and Murray, S. M.: Nasopalatine cysts. J. Laryngol. 81:37, 1967.
55. Abrams, A. M., Howell, F. V., and Bullock, W. K.: Nasopalatine cysts. Oral Surg. 16:306, 1963.
56. Hatziotis, J.: Median palatine cyst: report of case. J. Oral Surg. 24:343, 1966.
57. Tilson, H. B., and Bauerle, J. E.: Median mandibular cyst: report of case. J. Oral Surg. 28:519, 1970.
58. Standish, S. M., and Shafer, W. G.: The lateral periodontal cyst. J. Periodont. 29:27, 1958.
59. Seward, M. H.: Eruption cyst: an analysis of its clinical features. J. Oral Surg. 31:31, 1973.
60. Bhaskar, S. N.: Oral Surgery—Oral Pathology Conference, No. 13, Walter Reed Army Medical Center. Oral Surg. 19:796, 1965.
61. Gardner, D. G., Sapp, J. P., and Wysocki, G. P.: Epithelial cysts of the jaw. Bull. Int. Acad. Pathol. 17:6, 1976.
62. Robinson, H. B. G.: Primordial cyst versus keratocyst. Oral Surg. 40:362, 1975.
63. Eversole, L. R., Sabes, W. R., and Rovin, S.: Aggressive growth and neoplastic potential of odontogenic cysts with special reference to central epidermoid and mucoepidermoid carcinomas. Cancer 35:270, 1975.
64. Toller, P.: Origin and growth of cysts of the jaws. Ann. R. Coll. Surg. Engl. 40:306, 1967.
65. Main, D. M. G.: Epithelial jaw cysts: a clinicopathological reappraisal. Br. J. Oral Surg. 8:114, 1970.
66. Toller, P. A.: Autoradiography of explants from odontogenic cysts. Br. Dent. J. 131:57, 1971.
67. Wysocki, G. P., Sapp, J. P.: Scanning and transmission electron microscopy of odontogenic keratocysts. Oral Surg. 40:494, 1975.
68. Attenborough, N. R.: Recurrence of an odontogenic keratocyst in a bone graft: report of a case. Br. J. Oral Surg. 12:33, 1974.
69. Philipsen, H. P.: On "keratocysts" in the jaws. Tandlaegelbladet 60:963, 1956.
70. Gorlin, R. J., and Goltz, R. W.: Multiple nevoid basal cell epithelium, jaw cysts and bifid rib: a syndrome. N. Engl. J. Med. 262:908, 1960.
71. Mason, J. K., Helwig, E. B., and Graham, J. H.: Pathology of nevoid basal cell carcinoma syndrome. Arch. Pathol. 79:401, 1965.
72. Gorlin, R. J., Pindborg, J. J., Clausen, F. P., and Vickers, R. A.: The calcifying odontogenic cyst—a possible analogue of the cutaneous calcifying epithelioma of malherbe. Oral Surg. 15:1235, 1962.
73. Chen, S. Y., and Miller, A. S.: Ultrastructure of the keratinizing and calcifying odontogenic cyst. Oral Surg. 39:769, 1975.
74. Freidman, P. D., Loumerman, H., and Gee, J. K.: Calcifying odontogenic cyst. Oral Surg. 40:93, 1975.
75. Gorlin, R. J., Pindborg, J. J., Redman, R. S., Williamson, J. J., and Hansen, L. S.: The calcifying odontogenic cyst: a new entity and possible analogue of the cutaneous calcifying epithelium of Malherbe. Cancer 17:723, 1964.
76. Angelopoulos, A. F., Tilson, H. B., Stewart, F. W., and Jaques, W. E.: Malignant transformation of the epithelial lining of the odontogenic cysts. Oral Surg. 22:415, 1966.
77. Faulkner, S., Herberts, H., and Olyen, S.: Carcinoma arising in odontogenic cysts of the jaws. Odontol. Tidskr. 65:220, 1957.
78. Kay, L. W., and Kramer, I. R. H.: Squamous-cell carcinoma arising in a dental cyst. Oral Surg. 15:970, 1962.
79. Morrison, R., and Deeley, T. J.: Intra-alveolar carcinoma of the jaw: treated by supravoltage radiotherapy. Br. J. Radiol. 35:321, 1962.
80. Bhaskar, S. N.: Synopsis of oral pathology, p. 190. 2nd Ed., C. V. Mosby Co., St. Louis, 1965.

Index

563